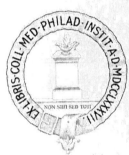

50TH ANNUAL MEETING ... APRIL 22, 23, 24 ... TULSA

THE *Journal*

OF THE OKLAHOMA STATE MEDICAL ASSOCIATION

VOLUME XXXV • OKLAHOMA CITY, OKLAHOMA, JANUARY, 1942 • NUMBER 1

★ *Published Monthly at Oklahoma City, Oklahoma, Under Direction of the Council*

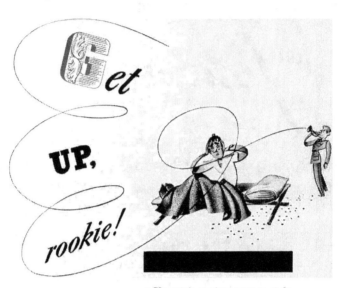

Get UP, rookie!

● The strictly regulated program of the Army helps to harden the soft, lackadaisical rookie. But what about the men who remain in civilian life?

When the deleterious effect of a soft civilian life—irregular habits, lack of exercise, faulty diet—leads to constipation, the use of Petrogalar* is frequently indicated.

Petrogalar adds bland, unabsorbable moisture to the stool to induce a soft, easily passed mass.

Consider its use for the treatment of constipation. Petrogalar is pleasant to take and economical to use.

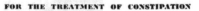

FOR THE TREATMENT OF CONSTIPATION

Petrogalar•

Trade Mark. Petrogalar is an aqueous suspension of pure mineral oil each 100 cc. of which contains 65 cc. pure mineral oil suspended in an aqueous jelly containing agar and acacia.

Petrogalar Laboratories, Inc. · 8134 McCormick Boulevard · Chicago, Illinois

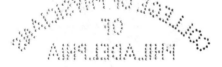

THE JOURNAL

OF THE

OKLAHOMA STATE MEDICAL ASSOCIATION

| VOLUME XXXV | OKLAHOMA CITY, OKLAHOMA, JANUARY, 1942 | NUMBER 1 |

The Relation of the Mental Hospital Physician to the Patient and His Relatives[*]

JOHN L. DAY, M.D.

SUPPLY, OKLAHOMA

In this day and age we are apt to think we are pioneering, but a little reflection will remind us that there is "nothing new under the sun." Primitive man believed that disease afflicted him because of the wrath of evil spirits and the healing art therefore consisted in the use of such methods as would repel or propitiate such evil influence. The insane was one who was possessed by an evil spirit. Jesus of Nazareth went about "healing the sick and casting out devils." It is not surprising therefore that the treatment of mental disease was in the hands of priests, and that this treatment consisted in great measure of religious ceremonies. In Greece the medical priests were in charge of temples where sick people were treated. These temples were quite numerous and while they were not devoted exclusively to the care of the mentally ill, definite provisions were made for such care and were the forerunners of the modern general hospital. The ceremonies having to do with treatment of the mental cases have been described by Hippocrates. Celsus in A. D. 5 wrote upon the subject of the treatment of mental disease and gave us some wise rules as to hygienic and moral management. The accounts of Coelius Aurelianus, A. D. 195 are the most complete of any writers of that period. He has the following to say about the management of difficult and disturbed patients: "If the sight of other persons irritates them and only in very rare cases, restraint may be employed, but with the greatest precautions, without any unnecessary force and after carefully protecting all joints and with special care to use only restraining apparatus of a soft and delicate texture, since means of repression employed without judgment increase and may even give rise to furor in-

stead of repressing it." It is well that we follow these rules today.

For many years however there was little provision made for the mental patient. He was allowed to roam about or was placed in jail or an almshouse. The point is that in spite of mystery and superstition he was considered a medical problem. The first mental hospital was Bethlehem or Bedlam as it was called, founded by Simon Fitz Mary, sheriff of London in 1247. In 1660 the Hotel Dieu in Paris set aside two wards for the insane. The York Retreat was founded in 1796 by William Tuke. Philip Pinel became physician for the insane in 1793. He advocated many administrative procedures which are used in our present mental hospitals. The emphasis was upon "moral treatment" yet the necessity for a medical atmosphere was recognized. They also had their difficulties with unsatisfactory employees. The personality of the attendant was considered of prime importance, he was urged not to be familiar with his patients, yet to do everything possible to arouse their affection and confidence. He was not to reason with them during moments of stress, nor was he to speak condescendingly to them in lucid intervals.

The first organized psychiatry in this country was confined to the mental hospital. In the beginning the humanitarian idea was in the foreground. Psychiatry was therefore based largely on kindly care, and hospitals were built with the purpose of providing good physical attention and segregating these individuals from the community. Improvement in all cases and recovery in some was noted and thus the idea of therapy was born. Many problems arose and progress in the care of the insane was not always uniformly advanced. Private hospitals came into being and the state hospitals in some cases fell into disrepute. The National Committee

[*]Read before the Section on Neurology, Psychiatry and Endocrinology, Annual Session, Oklahoma State Medical Association, May 21, 1941, in Oklahoma City.

for Mental Hygiene founded at about the beginning of this century came into being largely because of evils existing in the state hospitals. This Committee has been a potent factor in the development of psychiatry in America. It attempts to dispel the idea that there is a stigma connected with mental disease. It emphasizes the medical side of the problem. The relationship of psychiatry and the law has received attention. It has recognized the necessity for highly trained specialists in various fields of psychiatry. It aims to secure for the mentally ill the same medical attention as that accorded the physically ill.

While much has been accomplished and the attitude of the public has changed and the medical profession has made great strides in the matter of treatment of the mentally afflicted there yet remain many things to do. For example, let us consider the method of commitment to a state hospital, which at least in the beginning seems far removed from a medical procedure. First, someone, a relative or perhaps an officer of the law, signs a petition setting forth the complaint. This is presented to the County Judge who then, if he deems the case worthy, appoints two regularly licensed physicians to examine the person suspected of being insane. A time for hearing is set; notice of hearing is given and the physicians with the judge sitting as a sanity board interview the patient, hear evidence from friends, relatives and neighbors. The physicians fill out the prescribed blanks and make a certificate that this person is insane and a fit subject for treatment in a hospital for the insane. The judge then makes an order for admission to a hospital for the insane and instructs the sheriff or some of his force to transport the individual to the superintendent of the hospital there to be kept until he is legally discharged. In many instances the sick person has been confined in the jail until the foregoing procedure could be got under way. He is accompanied to the hospital by armed guards. It is essential that no individual be deprived of his liberty without due process of law but there should be some modification of the legal process and I am glad to say that frequently there is a deviation from the foregoing even if not strictly within the letter of the law.

Immediately upon admission however the individual should and does become a medical problem. He is received by a physician. He should be greeted as a sick person. His health should be inquired into briefly and he should be made to feel that he has arrived at a hospital and that his case will have careful attention and that when he is well he will be able to return home. The manner of his reception and the consideration given him during the first few days are of extreme importance. If relatives accompany the patient, they are interviewed, the method of reports and correspondence are explained to them. A guarded prognosis is given. They should be impressed with the idea that this is a medical case and therefore no absolute prediction can be made. It should be explained to them that mental disease unlike physical disease requires time for recovery or improvement, that they must think in terms of months rather than weeks, that medicine or drugs is only a part of the treatment provided, that the mere separation of the patient from his former environment and close relatives constitutes a method of treatment in itself.

The examination begins at once. I cannot too strongly emphasize the importance of careful, considerate observation. Notes are at once made to be transcribed later on the patient's record. It goes without saying that a thorough physical examination is made beginning as soon as the patient is sent to his ward. This of course includes various laboratory procedures and an accurate record is made of all essential details. All the while this is going on the examining physician is taking cognizance of mental symptoms. All members of the staff should become acquainted with the patient so when his case is worked out and presented to the staff meeting in regular session, each member will have a personal opinion based on observation and examination and will not depend on the history as read. The matter of diagnosis and classification is of relative value only, the important thing is to know the patient and treat him, not some specifically named disorder.

As the patient is becoming accustomed to his new surroundings the physician visits him frequently, he learns something of his delusions or hallucinations, the attendant is informed of some of his symptoms and is instructed as how best to manage him. Specific instructions are given the attendant remembering always that he (the attendant) is just that and not often a trained nurse. As the days pass the physician endeavors to gain the confidence of the patient, he should know his thoughts, why does he act as he does, there is generally a reason. The patient should be made to feel that the physician considers his case of paramount importance. He never makes light of his delusions, he listens to his story.

Each case is different, there is no set time for the patient to be transferred from the receiving ward, no set time to be assigned a task, each is treated as an individual. The physician should constantly study the varying moods of the patient, he should be cheerful without wisecracking, dignified without coldness, sympathetic but not sentimental. To those who are accessible talk over their troubles with them. Do not argue, be frank, tell him his thoughts are unusual and unreasonable, that at times many people do things or have thoughts which to them seem normal but to others are abnormal. I believe the definite turning point in the progress of a woman patient came when she said "Doctor, I will try to believe you are right."

We are all in accord with the idea that no mechanical restraint should ever be used but at times it is better to use some restraint rather than to have the excited, irritable, maniacal patient injured or injure others. There should be no standing order but the physician should give permission in writing with stated reasons for a specified form of restraint. The physician should know the individual patient well enough that he is able properly to prescribe restraint or seclusion.

There should be no routine about medication. If sedation is indicated it should be prescribed. It may consist of varying forms for various patients. If the new patient needs a laxative he should have it but not just because he is a recent admission. Likewise there should be no set procedure with respect to treatment of syphilitic cases. Does this particular individual require arsenical and mercury, if so in what form? Is he a fit subject for malaria? Is shock treatment indicated? The point I am trying to make is that each patient should be individualized and medical treatment outlined accordingly. This requires careful observation and definite study for each one.

The chronic case also should be individualized. Do not give a black pill to a certain number of cases on Ward X on Saturday and a green pill on Tuesday. There is no virtue in giving magnesium sulphate on Wednesday night. Such practices have been known to prevail. The physician has a complete drug stock at his disposal, he should give what the patient needs at the time or from day to day. This can only be done if he knows his patient individually and personally.

The relation of the physician to the relatives is of great importance. Consideration and tact is required as well as an infinite amount of patience. Your prognosis should be guarded yet as optimistic as the case warrants. Never say "never." How many of us recall, after having carefully and at length explained the situation to the relatives, hearing them say, "Doctor, just what is the matter with ———?" Remember that this situation is a trying one, attempt to put yourself in the relatives' place. Explain your method of making reports, your practice with respect to correspondence, the regulations regarding visiting.

All inquiries should be answered promptly but no letter should be written unless that particular patient is seen personally that day. Obviously it is impossible to make routine reports on all patient at stated intervals but the relatives should be notified by phone if necessary if a patient's condition becomes serious or critical. Arrangements should be made in advance for disposition of the body in case of death. All injuries should be reported to the relatives giving frankly the circumstances connected with the injury.

The hospital physician should take advantage of every opportunity to appear before medical and lay groups to explain about the modern methods of treatment for the mentally ill, the old asylum idea is still too prevalent among the people. Meet the press more than half way. Encourage visits to the hospital of highschool and college groups. I have endeavored not to set forth a set of rules to be followed literally, but to present the idea that individual, personal attention on the part of the physician is the important thing.

It has been said that the mentally ill needs a friend, that is true but it is also true that he needs a physician, one who stands in the relationship of the old family doctor to the physically sick. Even though he is working for the State the mental hospital physician should be imbued with the idea of rendering a personal service to the mentally afflicted and his relatives. In giving of himself unstintedly to this task he will be compensated in a far greater measure than that indicated by his salary. He should be as genuinely interested in his patients' recovery as is the private physician.

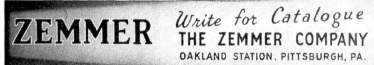

Hemorrhoidectomy with Special Reference to a New Technique and the Avoidance of Pain

ELLIS MOORE, B.S., M.D.

OKLAHOMA CITY, OKLAHOMA

Cursory investigation of recent literature reveals marked advancement in determining the operability of many diseases of the rectum and colon, including malignancy. However, very little change in operation for hemorrhoids has been developed, yet it is probably the most common complaint in the ano-rectal region. Hemorrhoids are often very painful. It is a condition which affects all races of people.

HISTORICAL

Hemorrhoidectomy is an ancient operation. It was Galen who first ligated the pile and allowed the mass to slough away. Hippocrates, it is claimed, was the first to practice excision. Since this early day, many ways of treating and operating hemorrhoids have been devised and much of the technique used today had its origin generations ago.

INCIDENCE

A statistical report recently published by a large insurance company gives the incidence of hemorrhoidal disease as one-fifteenth of the total population of the United States, but if this report could be broken down to individual case records and each case studied, it is highly probable that it would be found that many allied ano-rectal diseases were included in the original survey. At any rate the report gives evidence of the frequency of hemorrhoidal diseases.

In the following paragraph or two, I want to mention some of the present day methods and techniques and point out why there is so much complaint from the laity concerning postoperative pain and fear of operation for "piles." Medical charlatans have found this to be a fertile field and have capitalized on certain easy office procedures for the relief of hemorrhoids. For many years this subject has been inadequately taught in our medical schools, and much of the treatment and operative procedures in our hospitals have been turned over to junior surgeons, residents and interns whose efforts frequently result in unsatisfactory cures and unfortunate complications. Non-surgical or office procedures are always more appealing to people than hospital confinement. Therefore, the injection treatment has been devised and carried to all parts of the world and probably too often to the extremes. The fact that men with little skill can use the injection method with such ease is in itself a condemnation of it. A few skillful men of high calibre have brought the art of injection to its present high standard. I believe only a relatively few expert proctologists can wisely select and properly inject hemorrhoids. Injection is contraindicated in many instances, for example, in the presence of infection, fissure, ulcer, abscess, cryptitis, papillitis and in extensive prolapse; last, but not least, in cases of large external hemorrhoids or skin tabs. Doctor Buie and Doctor Rankin mention idiosyncrasy to certain drugs as a real danger to the injection method. Less than a month ago I was called to a doctor's office to see a frightful case. The doctor had used a quinine compound in a case who had an idiosyncrasy to this drug.

It is my experience, which is corroborated by that of Mayo Clinic and others, that it is rare to find internal hemorrhoids in the absence of external ones and similarly it is rare to fine external hemorrhoids in the absence of internal ones. Unless acute thrombosis or infection is present I always remove both types of hemorrhoids at the same time.

Experienced proctologists have found uncomplicated hemorrhoids to be productive of very little, if any, pain or discomfort. Pain is the symptom of a complication, usually infection or thrombosis.

Undoubtedly the clamp and cautery method of hemorrhoidectomy is the one most commonly used. Frankly it is not the technique of the trained proctologist. There are many objections to it, most of which have been described by other proctologists. One of the main objections is the failure to remove associated pathological lesions in the ano-rectal region at the time of the operation. There is often present a deformity about the anal margin due to a piling up of skin and the presence of large varicosities beneath the surface. Now, when the clamp and cautery operation is done, usually little effort is made to dissect out these varicosities, before the clamp is applied. Postoperative pain is nearly always a feature of no small moment to the patient who has had the cautery operation.

Lockhart-Mumery claim that the clamp and cautery operation is not complete, and that recurrence is common. Secondary hemorrhage is always a danger. Hirchman claims that the use of a hot iron in a mucous cavity is prone to be followed by stricture.

Over-sewing and burying stumps of muco-cutaneous tips of tissue is a violation of good surgical principles, especially if infection is present. The ano-rectal region is constantly bathed with infected material. Bruised skin and membranes always slough. This serves as an incubator, developing virulent infection and abscess formation.

Doctor Buie and Doctor Smith of the Mayo Clinic make use of a small clamp but their extreme skill and postoperative care accounts for their low number of complications. The management of postoperative hemorrhage is always much more difficult in the presence of clamped off and over-sewed surfaces. Cutting circularly around the anal orifice is violating one of the fundamentals of surgery as it tends to produce stricture.

Except on thrombotic, external hemorrhoids demanding immediate attention, I do not advise local infiltrating anesthetic. This tends to distort the tissue and renders it difficult for the operator to judge the original pathological land marks.

In my opinion cases presenting sloughing, gangrenous internal hemorrhoids should be operated. However, this is a moot question and treatment should be selected according to the merits of each individual case.

Thorough examination and history-taking form the basic ground work for diagnosis and proper treatment for all ano-rectal disorders. A carefully written history is of great importance. A description of the complaints, their association with bowel movements and any change in bowel habits are recorded. Probably the most important observation is the one pertaining to a change of bowel habit, from regularity to constipation or from regularity to an increase in the number of stools. Also the character of the stool is important. The patient should be asked about the presence of blood or mucus and its distribution.

Digital examination should not only include the anus and lower rectum, but also palpation of the coccyx, prostate and seminal vesicles. In female patients the examiner should know something of the conditions of the pelvic organs. The introduction of the anoscope, and subsequently the proctoscope, should be made very gently. If a spasm of this sphincter is encountered, the examination is stopped until the patient can relax. While hemorrhoids can be seen through a proctoscope, they can be studied and outlined best through the anoscope.

While much has been said of the various methods to be selected for the treatment of hemorrhoids, certain medical groups are inclined toward non-operative procedures, while others swing to surgery on all types.

Unfortunately, many well established and tried treatments are improperly given.

The method I advise is not particularly mine nor any one proctologist's. It is a method I have chosen to accomplish perfect results with the minimum of complications and discomfort. Some of the essential features of my technique are:

1. Results are uniformly more efficient and complete.
2. No postoperative pain.
3. No slough and a minimum of infection.
4. No danger of postoperative bleeding.
5. Period of convalesence lessened with greater and earlier activity.
6. Morbidity is diminished.

Regarding the preoperative care, the usual routine is carried out. Digital, anoscopic and proctoscopic examination in all cases and X-ray and laboratory examination when necessary.

The patient enters the hospital on the night before the operation. The usual urinalysis, blood count, coagulation and clotting time is taken. A blood Wasserman is usually included in the laboratory work unless a recent test has been made. Two plain water enemas are given the night before the operation, two hours apart. One enema in the morning two hours prior to the surgery—one seconal or nembutal capsule at 10 p.m. The usual preparation for any surgical operation before retiring. Morphine one-fourth to one-sixth gr., or dilaudid 1/32 gr. one hour prior, and one and one-half gr. seconal an hour and a half before operation.

The anesthetic of choice is caudal or sacral block given in the usual manner. A low, or so-called "Sitting Bull" spinal is excellent. Unless the patient refuses the above types, I never use a general.

The patient lies prone with hips elevated to the extreme, the Jack Knife position, with arms and shoulders comfortably resting on an arm board. In this position there will be no over-engorgement of the hemorrhoidal area with resulting removal of too much tissue, and the surgeon can be assured of sufficient room for assistance.

The anus and perineum for about a six inch radius is painted twice with tincture merthiolate, and drapes are placed. Before starting the operation I always test the anal tissue for anesthesia, using preferably a toothless hemostat. When anesthesia is complete the anal canal is dilated with an anoscope only and not divulged as advised in older text books. I first use two or three strips of rolled gauze passed through the anoscope to bring down gently all hemorrhoids. A small piece of gauze attached to a tape may be rolled and pushed high in the midrectum to prevent stool seepage and blood back flowing, since the patient is lying prone.

Regardless of the theories and ideas of a few good proctologists concerning the main hemorrhoidal masses and their constant location in all cases, the main idea is surgically to approach these masses in the easiest and most convenient way to remove them successfully. The following procedure is usually advisable; however, I want to say here that there are two things to keep in mind: first, select the hemorrhoid which, when removed, will allow the operator to approach better each consecutive one, and, secondly, at the same time not be hampered by the oozing of blood from the site of a freshly operated field.

To expose the hemorrhoid to the best advantage, grasp the skin with a five inch Kelly forcep about one inch from the base of the selected hemorrhoid to be removed. The forcep is so placed as to make traction of the skin in line with the hemorrhoid mass and be pointed toward the anus. By traction and retraction in opposite directions, the internal and external hemorrhoid then present themselves as one defect and are removed in one mass. In chronic fissures sometimes you may find the anal contracture so marked that even the finger is not easily admitted. In such cases the sphincter is divided in the mid line posterior. By all means never dilate the anal canal by force. Painful hematoma, muscle destruction with formation of scar tissue, and incontinence are the results. With another five inch curved Kelly forcep, I grasp the top and uppermost pole of the hemorrhoid mass and include in this pick-up the mucous membrane as far as one-half an inch superior to the pectinate line. All of the hemorrhoidal mass, both internal and external, is gently manipulated for exposure.

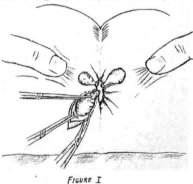

FIGURE I

Figure 1: The hemorrhoids have been drawn outside the anus in their respective quadrants. The most dependent one is selected and an elliptic incision is made on each side including all the hemorrhoidal mass.

This having been accomplished, the next step is the removal. With curved scissors, I start the incision just below the first pair of forceps on the skin toward the hemorrhoid incise the skin and mucous membrane around the mass on both sides, reaching the apex or upper angle at such a distance that it would circumscribe all the mass including the veins, but much care is taken not to dip down too far to include any fibers of the sphincter muscle. The mass is now lifted away and upon inspection we find an open eliptical wound, the outer angle of which is just below where the first skin forceps was anchored and the inner angle just above the pectinate line. With a plain cat gut suture on a small, full curve cutting needle, all bleeding points are brought up and included in a continuous locked suture along the cut edge of the upper portion of the wound but leaving the lower skin portion of the wound gaping for drainage. This point is very essential because all

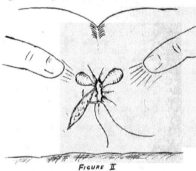

FIGURE II

Figure 2: The hemorrhoidal mass has been dissected out and the suturing started. All bleeding points are caught up in this procedure.

tissue about the anal canal is constantly bathed in bacteria. Attention is called to the fact that I do not have any buried sutures in any part of the wound to invite abscess and the stumps of the hemorrhoidal veins have been caught up and sutured under the cut edge of the mucosa.

After the hemorrhoid is removed and suturing completed the traction released there should be a falling together of the edges of the mucosa. The skin edges almost fall together also but are gaping just enough to furnish a trough for drainage. This completes the removal of one hemorrhoid. All others are removed in the same manner, but care is taken to leave strips of mucous membrane between each operative field to prevent stricture.

Inspection of the anal canal is very important following this technique—removing any clots and not overlooking any inflamed

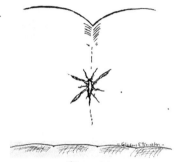

FIGURE III

Figure 3: All hemorrhoids have been removed and suturing completed. The edges of the upper portion of the wound fall together while the outer portion gaps just enough for drainage.

papilla or fissure. Should such be found they are excised at this time. If any postoperative bleeding occurs the operator will know a fresh hemorrhage has taken place.

With the speculum inserted, a sponge saturated with tincture merthiolate is placed in the anal canal and the speculum withdrawn. At the end of one minute the sponge is removed and again the canal is observed through a speculum. All excess merthiolate is taken up with a dry sponge. Anesthetic ointments never prevent postoperative pain appreciably. Gentleness in handling the tissue and the proper care of all anal lesions have been found to be more effective.

Fissures and ulcers have been reported in patients as high as 30 percent by some operators. They are usually found in the mid line posterior. These should be excised deep enough to include the indurated, infected tissue surrounding them. Small fistulae are dissected out after the hemorrhoidectomy is completed. Large fistulae are dealt with separately and in the lithotomy position if they extend over the perineum.

The next step is to prevent postoperative pain. Tincture merthiolate is now painted over the area for a four inch radius about the anus and, with the index finger of the left hand in the ano-rectal canal as a guide, I inject with the right hand an anesthetic agent in oil in fan shape about the anal canal deep in the perianal fat. This is evenly distributed so that all nerves will be anesthetzed by its effect. The duration of the anesthesia is about 14 to 21 days. This part of the operation is so very important, to prevent pain, sphincter spasm and discomfort. Caution must be exercised here not to pool the anesthetic in the ano-rectal fat nor to puncture the rectum. Two strips of vaseline gauze are carefully placed in the anal canal and the outer ends smoothed in and out over

the wounds. This gauze is removed on the second postoperative day. A sterile gauze dressing is applied over the wound and the buttocks brought close together with two two-inch adhesive straps applied from side to side.

IMMEDIATE POSTOPERATIVE CARE

The patient is removed from the operating room in a prone position on a carrier and kept in this position in bed for three hours. After this time the pelvic musculature will have regained its tonicity and the patient may turn from side to side. The patient should not be turned on the back too soon because of pressure effect on the operative field. When the patient first notices a slight burning in the ano-rectal region he is given a hypodermic of one-fourth gr. morphine, or 1/32 dilaudid. This is repeated every four hours if necessary. As a rule no hypodermics are needed after the first day. Hot boric packs are continuously applied unless the patient is sleeping. This is essential to relax the sphincter and prevent painful spasms. On the fourth day the patient gets a laxative of one ounce of milk of magnesia. I order no mineral oil to the patient while in the hospital unless he wants it or his mind will be eased by taking it.

Regarding the diet, the following is most satisfactory to my patients:

First day: Liquids, i.e. Coca Cola, tea and broth.

Second day: A full tray with orders to eat only half the amount on the tray. (In this way they get a better variety of dishes.)

Third day: A full tray and they may eat all they want of it.

After the patient leaves the hospital, the care may be given by the home physician. This consists of daily office dressing for the first week. A dressing every third day for ten days. At the end of this time, the gloved finger should explore the anal canal to determine the presence of forming adhesions and the size of the canal. If a contracture is detected, gentle massage should be given twice weekly for a few weeks. Hot sitz baths are recommended daily for a while if there is any discomfort. A full, well-cooked, bland diet and doses of mineral oil over a period of time as seems necessary is advised. A final check-up examination should be made by the surgeon at the end of the third month.

Advantages of this technique:

1. Hemorrhoidal recurrences are eliminated.
2. Postoperative pain and hemorrhages are prevented.
3. Infection is very rare following this technique.
4. Trauma is lessened.
5. Systematic division of the field is accomplished.

SUMMARY

1. A new technique for hemorrhoidectomy has been described in detail. This technique reveals the simplicity and completeness of a procedure which neatly removes all hemorrhoids and allows for drainage, prevents infection, sloughing and secondary hemorrhage, rendering postoperative surgery negligible.

2. Included in this new technique is the use of anesthetic agents in oil which has for its purpose a prolonged anesthesia until the patient has completely recovered from surgery.

3. The postoperative or convalescent period in the hospital is notably shortened and painless. Last but not least, the "final end results" are most gratifying.

BIBLIOGRAPHY

Jackson, Raymond J.: Preoperative and Postoperative Care in Ano Rectal Surgery. Surgical Clinics of North America, August, 1940.

Bacon: Anus-Rectum-Signoid Colon. Lippincott, Philadelphia.

Baumeister-Moon: A Complete Technique for Hemorrhoidectomy. Surgery-Gynecology and Obstetrics, September, 1940.

Buie, Louis A.: Preoperative and Postoperative Care in Ano-Rectal Surgery. Reprint from Archives of Surgery, June, 1940.

The Present Day Conception of Convulsive Disorders*

CHARLES R. RAYBURN, M.D.

NORMAN, OKLAHOMA

May it be called to the attention of those interested in this subject, at the very outset, the exact title of this paper. The expression, "Convulsive Disorders," is used rather than the word epilepsy. The word epilepsy means in Greek—seizures. There are many types of seizures or convulsive disorders. Convulsions are symptoms and there is no disease entity epilepsy, as there is pneumonia, diabetes, brain tumor, encephalitis, chorea, etc. Whenever the word epilepsy is used, it should convey solely the idea that a symptom is being considered, just the same as headache, temperature, leukocytosis, etc. The word "epilepsy" has been handed down for generations and in the past has been applied to conditions often considered hereditary in nature and from a prognostic standpoint more or less hopeless. Therefore, when this word is used today, because of the way it has been interpreted for past generations, it is really unfair to the patient and to the patient's relatives. They have a tendency to consider a diseased condition labled by the doctor or any one else as "epilepsy" with the wrong perspective. Therefore, throughout the remainder of this paper the expression convulsive disorder will be used except in special instances. In Anglo-Saxon terminology, an "epileptic" is a person subject to fits. Specifically, and more accurately, epilepsy or a convulsion is a symptom of a disturbance in the electrical activity of the brain, with a tendency for this disturbance, from time to time, to vary in degree.

The symptom complex of any type of convulsion is manifested usually by:
1. Impairment of consciousness
2. Autonomic and nervous manifestations
3. Convulsive (motor) disturbances
4. Psychic (mental) disturbances

Convulsions occur only when and after the brain is involved. This is true whether the convulsions are associated with high temperature, head trauma, alcohol, idiopathic convulsions or intestinal parasites. In any of these or similar conditions, there is usually an edema of the brain which in turn has developed from either mechanical obstruction in the fluid pathways of the brain or from a toxic irritation of the brain tissue.

First divide convulsions into two groups:
1. Essential (idiopathic, cryptogenic) convulsions
2. Symptomatic convulsions

In the first group, namely, the essential, no actual blemish of the brain may be demonstrable. In the second group demonstrable lesions of the brain may exist or else etiological causes of cerebral edema may be found elsewhere in the body. In the last group, namely, symptomatic, there is usually found:
1. Congenital brain defects
2. Trauma or brain injury occurring before birth, at birth or subsequent to birth
3. Systemic diseases and intoxications as uremia, pernicious anemia, tetany, disease of glands of internal secretion, etc.
4. Drug irritation or edema of the brain and central nervous system,—as cocaine, caffeine, ergot, nicotine, lead, carbon monoxide, etc.

For an individual to have convulsions, of either the essential or symptomatic types, the electrical activity of the cells of that individual's brain must be such as to permit the convulsion. The electrical activity of the brain varies in people just the same as blood pressure varies, or the same as pulse rate,

*Read before the Section on Neurology, Psychiatry and Endocrinology, Annual Session, Oklahoma State Medical Association, May 20, 1941, in Oklahoma City.

blood sugar, leukocyte count, etc., varies. No two people can be expected to have just the same of any of these. Two people may have exactly the same tumors of the brain or the same injury to the brain, and one of these might have convulsions and the other not. In the one the electrical activity of the brain cells could be more easily disturbed than in the other. It is this element of convulsions namely, "easily disturbed electrical activity of the brain cells," which may be inherited and it is the only element outside of organic and anatomical abnormalities which plays any part in the so-called "hereditary phase of epilepsy or convulsive disorders."

Briefly stating, to have convulsions two things must exist:

1. The brain whose cells are such that the normal electrical activity can easily be disturbed.
2. Something to disturb this electrical activity. This may be a lesion of the brain or chemical irritant. Such irritant may be taken in from outside of the body or it may develop within the body, as from a disturbed metabolism or disturbed physiology and such may be to the degree that it is difficult to determine that it actually exists.

To determine the electrical activity of the brain cells there has been developed the electro-encephalogram. This instrument measures the electrical potentials of the brain which in turn can be obtained from the brain by simply placing electrodes on the intact skull. The instrument amplifies the electrical potentials much in the same way as the electrocardiograph records the cardiac potential on a moving film as the electro-cardiograph records the cardiac picture. This instrument has been developed by the two Dr. Gibbs and Dr. William G. Lennox of Boston. A very good explanation of this is found in Tice's "Practice of Medicine," Vol. 10, Chapter 12. By the use of the electro-encephalogram to determine the electrical activity of the brain cells and the use of the pneumo-encephalogram to determine the organic lesions of the brain the various convulsive disorders can well be analyzed and understood. However, as in any disease, the history and the physical examinations are important features in interpreting convulsive disorders.

Convulsions occurring in adult life are nearly always based upon either some prominent organic brain condition as brain tumor, head trauma, cerebral hemorrhage, cerebral arteriosclerosis and the like, or some easily located physical illness as uremia, blood sugar disturbances, etc.

Convulsive states having their onset in infancy, childhood and youth are the ones which so often bother the family doctor, the internist and even the neuro-psychiatrist, and so often in this group when they occur around puberty and adolescence are referred to as "epilepsy of the idiopathic type." As a matter of fact, if a careful history of birth and childhood is obtained, and if electro- and pneumo-encephalograms are taken, organic brain conditions will be found to exist. There are of course exceptions, for children may have disturbed metabolisms and disturbed physiology the same as adults. However most of these convulsions which occur in infancy, childhood and early youth, are based upon either anatomical abnormalities which may be inherited or upon injuries occurring at birth (which is very frequent), or injuries occurring in early infancy and childhood, either from head trauma or cerebral infection. It has been reported in the literature of our obstetricians that 40 percent of the babies having apparently perfectly normal deliveries have sufficient trauma of the head, that red blood cells can be obtained from cerebro-spinal fluid by doing a lumbar tap immediately after birth; and in 60 percent of the babies born by difficult labor which includes either precipitate or prolonged labor, and forceps delivery. Some of the common physical and anatomical abnormalities which have a tendency to be inherited and may play a part in considering convulsions of children are:

1. Congenital malformations of the brain tissue
2. Congenital malformation of the cerebro-spinal fluid pathways
3. Angiomatous (birthmark), or blood vessel abnormalities in and about the brain.
4. Congenital malformations of the skull bones, particularly small jugular forminae.

There are two outstanding periods in a child's life in which convulsions are prone to have their onset, when such convulsions are a result of birth injury or an injury occurring in early infancy or childhood. The first period is between the ages of birth and four years, while the second is around puberty between the ages of ten and fifteen. In the first group, quite often there is sufficient injury to the brain tissue or the blood vessels of the brain that mental deficiency or spastic paralyses, one or both, are in appreciable evidence. In the second group, however, the child is considered normal in every respect until its first convulsion. In this group it is evident from recent studies in the past few years that the arachnoid granulations, which at the age of puberty rapidly develop into Pacchionian bodies, have failed to develop, and it is now known that red blood cells, as a result of injury getting into the sub-arachnoid space in and around the arachnoid granulations ,at birth, in infancy and childhood, cause so much scar tissue in these structures that they will not develop into the Pacchionian bodies. Since it is through these latter structures that most of the cerebro-spinal fluid enters back into the blood circulation and since, when they are impaired, this function will not be properly carried out and the cerebro-spinal fluid will be dammed up into its pathways, mild or severe edema of the brain tissue takes place. When the body is in a prone or dependent position, a slowing up of the cerebrovascular circulation occurs and this is why so many of the convulsions occurring at this period in life manifest themselves either at night, and are thus called nocturnal convulsions, or else early in the forenoon after a night's rest with the body in a normal prone position.

In obtaining the history of such cases, namely, convulsions based upon birth injury, either a few or several of the following informational data relative to the individuals may be obtained:

1. The child was cyanotic, breathed with difficulty or had to be resuscitated, immediately after birth
2. The child did not cry out immediately after birth
3. The labor was precipitate, prolonged or unusually difficult
4. Forceps were necessary
5. The child was premature, or perhaps of very large size
6. It was the first child and perhaps the mother was well advanced in years, before the child was born.

In this connection, the first convulsion may have been petit mal and, either petit mal or grand mal in type occurs usually when the body is in a dependent position or shortly after it has been in such position. Convulsions occurring most frequently at night or in the early morning are nearly always based on impaired cerebro-spinal fluid circulation and an organic brain condition.

In addition to all of these causative factors of convulsions, it should be borne in mind that the convulsive potential, namely, the ability of the brain cells to have their electrical activity easily disturbed, must be co-existing.

The whole field of convulsive disorders may be outlined by the following diagram:

On the right side we have those factors which swing the pendulum into the convulsive field, while on the left side of the balances we have those factors which help counterbalance the convulsive features and swing the pendulum to the non-convulsive field or the safe zone. Most of these are therapeutic procedures which may be estab-

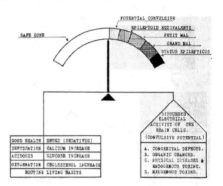

lished. Furthermore by establishing these procedures or eliminating any of those listed on the convulsive side under the letters, A, B, C, and D will help prevent the actual occurrance of convulsive attacks. The convulsive potential on the right side of the balance is the one factor which cannot be eliminated. Subdivisions of the other factors on the convulsive side of the balances are here listed:

CAUSATIVE FACTORS

A. Congenital Defects
  1. Cerebral Aplasia
  2. Cerebromocular Degeneration
  3. Congenital idiocy
  4. Tuberous sclerosis
  5. Cranial Bone Anomalies
  6. Blood Vessel Anomolies

B. Organic Changes
  1. Trauma-Hemorrhage at birth
  2. Sinus Thrombosis
  3. Encephalitis, Meningitis
  4. Gliosis, scars, multiple sclerosis
  5. Senility Arteriosclerosis
  6. Tumors, Cysts
  7. Others

C. Physical Diseases and Endogenous Toxins
  1. Uremia, Eclampsia, Asphyxia
  2. Polycythemia, Anemia, Alkalosis
  3. Decreased oxygen, Calcium, Glucose
  4. Hypertension, Hypotension, Unstable emotions
  5. Craniofacial Hemiatrophy
  6. Raynaud's Disease, Stokes-Adams Syndrome
  7. Tetanus, Acute Fevers

D. Exogenous Toxins
  1. Alcohol, Water, Insulin
  2. Picrotoxin, Absinth, Thuzone

3. Camphor, Metrazol, Protein
4. Caffeine, N i c o t i n e, Adrenalin, Strychnine
5. Carbon Monoxide, Lead, Ergot

Allied or mild convulsive states as classified by Lennox in Tice's "Practice of Medicine" are:

1. Effecting Consciousness
   Petit mal
   Pyknolepsy
   Narcolepsy
   Somnambulism
   Bad temper or temper tantrums
2. Overactivity of Muscles
   Grand mal seizures
   Jacksonian seizures
   Tonic epilepsy
   Epilepsy partialis continua
   Hysterical convulsions
   Tetany
   Eclampsia
3. Loss of Muscle Activity or Tone
   Syncope
   Akinetic epilepsy
   Cataplexy
   Catalepsy
   Periodic familial paralyses
   Carotid sinus reflex
4. Sensory
   Reflex epilepsy
   Sensory epilepsy
   Migraine
   Vertigo
5. Autonomic System
   Vasovagal seizures
   Sympathetic seizures

CARE AND TREATMENT

When a convulsive seizure starts in any individual it is good treatment, from a medical standpoint, to protect the individual in his fall if such can be done. Then permit him to lie where he has fallen or where he has been placed until the muscular spasms have passed. If possible one should insert a small piece of wood or a rolled piece of cloth in between the teeth to prevent biting of the tongue. Loosening of all bands around the body such as collars or belts is advantageous to oxygenation. To decrease the number of convulsions as a result of treatment increases the chances of an individual making a better social adjustment. The more convulsions an individual has the more he is likely to have, and the more he is likely to be incapacitated as a result of mental deterioration and other complications associated with this type of illness. Conversely, if the number of convulsions can be decreased, the less number of convulsions one is likely to have. Treatment should be instituted with this view in mind even though one cannot expect the elimination of all convulsions.

While no treatment is available, as yet, which will definitely and permanently alter the electrical activity of brain cells, some drugs such as luminal and dilantin, and the bromides will raise the convulsive threshold. Conditions which have a tendency to lower the convulsive threshold such as brain tumor, scar tissue on the brain, "birthmarks" on the brain, physical diseases, disturbed physiology, and metabolism, should be corrected.

Those convulsions in which birth injury has played a part, in particular those which have the first convulsive symptoms between the ages of ten and 14 are very amenable to the following treatment:

1. Limitation of fluid intake with copius watery bowel evacuations using saline cathartics, once or twice weekly.
2. Regular living habits, eating and sleeping
3. Elevation of the head of the bed when resting or sleeping
4. High sugar carbohydrate diet
5. Establishing a mild state of acidosis
6. Increase of calcium and cholesterol intake
7. High oxygenation
8. Using anti-convulsants such as phenobarbital, dilantin, and the bromides.

The above eight procedures may often be worthwhile in convulsions due to any and all etiological factors.

CONCLUSIONS

1. There is no disease entity epilepsy.
2. The term "seizure" or the term "convulsive disorder" is more accurate and more appropriate than the word epilepsy.
3. The causes of convulsions are many and varied.
4. Convulsions are not inherited.
5. Only a very varying convulsive threshold demonstrated by a disturbed electrical activity of the brain cells has a tendency to be inherited as a recessive Mendelian characteristic.
6. One should not speak of curing a convulsive state even though actual unconsciousness and muscular convulsions are eliminated.
7. Treatment is worthwhile. Occasionally an individual may have his convulsions eliminated. Frequently convulsions can be decreased in number and frequency.
8. With proper care and attention it is seldom necessary to confine individuals having convulsions to a state institution. Although in long standing cases with mental deterioration or in those which develop an actual psychosis or mental sickness, institutional care may be advisable.

Experience with Amebic Dysentery in Northeastern Oklahoma[*]

GEORGE K. HEMPHILL, M.D.

PAWHUSKA, OKLAHOMA

It is not my intention in this paper to give an extensive review of either the latest methods of diagnosis of amebic dysentery or the latest methods of treatment as the time allotted does not permit such a review, and besides, it is available to any of you in your books and journals once you have suspected the condition.

This paper is, rather, an effort to call to your attention the frequency of amebic dysentery or amebiasis in the average practice of the general practitioner. My interest in amebiasis was first aroused, as I think is often true, by a case in which I failed to make the diagnosis. I failed even to suspect amebic dystentery, in spite of the fact that I had been called in after two other doctors had failed to give satisfaction because they had failed to produce any improvement of symptoms, and in spite of the fact that the case was almost a textbook picture of amebic dysentery.

Two days later after I also had failed to get any improvement in the case, she was taken to Oklahoma City, 150 miles by ambuance, and when I was told a week later that amebic dysentery had been diagnosed almost immediately and that she had improved markedly following the institution of specific treatment, I resolved at least to examine a stool specimen of any case of diarrhea that did not respond to the usual treatment within 24 hours.

Although I did this for about two years, I was not rewarded with a great deal of success until I found a small detail that has been important in my finding motile ameba in a specimen. I had been having this specimen brought to the office after being passed at home, when I would get a report that there were several suspicious looking objects, but they were not motile so a positive report could not be given. On this particular day a three-year-old boy was brought in with a history of eight or ten bloody bowel movements daily. He did not look as ill as he should have with that history, but expressed a desire for a bowel movement while he was in the office, so a specimen was saved and examined at once. It was positive. My technician remarked how easy it was to examine

a specimen immediately after it was passed, as then the ameba were very motile and easily identified.

Since that time I have tried in any case in which I suspected amebiasis to obtain a specimen in the office and examine it at once. Since doing this, I find a greater number of positive specimens. It is usually easy to obtain a specimen either with a proctoscope or a sigmoidoscope in any case that is having acute diarrhea or dysentery. However, in the chronic case where it is suspected, it is usually necessary to give a saline cathartic in order to bring them into the lumen of the bowel. So much for method of diagnosis.

Next, I would like to list a few cases that have come under my care in the last year as examples of the fact that there are many cases in which ambiasis is apparently not even considered, and as a result, the diagnosis is missed.

About a year ago a five-year-old boy came under my care. He had been ill at intervals since the age of two years. A diagnosis of coeliac disease was made at one time as a cause of the intermittent diarrhea. He had had Neoprontosil and Sulfanilamide at intervals and was improved temporarily. He had had several blood transfusions. A diagnosis of colitis due to malaria had also been made, although there never had been a report of a blood smear for malaria. During this entire three years he had had a secondary anemia for which he had had medicine given him in addition to the transfusions. He was first seen by me about a year ago. At that time the stool was positive for round worms and he was given two weekly courses of gentian violet. Subsequent to this time he improved markedly for a period of a month or six weeks, following which he had a relapse of diarrhea and foul smelling stools. At this time a stool specimen was examined warm, and was positive for ameba. It so happened that he was the most difficult case I have ever had to treat and would relapse each time after the usual type of treatment, until finally on December 11, I gave him a course of combined treatment of Carbarsone by mouth and chiniofon retention enemas. Since that time he has apparently remained well, but only last month his father came in with an acute dysentery in which the first specimen

*Read before the Section on General Medicine, Annual Session, Oklahoma State Medical Association, May 21, 1941, in Oklahoma City.

was found to be positive for ameba, so that it is possible he is now in the chronic or carrier state. I think it will probably be advisable to have a recheck on his stool specimen.

I cite this case to illustrate the fact that this boy had been treated over a period of three years by several doctors, giving symptoms of frequent bloody stools, secondary anemia, and a failure to respond to the usual treatment for either the diarrhea or the specific treatment which was given for malaria, all of this for three years without a stool specimen ever having been examined.

Another case I would like to mention was a woman about 30 years of age, a beauty operator, who gave a history of having been in a hospital in Missouri for two months with a diagnosis of mucous colitis. She thought she had improved sufficiently to return to work but had only worked three days when the diarrhea returned with severe tenesmus and abdominal cramps. The first specimen examined was positive for ameba and after a course of treatment her symptoms left and have not recurred in the six months since. As far as I know a stool specimen was never examined during her two months' treatment in the hospital in Missouri.

We would think a physician grossly negligent who treated a case of frequency, dysuria, and polyuria two months empirically for cystitis or pyelitis without examining the urine to eliminate diabetes, and yet it is not uncommon to find a case of diarrhea or dysentery treated for a month or two without specimens ever having been examined.

It might be of interest to you to know the state health department will send specimen containers in which you may send stool specimens to them for culture and examination for ova, bacillary dysentery, etc., in case a trained technician is not available to you. Also I might mention that the Eli Lilly company has a very excellent film on amebic dysentery, with some very good motion pictures filmed through the microscope, which give you a good picture of the ameba in motion. They are obtainable free by any medical society, for showing.

Let me close by adding a few general statements about amebiasis which some of you may have forgotten.

1. Only two percent or less of cases harboring ameba even have a diarrhea.

2. It has been found in every state in the Union.

3. The incidence is probably around four to eight percent of the general population.

4. It is spread by infected vegetables such as lettuce, cabbage, etc., and by flies.

5. Many chronic cases give symptoms which are often interpreted as indicating the so-called chronic appendicitis, chronic gall bladder disease or sub-acute gastric ulcer.

6. It may be necessary to give a saline to bring the organisms into the lumen of the bowel in the subacute or chronic cases, as they tend to become imbedded in the wall of the bowel.

A good method of examining this type of case is to have them come to the laboratory or office and give them two tablespoonfuls of Magnesium Sulphate and then examine each stool as passed immediately, keeping it warm on a warm stage until four or five stools have been passed.

One man by using this technique reported the finding of 53 patients infested with this organism in five years, none of which had dysentery and none being confined to bed because of the presence of the ameba, with the exception of one patient who had a perforation of the bowel. Many of these had been previously treated for intestinal flu or generalized gastrointestinal disturbances.

Generalized symptoms of the chronic cases have been listed as: constipation, evanescent attacks of diarrhea, anorexia, nausea before or after eating, loss of weight, frontal headaches, sleeplessness and disturbed slumber, poor memory, fever or subnormal temperature, the symptoms being insidious.

I realize that this paper has been somewhat sketchy and perhaps overfilled with a few individual cases, but I did this intentionally in order to impress upon you how easily these cases are treated over long periods of time without the physician's suspecting and ruling out or finding the infection. I think it is very true with this infection, as is said with many others, that it is not in not knowing, but in not looking, that we find our failure, and so if this short talk will result in some of you at least thinking of and finding or ruling out the presence of ameba by the examination of a warm stool specimen on patients giving these symptoms in your practice in the future, I will feel that its presentation has been worthwhile.

DISCUSSION

S. C. SHEPARD, M.D., F.A.C.P.
TULSA, OKLAHOMA

Amobic dysentery is an acute ulcerative disease of the large intestine, caused by entameba hystolyca, producing bloody mucus stools, likely to be intermittent in character. It is liable to cause the formation of hepatic subphrenic or pulmonary single abscesses.

Amobic dysentery was for a long time considered to be a tropical disease. However, it is now found in all parts of the United States. It seems to be becoming more prevalent throughout the country, quite probably because of the increased consumption of raw vegetables. Most truck gardeners fertilize with raw manure which may be contaminated with human secretions. Or the washing of such vegetables in preparation for market may be done in small puddles which may be contaminated. Also it may be spread from contaminated sources by means of house flies. A food handler, who is a carrier, may contaminate several hundred individuals by careless handling of the food.

The diagnosis may best be made by finding motile ameba or the cysts in a stool. A fresh stool or scrapings from an ulcer are the best media in which to look for the ameba. The cysts must be classified by one who is experienced in differentiation of various amebic cysts.

The ameba must live in or on tissues under the mucous membranes of the intestines, or other tissues. They exert a proteolytic effect and dissolve out a cavern. This causes a small grayish ulcer with ragged undermined edges, which are often necrotic in appearance. They have a characteristic musky odor.

Any one of three forms of amebic dysentery is usually seen.

First: Acute, which begins suddenly with severe abdominal pains, bloody mucus stools with a fetid odor, and followed by secondary infection with streptococcic or dysentery bacillus. Chills and fever occur, and usually alternate diarrhea and constipation.

Second: Mild, which has a slow insidious onset and may go for a long period undiagnosed. There are vague signs of indigestion, dyspepsia, abdominal discomfort, loss of strength, and possible loss of weight. There is either moderate diarrhea or constipation.

Third: Chronic, which manifests vague dull distress in the abdomen. The health is below par. There is weakness, nervous symptoms, a low blood count, and the patient may have 15 stools a day. This often simulates pellagra.

Treatment consists of a bland diet and drugs. Probably the most commonly used and most effective of the drugs is emetine, with a dosage up to ten grains used hypodermically. Chiniofon, carbarsone, acetarsone, and vioform are probably among the most frequently used. Irrigations may be employed, consisting of a wide variety of drugs and solutions. This depends on each individual treating the disease, as to the choice of such.

In conclusion, then, amebic dysentery is a disease which occurs rather frequently, and should be looked for at all times.

Mastoiditis: A Case History[*]

FRANK VIEREGG, M.D.

CLINTON, OKLAHOMA

In presenting this case before this body I am well aware of the limitations and shortcomings of this paper. I have never liked to hear a paper in which the essayist was not able before the end of the paper to give his audience all of the conclusions that should be deduced from a study of the case at hand, but in this case I am not able to do that. Had I been able to diagnose this case correctly before operation, I am not positive that I would have had the temerity to start any operative procedure. But the results, evidently, justified what I did do.

This patient, Mrs. KWA, aged 32, presented herself to the Western Oklahoma Charity Hospital, February 6, 1941. Her chief complaint was of "pain, tenderness, and swelling behind the left ear." Her present illness began about eight weeks ago with an influenzal-like attack which ran a course of two to three weeks. This attack left her weak and exhausted. About that time she began to have an attack of bilateral ear ache. In several days the left ear drum ruptured

*Read before the Section on Eye, Ear, Nose and Throat, Annual Session, Oklahoma State Medical Association, May 21, 1941, in Oklahoma City.

spontaneously and discharged pus. This ear discharged for about two weeks with a gradual decrease in amount. As the discharge decreased the pain and tenderness behind the ear gradually developed. This swelling and tenderness increased until the time of admission to the hospital. She thinks that she had had a gradual loss of hearing extending back for about a year. During this time she has had no fever to her knowledge, and to my knowledge did not have any medical attention.

Her general health has never been good since she was about 15 years of age. She has had much lower abdominal distress and lower back ache and a marked vaginal discharge for years. At time of admission she thought she was about three months pregnant. In talking with her family physician I found that she had been on antisyphilitic treatment for some time, but just how thorough this was I don't know.

At the time that I first saw her she had the appearance of being much older than her admitted age of 32. Her temperature was 99.4 and respiratory rate of 20.

The chest examination was essentially negative.

Abdomen: Slight tenderness of the entire lower abdomen with a mid-line mass about the size of a grapefruit.

Head: The first thing one noticed about the head was the position of the left ear. It stood at almost a right angle from the head. There was marked swelling over the entire mastoid region which had a tendency to run downward over the sterno-cleido. mastoid muscle. This mass was tender, reddened, with the mushy sort of feeling you could elicit over a subperiosteal edema. This mass also extended backwards over what I would have called an enlarged mastoid region. The canal of the ear was filled with a foul smelling sero-purulent discharge. However, the patient declared that the ear had not discharged for several days. The posterior superior quadrant of the canal presented a characteristic "sagging." The drum was inflamed, lacked lustre, but did not seem to be bulging. There was a small hole in the drum membrane. A rather superficial tuning fork test done on the two ears in the hospital ward did not show any marked reduction of hearing on this left side. The Meber test did not lateralize. The X-ray examination did not show much difference on the two sides, but showed both sides to be markedly sclerosed, throughout the entire mastoid processes. The report from the X-ray laboratory read, "Both mastoid areas equally cloudy."

The Wasserman report showed a negative Wasserman reaction. The spinal fluid Wasserman was negative. The Kahn Reaction was negative. The urinalysis showed only a trace of albumin that was in any way out of line. There were 3,800,000 RBC. The white count showed 16,800 with 84 percent polys.

I made the usual mastoid incision in this case, that is, parallel and posterior to the attachment of the pinna and about one-fourth an inch away. As soon as the periosteum was opened there was a great amount of pus that showed in the wound, together with a large amount of old blood clots, which was a rather unusual finding. As is my custom in such a case, I removed the cortex from an extremely hard, eburnized, mastoid process. The mastoid process instead of being very cellular and full of pus, had only a small amount of a serous-appearing, straw-colored fluid, and this was not under pressure. The bone was very hard, concrete-like in texture, and I could not say that it either was or was not infected. I cleaned out this area down to the tympanic antrum and the tip cells of the mastoid.

When I had reached what I thought was the posterior margin of the mastoid cells I found an area that looked like a few more

cells that apparently were filled with something, that had it not been in the mastoid area, I would have called polypoid tissue. I pushed on this area with a curette and the bowl of the curette passed out of sight in the direction of the occipital bone. This was followed by another gush of pus and a large amount of old blood clots. After this area was exposed by a counter incision, I found an area about one and one-half inches in diameter that was filled with this same sort of thing, that is, a substance that had all the appearances of nasal polypoid material, blood clots and pus. I cleaned this all out and found that it extended through both tables of the skull and was but loosely adherent to the underlying dura.

The dura was but very slightly inflamed, if at all, and the mass of stuff easily curetted off. I had some of this sent to the laboratory for examination. The report came back: "The gross specimen consists of two soft, red, ragged, irregular pieces of tissue, each about eight mm. Microscopic examination shows a very vascular, granulomatous structure intensely and diffusely infiltrated with leucocytes throughout. No evidence of malignancy and no definite evidence of any specific type of inflammation. Diagnosis: Subacute suppurative inflammation and granulation. Gumma can not be entirely excluded."

I filled this wound with one-half inch iodoform gauze packer strip and placed only three silkworm sutures. As a glance at this woman's postoperative temperature chart will show, she had a most uneventful recovery—her temperature never going above 99 during the rest of her stay in the hospital.

Whether this condition originated in the mastoid and spread to the occipital bone, or originated in situ, I am unable to say. I am not even positive that she ever had any mastoid trouble, but certainly she had a middle ear infection. And if I had known what that dark area behind the mastoid process in the X-ray was, I might not have had the nerve to operate.

In this case I am not able to come to any definite conclusion as to what the real nature of this thing was. I have never heard of a polypoid degeneration of a skull bone but that is what is most nearly resembled. It might have been a gumma, or doesn't one have a gumma of a flat bone? Could it have been an infected bone cyst, or doesn't one have a cyst of a flat bone? Certainly it did not have any of the markings of a bony tumor, and the microscopic examination also seemed to rule that out. Might it be a thrombosis of a terminal artery at this point? If so, why the polypoid appearance of the bone involving both tables?

· THE PRESIDENT'S PAGE ·

Happy New Year

Nineteen hundred forty-one is now past history; have the accomplishments of our profession been what we would desire? A correct inventory of the achievements of the medical profession in America will show that there is much for us to be proud of. The whole-hearted cooperation with the Federal Government in preparing for the present emergency has been surpassed by no group, there has been full and complete aid given to induction boards, this fully and with no compensation and at much personal sacrifice in many instances. While the Army Medical Corps are still in need of more medical officers, there is no question that this demand will be met and that the efficiency of the United States Army will not suffer on account of a shortage of medical men.

Let us redouble our efforts to make 1942 a record year in American Medicine. We must see that this emergency does not reduce the high standards of medical education. It goes without saying that every member of the Oklahoma State Medical Association will do his full part.

May each member of our profession enjoy a most happy and prosperous New Year.

Finis. B. Ewing
President.

• EDITORIALS •

PROCUREMENT AND ASSIGNMENT

The Procurement and Assignment Service was established by the President on October 30, 1941. Today we are at war. Every doctor will be asked to register with the Office of Procurement and Assignment; all men under 45 are subject to service under the order of the Selective Service Boards.

The address of Dr. Sam F. Seeley before the recent meeting of the Secretaries Conference, sponsored by the Oklahoma State Medical Association, appears in this issue of the Journal. Every doctor in the State should read this address before filling out the accompanying enrollment form addressed to Doctor Seeley. The prompt execution and return of this blank will save delay and expense and, for some, possibly the embarrassment of being ordered into service. *See insert following Page 26.*

The doctors of Oklahoma are to be commended for their relatively high response to the A.M.A. questionnaire. It is doubtful if the doctors of any other state in the union surpassed them. But because of procrastination or indifference on the part of some, the immediate response was not more than 60 percent. The State Association office spent much time and considerable money to bring the registration to approximately 99 percent. The A.M.A. questionnaire represented a deliberate effort to accumulate valuable data in anticipation of war. Much additional biographical and professional information has been gathered and made available. This comprehensive appraisal of each member of the medical profession and his relation to the civilian medical needs of his community makes equable selection and placement more nearly possible than it could be otherwise.

If we act promptly, it is possible, under the Procurement and Assignment Service, for the medical profession to make use of this accumulate knowledge in the assignment of the individual doctor to the service for which he is best suited, whether it be civilian or military. For those who procrastinate, such a selective assignment may be impossible. Likewise, delay may lessen the assurance of a commission in keeping with age, experience and abilities.

Of all the doctors in the United States responding to the A.M.A. questionnaire, approximately 60 percent volunteered their services. Now is the time to make this offer good. We are no longer deliberating in anticipation of war. We are facing an emergency and it is time to act.

The present estimate indicates that the army alone now needs 3,000 doctors. Approximately 4,000 internes are eligible for reserve commissions, but current reports indicate that not more than 50 percent have made application for a commission. We cannot wait for them to complete their intern services. They will be needed at home or in the army and navy as soon as they are ready. Medical students who become over-zealous in their desire to fight should be convinced that they can serve best by remaining in medical school in order that they may conserve the man hours they have devoted to medical education, and that they may be ready to fill the breach which must arise through the exigencies of a hard fought war for the duration.—L.J.M.

WAR AND OPPORTUNITY

In spite of our cherished way of life, the time has come when all professions, all industries and agencies must accept a certain degree of managerial direction. The medical profession may find comfort in the fact that the regimentation arising through the exigencies of war leave the doctor more initiative and freedom in the pursuit of his art than is vouchsafed to the members of any other participating group.

Though working under orders for the benefit of all mankind, the time-honored relationship between doctor and patient affords moments of intimate contact, which are vitally individualistic and productive of spiritual values wholly beyond the realm of military control. Though these moments of contact may be stressful and fleeting, they are charged with the unquenchable realities of life which give men strength to die for others. These are moments which merit a sympathetic touch of the hand, a kind word, and a swift interchange of heart searching appraisal. Skill without compassion is a cold impersonal thing, justifiable on the battle front, but out of place in the medical service.

The doctor in the service of his country should never lose sight of the fact that he has a rare opportunity to make the word "service" a living reality to sick and wounded soldiers. By thus preserving the cherished relationship between doctor and patient under the stress of war, it may become more worthy of preservation in time of peace.—L. J. M.

HOW A GREAT DIAGNOSTIC BOON MAY BECOME A BOOMERANG

Though we have had nearly forty years experience with x-ray as a diagnostic agent in diseases of the chest, attention should be called to the fact that doctors too often expect the x-ray to give the final word in doubtful cases, especially if tuberculosis is the disease in question. A careful consideration of the most authoritative knowledge available seriously disturbs this unwarranted faith.

The report of the roentgenologist may or may not contain all available information. This depends upon the training, experience and judgment of the roentgenologist and the ever present vicissitudes of x-ray interpretation. He must recognize the known wide variations of the normal. He knows that pathology may be present without making an impression on the x-ray, and that the significance of existing x-ray shadows may be difficult to determine.

The unwarranted dogmatic diagnosis occasionally reported by the roentgenologist, if accepted by the attending physician, may lead to disaster. From the general practitioner's standpoint, with few exceptions, an x-ray of the chest should not be requested until a thorough physical examination and all indicated available laboratory tests have been made. Such a procedure suggests the x-ray's limitations and places it where it belongs, namely, among other valuable diagnostic aids. This will help overcome an unfortunate fallacy which often leads the layman to believe that the diagnostic x-ray will seal his fate, whether it be good or bad.

In support of the above discussion, the writer quotes from some of the most authoritative sources: Osler[1] once said, "More than any others, radiographers need the salutary lesson of the dead house to correct their visionary interpretation of shadows, particularly those radiating from the roots of the lungs."

These are living words, vibrant with Osler's wisdom and foresight. Though they were recorded more than twenty years ago, they serve as a timely warning against the present danger of lack of knowledge, overenthusiasm and undue confidence.

This, from Allen K. Krause[2] in 1924, is equally significant: " 'Enlargement of the mediastinum' or 'chronic mediastinitis' runs through the x-ray reports, especially those of children's examinations, like a song; with a monotony that makes one wonder whether mediastinal changes are not the normal in the young."

The following quotation from the National Tuberculosis Association[3] Diagnostic Standards, 1926, implies special knowledge for the proper interpretation of x-rays of the chest

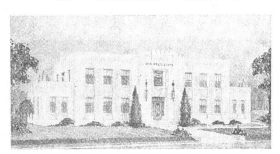

in children. "Interpretation of films should be made by an experienced physician, who is familiar not only with chest films in general, but with films of children's lungs in particular. He should also have a clinical background, and the interpretation should not be independent of careful consideration of history, symptoms and physical examination."

John A. Bigler[4] makes this significant statement: "It must be remembered that many types of pathologic changes may give shadows of the same opaqueness, etc., and that differentiation can be obtained only by consecutive roentgenograms, by the knowledge of other laboratory data and by the history and clinical and physical observations. . . . It is in the borderline cases that the most mistakes are made; the clinician reaches out for all available laboratory data and is given a positive diagnosis by the roentgenologist."

The following is from the report of a special committee appointed by the National Tuberculosis Association[5]. "To one observer, shadows noted are indicative of disease; to another, they are not evidence of a pathological process; to one they represent lesions of clinical significance; to another they suggest changes of no moment. . . . The normal chest from a radiographic standpoint is subject to such wide variations within normal limits as to be beyond possibility of exact description."

This very limited discussion and these references are offered with the hope of bringing about a consciousness of the diagnostic limitations of the x-ray and the danger of blindly accepting the roentgenologist's diagnostic report. It should be distinctly understood that they should not discourage the use of this valuable diagnostic agent which is ever becoming more important in the practice of medicine.—L. J. M.

(1) Osler, William; and McCrae, Thomas: The Principles and Practice of Medicine, New York: Appleton and Century, 1920, p. 208.
(2) Krause, A. K.: The Spread of Tuberculous Infection in the Body, Am. Rev. Tuberc. 9:83, April, 1924.
(3) National Tuberculosis Association: Diagnostic Standards. 1926.
(4) Bigler, John A.: Interpretation of Roentgenograms of the Chest in Children Based on Observations at Necropsy. Am. Jr. Diseases of Children, Vol. 38, Nov., 1929.
(5) National Tuberculosis Association: Clinical and Roentgen-Ray Findings in the Chests of Normal Children. Am. Rev. Tuberc. 6:331, 1922.

"CAVITIES IN THE SILICOTIC LUNG"

Under this title, Arthur J. Vorwald[1] points out the fact that the silicotic lung may present three distinct types of cavities:

"(1) Cavities associated with a *typical tuberculosis* that is little modified by coexistent silicosis.

(2) Cavities occurring in areas of *tuberculo-silicosis*, an extremely chronic condition resulting from the combined local effect of tubercle bacilli and silica dust. In them, the results of infection are obvious and tubercle bacilli are usually demonstrable.

(3) Cavities of the so-called *anemic type* which develop within areas of massive fibrosis, but show no evidence of causative organisms or cellular reaction."

Typical cavities are usually found in cases of first degree silicosis or in those with slight nodulation. In such cases the behavior of tuberculosis is essentially the same as in those who have not been exposed to silica. The phenomena accompanying such cavities are well known to those who follow the course of uncomplicated pulmonary tuberculosis. Tubercle bacilli are readily found in the sputum coming from such cavities.

Tuberculo-silicotic cavities occur in the more advanced silicotics. The cavities are usually unilocular and they are found in the dense fibrotic masses so common in advanced silicosis. These cavities are limited by the firm fibrotic tissue which discourages the usual softening and extension with multilocular formation. The content of such cavities is purulent, but quite black. Tubercle bacilli are much less numerous and intrapulmonary and extrapulmonary complications are less frequent than in the non-silicotic. On account of obliterative arteritis and phlebitis accompanying the dense fibrosis, pulmonary hemorrhage is less frequent than in uncomplicated pulmonary tuberculosis. For the same reason hematogenous spread is uncommon and the symptoms of toxemia are less obvious. Physical signs are not so easily elicited and the x-ray may not reveal the presence of cavities unless the technique calls for more than the average penetration.

Anemic cavities also occur in the conglomerate fibrotic masses found in advanced silicosis. They are due to the obliterative changes in the blood vessels, giving rise to avascular areas with necrosis, autolysis and liquefaction. The cavities are usually small, oval or button-hole in shape. The content is thin, black, nonpurulent; tubercle bacilli are not found even by animal inoculation. The diagnosis of this type of cavity presents the same difficulties found in the tuberculo-silicotic type.

This discussion of lung cavities in the silicotic supplies a good example of the varied clinicopathological problems arising in the slowly moving course of a very interesting and important disease.—L. J. M.

1. Vorwald, Arthur J.: Cavities in the Silicotic Lung. A Pathological Study with Clinical Correlation. The Amer. Jr. of Path., Sept., 1941. P. 709, Vol. XVII, No. 5.

No Lack in Biolac!

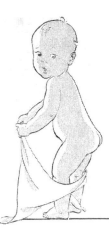

WITH THE sole exception of vitamin C, Biolac provides completely for the formula needs of normal infants throughout the entire bottle period. From the time when infants consume a full quart of formula per day, here's how certain essential food factors supplied by Biolac feedings compare with the minimal nutritional requirements recognized by the U. S. Food and Drug Administration.

	MINIMAL REQUIREMENTS	BIOLAC FEEDINGS
PROTEIN (gms./lb. body weight)	1.4 to 1.8*	2.2†
CALCIUM (gms./day)	1.0*	1.0
IRON (mgms./100 calories)	0.75	1.25
VITAMIN A (U.S.P. Units/day)	1500.	2500.
VITAMIN B₁ (U.S.P. Units/day)	83.	85.
VITAMIN B₂ (mgms./day)	0.5	2.
VITAMIN D (U.S.P. Units/100 calories)	50.	63.

*The Food & Drug Administration has not promulgated minimum requirements for protein and calcium in infancy. The values shown are those recommended by the National Nutrition Conference.
†When Biolac formulas are fed in the amount of 2½ fl. oz./lb. body weight.

Biolac is prepared from whole milk, skim milk, lactose, vitamin B₁, concentrate of vitamins A and D from cod liver oil, and ferric citrate. Evaporated, homogenized, *sterilized*.

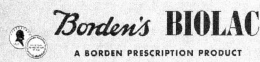

MEDICAL PREPAREDNESS

The Association has for the past month been giving complete cooperation to the American Medical Association and all Governmental Agencies, both military and otherwise, on Medical Preparedness. In order that the profession may have the latest information available concerning the Medical Preparedness program of the Association, the duties of the County Societies, and the present situation concerning the profession and military duty, as well as the program of Civilian Defense, that information is herewith reported as of January 15.

Oklahoma State Medical Association Medical Preparedness Committee

In July of 1940, the Council of the Association established the Committee on Medical Preparedness. The purpose of this committee was to correlate the efforts of the County Societies in securing a 100 percent return of the A.M.A. Medical Preparedness Questionnaire and to act in any other capacity that might be related to the Association and National Defense.

It will be this committee plus the committees of the County Societies that will act as liaison contacts between the Office of Procurement and Assignment, the Association and the membership of the County Societies.

The State Committee, composed of a chairman, vice-chairman, and a representative from each Councilor District, is listed below:

Chairman—Henry H. Turner, Oklahoma City

Vice-Chairman—L. S. Willour, McAlester

Councilor District Representatives:

One..John L. Day, Supply
Two...J. M. Bonham, Hobart
Three..J. M. Watson, Enid
Four......................................Tom Lowry, Oklahoma City
Five..J. L. Patterson, Duncan
Six..W. Albert Cook, Tulsa
Seven.................................Robert M. Anderson, Shawnee
Eight......................................F. L. Wormington, Miami
Nine.......................................J. M. Harris, Wilburton
Ten..John A. Haynie, Durant

Advisory Members

Robert U. Patterson, Oklahoma City

Grady F. Mathews, Oklahoma City

Louis H. Ritzhaupt, Oklahoma City-Guthrie

The Chairmen of the County Committees are as follows:

Alfalfa.............................L. T. Lancaster, Cherokee
Atoka-Coal.............................J. S. Fulton, Atoka
Beckham.........................E. S. Kilpatrick, Elk City
Blaine...................................L. R. Kirby, Okeene
Bryan...............................R. E. Sawyer, Durant
Caddo...........................R. E. Johnston, Anadarko
Canadian...............................J. T. Phelps, El Reno
Carter.............................F. W. Boadway, Ardmore
Cherokee.......................J. S. Allison, Tahlequah
Choctaw...............................E. A. Johnson, Hugo
Cleveland.......................W. T. Mayfield, Norman
Comanche...................Fred W. Hammond, Lawton
Cotton............................M. A. Jones, Walters
Craig.............................Paul G. Sanger, Vinita
Creek..........................G. C. Croston, Sapulpa
Custer.......................McClain Rogers, Clinton
Garfield.............................J. R. Walker, Enid
Garvin...................John R. Callaway, Pauls Valley
Grady...........................L. E. Woods, Chickasha
Grant.............................E. E. Lawson, Medford
Greer.............................J. B. Hollis, Mangum
Harmon.........................S. W. Hopkins, Hollis

Hughes...........................A. L. Davenport, Holdenville
Jackson...............................E. S. Crow, Olustee
Jefferson..............................L. L. Wade, Ryan
Kay...............................L. H. Becker, Blackwell
Kingfisher...............John W. Pendleton, Kingfisher
Kiowa............................B. H. Watkins, Hobart
Latimer.......................J. S. Callahan, Wilburton
LeFlore.........................O. M. Woodson, Poteau
Lincoln.......................John S. Rollins, Prague
Logan.........................W. C. Miller, Guthrie
Major.......................M. R. McCroskie, Fairview
Marshall.........................J. L. Holland, Madill
Mayes..........................V. D. Herrington, Pryor
McClain......................W. C. McCurdy, Purcell
McCurtain..................W. B. McCaskill, Idabel
McIntosh.......................D. E. Little, Eufaula
Murray.....................Paul V. Annadown, Sulphur
Muskogee..................H. T. Ballantine, Muskogee
Noble...........................T. F. Renfrow, Billings
Okfuskee........................A. S. Melton, Okemah
Oklahoma..................Horace Reed, Oklahoma City
Okmulgee...................R. L. Alexander, Okmulgee
Osage...............................C. H. Guild, Shidler
Ottawa.......................F. L. Wormington, Miami
Pawnee..........................R. E. Jones, Pawnee
Payne.......................R. E. Waggoner, Stillwater
Pittsburg.................R. K. Pemberton, McAlester
Pontotoc.........................M. M. Webster, Ada
Pottawatomie..................James M. Byrum, Shawnee
Pushmataha.................D. W. Connally, Antlers
Roger-Mills...............J. Worrall Henry, Cheyenne
Rogers........................R. C. Meloy, Claremore
Seminole..................Claude S. Chambers, Seminole
Stephens...........................W. S. Ivy, Duncan
Texas............................R. B. Hayes, Guymon
Tillman.......................J. D. Osborn, Frederick
Tulsa.............................James L. Miner, Tulsa
Wagoner.......................J. H. Plunkett, Wagoner
Washington-Nowata............J. V. Athey, Bartlesville
Washita.......................A. H. Bungardt, Cordell
Woods............................O. E. Templin, Alva
Woodward...........................John L. Day, Supply

Any member who desires to secure information concerning Medical Preparedness should contact the chairman of his county society's committee.

Office of Procurement And Assignment

On October 30, 1941, the President of the United States approved the establishment of the Office of Procurement and Assignment for the medical, dental, and veterinary professions. The Directory Board is composed of:

Dr. Frank H. Lahey, Chairman, President, American Medical Association, Boston; Dr. C. Willard Camalier, Chairman, Dental Preparedness Committee, American Dental Association, Washington, D. C.; Dr. Harold S. Diehl, Dean, Medical Sciences, University of Minnesota, Minneapolis; Dr. James E. Paullin, Atlanta Ga.; Dr. Harvey B. Stone, Associate Professor of Surgery, Johns Hopkins University School of Medicine, Baltimore; and Dr. Sam F. Seeley, Executive Officer, Washington, D. C.

IMPORTANT ANNOUNCEMENT

YOUR ATTENTION IS DIRECTED TO THE INSERT WHICH FOLLOWS PAGE 26, AS IT PERTAINS TO THE PROCUREMENT AND ASSIGNMENT QUESTIONNAIRE WHICH HAS APPEARED IN THE DECEMBER 27, 1941 AND JANUARY 3, 1942 JOURNAL OF THE AMERICAN MEDICAL ASSOCIATION AND TO WHICH REFERENCES HAVE BEEN MADE IN THIS ISSUE.

THE OFFICE OF PROCUREMENT AND ASSIGNMENT, IT SEEMS, WILL CONTINUE TO OPERATE AS EXPLAINED IN THE FOLLOWING PARAGRAPHS, BUT A NEW QUESTIONNAIRE FOR MEMBERS OF THE PROFESSION TO COMPLETE WILL BE MADE AVAILABLE IN THE NEAR FUTURE.

OPERATION

The existing facilities of the American Medical Association, American Dental Association and American Veterinary Medical Association have been graciously offered to the Procurement and Assignment Service. A regional office has been set up in Chicago in which questionnaires, rosters and punch card data pertaining to all physicians, dentists and veterinarians will be maintained and kept up to date. The Committees on Medical Preparedness of the American Medical Association, American Dental Association and American Veterinary Medical Association will be utilized in the conduct of surveys, dissemination of information to the professions and the recruitment of personnel as requisitioned by various governmental agencies. The Procurement and Assignment Service will maintain a central office in Washington, D. C. The regional office in Chicago will maintain the rosters. A board in each of the nine corps areas will consist of representatives of medical education, hospitals, the Medical Preparedness Committee of the American Medical Association and two civilian practitioners in each corps area. These boards will act in an advisory capacity with the view of assuring adequate professional care of the civilian and industrial populations within the area and in the selection of those professional people within the area who can be spared for service with the armed forces. They will function through the existing state, district and county committees on medical preparedness. The medical, dental and veterinary medical needs will be considered by committees of each of the respective professions.

After a complete survey has been made and the availability of personnel has been determined, the central office will then be prepared to furnish to all requisitioning agencies rosters of those available for duty within their organizations. The result of questionnaires clearly indicates that large numbers of physicians, dentists and veterinarians will voluntarily make themselves available for positions which will guarantee adequate professional care to the civil, industrial and military requirements. It is planned that in the very near future every physician, dentist and veterinarian will receive a questionnaire from the Procurement and Assignment Service on which he will be asked to designate his preference regarding the capacity in which he desires to contribute his maximum efforts to the successful culmination of the present national emergency. Alternate preferences will be stated and every professional man will be certified by the Procurement and Assignment Service as having volunteered his services.

From rosters maintained as a result of the foregoing information, requisitioning agencies will be furnished the names of those available as the needs arise, should expansion of the defense program require additional professional personnel. This plan is designed primarily to assure adequate personnel for the armed services and to avoid unwarranted dislocation of professional people from their present localities.

Address of Dr. Sam F. Seeley, Executive Officer

At the Second Annual Secretaries Conference of the Association, the principle speaker was Dr. Sam F. Seeley, Executive Officer of the Office of Procurement and Assignment. Because of the importance of the Office of Procurement and Assignment and its relation to every physician, Doctor Seeley's speech is hereby printed in full. Every member of the Association should read it to its conclusion.

Ladies and Gentlemen: Before entering upon a discussion of the functions of the new Procurement and Assignment Service of the Office of Defense Health and Welfare Services, recently organized in Washington, D. C., I wish to convey to you the appreciation of the Directing Board of the Procurement and Assignment Service for your splendid and whole-hearted cooperation in arranging this meeting on such a short notice. Dr. Frank Lahey of Boston, Chairman of the Directing Board of the Procurement and Assignment Service has requested that I appear before you, in order that I may explain to you the mission of the Procurement and Assignment Service.

I am certain that it will be a great source of satisfaction to you to know that the medical profession of this country anticipated many months ago the necessity of formulating a program which would ensure the best professional care of the armed forces, the industrial and civil agencies of our country. Under the direction of the President, the Office for Emergency Management has set up three distinct agencies charged with mobilization of our national resources in order that the best possible medical care may be given to every member of our country. These three agencies are as follows: (1) The Health and Medical Committee of the Office of Defense Health and Welfare Services, which functions in an advisory capacity; (2) The Office of Scientific Research and Development, which is conducting a broad program of medical research under the auspices of Doctor Richards of Pennsylvania, Chairman of the Committee on Medical Research, and (3) The Procurement and Assignment Service of which I will speak later.

The Health and Medical Committee is composed of a "main" committee, consisting of Doctor Abell of Louisville, Ky., the Surgeons General of the U. S. Army, U. S. Navy, the U. S. Public Health Service, and Doctor Richards. Subcommittees under the Health and Medical Committee assist in formulating national policies in reference to Medical Education, Hospitalization, Industrial Health and Medicine, Nursing, Negro Health and Dentistry.

All matters pertaining to medical research are carried out by the Medical Division of the National Research Council of the National Academy of Sciences. Doctor Weed, who is Chairman of the Medical Division of the National Research Council, has organized ten major committees with the necessary subcommittees, which are engaged in carrying out every conceivable angle of medical research which will contribute to the national emergency program. More than 200 of the most noted scientists of this country are engaged in carrying out research problems under the auspices of the National Research Council. Liaison officers from the Army and Navy carry problems from the Professional Service Division of those Services to the various committees of the National Research Council. These committees transmit to the Surgeons General resumes of the best known method of treatment of all diseases and injuries. Research problems are drawn up and allocated to laboratories throughout the entire country. The National Research Council committees assist in drawing up of memoranda which are transmitted to the medical officers of the Army and the Navy and which may be used as a basis for treatment along the most modern lines.

As early as June, 1940, the Surgeon General of the United States Army requested that the American Medical Association assist in the procurement of the necessary personnel for an Army of one and one-half million men. The American Medical Association started immediately in the drawing up of rosters of all of the physicians of the United States. Shortly after this, the American Dental Association also drew up rosters of the dental profession. At the present time the American Veterinary Medical Association is engaged in drawing up rosters of all of the practicing veterinarians of the country. These rosters have served to assist the Surgeon General of the Army in obtaining medical department personnel to carry out the duties incident to the maintenance of an Army of 1,700,000 men.

In April, 1941, the Subcommittee on Medical Education of the Health and Medical Committee passed a resolution to the "main" committee recommending that a central agency be set up for the purpose of procuring and assigning medical, dental and veterinary personnel to the armed services with a view of maintaining adequate professional care for the industrial population and the civilian population of this country. This resolution was accepted by the Health and Medical Committee, and at the meeting of the American Medical Association in Cleveland in June, 1941, this resolution was endorsed and passed back to the Health and Medical Committee. This Committee met on October 22 to initiate the development of a Procurement and Assignment Service. At that meeting the members of the Health and Medical Committee sought the consultation and advice of the leading medical and dental people of the United States. Liaison officers from practically every Government agency, including Selective Service and the Office of Civilian Defense, aided in drawing up this program. At this meeting a Commission was appointed by the Health and Medical Committee which was requested to draft a program for a Procurement and Assignment Service. At this point development moved rapidly forward. The Commission met on October 28 and recommended the setting up of the Procurement and Assignment Service. Their recommendations were forwarded to the President, to the Director of the Office of Defense Health and Welfare Services, and were approved by the President on October 30. The President has named the following members to serve on the Directing Board: Dr. Frank H. Lahey of Boston, Chairman; Dr. C. Willard Camalier, Washington, D. C.; Dr. Harold S. Diehl, Minneapolis, Minn.; Dr. James E. Paullin, Atlanta, Ga., and Dr. Harvey B. Stone, Baltimore, Md. Dr. Sam F. Seeley, at that time on duty in the Office of the Surgeon General, was named as Executive Officer to the Directing Board and by direction of the President, has been transferred from the War Department to serve as Executive Officer in a full-time capacity. Committees were formed immediately on Dentistry, Hospitals, Industrial Health, Information, Medical Education, Negro Health, Public Health, Veterinary Medicine, and Women Physicians. Liaison officers have been assigned by the Army, Navy, U. S. Public Health Service, Veterans Administration, Selective Service System, U. S. Civil Service Commission, Office of Civilian Defense, and the Division of Health Services, Children's Bureau, Washington, D.C.

The primary objective of the Procurement and Assignment Service is to maintain a complete list of all physicians, dentists, and veterinarians of the entire country with detailed information as to age, physical condition, professional qualifications, and availability for service in the various military, civil and industrial agencies of the country. This information has been tabulated on the punch card system. All agencies of the Government which utilize the services of physicians, dentists and veterinarians will make requisitions upon the Procurement and Assignment Service for personnel. These requisitions will state the age, professional qualifications, and the physical condition of those professional people whose services are desired by these agencies. Lists will be prepared from the rosters and forwarded to the requisitioning agency. These agencies will then enlist the services of these professional people. At the same time, the Procurement and Assignment Service will notify the people whose names have been tendered to the requisitioning agency that they have been chosen to enter upon their new duties.

Through the various committees serving the Procurement and Assignment Service, surveys are rapidly being made of all of the facilities of the United States. For example, every hospital will be canvassed and they will be asked to state the minimum number of professional people required to maintain adequate care of the sick of these institutions. In the same manner, the needs of school faculties, industrial organizations, national, state and county health organizations, and other agencies, both military and civil, will be surveyed.

The organization of the Procurement and Assignment Service is practically complete. The central office in Washington, D. C., has been set up, and a Regional Office is being set up in Chicago, which will maintain the rosters of the American Medical, Dental and Veterinary Medical Associations. Committees are being named in each of the nine Corps Areas, which will serve in an advisory capacity to the Corps Area Commander. Incidentally, these geographical Corps Areas of the Army coincide exactly with the Defense Areas set up by the Office of Civilian Defense. The Committees serving in each Corps Area will consist of a representative of medical education, a representative of hospitals, a representative of the national preparedness committee, and at least two well-known civilian practitioners of that territory who are acquainted with the professional people and with the needs of those areas. At present the committees are being set up within the Corps Areas in each of the States and these State Committees will be asked in the very near future to develop committees within their districts and counties in order that the many functions of the Procurement and Assignment Service may be carried down to the last county of the country. I am now en route to Chicago where, on December 18, the Directing Board will meet with the members of the Committees on Preparedness of the American Medical, Dental, and the Veterinary Medical Association, at which time a program will be drawn up and shortly thereafter the States will be asked to complete the organization within their area.

The functions of this Service are broadly two in character, procurement and assignment. In order to maintain the existing rosters and to determine the professional qualifications of professional personnel, also to determine the needs of the medical training institutions, hospitals, the health departments, industrial organizations and civil communities, the committees of each county will forward to the central office through their State committees information which will serve to ensure proper distribution of professional personnel in every capacity. These committees will be asked to serve in the conduct of surveys by the various committees of the Procurement and Assignment Service. To date, more than 1,900 of the more than 3,000 counties of the United States have been completely surveyed and reports are now on file in the office upon which the needs of the community and the availability of personnel of those communities may be judged.

Assignment of professional personnel will be based upon the information gained through these various com-

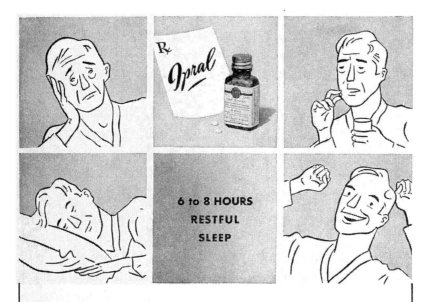

munities. As far back as July of 1940 more than 50 percent of the first 150,000 physicians who answered questionnaires volunteered for military service in case of war. Under the present circumstances and in view of recent military developments, it is anticipated that the majority of all physicians, dentists and veterinarians are now ready to volunteer for active military service in any capacity which may be best suited to the national defense program. It is hoped that the functions of the Procurement and Assignment Service may be facilitated by the early volunteering of the professional people throughout this country. It is our hope that so many will volunteer to serve in any capacity which the Service may predetermine that we will be able to satisfy at an early date the needs of the military service and may turn our attention to an equally important function, that of avoiding disproportionate dislocation of professional people from communities where their services are needed. In this way, the Procurement and Assignment Service expects to minimize the dislocation of professional people from key positions in the civil and industrial communities.

Let us turn for a moment to the assets in terms of professional people of our country today. At the present time, any man under the age of 28, if physically able, is required to enter the military service. Approximately 60 percent of those graduating after 12 months of internship are under the age 28. The majority of these men are physically fit and must enter upon military service. The Selective Service System has deferred these men for a time sufficient to guarantee graduation from medical school and the completion of 12 months of internship. These students have been asked that during the last two years of medical school training they join the Medical Administrative Corps Reserve or a Reserve Corps in the Navy of a like nature. After graduation from college, they are asked to join the Medical Corps Reserve of the Army or the Navy in order that they may be sent to active duty immediately upon completion of the 12 months internship. It becomes apparent that if a medical student has not identified himself with the Army or the Navy after the completion of 12 months of internship, and he is under the age of 28, he may be drafted as a private. For this reason, it is necessary that all men engaged in medical education must seek a Reserve Commission in the Army of the United States or in the Reserve Corps of the Navy, in order that their induction into the military service will result in the utilization of their medical training. During the World War of 1917, the draft age was higher than 28. At the present time, we are unable to state whether the draft age will be raised and we are unable to surmise what age will be set if the draft age is raised. For this reason, the Directing Board of the Procurement and Assignment Service recommends that every doctor who is physically able identify himself as willing to enter the military service in case he is needed. It is anticipated that within the next 60 days every physician, dentist and veterinarian of this country will be canvassed and will be asked to return a questionnaire to the central office of the Procurement and Assignment Service. At that time an estimate will have been made of the number of professional people required by each of the Government agencies, the civil and industrial agencies, and the civil communities. It is anticipated that the names of professional people will be set aside so that they may be forwarded as the needs of the military service expand. Each recipient of a questionnaire will be asked to state his first, second, third and possibly more choices as to what type of service he would prefer to render. Upon analysis of these questionnaires, it is hoped that a sufficient number will have volunteered to serve in the armed forces, in the industrial plants, and in other agencies which would require dislocation from their present locality, so that a minimal disruption of the present conditions will result.

In closing, I wish to impress upon you the necessity of all of those physically fit volunteering to serve in the military services. It is obvious that there are not enough physicians, dentists and veterinarians in the age group under 28 to satisfy the military needs. Let us hope that voluntary enlistment will be sufficient that the draft age will not have to be raised and above all let us hope that it will not become necessary to consider legislation which would make it mandatory that professional people who are physically fit be forced into the military service against their will.

A Call to Service

DR. FRANK H. LAHEY
President of the American Medical Association

The establishment by the government of a Procurement and Assignment Agency properly places the responsibility for obtaining medical personnel in the hands of the medical profession. The success of this agency depends entirely on a few basic features: the complete cooperation of medicine in what even the most doubting must now admit is a truly national emergency; an unqualified willingness to serve the country however, whatever and whenever required; and a firm purpose to establish the fact that medicine intends to maintain its place in the forefront as it always has when a patriotic example is of such significance.

ATTENTION

Should any physician desire to make application for a commission in the Medical Corps, he should address his communication to: Headquarters, Second Military Area, 825 Federal Building, Oklahoma City, and for commissions in the Naval Reserve to Naval Recruiting Station, 3rd Floor, Post Office Building, Oklahoma City.

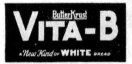

Emergency Medical Service
For Civilian Defense

Emergency Medical Service for Civilian Defense has been established on a uniform basis in each state under the direction of the Office of Civilian Defense, Washington, D. C., F. H. LaGuardia, Director. Emergency Medical Service, will be maintained upon the local level of the county unit with a chief of emergency medical service in each county. In Oklahoma, Dr. Grady F. Mathews, Commissioner of Health, has been appointed to the State Committee on Health and Housing, which in turn will supervise and coordinate the work of the Emergency Medical Care committees after their appointment by the local County Director of Civilian Defense.

Doctor Mathews' address on the subject of Emergency Medical Care, given before the Second Annual Secretaries Conference, graphically details the working of this committee. It is herewith reprinted in full. It should be expressly understood that the State Medical Association is in no way connected with the establishment, appointment, or operation of emergency medical care in the county setup other than the Association's representation on the State Committee on Emergency Medical Care in an advisory capacity by Dr. Finis W. Ewing, President of the Association, and Dr. Henry H. Turner, Chairman of Medical Preparedness.

Dr. Grady F. Mathews' Address
On Emergency Medical Care

Gentlemen: There is no longer any need to explain that conditions facing this country and this state are today most serious. The vicious, unexpected attack of axis bombers has made only too clear what was but remotely realized by most of us a short time ago.

Up until a week ago today what thinking had been done about preparedness was geared to the motto "National Defense." Considerable thinking was done in an effort to devise a method for protecting the lives of civilians. Rather detailed arrangements were worked out, on paper. Since last Sunday, those plans have been brought into the open, so to speak, carefully considered, discussed and vitalized into a plan of action which is being set into motion with surprising speed.

Members of the medical profession have for the past few months heard and read many hints as to the role they would play in defense activities. They themselves have realized that they would have many, responsible duties—but just what those duties would be and when and where has been quite vague.

I would like at this time to give you a word picture, if I can, of some very definite, very important duties which must have the cooperation and work of members of the medical profession.

I have been made state chairman of the committee on health and housing, which is one of the state defense committees. Mr. J. William Cordell is executive chairman of the state defense committee, and health and housing is one of the subordinate groups under the general, all inclusive plan for defense activities among civilians in Oklahoma. You understand of course that a similar setup is being put into operation in all states, under the nation-wide direction of Mayor LaGuardia of New York.

May I at the start emphasize this fact. The work of the health and housing committee, both the state committee and the county committees, has been prepared in order that the state may have a *unified* method to meet any emergency. Such plans have been coordinated with other important state defense committee programs. We are prone at a time like this to begin and think along many lines, all seeking the common goal and all worthy of commendation, but resulting in confusion because of so many different groups and plans. We must think and work together—using one feasible plan. The simple truth is that we must get together, because there is much for each of us to do while carrying on in our everyday task.

As you no doubt know, many counties have already taken steps for civilian defense, forming county organizations which are to perform the same duties as outlined by the State Defense Council.

However, what is not generally known is the fact that the State Defense Council is a legally authorized organization, the result of a law passed by the last state legislature. The reason of this action was obvious—to give the state a unified, simplified plan so that all groups could take the same steps. Thus this plan is the only legally authorized system of organization for civilian defense, and it is so arranged that previously made, locally organized, defense plans can be easily "dovetailed" or adopted into the accepted plan. I feel sure that all counties will take this step, in the interest of harmony and unity.

The state health and housing committee can of necessity work primarily only as an advisory, guiding organization, a clearing house, if you please, for the work of the committees organized in the counties. It is that group which I want to explain to you.

The county defense committee will have three very important functions: emergency medical and hospital service, sanitation, and housing. Those three items will be its responsibility, and with only a moment's reflection, you can realize that the committee has a job which will be a big one.

I am going to try to "break down" the functions of the committee for you, so that you may have a better idea of just how the plan will work.

Each county defense committee, which is charged with many responsibilities other than those of health and housing, will have what is to be known as a county report center. Here is how that will operate.

Plans have been worked out whereby in case of air raids, or other emergency action, interceptor stations will flash a warning to seven district offices, which are the radio transmittors of the state highway patrol. The highway patrol will notify the county report center that danger is imminent. It is agreed that the county sheriff's office will be the report center for each county.

In other words, the report center will be the county clearing post, whether the emergency is within the county, and help is needed, or whether the danger is expected somewhere else.

The person on duty at the report center will call the county air raid warden, who will then call in for action the emergency medical officer, the county fire chief, senior air raid wardens, the sheriff or head of the police protection committee, and messenger and rescue squads.

These people will immediately assemble at the report office and stand by until the emergency is over, or in case the disaster has already happened, they will direct the various units to the scene of action. Thus in a very short time all committees should be functioning in a coordinated manner in accomplishing the purposes for which they were organized.

The county chairman of the health and housing committee will have three particular groups working under his general direction: the emergency medical and hospital service, sanitation, and housing. In addition, his group will work with other emergency agencies, such as fire and police, and voluntary agencies such as the Red Cross, health and nursing organizations.

You are of course most interested in the work of emergency medical and hospital service.

Here is the organization plan for that group. There will be a local chief of emergency medical and hospital service. He must be a physician of broad experience and administrative capacity. He should be responsible to the county defense committee. It should be his duty to survey immediately the medical resources and hospital facilities of the community, and to prepare local plans, develop organization and provide for training of personnel. Happily, some of the counties have already classified members of the medical profession. Those counties are just that much farther along on the road to preparation.

The chief of emergency medical and hospital service should be chairman of a medical advisory committee. Suggested membership for the committee might include the local health officer, hospital administrators, a physician recommended by the county medical society, a registered nurse, and representatives of the Red Cross and other agencies.

The plan calls for the chief of emergency medical and hospital service to organize or have organized what are to be known as emergency medical and hospital field units. To do this, general hospitals, both voluntary and governmental, should organize and assemble basic equipment. A field unit should consist of two or more squads under the direction of a physician. Squad leaders should be named, and be thoroughly trained in first aid.

Based on a 200 bed hospital and 25,000 population, it is recommended that the emergency field unit consist of two squads, one for each 12 hour shift. Each squad sould consist of two physicians, two or more nurses and two or more orderlies, and it should be capable of functioning, if necessary, as two separate teams. In areas where there are no hospitals, churches, schools and public buildings may be designated as headquarters.

Transportation is another problem for this group. A hospital ambulance, small truck, station wagon or even a passenger car will be adequate to transport personnel of a squad, and on return trips to transport casualties. Recruited private vehicles may be assigned to a hospital or parking center under control of a transport officer, who will work under direction of the chief of emergency medical and hospital service.

A working supply of medical and surgical equipment for use in the field should be available for each physician in portable case or bag with generous packs or drums of extra supplies.

Casualty stations and first aid posts are to be set up near the scene of trouble. The work of these two stations is to be limited to emergency first aid procedure and the preservation of morale. The seriously injured will be evacuated rapidly to a hospital. Those with minor injuries will go to their homes or temporary shelter.

The emergency field unit rescue squads and stretcher teams will have the task of getting casualties to the nearest station. Each squad should have a trained leader, using volunteer rescue workers. There, in briefest form is the general outline of the work in emergency medical and hospital service. The plan will work in this fashion:

A first aid post will be set up near the field of emergency. Victims can be taken by ambulance service direct from the first aid station to evacuation or clearance hospitals, or they can be routed to the casualty station, then by ambulance to the hospital. Backing up this organization will be the base hospital, which is the well established, operating hospital. A transport officer is in charge of arrangements for moving casualties—and the chief of emergency medical and hospital service will be in general direction.

Now let us consider the duties of the local chief of emergency medical and hospital services—just how will he go about getting the work I have outlined actually performed?

You remember I mentioned previously that he must be an outstanding medical leader and should be carefully selected after conferring with the state defense council, the local medical society and others in a position to know. He should be assisted by a medical advisory council. The physician in each county who has the job of emergency medical and hospital service chief has one of the most responsible, most difficult tasks of any civilian in our program for protecting the lives of our citizens.

Here, in brief form, is the outline of duties for the chief of medical and hospital services:

1—He should determine the scope of the activities of all official and voluntary organizations which are to participate in the emergency medical program, to integrate these organizations into the comprehensive local program. In other words, find out what his county has to suit the needs.

2—He should assist hospitals in the locality to organize, equip and train field units. In other words, get his field force in shape to work.

3—He must inspect and select sites for the establishment of casualty stations.

4—He should make a spot map of the locality, indicating the locations of hospitals, appropriate sites for casualty stations, depots for storage of stretchers, blankets and collapsible cots, and the locations of rescue squads. The map should indicate the number of emergency medical and hospital squads in each hospital. This information should be given to the control center and other groups working in the defense group.

5—He should work out a plan for transportation with local governmental departments, so that medical personnel may be able to get to the scene of trouble.

6—Field drills for the rescue squads should be held as a training project.

7—He should make an inventory of hospital beds in the locality and of the possibilities for emergency expansion in bed capacity.

8—This physician should assist in the preparation of plans for evacuation; he should assist in establishing courses for volunteers in the recruiting of volunteers for nurses' aid courses of the American Red Cross.

9—One of his duties is to stimulate and guide extension of first aid training courses as widely as possible among the local population.

10—He should stimulate and guide industrial plants, business establishments and governmental bureaus in the locality in the training and organization of effective first aid detachments among the employees.

You get the idea from these duties that he should be a leader in all activities to awaken his community to the dangers ahead, and help them become better prepared.

I don't intend to discuss the work of the sanitation and housing divisions of the county defense committee, except for these brief, general statements. The supervisor of sanitation will be responsible for increased protection over the water and food supplies; and more attention to garbage, sewage and incineration. He will have the duty of providing alternate workers to take over the duties of those in charge of operations, so that this important work can go on in case of accident. This group will have charge of plans to protect water and food supplies against sabotage. Naturally its work will begin with the regularly employed people, and will be merely a civilian effort to assist them.

The director of housing will have duties of providing shelter, supervising construction of bomb proofing, protecting railroads and airports, streets and highways, power and utility plants.

You are more concerned with the medical aspects of our civilian defense effort.

Once again the medical profession is challenged to perform a difficult, important task. I hope you realize from my remarks that the position of chief of the emergency medical and hospital service is a tremendous responsibility.

I hope further that you realize that it is not a one man job, this business of providing adequate medical care for emergencies. Every physician in the county will have something to do. The chief can actually do little himself, because of his administrative duties. Everyday, practicing physicians must face the emergency and work to overcome it. We hope that the plan outlined here will enable the work to be done efficiently, quickly and thoroughly. I feel sure that the county plan will be put quickly into operation, and that the medical societies stand ready to take their places.

And now, in closing, just a word about the value of

such a plan. Up until last Sunday, it was hard to visualize the need for such an organization. Being traditional lovers of peace, we had heard often that America could not be—would not be attacked. We know today that those statements were but the wishful thinking of those who did not understand modern warfare.

If our west coast and east coast can be menaced—so can our great interior regions—our state of Oklahoma.

We must assume this condition—we must realize that Oklahoma can need the services of just such an organization as I have outlined for you this morning. Realizing this—we must be ready.

"WHAT CAN I DO?"*

MAJOR LOUIS H. RITZHAUPT
State Medical Officer

*Read before the Second Annual Secretaries Conference, Oklahoma State Medical Association, December 14, 1941, in Oklahoma City.

Since the closing days of the last World War, through the few carefree years of plenty, the people of our nation developed false security which was finally terminated with the economic crisis of 1929. The following ten years brought the people a type of living to which they were not accustomed. There was a radical change in the economic, social, moral and physical mode of living which produced a constant state of fear and apprehension; and the mighty sequence of world events were converging upon this crowded climax of human history in which we live.

Wars, and rumors of wars caused a complete transformation of the entire international situation. Governments were overthrown, solemn treaties violated, vast territories occupied by invading armies; great cities destroyed, and multitudes driven into exile or placed in bondage. The liberty of the entire universe was never in greater peril. The very earth shook with these constant upheavals, and the American people stood wondering what fresh surprises were to come in the days ahead. Then on Sunday afternoon, December 7, the great radio stations electrified the nation with the word that a cunning foe, under cover of an offer of Peace had attacked a United States' possession; evidently the storms from abroad were directly challenging our institutions. The period of uncertainty, disunion and apprehension was terminated. War was declared against us, and we in turn, through our constitutional government, declared war against our enemies. The voices of the patriotic and unselfish American people rose in one grand chorus, asking "What Can I Do?"

This is the question that is uppermost in the minds of the medical profession of our State and our Nation. Those who are educated in the science of medicine have been the guardians of civilization, even greater than the armies or the statesmen of the years which have passed or the years which are to follow. In this crisis, it is well that we maintain our consistency of thought and ability to act as if we were meeting the crisis at the bedside of a patient. We have been taught to function during emergencies.

Our plan of organization cannot be created to advance ourselves individually. It must be planned through the government, through the American Medical Association, through the Oklahoma State Medical Association and its various county branches, so that we may protect and administer to those who remain at home and to those who are fighting for our soil and democratic way of life.

It is well that this crisis did not come upon us without previous schooling. The necessity of selecting, training and equipping the Army of the United States became more important by the Declaration of War. Every member of the medical profession who has been called upon, has given freely of his time and energy in examining the young men of this state registered under the Selective Training and Service Act of 1940. The rigidity and exactness which have been required in selecting those in the armed forces of the United States is recognized by us all. Sometimes we have felt that the Army Induction Station and its examining physicians have been too rigid in their requirements, but we do know that all those young men who have been selected are mentally and physically qualified to lead an army against our foes. This fact should give to our people a feeling of confidence and security. Our work has just begun.

The outstanding tasks that our profession must accomplish are:

1. To aid in the selection of the armed forces.
2. To rehabilitate those with correctable physical defects so they may be qualified for general military duty.
3. To provide medical and surgical care for the armed forces, supervising the sanitation and preventive medicine, evacuation of the sick and injured and the professional care and treatment of the soldiers after evacuation.
4. To see that the civilian population has adequate and sufficient medical and surgical assistance.
5. To aid in the rehabilitation of those who may be injured at the battlefront.

After January 1, 1942, the examining physicians for the various local boards will be required to make a cursory inspection of all registrants in Class I. It will not be necessary to make a detailed examination or any laboratory tests. It is estimated that this procedure will eliminate not more than ten percent. The remaining 90 percent will be sent to the Army Examining Station where a complete and detailed physical examination will be made. The Medical Advisory Boards will be required to function in connection with the Army Examining Station, no case will be referred to them by the local board. If the demand for the army personnel should be more acute, the entire task of selecting the army may revert back to the local board examining physicians, requiring them to make the final examination. I state this now so that you will not be unprepared if you should again be required to take up the tedious task which you so faithfully performed the past year.

The President of the United States, in his recent proclamation, ordered National Headquarters, Selective Service System, to formulate rules and regulations by which registrants who have been certified by the Army Examining Board to have a physical defect that is remediable, are referred to the local board. At this time it is contemplated that the registrant, the local board, and the physician and dentist whom the registrant may select, will confer together, in order that the proper correction can be made. The doctors, dentists and hospitals in the registrant's own community will be used. The expense will be borne by the government, but I have no information as to the basic fees. I wish to encourage and urge doctors to accept the government compensation and not offer their services without any financial remuneration. Permit me to suggest that it would be far better to buy Defense Bonds than to donate your services.

The Office of Civilian Defense, through the State Defense Committee and its Sub-Committee on Health and Housing, with Dr. G. F. Mathews as Chairman, has laid plans for organizing the medical and hospital facilities, the creation of sanitary and housing units and other agencies which are essential to the protection of the civil and industrial population. The last Legislature authorized the Governor to organize a Woman's Home Guard, which under the law, can only be a medical unit, and should be able to function in cases of catastrophies or emergencies, when organized. Those physicians who have restricted their practice to some specialty may be required to devote more time to the practice of general medicine and return to the "country doctor's" style of attending patients.

Who will be medical officer in the United States Army? The Surgeon General has frequently made the statement that the medical personnel is now inadequate. All but 12 of the doctors of this state have completed the personnel questionnaire that was sent out by the American Medical Association.

Under the direction of the President of the United States, the Office for Emergency Management has set up three distinct agencies, charged with the mobilization of our natural resources. They are:

1. The Health and Medical Committee of the Office of Defense, Health and Welfare Services. This Committee is composed of Dr. Abell, of Louisville, Ky., the Surgeon General of the United States Army, the United States Navy, the United States Public Health Service, and Dr. Richards, of Pennsylvania.

2. The Office of Scientific Research and Development, which is conducting a program of medical research.

3. The Procurement and Assignment Service, which is a central agency set up the purpose of procuring and assigning medical, dental and veterinary personnel to the armed services, with a view of maintaining adequate professional care for the industrial and civil population of this country. President Roosevelt named Dr. Frank H. Lahey, of Boston, as Chairman of the Directing Board. Dr. Sam F. Seeley, Major of the Medical Corps out of the office of the Surgeon General, was named as Executive Officer to the Directing Board. The personnel questionnaire submitted by the American Medical Association to the doctors of the United States has been made available to the Procurement and Assignment Service, and all agencies of the Government which utilize the service of the physicians, dentists and veterinarians, will make requisition upon the Procurement and Assignment Service for personnel. Out of the first 159,000 questionnaires returned to the American Medical Association, 60 percent of the doctors designated their willingness to serve in the armed forces. All of these are not physically qualified for active duty.

The question may arise in the minds of some of us as to which is our greatest obligation—administering to the civilian population, or selecting and caring for the armed forces? They are both of equal importance. And fortunately the cycle of life has divided us into three groups—the young, the middle-aged, and the old. This classification is not necessarily by years, but may be according to ability and accomplishments, activity and physical status, and above all, our feeling of patriotism and sacrifice.

During the past decade the physicians of this State and Nation, as a whole, have seen economical reverses. We have felt the threat of socialized medicine which would subjugate the scientific mind to political influences. The government has prosecuted some of those who tried to thwart organizers of unions and groups who would deprive a citizen of selecting his own physician. This, yes more than this, in a twinkle of an eye, must be, and is forgotten. Before we can conclude the task that lies before us, individually, we must forget the thought of financial gain or advancement. As a profession, collectively we must see that the selfish individual does not profit. There is a bronze image in the rotunda of the Capitol Building at Washington, erected by the State of Georgia to the memory of Crawford W. Long, M.D., the discoverer of ether in 1842. Upon the base of the statue are inscribed these words:

"My profession is to me a ministry from God."
In this hour of crisis we should recognize the truth of this statement. Every physician who is divinely blessed and whose knowledge is enhanced by scientific training will respond to the call of his country, accepting that task which he best can perform or to which he is assigned. We must carry on and do with all our might and mind that which our hands find to do.

MEDICAL CHANGES IN BRITAIN*

*Reprinted from the December 13 issue of the American Medical Association Journal.

Bombing and overcrowded insanitary shelters led the British to anticipate epidemics, says Ritchie Calder in John O'London's Weekly (April 25, 1941). But when a body of American experts under Prof. J. E. Gordon of Harvard arrived they found that the expected epidemic had failed to materialize.

In fact, the shelters had a lower disease rate than the average for the country. And the country as a whole, apart from the war epidemic of "spotted fever," or cerebrospinal menigitis, due mainly to the bringing together of young people under dormitory conditions, in the army and other ways, could show a bill of health comparable with the good years immediately before the war.

Although the war has not yet brought epidemics, it has created problems in the organization of medical services. There have been many proposals for changes in the panel system, which this writer says "no one would dare to pretend . . . has been satisfactory." It is generally agreed that the "approved society" system is wasteful. The British Medical Association has proposed the panel system to dependents, but the first effect of this would be to make nearly double the sales value of existing practices, which would compel physicians to pay some $10,000 to start in practice.

The voluntary hospital system has been heading for bankruptcy for several years—a fate which increased gifts and hospitalization insurance have only postponed.

As a result of the war, some of these hospitals began, for the first time in history, to bank money. They were paid by the state to keep the beds empty for casualties. The government leased these beds at anything from two and a half guineas to seven guineas a week (about $8 to $25). The hospitals were then able to lease emergency hospitals, built by the state, with the help of the bed rent from the state. This paradoxical device maintained the facade of the voluntary system. And since the war began, hospitals have been among the main targets of the Nazi air raiders, and an essential part of the postwar replanning will have to deal with their rebuilding.

Private practice has been hard hit. Large numbers of doctors have been recruited for the forces and others taken into the government's hospital scheme. Expansion of industrial practice and special shelter service have taken others, and evacuations and the creation of "defense areas" have caused widespread dislocations. It has also brought some steps toward reorganization and numerous proposals for reconstruction after the war. A "regional plan" for hospitals to include both voluntary and government operated hospitals has been developed, and there seems to be a trend toward state medicine with salaried physicians as part of an integrated system.

Manifestly the old order in medicine is finished. One thing is certain: We shall have the right to demand after this not the sickness service, which is all we have got at the moment, but a health service, embracing the whole population, irrespective of income, and providing medical care from birth to death, not as a purchasable commodity, but as an inalienable right. That service would conceive health as a biological trinity—protective medicine, which includes nutrition and environment (positive health); preventive medicine, which is the public health services, our pickets against disease; and curative medicine, including early diagnosis and highly skilled treatment, with all the resources of modern medical science and practice.

Flying Service Offers Ambulance Plane

Worthy of the attention of all members of the Association is the Pavey Flying Service in Tulsa, which furnishes to physicians a completely equipped ambulance plane for transporting patients.

The Pavey Service is one of three such services available in the Southwest, the other two being located in Wichita, Kan., and Lubbock, Tex.

Survey Made of Physicians In Active Service

A recent survey taken by the Indiana State Medical Association concerning the percentage of doctors in the states who have been called into military service was made, and an incomplete analysis of this survey is shown in the accompanying table.

Since the figures were given on the survey by the Association, 18 more Oklahoma physicians have been called to duty and on the basis of this figure, Oklahoma percentage now stands as of December 15 at approximately seven percent. This figure is based on an approximate 2,000 doctors in the state of Oklahoma and not on the membership of the Association.

PERCENTAGE OF PHYSICIANS IN ACTIVE SERVICE

STATE	Number of Physicians in State	Percentage of Total
Alabama	67	4.25%
Arizona	Not over 20—membership 360	
Arkansas	Around 75	4%
California	285	4.2%
	(These figures apply only to members of Cal. Medical Association).	
Colorado	73	About 5%
Connecticut	125	5%
District of Columbia	66	5%
Georgia	Not available	Do not know
Idaho	21	5%
Illinois	Exact number not available	
Indiana	Around 300	7.3%
Iowa	129	5%
Kansas	104	.052%
Kentucky	104—about 2,200 physicians	
Louisiana	in state	
Maryland	173	8¾%
Michigan	No information	
Mississippi	113	1.7%

Missouri	61 of 1,302 white physicians		4.68%
Montana	50 negro phys., none inducted		
Nebraska	No definite information		
New Hampshire	No definite information		
New Jersey	116		8%
New Mexico	30		4.5%
Ohio	347		5.59%
Oklahoma	8??		3.1%??
Pennsylvania	Approximately 550	Approximately	5.9%
Rhode Island	122		6½%
South Carolina	Approximately 650		.06%
Tennessee	36		3.7%
Texas	95		8.9%
Utah	176		.074%
Vermont	No definite information		
Virginia	26		5%
Washington	Approximately 50	Membership	400
West Virginia	225 to 250		
Wisconsin	76		19%
Wyoming	74		5.28%
	About 120		3%
	Approximately 30		

Novel Use of Sponge Rubber

Another novel use of sponge rubber as a medium to absorb vibration is reported by The B. F. Goodrich company, Akron, Ohio. One of the leading nose and throat specialists of the company has a laboratory located 20 feet from railroad tracks, where the accurate photographing of bacteriological specimens was impossible because of the vibration.

The problem was solved by the construction of piers sunk into the ground, supporting the camera with a magnifying ratio of 1,000 to one. The sponge rubber, used in conjunction with cork and concrete in the construction of the piers eliminated the vibration.

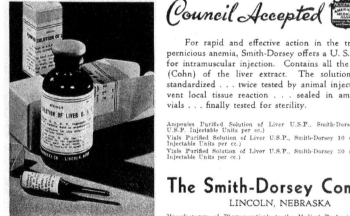

ASSOCIATION ACTIVITIES

Postgraduate Committee Ends Pediatric Course

Physicians throughout the state will be interested to know that the pediatric course in Oklahoma, by Dr. James G. Hughes, closed the first week in January. Dr. Hughes has completed two years of teaching in the state. Everyone knows by this time that the course was well received and Dr. Hughes has been warmly complimented by physicians everywhere by reason of his practical instruction. Likewise, his consultations among the physicians have been much appreciated.

The following teaching centers were used. The number opposite each center indicates the enrollments: (Circuit No. 1 was given by Drs. Rupe, Danis, and Harrison of St. Louis.)

Circuit I	No.	Circuit V	No.
Tulsa	50	Okla. City	59
Bartlesville	23	Shawnee	23
Miami	22	Norman	16
Vinita	13	Wewoka	16
Claremore	10	Pauls Valley	12
Tulsa (Col.)	8		
		Total	126
Total	126		
Circuit II	No.	Circuit VI	No.
Ada	27	Chickasha	20
Durant	18	Lawton	20
Sulphur	12	Duncan	18
Idabel	11	Ardmore	14
Hugo	10	Frederick	10
Total	78	Total	82
Circuit III	No.	Circuit VII	No.
McAlester	20	Enid	33
Muskogee	19	Woodward	20
Okmulgee	17	Guymon	11
Poteau	13	Alva	9
Tahlequah	11	Fairview	6
Total	80	Total	79
Circuit IV	No.		
Cushing-Stillwater	23	Circuit VIII	No.
Sapulpa-Bristow	15	Clinton	23
Ponca-Blackwell-		El Reno	20
Tonkawa	19	Guthrie	13
Pawhuska	14	Watonga	9
Pawnee	12	Okla. City (Col.)	9
Total	83	Total	74

Circuit IX	No.
Anadarko	15
Elk City	14
Hollis	6
Altus	1'
Hobart	8
Total	54

Total number of enrollments	782
Total number of consultations	979
Total number of lay lectures	50

Many will be interested to know that Dr. Hughes is being called immediately into Military Service, and further that the Army authorities were liberal minded in assisting the State Medical Association to keep alive this postgraduate program by permitting Dr. Hughes to remain with the program until he had finished instruction within the state. The Postgraduate Committee and the State Medical Association, therefore, wish to express publicly their appreciation to the 8th Corps Area Medical Department and the Surgeon General's office for the deferment given Dr. Hughes in behalf of this program and for permitting its completion.

The Commonwealth Fund of New York has appropriated funds for a two-year program in Internal Medicine, and your Committee is now attempting to complete plans to open this program, which has been requested by so many physicians in the state, and is negotiating with several possible instructors from which one will eventually be chosen.

Our appreciation is again expressed to The Commonwealth Fund of New York, and to the State Health Department and Dr. Grady Mathews, for their financial assistance given to the Association in this program of higher education.

"DOCTORS AT WORK"

"Doctors at Work," the dramatized radio program broadcast by the American Medical Association and the National Broadcasting company, began its second season on the air, December 6, 1941, and was brought to Oklahoma listeners at 4:30 p.m. (Oklahoma time) through the studios of Station WKY, Oklahoma City, and KVOO, Tulsa.

This program, which deals with the experiences of a fictitious but typical young American doctor, will be broadcast regularly every Saturday afternoon at 4:30 p. m., Oklahoma time, over WKY and KVOO as long as Oklahomans demand it.

Last year, "Doctors at Work" portrayed the experiences of Tom Riggs choosing medicine for his vocation and proceeding to acquire the necessary education and hospital training for the private practice of medicine. This year's serial will depict the subsequent life of Dr. Tom Riggs and his wife in time of national emergency in a typical medium sized American city.

Ten Oklahoma Doctors Receive Commonwealth Fellowships

The Commonwealth Fund of New York City has announced the granting of fellowship awards for 1942 to ten Oklahoma doctors.

The names of these doctors and the branch of medicine in which they were awarded their fellowships are as follows:

Dewey Lee Mathews, Tonkawa, Medicine; Addison B. Smith, Stillwater, Surgical Diagnosis; Orville M. Woodson, Poteau, Surgery, Obstetrics and Gynecology; F. Keith Oehlschlager, Yale, Surgery and Medicine; Lee Roy Wilhite, Perkins, Medicine, Obstetrics and Gynecology; Raymond O. Smith, Hominy, Medicine; A. C. Little, Minco, Medicine; and Ernest Rose, Sulphur, Obstetrics and Gynecology.

Southwest Oklahoma Medical Society Meets

Members of the Southwest Oklahoma Medical society met December 15 at the Country club in Hobart for a dinner meeting and scientific program.

Three speakers, Dr. R. M. Slabaugh, Sayre; Dr. Louis H. Ritzhaupt, Oklahoma City, and Dr. Paul H. Dube, Shattuck, were heard on the program. Doctor Slabaugh discussed "Differential Diagnosis of the Anemias;" Doctor Ritzhaupt, "Position of the Medical Profession in National Defense," and Doctor Dube, "Surgical Treatment of Arthritis of the Knee Joint."

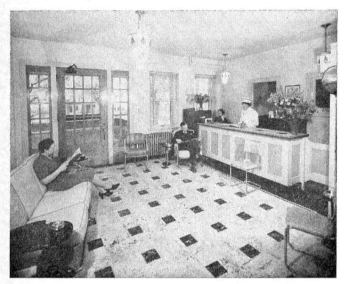

NEWS FROM THE COUNTY SOCIETIES

Most of the county medical societies finished their 1941 meeting year with the election of 1942 officers. Such lists of new officers that were available at the time of this printing are reported on this page.

Dr. R. Q. Goodwin, Oklahoma City, was elected president of the Oklahoma County Medical association, and Dr. Walker Morledge, Oklahoma City, vice-president. Dr. W. E. Eastland, Oklahoma City, was elected secretary-treasurer. Delegates to the 1942 Annual Meeting are Dr. W. F. Keller, Dr. Onis G. Hazel, Doctor Morledge, Dr. L. C. McHenry, Dr. C. R. Rountree, Dr. O. A. Watson, Dr. J. B. Snow, Dr. D. H .O'Donoghue, Dr. C. M. Pounders, Dr. George Garrison and Dr. Allen Gibbs. Alternates chosen include Dr. W. W. Rucks, Jr., Dr. Neil Woodward, Dr. R. H. Akin, Doctor Eastland, Dr. M. R. Jacobs, Dr. R. L. Murdoch, Dr. R. L. Noell, Dr. W. K. West, Dr. Harper Wright, Doctor Goodwin, and Dr. George Kimball.

New president of the Pontotoc county society is Dr. R. E. Cowling, Ada. Dr. M. M. Webster and Dr. E. R. Muntz, both of Ada, were elected vice-president and secretary-treasurer, respectively. Delegates for the society are Dr. E. M. Gullatt, Dr. E. A. Canada, Dr. Ollie McBride and Dr. Sam A. McKeel. Dr. M. L. Lewis and Dr. W. F. Dean were chosen as censors. and Doctor Webster, Doctor Muntz and Dr. R. E. Cowling were appointed to the Scientific Program committee.

Dr. Shade D. Neely, Muskogee, was elected president of the Muskogee county society, at a meeting, December 1, in Muskogee. Other Muskogee county officers were Dr. L. S. McAlister, vice-president; Dr. J. T. McInnis, secretary-treasurer; Dr. M. K. Thompson, censor; Dr. C. E. White and Dr. J. H. White, delegates; and Dr. I. B. Oldham, Jr. and Doctor McAlister, alternates.

Dr. W. M. Browning, Waurika, will head the Jefferson County Medical society as president. Elected to serve with him as secretary and delegate respectively were Dr. J. I. Hollingsworth, Waurika, and Dr. L. L. Wade, Ryan.

1942 President of the Okmulgee County Medical society is Dr. J. G. Edwards of Okmulgee. Other newly elected officers are Dr. Robert L. Alexander, vice-president; Dr. John R. Cotteral, secretary-treasurer; Dr. I. W. Bollinger, delegate, and Dr. J. C. Matheney, alternate.

Dr. Ralph W. Rucker, Bartlesville, was elected president of the Washington-Nowata county society, December 10, at the regular meeting of the society. Dr. R. K. Davis, Nowata, will serve as vice-president; Dr. J. V. Athey was re-elected as secretary-treasurer; and Dr. R. C. Gentry was chosen as censor. Dr. R. L. Kurtz was re-elected trustee for the society.

Delegates are Dr. S. A. Lang, Dr. L. D. Hudson and Dr. H. C. Weber, and alternates are Doctor Davis, Dr. E. E. Beachwood and Dr. J. P. VanSant.

Dr. D. S. Harris of Drummond was elected president of the Garfield county society, and Dr. John R. Walker, Enid, was re-elected to serve as secretary for the fifteenth consecutive year. Other officers elected are Dr. Bruce R. Hinson, Enid, vice-president; Dr. V. R. Hamble and Dr. W. P. Neilson, both of Enid, delegates; and Dr. Wendell J. Mercer, Dr. Evans E. Talley and Doctor Hinson, censors.

Dr. J. B. Clark, Coalgate, and Dr. J. S. Fulton, Atoka,

were re-elected as president and secretary-treasurer, respectively, of the Atoka-Coal County Medical society, with Dr. J. C. Canada, Atoka, serving with them as vice-president. Other officers include Doctor Clark and Doctor Canada as delegates; Dr. W .W. Cotton, Atoka, and Dr. R. C. Henry, Coalgate, as alternates; and Dr. R. D. Cody, Centrahoma, Doctor Cotton, and Doctor Henry as censors.

New president of the Pittsburg County Medical society is Dr. Austin R. Stough, McAlester. Serving with him during 1942 will be Dr. Will C. Wait, McAlester, vice-president, and Dr. Edward D. Greenberger, McAlester, re-elected as secretary-treasurer of the society.

Delegates are Dr. T. H. McCarley and Dr. L. S. Willour, both of McAlester, and their alternates include Doctor Wait and Dr. Frank Baum, McAlester. Doctor Greenberger, Doctor Baum, and Dr. R. K. Pemberton, McAlester, will serve as censors, and Doctor Willour, Doctor Greenberger and Dr. Floyd Bartheld, McAlester, will serve on the Scientific Program committee.

Dr. J. M. Allgood of Altus will preside over the Jackson county society in 1942, and Dr. C. G. Spears, Altus, will serve the society as vice-president. Re-elected as secretary-treasurer was Dr. Willard D. Holt of Altus.

Dr. E. S. Crow, Olustee, was chosen as delegate, with Dr. E. W. Mabry, Altus, as alternate. Censors are Dr. J. R. Reid, Doctor Spears and Doctor Mabry, all of Altus.

Re-elected as president of the Noble county society was Dr. J. W. Francis of Perry. Also re-elected as secretary-treasurer was Dr. C. H. Cooke, Perry. Delegates include Dr. A. M. Evans, Perry, and Doctor Cooke, and Dr. T. F. Renfro, Billings, was chosen as alternate.

Dr. John Carson, Shawnee, was elected president of the Pottawatomie county society; Dr. Paul Gallaher, Shawnee, was elected vice-president, and Dr .Clinton Gallaher, Shawnee, was re-elected secretary-treasurer. Delegates are Dr. G. S. Baxter and Dr. W. M. Gallaher, both of Shawnee, and alternates are Dr. E. E. Rice and Dr. R. M. Anderson, both of Shawnee. Dr. M. A. Baker and Dr. A. C. McFarling, both of Shawnee, and Dr. R. C. Kayler, McLoud, are censors, and Doctor Carson, Dr. Paul Gallaher and Dr. Clinton Gallaher will serve on the Scientific Program committee.

At the December 20 meeting of the society, it was planned to have the Annual Meeting and Ladies Night January 17 in the Aldridge hotel, Shawnee. Dr. G. S. Baxter was appointed Chief of the Emergency Medical and Hospital services on the County Civilian Defense committee, and the society directed its president to appoint a Medical Protective committee to act in the interest of all physicians in Shawnee who may be dislocated from their practices in the interest of national defense.

It was also voted to reduce dues of out-of-town members to a total of twelve dollars a year, with two dollars going to the county society and ten dollars to the Association. It was also voted that the regular monthly Bulletin be made the official organ of the society, and that the regular weekly radio programs under the direction of Dr. R. M. Anderson be continued.

The Woods County Medical society has elected Dr. W. F. LaFon, Waynoka, as its 1942 president and Dr. C. A. Traverse, Alva, as vice-president. Dr. O. E. Templin, Alva, was re-elected secretary-treasurer, and Dr. D. B. Ensor of Hopeton was elected to serve for three years as censor and delegate. His alternate is Dr. I. F. Stephenson, Alva.

Dr. J. B. Hampton, Commerce, was elected president of the Ottawa county society, and Dr. M. M. DeArman, Miami, was elected vice-president of the Middle district; Dr. J. R. Barry, Picher, vice-president of the Northern district, and Dr. J. H. L. Staples, Afton, vice-president of the Southern district. Secretary-treasurer is Dr. Walter Sanger of Picher, and censors are Dr. M. A. Connell, Picher, and Dr. W. J. Craig and Dr. W. G. Chesnut, both of Miami. Delegates to the Annual meeting and their alternates will be appointed at the February meeting of the society.

At the December 17 meeting of the Garvin County Medical society, Dr. T. F. Gross, Lindsay, was elected president, Dr. A. H. Shi, Stratford, vice-president, and Dr. John R. Callaway, Pauls Valley, was re-elected secretary-treasurer. Dr. G. L. Johnson, Pauls Valley, was chosen as delegate, and Dr. Morton E. Robberson, Wynnewood, as censor for 1942-43.

Dr. J. H. Plunkett, Wagoner, was elected 1942 president of the Wagoner county society, with Dr. S. R. Bates, Wagoner, serving as vice-president and Dr. H. K. Riddle, Coweta, as secretary-treasurer. Doctor Riddle will serve also as delegate to the Annual meeting, and Doctor Plunkett as his alternate.

University of Oklahoma School of Medicine

Dr. Lewis L. Reese, Medical Director of the State University and Crippled Children's hospitals resigned on November 20, 1941, and Dr. George N. Barry was appointed Acting Medical Director.

On the afternoon of December 4, the School of Medicine was closed as a tribute to Dr. R. C. Lowry, professor of clinical obstetrics, who died suddenly on December 2, 1941. The faculty and student body lost a sincere and true friend and an excellent teacher.

General Robert U. Patterson, Dean of the School of Medicine, was guest speaker at the meeting of Alpha Epsilon Delta, premedical fraternity at the University of Oklahoma, on November 19. His subject was "The Army and its Relation to Medicine."

Dr. H. A. Shoemaker, Assistant Dean, spoke to members of the Physiology Club of the University of Oklahoma on November 25. His topic was "Physiology of Anesthesia."

The following members of the Faculty were on the program of the meeting of the Oklahoma Academy of Science at Edmond, Oklahoma, December 5 and 6: Dr. Donald B. McMullen, Dr. H. D. Moor, Dr. Paul W. Smith, Dr. Irwin C. Winter, Dr. Arthur A. Hellbaum, Dr. H. A. Shoemaker, Mr. Clark Ice, Dr. Carl A. Bunde, Dr. M. R. Everett, Dr. Irvin S. Danielson, and Miss Fay Sheppard.

Dr. Henry G. Bennett, Jr., recently appointed assistant in Gynecology on the faculty of the medical school, has been called to active duty with the United States Army.

Several members of the Faculty will attend the meeting of the A. A. A. S. at Dallas, Texas, December 29 to January 3.

The annual Christmas party of the School of Medicine was held at 8:00 P. M., December 18, 1941.

A total of 74 junior and senior students have applied for commissions in the Army or the Navy; 59 as 2nd Lieutenants in the Medical Administrative Corps of the Army of the United States, and 15 as Ensigns H. V. (P.) in the Naval Reserve. There are a total of 58 men and two women in the junior class, and 52 men and three women in the senior class.

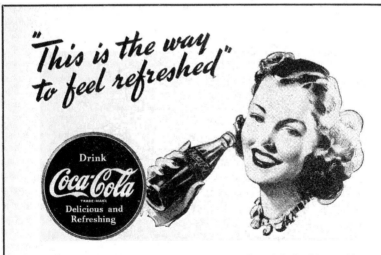

News From The State Health Department

Well developed methods of tuberculosis case finding are outlined in the report of a study made by the subcommittee on case finding procedures in tuberculosis of the American Public Health association, and now used by the Oklahoma State Health department.

The committee members were named because of recognized authority in this field and were given a free hand to determine the best case finding methods as an aid to physicians and health departments throughout the nation. Conclusions of the committee were accepted as the belief of experts in this phase of work. Among those on the committee were Bruce H. Douglas, M.D., tuberculosis controller, Detroit Department of Health; Esmond R. Long, M.D., director, Henry Phipps Institute, Philadelphia and Robert E. Plunkett, M.D., general superintendent, tuberculosis hospitals, New York State Department of Health.

Contrary to common understanding, the report terms the age period between five and 15 years as latent in the pathogenesis of tuberculosis. The most productive and important work to be done in tuberculosis control is among those 15 years of age and over, whether they be considered as contacts to known cases or on the basis of mass surveys, the report states.

Experience indicates that the incidence of significant pulmonary tuberculosis will be about one in 3,400 grade school children examined, whereas the ratio in high school students is about one in 700.

"There is a definite trend today away from mass surveys of grade school populations and a greater emphasis on high schools and colleges," the report says. In the past the emphasis has been on finding tuberculosis in youngsters so as to give early treatment, but the committee report, based on wide experience, maintains that the incidence is too low to justify the cost of widespread searching.

The report also defends the value of the tuberculin test, stating that "experience indicates that the overwhelming majority of patients with active tuberculosis of the reinfection type react positively to tuberculin." The study continues, "It is our opinion that the tuberculin test is an instrument of high efficiency in detecting active reinfection tuberculosis and that only an occasional case of tuberculosis of the type will be missed by the test."

The report deals primarily with large scale efforts to find tuberculosis cases, such as those undertaken by the state tuberculosis association and the state health department. "The selection of a suitable population for mass surveys is of utmost importance. From data now available it is possible to draw certain broad generalizations as to the basis for selecting the group to be surveyed. Primarily it will be an adult population above 20 years of age," the report states.

"The peak of tuberculosis mortality for women has been at the age period 25 to 29; for men the peak has been pushed along from the age period 35 to 39 in 1900 to the age period 65 to 69 in 1937," according to the report.

Diagnostic facilities listed in order of importance for the examination of adult groups are: x-ray; examination of sputum; case history; physician examination and tuberculin test.

The health department recognizes the value of an x-ray for everyone as the best means of diagnosis for tuberculosis, whether an adult or a grade school child, and recommends this procedure where it is possible on an individual basis.

"Operating as we are, with limited funds and personnel, the state health department finds it wise to give more attention to young adults in our case finding efforts, and concentrate less on those under 15 years of age, as studies of the best authorities have proved that the young age group is far less likely to have the disease than are older people. This same procedure might well be followed by the private physician in his search for tuberculosis," Dr. G. F. Mathews, commissioner, commented.

The study also contains a detailed section on case finding methods as they apply to the practicing physician. Copies of the study may be obtained from the tuberculosis association for a nominal sum.

Four staff members of the state health department are now in school, taking nine month courses which will give them their degrees in public health.

They are Dr. John Y. Battenfield, Dr. M. L. Peter, Harold Malone and Bill Lanphere. Doctor Battenfield, epidemiologist stationed in the central office, is in Johns Hopkins university's School of Public Health, while his duties are being assumed by other members of the staff. Doctor Peter, director of the Payne County Health department, Stillwater, is also at Johns Hopkins. Dr. Perry Hewitt is in charge of the Stillwater department.

Mr. Malone, engineer in the field advisory unit stationed at Oklahoma City, is in the University of Michigan School of Public Health. His duties are being handled by G. T. McNew, engineer formerly stationed at Woodward. Lanphere, sanitarian in the Carter County Health department, Ardmore, is also at Michigan, and has been succeeded by Spencer Barnhill, formerly of Tulsa.

The newest division of the state health department, industrial hygiene, is now hard at work in a field which has assumed unusual importance because of the national emergency.

Studies of working conditions have been made in over 40 plants in Oklahoma which are at work on defense contracts. In some instances recommendations made as a result of the studies have led to the removal of working conditions which were hazardous to the health of the workers.

Particular attention is being given to dust, gas, vapors and mists and similar conditions in work areas which might be considered dangerous.

The division has also completed a detailed study of the working conditions in typical mines of the tri-state lead and zinc mining region of Miami. A comprehensive report, including recommendations has just been completed and turned over to the industry. E. C. Warkentin and Bob Ady, engineers, do the work of this division.

Full time, local health service continues to develop in Oklahoma, with 40 counties now having the benefit of trained public health workers on duty.

Newest counties to provide a well planned public health program of disease prevention are Okmulgee, Stephens and Jefferson, making an all-time high in the development of this work.

Six Washington-Nowata Society Members Have Perfect Attendance Records

A chart of the 1941 attendance record of members of the Washington-Nowata County Medical society has been received in the office of the Association from Dr. J. V. Athey, Secretary of the society.

With a total average attendance of 63 percent for the whole group, the chart shows that six doctors had records of 100 percent attendance, eight had records of 90 percent, three had records of 80 percent, and five had records of 70 percent.

The six members whose attendance was 100 percent were Doctor Athey, Dr. E. E. Beechwood, Dr. Forrest S. Etter, Dr. O. I. Green, Dr. S. M. Parks, and Dr. Thomas Wells.

Smokers Can't Help Inhaling—but

they can help their throats!

ALL those who smoke inhale — at least sometimes. And *when* they inhale, the danger of irritation increases. Therefore, the importance of this Philip Morris advantage:

The irritant quality in the smoke of four other leading brands was shown in recognized laboratory tests* to average *more than three times that of the strikingly contrasted Philip Morris.*

Further—the irritant effect of such cigarettes was observed to last more than 5 times as long!

A change to Philip Morris cigarettes will minimize irritation due to smoking.

PHILIP MORRIS

PHILIP MORRIS & CO., LTD., INC.   119 FIFTH AVE., NEW YORK

**Facts from: Proc. Soc. Exp. Biol. & Med., 1934, 32, 241-245; N. Y. State Jrl. of Med. Vol. 35, No. 11,590; Arch. of Otolaryngology, Mar. 1936, Vol. 23, No. 3,306.*

Group Hospital Service News

N. D. Helland Is New Executive Director

Mr. N. D. Helland is now Executive Director of GROUP HOSPITAL SERVICE, Oklahoma's approved "Blue Cross Plan" for hospital care. He succeeds Mr. Walter R. McBee, who was "drafted" by the State of Texas in August. Mr. Helland comes here from Milwaukee, Wisconsin, and was selected for Oklahoma after a number of executives from various approved plans had been interviewed by the Board of Trustees. Helland first affiliated with the "Blue Cross Plan" at Minneapolis, later going to Milwaukee with the "Blue Cross Plan." His wife and two children, Nancy, 12, and Dennis, 7, moved with Mr. Helland to Tulsa December 1.

Mr. Helland, widely known throughout the nation's non-profit plans for his sales ability, comes to Oklahoma with an ambitious program for extending this voluntary community service throughout the state. Back of his good intentions is the record of the "Blue Cross Plan" in Milwaukee, where 75,000 members were enrolled in 23 months.

Mr. Helland has stated that it is becoming increasingly difficult to point out big names in American industry which do not participate in the community service plans. The reason is not only because of the benefits derived, but because the "Blue Cross Plans," in fulfilling their functions, do so in such a manner as to preserve the presence of individual freedom and self-help and the existing voluntary hospital system and private practice of medicine—the very foundations on which America has built the finest health standards the world has ever known.

This community service plan will progress in Oklahoma in direct proportion to the interest and cooperation of the Oklahoma State Medical Association. The continued whole hearted support of every member of the Association is earnestly solicited in extending this service. The personnel of your "Blue Cross Plan" is eager to assist you in every way possible to serve the people of your community.

Fifth Neuropsychiatric Institute Planned

Under the sponsorship of the American Psychiatric Association the fifth interstate Neuropsychiatric Institute will be held March 22 to April 4, 1942, at State Hospital No. 2, St. Joseph, Mo.

The Institute, which will be conducted under the Association's sponsorship through its committee on psychiatry and medical education, will present many interesting lectures on neuroanatomy, neuropathology, psychobiology, psychotherapy, neuroroentgenology, neurosurgery, and electro-encephalography, together with a presentation of clinical psychiatric and neurologic problems and related subjects.

Resolution on Postgraduate Course

The Blaine County Medical Society, on this 20th day of November, in regular session assembled in the city of Watonga, Okla., does hereby offer the following resolution:

(1) We approve the two schools of postgraduate work conducted by Drs. Smith and Hughes, respectively. We hereby express our appreciation to the Foundation, the State Medical Association, Dr. Smith and Dr. Hughes and any and all others who have assisted in bringing to us these interesting and instructive courses of study.

(2) The suggestion has been made that another course in "Internal Medicine" would possibly be offered. This meets with our hearty approval and should it be offered we believe that each and every member of the Society will support it and attend the lectures as we have done with the previous courses.

The above resolution is approved by unanimous vote.

W. F. Griffin, M.D., Secretary.

• OBITUARIES •

Dr. J. B. Hix
1878-1941

Joseph Bedford Hix was born in Whittleyville, Tenn., December 11, 1878. His old home community was his home until he was grown and had secured his education and prepared to serve his fellow men as a physician.

Doctor Hix received his A.B. degree at Peabody college in Nashville, Tenn., and taught for a number of years in Tennessee, Kentucky and Louisiana before he began his study of medicine. After he had graduated with an M.D. degree from the University of Tennessee, he practiced medicine in Jackson county in that state for six years.

In 1914, Doctor Hix and his wife moved to Oklahoma, where he continued his practice in Tipton until 1917. At that time, they established their home in Altus. In 1922, Doctor Hix began to specialize in skin and x-ray treatment, a specialty which he continued until his death.

He died, following illness from a heart disease, December 13, 1941.

Survivors include his wife of the home address, a brother, W. M. Hix, Redlands, Calif., and several nieces and nephews of Tennessee and California.

Resolution

WHEREAS, Doctor Joseph B. Hix was, for many years, an active and respected member of the Jackson County Medical Society, and,

WHEREAS, during that period of time he was a respected and honored member of the Jackson County Medical Society, co-operating in every way for the good of the Society and his community, giving freely of his time and efforts to promote the betterment of the medical profession and his colleagues, and,

WHEREAS, the said Doctor Joseph B. Hix has departed this life, and the Jackson County Medical Society wishes to commemorate his passing by an appropriate resolution.

NOW, THEREFORE, BE IT RESOLVED BY The Jackson County Medical Society, this 29th day of December, 1941, that the death of Doctor Joseph B. Hix is considered a great loss to this Society and the community in which he lived.

BE IT FURTHER RESOLVED that the Jackson County Medical Society takes this method of expressing to the Medical profession and to Mrs. Hix its regret at the passing of our friend and colleague.

BE IT FURTHER RESOLVED that a copy of this resolution be sent to Mrs. Joseph B. Hix and that a copy also be forwarded to the State Medical Journal for publication.

Raymond H. Fox
Willard D. Holt
E. W. Mabry
Committee on Resolutions

Dr. Jesse Bird 1875-1941

Dr. Jesse Bird, a practicing physician in Oklahoma for 39 years, died December 9 in an Oklahoma City hospital, where he had been admitted after suffering a heart attack.

Doctor Bird was born March 4, 1875, in Gainseville, Tex., and was graduated from the Louisville university school of medicine in 1897. He practiced medicine first in Texas, then in Dougherty, Okla., and finally in Oklahoma City, where he made his home till his death.

Survivors include his wife at the home address, a son, Jesse Dale Bird, Oklahoma City; three daughters, Mrs. Harry Weston, Guernsey, Wyo., Miss Anna Grace Bird, Hydro, and Mrs. Margaret Fulton of the home address; three brothers, Edgar Bird, Arlington, Tex., George Bird, Alvarado, Tex., and Tom Bird, Chickasha; and five grandchildren.

Tons of Liver reduced to
thimble-fuls of concentrate for the —

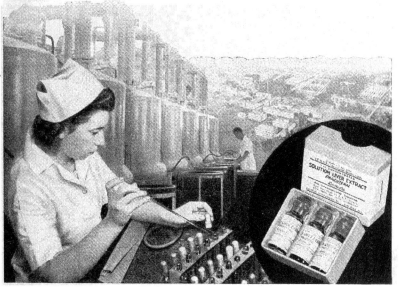

BOOK REVIEWS

"The chief glory of every people arises from its authors."—Dr. Samuel Johnson.

"PERSONAL AND COMMUNITY HEALTH." C. E. Turner, A.M., Sc.D., D.P.H., Professor of Biology and Public Health, Massachusetts Institute of Technology. Fifth Edition. The C. V. Mosby Company, St. Louis, 1939.

This book is well written and arranged so that the topics appear in a logical sequence. Throughout the book the discussion of hygiene is based on normal physiology. The first part is devoted to personal health, with discussions of the hygiene of the various systems and organs of the body. The second part deals with community health. The material on disease prevention is well organized and the basic principles of immunity are discussed. The chapters on the relationship of water supply, waste disposal, ventilation, maternal and child hygiene, school hygiene and industrial hygiene to the health of the community are well adapted to give the student a clear-cut concept of their importance.

The report (1935) of the American Health Association on the control of communicable disease appears in the appendix. A revised report (1940) has appeared since the publication of this book but the former still serves as an excellent reference and summary of some 62 diseases.

The stated purpose of this book is to place health instruction on a college and university level. The author is well qualified, with his practical and teaching experience, to write such a book. The book is well suited in beginning courses of chemistry and biology. Students interested in physical education, predental or premedical courses would find it of practical value. Used as a background for those who are going to teach hygiene in the public schools this book would be excellent. It would also serve as a text and reference book for nurses—Donald B. McMullen.

———

"CANCER OF THE FACE AND MOUTH." Diagnosis, Treatment, Surgical Repair, Vilray P. Blair, M.D., Sherwood Moore, M.D. and Louise T. Byars, M.D., St. Louis, Mo. C. V. Mosby Company, St. Louis, 1941.

Vilray P. Blair has often spoken and written his opinions in regard to how cancer of the face should be treated. These opinions have been widely accepted and respected. This volume represents an enormous amount of labor and effort upon his part in gathering together in a systematic manner his ideas and showing the results both good and bad in a group of 1,500 cases. He has been ably assisted by Dr. Sherwood Moore, Professor of Radiology in the Washington University School of Medicine and Director of the Edward Mallinckrodt Institute of Radiology, and Dr. Louis T. Byars of the Plastic Surgery Department of the Washington University School of Medicine.

They show conclusively that if cancer of the face is to be treated successfully there must be close correlation of the pathologist, surgeon and radiologist.

They postulate the following principles which they think should govern the management of any case of malignancy:

1. Early recognition and treatment.
2. Selection of a rational plan of treatment.
3. Adequate execution of the selected plan.
4. Adequate observation and care of the patient before, during, and after treatment.

The work is made especially enlightening by the wealth of good photographs and diagrams.

This volume can be read to an advantage by all classes of practitioners since it is written in clear, concise and straightforward language, laying down definite criteria for diagnosis, treatment and prognosis.—John F. Burton.

"DISEASES OF THE BLOOD," an Atlas of Hematology. Roy R. Kracke, M.D., Professor of Bacteriology and Laboratory Diagnosis, Emory University School of Medicine; formerly Director of the Hematology Registry. Second Edition. Cloth. Price $15.00. 692 pages. 54 colored plates and 45 other illustrations. J. B. Lippincott company, Philadelphia.

Throughout the ages the role of the blood in health and disease has had a prominent place in all discussions and treatises on medicine. One of the first objects to be examined with the compound microscope was the blood. Thus were the corpuscles discovered. From that day to this the study of the blood has had a prominent place in all sciences dealing with life, health, and disease. One after another, characteristic changes in the blood have been recognized as part if not the most important manifestation of this or that disease, so there came to be listed certain blood diseases, as anemias and leukemias, as well as blood changes concomitant with other pathologies such as infections and parasitic infestations. In determining these changes a great many technical procedures have been developed. And with the realization of the importance of laboratory procedures as an aid to clinical examination in diagnosis and guide in treatment, a specialty of medicine, clinical pathology, has developed to a high degree and is an essential part of any clinical setup. Most frequent of all laboratory procedures is examination of the blood, and a knowledge of the normal and pathological blood or hematology requires perhaps the widest as well as the most detailed study and a knowledge of variety of exacting techniques of any laboratory procedures except tissue pathology.

Unfortunately, due to a somewhat meager knowledge of biological principles and variations of these in complex organisms, and also different points of view or insufficient study of embryology, cytogenesis, and tissue differentiation there has been developed an argument as to the origin, relation, and propagation of the various blood elements. A veritable library has grown up on the facts of hematology interpreted on the basis of the views of this or that "school" of hemocytologists.

Dr. Kracke's book is a decided contribution to the library of hematology. His book is not written on the assumption that the reader has an advanced knowledge of the subject, which is a defect of some very excellent books. Dr. Kracke begins with the fundamentals, even with definitions of terms. He present the gist of the theories of the various "schools" of hematogenic thought. His book is valuable to the student of hematology because of his discussion of fundamentals of hematology. It is valuable to the clinician because of his discussion of the etiology and treatment of blood diseases as well as the pathology and interpretations of the blood pictures. It is valuable to the technologist because of the directions for laboratory procedures. Dr. Kracke has added another valuable section on the blood pictures of various animals which will be an aid to the research worker.

The colored plates are a little too highly colored and the colors do not match those seen in prepared specimens, but the morphology of the cells both individual and relative is faithfully true. Dr. Kracke's book should be in the library of all physicians, pathologists and technologists.—L. A. Turley, Ph.D.

Dr. Brewer Returns to Oklahoma City

Dr. A. M. Brewer has returned to Oklahoma City after several weeks in Baltimore, Md., where he was enrolled in a graduate course in Urology at the Johns Hopkins hospital.

Doctor Brewer has reopened his office in the Perrine Building, where his practice will be limited to Urology.

REVIEWS and CORRESPONDENCE

SURGERY AND GYNECOLOGY

Abstracts, Reviews and Comments From
LeRoy Long Clinic
714 Medical Arts Building, Oklahoma City

"THE RIGHT LATERAL RECTUS INCISION IN ACUTE APPENDICITIS." C. Grant Bain, M.D., Chehalis. Wash. The American Journal of Surgery, November. 1941, Vol. LIV. No. 2, Page 388.

In recent years the McBurney incision for appendectomy has been recommended highly. Its advantages are unquestioned but its disadvantages suggest themselves when the advantages of the right lateral rectus incision (not the right rectus "splitting" incision) are considered especially in acute cases which may have developed complications. Moreover, in those acute cases in which the diagnosis is not completely clear and in those so-called chronic cases in which some exploration may be desirable at operation, these advantages become even more apparent. The right lateral rectus incision is more directly over the site of the appendix, the meso-appendix and localized complications. The incision avoids damage to anatomical structures; it lends itself to extension readily in either direction; it permits a firm closure, even when drainage has to be employed and it facilitates the operative procedure.

The right lateral rectus incision is a slightly oblique incision just lateral to the lower right rectus muscle or just over the lateral edge of the muscle through the rectus sheath; then using some slight displacement of this muscle edge mesially, the posterior sheath is exposed. This is not a muscle splitting incision. The muscle is disturbed only by temporarily retracting the lateral edge mesially, and in closing it resumes its original position between the two layers of fascia. There is no injury to nerves or blood vessels as a rule. It is usually possible to limit the incision to the space between the eleventh and twelfth intercostal nerves.

COMMENT: My personal preference remains the McBurney incision, but there are certainly instances in which the right lateral rectus incision is of distinct value. Although the author has had only one incisional hernia after using this incision in 50 cases, it is my opinion that incisional postoperative hernia is more apt to occur after this type incision than after McBurney incision. For example, I have had no postoperative incisional hernias in the past 50 appendectomies through McBurney incision.—LeRoy D. Long.

"TOTAL HYSTERECTOMY, ABDOMINAL AND VAGINAL." W. C. Danforth, M.D., Evanston, Ill. American Journal of Obstetrics and Gynecology, October. 1941, Vol. 42. No. 4, Page 587.

This is a report of hysterectomies done on Dr. Danforth's service at the Evanston hospital.

There were 744 subtotal hysterectomies with a mortality rate of 0.8 percent. There were 150 total abdominal hysterectomies with a mortality rate of 0.66 percent and there were 425 vaginal hysterectomies with no mortality.

COMMENT: The authors of both of the above articles prefer the total hysterectomy where the mortality rate can be kept low because of the removal of the cervix from any possible future danger of cancer in it but also they feel that the removal of the cervix prevents not infrequent postoperative leukorrhea and chronic foci of infection.

It should be mentioned that the mortality figures of Danfroth are extremely good while those of Miller and his associates are slightly less than the average of large reported series. It may be interesting to remember that we reported in 1938 on 1,000 consecutive hysterectomies done at St. Anthony hospital in Oklahoma City with a mortality rate for the entire group done by the various surgeons there of 0.9 percent.

The old question of total or subtotal hysterectomy is again raised and, naturally, will be considered many times in the future. Total hysterectomy, either abdominally or vaginally, is undoubtedly a better operation than a subtotal hysterectomy when there is any disease of the cervix, and it may be even argued that it is a better operation in any patient in whom a hysterectomy is indicated whether the cervix is diseased or not. However, this question of total or subtotal hysterectomy cannot be settled as a broad basis for action by all men who do pelvic surgery or for all patients. Realizing the advantages of a total hysterectomy over a subtotal hysterectomy, an individual surgeon must consider an individual patient and decide in each instance whether or not he feels that the total operation is advantageous in that particular situation.—Wendell Long.

EYE, EAR, NOSE AND THROAT

Edited by Marvin D. Henley, M. D.
911 Medical Arts Building, Tulsa

"INFLUENCE OF THE EMOTIONS UPON ESOPHAGEAL FUNCTION:" A Comparison of Esophagoscopic and Roentgenologic Findings. William B. Faulkner, F. H. Rodenbaugh and John R. O'Neill. Radiology, Vol. 37, page 443-447, October. 1941.

Psychiatrists have known that emotions can so disturb organic function as to produce severe symptoms which are indistinguishable from those of definite organic disease. The authors observed during an esophagoscopic investigation that the severe esophageal spasm of a patient disappeared by a chance statement of the examiners. They could bring about spasm by the discussion of unpleasant subjects and the arousing of undesirable emotions, and they could cause them to disappear by pleasant and wished-for talk.

Similar psychosomatic changes have occurred in at least 25 other patients, and the changes could be demonstrated by roentgenological examinations. There was, for instance, a woman with severe cardiospasm. When suggestions were made to arouse pleasant emotions, the barium instantly ran into the stomach, all signs of cardiospasm disappeared, and further immediate ingestion showed no esophageal spasm. As soon as the woman began to talk about her family difficulties, the spasm of the cardia returned.

The authors mention other examples of such emotionally controlled esophageal spasm: the salesman whose cardiospasm came from the feeling of insecurity; the married woman with a spasm from economic and social difficulties; a man who was afraid that he would be dropped from "relief." In the existence of such emotional esophageal spasm, one should be very careful in excluding the possibility of stricture, ulcer, carcinoma, foreign body, or other possible cause of the spastic symptom.

"TREATMENT OF SPASMODIC RHINITIS BY GENERAL NON-SPECIFIC DESENSITIZATION." P. de Gunten. Geneve. Schweizerische medizinische Wochenschrift. Vol. 71. page 958-961. August. 1941.

The large number of people who are suffering from spasmodic rhinitis and in whom all measures for cure were ineffective proves that mostly the symptomatic present treatment is insufficient, and that there is a necessity of replacing it by a method based upon our present knowledge of the pathogenesis of this affection. Owing to the fundamental work of Widal and Besredka, spasmodic rhinitis was declared an allergic disease, but, ever since, it has been a disease very reluctant to the therapeutic measures of specific desensitization. The inconstancy of results of vaccinotherapy showed that there are other etiological factors beside the allergenes. The frequency of spasmodic rhinitis in patients of a vagotonic or sympathicotonic habitus and the association of hayfever with asthma make it evident that the role of humoral and nervous constitution is important in the pathogenesis of this affection.

The complexity of pathogenesis requires a total aid by all available procedures and desensitization, disintoxication, and the use of drugs bringing the neurovegetative system into equilibrium. It also requires the use of opotherapeutic measures. It has been only recently that Halphen and Maduro pointed out the importance of endocrine disorders in the genesis of hayfever.

For non-specific desensitization the author recommends two substances: calcium thiosulfate, and jaborandi, both of which he has been using for the last three years in cases of intractable seasonal or perennial hayfever.

Calcium thiosulfate has an anti-shock and anti-allergic effect. It is also a desensitizing agent by its calcium component. Calcium is also an old-established regulator of the neuro-vegetative system. The author used a 20 percent solution of calcium thiosulfate ("Thiocalcium") for intravenous injections. The immediate effect is a sensation of heat; the intensity of this sensation varies according to the sensitiveness of the patient and the rapidity of the injection. After three or four injections, there is a definite improvement in the cases which will benefit; further six to eight injections may be given at two to three days' intervals. For the next three to four weeks, weekly injections are needed for maintaining the improvement. Simultaneous oral administration of calcibronat, or administration of ephedrine is recommended.

The other agent recommended is jaborandi (Neopancarpine), the active principle of which is an alkaloid, the pilocarpine. It is generally used as a sudorific and sialagogue agent, and for its action on the vagus nerve. It is used for intranasal instillation in isotonic solution (Rhinofluine), for subcutaneous injections, and perorally in drops or tablets. The injections are daily, and the tablets are taken for several months at the seasonal appearance of hayfever.

The author recommends the non-specific desensitization treatment in all cases of seasonal or perennial spasmodic rhinitis. First, the calcium thiosulfate treatment should be tried. If it fails to cure or improve the condition, the jaborandi treatment should begin. The author claims that the thiosulfate injections cured or improved 85 percent of the perennial hayfever cases.

CARDIOLOGY

Edited by F. Redding Hood, M. D.
1200 North Walker, Oklahoma City

"STUDIES ON CONGESTIVE HEART FAILURE, THE IMPORTANCE OF RESTRICTION OF SALT AS COMPARED TO WATER." Henry A. Schroeder, M.D., New York. Condensed from the American Heart Journal.

There is fairly general agreement as to the importance of restricting fluids in the treatment of congestive heart failure, but in the matter of the restriction of sodium chloride, and to what extent it should be restricted, there is difference of opinion.

Twenty-three patients were selected for study, and an attempt was made to find the most obstinate cases of congestive heart failure. Patients were given weighed diets, in which the content of sodium chloride, the caloric value, the protein content, and the intake of fluid were constant for definite periods. Factors such as activity and digitalis therapy were carefully controlled. The output of chloride in the urine was measured daily.

The Action of Sodium Chloride: It was observed in all cases that a reduction in the amount of ingested salt was followed by a loss in weight and in edema fluid. Often diuresis and loss of weight began immediately when the intake of sodium chloride was reduced from 2.0 Gm. in 24 hours to 1.0 Gm. In obstinate cases in which the edema was of long standing, it was always possible to prevent the accumulation of fluid by restriction of salt, although occasionally this necessitated a diet containing as little as .5 Gm. in 24 hours. The addition of a small amount of salt to the diet (1.0 Gm. to 2.0 Gm.) was followed, on the other hand, by an immediate gain in weight.

The Action of Fluid: It was found that the intake of fluids had little relation to the accumulation or disappearance of edema when the intake of salt was low enough. On the administration of a minimal amount of sodium chloride, weight was lost and edema disappeared as rapidly on a regime of restriction of fluids as on one in which water was freely given. There was, in fact, no effect on varying intake of fluids even in cases of severe chronic congestive heart failure.

The Choice of a Diet: In most instances 1.0 Gm. of sodium chloride in the diet was found to be low enough to prevent edema, but in a few cases, in which the heart failure was of long duration and the edema continuous, it was necessary to reduce the intake of salt to 0.5 Gm. per day. By measuring the excretion of chlorides in the urine it was possible to estimate the degree of restriction of sodium chloride which would be necessary for an effect, and a diet containing less than the amount excreted was used.

A diet containing 0.5 Gm. of sodium chloride per day is inadequate in its protein content and cannot be given for a long period of time. A diet in which the salt content is 1.0 Gm. is adequate except for vitamins, and these should be added.

DISCUSSION. There is good reason for rigid restriction of sodium chloride in chronic congestive heart failure. Edema fluid is composed principally of water and salt. Considerable water is necessary in the economy of the organism, but excess salt is not. Water cannot be deposited in the tissue spaces without salt. Salt is, therefore, necessary for the formation of this type of edema.

The rationale for the rigid restriction of fluids is not clear. If the intake of water is limited and the patient dehydrated, the deposition of edema should be lessened. Although dehydration can result from this procedure, it is uncertain that diuresis is thereby initiated. In these cases the output of urine was markedly depressed when the intake of fluids was low, and diuresis was not established until an adequate amount of fluid was administered. Furthermore, a certain volume of urine is necessary for the optimum excretion of chlorides (approximately 60 cc. per hour). If the volume is permitted to shrink below this, the output of chlorides is lessened. The opposite course is, therefore, preferable. If the output of urine can be increased by the administration of water, accompanied by rigid restriction of salt, the depletion of chlorides would be accelerated. On this plan, in no case did the output of urine fail to increase when extra water was added and sometimes an increase in the amount of water taken actually initiated loss of weight.

It is evident from these data that the administration

of comparatively large amounts of fluid to cardiac patients does not increase the rate of formation of edema, provided the intake of salt is low enough. Limitation of the ingestion of salt, including limitation of those foods in which the salt content is high, imposes little hardship upon the patient, whereas restriction of fluids to the degree necessary to produce an effect may be difficult, hazardous and uncomfortable. The occasional diuresis, with loss of weight, which has been observed when fluids were given, suggests that sometimes water is beneficial in this condition. For practical purposes it appears wise to allow patients with heart failure to drink as they please, provided the intake of sodium chloride (and other sodium salts) is carefully limited.

Compared to the amount of salt in the diets used in this study, the amount in the usual ''salt-free'' or ''cardiac'' diet is relatively high. An ordinary ward diet to which no extra salt and no salty foods have been added contains approximately 4.0 Gm. of sodium chloride; one cooked without salt contains 2.0 to 3.0 Gm. Since it has been shown that some patients may gain weight when taking 2.0 Gm. and remain at the same weight when taking 1.0 Gm. of salt in 24 hours, the kind of food given in the treatment of this type of edema assumes importance. The beneficial effects of the Karell diet (800 cc. of milk in 24 hours) may be due to the low content of fluid and of food, but especially to the fact that the salt content is also reduced to 1.0 Gm.

Few complaints were made about these diets when the food was properly seasoned. Patients were able to take them at home with less hardship than would be caused by the restriction of fluids.

ORTHOPAEDIC SURGERY

Edited by Earl D. McBride, M. D., F. A. C. S.
605 N. W. 10th, Oklahoma City

"CAUSALGIC BACKACHE." Otho C. Hudson, Carl A. Hettesheimer and Percival A. Robin. Amer. Jr. of Surg., LII, 297, May 1941.

The authors describe a type of back pain that involves the lumbar muscles, especially the quadratus lumborum. This pain is due to irritation of the twelfth thoracic and first lumbar nerves and radiates along the twelfth rib. A clinical picture of asymmetrical muscle imbalance occurs. This group of cases makes up another definite clinical entity, which can be separated from that vast group of patients suffering from back pain. The treatment is simple and effective.

This type of backache is produced by muscle imbalance and muscle spasm, which increase the tension within the quadratus lumborum fascia with direct pressure on the twelfth thoracic nerve, as in the scalenus anticus syndrome. The irritation is manifested by pain with radiation along the course of this nerve. The abdominal muscles become weakened by lack of use, and the overworked sacrospinalis muscles become contracted with an increase of lumbar lordosis and anterior inclination of the pelvis.

The history given by the patient is quite characteristic. It is the history of low-back pain of several years' duration, which is localized in the crest of the ilium and is unilateral. If the pain is right-sided, in many cases appendectomy, gall-bladder surgery, or urological instrumentation have been resorted to without relief. The discomfort continues at night as well as during the day.

Examination reveals increased lumbar lordosis, postural scoliosis, and tilting of the pelvis with abduction of the lower extremity, internal rotation of the thigh, and marked pronation of the foot. There is often hyperaesthesia over the cutaneous distribution of the twelfth thoracic and first lumbar nerves. Tenderness along the twelfth rib is elicited. Tenderness and hyperaesthesia

are observed parallel to Poupart's ligament, the upper inner aspect of the thigh, and paravertebrally over the twelfth thoracic and first lumbar transverse processes.

The treatment is rather simple and consists of raising the heel of the abducted extremity to overcome the pelvic tilt. This relaxes the quadratus lumborum and allows the rib to return to normal position, resulting in correction of the scoliosis and disappearance of the internal rotation of the thigh. Exercises for the development of the abdominal muscles and the sacrospinalis group are given.

"THE MANAGEMENT OF SCOLIOSIS." Frederick vom Saal. Amer. Jr. of Surgery. LII, 433, June 1941.

Etiological factors in the various types of scoliosis are discussed as paralytic, idiopathic, thoracogenic, neuropathic, and congenital. In the treatment of the postpoliomyelitic curves, it was found that if the curve was progressing before application of the brace, it would continue to do so after application of the brace. The majority of curves in the idiopathic group stopped progressing before cessation of growth. Fusion was done in 41 patients in a group of 174 with the various types, the patients with postpoliomyelitic scoliosis predominating. Many of these will need fusion for the prevention of deformity. The author uses the Risser type of jacket, with certain modifications. The jacket is applied with the patient in the maximum bending position toward the concave side of the primary curve, thus straightening the compensatory curves, producing one long curve, and derotating the secondary curves, making the patient straighter and more comfortable. Hinges and turnbuckles are then used for correction. A second modification consists of later rotating the upper part of the cast, so as to bring the shoulder on the convex side of the primary curve foward, after first removing the hinges and turnbuckles. This aids in the correction of rib deformity and brings the spinous processes into a more nearly vertical position—allowing greater ease of operation in the later spine fusion, and better cosmetic results. This does not apply in long-standing cases with severe rotation of the vertebral bodies. The fusion area is determined by studies of the immediately preoperative roentgenogram.

The operation is performed in the usual manner, using the modified Hibbs or Mackenzie Forbes technique, fusing six or seven vertebrae at one time, and using additional bone chips in all cases. Preoperative and postoperative care are discussed.

INTERNAL MEDICINE

Edited by Hugh Jeter, M. D., F. A. C. P., A. S. C. P.
1200 North Walker, Oklahoma City

"NERVES OF THE ADULT HUMAN ENDOMETRIUM." David State, M.D. and Edwin F. Hirsch, M.D.. Chicago. Archives of Pathology. Volume 32, Number 6, December, 1941.

The authors have reviewed published reports regarding the distribution of nerves in the human uterus and found limited information regarding their distribution. The results of this investigation are briefly abstracted. Evidence is presented to indicate that the presence of nerve fibers in the endometrium has lead to confusion because of inadequacy of staining methods employed. A method of staining is given and several photomicrographs are included.

As a result of their investigation with improved methods, they conclude that the distribution of the nerve supply of the spiral and that of the basal arteries of the endometrium apparently are distinct. The spiral arteries are innervated in the inner fourth of the myometrium near their bifurcation; the basal arteries are supplied by nerves in the basilar portions of the endometrium or in the immediately underlying myometrium.

A vasomotor nervous mechanism in the control of the vascular reactions of the endometrial arteries during the menstrual cycle is suggested by this anatomic study.

"INFLUENCE OF SODIUM BICARBONATE IN PREVENTING RENAL LESIONS FROM MASSIVE DOSES OF SULFATHIAZOLE." David R. Climenko, M.D., Ph.d., Rensselaer, N. Y. and Arthur W. Wright, M.D., Albany, N. Y. Archives of Pathology. Volume 32. Number 6, December, 1941.

In this, the authors have experimentally, in monkeys, administered large doses of sulfathiazole and found that by such large doses the animals would invariably develop renal lesions and die. The experimental results would seem to indicate that the major pathological changes were traumatization of the collecting tubules due to the precipitation of crystalline material in the renal parenchyma.

They, therefore, suggest that in clinical practice, use should be made of bicarbonate, or other suitable alkali, sufficient to maintain the urine on the alkaline side, and point out that Bridges and Mattice have shown that the amount of alkali will vary from patient to patient and from time to time in the same patient.

When a dose level of sulfathiazole is used which kills the major portion of experimental animals and produces severe renal lesions in all experimental animals, it is possible to prevent fatalities and also to inhibit the formation of the multiple local inflammatory lesions in the kidney by the administration of large quantities of sodium bicarbonate.

This action of bicarbonate can be accounted for by the fact that both sulfathiazole and its conjugated derivative acetylsulfathiazole are many times more soluble in alkaline mediums than they are in acid mediums and that the maintenance of an alkaline urine prevents precipitation of the drug in the kidney and thereby prevents formation of the local lesions.

UROLOGY
Edited by D. W. Branham, M. D.
502 Medical Arts Building, Oklahoma City

"TEN YEARS' EXPERIENCE IN THE MANAGEMENT OF CRYPTORCHIDISM." Virgil S. Counseller, M.D. The Journal of Urology.

The author presents a valuable contribution that sums up our present day concept of the undescended testes. Of interest is the fact that he does not feel that hormone therapy is as effective as some of the reports show. In his opinion the administration of gonadotropic harmone is indicated in but a small percentage of patients, and that with the majority, surgical treatment is advisable. The time of surgery should be delayed to the age of puberty, in most instances the type of operation performed depends entirely on the physical characteristics present; position of the testes, size of scrotum, etc. Castration is done in only adult patients, or on patients where it is impossible to replace the testes satisfactorily by orthodox surgery.

"SPASTIC URETERITIS (URETERAL STRICTURE)? ESSENTIAL CLINICAL CONSIDERATIONS." Henry W. E. Walther and Robert M. Willoughby, M.D. The Journal of Urology.

I was particularly interested in this article on a subject that has had comparatively little attention the past few years. Yet in my opinion it is a clinical condition that is comparatively common and productive of much distress referable to the abdomen. In a questionnaire issued to a large number of urologists, the returns proved to him that the majority of the urologists feel there is such a condition as painful stenosis or spastic conditions of the ureter. Opinions differ as to its frequency and its causation. There is little difference of opinion, however, as to the clinical picture, regardless of the causative factors, and there is a rather general belief in the efficacy of ureteral dilatation as a means of relief.

"FOUR SIMPLE RULES FOR A SUCCESSFUL RESECTION." Henry S. Brown, M.D. Transactions of the South Central Section of the American Urological Association, Denver, Colorado, 1940.

Dr. Brown has contributed to the surgery of prostatic resection four basic rules that if followed will aid the Urologist in determining whether a satisfactory resection has been performed.

1. With the sheath carefully centered and the verumontanum just visible, there should be no tissue observed to fall into the open end of the sheath when it is rotated in a complete circle.

2. On examination with the retrograde telescope, the entire circumference at the junction of the operated area and the bladder should show no prostatic tissue projecting into the bladder at any point.

3. On examination of the prostatic cavity with the retrograde telescope no tissue should be seen projecting into this cavity.

4. The verumontanum should be completely visible with the retrograde telescope.

Hotel Offers Rates for A. M. A. Meeting

Announcement of special rates to be granted physicians attending the American Medical Association meeting in June, 1942, in Atlantic City, has been made by the Ritz-Carlton hotel.

Any doctor who is interested in obtaining information about the rates and reservation cards should contact the Executive Office at 210 Plaza Court, Oklahoma City.

Vitamins were there all the time!

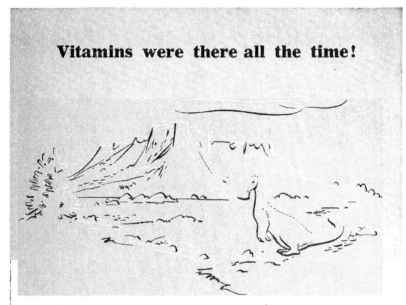

Vitamins have performed their vital functions for untold ages—but modern science has accomplished something new. It has revealed specific functions of vitamins, isolated many of them, and taught us how to make some of them synthetically. As a result, we can now make from the pure vitamins pharmaceutical preparations of great potency appropriate for the treatment of each of the various clinical syndromes caused by lack of one or more of these essential food factors.

Fifty-five years of experience in making fine pharmaceuticals equip The Upjohn Company to prepare these vitamin products for you.

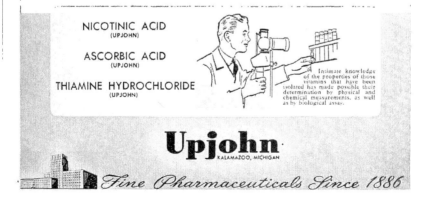

NICOTINIC ACID
(UPJOHN)

ASCORBIC ACID
(UPJOHN)

THIAMINE HYDROCHLORIDE
(UPJOHN)

Intimate knowledge of the properties of those vitamins that have been isolated has made possible their determination by physical and chemical measurements, as well as by biological assay.

Upjohn
KALAMAZOO, MICHIGAN

Fine Pharmaceuticals Since 1886

OFFICERS OF COUNTY SOCIETIES, 1942

COUNTY	PRESIDENT	SECRETARY	MEETING TIME
Alfalfa			
Atoka-Coal	J. B. Clark, Coalgate	J. S. Fulton, Atoka	
Beckham	H. K. Speed, Sayre	E. S. Kilpatrick, Elk City	Second Tues. eve.
Blaine	Virginia Olson Curtin, Watonga	W. F. Griffin, Watonga	
Bryan			
Caddo			
Canadian			
Carter	Walter Hardy, Ardmore	H. A. Higgins, Ardmore	
Cherokee			
Choctaw			
Cleveland			
Comanche			
Cotton			
Craig			
Creek	Frank Sisler, Bristow	O. H. Cowart, Bristow	
Custer			
Garfield	D. S. Harris, Drummond	John R. Walker, Enid	Fourth Thursday
Garvin	T. F. Gross, Lindsay	John R. Callaway, Pauls Valley	Wed before 3rd Thurs.
Grady			3rd Thursday
Grant	I. V. Hardy, Medford	E. E. Lawson, Medford	
Greer	S. W. Hopkins, Hollis		
Harmon		W. M. Yeargan, Hollis	First Wednesday
Haskell		N. K. Williams, McCurtain	
Hughes	Wm. L. Taylor, Holdenville		
Jackson	J. M. Allgood, Altus	Willard D. Holt, Altus	Last Monday
Jefferson	W. M. Browning, Waurika	J. L. Hollingsworth, Waurika	Second Monday
Kay	J. C. Wagner, Ponca City	J. Holland Howe, Ponca City	Third Thurs.
Kingfisher			
Kiowa			
LeFlore			
Lincoln	E. F. Hurlbut, Meeker	C. W. Robertson, Chandler	First Wednesday
Logan			
Marshall			
Mayes			
McClain			
McCurtain	R. D. Williams, Idabel	R. H. Sherrill, Broken Bow	Fourth Tues. eve.
McIntosh			
Murray			
Muskogee	Shade D. Neely, Muskogee	J. T. McInnis, Muskogee	First & Third Mon.
Noble	J. W. Francis, Perry	C. H. Cooke, Perry	
Okfuskee	J. M. Pemberton, Okemah	L. J. Spickard, Okemah	Second Monday
Oklahoma	R. Q. Goodwin, Okla. City	Wm. E. Eastland, Okla. City	Fourth Tuesday
Okmulgee	J. G. Edwards, Okmulgee	John R. Cotteral, Henryetta	Second Monday
Osage	C. R. Weirich, Pawhuska	George K. Hemphill, Pawhuska	Second Monday
Ottawa	J. B. Hampton, Commerce	Walter Sanger, Picher	Third Thursday
Pawnee			
Pittsburg	Austin R. Stough, McAlester	Edw. D. Greenberger, McAlester	
Pontotoc	R. E. Cowling, Ada	E. R. Muntz, Ada	Third Friday
Pottawatomie	John Carson, Shawnee	Clinton Gallaher, Shawnee	First Wednesday
Pushmataha	P. B. Rice, Antlers	John S. Lawson, Clayton	First & Third Sat.
Rogers			
Seminole			
Stephens			
Texas			
Tillman			
Tulsa	H. B. Stewart, Tulsa	E. O. Johnson, Tulsa	Second & Fourth Mon. eve.
Wagoner	J. H. Plunkett, Wagoner	H. K. Riddle, Coweta	
Washington-Nowata	R. W. Roeker, Bartlesville	J. V. Athey, Bartlesville	Second Wednesday
Washita	A. S. Neal, Cordell	James F. McMurry, Sentinel	
Woods	W. F. LaFon, Waynoka	O. E. Templin, Alva	Last Wednesday
Woodward			

THE JOURNAL
OF THE
OKLAHOMA STATE MEDICAL ASSOCIATION

| VOLUME XXXV | OKLAHOMA CITY, OKLAHOMA, FEBRUARY, 1942 | NUMBER 2 |

Electro-Surgical Treatment of the Pathologic Cervix*

KENNETH J. WILSON, M.D.

OKLAHOMA CITY, OKLAHOMA

Cervical disease is the most frequent source of gynecologic pathology. The histological nature of this portion of the uterus, subjected to trauma of parturition, exposure to infection from the vaginal, urinary and alimentary tracts, as well as that of the male consort, entails a liability to pathologic alteration not exceeded by that of any other organ. It is estimated 70 to 80 percent of all multiparous women, and some 20 percent of virgins and nulliparous females, are afflicted with the malady. The trend in medical thought of a solution to this problem is toward a more conservative method of approach that would be a little more acceptable to a greater number of victims. With this in view, electrical procedure has gained much favor through success attending its use.

Satisfactory treatment of the diseased cervix is contingent on familiarity with histological structure and pathologic alteration. As we recall histology of the cervix we are reminded of the downward continuation of the muscular corpus, with rather sudden blending into fibro-elastic tissue that looses muscle elements at the portio. A narrowing of the canal at this junction is designated the internal os. It widens again to form the isthmus, as it becomes less constricted in the external os. Membrane lining the canal is gathered up in minute folds, forming a sort of rugae, that is studded with innumerable racemose glands, horizontally situated with slight upward trend of the ducts, that evince a marked susceptibility to bacterial invasion. The most important factor in dissemination of infection is its rich lymphatic system that ramifies every part of the corpus and adjacent structures before terminating in larger collecting trunks that traverse the utero-

sacral and broad ligaments. Branched racemose glands with high columnar epithelial lining and narrow outlet are most conducive to the production of lesions found.

Classical differentiation of pathologic changes is not so important if we bear in mind the beginning is always in endocervical tissue. Erosion is loosely applied to the varying picture, but should be restricted to designation of those areas with macerated epithelia that do not penetrate the basement membrane. Eversion indicates a simple pouting of a lining membrane or turning out of raw surfaces of laceration. Ectropion is a more extensive hyperplasia of tissue that may embody any or all the other lesions. If there is extensive focalized hyperplasia it may result in formation of polyps. Distention of occluded tubules with the products of inflammation accounts for nabothian cysts, that may become sterile, but most often continue as chronic foci of infection. Fairly recently it has been noted that deposits of fibrous tissue in the cervix and corpus is due to a compensatory effort to withstand long continued inflammatory reaction. In view of this granulating profusion of cellular disorder one must appreciate its importance in the incidence of cancer. Accumulated statistical data indicates that 80 percent of pelvic malignancies may be charged to neglected, or improperly treated, cervical disease. Furthermore, 90 percent of these arise in the squamous epithelial covering of the portio, usually in or near the os, easily accessible, and highly responsive to therapy. Is it unreasonable, therefore, to assume credit for thermal destruction of many cervical epitheliomata, in their incipiency, as is accomplished in other epithelial locations?

A major portion of the responsibility for continued cervical disease rests with the attendant accoucheur, and can hardly be excus-

*Read before the Section on General Surgery, Annual Session, Oklahoma State Medical Association, May 20, 1941, in Oklahoma City.

ed in the light of present methods of control. I think it generally conceded there is always traumatic damage to the cervix in parturition, that may be amenable to self restitution, but more often necessitates therapeutic measures designed to restore cervical parity. Experience teaches us that most of these injuries, if left to the favor of fortune, will ultimately confront us with a chronically infected organ that may have a far reaching influence on the health of its possessor, After complying with the principles involved in minimizing cervical injury let us anticipate sequelae sure to accompany unhealed separation of mucosa. With the advent of new therapy for restoration of the lacerated cervix there has been a growing inclination to defer immediate surgical repair, with added risk and uncertain results, until more elective methods are exhausted.

As many of these conditions do not present symptoms it is all the more important that the cervix be visualized. Palpation alone is often misleading, although it is an essential part of examination. In those who seek relief there is usually a history of a sense of weight or dropping down of the pelvic structures and perineum, leucorrheal discharge, backache that may extend down the thighs, particularly if the utero-sacral ligaments are involved, dyspareunia, bladder and rectal discomfort, menstrual anomalies, sterility, occasionally remote neuritic and rheumatic pains and finally nervous invalidism. This remarkable chain of symptoms is produced largely by lymphatic extension of infection, lymphangitis and lymphadenitis, that may involve any part or all the pelvic lymphatic system. Marked erosion may be attended with sanguineous discharge, as may that of malignancy, precipitated by the slightest trauma. My observation of these lesions leads me to believe fully half the pelvic disturbances seen are directly attributable to cervical disease, that could be relieved with office treatment. One has only to recall lymphatic extension of tonsil infection, and modes of cure to appreciate the same phenomenon in infected cervices. Leucorrhea is the most frequent symptom encountered in gynecologic practice and fully three-fourths of these are due to cervicitis. Uterine bleeding is many times from small granulations situated in the cervical canal, that may escape notice. A preponderance of cases consulting the gynecologist are of long duration that have been neglected or inadequately treated. Too often having been subjected to ill advised laparotomy, in spite of gross cervical pathology that might have accounted for the pelvic symptoms. Rarely is the need for exploration so pressing it could not await conservative treatment of the cervix. It is my impression that more than half the indi-

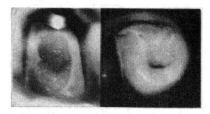

E-1   E-3

E. Cervical laceration, eversion and follicular infection. Mrs. M., 34 years of age, para two, 16 and 13 years of age Symptoms present for several years; pelvic weight and soreness, backache, moderate discharge and nervous invalidism. 1. Sept. 24, 1939, cervix treated. 3. Oct. 25, 1940, all symptoms relieved, marked diminution of uterine hypertrophy.

cations for radical treatment could be obviated with proper electrical therapy. The possibility of cancer must be paramount in diagnosis and whenever suspected, microscopic study made.

In the treatment of cervical disease by electro-thermal methods there is no consideration of acute infection, as contraindications are clear. It is the chronic type, in which we have all seen the futility of medical application and injection, that give spectacular results with this procedure that has supplanted scalpel plastics. Time will not permit a detailed comparison of cautery and coagulation therapy, but the results parallel the generally undestood effect in dealing with skin lesions; moles, warts and epithelioma. Disappointments with the cautery have been largely due to failure to recognize its limitations. For superficial erosion and early post-partum mutilations of the cervix its application is to be commended.

Different methods of coagulation have their advocates and are meritorious in the hands of their respective operators. My experience with the various modalities, used in several hundred cases, teaches me there is some option, but unipolar coagulation with an ordinary spark-gap diathermy has many advantages. In the first place, contour, depth and distribution of cervical lesions are notoriously irregular. Therefore, uniform excision by conization or bipolar coagulation is only applicable in those symmetrically encircling the cervical canal. While the single electrode may be minutely applied to any lesion or multiplicity of them. It promotes conservatism, which is of great importance, in that one may attack different locations without destruction of intermediary structure. It makes a safe office procedure out of a formidable surgical problem, because it may be administered in fractional doses

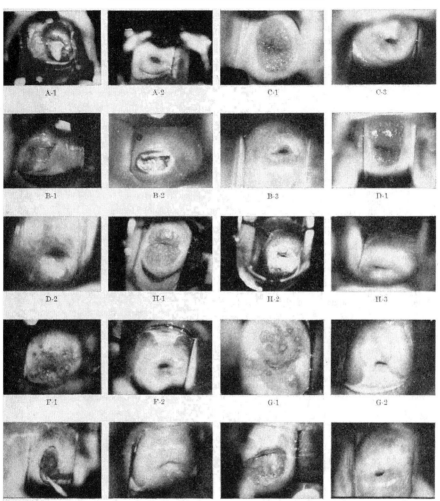

A-1   A-2   C-1   C-3

B-1   B-2   B-3   D-1

D-2   H-1   H-2   H-3

F-1   F-2   G-1   G-2

I-1   I-2   J-1   J-2

A. Chronic endocervicitis, in patient Mrs. R., age 22 years., nulliparous, married 18 months, complaining of leucorrhea and occasional dyspereunia. 1. Before treatment, Aug. 3, 1939. 2. After healing, Oct. 6, 1939, complete relief of symptoms.—B. Post partum laceration and contusion. Mrs. O., age 18 years., three months after a normal delivery, no symptoms 1. Cervix visualized before treatment, Nov. 15, 1939. 2. After coagulation, Nov. 15, 1939. 3. Almost complete resolution, Jan. 3, 1940.——C. Chronic polypoid erosion. Mrs. D., age 20 years para three, all the cardinal symptoms of pelvic inflammation, retroversion. 1. Before treatment Dec. 30, 1939. 3. April 27, 1940, lesion healed, marked amelioration of symptoms.—D. Ectropion, with chronic cystic cervicitis. Mrs. L., age 26 years, para two, five and two years, of age, cautery treatment following first birth. Delayed menses, two weeks to two month, dysmenorrhea, leucorrhea, marked tenderness of the utero-sacral ligaments, pelvic, back and thigh ache, scant flow, urinary and rectal discomfort. 1. Aug. 4, 1939, electrocoagulation treatment, followed by administration of thyroid. 2. Appearance of cervix on Oct. 21, 1940. Relief of symptoms, with reestablished normal menses.—F. Chronic cystic cervicitis. Mrs. D., aged 36 years, Para one, 17 years previous. Very nervous, pelvic pain, leucorrhea. Two years previous had been treated for several weeks for urinary tract infection. One year ago, exploratory pelvic operation. No pathology amenable to surgical correction. 1. Cervix treated on Nov. 25, 1939. March 14, 1940, small endocervical polyp, about the internal os coagulated. 2. Jan. 9, 1941, patient has complete relief from symptoms.—G. Chronic cystic cervicitis. Previously inadequately treated by cautery. Mrs. D., age 24 years, no symptoms. One child four and one two years of age. 1. Follicular infection behind fairly normal appearing vaginal covering that has bridged the ducts, from previous cautery application. 2. Healed cervix, Nov. 25, 1940, with marked reduction of hypertrophy.—H. Chronic erosion, eversion and ectropion. Mrs. P., age 23 years, para four, one abortion. Exaggerated cardinal pelvic symptoms. Menorrhagia and Invalided. 1. Cervical lesion July 29, 1939. 2. Coagulation. 3. Oct. 18, 1939, a normal cervix with disappearance of all symptoms.—I. Cervical polyp, chronic endocervicitis. Mrs. W., age 46 years, para seven, menopausal state, sense of prolapsus and pelvic soreness. 1. Cervix before coagulation of canal and polyp, May 2, 1940. 2 Appearance Dec. 6, 1940. Symptoms free.—J. Post partum contusion, laceration and eversion. Mrs. W., 27 years of age, para one, six months post partum, continuous backache. 1. Appearance of untreated cervix Nov. 25, 1940. 2. After healing Aug. 29, 1941, backache relieved shortly after treatment.

without troublesome bleeding sometimes attending massive sloughing. It gives an even desiccation and much less scar formation. The single needle lends facility for control of depth and distribution of current, with minimum destruction at the point of entry. It yields a good functional result; soft elastic structure that dilates without tearing in subsequent deliveries. Several years experience in these cases, with every type of lesion and modalite, has led me to adoption of the coagulation method in all instances. I do not mean to imply that occasional complication does not arise, nor that all patients will fully cooperate, but these imperfections are no greater than those of other methods of medical or surgical endeavor. Careful estimation of quiescence of infection will eliminate the hazard of this treatment, (having in mind the occasional occurrence of pelvic peritonitis sometimes attending slight trauma to an infected cervix.) Fineness of surgical judgment and familiarity with surgical liability of infection is as essential in electro-surgical procedure as that of any other.

It is my custom to impress the patient with the importance of prolonged observation following coagulation of the pathologic process, anticipating vaginal discharge for several days as the slough separates and forewarn them of shrinking and contraction of the cervical canal that prevails throughout the healing period. Moderate erosions and simple lacerations are lightly coagulated in their entirety. Extensive lesions are treated in a similar manner, but depth of inflammatory reaction, presence and situation of cysts, hyperplasia, size, depth and contour of canal and possibility of endometriosis or malignancy must be considered in estimating depth and distribution of coagulating current required.

Conservative destruction of tissue is preferable to over-treating, as it minimizes constriction and may be repeated at eight week intervals, if necessary. Insertion of an applicator into the canal, at intervals determined by its size, will prevent bridging of the aperature by proliferating squamous epithelial covering and help to direct its extension into the canal. If there is too much contraction in spite of repeated dilations or failure of cooperation, insertion of stem pessary for a few days, or negative galvanism, will insure relaxation. Cases of long standing that have had inadequate treatment, in which much of the granulation tissue and more accessible glands have been removed, with resultant decrease in cervical discharge that has permitted vaginal epithelium to bridge the aperatures of deeply infected glands; so that persistent infection is hidden by a fairly normal vaginal covering, are problematic. They tax the ingenuity of the operator and require patience and persistence. The remedy is deep coagulation with a very fine needle producing slender coagula that reach remote recesses of infected glands. Marked hypertrophy is reduced through this medium. It is gratifying to note in the results of this therapy, in many instances, a marked diminution in the size of a so-called subinvoluted or fibrous uterus.

In closing, I should like to encourage wider application of electro-thermal treatment of early and moderate cervical lesions and emphasize importance of thorough training in assuming responsibility for older extensive ones. With the great possibilities afforded by electrical treatment of the cervix for the relief of gynecologic symptoms and its far reaching influence in the prevention of cancer, it is lamentable that greater interest in this subject is not manifested. I submit a few color- film slides, from my collection, in substantiation of the efficacy of this therapy.

BIBLIOGRAPHY

1. Black, William T. Good and Bad Results in Treatment of the Cervix Uteri J-A.M.A. 1939 Vol. 112-2.

2. Baumrucker, O. Z. and G. O. Cervical Erosions. J-Surg, Gyn, and Ob. July 1938 Vol. 67-1.

3. Baer, Joseph L. Cervix in Obstetrics and Gynecology. J-A.M.A. 1938 Vol. III-26.

4. Davis, Carl Henry. Gynecology and Obstetrics. (W. F. Prior). Vol. I, 1-25. Vol. II, 11-I Vol. III, 7-29.

5. Frost, Inglas F. Erosion and Infection of the Antepartum Cervix and their Treatment by Electrocoagulation. American J-Surgery. Vol. 45-1.

6. Kleegman, Sophia J. American J-Surgery. April 1940. 68:294-310.

7. Miller, Norman F. and Todd, Oliver E. Conization of the Cervix. J-Surg, Gyn, and Ob. Sept. 1938. Vol. 67:265-268.

8. Greenhill, J. P. Comparison of End-Results of Treatment of Endocervicitis by Electro-Physical methods. Year book Ob, and Gyn., 1938. Page 353.

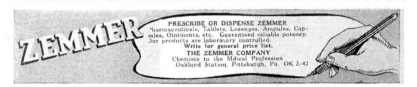

Hypertrophic Arthritis and Physiotherapy

E. GOLDFAIN, M.D.

OKLAHOMA CITY, OKLAHOMA

It is in hypertrophic arthritis that physio-therapeutic measures should be employed to the utmost but with a well-informed and pre-conceived idea of their physiologic value and applicability.

Usually beginning near or after the age of forty, insidious in its onset, more common in women than in men, it constitutes one of the major problems of middle and old age. Most often it will appear in the distal phalangeal joints of the fingers, with the development of the Heberden's nodes. Mild tenderness of the finger joints is often noted before bony nodes appear. The bony nodes may remain stationary for varying periods of time or they may progressively enlarge and appear in additional joints. The knee joints quite regularly become involved. The disease process may start and remain limited there for a long time. Because the knees have to with-stand body weight they are subjected to a great deal of physical wear and tear. There-fore knee involvement is a serious localiza-tion of the disease process.

There is associated with practically every case of hypertrophic arthritis, to a lesser or greater degree, secondary fibrositis. This condition reveals itself by the symptoms and signs of stiffness, jelling phenomena, pain on motion, tenderness on pressure at joint margins, fibrous tissue swellings in the form of puffiness, effusions and indurations of ligamentous, capsular and tenosynovial tis-sues plus joint enlargement.

The diagnosis is established upon the above findings plus essentially always pres-ent X-ray findings consisting of lipping, moth-eaten like shadows, spicule shadows, beak-like formations and irregularity of joint surfaces caused by degenerative changes and disappearance of the articular cartilage.

The pathologic picture of the fibrous tis-sues in a case of hypertrophic arthritis ex-plains the reason for the stiffness and loss of resiliency of the locomotor system. Fi-brous tissue thickenings, adhesions, reduc-tion of elasticity, contracture tendencies, crepitations of joints, stiffness on arising with limberness on moderate exercise are a quite direct result of fibrositis pathology.

The symptomatology and the underlying pathology in hypertrophic arthritis in due time cause definite limitation of motion of the involved joints. Such result initiates a series of events that makes for faulty mechanics, improper posture, serious seque-lae in the way of invalidism with its vicious results on physiology of the locomotor sys-tem as a result of reduced or non-use of same. This process may take place slowly or quite rapidly.

Even though bony ankylosis does not take place except occasionally in the spine the adverse effects upon the circulatory, gastro-intestinal, respiratory and other important systems of the body by fibrosis, subluxa-tions, bony overgrowths, localized redden-ings and swellings, joint pains, articular cartilage loss with resultant bony eburnation and overgrowth may be as serious as in a case of atrophic arthritis.

Hypertrophic arthritis may express itself in hip joint involvement and in older people is known as malum coxae senilis. Often these affected individuals have an amount of motion at the hip out of all proportion to the bony overgrowth present. This re-sult is due in great part to the slow develop-ment of the bony changes which consequently allows gradual adjustment of the local fibro-muscular and joint tissues and the retention of a greater degree of motion.

It is in the prevention of such limitation of function of involved joints and its ensuing sequelae that physiotherapy and orthopedic measures reach their fullest scope. This paper concerns itself with the physiothera-peutic management of these cases.

The use of physiotherapy measures for the relief of human ills, especially rheumatic con-ditions, goes back into the dim reaches of antiquity. From those days down to the present an appreciation of the importance of these measures in treatment has grown very slowly, but at a more rapid rate lately.

The aim of such treatment should be to overcome the ill-effects of dysfunction and non-use on the bones, muscles, joints, and fibrous tissues. This can best be accomplish-ed by a properly outlined regime of rest with balanced activity (active and/or passive ex-ercise), application of heat, massage, post-ural exercise, fresh air, sunshine.

It is not within the purview of this paper to quote the manner of carrying out the physiotherapy treatment measures.

A brief summary of the objectives to be obtained by each therapeutic measure, however, needs to be stated:

Heat exerts its favorable influences by promoting:

1. Perspiration.
2. Warming the tissues.
3. Inducing vasodilation of superficial venous vessels.
4. Increases arterial blood supply to the tissues.
5. Stimulates the pulse rate.
6. Relieves tissue edema.
7. Mobilizes stagnant blood pools.
8. Stimulates metabolism.
9. Induces temporary relative systemic alkalosis.
10. Relaxes tissues.
11. Prepares the patient for massage.

Massage is one of the oldest and most valuable of measures. It is a two-edged weapon and its use by uncritical hands needs to be strongly curbed. Its action is multifold, viz.:

1. Relaxing effect on central nervous system.
2. Mobilizes stagnant blood pools in the capillary bed of superficial and deep muscular structures.
3. Lymphatic circulation is stimulated.
4. May correct relative secondary anemia by mobilizing non-functioning red blood cells.
5. Especially valuable in correcting circulatory system dysfunctions, venous and arterial, due to inactivity in fibro-muscular tissues.
6. Helps to increase absorption of exudates about joints.
7. Prevents and delays tissue atrophy.
8. Stimulates general and local metabolism.
9. Relieves muscle pain.
10. To some degree a substitute for exercise.

Exercise of active and/or passive type is indicated for the purpose of keeping the patient ambulatory, overcoming the ill-effects of the hypertrophic arthritis, preventing circulatory system dysfunction, stimulating metabolism of the entire body, preventing contracture, keeping the body tissues in good tone and promoting resiliency of locomotor system tissues, as the best arthritic syndrome corrective, and a final antidote for same.

Sun bathing, when it is possible to secure same, is preferable to ultra-violet ray treatment. Ultra-violet ray treatment is of value as a substitute during the fall, winter, and early spring seasons. The movement of air currents, while sun bathing, and the fresh air available at such times add value to the sun bath. Skin function is improved. Undernutrition, secondary anemia, general reduced bodily vigor are all favorably affected by sun or ultra-violet ray baths. They act as a whip to the general body metabolism. Improvement in skin circulation, relief of muscular aching, and a tonic systemic effect are also obtained.

Rest is a physical treatment measure even as those already mentioned. Its objective should be to obtain:

1. Elimination of fatigue.
2. Reduce wear and tear effect on the general body economy.
3. Sedate the central nervous system.
4. Reduce the ill-effects of daily activities on the central nervous system.
5. Keep patient from overstepping his particular sum total of nervous and physical energy reserve.
6. Help body to respond to treatment measures by reducing load under which it is carrying on.
7. As a proper counterbalance to exercise measures.
8. Can be applied locally by intermittent splinting as necessary.
9. A two to six week hospital rest period, in the more active cases, should precede when possible comprehensive management of patient along general medical and physiotherapeutic lines.

CONCLUSION

It is best to close on a note of caution. He who treats hypertrophic arthritis or the rheumatoid syndrome should not put all his eggs in one basket.

The rheumatic patient needs to be considered as an entity. To view an arthritic case from a narrow bone and joint point of view is to invite a lesser degree of success from medical management.

Physiotherapy is only one weapon, though an important one, in the armamentarium of the physician. Sound common sense medical measures, viz.; medicinal, dietetic, focal infection correction, readjustment of gastro-intestinal dysfunction, vaccine and nonspecific protein injections, and X-ray exposures, either singly, severally, or all together should be used in each arthritic case.

BIBLIOGRAPHY

1. Pemberton, Ralph: Arthritis and Rheumatoid Conditions: Their Nature and Treatment, 1935, Lea and Febiger, Philadelphia.
2. Krusen, Frank Hammond: Physical Therapy in Arthritis, 1937, Paul B. Hoeber, Inc., New York.
3. Goldthwait, Brown; Swaim; Kuhn: Body Mechanics in the Study and Treatment of Disease, 1937, J. B. Lippincott Co., Philadelphia.
4. Year Book of Physical Therapy:
   a. Diagnosis and Treatment of Hypertrophic Arthritis, J. Albert Key, Herman J. Rosenfeld, O. E. Tjoflat (Washington Univ.) pp. 246-248.
   b. Manipulation and Exercise in Osteoarthritis, A.M.A. Moore (London) pp. 265-266.
   c. Exercise in Treatment of Arthritis: Stella S. Bradford, Montclair, N. J., pp. 266-269.

Syphilis: A Problem for the Internist*

W. C. THOMPSON, M.D.

STILLWATER, OKLAHOMA

During recent years, the magnitude of the problem of combatting syphilis has been made apparent to the medical profession and to the public principally through the efforts of the Surgeon-General of the United States Public Health Service. The combined energy of all the branches of the practicing profession and of the public health officers is needed. It is particularly the duty of the internist to lead in the instruction of medical students and internes in the field of syphilology. First, the training of the internist fits him to understand the significance of generalized infection; second, his knowledge of chronic disease makes him familiar with the potential dangers of latent syphilis. Indeed, syphilis in all its ramifications may tax the keenest diagnostic abilities.

The association of syphilology with internal medicine has not been as close as it deserves. Moore[1] has described the situation which existed 30 years ago. The management and teaching of syphilis were undertaken in practically all divisions of large hospitals. Patients with suspected primary lesions appeared in the urologic or gynecologic clinic, according to sex; and when the eruption had appeared, went to the department of dermatology, or to that of otolaryngology with sore throat, or of ophthalmology with iritis. Each clinic reached a correct differential diagnosis, and in one or more clinics antisyphilitic treatment after a fashion was administered. There was no systematic treatment or follow-up over the long period necessitated in the days of mercury. After a long latent period, with the appearance of tertiary lesions, the unfortunate patient turned up in the medical department with cardiovascular syphilis, or spent his final days as a hopeless wreck in the care of the department of neuro-psychiatry.

Moore relates that the discovery of the causative organism, the development of the Wassermann test, and the discovery of arsphenamine served to place the practice of syphilology on a firmer basis. The technical knowledge involved in the diagnosis and treatment of syphilis required radical

changes in hospital organization. It became necessary to centralize these activities in a single department. Into whose hands was this to be entrusted? This has constituted a subject of debate for many years.

The outstanding German and French dermatologists were responsible for the association of dermatology and syphiliology nearly half a century ago. This probably resulted from the fact that most of the recognizable syphilis in those days presented cutaneous manifestations. In fact, within recent years, I served on the staff of a foreign hospital in which a German-trained physician was in charge of the Department of Dermatology, Syphilology and Urology. With the advent of the Wasserman test, the possibility of darkfield diagnosis, and the increased knowledge of the pathology of syphilis, as related to visceral, cardiovascular and neurologic complications, the cutaneous aspects of syphilology were overshadowed.

In 1914, the Syphilis Division of the Medical Clinic of the Johns Hopkins Hospital was organized as a separate entity by Dr. Albert Keidel. The treatment of syphilis had been practiced previously in a dozen or more clinics of that large hospital, by varying methods. There had been no possibility of co-ordinating the treatment or study of syphilis, nor had the epidemiologic and sociologic aspects of the problem been considered previously. This pioneer syphilis clinic, the well-known "Department L" of Johns Hopkins, has continued to function with a staff of physicians trained primarily in internal medicine. Other institutions which have placed the teaching of syphilis in the department of medicine include Yale, Vanderbilt, Duke, Stanford, Cornell, Georgia, New York and Harvard universities.

Regardless of where the responsibility is placed for teaching this most important branch of medicine, there are certain outstanding fundamentals that must be observed in practice and passed on to the medical student and intern. I wish to enumerate a few of these facts.

I. DIAGNOSIS.

The diagnosis of primary syphilis is essentially a laboratory problem. Every genital

*Read before the Section on General Medicine, Annual Session, Oklahoma State Medical Association, May 20, 1941, in Oklahoma City.

lesion and every suspicious extragenital one deserves darkfield examination.

We are well aware that a negative serologic test does not rule out syphilis. Particularly should this be remembered in connection with a suspected primary lesion. It is important that prospective blood donors be examined physically as well as tested serologically.

The so-called therapeutic test in early syphilis is fallacious, for non-syphilitic lesions frequently heal spontaneously and rapidly. Likewise the provocative test in suspected late syphilis is not reliable and is not to be depended upon.

The diagnosis of secondary syphilis may be confusing upon occasion, and may require consultation with the dermatologist. It is of great help to recall that the blood Wassermann is essentially 100 percent positive at this stage.

II. TREATMENT

It is to be emphasized that the treatment of early syphilis has been standardized in the reports of the Cooperative Clinical Group, and that one assumes considerable responsibility in departing to any degree from the recommended procedure of alternating courses of arsenical and heavy metal, in continuous treatment. On the other hand, the treatment of late syphilis must be individualized.

While we have been taught that old arsphenamine is superior in the treatment of early syphilis with respect to percentage of cures and chance of relapse, the technical difficulties attending its preparation have caused its use to be confined generally to large clinics. It appears that mapharsen is the equal of, and perhaps may be superior to, neoarsphenamine. Sulpharsphenamine had best be reserved for intramuscular use in children who tolerate it well, and for only those rare adults who have no accessible veins. Tryparsamide is of no value in early syphilis, and is of greatest value following fever therapy in central nervous system syphilis.

With regard to heavy metals, bismuth is superior to mercury. For general purposes, the insoluble bismuth subsalicylate in peanut or olive oil (10 percent weight to volume) is preferable. If administered properly, it is not painful and one injection weekly is sufficient. Oil-soluble preparations require injection at five-day intervals, and water-soluble bismuth must be given twice weekly. The new oral preparation probably will be most useful for patients on vacation, or for other reason not having access to a physician for a short period. Certainly the risks of self-medication should make it unwise to substitute oral bismuth for intramuscular therapy under usual circumstances.

The chemotherapy of syphilis by massive doses or arsenical administered by intravenous drip over a five-day period was announced about three years ago. The Council on Pharmacy and Chemistry, in its preliminary report last year[2], expressed the opinion that this mode of therapy must still be considered as in the experimental stage, and that its use should be confined to large university and public health clinics.

Fever therapy generally is not of value in early syphilis although in drug-resistant early syphilis it may be desirable.

Examination of the cerebrospinal fluid is indicated for every patient with syphilis. In early syphilis, when the blood serologic findings remain positive after six months' treatment, invasion of the central nervous system is a strong possibility and lumbar puncture is indicated. That is, asymptomatic neurosyphilis may exist. On the other hand if the course of the patient proceeds normally during treatment for early syphilis, lumbar puncture may be delayed until a year's treatment is completed. Some syphilologists, notably Lange, advocate waiting until treatment has been completed, giving this as a "final blessing," to use Lange's words. If the patient is first seen in late latent syphilis, or if the duration is unknown, spinal puncture at the first opportunity will be of value. Unsuspected asymptomatic neurosyphilis may be detected.

Hyperpyrexia is the treatment par excellence for some forms of neurosyphilis, particularly paresis and optic atrophy. Its use involves danger, and it is to be regarded as entailing risk even under ideal hospital conditions. Although statistical evidence offered by O'Leary[3] would indicate that artificial fever is superior to malaria with respect to mortality and chance of relapse, the latter is decidedly in favor with certain of the Eastern syphilologists.

The oft-repeated dictum, that we must treat the patient and not his serologic reaction, is perhaps the most disregarded teaching which the syphilologist attempts to convey. The subject of Wassermann-fastness is too extensive to discuss here, and has been covered adequately by Moore in his writings. By way of summary, let these few remarks be made. If the serologic reaction in early syphilis remains positive after six months' active treatment, asymptomatic neurosyphilis must be suspected, and examination of the cerebrospinal fluid is indicated. In late syphilis, where the serologic reaction remains positive, in spite of adequate treatment (18 to 24 months), examination of the central nervous system, the cardiovascular system, and of the bones and mucous membranes is indicated. If these investigations are negative, it is proper to suspend active treatment, and to place the patient under prolonged observation.

Asymptomatic neurosyphilis is best treated by adequate routine methods for a reasonable period. If the cerebrospinal serologic reaction is resistant to ordinary methods, we may add intraspinal treatment or tryparsamide. Malaria is to be reserved for those patients who fail to derive serologic negativity from other methods.

Morgan[4] reminds us that treatment although far from ideal, if properly applied, is effective in (1) curing and rendering noninfectious the vast majority of patients with early syphilis; (2) preventing congenital syphilis; (3) protecting patients with latent syphilis from the sequelae of chronic infec-tion; and (4) prolonged life and comfort in the established chronic disease.

Finally, the physician who treats and teaches syphilis must be one who knows something of syphilis in all its phases. He must understand its diagnosis, treatment and public health aspects. It is my opinion that the physician with a sound training in internal medicine is the one most able to acquire a thorough knowledge of syphilis, and is best qualified to teach this branch of medicine.

BIBLIOGRAPHY

1. Moore, J. E. The Teaching of Syphilis. Journal of the Association of American Medical Colleges, May, 1939.
2. Preliminary Report, Council on Pharmacy and Chemistry. J.A.M.A., 115: 857-9, 1940.
3. O'Leary, P. A.: J.A.M.A., 115: 677-661, 1940. Malaria and Artificial Fever in the Treatment of Paresis.
4 Morgan, Hugh J. The Internist and the Syphilis Control Program. Ann. Int Med. 11: 469-473, 1937.

Some Common Diseases That Can Be Helped By X-Ray[*]

C. M. MING, M.D.

OKMULGEE, OKLAHOMA

It is with some hesitation that I take the liberty of discussing radiation therapy before the General Medical section of our State Society. However, this is the place that such a discussion should bear the best fruit.

In strictly X-Ray meetings and circles the facts that I shall present are well known and freely discussed in a matter-of-fact way. But it is possible that some of you do not attend these meetings and do not follow X-Ray literature closely. A great deal of this literature does not reach your more familiar journals. What radiologists believe are facts may not be absorbed with conviction by the general practitioner.

The results of X-ray therapy in the inflammatory field are so good, the theraputic value has been so thoroughly established, and the testimony so favorable it is surprising that it is not more widely used. There are many well-qualified men doing this work and the apparatus for its use is easily accesible. The old adage: "A workman must be familiar with his tools," applies here in its strictest sense.

Let us consider now the common diseases which we see every day. Where shall we start? It might not be amiss to begin with infections of the face, around the nose and the upper lip, the so-called dangerous area.

These infections, mostly staphylococcic, are often considered unimportant and therefore neglected or mistreated. They are definitely not surgical cases. The treatment should be conservative, a hands-off policy we might say, consisting of rest, warm compresses, radiation therapy and possibly sulfonamides. X-ray should be regarded here as the treatment of choice, the rest merely aids.

Felons, paronychia, cellulitis and the lowly carbuncle fall in this same group. Irradiation remains the most effective treatment of acute parotitis. It also gives good results in the suppurative type. No other is so effective and none gives as good results. Patients usually experience reduction in temperature and there is a general improvement in the clinical picture.

Infected cervical adenitis (or adenitis anywhere) is usually slow in progress. The predominating germ is usually staphylococcus. Sulfonamides are helpful in such cases, but the treatment is more efficacious when used in conjunction with radiation. The more acute the case of adenitis the better the response is to treatment. The fact that radiation is not bactericidal may prevent some men from using it, but such should not be the case.

I know that you are wondering about using sulfonamides and X-ray together. In cases of malignancy where large doses of both might have been administered this could

*Read before the Section on General Medicine, Annual Session, Oklahoma State Medical Association, May 20, 1941, in Oklahoma City.

be a problem. But the cases under discussion require such small comparative doses of radiation that it is most likely that the two can be used together successfully. It is being done all over the country. I have been keeping this point under observation and believe this to be the conclusion reached in most of the clinics in this country.

Radiation is a great aid in treating early pneumonia, delayed resolution in pneumonia, impending empyema, in fact in most cases where inflammatory processes exist. Used pre-operatively or post-operatively the goals easily attained are: inhibition of multiplication of bacteria, lessened pain, relief of muscular spasm, reduced temperature, a better general condition of the patient and a more rapid recovery. Add this to whatever treatment you are doing for one year and you will be more than pleased with the results.

In dermatology are some 80 diseases which are benefited by X-ray treatment. Time does not permit listing them here.

In the case of the carbuncle it may be difficult to withhold the hand of the eager surgeon. So it is probably best to make a joint assault on this lesion by the electro-surgical knife, cautery, free puncture, sulfathiazole and radiation therapy. The latter is very, very important.

Ayers summarizes answers to 1,000 questionnaires sent to surgeons and dermatologists as follows: more surgeons favor cautery, more dermatologists favor conservatism including X-ray.

The duration of treatment under surgery is almost twice as long as when radiation is used. Mortality is low in both but it is three times as great under surgery as under dermatologic treatment. Cosmetic results are infinitely superior under the conservative treatment.

Cellulitis is a rather common condition, usually passed by without due respect to its possible serious complications, following extraction of teeth and similar infections. These cases often present alarming symptoms such as dysphagia. Patients are unable to swallow, or have dyspnoea. A light dose of X-ray followed by a second one in a day or two is all that is recommended.

Massive cellulitis, it goes without saying, should have all the remedies usually used, each in its place; drugs, heat and cold, drainage, inductotherm, X-ray. Co-operation between surgeon, internist and radiologist should be at all times complete for the best results.

I have a firm conviction that Otolaryngologists and Ophthalmologists and other high class specialists are using radiation treatment more and more in the past few years.

Take as an example an early mastoid infection. In this condition radiation may be of great value. Very often it will obviate the necessity for radical surgery. Mastoiditis differs from soft tissue infections, in that the bony structure definitely limits distension. Here even a slight relief of pressure may be a decisive factor. X-ray may do this.

I am thinking of a case with which I had some contact, a mastoid. The specialist of choice was out of town, so another was called in. After some delay, and usually there is a pro and con period, trying to decide whether or not to operate, he decided that an operation was imperative. There was more delay waiting for the family to agree. By that time the first doctor had returned and on seeing the case said that in his opinion an operation was not necessary. Later an operation was done, but the result was bad.

During all this delay X-ray might well have been used. A rational procedure would be to use X-ray as early as possible. It need not interfere with any other treatment but could be used in conjunction with all others. The results often are amazingly favorable.

Consider otitis media, acute and chronic. With X-ray myringotomy is frequently lessened, relief from pain is almost immediate, the discharge is lessened and often in chronic cases the hearing is improved. This treatment may also be used when surgery is contraindicated. Such small doses as from 60 to 100 R. units may suffice.

Stepping ever so lightly into the sinus infection field, my experience has been that in many cases headaches and nasal discharge often recede rapidly after radiation. The first dose may increase the symptoms for a few hours, then relief is the rule. A high percentage of improvement is obtained.

It is a valuable adjunct to nose and throat therapy. Better results are obtained in infected antra where puncture-irrigation and X-ray are used than by either method alone.

These infections are highly radio sensitive, consisting mostly of lymphocytes and polymorphonuclears. A choice of cases should be made. Most sinus infections respond to the usual suction and local treatment but as they become sub-acute these measures may prove ineffective. Then also radiation is indicated.

A clinician believes only what he sees and he is going to see more cures in this field than in previous years. Please do not misconstrue my enthusiasm to indicate that one

Short Summary Sinus Technique:
4 bi-weekly doses 100R each
125 Kilo Volt
5 ma
35 c.m. skin focal distance
4 m.m. al filter
45 percent of amount to produce slight erythema
Most prefer this fractional dosage.

or two X-ray treatments will suffice to the exclusion of other methods. A feature that is often overlooked is that the treatment of acute sinus conditions by radiation therapy often prevents development of chronic infected sinus disease.

The dose for this is usually very small. This should be explained as patients are often afraid of X-ray and radium. X-ray has not yet been entirely deleted of its air of mystery.

The above mentioned good results are also being obtained in the so-called "red throat," "flu throat" or streptococcus throat infections. Not commonly used but as favorable reports accumulate, this treatment is daily becoming more popular.

In cases where pus has formed the pathology may be classed as chronic and there therapy is least valuable. The biological conclusions are: here fibroblast and much connective tissue are present and these cells are the more resistant type. These cells retard the action of the rays and render treatment less effective.

On the other hand, early in acute infections, the leukocytes are present in great numbers. They probably are least resistant to radiation and a small amount of treatment causes great destruction of these cells. The radiation liberates anti-bodies and ferments which in turn are used by the body as defense mechanisms.

Decreased tension and drainage are facilitated and there is a gradual return to normal of infected tissues. Glandular hyper secretion and increased vascularity are reduced. Radiation is most beneficial during the infiltrative stage and moderate doses are sufficient or even preferbale to larger doses.

Sub-acromial bursitis often responds to treatment by relief of pain within 48 hours. Here another factor is at work, the regression of calcification. Here again the disappearance of the deposit is rapid and pain quickly relieved. Acute cases respond rapidly while sub-acute ones are slower, because, in these chronic cases thickening, induration and adhesions are present.

In the arthritis group we might place arthritis first, then trigeminal neuralgia, lumbago, muscular rheumatism, gonorrheal joint diseases, metetarsalgia, torticollis, various herpes and spondylitis. Radiation should be applied locally over the involved area, the treatment given two or three times weekly from twice to 12 times, depending on the other treatment factors involved in each case. Also, sometimes, the spinous roots and ganglia of the offending region are rayed. The results in arthritis and neuritis are dependent on reduced irritation on nerve sheaths, causing lessened pressure which is the pre-

viously described effect on leukocytes and the analgensic effect of the ray.

The U. S. Army has purchased and is using a large number of mobile Therapy X-Ray units, a type of apparatus unknown in the World War. Mortality in the A.E.F. from gas gangrene is reported having been as high as 48 percent. In similar cases now the diagnosis will be greatly facilitated by X-ray films which will reveal even a small amount of gas in the tissues. In this way treatment may be given much earlier and should result in a much decreased mortality.

May I enumerate some rational, sensible reasons for radiation therapy:

1. Small dose
2. No complications (when properly administered)
3. Causes no pain
4. Relieves pain by its analgesic effect
5. May be used with other treatments
6. Not necessarily expensive
7. Causes regression of inflammatory processes
8. Inhibits multiplication of bacteria
9. Fosters absorption and liquefaction
10. Causes less scarring
11. Has analgesic effect—no anesthetic needed
12. Relieves muscular pains
13. Relieves pressure on nerve sheaths
14. Influences regression of calcification
15. No hospitalization usually needed
16. Softening of the fibrotic scar tissue
17. Aborts many lesions
18. Direct effect on lymphocytes and leukocytes
19. Establishes better blood supply

I hesitate to enumerate all the conditions where the X-ray is being used successfully because the list is so long. Suffice it to say, that wherever infection and inflammation exist, there is a possible field. It should not be used as a last resort where other treatment has been ineffective. X-ray should take its place along with surgery, medicine, serums, sulfonamides, oxygen therapy, transfusions, Wangensteen suction and other well-known procedures.

Every one, of course, knows that radiation therapy means either radium or X-ray.

In closing may I observe that with a better understanding and appreciation, a more universal application by Radiologists and other physicians, radiation therapy will soon be recognized as one of the most important theraputic agents of defense in the treatment of infections.

BIBLIOGRAPHY

Journal A.M.A. 108:11, 858 March, 1937.
1940 Year Book, page 401.

DISCUSSION

W. S. LARRABEE, M.D.
TULSA, OKLAHOMA

I have listened to Dr. Ming's paper with great satisfaction. It is timely and certainly it belongs in the general session.

It has long been a mystery to me why the internist, the surgeon, and the general practitioner hesitate to refer a carbuncle, shingles or whooping cough to the roentgenologist when they call in the other special men routinely.

I am sure it isn't that they do not know that X-irradiation is indicated, because after every other form of therapy has been unsatisfactory, they call on us. It is not that they just don't think of X-ray as a theraputic agent; because often they own a diagnostic X-ray machine, and not being acquainted with the therapy end, they have tried the diagnostic unit and failed to get results. I leave this question to those skilled in human behavior.

Who wants to see a corneal ulcer waiting as he comes in the door—try X-irradiation on the next one. I pledge you relief of pain in four hours and marked improvement in 24 hours. Who likes to be called at two o'clock A.M. because the child is whooping his head off and his mother thinks he is strangling? Relief from whooping cough in 24 hours is not unusual and in over 300 cases I have had but two failures to give cessation of cough and fever, stop the nausea and vomiting and have the child comfortable after the first three treatments. Treat your next case of Strep sore throat (whether acute or chronic) by X-irradiation. You will be surprised.

Taken early, a large percentage of boils and carbuncles can be aborted by X-irradation, if they do progress to the formation of pus, the X-irradiation will shorten the course and relieve the pain.

I feel that I should mention something that Doctor Ming was too modest to say: *You cannot* do X-ray therapy with a diagnostic equipment. Don't do as a friend of mine did, use a small diagnostic unit to treat Herpes-Zoster—you'll only add some more blisters to a skin already insulted.

No one here will prescribe morphine, sulphathiazole or what not unless he designates the dose, yet many (not of you all but of others) have said, "I gave her some X-ray but it didn't do any good." How much? What kind? How filtered? The number of R units? How should I know? I just turned it on for a few minutes!

Gentlemen, it is just as important to know the voltage, filter, milly amperage, distance and number of roentgens as it is to know whether you use a 64th or a five grain dose of morphine. Unless you have X-ray produced from 140 to 200 K.V. and know the other factors, don't use it. Your roentgenologist has the proper type of equipment and he knows how to use it. Send your X-ray therapy to him and use him as you do your other specialist. You will be happy.

As a general rule:

Where there is pain

Where there is swelling

Where there is infection

There also should be X-irradiation.

Functional Symptoms in Skin Disorders

ONIS GEORGE HAZEL, M.D.

OKLAHOMA CITY, OKLAHOMA

There is an increasing evidence of and literature on the influence of the subconscious mind on skin disorders. Stokes[1] has written on functional disorders for more than a decade and has lived to see much of his earlier and ridiculed impressions accepted.

The neurotic state does in some, yet poorly understood, way produce skin lesions that are difficult to differentiate from those due to organic conditions. I only wish to add my own observations which in well studied cases have led me to believe that functional skin disorders represent a much larger group than most dermatologists have believed. I have seen urticaria, lichen planus, pruritis ani, pruritis vulvae, generalized pruritis with excoriations, neurodermatitis and eczematoid dermatitis appear suddenly after painful reality situations, frustrations, marital difficulties, extra marital relationship, neurotic impotency, and other manifestations of infantile behavior too often to be a matter of coincidence.

Functional disorders of the heart, gastro-intestinal and genito-urinary systems have been long acknowledged, but, unfortunately, dermatologists have been organists. We have blamed allergy, contact factors and excessive bathing in conditions for which we could not find a satisfactory explanation. I now, also, add neurosis, but the proof will lie in the satisfactory application of psychosomatic medicine therapy.

Chronic urticaria offers the most clear cut case histories that I have observed:

CASE HISTORY

Case No. 1. Miss M. aged 37, has been employed by one company for 17 years. On-set of urticaria was one year ago. All tests have been negative and all previous therapy unsuccessful. I saw her in consultation and asked her what happened in her life one year ago. After leading questions she stated that her brother had lost his job and that her mother and her brother's two children had come to live with her. She felt inadequate to meet the new responsibilities. The children, who had lived in a small town, found in the City an opportunity to express their previously restricted inhibitions. She arranged for the children to live with another relative, and without another dose of anti-allergic drugs was fully recovered and has remained well.

Case No. 2. Mr. R., aged 40, had his first attack of urticaria two months ago after sexual relationship. His wife had died six months previous to this experience. His urticarial lesions were confined to the lower abdomen and anterior thighs. He had a recurrence with each sexual experience. He felt a deep sense of guilt for his behavior. He was asked not to have sexual relationship for a period of one month, and during this time he did not have any difficulty. He has now returned to his sexual activity and has an attack with each experience.

Pruritis ani and vulvae also are often precipitated by emotional shock.

Case No. 3. Mrs. C., aged 36, a widow for two years had her first attack of pruritis vulvae two weeks after her husband's death. She had enjoyed a very active sexual life with her husband and said that she felt that she would get well if she could lead a normal sexual life. All skin tests were negative and all therapy unsuccessful. She drives 200 miles a week to have the vulvae irritated with local applications.

Case No. 4. Mrs. K., aged 38, has had pruritis vulvae for one year and it was so severe that she pounded the external genitalia with her hands at night and scratched until the skin would bleed. Her husband was a drunkard and treated her as his mother

and went away for days when provoked by his wife. Weak solution of salicylic acid gave relief for 24 hours. I saw her three weeks later and applied a strong solution of salicylic acid and tar. The pain was excruiating. She called me the next day and denounced me for burning her. She returned a week later to tell me that she was entirely well.

Neurodermatitis is a chronic skin disease with a strong functional component:

Case No. 5. Mrs. M., aged 35, a business woman who as a girl had had an unhappy marriage to an older man. He was killed in an automobile accident three years ago. Her sister also died about this same time with what the patient described as difficulty in breathing. She married two years ago and on the day of her wedding went to a hospital with a severe asthmatic attack. She improved after a few days but developed an eczema on the arms and neck. This neurodermatitis responded at first to x-ray therapy, but later was not benefited. She was thoroughly investigated for all possible allergic reactions. Two months ago she came to the office crying and said that if the eczema spread she felt that she must end it all. I asked about different possible sources of psychic trauma and she at last told me that she was afraid she would die with a choking attack as did her sister. I tried suggestive therapy. Three days later she received a letter from her mother who also suggested fear as the cause of her trouble. She is now greatly improved.

SUMMARY

I could repeat scores of similar or even more dramatic case histories, but I do not well understand the mechanism that produces so bizzare and different type of lesions. I leave it to you who are psychiatrists and to our guest speaker, Dr. Lauren H. Smith, to explain the dynamic of such phenomenon.

CONCLUSIONS

1. Many skin disorders can in part or in whole be produced by a neurotic state.

2. The treatment of such conditions lies in the field of psychoanalysis and psychosomatic medicine. The medical profession has awakened to the necessity of studying systematically what is commonly referred to as the "art of medicine," the better understanding of the therapautic use of the psychic component in the disease process. This implies an understanding of the emotional relationship between physician and patient. We must understand the patient as a human being who has his anxieties, fear, hopes, and dispairs, even as you and I, and these can make him ill.

REFERENCES

1. The Effect on the Skin of Emotional States: II Stokes, John H. Archives of Dermatology and Syphilology, Nov., 1930, No. 5, P. 803.
2. The Effect on the Skin of Emotional and Nervous States: III, Stokes, John H., and Pillsbury, D M., Arch Derm. and Syph. Nov., 1935, No. 5, p 803.
3. The Effect on the Skin of Emotional and Nervous States; Stokes, John H., and Kulchar, George V., and Pillsbury, D.M., Arch Derm. and Syph. April, 1935, No. 4, p 470.

TUBERCULOSIS AND GENIUS

The following paragraphs are reprinted from the "Billy Phelps Speaking" page of the February, 1942 issue of The Rotarian. The "Billy Phelps" page contains comment on recent books by William Lyon Phelps, well-known educator, reviewer and author.

"When I was in Oklahoma City, Oklahoma, in 1940, I had a good time at the Men's Dinner Club; now I welcome an original work by one member, Dr. Lewis J. Moorman. It has the interesting title *Tuberculosis and Genius*. Although I myself have never had either tuberculosis or genius, I am not in favor of killing those with the former, for fear they might have the latter; and I do not think the *chief* end of man is to be healthy. Dr. Moorman's book, after a very instructive introductory chapter, takes up 11 famous 'cases'—Stevenson, Schiller, Marie Bashkirtseff, Kathrine Mansfield, Voltaire, Moliere, Francis Thompson, Shelley, Keats, St. Francis of Assisi; and the volume closes with a bibliography.

"The author is a practicing physician with especial interest in tuberculosis; for 25 years he has conducted a private sanatorium, but he has been as much interested in human nature as in this disease, and has had many opportunities to observe it, having had 20 years of teaching in the medical department of the University of Oklahoma and three years of deanship. This book will interest lovers of literature as well as pathologists, and I suggest that in the next edition Dr. Moorman add a chapter on Emily Bronte."—R. H. G.

DO YOU MEAN ME?

Are you an active member, the kind that would be missed,
Or are you just contented that your name is on the list?
Do you attend the meetings, and mingle with the flock,
Or do you stay at home and criticize and knock?
Do you take an active part to help the work along,
Or are you satisfied to be the kind that "just belong?"
Do you ever go visit a member that is sick?
Or leave the work to just a few and talk about the "clique"?
There's quite a program scheduled that I'm sure you've heard about,
And we'll appreciate if you, too, will come and help us out.
So come to the meetings often, and help with hand and heart.
Don't be just a member, but take an active part.
Think this over, member, you know right from wrong,
Are you an active member, or do you just belong?
　　　　　　　　　　　　　　　　—Anon.

(From Rocky Mountain Medical Journal, Sept., 1941.)

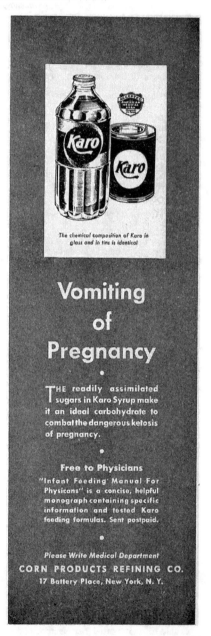

Another defense problem solved—

the American soldier's identification tag now carries his blood type.

"TYPE THE BLOOD OF EVERY SOLDIER" was the recent order issued by American Army officers.

To aid the Army surgeons in fitting such a vast blood grouping program into their schedule, Lederle developed a new dried blood serum with important advantages over human serum. Less costly and more stable, this new serum is derived from immunized rabbits. Large amounts of rabbit serum are reduced to small quantities of a stable and uniformly potent powder. The new product results in much greater speed in the agglutination reaction. Now, in an incredibly short time, clumping of the A, B and AB cells is visible to the naked eye.

Among other qualities found in the blood grouping sera are greater accuracy and uniformity of results. Stability is assured; the product lasts indefinitely. The Lederle serum has received Army surgeons' approval. "Blood Grouping Sera (Powdered) *Lederle*" are in extensive use in the Army camps.

LEDERLE LABORATORIES, INC.
30 ROCKEFELLER PLAZA   NEW YORK, N.Y.

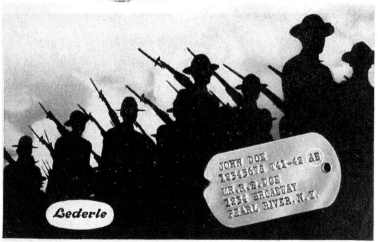

· THE PRESIDENT'S PAGE ·

By the time this appears there will undoubtedly have been much progress made with reference to the Procurement and Assignment of Medical Men in the United States Army and Navy and Civilian Defense. There will certainly be some mistakes made, but in the final analysis this method of making proper assignment of doctors the greatest good to the greatest number will be served and will help to win the war.

It is a well known fact that the distribution of doctors is very unequal, and in time of peace this condition might be overlooked and little or nothing done about it. Now, this great country of ours is engaged in an all-out war and we cannot lose sight of the fact that it is just as important to conserve health in the rural districts and in the smaller towns as in cities, and it must be remembered that one doctor in a city with adequate hospital and nursing facilities can serve a much larger population than if he were located in a more sparsely populated community. In the selection of medical men for our armed forces we must not lose sight of the needs of our civilian population.

This may be a long war and the nation that conserves her natural resources and raw materials and makes proper distribution will win the war. Let us lend our every effort to this end.

Finis. B. Cuning

President.

• EDITORIALS •

YOUR STATE MEETING

Regardless of the present unrest and the uncertainty concerning the future of medicine, every doctor remaining at his post in civilian practice should be thinking about the approaching State Medical Association meeting which convenes in Tulsa, April 22 to 24. It is our duty to faithfully uphold organized medicine and to safeguard the principles for which it stands. This is one of the debts we owe to those who have given up all in favor of military service. With this obligation in mind, we should gird up our loins and pay the price like men, otherwise we may "repent in dust and ashes."

If you should be requested to participate in the program of the State meeting, or to serve on a Committee, please respond promptly. Whether or not you receive a request, the meeting, in part, is your responsibility and you can make a valuable contribution by lending your presence and your participation in the open discussions. Mark the dates on your calendar and plan to be away from your practice two or three days.

Finally, we owe it to ourselves and our patients to attend this annual meeting because we need the professional intercourse it offers, the knowledge it provides and the stimulus which comes through contact with those who are striving to keep up with the rapid progress of medical science. Nothing but dire emergency should be permitted to come between us and this meeting. In the last analysis, it is merely a matter of three profitable days in pursuit of knowledge and pleasure, or 365 unhappy days of living with a guilty conscience.—L. J. M.

PERTINENT ISSUES

In a letter to officers, staff and members of the Chamber of Commerce of the State of Oklahoma, released December, 1941, attention is called to a "project for the federal government to take over the complete control and administration of Unemployment Compensation Insurance, a drafted bill in a pigeon-hole somewhere in Washington, and ready to be introduced whenever the pressure-groups behind it, now drumming-up Congressional support, think it can be enacted.

Tied up with the proposed federalization of Unemployment Compensation are the following issues:

1. States rights;

2. More centralization of power in Washington;
3. Elimination of Merit Rating;
4. More and greater federal payroll taxes;
5. More federal bureaucracy;
6. Deadly uniformity over the whole country in taxes and benefits;
7. Use of unemployment compensation as a national political racket."

It seems unnecessary to stress the importance of these seven issues. Thinking people will readily recognize the ominous portent of each, but the financial phase of Number 3 justifies a further quotation from the above mentioned letter.

"If a federal bureau takes it over, the payroll tax in Oklahoma will never have a Chinaman's chance of being lowered to meet local conditions and Merit Rating will be definitely out. Oklahoma has about 6,000 firms paying unemployment payroll taxes. About 45% are now eligible for Merit Rating at a saving of $2,500,000 per year. Federal Control would eliminate Merit Rating."

This proposed legislation is of vital interest to everyone, professional men included, who employs one or more persons. But in the last analysis, it is of even greater interest to every citizen of the State because it implies further infringements upon our personal liberties and places the solution of our local problems in the hands of federal bureaucracies.

Talk to your friends and write to your Representatives.—L. J. M.

"CRACKING UP"

The American Medical Association now has ready for distribution at a very low quantity price, reprints of "Cracking Up Under the Strain," by Edgar V. Allen.

Following the first paragraph, which defines the meaning of the term "Business Executive," and which includes many doctors, the author says: "In caricature and in comedy the business executive is frequently portrayed as big at the waist, bald on the head, and soft in the heart for pulchritudinous females. This is too superficial a characterization. Physicians are much more interested in the facts that too frequently the executive's blood pressure is high, his arteries are hard and his temper is short. He is commonly irritable, nervous and melancholic. His brain is weary, his muscles are tired, his bowels are constipated and his stomach is acid. All too frequently, he lies mumbling and muttering in a hospital bed, panting his life away as a result of high blood pressure and hardening of the arteries. When he stumbles and falls from apoplexy, or after a shudderingly severe episode of cardiac pain, he is hurried off to the sleep from which there is no awakening. These are inevitable ends, for in spite of man's eternal struggle for life and for longer life, he cannot avoid death. But life might have been fuller and death delayed."

The above quotation indicates the appealing style employed for the purpose of placing before your patients valuable information concerning various sub-topics, such as, "Food, Smoking, 'The Strenuous Life,' The Failure to Define Objectives, Ambition and Alcohol."

Finally, the closing paragraphs are devoted to "Suggested Remedies." These fit the average doctor so snugly he would never suspect that the cloth was cut for the "Business Executive."

The American Medical Association also offers an interesting monograph on "Clinics for the Childless" by J. D. Ratcliff.

Every doctor should have a supply of these pamphlets for distribution to well chosen friends and patrons. Through such a dispensation of knowledge and advice, he can render genuine service and build valuable friendships.—L. J. M.

THE UNIVERSITY HOSPITAL

The ever present pressure of a long waiting list and the daily disappointment of new applicants because admission to the hospital is not promptly granted, often lead to unwarranted criticisms. Even though the hospital authorities do everything within their power to extend the service and to deal fairly with every applicant, disappointments and misunderstandings are inevitable.

If all the doctors in the State, all the County Judges and County Commissioners were fully aware of the existing conditions and cognizant of the difficulties constantly facing the management of the hospital under these conditions, the misunderstanding and criticism would be reduced to a relatively unimportant minimum. The waiting list now averages above two thousand. Some individuals have been on this list ten years, some have died while waiting for admission. The indigent sick in need of hospitalization in Oklahoma will approximate an average of fifty thousand. With all beds constantly occupied, the University and Crippled Children's Hospitals can accommodate approximately seven thousand annually.

These figures merely emphasize some of the problems mentioned above. Even though the hospital had been originally designed for the sole purpose of caring for the State's indigent sick, the task would be an impossible one.

In order that we may have a better understanding of the functions and limitations of the University Hospital, the following is quoted from an opinion rendered by the Attorney General's office March 21, 1927:

"Chapter 170, Session Laws of Oklahoma, 1917, authorized the building of the University Hospital as a part of the medical department of the State University. Said hospital was built not for the purpose of providing hospital facilities for persons who might endanger the health or safety of other citizens of the State or for the purpose of making better citizens of its patients, or even for the purpose of giving hospital attention to destitute county charges, but it was built for the express purpose of giving practical training to the medical students of the State University. This is clearly revealed by the title of said Act, which, in part, is as follows: 'An Act providing for the construction of a hospital and buildings for the medical department of the University of Oklahoma . . .'"

"Under the constitutional authority contained in Section 3 of Article 17, the Legislature has provided by law, the manner in which counties shall take care of its aged, infirm and unfortunate citizens who have claims upon the sympathy and aid of said counties. Section 8211 to 8234, inclusive, compiled Oklahoma Statutes 1921, provide that the County Commissioners, as overseers of the County poor, shall take care of its poor and indigent citizens and even needy strangers who are sick or distressed in their county. Sections 5659 to 5671, inclusive, as amended by Chapter 205, Oklahoma Session Laws, 1923, authorize counties to erect county hospitals where destitute county patients are treated and cared for at the expense of the county, which hospitals are under the supervision of the Board of Control appointed by the County Commissioners."

No doubt this interpretation of the law with reference to the University Hospital will be a surprise to many doctors in the State. Under this interpretation, it would appear that the doctors who are interested in medical education, instead of urging the acceptance of the routine indigent case, should be choosing from among the indigent sick the most interesting cases to be admitted to the University Hospital for teaching purposes.

Considering the provision for county hospitals, it would further appear that the doctors in each county should strive to bring about the building of county hospitals for the care of the indigent sick. Under such a plan, the great majority of the indigent sick could be cared for by local doctors and the expense, including a reasonable fee for medical and surgical care, could be met by funds provided by local taxpayers and the University Hospital's pathetic waiting list could be reduced. Through cooperation with county hospitals, the University beds could be filled with cases suitable for teaching purposes and to that extent the burden of the county hospitals would be lightened.

Every doctor in the State should be interested in the above proposals.

First, because they provide for adequate local care of the indigent sick.

Second, because they would relieve the unwarranted pressure on the University Hospital.

Third, because they seek to provide more suitable teaching material for the Medical School.

Fourth, because the proper execution of these proposals would elevate the standards of medical education in the State and thus tend to perpetuate better medical care for all the people all the time.

With these possibilities in mind, the doctors of the State are urged to become public spirited and, if necessary, politically minded to such an extent that they shall strive to bring about the election of County and State officials who will see "eye to eye" with the doctors in matters pertaining to public health, medical education, and, finally, socialized medicine. Every politican knows that the average doctor has a powerful community influence and every good citizen knows that he is relatively unselfish in the exercise of this influence. Concerted effort on the part of the medical profession in the proper use of this powerful agent would make candidates for office "sit up and take notice," and result in great public good.—L. J. M.

METHUSELAH

Methuselah ate what he found on his plate,
And never, as people do now,
Did he note the amount of the calory count;
He ate it because it was chow.
He wasn't disturbed as at dinner he sat,
Devouring a roast or a pie,
To think it was lacking in granular fat
Or a couple of vitamins shy.
He cheerfully chewed each species of food,
Unmindful of troubles or fears
Lest his health might be hurt
By some fancy dessert;
And he lived over nine hundred years.
—Unknown.
(From Rocky Mountain Medical Journal, Oct., 1941.)

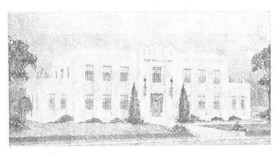

ASSOCIATION ACTIVITIES

Seven Guest Speakers Accept Annual Meeting Invitation

The Scientific Work committee at its meeting in Oklahoma City, January 25, completed tentative plans for the Scientific Program of the Annual Meeting.

The Committee has been confronted with a difficult task in securing guest speakers, as the National Emergency has placed added responsibilities and duties on the staffs of clinics and medical schools which usually are available for state meeting programs.

So far, seven speakers have accepted invitations, and their prominence in their respective fields of medicine has already assured the meeting of an outstanding Scientific Program.

Those who have accepted are as follows:

Dr. Charles C. Dennie, Kansas City, Mo.—Dermatology and Radiology.

Dr. George Herrmann, Galveston, Tex.—Medicine.

Dr. John C. Burch, Nashville, Tenn.—Obstetrics and Gynecology.

Dr. T. Leon Howard, Denver, Colo.—Urology and Syphilology.

Dr. Titus H. Harris, Galveston, Tex.—Neurology, Endocrinology and Psychiatry.

Dr. M. Edward Davis, Chicago, Ill.—Public Health.

Dr. A. B. Reese, New York City.—Eye, Ear, Nose and Throat.

1942 Annual Meeting Scientific Program Approved

The Scientific Work committee, the Annual Meeting committee and officers of the Tulsa County Medical society met January 27 in Tulsa for formal approval of the Scientific Program for the 1942 Annual Meeting of the Association.

Present at the meeting were Dr. H. B. Stewart, president of the Tulsa County Medical society; Dr. E. Rankin Denny, chairman of convention arrangements; Dr. W. A. Showman, chairman of the Commercial Exhibit committee: Dr. I. A. Nelson and Dr. J. E. McDonald, co-chairman of the Scientific Exhibits committee; and Dr. R. C. Pigford of the Scientific Work committee.

Also, Jack Spears, Executive Secretary of the Tulsa County Medical society; Dr. Finis W. Ewing, Muskogee, president of the Association; Dr. Lewis J. Moorman, Oklahoma City, secretary-treasurer of the Association, and R. H. Graham, Oklahoma City, Executive Secretary of the Association.

Scientific Exhibitors to Apply For Space at Annual Meeting

The Scientific Work committee of the Association at its last meeting adopted the application blank on page 69 of this issue of the Journal for the use of those who desire to have a scientific exhibit at the Annual Meeting in Tulsa, April 22, 23 and 24.

In the past, the arrangements for the scientific exhibits have been far from satisfactory, and this has been occasioned mainly through insufficient information as to the needs of the exhibitors.

During the discussion of the problems related to the scientific exhibits, it was the unanimous opinion of those present that every encouragement possible should be given to members of the Association to participate in this feature of the Annual Meeting. The Committee is particularly desirous of having exhibits from all parts of the state, as well as exhibits covering studies in fields of medicine other than the specialties.

As there is no charge for Scientific Exhibits space, there is little reason why the exhibits should not be a major attraction.

Anyone desirous of exhibiting should send his application to the Chairman of the Scientific Exhibits committee, 210 Plaza Court, Oklahoma City, as soon as possible, as applications under the new arrangements cannot be considered after April 1.

Delegates and Alternates to Annual Meeting Are Announced

In compliance with the by-laws of the Oklahoma State Medical Association, the delegates and alternates of the county societies who have been certified to the office by the local county societies are hereby announced.

All delegates and alternates will be seated in accordance with the membership certified as of March 22.

COUNTY	DELEGATE	ALTERNATE
Alfalfa	H. E. Huston, Cherokee	
Atoka-Coal	J. C. Canada, Atoka	W. W. Cotton, Atoka
	J. B. Clark, Coalgate	R. C. Henry, Coalgate
Beckham	H. K. Speed, Sayre	E. S. Kilpatrick, Elk City
Blaine	Virginia Olson Curtin, Watonga	L. R. Kirby, Okeene
Bryan	J. T. Colwick, Durant	J. A. Haynie, Durant
Caddo		
Canadian	J. T. Phelps, El Reno	M. E. Phelps, El Reno
Carter	G. E. Johnson, Ardmore	F. W. Boadway, Ardmore
	J. L. Cox, Ardmore	Walter Hardy, Ardmore
Cherokee		
Choctaw		
Cleveland	F. C. Buffington, Norman	O. E. Howell, Norman
	Phil Haddock, Norman	W. B. Carroll, Norman
Comanche		
Cotton	George A. Tallant, Walters	A. B. Holsted, Temple
Craig	F. M. Adams, Vinita	Lloyd H. McPike, Vinita
Creek	C. R. McDonald, Mannford	Charles Schrader, Bristow
Custer	McLain Rogers, Clinton	Gordon Williams, Weatherford
	Ellis Lamb, Clinton	Ross Deputy, Clinton
Garfield	V. R. Hamble, Enid	
	W. P. Neilson, Enid	

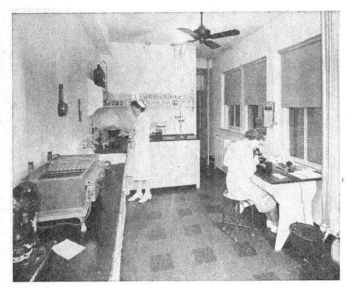

Garvin	Galvin L. Johnson, Pauls Valley	
Grady	W. H. Cook, Chickasha	
Grant	E. E. Lawson, Medford	
Greer	L. E. Pearson, Mangum	J. B. Hollis, Mangum
Harmon	W. G. Husband, Hollis	Russell Lynch, Hollis
Haskell		
Hughes	W. L. Taylor, Holdenville	
Jackson	E. S. Crow, Olustee	E. W. Mabry, Altus
Jefferson	L. L. Wade, Ryan	
Kay		
Kingfisher	F. C. Lattimore, Kingfisher	John R. Taylor, Kingfisher
Kiowa	J. M. Bonham, Hobart	
LeFlore	F. P. Baker, Talihina	
Lincoln	Ned Burleson, Prague	Carl Bailey, Stroud
Logan	L. A. Hahn, Guthrie	J. L. LeHew, Jr., Guthrie
Marshall		
Mayes		
McClain	O. O. Dawson, Wayne	G. S. Barger, Purcell
McCurtain	R. B. Oliver, Idabel	W. W. Williams, Idabel
McIntosh	Wm. A. Tolleson, Eufaula	D. E. Little, Eufaula
Murray		
Muskogee	C. E. White, Muskogee	I. B. Oldham, Jr., Muskogee
	J. H. White, Muskogee	L. S. McAlister, Muskogee
Okfuskee	C. M. Cochran, Okemah	M. L. Whitney, Okemah
Oklahoma	W. F. Keller, Okla. City	W. W. Rucks, Jr., Okla. City
	Onis G. Hazel, Okla. City	Neil Woodward, Okla. City
	Walker Morledge, Okla. City	R. H. Akin, Okla. City
	L. C. McHenry, Okla. City	W. E. Eastland, Okla. City
	C. R. Rountree, Okla. City	M. F. Jacobs, Okla. City
	O. A. Watson, Okla. City	R. L. Murdoch, Okla. City
	J. B. Snow, Okla. City	R. L. Noell, Okla. City
	D. H. O'Donoghue, Okla. City	W. K. West, Okla. City
	C. M. Pounders, Okla. City	Harper Wright, Okla. City
	George Garrison, Okla. City	R. Q. Goodwin, Okla. City
	Allen Gibbs, Okla. City	George Kimball, Okla. City
Okmulgee	I. W. Bollinger, Henryetta	J. C. Matheney, Okmulgee
Osage	G. I. Walker, Hominy	Roscoe Walker, Pawhuska
Ottawa		
Pawnee		
Payne	A. B. Smith, Stillwater	R. E. Waggoner, Stillwater
Pittsburg	T. H. McCarley, McAlester	W. C. Wait, McAlester
	L. S. Willour, McAlester	Frank Baum, McAlester
Pontotoc	E. M. Gullatt, Ada	E. A. Canada, Ada
	Ollie McBride, Ada	Sam A. McKeel, Ada
Pottawatomie	G. S. Baxter, Shawnee	E. E. Rice, Shawnee
	W. M. Gallaher, Shawnee	R. M. Anderson, Shawnee
Pushmataha	P. B. Rice, Antlers	E. S. Patterson, Antlers
Rogers	R. C. Meloy, Claremore	
Seminole	Claude S. Chambers, Seminole	Mack I. Shanholtz Wewoka
Stephens	C. N. Talley, Marlow	Claude B. Waters, Duncan
Texas		
Tillman	T. F. Spurgeon, Frederick	J. E. Childers, Tipton
Tulsa	R. A. McGill, Tulsa	E. Rankin Denny, Tulsa
	George Osborn, Tulsa	T. J. Hardman, Tulsa
	W. A. Showman, Tulsa	Eugene Wolff, Tulsa
	M. J. Searle, Tulsa	Carl Simpson, Tulsa
	Marvin D. Henley, Tulsa	W. A. Walker, Tulsa
	W. Albert Cook, Tulsa	W. R. Turnbow, Tulsa
	R. C. Pigford, Tulsa	M. D. Spottswood, Tulsa
	W. S. Larrabee, Tulsa	
Wagoner	H. K. Riddle, Coweta	J. H. Plunkett, Wagoner
Washington-Nowata	S. A. Lang, Nowata	K. D. Davis, Nowata
	L. D. Hudson, Dewey	J. P. Vansant, Dewey
	H. C. Weber, Bartlesville	E. E. Beechwood, Bartlesville
Washita	A. H. Bungardt, Cordell	James F. McMurry, Sentinel
Woods	D. B. Ensor, Hopeton	C. A. Traverse, Alva
Woodward	Joe L. Duer, Woodward	
	H. Walker, Buffalo	
	Duke Vincent, Vici	
	J. C. Duncan, Forgan	
	O. C. Newman, Shattuck	

At the January 28 meeting of the Okahoma County Medical auxiliary, which meets at the Y.W.C.A. at 9:30 A.M., a layette shower was held by members. The layettes will be distributed to needy cases.

Mail to I. A. Nelson, M.D., Chairman Scientific Exhibits,
210 Plaza Court, Oklahoma City.

Application for Space in the Scientific Exhibit
of the
Oklahoma State Medical Association

Application is hereby made to the Committee on Scientific Exhibits for space at the Annual Session, Tulsa, Oklahoma

(1) ....
(State exact title of exhibit for the program and the Journal announcement).

(2) Brief description of exhibit ....
....
....
....

(3) Exhibit will consist of the following: (check which)

charts and posters............................ photographs................................

photomicrographs................................ drawings................................

roentgenograms................................ specimens................................

other material ....

(4) The following equipment will be used: (check which)

cabinets................................ view boxes................................

microscopes................................ other equipment................................

(5) Booth requirements:

Length of back wall desired..

Minimum requirement..

(6) Description of booth: The side walls are five feet, the back walls five feet or in multiples thereof, and a shelf twelve inches wide two and one-half feet from the floor will be provided. The back wall of each booth is of veneer which will permit the use of thumb tacks, etc.

Signed: ...., M.D.

....
City

Applications for Exhibit Space Cannot Be
Considered After April 1

Discussion of 1941 Income Tax
By Association's Auditors

The following discussion on the 1941 Revenue Act was compiled by the H. E. Cole Company of Oklahoma City, auditors for the Association, and is published for the benefit of members of the Association in making out their 1941 Income Tax returns. The report was also delivered before the Annual Secretaries Conference of the Association, December 14, in Oklahoma City.

Should any doctor like to retain the services of the H. E. Cole Company, he should correspond directly with them at their office address, which is 214 Plaza Court Building, Oklahoma City.

The Revenue Act of 1941 is not a complete taxing statute by itself, but consists of amendments and additions to the Internal Revenue Code. Effective changes in the Internal Revenue Code bring forth new developments relating to those individuals already filing federal income tax returns and to the larger group of individuals who, affected by such changes, will begin filing returns for the calendar year 1941.

For the most part, the Revenue Act of 1941 concerning individuals consists of (1) Increase in Rates and (2) Changes in the Base to which Rates are Applied. Administrative changes in the law are few, because it is expected that a new bill will be introduced in Congress before the end of the current year which will concern such changes. However, it is believed that these further changes will affect the year 1942 and thereafter.

The 4 percent normal tax on individuals has not been changed.

The earned income credit which is 10 percent of the earned net income, but not in excess of 10 percent of the amount of the entire net income not to exceed $1,400.00 is still in effect. (Example: Professional income $5000.00, rental income $500.00, total gross income, $5,500.00. You have deductions amounting to $300.00, leaving a net income of $5,200.00. The earned income credit, then, would be $500.00—10 percent of $5,000.00 which is earned income, since it is less than 10 percent of the net income, $5,200.00, which would be $520.00. On the other hand, if the gross income is $5,500.00 and your deductions amount to $800.00, leaving a total of $4,700.00 net income, the earned income credit would be 10 percent of the net income, $4,700.00 or $470.00, since it is less than 10 percent of the earned income.)

Credit for interest on obligations of the United States and its instrumentalities is likewise unchanged. With the exception of interest on (1) United States savings bonds and Treasury bonds owned *in excess of $5,000.00* and (2) Obligations of instrumentalities of the United States, which is subject to surtax, the interest on (1) obligations of a State, Territory, or political subdivision thereof, or the District of Columbia, or United States possession; (2) obligations issued under Federal Farm Loan Act, or under such Act as amended; (3) obligations of the United States issued on or before September 1, 1917; and (4) Treasury notes, Treasury bills, Treasury certificates of indebtedness, postal saving obligations, adjusted service bonds, etc., *is entirely exempt from tax.*

The amount of credit for dependents, $400.00, is unchanged, although the allowance is restricted in certain cases to the head of a family—that is, when the taxpayer's status as the head of a family depends solely upon the existence of a person from whom he is also entitled to the credit for a dependent. For example: A widower maintaining a home for one child which also qualifies as a dependent is entitled to $1,500.00 exemption as the head of a family. However, if he supports two children, only one of whom qualifies as a dependent, his status as the head of a family is not occasioned solely by the existence of the dependent child and he is entitled to $400.00 credit for the dependent in addition to $1,500.00 exemption as the head of a family.

Changes in Income Tax Laws

The following changes have been made: (1) Elimination of the separate 10 percent defense tax and its inclusion in the respective rates to which it was previously added. (2) Reduction of personal exemption of a married person or the head of a family from $2,000.00 to $1,500.00 (3) Reduction of personal exemption of a single person or married person not living with husband or wife from $800.00 to $750.00 (4) Surtax rates have been substantially increased in all brackets. The surtax rate apply to the entire surtax net income, differing from the prior law under which the first $4,000.00 was free from surtax. The new surtax rates are scheduled in the following table as compared with previous surtax rates:

Surtax Net Income (A)	Surtax on Amount in (A) (B)	Amount in Excess of (A) but not in Excess of (C) is taxed at Rate shown in (D) (C)	(D)	Prev. Rate (1940)
$ 0	$ 0	$ 2,000	6%	
2,000	120	4,000	9%	
4,000	300	6,000	13%	4%
6,000	560	8,000	17%	6%
8,000	900	10,000	21%	8%
10,000	1,320	12,000	25%	10%
12,000	1,820	14,000	29%	12%
14,000	2,400	16,000	32%	15%
16,000	3,040	18,000	35%	18%
18,000	3,740	20,000	38%	21%
20,000	4,500	22,000	41%	24%

*Table continues on to $5,000,000.

TABLE SHOWING TOTAL FEDERAL TAX ON INDIVIDUALS BY REVENUE ACT OF 1941
Married Person, All Earned Income, No Dependents

NET INCOME*	TOTAL TAX
$ 1,500	————
1,600	$ 6
2,000	42
2,500	90
3,000	138
4,000	249
5,000	375
6,000	521
7,000	687
8,000	873
9,000	1,079
10,000	1,305
15,000	2,739
20,000	4,614
25,000	6,864
30,000	9,339
50,000	20,439

*Figures in this column represent net income before deducting personal exemption.

TABLE SHOWING OKLAHOMA STATE TAX RATE

Tax on FIRST $1,000.00	1%
Tax on NEXT $1,000.00	2%
Tax on NEXT $1,000.00	3%
Tax on NEXT $1,000.00	4%
Tax on NEXT $1,000.00	5%
Tax on NEXT $1,000.00	6%
Tax on NEXT $1,000.00	7%
Tax on NEXT $1,000.00	8%
Tax on BALANCE	9%

As in 1940, the gross income rather than the net income determines the liability of an individual for filing a return. So, a single individual or married individual not living with husband or wife must file a return on a gross income of $750.00, and married individuals living together must file a return on a combined gross income of $1,500.00.

The State exemption for married persons, or head of

a family is $1,700.00 and $300.00 for each dependent. The exemption of a single individual or married individual not living with husband or wife is $850.00.

The Community Property Act of 1939, which allows the income to be divided between husband and wife after declaration of intention to come under such act is filed, affects quite a saving, especially on net incomes of $3,000.00 or over. This Act has been ruled constitutional by the State, but it is still in controversy with the Federal Internal Revenue Department.

Deductions of Medical Profession

You will perhaps be interested in knowing what some of the deductions common to the medical profession are and we list here the principal ones:

(1) Salaries of all employees.
(2) Social Security Tax (one percent paid by employer for employee).
(3) Licenses, such as narcotic license.
(4) Office rent, expense and supplies.
(5) Collection fees.
(6) Medicinal drugs and supplies purchased.
(7) Dues to medical organizations and subscriptions to medical journals and periodicals.
(8) Insurance premiums—professional, auto, equipment, etc.
(9) Auto expense and depreciation—depends upon ratio of business use to personal use.
(10) Traveling expense—medical meetings, etc.
(11) Entertainment expense.
(12) Chamber of Commerce dues.
(13) Depreciation on equipment and fixtures—usually based on a life of ten years, or 10 percent depreciation.

Other deductions you are entitled to, not classified as business deductions are:

(1) Contributions to any organized charity.
(2) Taxes—Auto license and gasoline tax on auto other than business auto, ad valorem, personal, intangible, sales and state income tax.
NOTE: These items are deductible on the federal return. In addition to these items, the federal income tax is also deductible on the state return.
(3) Interest paid.
(4) Losses from fire, storm, shipwreck, theft or other casualty.
(5) Bad debts.

Just to elaborate on the item of auto depreciation and expense in business deductions and the auto license and gasoline tax on auto other than business auto, let us explain further that the entire expense and depreciation may be taken as business expense on one car when there are two cars in the family and one is used principally for business purposes. Then, on the other car, or family car as we shall call it, you are entitled to take the gasoline tax which is five and one half cents per gallon on the federal return and seven cents per gallon on the state return, and the auto license for this car.

Forty-Six Doctors Attend Meeting Of Fifth Councilor District

Highlighted by the talks of five guest speakers and with an attendance figure of 46, the Annual Meeting of the Fifth Councilor District was held the evening of January 12, at the Hotel Ardmore, in Ardmore. The meeting was held under the auspices of the Carter County Medical society.

Dr. Walter Hardy, Ardmore, President of the Carter county society, presided as toastmaster during the dinner and the program.

The speakers were Dr. Finis W. Ewing, Muskogee, President of the Association; Dr. James D. Osborn, Frederick, Secretary-Treasurer of the State Board of Medical Examiners; Dr. Louis H. Ritzhaupt, Guthrie, State Medical Director; R. H. Graham, Oklahoma City,

Executive Secretary of the Association; and Dr. J. I. Hollingsworth, Waurika, Councilor of District 5.

Members of the Program committee for the meeting included Doctor Hardy, Dr. H. A. Higgins and Dr. T. J. Jackson, all of Ardmore. The repection committee included Dr. G. E. Johnson, Dr. Joe N. Moxley and Dr. J. L. Cox, all of Ardmore, and the Entertainment and Refreshment committee consisted of Dr. F. W. Boadway and Dr. J. Hobson Veazey, both of Ardmore, and Dr. D. E. Cantrell, Sr., of Healdton.

Postgraduate Study Continued Internal Medicine

Physicians of Oklahoma will be interested to learn that postgraduate instruction will be continued, this time in Internal Medicine. A telegram from Dr. Henry H. Turner, Committee Chairman, who was in New York where he went to revise the budget in conference with officials of The Commonwealth Fund, assures the state office the Fund will give financial assistance again. The Oklahoma State Medical Association is grateful for the interest of the Foundation in their program. Particularly is this true at this time for those physicians left to care for a heavy civilian practice, while so many doctors have been called to serve in time of War in military service. Many advise this is their only opportunity for doing postgraduate work, during this War period.

The Postgraduate Committee, in a called meeting in Oklahoma City at noon February 8, gave the appointment of the instructorship for the course to Dr. L. W. Hunt, Assistant Professor of Medicine, University of Chicago. Doctor Hunt is also on the staff of the University of Chicago clinic, and Billings Hospital. He has an enviable record in research and a list of publications in the field of medicine to his credit. He also has been certified by the American Board of Internal Medicine. Instruction will open with the first circuit in Northeast Oklahoma the week of March 9, in the cities of Miami, Vinita, Bartlesville, Claremore and Pryor. Doctor Hunt is now preparing his lecture manual for the course covering his lectures, which will be given to all physicians who register into the course. Dr. Grady Mathews Commissioner of Health and Dr. J. T. Bell assured the Committee of their willingness to assist in sponsoring the course, with finances from the U. S. Public Health Department, if Washington officials grant the funds.

The following subjects will be included in the course: Some tentative changes may be made at the point where instruction begins:

1. Disorders of the Heart.
2. (a) Cardio-Vascular-Renal Disease.
   (b) The Management of Heart Failure and Renal Failure.
3. Nutritional Diseases and Deficiency States.
4. The Anemias and Blood Dyscrasias.
5. Diabetes Mellitus.
6. Chronic Non-Tuberculosis Pulmonary Diseases.
7. (a) The use and abuses of Sulfonamide Drugs.
   (b) The Pneumonias.
8. Gastrointestinal Diseases.
9. The Arthritides.
10. Endocrine Disorders—a discussion of the presently recognized endocrinopathies and their treatment.

(If timely, the schedule may be altered to include lectures pertinent to civilian health during the National Military Emergency.)

The course will cover a period of ten weeks as did obstetrics and pediatrics. County societies or others wishing specific information should address the Postgraduate Committee, 210 Plaza Court, Oklahoma City, Oklahoma.

MEDICAL PREPAREDNESS

Procedures Outlined for Role of Physicians in War Program

Detailed explanations of the war status of medical students, interns, residents and physicians are contained in *The Journal of the American Medical Association*, for January 24 in an editorial and in an official statement by the Procurement and Assignment Service for Physicians, Dentists and Veterinarians. Referring to the official statement, published in the Medical Preparedness Section of *The Journal*, the editorial says:

"Here are recommendations to all physicians with reference to the places they may occupy in the national emergency. There are directions addressed specifically to (1) medical students, (2) recent graduates, (3) interns who have completed twelve months in a hospital, (4) members of staffs of hospitals, (5) all physicians under 45 years of age and (6) all physicians over 45 years of age.

"These recommendations, it will be observed, do not state specifically that any group, either medical students, interns or physicians, will be deferred by draft boards. Congress did not provide for blanket deferment of any group. However, authorities in the Selective Service have indicated their desire to cooperate with the Procurement and Assignment Service; any bona fide medical student in good standing or any physician called by the draft board may file an appeal.

"The offices of the surgeon generals of the Army and of the Navy have arranged to permit junior and senior students who have enrolled in the medical administrative corps in the Army or who have obtained ensign commissions in the United States Naval Reserve to complete their medical education. Obviously the Procurement and Assignment Service must depend on the assurances of the Selective Service System and of the Army and Navy for proper action in these matters.

"Apparently some physicians, perhaps even many, have been confused by the publication of the enrolment blanks which appeared in previous issues of *The Journal of the American Medical Association* and in the state journals and by subsequent changes in procedure. Let us bear in mind that conditions change from week to week, almost from day to day. A procedure is initiated

to obtain a certain effect and to supply a certain need. When the effect is obtained and the need is satisfied, that procedure becomes obsolete. The blanks which were published in *The Journal* served to bring in enough applications to meet the immediate needs of the Army and Navy Medical Corps. Every one of the men under 36 years of age who filled out that blank has been considered to be a volunteer available for immediate service. Nevertheless, all names are being checked with the roster at the headquarters office of the American Medical Association. Those who are especially qualified in certain specialties are being given special consideration for the kind of work for which they are particularly fitted.

"Apparently a number of physicians, even some of advanced age, felt that in filling out these blanks they were making themselves available for immediate service with the Army or Navy or in some civilian capacity. Some are resentful that they have not been called; others are fearful that they may be called. Hence it is recommended that every physician, whether or not he has filled out any enrolment blank previously, should read most carefully the announcements which appear in this issue and which are specifically directed to physicians of definite age groups. Within the near future an enrolment blank will again be sent to every physician in the United States under the auspices of the Procurement and Assignment Service. This will give opportunity to every physician in the United States to enroll himself with that service as ready to serve a specific need for which he is fitted. The Procurement and Assignment Service proposes also to make available to every physician who does enroll a certificate and a numbered button which will indicate to every one that he is a man who has offered to do his utmost for our government in this time of emergency.

"Also under preparation is a statement consisting of questions and answers which have come from many physicians in many parts of the country. This statement will be published in *The Journal* just as soon as it is available, and reprints will be made available for those who wish to secure them."

Recommendations to All Physicians With Reference to the National Emergency

Under the heading, "Recommendations to All Physicians with Reference to the National Emergency," the official statement of the Procurement and Assignment Service says:

I. MEDICAL STUDENTS

"A. All students holding letters of acceptance from the dean for admission to medical colleges and freshmen and sophomores of good academic standing in medical colleges should present letters or have letters presented for them by their deans to their local boards of the Selective Service System. This step is necessary in order to be considered for deferment in class II-A as a medical student. If local boards classify such students in class I-A, they should immediately notify their deans and if necessary exercise their rights of appeal to the board of appeals. If, after exhausting such rights of appeal, further consideration is necessary, request for further appeal may be made to the state director and if necessary to the national director of the Selective Service System. These officers have the power to take appeals to the President.

"B. Those junior and senior students who are disqualified physically for commissions are to be recommended for deferment to local boards by their deans. These students should enroll with the Procurement and Assignment Service for other assignment.

"C. All junior and senior students in good standing in medical schools who have not done so should apply immediately for commission in the Army or the Navy. This commission is in the grade of Second Lieutenant, Medical Administrative Corps of the Army of the United States, or Ensign H. V. (P.) of the United States Navy Reserve, the choice as to Army or Navy being entirely voluntary. Applications for commission in the Army should be made to the corps area surgeon of the corps area in which the applicant resides, and to the commandant of the naval district in which the applicant resides. Medical R. O. T. C. students should continue as before with a view of obtaining commissions as First Lieutenants, Medical Corps, on graduation. Students who hold commissions, while the commissions are in force, come under the jurisdiction of the Army and Navy authorities and are not subject to induction under the Selective Service Act. The Army and Navy authorities will defer calling these officers to active duty until they have completed their medical education and at least twelve months of internship.

II. RECENT GRADUATES

"On successful completion of the medical college course, every individual holding commission as a Second Lieutenant, Medical Administrative Corps, Army of the United States, should make immediate application to the Adjutant General, United States Army, Washington, D. C., for appointment as First Lieutenant, Medical Corps, Army of the United States. Every individual holding commission as Ensign H. V. (P.), U. S. Navy Reserve, should make immediate application to the commandant of his naval district for commission as Lieutenant (J. G.) Medical Corps Reserve, U. S. Navy. If appointment is desired in the grade of Lieutenant (J. G.) in the regular Medical Corps of the U. S. Navy, application should be made to the Bureau of Medicine and Surgery, Navy Department, Washington, D. C.

III. TWELVE MONTHS' INTERNS

"All interns should apply for a commission as First Lieutenant, Medical Corps, Army of the United States or as a Lieutenant (J. G.), United States Navy or Navy Reserve. On completion of twelve months' internship, except in rare instances in which the necessity of continuation as a member of the staff or as a resident can be defended by the institution, all who are physically fit may be required to enter military service. Those commissioned may then expect to enter military service in their professional capacity as medical officers; those who failed to apply for commissions are liable for military service under the Selective Service acts.

IV. HOSPITAL STAFF MEMBERS

"Interns with more than twelve months of internship, assistant residents, fellows, residents, junior staff members and staff members under the age of 45 fall within the provisions of the Selective Service acts, which provide that all men between the ages of 20 and 45 are liable for military service. All such men holding Army commissions are subject to call at any time and only temporary deferment is possible, on approval of the application made by the institution to the Adjutant General of the United States Army certifying that the individual is temporarily indispensable. All such men holding Naval Reserve commissions are subject to call at any time at the discretion of the Secretary of the Navy. Temporary deferments may be granted only on approval of applications made to the Surgeon General of the Navy.

"All men in this category who do not hold commissions should enroll with the Procurement and Assignment Service. The Procurement and Assignment Service under the executive order of the President is charged with the proper distribution of medical personnel for military, governmental, industrial and civil agencies of the entire country. All those so enrolled whose services have not been established as essential to the Army, Navy, governmental, industrial or civil agencies requiring their services for the duration of the war.

V. ALL PHYSICIANS UNDER FORTY-FIVE

"All male physicians under 45 are liable for military service, and those who do not hold commissions are subject to induction under the Selective Service acts. In order that their service may be utilized in a professional capacity as medical officers, they should be made available for service when needed. Wherever possible, their present positions in civil life should be filled or provisions made for filling their positions, by those who are (a) over 45, (b) physicians under 45 who are physically disqualified for military service, (c) women physicians and (d) instructors and those engaged in research who do not possess an M.D. degree but whose utilization would make available a physician for military service.

"Every physician in this age group will be asked to enroll at an early date with the Procurement and Assignment Service. He will be credited for a position commensurate with his professional training and experience as requisitions are placed with the Procurement and Assignment Service by military, governmental, industrial or civil agencies requiring the assistance of those who must be dislocated for the duration of the national emergency.

VI. ALL PHYSICIANS OVER FORTY-FIVE

"All physicians over 45 will be asked to enroll with the Procurement and Assignment Service at an early date. Those who are essential in their present capacities will be retained and those who are available for assignment to military, governmental, industrial or civil agencies may be asked by the Procurement and Assignment Service to serve those agencies.

"The maximal age for original appointment in the Army of the United States is 55. The maximal age for original appointment in the Naval Reserve is 50 years of age."

The statement is signed by: Frank H. Lahey, M.D., Chairman; Harvey B. Stone, M.D.; James E. Paullin, M.D.; Harold S. Diehl, M.D.; C. Willard Camalier, D.D.S., and Sam F. Seeley, M.D., Executive Officer.

Accompanying the statement is the request that "All inquiries concerning the Procurement and Assignment Service should be sent to the Executive Officer, 5654 Social Security Building, Fourth and Independence Avenues S.W., Washington, D.C., and not to individual members of the Directing Board or of committees thereof."

More County Medical Preparedness Chairmen Are Announced

The February issue of the Journal of the Association carried a list of the Chairmen of the Association's Medical Preparedness committees from the different counties in Oklahoma.

The following list contains additions to that published in the February issue.

Adair	Warren A. Beasley, Stilwell
Beaver	Theodore D. Benjegerdes, Beaver
Coal	J. B. Clark, Coalgate
Delaware	C. F. Walker, Grove
Dewey	W. E. Seba, Leedey
Ellis	O. C. Newman, Shattuck
Haskell	N. K. Williams, McCurtain
Johnston	J. T. Looney, Tishomingo
Nowata	S. A. Lang, Nowata

Dr. Fred Rankin Called to Service

Dr. Fred Rankin, Lexington, Ky., president-elect of the American Medical Association, has been called to active duty in the Office of the Surgeon General of the United States Army.

With the rank of Colonel, Doctor Rankin will serve as consulting surgeon. He assumes active duty on March 1.

Industrial Physicians and Industrial Hygiene Association Plan Joint Meeting

The American Association of Industrial Physicians and Surgeons and the American Industrial Hygiene Association will hold their joint Annual Convention in Cincinnati from April 13 to 17, 1942. A program is in preparation in which important medical and hygiene problems associated with the present huge task of American industry will be presented and discussed in clinics, lectures, symposia, and scientific exhibits.

The central purpose of the meeting will be to provide a five-day institute for the interchange and dissemination of information on new problems as well as for the consideration of up-to-date methods of dealing with those that are well known.

Emergency Medical and Hospital Service Chiefs Appointed

The office of William Cordell, Executive Secretary of Civilian Defense for the state of Oklahoma, has announced the local appointment of the following physicians as Chiefs of Emergency Medical and Hospital Service for their respective counties:

COUNTY	CHIEF
Adair	Dr. R. M. Church, Stilwell
Alfalfa	Dr. H. E. Huston, Cherokee
Atoka	Dr. J. C. Canada, Atoka
Beaver	Dr. T. D. Benjegerdes, Beaver
Beckham	Dr. V. C. Tisdal, Elk City
Blaine	Dr. W. F. Bohlman, Watonga
Bryan	Dr. J. T. Colwick, Durant
Caddo	Dr. Fred L. Patterson, Carnegie
	Dr. G. E. Haslam, Anadarko
Canadian	Dr. J. T. Phelps, El Reno
Carter	Dr. F. W. Boadway, Ardmore
Cherokee	Dr. R. K. McIntosh, Jr., Tahlequah
Choctaw	Dr. E. A. Johnson, Hugo
Cimarron	Dr. Harry B. Hall, Boise City
Cleveland	Dr. William A. Loy, Norman
	Dr. W. T. Mayfield, Norman
Coal	Dr. J. B. Chark, Coalgate
Cotton	Dr. George Baker, Walters
Craig	Dr. J. B. Darrough, Vinita
Creek	Dr. W. L. Piekhardt, Sapulpa
Delaware	Dr. C. F. Walker, Grove
Dewey	Dr. E. M. Loyd, Taloga
Ellis	Dr. Roy Newman, Shattuck
Garvin	Dr. Ray Lindsey, Pauls Valley
Grady	Dr. H. M. McClure, Chickasha
Greer	Dr. G. F. Border, Mangum
Harmon	Dr. L. E. Hollis, Hollis
Haskell	Dr. J. C. Rumley, Stigler
Hughes	Dr. H. A. Howell, Holdenville
Jackson	Dr. E. S. Crow, Olustee
Jefferson	Dr. D. B. Collins, Waurika
Kay	Dr. G. H. Yeary, Newkirk
Kiowa	Dr. J. M. Bonham, Hobart
Latimer	Dr. J. M. Harris, Wilburton
LeFlore	Dr. Neeson Rolle, Poteau
Lincoln	Dr. J. S. Rollins, Prague
Logan	Dr. R. F. Ringrose, Guthrie
McClain	Dr. W. C. McCurdy, Jr., Purcell
McIntosh	Dr. W. A. Tolleson, Eufaula
Major	Dr. M. R. McCroskie, Fairview
Marshall	Dr. J. L. Holland, Madill
Mayes	Dr. E. H. Werling, Pryor
Murray	Dr. F. E. Sadler, Sulphur
Muskogee	Dr. S. D. Neely, Muskogee
Noble	Dr. J. W. Francis, Perry
Nowata	Dr. S. A. Lang, Nowata
Okfuskee	Dr. A. S. Melton, Okemah
Oklahoma	Dr. Chester L. McHenry, Oklahoma City
Okmulgee	Dr. I. W. Bollinger, Henryetta
	Dr. J. G. Edwards, Okmulgee
Pawnee	Dr. R. L. Browning, Pawnee
Payne	Dr. C. W. Moore, Stillwater
Pittsburg	Dr. L. S. Willour, McAlester
Pontotoc	Dr. M. M. Webster, Ada
Pottawatomie	Dr. G. S. Baxter, Shawnee
Pushmataha	Dr. P. B. Rice, Antlers
Roger-Mills	Dr. J. Warrall Henry, Cheyenne
Rogers	Dr. R. C. Meloy, Claremore
Seminole	Dr. John P. Grimes, Wewoka
Sequoyah	Dr. W. H. Newlin, Sallisaw
Stephens	Dr. C. B. Waters, Duncan
Texas	Dr. L. G. Blackmer, Hooker
Tillman	Dr. O. G. Bacon, Frederick
	Dr. C. C. Allen, Frederick
Tulsa	Dr. D. L. Garrett, Tulsa
Wagoner	Dr. J. H. Plunkett, Wagoner
Washington	Dr. S. G. Weber, Bartlesville
Washita	Dr. A. H. Bungardt, Cordell
Woods	Dr. O. E. Templin, Alva
Woodward	Dr. C. W. Tedrowe, Woodward

All Chiefs of Emergeny Medical and Hospital Service and the Chairmen of the Health and Housing committee will meet with Colonel W. B. Russ, San Antonio, Tex., Director of Emergency Medical Care in the Eighth Corps Area, for discussions and classification of their duties. The meetings will take place February 5 in Tulsa, and February 6 in Oklahoma City.

Insignia Prepared for Medical And Nurses' Aides Corps

The Office of Civilian Defense has prepared insignia for volunteer civilian defense workers to wear after they have been enrolled and trained. The designs have been patented by the OCD, and only enrolled civilian defense workers are entitled to wear them as part of uniforms or of any clothing that may simulate official wear.

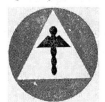

MEDICAL CORPS

Physicians and nurses serving in emergency medical field units will be identified by a red caduceus in a white triangle set in a blue circle. In the event of a war emergency such as an air raid, the problem of caring for the sick and injured will be handled by the Emergency Medical Service.

NURSES AIDES CORPS

Volunteer nurses' aides will be identified by a red cross within a white triangle set in a blue circle. This indicates that the volunteer has been enrolled and trained by the American Red Cross for service in civilian defense . This insigne must not be worn until the aide has completed her course of training, which she will receive from the Red Cross and from hospitals designated as training centers.

Dr. Taylor to Serve Seventh Term As President Hughes County Society

Dr. William L. Taylor of Holdenville has been elected to serve as president of the Hughes County Medical society for the seventh consecutive time. The society met January 2, in Holdenville, for dinner and a scientific program.

Among the guests were Dr. Finis W. Ewing, Muskogee, President of the Association; Dr. L. C. Kuyrkendall, McAlester, and R. H. Graham, Oklahoma City, Executive Secretary of the Association. There were also guests present from the Pottawatomie and Pontotoc County Medical societies.

Protection of Civil Rights of Persons in Military Service*

Designed to protect from impairment the civil rights of all members of the Army, Navy, Marine Corps, Coast Guard and all members of the United States Public Health Service detailed by proper authority for duty with the Army or Navy, a law was approved by the President, October 17, 1940, commonly referred to as the Soldiers' and Sailors' Civil Relief Act of 1940. In substance, this law is an up-to-date revision of a similar enactment passed during the first world war, and its fundamental purpose is to free persons in the military service from harassment and injury to their civil rights during their term of military service and thus to enable them to devote their entire energy to the defense needs of the nation.

The provisions of the law, broadly stated, apply to persons on active duty with any branch of the services mentioned and to those in training or undergoing education under the supervision of the United States preliminary to induction into the military services who (1) may become defendants in a court action, (2) have dependents occupying a dwelling for which the agreed rent does not exceed $80 a month, (3) may have contracted, prior to entry into service, for the purchase of real or personal property on the instalment plan, (4) may have obligations relative to mortgages on real or personal property, (5) may hold policies of life insurance of a face value not in excess of $5,000, (6) may have taxes or assessments on real property falling due, (7) may have initiated or acquired a right to lands owned or controlled by the United States or (8) may become liable for income taxes. Generally the law provides remedies in the form of suspension of proceedings and transactions during the time a person is in the military service only when, in the opinion of the court, such person's opportunity and capacity to perform his civil obligations are impaired by reason of his being in military service.

GENERAL RELIEF

Before any judgment in default may be entered in any court, the plaintiff must file an affidavit showing either that the defendant is not in military service, that he is in such service, or that the plaintiff is unable to determine whether or not the defendant is in service, as the case may be. If the absent defendant is in military service, the court must appoint an attorney to represent him and protect his interest. This attorney, however, will have no power to waive any right of the absent defendant or bind him by his acts. Unless it appears that the defendant is not in service, the court may require, as a condition before any judgment is rendered, that the plaintiff file a bond conditioned to indemnify the defendant, if in military service, against any loss or damage that he may suffer by reason of any judgment should the judgment be thereafter set aside in whole or in part.

If judgment is entered against a person while he is in service or within 30 days thereafter, application may be made for a reopening of the case not later than 90 days after the termination of the service, at which time any meritorious or legal defense may be interposed. Vacating, setting aside or reversing any judgment, however, will not impair any right or title acquired by an bona fide purchaser for value under such judgment.

At any stage thereof, any action or proceedings in any court in which a person in military service is involved, as either plaintiff or defendant, may be stayed by the court during the period of such service or within 60 days thereafter. Likewise the execution of any judgment or order entered against a defendant in service may be stayed and any attachment or garnishment of property, money or debts in the hands of another may be vacated

*Prepared by the Bureau of Legal Medicine and Legislation, and reprinted from the Journal of the A. M. A., January 24, 1942.

or stayed. If an action for the compliance with the terms of any contract is stayed, no fine or penalty will accrue by reason of failure to comply with the terms of such contract during the period of stay.

Any stay of any action, proceeding, attachment or execution ordered by the court may be ordered for the period of military service and three months thereafter and subject to such regulations as he may prescribe, to order payment of instalments in such a manner and at such times as the court may fix or otherwise. Where the person in military service is co-defendant with others, the plaintiffs may nevertheless by leave of court proceed against the others. The period of military service, the law provides, shall not be included in the running of any statutes of limitations.

RENTS

No eviction or distress may be made during the period of military service with respect to any premises for which the agreed rent does not exceed $80 a month, occupied chiefly for dwelling purposes by the wife, children or other dependents of the person in service, except on leave of court. The Secretary of War or the Secretary of the Navy, as the case may be, is empowered, subject to such regulations as he may prescribe, to order an allotment of the pay of a person in military service in reasonable proportion to discharge the rent of premises occupied for dwelling purposes by the wife, children or other dependents of such person. This provision, it will be noted, applies only in connection with the rental of property used chiefly for dwelling purposes. It would seem to be inapplicable to premises used chiefly for office purposes. Legislation has been proposed to extend relief to persons in service in connection with leases executed for offices, but Congressional action on such legislation has not been completed.

INSTALMENT CONTRACTS AND MORTGAGES

No person who prior to the date of approval of the law has received a deposit or instalment of the purchase price under contract for the purchase of real or personal property from a person who after the date of payment has entered military service may exercise any right or option under the contract to rescind or terminate it or resume possession of the property for nonpayment of any instalment falling due during the period of military service, except by action in a court of competent jurisdiction. The law, however, does not prevent the modification, termination or cancellation of any such contract or prevent the repossession or retention of property purchased or received under the contract, pursuant to a mutual agreement of the parties if such agreement is executed in writing subsequent to the making of the contract and during or after the period of military service of the person concerned. In any court action based on such contract, the court may order the repayment of prior instalments or deposits as a condition of terminating the contract and resuming possession of the contract, may in its discretion order a stay of proceedings for the period of military service and three months thereafter, or may make such other disposition of the case as is equitable to conserve the interests of all parties.

The law specifically provides, however, that no court may stay a proceeding to resume possession of a motor vehicle, tractor or the accessories of either, or for an order of sale thereof, where the property is encumbered by a purchase money mortgage, conditional sales contract or a lease or bailment with a view to purchase, unless the court finds that 50 percent or more of the purchase price of the property has been paid. In any such proceeding the court may, before entering an order or judgment, require the plaintiff to file a bond to indemnify the defendant against any loss or damage that he may suffer by reason of the judgment should it be set in whole or in part.

Similar relief is afforded persons in service in connection with mortgages. The law applies only to obligations originating prior to its approval date and secured by mortgage, deed or trust or other security in the nature of a mortgage on real or personal property owned by a person in military service at the commencement of the period of service and still so owned by him.

INSURANCE PREMIUMS

With respect to life insurance policies, the law provides that on application by a person in military service the Administrator of Veterans' Affairs may guarantee payment of premiums in order to prevent lapsing or forfeiting of policies. Such persons may, within one year after leaving military service, pay up premiums unpaid by them and resume payment of regular premiums. If they fail to do so, the policy lapses and the cash surrender value accrues to the government to the extent necessary to meet the cost of premiums which it has guaranteed. The Veterans' Administration is required to issue through suitable military and naval channels a notice for distribution to persons in military service explaining the benefits provided by the law in connection with life insurance policies and to furnish forms to be distributed to those desiring to apply for benefits.

The benefits are applicable to contracts of life insurance up to but not exceeding a total face value of $5,000, irrespective of the number of policies held by the person, when the contracts were made and the premium was paid thereon before the approval date of the law or not less than 30 days before entering service. The benefits do not apply to any policy on which premiums are due and unpaid for a period of more than one pear at the time when application for benefits is made, to any policy on which there is outstanding a policy loan or other indebtedness equal to or greater than 50 percent of the cash surrender value of the policy, to any policy which is void or which may at the option of the insured be voidable in case of military service, or to any policy which as a result of military service provides for the payment of any sum less than the face thereof or for the payment of an additional amount of premium.

TAXES ON PROPERTY AND INCOME

If a person in service, or any person in his behalf, files with the collector of taxes, or other officer whose duty it is to enforce the collection of taxes or assessments, an affidavit showing (1) that a tax or assessment have been assessed on property as described below, (2) that such tax or assessment is unpaid and (3) that by reason of service the ability of the person to pay the tax or assessment is materially affected, no sale of the property may be made to enforce the collection of the tax or assessment, or any proceeding or action for such purpose commenced, except on leave of court granted on application made by the collector or other officer. The court is authorized to stay such a proceeding or sale for a period extending not more than six months after the termination of the period of military service of such a person.

When by law, however, such property may be sold or forfeited to enforce the collection of the tax or assessment, the person in military service has the right to redeem the property at any time not later than six months after the termination of service, but in no case later than six months after the date when the Soldiers' and Sailors' Civil Relief Act ceases to be in force. If any tax or assessment shall not be paid when due, such tax or assessment due and unpaid will bear interest until paid at the rate of six percent per annum.

The benefits here discussed apply when any taxes or assessments, whether general or special, falling due during the period of military service in respect of real property owned and occupied for dwelling, agricultural or business purposes by a person in military service or his dependents at the commencement of the period of military service and still so occupied by his dependents or employees are not paid. The Secretary of War and the Secretary of the Navy are required to make provision, in such manner as each may deem appropriate for his respective department, to insure notice to persons in military service of the benefits accorded with respect to taxes and the action made necessary to claim those benefits in each case.

With respect to income taxes, the law provides that the collection from any person in military service of any tax on his income, whether falling due prior to or during his period of service, shall be deferred for a period extending not more than six months after the termination of his period of service, if the person's ability to pay the tax is materially impaired by reason of service. No interest on any amount of tax, collection of which is deferred, and no penalty for nonpayment of such amount during such period, will accrue for the period of deferment by reason of such nonpayment.

PUBLIC LANDS

The law provides, in general, that no right to any land owned or controlled by the United States initiated or acquired under the laws of the United States, including the mining and mineral leasing laws, by any person prior to entering military service shall during the period of service be forfeited or prejudiced by reason of his absence from the land or his failure to perform any work or make any improvements thereon or his failure to do any other act required by or under such laws. Special provisions relate to homesteads, desert land entries, mining claims, mineral leases and irrigation rights. The Secretary of the Interior is required to issue through appropriate military and naval channels a notice for distribution to persons in service explanatory of the benefits of the law in connection with public lands and to furnish forms for use by persons desiring to apply for the benefits.

ADMINISTRATIVE REMEDIES

If in any proceeding to enforce a civil right in any court it is made to appear that any interest, property or contract has since the approval date of the law been transferred or acquired with intent to delay just enforcement by taking advantage of the benefits of the law, the court will enter such judgment or order as might lawfully be entered, the provisions of the Soldiers' and Sailors' Civil Relief Act to the contrary notwithstanding.

In any proceeding under the law a certificate signed (1) by the Adjutant General of the Army as to the persons in the Army or in any branch of the United States service while serving pursuant to law with the Army, (2) by the Chief of the Bureau of Navigation of the Navy Department as to persons in the Navy or in any other branch of the service while serving pursuant to law with the Navy, (3) by the Major General Commandant, United States Marine Corps, as to persons in that corps or in any other branch of service while serving pursuant to law with the Marine Corps, or signed by any officer designated by any of them respectively, shall when produced be prima facie evidence as to any of the following facts stated in such certificates: That the person named has not been, or is, or has been in military service; the time when and the place where such person entered military service; his residence at that time, and the rank, branch and unit of such service that he entered, the dates within which he was in military service, the monthly pay received at the date of issuing the certificate, the time when and the place where such person died in or was discharged from such service.

This law will remain in force until May 15, 1945. If at that time the United States is engaged in war, the law will remain in force until such war is terminated by treaty of peace proclaimed by the President and for six months thereafter.

Work eight hours a day and don't worry. Some day you may be the boss. Then you will work 18 hours a day and do all the worrying.—Bulletin, Garfield County Medical society.

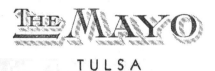
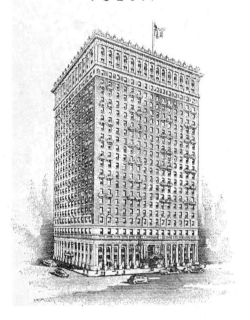

NEWS FROM THE COUNTY SOCIETIES

About ten members were present for the meeting of the Garvin County Medical society, January 14, in Pauls Valley. Dr. Clinton Gallaher, Shawnee, a guest from the Pottowatomie county society, talked on "Trachoma," and a discussion of his subject followed his talk.

The society will meet February 18 in Pauls Valley, with Dr. R. M. Alley, Shawnee, as guest speaker. His subject will be "Differential Diagnosis of Pulmonary Tuberculosis."

The Thirty-Seventh Annual Meeting and Ladies' Night was held by members of the Pottawatomie County Medical society, January 17, at the Aldridge hotel in Shawnee. About 90 members and guests were in attendance.

Following dinner, Rev. Donald Hyde of the First Presbyterian church of Shawnee, gave the invocation, guests and new officers of the society were introduced, and Gus Nelson, accompanied at the piano by Mrs. Paul Gallaher, gave a vocal colo.

Then, Dr. R. M. Anderson, toastmaster for the occasion, introduced the speaker of the evening, C. W. Patton, Professor of Modern History at O. B. U., who addressed the meeting on the "Impact of War."

Guests included Dr. Finis W. Ewing, Muskogee, President of the Association; Dr. R. Q. Goodwin, Oklahoma City, President of the Oklahoma County Medical association; Dr. Ned R. Smith, Tulsa, President of the Tulsa County Medical association; and R. H. Graham, Oklahoma City, Executive Secretary of the Association.

Dr. Alfred R. Suggs, Ada, discussed "New Developments in Urology" at the meeting of Okmulgee and Okfuskee county societies, January 12, in Okmulgee.

About 24 members were present for the dinner meeting and program. The group will meet February 9 in Okemah.

The Annual Inaugural Banquet and installation of new officers was held by the Washington-Nowata County Medical society, January 14, in Bartlesville, with about 54 members and guests present.

"The Intimate Relations Between the Three 'Learned Professions,' Clergy, Law and Medicine" was the topic of the address given by Attorney L. A. Rowland of Bartlesville, who was the speaker of the evening. The program also included music and readings.

The society will meet February 11 in Bartlesville, when Dr. H. C. Weber will talk on "Surgical Treatment of Infections of the Hand," and Dr. S. A. Lang will discuss "Allergy in Children." Dr. R. C. Gentry and Dr. L. D. Hudson will lead the discussion of the two talks.

Dr. L. S. Willour, McAlester, was the speaker for the meeting of the Pittsburg County Medical society, December 19, in McAlester. About 20 members were present.

Doctor Willour presented a program on fractures, epiphyseal dislocations and spinal injuries, illustrating his presentation with numerous lantern slides and motion pictures of some of his cases. The use of Kirschner wires in intracapsular and intertrochanteric fractures was presented.

The society met January 29 in McAlester for its Inaugural Banquet, with the Auxiliary members as guests.

Inauguration of 1942 officers was held at a dinner dance, January 24, given by the Oklahoma County Medical association at the Oklahoma City Golf and Country club, Oklahoma City.

Officers were elected at the December 18 meeting, following a buffet supper. The Oklahoma City Clinical society met during a recess at this meeting and reported on the 1941 clinical conference.

Dr. Walker Morledge and Dr. Charles M. O'Leary, both of Oklahoma City, were the speakers at the meeting, January 27, at the Medical school in Oklahoma City.

Dr. Tom Lowry and Dr. Lewis J. Moorman, both of Oklahoma City, were guest speakers at the January 12 meeting of the Osage County Medical society in Pawhuska. About 13 members were present.

Doctor Lowry discussed "Diagnosis of Pulmonary Tuberculosis from the General Practitioner's Standpoint," and Doctor Moorman discussed "Treatment of Tuberculosis."

Members of the Wagoner County Medical society have decided to consolidate with the medical societies of Muskogee and Sequoyah counties. New officers of the Wagoner society are Dr. J. H. Plunkett, Wagoner, president; Dr. S. R. Bates, Wagoner, vice-president; and Dr. H. K. Riddle, Coweta, secretary.

Dr. Ollie McBride of Ada presented an extensive case report for discussion before members of the Pontotoc county society, January 21, at the Aldridge hotel in Ada. About 19 members attended the meeting. Doctor McBride's report concerned a case of periarteritis nodosa and gastric ulcer.

Guest speaker for the December meeting of the Beckham county society was Dr. Finis W. Ewing, Muskogee, president of the Association. Following a banquet, Dr James G. Hughes, speaker for the Postgraduate Committee's Pediatrics program, lectured, and election of 1942 officers was held.

Dr. H. K. Speed, Sayre, was re-elected president, and Dr. E. S. Kilpatrick, Elk City, was elected secretary. It was planned to rotate monthly meetings of the society from Elk City to Sayre and to Erick.

Dr. J. C. Wagner, Ponca City, read a paper entitled "Eclampsia" for members of the Kay county society at a meeting, January 14, in the Larkin hotel, Blackwell. Seventeen members and two guests were present.

Discussion of the paper was led by Dr. Merl Clift, Blackwell and Dr. C. W. Arrendell of Ponca City, and a general discussion of Malpractice Insurance followed. An informal dinner preceded the meeting and program. The society will meet February 19 at Tonkawa.

A committee on Health and Housing for the Civilian Defense Movement was appointed at the January 15 meeting of the Blaine county society. The county also reported that this committee will also act as the committee on Emergency Medical and Hospital Service.

Dr. F. C. Buffington of Norman has been elected president of the Cleveland county society, with Dr. M. P. Prosser and Dr. Phil Haddock, both of Norman, serving as vice-president and secretary respectively.

The Cleveland county society election was held at a meeting, January 8, in Norman. Delegates elected were Doctor Buffington and Doctor Haddock, with Dr. O. E. Howell and Dr. W. B. Carroll, both of Norman, serving as alternates. Censors are Dr. M. M. Wickham and Dr. Gertrude Nielsen, both of Norman, and Dr. W. C. McCurdy, Jr., of Purcell. Dr. William A. Loy, Norman, will head the Scientific Program committee for 1942.

The Logan County Medical society elected Dr. William C. Miller, Guthrie, as its president, Dr. C. L. Rogers, Marshall, as vice-president, and Dr. J. L. LeHew, Jr., Guthrie, as secretary. Dr. L. A. Hahn, Guthrie, was elected delegate, with Doctor LeHew as his alternate. Censors are Dr. J. E. Souter, Dr. Roy W. Anderson and Doctor Miller, all of Guthrie.

At the society's January meeting in Guthrie, a discussion of Scarlet Fever was held, and tentative plans to visit the Oklahoma County Medical association meeting in February were made.

Several case history reports by members made up the scientific program of the Creek county society meeting, January 13, in Sapulpa. Thirteen members of the society were present to hear the reports.

Dr. W. P. Longmire, Jr., Sapulpa, presented a case of hemorrhagic encephalitis, and Doctor Wharton reported a case of encephalitis in a nine-year-old boy. Dr. J. F. Curry of Sapulpa, presented an unusual obstetrical case, and Dr. Frank H. Sisler, Bristow, a case of cancer of the gall bladder and liver. Dr. O. H. Cowart's case was one of virus pneumonia.

Blood Bank Is Project in Ottowa County

Dr. Walter Sanger of Picher, secretary of the Ottowa County Medical society, has announced that the Picher Lions club is sponsoring and donating to a blood plasma bank to be used by the whole of Ottawa county. Dr. M. A. Connell of Picher has been designated as collector for the bank.

Those able to pay for blood will be charged a small fee for use of the bank, and those who are not able to pay will be expected to have friends or relatives donate blood to replace what they have used and more.

The Ottawa County Medical society met January 15 in Miami, with about 16 members present. Speakers at the meeting were Dr. Edward N. Smith, Oklahoma City, who spoke on "Shock," and Dr. J. Moore Campbell, Oklahoma City, who discussed "Peritonitis."

Dr. Templin Serves 22nd Term as Secretary Of Woods County Medical Society

It has been reported that Dr. O. E. Templin of Alva, who was recently re-elected secretary of the Woods County Medical society, is beginning his twenty-second consecutive term as secretary of his county society.

Following an informal dinner for members and their wives, a business and scientific meeting was held, January 27, in Cherokee by the Woods-Alfalfa County Medical society.

On the scientific program were Dr. Coyne Campbell and Dr. Patrick Nagle, both of Oklahoma City, guests of the society. Doctor Campbell spoke on "Insulin Shock-Metrazol and Electrical Therapy in Treating Psychiatric Diseases," and Doctor Nagle on "Intestinal Obstruction Complicating Appendiceal Peritonitis."

Joe Stone, an attorney, was guest speaker for the last meeting of the Muskogee County Medical society at the Baptist hospital in Muskogee. Mr. Stone discussed "The Physician as a Legal Witness."

Others on the program included Dr. F. B. Dorwart and Dr. Pat Fite, both of Muskogee. Doctor Dorwart discussed "Coronary Accident," and Doctor Fite, "Military Surgery."

The society will meet again March 2 at the hospital, with Dr. D. H. O'Donoghue of Oklahoma City as a speaker. His topic will be "Practical and Medico-Legal Orthopedics."

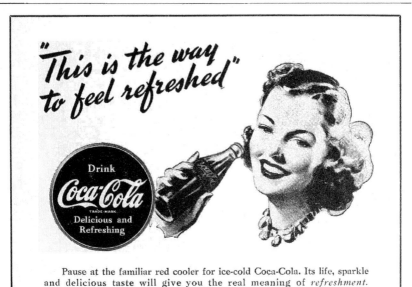

• OBITUARIES •

Dr. J. L. Adams
1877-1941

Dr. J. L. Adams, for 16 years a practicing physician in Kiowa county, died December 31, 1941, in Hobart in the hospital he founded and operated. His death was caused by a heart attack.

Born February 11, 1877, in Arkansas, Doctor Adams came to Hobart April 6, 1925, and began his practice of medicine. He was graduated from the University of Arkansas School of Medicine in 1910.

For ten years he served Kiowa county as health officer, and he was active in Red Cross first aid and school work.

He served the Kiowa County Medical society as president for two different terms, and as secretary several terms.

Doctor Adams is survived by his wife, and three sons, Dr. Sylva Adams of Oregon, Dr. Richards Adams of Tulsa, and Idus Adams of Hobart; and one daughter, Mrs. John Swoboda of Mangum.

Dr. J. W. Browning
1869-1942

Dr. J. W. Browning, one of Oklahoma's pioneer physicians, died at his home in Geary, January 9, following a long illness.

Doctor Browning had maintained offices in the First National Bank building in Geary since 1899. Born in Washington county, Tennessee, in 1869, he was graduated from Washington college in that state and began his study of medicine in 1894 at Baltimore Medical college, Baltimore.

When he had passed the Texas State medical examination, he began his practice at Whitesboro, Tex., then after a year of practice, he resumed his studies at Barnes Medical college, St. Louis, where he received his M.D. degree in 1899.

Doctor Browning was married to Ida E. Clarke at Wilson, Tex., April 20, 1899, and the couple moved to Geary in Oklahoma Territory.

He continued his medical studies through special courses at Chicago Polyclinic, the New York Postgraduate school, and Johns Hopkins university. He was active in the State Medical Association and the Blaine County Medical society, serving several times as president of the county society.

Ever active in organization work, Dr. Browning was a 32nd degree Mason, a member of the Geary Chamber of Commerce, and contributed to and sponsored many worthwhile civic enterprises in his community.

He is survived by his wife and four daughters, Mrs. Bryan Griffin and Mrs S. L. Pangburn, both of Lawton; Mrs. Charles R. Young, Tulsa, and Miss Grace Browning, Chicago.

Dr. Okey Nelson Windle
1882-1942

Okey Nelson Windle was born November 3, 1882, at Ripley, West Virginia. He received his M.D. Degree from the American Medical College at Baltimore, Md., in 1905, and practiced for awhile in Nowata county, Oklahoma. In November 1908, he moved to Sayre and entered a partnership with Dr. H. K. Speed, the partnership lasting for 12 years. Since that time he practiced alone in Sayre until his death, January 3, 1942. During his years spent in Oklahoma, he was an active member of the State and Beckham County Medical societies.

He leaves behind him his good wife, a daughter Mrs. Ross Dugger; a son, Bobby, and another daughter Laura Ann.

His death was caused by a coronary occlusion.

Dr. C. S. Bobo
1856-1942

Dr. C. S. Bobo, the first physician to register after Oklahoma obtained its statehood and therefore the receiver of Certificate Number 1 to practice medicine in Oklahoma, died February 3 at his home in Norman.

Known by every doctor in the state as well as hundreds of other citizens, Doctor Bobo had practiced medicine for almost 60 years. He served as president of the Oklahoma State Medical Association in 1907 and 1908, and held honorary memberships in the Association and the Cleveland County Medical society at the time of his death. In 1937, he was made a life member of the American Medical Association.

Born in Pickens county in Alabama, he was graduated in 1881 from the Louisville Medical college, Louisville, Ky., with honors including a gold medal for proficiency. For 15 years he practiced in northwestern Texas, then moved to Oklahoma in 1898, where for eight years he practiced in the Norman district, making his calls on horseback.

He became professor of forensic medicine in the University of Oklahoma School of Medicine in 1907, and a year later was named dean of the school. He established in 1910 the last two years of clinical medicine at Oklahoma City in the medical school which absorbed that of Epworth university.

He was chairman of the legislative committee which drafted the medical law governing the practice of medicine in Oklahoma, and was director of the student health service at the University and superintendent of the University infirmary from 1933 to 1937.

In 1937, when he retired from the health service, he was honored with a banquet on his birthday to commemorate his long years of service. Later after his retirement, he still accepted the work as city health officer of Norman.

His survivors include his wife, Mrs. Katie Bobo, of Norman; three sons, W. K. Bobo, of Oklahoma City, O. H. Bobo, of Tulsa, and Sidney Bobo, of Norman; a brother, Z. B. Bobo, of Rhome, Tex., and one sister, Mrs. Charles Poe, Fort Worth, Tex.

Dr. I. B. Oldham
1872-1942

On January 14, Dr. I. B. Oldham of Muskogee passed away at the Oklahoma Baptist hospital in Muskogee.

Doctor Oldham was 70 years old, a pioneer in Muskogee's medical, civic and church activities. A resident of Muskogee since 1903, Doctor Oldham held many positions of prominence in the city's affairs. He was chairman of the agriculture committee of the Chamber of Commerce for many years, and at the time of his death was an honorary director of the organization.

He was a deacon of the First Baptist church, a past director of the Oklahoma Baptist university at Shawnee, and aided in founding the Oklahoma Baptist hospital in Muskogee, where he died.

He was several times president of the Muskogee County Medical society, and was active in the State Association. He also served as president and committee member of civic groups such as the Optimist club and the Lions club.

He attended Central university at Richmond, Ky., and the Louisville Medical college, and began his practice of medicine at Kirksville, Ky. In 1895, he married Mary Lewland, and in 1903, they moved to Muskogee.

Doctor Oldham is survived by his wife; three sons, Dr. Brown Oldham, Jr. and Phil K. Oldham, both of Muskogee, and Newland Oldham, Carlsbad, N.M.; three daughters, Mrs. C. H. Zachary, Dallas, Tex., Mrs. C. W. Garrett, Fort Gibson, and Mrs. H. O. Williams of Muskogee; and nine grandchildren.

University of Oklahoma School of Medicine

The following members of the School of Medicine faculty attended the meeting of the American Association for the Advancement of Science in Dallas, Tex., December 29 to January 3: Dr. H. A. Shoemaker, Dr. Mark R. Everett, Dr. J. M. Thuringer, Dr. Donald B. McMullen, Miss Elizabeth Hall, and Miss Ruby Wortham.

Doctor Shoemaker represented the American Society for Pharmacology and Experimental Therapeutics at the Union of American Biological Societies and the Council of the American Association for the Advancement of Science.

Dr. M. R. Everett read a paper at the Chemical Section on the "Relations of Sugar Structure and of Salt Catalysis to Carbohydrate Oxidation." Dr. J. M. Thuringer read a paper on "Thick Walled Arteries in the Adventitia of the Aorta."

Dr. Paul C. Colonna attended the meeting of the American Academy of Orthopedic Surgeons in Atlantic City January 11 to 15, where he contributed to the program by taking part in the discussion of one of the papers presented.

Dr. M. R. Everett, Professor of Biochemistry, has recently completed a manuscript entitled "Medical Biochemistry," which will be published in book form by Paul B. Hoeber. It is expected that this book will be available very shortly.

Miss Helen L. Kendall, Registrar of the School of Medicine, has been confined to St. Anthony's hospital for several weeks.

Dr. Richard M. Burke, Superintendent of Western Oklahoma Tuberculosis Sanatorium, Clinton, visiting lecturer in medicine, has been elected a Fellow in the American College of Physicians.

Dr. John M. Parrish, Jr., until the first of the year a Resident in Obstetrics and Gynecology at the University hospital, has been appointed to the Obstetrical Service of the Outpatient Department of the Hospital. Doctor Parrish has entered the practice of medicine in Oklahoma City with Dr. Tom Lowry, with offices in the Osler Building.

Dr. J. William Finch, Hobart, has been appointed to the faculty of the Medical School as a Visiting Lecturer in Medicine. Doctor Finch is a graduate of this school in the class of 1931.

Dr. Lachman Speaks at Academy of Science

Among the faculty members who attended the meeting of the Oklahoma Academy of Science, December 5-6 in Edmond, was Dr. Ernest Lachman, Associate Professor of Anatomy.

Doctor Lachman read a paper entitled "X-ray Anatomy as Exemplified in the Thorax" for the December 6 meeting of the Academy.

On December 18, 1941, the Women's Auxiliary to the Cleveland County Medical society met at 7:30 P.M. at the Central State hospital, Norman. Of the 29 members, 12 were present. Mrs. Jim L. Haddock, president of this group, had charge of the meeting. The questions discussed and actions taken thereon were as follows: (1) Authorization of Red Cross Nurses' Training Course, and (2) Discontinuance of the dessert course.

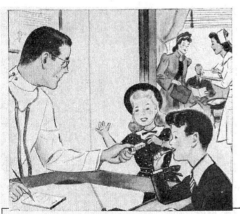

News From The State Health Department

The Oklahoma State Health department has recently adopted a new form for obtaining delayed birth certificates which conforms to all requirements of the United States Census Bureau, Dr. G. F. Mathews, Commissioner, has announced.

The "delayed" form is used to record the birth of a person born in Oklahoma whose birth was not recorded at the time of birth.

Those wanting birth certificates should write to the State Health department, Oklahoma City, enclosing the statutory fee of 50 cents in cash or money order, with the following information: applicant's full name; date and place of his birth; the father's full name and the mother's maiden name.

This information must be sent in first, so that a search of the 1,750,000 birth certificates now on file may be made to determine if the applicant's birth has been recorded. If it has been recorded, a certified copy will be returned.

If the birth has not been recorded, then the new form for a delayed certificate will be mailed to the applicant.

In addition to the usual requirements of affidavits by relatives and non-relatives, the new form requires documentary evidence giving proof of the date and place of birth and the parentage.

The new form requires one Class A and one Class B document or three Class B documents, before a perfect certificate can be issued.

A Class A document is one established before the applicant's fourth birthday. Documents of this class include a Baptismal record, Cradle Roll record, Biblical record or an insurance policy.

Class B documents are those established since the applicant's fourth birthday. They include those of Class A, and records such as military, employment, hospitalization, U.S. decinnial census report and a discharge from the army or navy. Class B documents must have been issued at least five years before the application for delayed birth certificates.

Those desiring birth certificates are being urged to write directly to the health department, and not to bother the private physician for this information.

"Private physicians can do a real service to their patients and the program of compiling vital statistics by filling out birth certificates at the time of birth," Doctor Mathews added.

Menninger Psychiatric Foundation Organization Completed

After several years of planning, the Menninger Foundation was organized and incorporated under the laws of Kansas in April, 1941, with headquarters in Topeka. The purposes of this new non-profit psychiatric foundation are fourfold:

1. Provision for psychiatric education, especially the training of young physicians in psychiatry. The shortage of well-trained psychiatrists will presently become acute in relation to the requirements of World War II and the post-war period.
2. Encouragement of research in psychiatric and psychological fields.
3. Making available psychiatric treatment for patients in the low income bracket.
4. Prevention of mental illness, especially through development of child psychiatry and application of psychiatric knowledge to education and child-rearing.

In addition to local officers, the following trustees have been elected: Dr. Winfred Overholser, St. Elizabeth's Hospital, Washington, D.C.; Mrs. Albert Lasker, New York and Chicago; Dr. John C. Whitehorn, Johns Hopkins University, Baltimore; Mrs. Lucy Stearns McLaughlin, Santa Fe, N. M.; Dean J. Roscoe Miller, Northwestern University Medical School, Chicago; Mrs. Sidney C. Borg, Jewish Board of Guardians, New York City; and George E. Hite, Jr., Milbank, Tweed and Hope, New York City.

The Menninger Foundation has already initiated several projects from its financial gifts. Grants have been made for a ten year study of the place of occupational therapy in psychiatric treatment, for a seminar and special Bulletin on Military Psychatry and the distribution of this information to physicians on the Medical Advisory Boards of the entire country, and for research in the use of hypnosis in emergency psychotherapy and in substantiatng newer psychiatric theories. Other projects are to follow.

American Board Obstetrics, Gynecology Announces Examinations

The general oral and pathological examinations (Part II) for all candidates (Groups A and B) will be conducted at Atlantic City, N.J., by the entire Board, prior to the opening of the annual meeting of the American Medical Association in Atlantic City, on June 8, 1942, the American Board of Obstetrics and Gynecology has announced.

Applications for admission to Group A, Part II, examinations must be on file in the Secretary's Office not later than March 1, 1942. It will greatly facilitate the work of the Board if applications are filed as far as possible in advance of the closing date for their receipt.

Formal notice of the time and place of these examinations will be sent each candidate several weeks in advance of the examination dates.

Candidates for *reexamination* in Part II must make written application to the Secretary's Office before April 15, 1942.

As previously announced in the Board booklet, this fiscal year (1941-1942) of the Board marks the close of the two groups of classification of applicants for examination. Thereafter, the Board will have only one classification of candidates, and all will be required to take the Part I examinations.

The Board requests that all prospective candidates who plan to submit applications in the near future request and use the new application form which has this year been inaugurated by the Board. The Secretary will be glad to furnish these forms upon request, together with information regarding Board requirements. Address Dr. Paul Titus, Secretary, 1015 Highland Building, Pittsburgh (6), Pennsylvania.

FWA Advises Hospitals to Arrange Own Financing Programs

Hospitals should go just as far as they can in arranging their own financing programs without waiting for hoped-for aid from Defense Public Works grants or loans, Assistant Federal Works Administrator Baird Snyder, III, has pointed out.

Mr. Snyder, acting for Federal Works Administrator Philip B. Fleming, made this statement by way of warning to a large number of hospitals which, he was informed, are delaying fund-raising or other financial programs for expansion of facilities while they await decisions on applications to FWA. Mr. Snyder said:

"In addition to the hospital projects which already have been approved, applications have been filed for additional hospital projects, the total estimated cost of which is more than $155,000,000. Under the new Lanham Act appropriation, only $150,000,000 was made available for Defense Public Works of all types.

"It is quite apparent that a number of these hospitals are not eligible under the Act by reason of the fact that their need for expansion is not based upon the defense program.

"With respect to those whose expansion is brought about by the pressure of the defense program, their chances of sharing in the funds would be greatly increased if they would arrange in advance of their applications their own share of the financing that will be necessary."

Woodward County Medical Society Announces 1942 Program

The scientific programs for the 1942 meetings of the Woodward County Medical Society have been announced.

Pulmonary Infections and Complications was the general topic of the program at the February 12 meeting, with Dr. H. Walker, Dr. T. B. Triplett and Dr. H. L. Johnson as speakers. Doctor Walker discussed "Influenza and Bronchitis;" Doctor Triplett, "Pneumonia," and Doctor Johnson, "Hydrothorax." The meeting was held in Woodward.

Other general topics for the future programs include Diseases of the Rectum, Diagnosis and Treatment of Fractures, The Sulfonamides, The Relation of Psychoneuroses to Schizophrenia, Disorders of the Heart, Ear, Nose and Throat Infections, Gallbladder Diseases and Complications, and Urology.

Guest speakers who will take part in programs during the year include Dr. R. L. Murdoch, Dr. Paul C. Colonna, Dr. Coyne H. Campbell and Dr. F. Redding Hood, all of Oklahoma City.

What Every Woman Doesn't Know— How to Give Cod Liver Oil

What Every Woman Doesn't Know is that psychology is more important than flavoring in persuading children to take cod liver oil. Some mothers fail to realize, so great is their own distaste for cod liver oil, that most babies will not only take the oil if properly given, but will actually enjoy it. Proof of this is seen in orphanages and pediatric hospitals where cod liver oil is administered as a food in a matter of fact manner, with the results that refusals are rarely encountered.

The mother who wrinkles her nose and "makes a face" of disgust as she measures out cod liver oil is almost certain to set the pattern for similar behavior on the part of her baby.

Most babies can be taught to take the pure oil if, as Eliot points out, the mother looks on it with favor and no unpleasant associations are attached to it. If the mother herself takes some of the oil, the child is further encouraged.

The dose of cod liver oil may be followed by orange juice, but if administered at an early age, usually no vehicle is required. The oil should not be mixed with the milk or the cereal feeding unless allowance is made for the oil which clings to the bottle or the bowl.

On account of its higher potency in Vitamins A and D, Mead's Cod Liver Oil Fortified With Precomorph Liver Oil may be given in one-third the ordinary cod liver oil dosage, and is particularly desirable in cases of fat intolerance.

Annual Washington's Birthday Clinics To Be Held by Internists Association

The Annual Washington's Birthday clinics of the Oklahoma City Internists Association will be held Monday, February 23, at the University hospital in Oklahoma City, Dr. Mary V. Sheppard, secretary of the Internists Association, has announced.

The clinics will start at 9:30 in the morning and will be in session until 4:00 o'clock in the afternoon. During the noon luncheon, a round-table discussion of current problems will be held.

Members of the Medical Association are invited to attend the clinics and luncheon as guests of the Internists Association.

BOOK REVIEWS

"The chief glory of every people arises from its authors."—Dr. Samuel Johnson.

"THE DOCTORS MAYO." H. B. Clapesattle. Price $3.75. Pp. 800, 57 illustrations, notes and index. Minneapolis: University of Minnesota Press, 1941.

Since this review is intended for members of the medical profession, it seems appropriate to quote freely from the Foreword by Guy Stanton Ford, President of the University of Minnesota.

"If there be a fixed point from which to reckon the origin of this volume and the relation of the University of Minnesota Press to it, it is perhaps the day in 1927 when I suggested to Dr. W. J. Mayo that he write his autobiography and let the Press publish it. Knowing him as I did, I had little hope of getting him to write his own story—if for no other reason than that the idea of anything like personal exploitation was beyond his own and his profession's code. Furthermore, the whole great achievement was so much the work of "my brother and I" that it could never be told in terms of an individual. Had he given my suggestion the slightest consideration the outcome would, I am sure, have been put under seal until he and Dr. Charlie were long beyond any misinterpretation or reasonable criticism of themselves or the institutions, Clinic and Foundation, that they created.

"There was nothing novel in my insisting as a historian rather than as chairman of the university committee on the Press that the story must be told. That it would be told whether the Drs. Mayo wished it or not and in terms they could not personally or professionally sanction was borne in upon them over and over again during the last decades of their lives. It was a story that many wanted to hear, many wanted to write, and that publishers would gladly print. The requests for the privilege of preparing and publishing a volume on their lives and on the Clinic were numerous, sometimes insistent, and always embarrassing whether they came from the competent or the incompetent. Even more distressing to the Drs. Mayo and their associates were the unauthorized articles and sketches that appeared with increasing frequency. It was evident to even the most reluctant of the group that some positive and constructive action must be taken."

In October 1936, with the above facts in mind, President Coffman and Guy Stanton Ford, then Dean of the Graduate School, "cornered the Drs. Mayo and their chief advisers in the cabin (of their yacht) and put before them the case for the publication of a volume on themselves and their work." "President Coffman and I ended the conference on our part by offering, on behalf of the university, to have prepared and published by the University Press an objective biography that would so far as possible meet the standards of a profession, that of history, whose ethical code is as definite and as high as that of the medical profession. Here at least I was speaking of what I knew, for my professorship was in history, my father was a country doctor of the old school, and as dean of the graduate school for over twenty years I had been directly and indirectly concerned with doctors and their education.

"The Drs. Mayo and their associates were evidently relieved to have the university assume the responsibility involved and stated frankly that on that condition and that alone would they willingly see the volume undertaken. They would do whatever they could in making their records available. Beyond that they wanted no part in it."

After spending three years at the difficult task of sifting a great mass of material, Helen B. Clapesattle, the author of this voluminous work, presents more than 800 pages of biographical and historical data so arranged as to give a colorful picture of the Drs. Mayo and a creditable account of scientific progress in the crowning century of all medical history. Here is a moving drama of accomplishment with the father and two sons holding the stage for more than a hundred years.

The author has skillfully revealed the significance of the period in which the Drs. Mayo lived and she has properly stressed the effect of local influences in the development of a remarkable family career. But the story does not fail to show that through individual and concerted alertness and farsighted industry, they were always ready when opportunity knocked. This is evident not only in the scientific phase of their progress, but in their ability to choose capable coworkers and to awaken in them an inspiration for accomplishment. And what is more remarkable, they manifested unusual executive, administrative and business ability. With a comprehensive vision they witnessed the gradual development of a clinic which has attracted the attention of medical men throughout the world and extended its service through teaching and practice to virtually every country on the globe.

The first part of the book presents the heroic story of "The Old Doctor." Here is a vivid picture of pioneer medicine on the middle border where service to the patient was akin to that given by Ian MacLaren's beloved Dr. MacLure; where hazards and hardships were welcomed as a part of the daily routine. No matter how difficult the task, it was accompanied by the unselfish spirit, characteristic of the country doctor before the softening influence of modern living.

Will and Charlie were born into this atmosphere of unselfish service which was so freely shared by their courageous mother. As they grew to maturity there was improved transportation; the resources of the surrounding country were marshalled; and the practice of medicine was undergoing a rapid change. They studied medicine and joined their father when medical science was entering a period of unprecedented evolution.

The second part of the book is devoted to this development under the title, "Will and Charlie." Time will not permit a detailed discussion of this phase of the story which occupies nearly 400 pages. It shows not only the development and rapid growth of the Mayo Clinic, but the world-wide progress which served as a stimulus for the Mayo brothers.

The third part deals with the "Clinic and Foundation," and shows how the management of the Clinic was divorced from family control; how a part of the Mayo fortune was devoted to endowment of the Foundation for the development of the fellowship plan through affiliation with the University of Minnesota; and finally, a provision for perpetuation of the Clinic through the regular income from the same.

In *The Drs. Mayo* we find an example of good biographical writing interwoven with a great store of related historical facts.—Lewis J. Moorman.

"THE MARCH OF MEDICINE," New York Academy of Medicine Lectures to the Laity, 1941. Pages xiii & 154. Price $2.00. Published November 24, 1941."

"These essays originated as lectures to the laity at the New York Academy of Medicine. Their purpose is twofold, first to show historically how medicine has developed, and second to reveal its social and cultural significance.

"'The lectures in this 1941 edition of 'The March of Medicine' range the whole history of the subject. At one end are discussions of the relation of humanism to science, and of philosopy as therapy. And, looking toward the future, are papers on cancer and the endocrine glands.''

Contents

Foreword by Malcolm Goodridge, M.D.; Introduction by Haven Emerson, M.D.

1. Humanism and Science, The Linsley R. Williams Memorial Lecture, by Alan Gregg, M.D.
2. Paracelsus in the Light of Four Hundred Years, by Henry E. Siegerist, M.D.
3. Psychiatry and the Normal Life, by William Healy, M.D.
4. Philosophy as Therapy, by Irwin Edman, Ph.D.
5. The Promise of Endocrinology, by Oscar Riddle, Ph.D.
6. What We Do Know About Cancer, by Francis Carter Wood, M.D.

Index

* (Condensed from a review from the Columbia University Press).

"SYNOPSIS OF ALLERGY." Harry L. Alexander, A.B., M.D., Professor of Clinical Medicine, Washington University School of Medicine, St. Louis; Editor of The Journal of Allergy. Cloth. Price $3.00. Pp. 246, with 22 illustrations, 29 tables. St. Louis. C. V. Mosby Co., 1941.

This book is a concise presentation of the various common allergic diseases and less common allergic conditions encountered in general and special practice. The various subjects are presented in a practical way and the reading is understandable. The chapter on atopy clarifies in simple language a very confusing subject. The nature of atopic antibodies is adequately and clearly discussed as well as the nature of hypersensitivities and the mechanism of sensitization.

In the early part of the book, there is an outline of diagnostic methods which has a special appeal because of the completeness and clarity of the various procedures. There is a discussion of the significance of skin testing, with indications and evaluation of the various techniques employed. The methods of passive transfer, ophthalmic tests, mucosal (nasal) tests, and leucopenic tests, are briefly outlined in sufficient detail for anyone to use these particular or special methods of investigation.

There are several tables of recommended schedules for hyposensitization which may be used as a guide in treatment. These schedules may be followed in desensitization of patients who are markedly sensitive as well as those who are only moderately sensitive. The author briefly discusses the problem of management in regard to foods with rather complete tables for elimination diets and methods of oral desensitization to foods.

There is a very interesting chapter on bronchial asthma in which the pathological changes are described in both the acute and chronic cases. Laboratory procedures recommended for asthmatic patients are discussed as well as the treatment and the drug management. There is a short discussion on the treatment of status asthmaticus, a very important addition to the book. The latter part of the chapter discusses the common complications of asthma, including sinusitis, bronchitis, bronchiectasis, and eczema. Two interesting pages offer considerable enlightenment on the subject of cardiac complications in asthma, based on 50 autopsies of chronic asthmatic sufferers.

In the chapter on hay fever, some discussion is lent to the matter of common pollinating plants, with fairly good pictures to aid in the identification of various plants, particularly weeds and grasses. The discussion of co-seasonal, pre-seasonal and perennial treatment is rather complete, with indications and recommendations for frequency of treatment and the dosage to be followed.

Chapters on atopic rhinitis, headaches, and conjunctivitis are briefly included in this synopsis. The chapter on allergic dermatoses is very good and considers all of the atopic involvements of the skin, including urticaria, both acute and chronic, allergic purpura, eczema, atopic and contact dermatitis. There is a table in this chapter which includes a standard list of contactants recommended by the author for contact testing, with the proper amounts or dilutions of the testing agent to be used. The discussion of contact dermatitis as well as the other skin problems of the allergic individual is very interesting and rich in practical information, diagnosis and methods of treatment. There are a number of prescriptions for lotions, emulsions, etc. A separate chapter on the subject of "Drug Allergy" is very informative, and the table of common drugs listing the usual symptoms and reactions produced by each is a valuable reference source.

Of considerable interest to clinicians desiring to do their own testing is the chapter which deals entirely with the preparation of extracts for both food and pollen testing and the author's method of standardization. Directions are also given for sterilization of products and formulas for the commonly used extracting fluids.

In the appendix there is a very interesting list of common household remedies, cosmetics, etc., showing their ingredients. The latter part of the appendix deals entirely with the diagnostic methods and the interpretation of both intradermal and scratch testing. There is a list of recipes for elimination diets.

This synopsis is an excellent treatise on the subject of allergy. The author has been very successful in keeping to the point throughout the entire book of 238 pages, adequately supplied with original tables and pictures. This book can be recommended to clinicians interested in the problems of allergy.—Wayne M. Hull.

"MANAGEMENT OF THE CARDIAC PATIENT." William G. Leaman, Jr., M.D., F.A.C.P. Cloth. Price $6.50. 705 pages. 255 original illustrations, two of which are in color. J. B. Lippincott company, Philadelphia.

In slightly less than 700 pages, the author has compounded an excellent treatise on heart disease. His approach to therapy is through an attempt to understand the etiology, diagnosis, pathology and disturbed physiology present. There is very little indulgence in the theoretical aspects of heart disease and little reference to controversial subjects so that there is "much meat but little gristle" to digest.

The discussion of so many case histories taken from the author's wide clinical experience gives a practical tone to the entire book. Especially interesting is the chapter on the Social Adjustment of the Cardiac Patient. The chapter on Electro-cardiography is well presented.

There is a very good discussion concerning Venous Pressure and its limitations but, unfortunately, there is an error. In giving the normal range, the author refers to 6-12 millimeters of water rather than centimeters. This is a small item and will cause little trouble.

All in all, the book is well composed and well edited. This reviewer recommends it highly to the general practitioner as well as the specialist.—Bert E. Mulvey, M.D.

Chicago Selected for 1942 Clinical Congress Of the American College of Surgeons

Because of the war, the thirty-second annual Clinical Congress of the American College of Surgeons will be held in Chicago October 19 to 23, instead of in Los Angeles as originally planned. Headquarters will be at the Stevens Hotel. The twenty-fifth annual Hospital Standardization Conference sponsored by the College will be held simultaneously. The programs of both meetings will be based chiefly on wartime activities as they affect surgeons and hospital personnel in military and civilian service.

REVIEWS and CORRESPONDENCE

SURGERY AND GYNECOLOGY

Abstracts, Reviews and Comments From
LeRoy Long Clinic
714 Medical Arts Building, Oklahoma City

"A COMPARATIVE ANALYSIS OF TOTAL ABDOMINAL, SUPRAVAGINAL, AND VAGINAL HYSTERECTOMIES." Hillard E. Miller, M.D., F.A.C.S., and Orin Prejean, M.D., New Orleans, La. American Journal of Obstetrics and Gynecology, October, 1941, Vol. 42, No. 4, Page 581.

This is a review of the hysterectomies done on the Tulane University Gynecological Service of Charity hospital during 1939 and 1940. There were a total of 828 consecutive hysterectomies divided as follows: 374 total abdominal with a mortality rate of 1.33 percent; 255 supravaginal with a mortality rate of 2.75 percent and 199 vaginal hysterectomies with a mortality rate of 1.0 percent.

"THE EFFECT OF GONADOTROPINS UNDER THE HUMAN OVARY." Samuel H. Geist, M.D., Joseph A. Gaines, M.D., and Udall J. Salmon, M.D., New York, N. Y. American Journal of Obstetrics and Gynecology, October, 1941, Vol. 42, No. 4, Page 619.

This study is well summarized by the authors as follows:

"The effect of a variety of gonadotropins upon the human ovary was studied in a series of 911 cases.

"The following gonadotropins were used: hypophyseal, chorionic, pregnant mares, serum; combination of chorionic and hypophyseal, chorionic and equine, and chorionic and stilbestrol.

"The histologic alterations in the human ovary caused by the various gonadotropins differed quantitatively rather than qualitatively. The intensity of reaction was most marked following the hypophyseal gonadotropins, decidedly less with equine, and least with the chorionic gonadotropins. The histopathologic ovarian changes in the majority of instances in which the hypophyseal gonadotropin was administered, included enlargement of cystic follicles, proliferation of the granulosa cells lining these follicles, proliferations and luteinization of the theca interna cells, perifollicular congestion and hemorrhage, and occasional edema and congestion of the ovarian parenchyma. With the equine gonadotropin, similar alterations were noted, but in a smaller precentage of cases and to a lesser degree. The only conspicuous effect of the chorionic gonadotropin was the production of perifollicular congestion and hemorrhage.

"No synergistic effects were observed with any of the gonadotropin combinations. The response to the hypophyseal and chorionic or the hypophyseal and equine gonadotropins did not materially differ from those following the use of the pituitary extract alone. The combination of equine and chorionic gonadotropins had no greater effect than that induced by the sum of the individual components. Stilbestrol was not found to enhance the activity of the chorionic hormone.

"In no instance was evidence of ovulation found which could be unquestionably attributed to the administered gonadotropins.

"The absence of any increase in the number of maturing Graafian follicles, the absence of ova or degenerative remnants of ova in the cystic follicles, and the absence of induced ovulations suggests that, while the available gonadotropins may stimulate those granulosa and theca interna cells, in follicles undergoing atresia, which are still capable of response, they apparently do not induce follicle maturation or stimulate the development of follicles containing normal ova to maturity and ovulation."

COMMENT: Recently, a series of articles upon this important subject were abstracted in these columns. At that time, we spoke of this excellent work of Geist and his associates which is most discuraging as far as the effect of our present gonadotropins. Since satisfactory effective gonadotropins must be found before many of the menstrual and ovulatory disturbances in women can be corrected, it is earnestly hoped that we will soon have such a product. From the work that has been done it is much more likely to be a direct extract of the anterior pituitary gland itself.

For the purpose of stimulating proper ovulation and menstruation, we must still rely upon general medical measures and desiccated thyroid extract therapy.—Wendell Long.

"PROLIFERATIVE CHANGES IN THE SENILE ENDOMETRIUM." Emil Novak, M.D., and E. H. Richardson, Jr., M.D., Baltimore, Md. American Journal of Obstetrics and Gynecology, October, 1941, Vol. 42, No. 4, Page 564.

This is a histological study of 137 endometriums obtained both by curettage and hysterectomy and all of these patients did not necessarily have postmenopausal bleeding.

Twenty additional cases were discarded because the endometrial curettings were insufficient for histological study and probably indicated a marked degree of atrophy.

This study was undertaken to demonstrate the frequency and clinical importance of hyperplastic endometrium after the menopause.

"A study was made of 137 endometriums from women ranging from 2 to 40 years after the menopause. Less than one-half of these, 62 cases, showed the atrophic changes usually looked upon as characteristic of the senile endometrium. Fully 42 presented pictures of proliferative activity, moderate in 14, while 28 showed considerable areas of outspoken hyperplasia similar to that seen so often during reproductive life. These findings are no doubt to be linked up with the well-known fact that estrogen may be produced long after the menopause. The source of this postmenopausal estrogen is not definitely known, though it seems reasonably certain that it is not in the ovaries, but rather in some of the other endocrine glands, probably the adrenals.

"The endometriums in this series were studied in age groups, showing a striking lack of correlation between the ages of the patients and the histology of the endometrium. The mucosa of some women show marked atrophy within a few months of the last period, while that of others, 30 or 40 years later, may show striking hyperplasia. The latter, for example, was found in 5 women of 70 or over, the oldest being 87 years.

"The clinical importance of these findings lies in the fact that postmenopausal bleeding is a not infrequent symptom in such cases, and it would seem likely that it is due to a hormonal mechanism like that involved in the common functional hemorrhage of the reproductive era.

"The remaining 33 cases of this series revealed a histologic picture which we consider to represent a retrogressed hyperplasia. It is characterized by a typical Swiss cheese pattern, but with obvious evidence of retrogression and inactivity, such as fibrosis of the stroma. The significance of this endometrial pattern is that the hyperplasia pattern found in a large proportion of menopausal women persists for many years thereafter, although the causative hormonal factor is no longer operative. Finally, our findings suggest that this residual hyperplasia, rather than inflammation or stromal cicatrization, is the most frequent explanation of the cystic gland distention so often seen in senile endometriums."

COMMENT: This investigation has a practical aspect in that it reveals again .the frequency of hyperplastic endometrium in postmenopausal uteri.

It should be stressed that this article in no way lessens the absolute necessity for thorough diagnostic curettage in all women who have bleeding from the uterus after the menopause. It is only by this means that carcinoma of the uterine body can be identified early enough to warrant hopes for good results from treatment.

There is an additional precaution which should be observed in the curettage of women who have postmenopausal bleeding. Some of these patients have uterine bleeding because of an ovarian tumor which is hormonally active as well as malignant, and the enlarged senile ovary can be identified only by careful pelvic examination under anesthesia at the time of curettage.

The intriguing question of the relationship between postmenopausal hyperplastic endometrium and adenocarcinoma of uterine body is not raised in this study but in former publications by Taylor and also Novak. One must agree that there is a reasonably frequent association of the two conditions whether or not it is cause and effect or different stages of the same disease. —Wendell Long.

EYE, EAR, NOSE AND THROAT
Edited by Marvin D. Henley, M. D.
911 Medical Arts Building, Tulsa

"SYMPTOMLESS PERIOD OF BRONCHIAL FOREIGN BODIES." Paul Bailey, Portland ,Ore. Northwest Medicine, Vol. 40, page 365-367, October, 1941.

After the aspiration of a potentially lethal foreign body, there nearly always follows a symptomless period during which the significance of an occasional wheeze or cough may be overlooked.

There is often no history of the aspiration of a foreign body. Foreign bodies are unknowingly inhaled during periods of emotion, excitement, in automobile collisions or even slight falls and during anesthesia. Alcohol in large doses produces a degree of anesthesia.

Cough and gagging are usually experienced at the moment of aspiration, but this is sometimes not the case. A shingler could inhale a full-sized nail and not cough at all. Such patients may be presented weeks or months after the accident at which time they may be symptomless.

The symptomless period is extremely variable and depends on the character, size and shape of the foreign body. If a vegetable irritant mass obstructs the bronchus, the symptomless interval may be a matter of moments, even seconds. On the other hand, the non-irritant metal nail may be quitely resident for months or even years, if there is left a by-pass for transfer of air and lung secretion.

Less than three percent of bronchial foreign bodies are coughed out again. Inhaled peanuts will not disintegrate; they are not digested by the lung. The only sign at the symptomless stage is elicitation of an asthmatoid wheeze at the end of forced expiration. It is clearest after secretion is expelled by coughing. Presence of this wheeze always suggests bronchial foreign body, and immediate examination and continued observation is justified.

Vegetable bodies are extremely irritating to the bronchial mucosa and they rapidly induce annular swelling of the mucosa. Soon the airway is obstructed, and a check valve mechanism is set up which traps the air in the lung distal to the obstruction. This condition is called "obstructive emphysema" and signifies the end of the symptomless period.

The obstructive emphysema is followed by atelectasis, and the continued mucosal swelling buries the foreign body so that even at inspiration no air can pass by. Secondary infection takes place rapidly, and high fever, toxemia as well as dyspnea, and prostration are added to the manifestations. Patients at this stage are very poor surgical risks, yet, bronchoscopic removal of the foreign body is urgent.

The proper time for the removal of bronchial foreign bodies is during the symptomless period and before the development of undesired sequelae. Careful examination during this period will result in correct diagnosis. Careful roentgen study will demonstrate a to and fro shift of the heart and mediastinum, which is characteristic of obstructive emphysema. With atelectasis, there is no respiratory to and fro mediastinal shift and the foreign body will be found on the side to which the heart is shifted, whereas with obstructive emphysema, the foreign body will be on the side from which the heart moves at expiration.

"CANCER OF THE LUNGS." A Ceballos, Buenos Aires. La Prensa medica Argentina, Vol. 28, page 1843-1855, September, 1941.

General observation in hospitals and private institutions shows that there is an increase in pulmonary cancer. Twenty-five years ago, the autopsy of a lung cancer was a rarity. At the Pathological Institute of Elizalde, there were 16 primary and seven metastatic lung cancer cases examined in 244 autopsies in 1939, while in the period of from 1905 to 1908, there has not been a single case of lung cancer found. In Roffo's Cancer Institute the rate of incidence of pulmonary carcinoma was 0.39 percent in 1926; it is now 3.03 percent. Sergent ,of Paris, asserted in 1939 that the increased incidence is only relative; he believes that much of the pulmonary cancer material was hidden formerly under such terms as chronic suppuration of the lungs. But most of the other investigators are certain that the increase is absolute. Roffo stated that, together with the increase in pulmonary cancer, the number of cutaneous cancer is also higher in Argentina.

The author himself has observed more and more lung cancer cases in recent years (after 1928), often in such a number that one could almost speak of an epidemic of pulmonary carcinoma. Most of the patients were inhabitants of cities, and it was very rare to find a person with lung cancer who has been living in remote districts of Argentina or in Patagonia.

Many factors have been suspected in the absolute increase of pulmonary cancer. Some authors thought that the great influenza epidemic of 1918 prepared the lungs of the whole world for the development of cancer. A group of scientists believes that the chief etiological factor is tuberculosis. There have been actual observations of cancer beginning in tuberculous cavities of the lungs. It seems, however, that the association of tuberculosis and cancer in the same lung is merely coincidental; in fact, tuberculosis has rather a regressive influence upon pulmonary cancer.

Successful or hopeful treatment depends on the early diagnosis: the lung cancer should be recognized before the lymphnodes become affected. Pulmonary cancer starts its development in the bronchial epithelium, and the best prognosis is for those tumors that develop in the peripheric subcortical bronchi. For a shorter or longer time, the cancer does not produce any symptoms, yet there are cases in which the development of lung cancer is so rapid that the disease is mistaken for lung abscess. The bronchus is plugged by the tumor, and the lung becomes atelectatic; soon, suppuration sets in, which will result in pleural adhesions.

The initial symptoms are not characteristic, and resemble those of ordinary chronic catarrhs. The most frequent symptom is cough with or without expectoration. There may also be pain, especially in case of cancer of the apex of the lung; the pain may irradiate to the arms and fingers. Other cases are symptomless, and the presence of tumor is only occasionally discovered at the time of a chest roentgenography. Some physicians distinguish a clinical, a roentgenological and a bronchoscopical stage in the development of pulmonary cancer.

The clinical phase of development includes such manifestations as cough, bloody sputum, hemoptysis, and pain in the chest. The diagnosis is chiefly based upon radiological examination, but the radiological signs are not pathognomonic. The roentgenogram varies according to the evolution and extension of the tumor. Recently, much effort has been made for the evaluation of cells found in the sputum. If cancer cells are found, the diagnosis of lung cancer is almost certain, but absence of cancer cells does not speak against such a diagnosis. Bronchography is of great important in the recognition of pulmonary malignant tumors. Other means of diagnosis are the thoracoscopy and the bronchoscopy, but bronchoscopy itself is not a great help.

Attempts for the treatment of lung cancer are either radiological or surgical. The surgical measures include the resection of the lung, the lobectomy and the pneumectomy. Bronchoscopic removal may be possible in a few cases. In the author's experience, radiotherapy was of little value; this is also the concensus of opinion of the majority of surgeons.

Surgical treatment of lung cancer is a rather new invention. The first pneumectomy, for bronchiectasis, was performed by Nissen in 1031. The first operation for lung cancer was done by Graham in 1933. Partial operations (cauterization, etc.) have been referred to by Sauerbruch. The total pneumectomy, which is the only surgical measure of any success, is a difficult operation with a considerable high mortality rate. Presence of infection almost certainly makes the operation a failure; there are also various accidents that may happen during the surgical intervention. Ligation of the pulmonary artery is only a palliative measure followed by a slight temporary relief.

"SUPRAORBITAL NEURALGIA OF MALARIAL ORIGIN." Boletin del Hospital Oftalmologico de Ntra. Sra. De lo Luz. Mexico. Vol. 2. page 209-214. June. 1941.

For many years the author has been studying eye patients coming from the vast malarial zones of Veracruz, Tabasco, and the isthmus of Tehuantepec. He has observed a great number of patients with ocular manifestations of malaria. He saw malaria patients with papillitis, neuroretinitis, retrobulbar neuritis, paralysis of the extrinsic muscles of the eye, transient increases in eye tension, etc., but the most frequent eye symptom in these patients was the neuralgia of the supraorbital nerve.

Neuralgia of the supraorbital nerve in malaria patients is usually coexistent with neuralgia of some other branches of the trigeminal nerve, the constant participation of the occipital nerve being characteristic. The condition occurs not only in cases of active malaria but also in patients whose malaria has been cured. It is strange that the ocular complications of malaria have been so little studied and so rarely mentioned in the literature.

Most of the malarial ocular complications affect the nervous system of the eye and its adnexa, which is explained by the neurotropic nature of the toxins of plasmodia. The symptoms themselves and the evolution of these manifestations resemble generally the development of toxic neuritis, especially the neuritis caused by intestinal parasites. The papillitis and the optic neuritis produce mostly congestive symptoms without inflammatory exudates or degenerative lesions.

Supraorbital neuralgia is very typical and very frequent in malaria patients. The very fact that someone was a resident in a malarial territory, and suffers from supraorbital neuralgia, may be used for the diagnosis of obscure fevers and may be the foundation of the diagnosis of malaria.

The patients consult oculists and otologists because they attribute the painful symptoms to ocular, nasal and auricular disturbances. It may happen that the specialist detects errors of refraction in the painful malarial eye, and, not suspecting malaria, prescribes eyeglasses, which very often will increase the patient's subjective complaints. Sometimes, especially in a case of unilateral supraorbital neuralgia, the frontal or the ethmoid sinus is blamed for the pain, or a carious tooth is searched for. This may result in needless surgery on the nasal sinuses, unnecessary extraction of teeth, etc.

The neuralgia is almost always unilateral, being most frequently on the left side. One important and relatively frequent form of ocular complication is a hyperemia of the papilla associated with slight ocular hypertension, and narrowing of the visual field, together with neuritis of the supraorbital nerve. There may be photophobia and slight loss of vision. All symptoms may quickly disappear after treatment of the neuralgic pain. Characteristic for the supraorbital neuralgic pain is its periodicity, and its change with the change of climate or altitude.

The supraorbital, and other malarial neuralgias may exist without positive laboratory findings of malaria. The best treatment is with quinine given intravenously. Plasmoquin and atabrine are less efficacious.

PLASTIC SURGERY
Edited by George H. Kimball, M. D., F. A. C. S.
912 Medical Arts Building, Oklahoma City

"URETRO-INTESTINAL IMPLANTATION." Southern Medical Journal Vol. 35 Jan. 1942. No. 1.

The author has perfected a plan for uretero-intestinal anastomosis, whereby he first places the ureters in the wall of the bowel without angulation, torsion, tension, or compression. He plants each ureter at the same time. Two weeks later he divides the lower end of the ureter and through the lumen at the distal end he passes an electrode to make the fistula between the ureter and the sigmoid. This plan allows for the ureter to become attached to the bowel aseptically. The second step allows the opening to be made without danger of contamination. The technic is very well illustrated by drawings and photographs.

The author reports seven cases by this technic. One case died suddenly about two months after the last operation, but an autopsy was not obtained.

The author did this type of operation on ten experimental animals with good results.

Comments: I believe that the technic described is a decided improvement in transplantation of the ureter into the bowel. Anyone interested in this operation should read the entire article. One of the principal objections to this plan is the finding of the lower end of the ureter following the second operation. This disadvantage, however, is not so great as the contamination which may occur by another method.

CARDIOLOGY

Edited by F. Redding Hood, M. D
1200 North Walker, Oklahoma City

"ENLARGEMENT OF THE HEART." P. D. White, New England M. Med. 225:571-574 (Oct. 9), 1941.

The causes of heart damage are widely known, but the significance of cardiac enlargement is not often enough appreciated, possibly because, in the early stages at least, it is not readily discernible. Heart murmurs, irregularities and arrhythmias are easily detected; the signs and symptoms of heart failure are not hard to recognize. The ease with which, by means of technical refinements in diagnostic methods, murmurs and arrhythmias may be elicited has lead to the neglect of the functionally more important condition of heart size.

The first cardiac abnormality of consequence to be described was enlargement of the heart. That was when palpation and percussion were the only means available for heart study. By the development of the technic of auscultation, attention was diverted from the more fundamental consideration of the size of the heart.

MacKenzie sought to lead clinicians back to first principles. He started with careful observation and painstaking manual and visual examination. After confirming thus gained opinions with the aid of mechanical devices, he returned to the use of his hands and eyes for knowledge applicable to diagnosis, prognosis and treatment. Paul D. White, M.D., of Harvard Medical school, Boston, also insists that the art of percussion be revived as a method of cardiac examination, useful in its own right and necessary as a corrective check of roentgenograms, or when elaborate diagnostic equipment is not conveniently at hand.

Cardiac enlargement is not to be considered an indication of heart strength; it means that the myocardium is not normal, that it has been under strain, is still overtaxed and, consequently, is likely to fail.

Enlargement of the heart may be due to acute dilatation—a designation often formerly used but more recently disdained—or to preponderant hypertrophy, or to both. Increase in the size of the heart probably starts as overstretching of the muscle with subsequent hypertrophy. The process may go on by stages, with arrest for long periods, over a great many years; it may stop at any point.

INTRINSIC CAUSES. Four conditions which lead to acute dilatation are: (1) Severe, acute rheumatic myocarditis; (2) Prolonged paroxysmal tachycardia, and; (3) Massive pulmonary embolism affecting the right ventricle.

The acute condition may cause early death or may remain stationary, to be followed by compensatory hypertrophy. With systemic or pulmonary hypertension or aortic stenosis, hypertrophy may occur first, dilatation coming on later as a manifestation of final failure.

Dilatation happens first with aortic regurgitation, but hypertrophy soon ensues to an extent warranting the designation "cor bovinum." Mitral valve disease and auricular fibrillation engender hearts of record breaking size, with enormous left and right auricles and right ventricles, but normal or small left ventricles. Which chamber shows initial changes depends upon the causal lesion, whether it be hypertension, pulmonary disease, or defects of one or more valves.

Enlargement of the left ventricle increases heart weight; a big left auricle displaces greater space. More attention should be given to the size of the right ventricle; if it alone is enlarged, it may easily be overlooked. The electrocardiagram may give the clue. The usual reason for enlargement of the right ventricle is failure of the left.

EXTRINSIC CAUSES. Extracardiac causes, such as anemia or myxedema, are often responsible for producing cardiac enlargement. Chronic pericarditis, once wrongly blamed for bringing about enlargement of the heart, is now known not to do so.

The range of normal heart size is exceedingly difficult to evaluate with certainty. Even the anatomist or pathologist cannot designate heart weights and volumes for normal persons within any practically useful limits. To say that the weight of the heart shall be 0.5 percent of the body weight is a very imperfect estimate indeed. Body build and hereditary tendencies must be considered.

PALPATION AND PERCUSSION. The simplest way to appraise heart size is to locate the position of the apical impulse by palpation. In those cases in which the maximum apex impulse lies in the fifth interspace within or on the midclavicular line, it may be declared that there is no significant cardiac enlargement. This maneuver must be supplemented by percussion of the left border of the heart, to determine undue prominence of the right ventricle, auricle or pulmonary vessels.

There is such great variation of heart size depending upon chest confirmation, age, height and weight that only the simplest diameters need be measured on seven foot roentgenograms.

FLUOROSCOPY. Actual visualization of the patient under the fluoroscopic screen is the best method for obtaining a comprehensive idea not only of the size but also the shape of the heart in relation to the thoracic cage. The "cardiothoracic" ratio has too wide a variation, 33 percent to 55 percent, to be an accurate index to heart size. A better judgment may be made by correlating the transverse diameter of the heart with height, weight and age by slide rule or nomograms (Hodges-Eyster).

The greatest skill, with full knowledge of all modifying factors, is required to ascertain with exactitude very slight enlargements; but discovery of early enlargement is the most important single prognostic finding. The prognosis of heart disease may be epitomized in the blunt statement, "The larger the heart, the worse the future."

TREATMENT. The implication for treatment is also inherent in cardiac size, even more surely than in the presence of murmurs or arrhythmias. Increase in size of the heart means that the organ is being overtaxed. Therefore, whatever the strain is, it should be relieved. Conversely, all hearts that are presumably under strain by reason of underlying intra- and extracardiac disease must be closely investigated for signs of enlargement.

It seems reasonable also to give one or one and one-half gr. of digitalis daily to patients with cardiac enlargement, although the value of the drug for this purpose has yet to be proved on other than empirical bases.

ORTHOPAEDIC SURGERY

Edited by Earl D. McBride, M. D., F. A. C. S.
605 N. W. 10th, Oklahoma City

"MALIGNANT TUMORS OF TENDON SHEATHS." E. S. J. King. The Australian and New Zealand Journal of Surgery. X. 338, 1941.

Seven cases of synovial sarcomata are described in detail to emphasize the peculiarities of the malignant type of synovial tumor.

In general, the tumors are well delineated and are attached to a tendon sheath originally. After a latent phase, they suddenly increase in size and invade neighboring tissues, occasionally metastasizing to regional lymph nodes, liver, and lungs.

Microscopically, the tumors present a varied appearance, but there is an abundance of closely spheroidal or spindle cells with mucoid interstitial material and synovial spaces. These have a lining of connective tissue resembling normal synovial membrane. This lining membrane compares with that found in osteoarthritic joints, and can be distinguished only by the presence of mitiotic figures and by examination of the adjacent tissue.

Local excision of these tumors is unsuccessful, since in six of the seven cases there were recurrences or metastases. Radium implantation, together with wide excision of the tumor mass, has given the only satisfactory results.

"THE SURGICAL TREATMENT OF LEG LENGTH DISCREPANCIES." Paul H. Harmon and William M. Krigsten. Illinois Med. Jr., LXXIX, 300, 1941.

The authors discuss the indications, operative technique, and relative value of three methods used for treatment of leg-length discrepancies: 1. epiphyseal arrest; 2. leg shortening; and 3. leg lengthening. Over 120 patients at the University of Chicago clinics have had operations for epiphyseal arrest, many having had more than one epiphysis closed. There were no postoperative infections or deaths. In two patients the short leg overgrew the sound leg, but in several, especially in girls, the operation was performed too late to be effective. The tendency has been to arrest growth at the knee in the femur only, but now the authors state they would also fuse the tibial and fibular epiphyses. Epiphyseal arrest should rarely be done after the age of 11 or 12 in girls, and 13 to 15 in boys, as very little or no growth can be expected in the long bones.

Thirty-five patients, with more than two inches of shortening, had operative shortening of the femur in the sound side. Except in one case in which infection was followed with loss of bone grafts and slight angulation, the results were excellent, with union in all cases. This method of leg-length equalization is mathematically accurate when properly done, and, although it carries greater operative risk than epiphyseal arrest, it has wide application.

In ten patients, 11 leg-lengthening operations were performed, four on the tibia and seven on the femur. One patient died from cellulitis and septicaemia. In two patients there was massive sequestration of the femoral diaphysis, and in one of these a stiff knee also resulted. Leg lengthening, the authors state, has limited application. They believe it is indicated in certain patients who are short of stature, but should be done only by a limited group of surgeons who have had experience with this method.

"OCCULT FRACTURES." Roland Hammond and Denis S. O'Connor. The Journal of Amer. Med. Ass'n. CXVII, 500, 1941.

The authors reemphasize the warning given in 1908 by Sir Robert Jones to the effect that clinicians must not depend solely upon roentgenograms for the diagnosis of fractures to the exclusion of clinical judgment.

In spite of the great improvement in roentgenographic technique and interpretation since that time, there yet remain cases in which a fracture cannot be demonstrated, although clinical evidence strongly suggests it and later roentgenographic evidence confirms it. Such fractures are defined by the authors as "occult fractures," and they present 12 cases.

The authors advocate continuation of the program of improved education of technicians and better training of practitioners in the interpretation of roentgenographic findings alone or in collaboration with the roentgenologist, but they point out that in case of doubt the clinical findings should always take precedence over negative or inconclusive roentgenographic findings.

INTERNAL MEDICINE

Edited by Hugh Jeter, M. D., F. A. C. P., A. S. C. P.
1200 North Walker, Oklahoma City

"RHEUMATISM AND ARTHRITIS." Review of American and English Literature for 1940. (Eighth Rheumatism Review). Philip S. Hench, M.D., F.A.C.P., Rochester, Minn., Walter Bauer, M.D., F.A.C.P., Boston, Edward Boland, M.D., Los Angeles, M. Henry Dawson, M.D., New York, Richard H. Freyberg, M.D., Ann Arbor, W. Paul Holbrook, M.D., F.A.C.P., Tucson, J. Albert Key, M.D., F.A.C.S., St. Louis, J. Maxwell Lockie, M.D., F.A.C.P., Buffalo, N. Y., and Currier McEwen, M.D., F.A.C.P., New York.

This is an annual review of a subject, pertinent abstracts of which are as follows. Snyder emphasized that more than 320,000 otherwise able persons in the United States are rendered unemployable for an entire year by these disorders; the greatest incidence occurs among persons without maintenance incomes.

Sulfanilamide in Treatment of Gonorrheal Arthritis. The treatment of gonorrheal arthritis with sulfanilamide was discussed. Sulfanilamide was generally preferred to other compounds. (Some of us prefer sulfathiazole.—Ed.)

According to Harris "an important, and perhaps large percentage of cases of run-of-the-mill arthritis are caused by Brucella infection." (With this we cannot agree. Harris gave no statistical proof. One of us, R. H. F., studied 25 cases of typical rheumatoid arthritis for evidence of brucellosis without success. Of 25 cases of rheumatism not typical of any common arthritis, in three active brucellosis was present and in six "possible brucellosis." It was concluded that rheumatic symptoms are common in brucellosis and temporary inflammation of joints may occur, but seldom if ever does brucellosis cause chronic, nonpurulent inflammation of joints.—Ed.)

Laboratory Data in Rheumatic Fever: Sedimentation Rate of Erythrocytes. This was again considered the most important single laboratory test of rheumatic activity.

Conclusions of Etiology. In Italy "the prevalent opinion is that rheumatoid arthritis is a true infectious disease: the fact that the causative agents has not yet been found does not mean that it does not exist." According to Pemberton and Scull the streptococcal antibodies present in the serums of patients with rheumatoid arthritis are "not to be dismissed from consideration, but their etiologic importance must be interpreted conservatively as non-specific until more direct evidence is at hand." Impressed by the ameliorating effect of jaundice and pregnancy on rheumatoid arthritis Osgood concluded that "the chances are better that the unknown etiologic of X factor which we know exists but which we have thus far been unable to discover will prove to be a biochemical rather than a bacterial factor." (Obviously the cause of the disease remains unknown.—Ed.)

Some of those who are now belittling the theory of focal infection (e.g., Cecil, Haden) were formerly among its staunchest advocates. (Their own frankness in explaining the reasons for their about-face is commendable and lends considerable weight to their current views. But if they were wrong once they may not yet be entirely right.—Ed.)

Still's Disease and "Felty's Syndrome." (Readers will be interested to know that Sir Frederick Still died just recently in London, aged 73 years.—Ed.)

UROLOGY

Edited by D. W. Branham, M. D.
502 Medical Arts Building, Oklahoma City

"TREATMENT OF GONORRHEA AT FITZSIMONS GEN-ERAL HOSPITAL." Donald B. Peterson and Eugene S. Beuchat. Journal of AMA. Jan. 10, 1942.

The authors detail some modification of diagnosis and treatment control in gonorrhea that may be interesting to the profession.

They modify the same technique of the usual gram stain to the effect that the safranin counter-stain is applied before decolorization. They state that such technique shifts the staining character of the pus cells to the blue side, and therefore, nuclei and cytoplasm are differentially stained.

In the management of patients who are on treatment for gonorrhea a study is made particularly of the character of the pus cell. Patients who show old necrotizing pus cells, even if secretion is present, are thought to be progressing satisfactorily to a cure with chemotherapy. If the pus cells are clear and discrete (young types) they change the therapy to fever. Fever therapy added to the treatment has increased the percentage of cures over those who have been given chemotherapy alone.

"THE USE OF POWDERED SULFANILAMIDE IN IN-FECTED GENITO-URINARY WOUNDS." Charles D. Donahue. Journal of Urology. Sept., 1941.

The authors present this article to show the beneficial effect of sulfanilamide in wounds that are infected. Four suprapubic prostatectomies were performed on patients with purulent residual urine. With the use of sulfanilamide the wounds healed by primary intention except for the area occupied by the suprapubic drains. Two of these patients were very obese and had very thick, fatty abdominal walls.

In every instance cystotomy wounds likewise healed by primary intention. Two of these patients were worse than poor operative risks, and had convalescence been other than smooth, these patients probably would not have survived.

One perirenal abscess also was operated on, with the postoperative drainage continuing only a short time. The wound around the drain closed by primary intention.

There was one ureteral transplant to the skin and one ureteral stone removed by open operation.

In conclusion, sulfanilamide powder has proven to be of value in wound healing, and may be used without fear of tissue damage. Further experimental work must be done in order to determine minimal amounts of sulfanilamide to be effective.

"CHANCROID — TREATMENT WITH SULFATHIAZOLE AND SULFANILAMIDE." Borris A. Kornblith. et al. Journal of AMA. 1941.

This report deals with 175 patients with chancroid, all of whom were treated with sulfanilamide or sulfathiazole. Before the advent of chemotherapy, surgical intervention in cases of chancroid included incision and drainage of fluctuant buboes, the dorsal slit of the prepuce, cauterization of open lesions and circumcision. Since the introduction of sulfanilamide and its derivities, radical elective surgical procedures have been eliminated. In all of the cases of inguinal adenopathy, with or without abscess formation, there was no necessity for incision. Aspiration was found sufficient when necessary.

All definitely proved chancroidal infections healed with chemotherapy. Local applications of sulfathiazole powder healed superficial chancroidal ulcerations. The use of sulfanilamide was so effective that it may be utilized as therapeutic tests in the differential diagnosis of chancroid.

Vitamin B Complex Literature Surveyed in New Abstract Book

Published as a convenience to physicians and others interested in the subject, the new Lederle Vitamin B Complex Abstract Book provides in compact form a topical survey of accomplishments in the development of Vitamin B components, and their application in a wide range of conditions.

Because the literature on the subject is already too extensive to be covered in full, this 62 page booklet presents in abstract form only the most salient of recent articles from leading medical journals and other sources. For convenience the studies pertaining to various diseases and Vitamin B Complex deficiencies are arranged alphabetically. The articles have been sufficiently condensed so that each seldom occupies more than a single page. Suggested references are included with each as a guide to more extensive reading and study.

This booklet, "Abstracts Selected from Published Articles on Vitamin B Complex and its Components" is being distributed to physicians and is available on request to Lederle Laboratories, 30 Rockefeller Plaza, New York, New York.

Quinine Sulfate Relieves "Night Cramps"

"Night cramps" were relieved in fifteen patients by means of quinine sulfate, Harold K. Moss, M.D., and Louis G. Herrmann, M.D., Cincinnati, report in The Journal of the American Medical Association.

The condition, which consists of painful spasms of muscles in the extremities, generally occurs in middle aged and elderly persons while they are at rest. On the basis of successful reports in the literature of the use of quinine in certain rare muscular diseases, the authors tried quinine sulfate for this more common condition. A beneficial effect was noted in all cases, complete cessation of pain being obtained sometimes within a few hours.

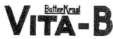

OFFICERS OF COUNTY SOCIETIES, 1942

COUNTY	PRESIDENT	SECRETARY	MEETING TIME
Alfalfa	Jack F. Parsons, Cherokee	L. T. Lancaster, Cherokee	Last Tues. Each 2nd Mo.
Atoka-Coal	J. B. Clark, Coalgate	J. S. Fulton, Atoka	
Beckham	H. K. Speed, Sayre	E. S. Kilpatrick, Elk City	Second Tues. eve.
Blaine	Virginia Olson Curtin, Watonga	W. F. Griffin, Watonga	
Bryan	A. J. Wells, Calera	W. K. Haynie, Durant	Second Tues. eve.
Caddo	Fred L. Patterson, Carnegie	C. B. Sullivan, Carnegie	
Canadian	P. F. Herod, El Reno	A. L. Johnson, El Reno	Subject to call
Carter	Walter Hardy, Ardmore	H. A. Higgins, Ardmore	
Cherokee			
Choctaw			
Cleveland	F. C. Buffington, Norman	Phil Haddock, Norman	Thursday nights
Comanche			
Cotton	George W. Baker, Walters	Mollie F. Scism, Walters	Third Friday
Craig	W. R. Marks, Vinita	J. M. McMillan, Vinita	
Creek	Frank Sisler, Bristow	O. H. Cowart, Bristow	
Custer	Richard M. Burke, Clinton	W. C. Tisdul, Clinton	Third Thursday
Garfield	D. S. Harris, Drummond	John R. Walker, Enid	Fourth Thursday
Garvin	T. F. Gross, Lindsay	John R. Callaway, Pauls Valley	Wed before 3rd Thurs.
Grady	D. S. Downey, Chickasha	Frank T. Joyce, Chickasha	3rd Thursday
Grant	I. V. Hardy, Medford	E. E. Lawson, Medford	
Greer	G. F. Border, Mangum	J. B. Hollis, Mangum	
Harmon	S. W. Hopkins, Hollis	W. M. Yeargan, Hollis	First Wednesday
Haskell	William Carson, Keota	N. K. Williams, McCurtain	
Hughes	Wm. L. Taylor, Holdenville	Imogene Mayfield, Holdenville	First Friday
Jackson	J. M. Allgood, Altus	Willard D. Holt, Altus	Last Monday
Jefferson	W. M. Browning, Waurika	J. I. Hollingeworth, Waurika	Second Monday
Kay	J. C. Wagner, Ponca City	J. Holland Howe, Ponca City	Third Thurs.
Kingfisher	C. M. Hodgson, Kingfisher	John R. Taylor, Kingfisher	
Kiowa	J. M. Bonham, Hobart	B. H. Watkins, Hobart	
LeFlore	G. R. Booth, LeFlore	Rush L. Wright, Poteau	
Lincoln	E. F. Hurlbut, Meeker	C. W. Robertson, Chandler	First Wednesday
Logan	William C. Miller, Guthrie	J. L. LeHew, Jr., Guthrie	Last Tuesday evening
Marshall			
Mayes			
McClain	B. W. Slover, Blanchard	R. L. Royster, Purcell	
McCurtain	R. D. Wilhnus, Idabel	R. H. Sherrill, Broken Bow	Fourth Tues. eve.
McIntosh	F. R. First, Checotah	William A. Tolleson, Eufaula	Second Tuesday
Murray			
Muskogee	Shade D. Neely, Muskogee	J. T. McInnis, Muskogee	First & Third Mon.
Noble	J. W. Francis, Perry	C. H. Cooke, Perry	
Okfuskee	J. M. Pemberton, Okemah	L. J. Spickard, Okemah	Second Monday
Oklahoma	R. Q. Goodwin, Okla. City	Wm. E. Eastland, Okla. City	Fourth Tuesday
Okmulgee	J. G. Edwards, Okmulgee	John R. Cotteral, Henryetta	Second Monday
Osage	C. R. Weirich, Pawhuska	George K. Hemphill, Pawhuska	Second Monday
Ottawa	J. B. Hampton, Commerce	Walter Sanger, Picher	Third Thursday
Pawnee			
Payne	John W. Martin, Cushing	James D. Martin, Cushing	Third Thursday
Pittsburg	Austin R. Stough, McAlester	Edw. D. Greenberger, McAlester	Third Friday
Pontotoc	R. E. Cowling, Ada	E. R. Muntz, Ada	First Wednesday
Pottawatomie	John Carson, Shawnee	Clinton Gallaher, Shawnee	First & Third Sat.
Pushmataha	P. B. Rice, Antlers	John S. Lawson, Clayton	
Rogers	W. A. Howard, Chelsea	P. S. Anderson, Claremore	First Monday
Seminole	H. M. Reeder, Konawa	Mack I. Shanholtz, Wewoka	
Stephens	E. C. Lindley, Duncan	A. J. Weedn, Duncan	
Texas			
Tillman	C. C. Allen, Frederick	O. G. Bacon, Frederick	
Tulsa	H. B. Stewart, Tulsa	E. O. Johnson, Tulsa	Second & Fourth Mon. eve.
Wagoner	J. H. Plunkett, Wagoner	H. K. Riddle, Coweta	
Washington-Nowata	R. W. Rucker, Bartlesville	J. V. Athey, Bartlesville	Second Wednesday
Washita	A. S. Neal, Cordell	James F. McMurry, Sentinel	
Woods	W. F. LaFon, Waynoka	O. E. Templin, Alva	Last Wednesday
Woodward	M. H. Newman, Shattuck	C. W. Tedrowe, Woodward	

THE JOURNAL
· OF THE
OKLAHOMA STATE MEDICAL ASSOCIATION

| VOLUME XXXV | OKLAHOMA CITY, OKLAHOMA, MARCH, 1942 | NUMBER 3 |

Practical Refraction*

JAMES P. LUTON, M.D.
OKLAHOMA CITY, OKLAHOMA

My purpose in presenting this paper is to set forth briefly the steps which I consider necessary in the routine refraction as related to every day practice. In outlining these procedures I am not laboring under the delusion that they are the ones which will give the best results in the hands of every practitioner because it has been proven many many times that equally good refractionists may arrive at the same conclusion by methods which are not the same. With full realization of this fact I shall enumerate my own methods and at the same time try to cite some of the reasons which justify their use.

The first step, and one which is not open to controversy is a good history, not only of the present complaints, but of the past history and family history as well. The history alone, when carefully taken and properly analyzed will often not only rule in or out the eyes as the offending organs, but it will also present some general idea in regard to the type of refractive error present. The history should include information concerning the general health, and particularly anything concerning the infections of the upper respiratory passages and the para-nasal sinuses. I'm sure we have all seen patients with symptoms apparently due to refractive errors present, but who were not relieved by correction of that error. Then with more careful history taking and possibly with the aid of the rhinologist we find pathology in the nose or sinuses which proves to be the real cause of the symptoms. In many of these cases time, money, and perhaps embarrassment might have been saved by more attention to the history. The same may be true, though less frequently, of certain gastrointestinal diseases and of certain types of pelvic pathology, not to mention numerous other possibilities. In my own experience this laxity in history taking is one of the

most frequent stumbling blocks, simply because it is too easy to listen to the patient say, "My eyes give me a headache." and to allow it to go at that.

Before beginning the second step we check the manifest visual acuity both with and without correction if the latter is worn. This is followed by inspection with more or less oblique illumination from an ordinary 60 watt electric light bulb equipped with a reflector, and attached to an arm so that it may be moved to any desired position. Although it would probably be advised I do not use the loupe or condensing lens unless there is some suspicion of pathology in the cornea or anterior chamber. In case of doubt or if any pathology is visible to the naked eye I use an ordinary binocular loupe and a small hand slit lamp of the Shahan type to complete the inspection. At the conclusion of inspection it is the rule to observe the movements of the eyes in the six cardinal directions, for gross abnormalities in actions of the extrensic muscles.

From inspection we progress to the third step, that of determination of the near point of convergence and the near point of accommodation of each eye. The former is determined by having the patient fixate a small object, usually the point of a pencil, and while he is fixing the object it is gradually brought nearer to the eyes. The patient is asked to state when the object becomes double. During this procedure the eyes are carefully watched and the point at which one eye lags in convergence or gives up fixation entirely is taken as the near point of convergence, or NPC. The patient's eyes must be watched because it will frequently be found that he suppresses with one eye the minute it ceases to fix and he does not see double. The NPC is recorded in millimeters. Other information gathered by this simple procedure is a rough estimate of the grade of fusion present, and an indication as to which is the dominant eye. The non-dominant eye

*Read before the Section on Eye, Ear, Nose and Throat, Annual Session, Oklahoma State Medical Association, May 20, 1941, in Oklahoma City.

will usually be the one which gives up fixation first. The near point of accommodation is taken with each eye separately. We use the smallest letters on the near vision test chart, have the patient fix one word, and with the other eye covered we bring the card up to the eye under examination until the letters begin to blur. This distance is recorded in millimeters as the patient's near point of accommodation or PP . For those patients who are presbyopic or sufficiently hyperopic to require it we interpose a plus sphere and test in similar manner. The strength of the sphere must be recorded along with the distance in millimeters. The two, sphere in diopters and distance in millimeters, can be changed to either one or the other and added, but in practice we have found it more simple to record the two in combination. Determination of the NPC and PP are not only valuable in the immediate examination but they also offer a quick method in subsequent examination for determining any changes which may have taken place in the patient's ability to accommodate, thereby indicating the probabilities of the patient requiring a change in lenses. The PP also serves as a check on anomalies of accommodation and may put the examiner on his guard in looking for some pathological condition which would not otherwise be apparent. The method described here for determining the PP is used because it is simple, quickly performed, and gives the information desired in the ordinary routine refraction. We do not feel that it is necessary in the average case to go into the finer points of determination of the PP with the eye corrected for refractive errors because the information gained here is sufficient in most cases and we have it in mind to assist us in making deductions during the subsequent steps of the examination. If for any reason it is found necessary to make a more accurate determination this can be done after the refraction has been completed.

Our fourth step is measurement of the corneal astigmatism with the ophthalmometer. I realize that use of this instrument is considered superfluous by many men because it does not take into consideration the astigmatism which may be present in the lens. It does have the very definite advantage of measuring corneal astigmatism both in strength and as to axis very accurately in a majority of cases, and this is a very valuable adjunct to other findings if given proper consideration. It allows us to determine whether or not lenticular astigmatism is present and if so, how much is present and whether or not it coincides with the corneal astigmatism or tends to neutralize the same. If these factors are all considered properly in the final determination of the total error we feel certain that the prescribed glasses are much

more likely to be comfortable and to serve the purpose for which they were intended. As a word of caution, there are three points at which the examiner is likely to be misled in use of this instrument if he is not constantly on his guard. I recall having allowed such errors to creep into my personal experience on more than one occasion. The first is that of placing too much confidence in the ophthalmometer reading and not searching carefully enough when the reading is negative. Relatively large errors may be overlooked if the examiner is lulled into a sense of false security in this way, and proper care is not exercised, both in the manifest and in the retinoscopic examinations. On the other hand it frequently occurs that the corneal astigmatism as recorded by the instrument is neutralized at least partially by accompanying lenticular astigmatism, and the patient may be over corrected. The third point of caution is the ability of some patients by the simple process of squeezing the lids to change the shape of the bulb, thereby changing the corneal curvature. I have seen this happen on numerous occasions while the measurement was being made, and the amount of such change may be very great. This of course may be prevented by asking the patient not to squint, and at the same time observing to see that he complys with the request.

Our fifth step is retinoscopic examination. I'm certain that we all agree that it is an indispensable part of every refraction, and particularly so in children who cannot tell us what they see. Even so, there is a wide variation of opinion as to the type of instrument used and the procedure to be followed. Due perhaps to my early training and habits developed at that time I have continued to use the plane mirror retinoscope electrically lighted from the handle. It is simple and convenient and seems to serve the purpose very well with the possible exception of inadequacy in the accurate determination of the axis of astigmatism. Users of the streak retinoscope seem unanimous in agreement that it is better for such determination, but until I have had more experience in its use the question will be left open in my mind. Our retinoscopic examinations are made with the refractor properly placed before the patient, the patient facing an object at 20 feet, in a semi-dark room. The working distance is about one meter. Examination is made with both eyes uncovered and at the start no lenses are present. From this point we determine whether the light reflex has a with motion in all meridians, if not, sufficient minus sphere is added to make the movements of the reflex with. Then plus sphere is gradually added until the first meridian shows a reversal. This is recorded and more plus is added until the reversal becomes complete in all meridians, and the amount of sphere used at this point is recorded. The difference between these two points is the strength of the astigmatism and the meridian of the first reversal is the axis. When the refractor contains minus cylinders as is the case with our instrument, the opposite meridian is of course used as the axis and a minus cylinder of the strength indicated above is placed before the eye in combination with the total sphere used in obtaining the last reversal. From this we deduct plus 1.25 diopters of sphere from the total sphere used in bringing about reversal in all meridians. In other words we do not simply try to neutralize the movements, but rather try to bring about a complete reversal in order to be sure that we have gone as far as we should. This accounts for the extra plus .25 diopter deducted from the total.

We are now ready for the sixth step, namely, manifest refraction, which is of course the real proving ground of every examination. The preceding steps have given us a close approximation of errors of refraction present and an incite into the condition of the patient's eyes together with some important information in regard to the ability of his eyes to overcome the amount of error present. In short it gives us grounds on which to base our judgment of the accuracy of the subjective findings. We have gone a step further, in that we have prepared the patient for examination by fogging him in to a considerable degree before the manifest examination has been started. This alone may uncover many cases of latent hyperopia.

Beginning with the retinoscopic finding placed before the patient and with one eye covered we procede in the usual manner to determine his manifest acceptance, first by attempting to add more plus sphere. If that is not accepted we try reducing the plus sphere or add more minus sphere as the case may be. As soon as the strength of sphere has been satisfactorily determined we turn to the cylinder, first testing the various strengths above and below that in the instrument, then by changing the axis to various points from five to 20 degrees in each direction from the original. At this point we resort to the use of a procedure which I feel is most valuable in the accurate determination of the strength and axis of the cylinder, that is the Jackson cross cylinder. A complete description of the method is not possible here because it is a subject which would take too much time. Since returning to its use some two or three years ago after throwing it in the discard for a year I have become so dependent upon the results that I would not like to be required to do a manifest examination without it. It has solved several

difficult problems for me which had remained virtually unsolved during that period of time in which the cross cylinder went unused. It is very valuable in getting away from overcorrection with minus cylinders and at the same time it is the most accurate and positive manifest method of determining the axis I have yet found. Following use of the cross cylinder we again check the sphere then re-check the patient's astigmatism on the radial chart, more perhaps through force of habit than for any real reason, because I cannot remember making any major change based on results gained from use of this chart. In all fairness to the method it may be said that the chart does occasionally cause one to return to the cross cylinder and other manifest examination in order to re-check the results. As a final check on the sphere chiefly in order to prevent fogging the patient, we always use the bichrome test. It has the advantage of being a very sensitive test, quickly and easily performed.

Following the manifest examination we determine the state of muscle balance with the Maddox rod and red glass, then the ductions by prisms and the muscle light at 20 feet. This phase of the examination will not be discussed here since it was taken up in some detail on a paper read before this group at the meeting last year. Suffice it to say that we consider it a routine procedure to be used in every case of refraction when two useful eyes are present.

In the eighth step we check by manifest examination, the near vision using the age of the patient, the amount of accommodation present as determined at the beginning of the examination, and our judgment based on past experiences as guides to the procedure. Some men have been able to use successfully dynamic retinoscopy as an aid here, but the reflex obtained has been too poor and too rapid in motion to be followed in practical work. There are only two conditions under which the manifest findings at near greatly influence our later decisions. The first is in presbyopes or in those patients who have marked weakness of accommodation from some other cause. The second is a reduction of cylinder strength in those cases of lenticular astigmatism which are reduced by the act of accommodation.

Following the above procedures we make an examination of the internal eye with the ophthalmoscope, then we are ready to decide whether the patient should be examined under cycloplegic or simply be re-checked on a later date. In general, all patients under 15 years of age are examined under atropine, those above 15 and up to 30 years are examined under homatropine, and those older are re-checked the following day. In the absence of glaucomatous states, paresis of accommodation and etc. we do not hesitate to use homatropine on older patients, even up to 45 or 50 years if conditions seem to indicate its use. For the most part a repetition of the retinoscopic and the manifest examinations is sufficient and this we always insist upon using, even though it may mean an out of town patient makes an extra trip. This second examination is made, if possible, early in the morning or at such time as the eyes have had plenty of rest, and the patient is not tired and nervous. If the findings at this examination do not agree reasonably well with those of the first examination we may resort to a cycloplegic or to a third examination, depending upon the conditions involved. If the findings do coincide, as is usually the case, we feel reasonably secure in our judgment as to the final prescription.

Pernicious Anemia

WANN LANGSTON, M.D.

OKLAHOMA CITY, OKLAHOMA

In the preface to his paper "On the Constitutional and Local Effects of Disease of the Suprenal Capsules" before the South London Medical Society in 1849, Thomas Addison said, "For a long period I had from time to time met with a very remarkable anaemia, occurring without any discoverable cause whatever—cases in which there had been no previous blood loss, no exhausting diarrhea, no chlorosis, no purpura, no renal, splenic, miasmatic, glandular, strumous, or malignant disease." This he designated as "Idiopathic Anaemia." To quote further: "The disease presented in every instance the same general character, pursued a similar course, and with scarcely a single exception, was followed, after a variable period, by the same fatal result." "It occurs in both sexes, generally, but not exclusively, beyond the middle period of life, and, so far as I, at present, know, chiefly in persons of somewhat large and bulky frame, and with a strongly marked tendency to the formation of fat. It makes its approach in so slow and insidious a manner that the patient can hardly fix a date to his earliest feeling of languor which is shortly to become so extreme. The countenance gets pale, the whites of the eyes become pearly, the general frame flabby rather than wasted; the pulse, perhaps, large, but remarkably soft and compressible. There is an increasing indisposition to exertion, with an uncomfortable feeling of faintness and breathlessness on attempting it; the heart is readily made to palpitate; the whole surface of the body present a blanched smooth and waxy appearance; the lips, gums and tongue seem bloodless; the flabbiness of the solids increases; the appetite fails; extreme languor and faintness supervene, breathlessness and palpitation being produced by the most trifling exertion or emotion; some slight edema is probably perceived about the ankles; the debility becomes extreme, the patient can no longer rise from his bed, the mind occasionally wanders, he falls into a prostrate and half torpid state, and at length expires."

Addison goes on to say that upon post-mortem examination he failed to find "any organic lesion that could properly or reasonably be assigned as an adequate cause of such serious consequences." He suspected some form of fatty degeneration, and in one case observed such a change in the heart, the semi-lunar ganglion and the solar plexus.

This classical description of the disease was not the first reference to the condition. J. S. Combe had in 1822 described what seems to have been a case, in which he referred to remissions of the symptoms.

In 1851 Barclay published a case in which he, for the first time, recorded soreness of the tongue. In 1870 Fenwick described atrophic changes in the mucosa of the stomach and intestines, and he related the blood changes to this atrophy. In 1871, Biermer apparently unfamiliar with Addison's report of 22 years before described a "new" disease which he named "Progressive Pernicious Anemia." Biermer, like Addison, stressed the point that the disease occurred without discoverable cause, but pointed out that it was especially prevalent among the poorer classes, an observation which William Hunter did not confirm. Hunter was equally in error when he made the statement that the condition is a "chronic infective disease." Hunter did, however, make an important contribution in stressing the atrophy of the gastro-intestinal mucosa, and in emphasizing the importance of Glossitis and Stomatitis. He went to considerable length in describing the glossitis even to the periodicity. We still speak of "Hunterian Glossitis" in connection with the diagnosis of Pernicious Anemia.

In 1874-75 Immerman made an important

contribution in separating a primary pernicious anemia for which no cause could be found as described by Addison and by Biermer, and a secondary, associated with other disease states. The latter group gradually grew to include the anemias associated with pregnancy, carcinoma of the stomach, parasitic infestation and dietary deficiencies.

In 1889 Leichtenstern described disseminated foci of degeneration in the posterior and lateral columns of the spinal cord in cases of severe anemias and designated the condition as "Anaemic Spinal Disease." Five years before he had reported three cases of pernicious anemia with tabes dorsalis.

In the last quarter of the last century the blood picture began to excite interest; macrocytosis and poikilocytosis were observed, and American workers noted hyperactivity of the bone marrow and the presence of nucleated red cells in the circulating blood. During the same period absence of hydrochloric acid was discovered in cases of pernicious anemia.

During the first quarter of the twentieth century no important contribution to our knowledge of pernicious anemia was made. And then, in 1926, came the announcement of the epoch making discovery of Murphy of the effect of liver feeding upon cases of pernicious anemia. The effect of this discovery was to stimulate investigation as nothing before had; a tremendous literature appeared; the entire field of hematology was intensively studied and a more complete understanding of blood dyscrasias was acquired than in all the previous years.

Thus, during the period of a hundred years, from Combe in 1822 to Murphy in 1926, gradually was constructed the picture of pernicious anemia as we know it today, namely, a progressive anemia with the constitutional disturbances associated with blood impoverishment, atrophy of the gastrointestinal mucosa, with achlorhydria; Hunterian Glossitis, and Stomatitis; the presence of macrocytosis; the presence of "Anaemic Spinal Disease," subacute combined degeneration of the spinal cord; and the characteristic response of the disease to specific therapy. A pernicious progressive fatal disease has been transformed into a benign condition, the most satisfactory to treat of all chronic incurable pathological processes.

RECOGNITION

The diagnosis of Pernicious Anemia depends mainly upon the recognition of abnormalities in three systems. The finding of such in one system leads to suspicion; in two, to diagnosis; in all three, to certainty. Finally, response to therapy removes all doubt if any exists.

First, the Digestive System: Anorexia, indigestion, nausea and vomiting; intermittent diarrhea; atrophy of the papillae of the tongue, glossitis and stomatitis; and the absence of hydrochloric acid in the gastric secretion. In former times the appearance of the tongue played a much greater part in diagnosis than now. In no other condition perhaps, is the appearance of the tongue so characteristic as in pernicious anemia; and in no condition, so far as I know, does the patient complain more bitterly. Often this glossitis and stomatitis constitute the very first abnormality noted. The edges and frequently the entire surface of the tongue are inflamed and have a beefy red or raw appearance; later the tongue may take on a perfectly smooth character, the entire dorsum being denuded of papillae. The buccal cavity may have the same appearance. Hunter called attention to the periodicity of this involvement of tongue and mouth, periodicity being a characteristic of the disease itself. Achlorhydria is said to occur universally.

Second, the Blood: The Anemia is characteristically hyperchromic and macrocytic. The hemoglobin is high, relative to the number of red cells. If one studies the stained smear he will be struck with the appearance of cells that are abnormally large, some that are smaller than normal, and many that are abnormally shaped—poikilocytes. Occasionally nucleated red cells will be seen. If a vital stain preparation is made reticulocytes will be seen in excess of the normal number, one percent. The mean corpuscular volume will be increased. There likely will be a leucopenia, and the neutrophils will be seen to have multilobular nuclei. The icteric index is frequently increased. Following specific and adequate therapy the reaction is characteristic—a rapid increase in reticulocytes, and slower rise in red cells and hemoglobin, with a drop in reticulocytes as red cells and hemoglobin approach normal. If the bone marrow is examined it will be found to be hyperplastic, and megaloblasts will be seen to predominate the picture.

At this point one may inquire as to a possible etiological relationship between these two systems, the blood and the digestive. In these last 15 years the investigations of Whipple, Castle, Minot and Murphy, Sturgis and Isaacs, and others have thrown much light upon this subject. Our present information may be summarized as follows:

The red cells are formed intravascularly in the capillary bed of the bone marrow, mainly lodged in the flat spongy bones. As the immature cells pass along the assembly lines at least two substances are added. One of these is hemoglobin, and if iron is not available iron deficiency anemia results. The other is a principle required for the proper maturing of the red cells. This has been designated the Erythrocyte Maturing Factor. If not available another type of deficiency anemia results, characterized by immaturity of the red cells. This is the anemia of Pernicious Anemia and the erythrocyte maturing factor has also been called the Anti Pernicious Anemia Factor or Principle. This principle normally is stored mainly in the liver and is supplied to the red cell factory on demand. If the storage be interfered with by extensive damage to the liver, an anemia resembling pernicious anemia may ensue. This Erythrocyte Maturing Principle is produced in the normal stomach by the interaction of two factors, one resident in the normal gastric mucosa and designated as Intrinsic Factor, and the other supplied in the food, principally protein, and called Extrinsic Factor. If the former is lacking due to atrophy or destruction of the gastric mucosa no Erythrocyte maturing factor is available; if there is deprivation of the necessary food elements there is also an insufficiency of the E. M. F. Such a deficiency may be corrected by the administration of adequate quantities of normal liver, in the form of food, as dried extracts administered orally, as more or less purified and concentrated extracts given parenterally, by the administration of normal gastric juice containing partially digested protein, or by the oral administration of preparations of normal gastric mucosa. Regardless of how it is supplied, E. M. F. is stored in the liver until required. The Intrinsic Factor seems to be lodged mainly in the mucosa near the pylorus. When this part of the mucosa is destroyed extracts of the liver fail to produce a reticulocyte response in pernicious anemia patients, while extracts from the livers of individuals in whom the entire gastric mucosa except near the pylorus is destroyed do produce such a response.

Thus there seems to be a relationship between the gastro-intestinal pathology in so far as it is the cause of deficiency in intrinsic factor, and the blood picture in Pernicious Anemia. Whether this same deficiency is responsible for the glossitis-stomatitis, I do not know. As will be pointed out later this seems a possibility; and the evidence seems to point to this gastro-intestinal pathology as the primary etiological factor.

The third system likely to be involved in Pernicious Anemia is the Neuro-muscular. Addison reported fatty degeneration of muscle and nerve plexuses. Leichtenstern recognized degeneration of the postero-lateral columns of the spinal cord in his "Anemic Spinal Disease." We now recognize signs of sub-acute combined degeneration of the spinal cord in nearly 50 percent of all cases

of primary pernicious anemia, and in some cases of other blood dyscrasias and secondary macrocytic anemias.

Sub-acute combined degeneration of the spinal cord may be defined as a progressive degenerative process affecting mainly the posterior columns and the pyramidal tracts of the cord, and usually associated with pernicious anemia.

The manifestations of involvement of the posterior columns are, first, paresthesias, numbness, tingling, sensations of coldness, burning and pricking, sometimes girdle sensations and back pain and varying degrees of anesthesia; second, ataxia and incoordination due to loss of tendon, joint or muscle sense, unsteadiness of gait particularly at night, loss of sense of position of the smaller, distal members, as the feet and toes; astereognosis with manual clumsiness, etc.; third, loss of vibratory sense, especially in distal members particularly below the knees.

Positive plantar reflex and exaggerated tendon reflexes and clonus indicating pyramidal tract involvement occur in a considerable percentage of cases; loss of sphincter control occurs in some. As the disease advances spasticity and contractures sometimes supervene.

This neurological syndrome must be differentiated from multiple sclerosis, tabes dorsalis, cord tumor and peripheral neuritis. This should not be difficult when one considers that this syndrome is usually associated with macrocytic anemia, achlorhydria and glossitis and stomatitis, findings not usually present in the others. Pernicious anemia then should not be difficult of recognition, since macrocytosis is practically always present by the time either neurological symptoms or findings appear.

At this point one may inquire as to the relationship of the nervous system lesion and the pathological processes in the other systems involved. The answer is not yet. It seems probable however that impairment in the function of producing Intrinsic Factor in the gastric mucosa precedes the other manifestations. In many cases glossitis and stomatitis are the first abnormal findings of which the patient complains, but upon investigation, achlorhydria and anemia with macrocytosis already are present. In other, and a large percentage of cases, the symptoms of anemia will be the first complained of, but again achlorhydria will be found. Again, in not a few cases neurological symptoms and signs will be the first obvious manifestations, but still the ever present macrocytic anemia and the achylia. Then this question arises: Just as the peculiar type of anemia must be due to the absence of anti-pernicious anemia principle, due in turn to absence of Intrinsic

Factor (in most cases), does it not seem likely that the glossitis and stomatitis on the one hand, the spinal cord degeneration on the other, may also be due to this deficiency?

MANAGEMENT

The modern streamlined treatment of the average case of pernicious anemia consists solely of the parenteral administration of adequate amounts of potent liver extracts to correct the deficiency—to maintain a blood count at normal level or a little above. This can be done by administering liver extract containing two units per cubic centimeter intramuscularly, six to ten units daily for a few days, then at gradually lengthening intervals, until finally only a dose a week or one in two weeks may be needed. More highly purified and concentrated extracts are now available, but one feels that perhaps they are not as effective as the cruder preparations. Iron is not required, and mixtures of iron and liver orally constitute an expensive, inconvenient, disagreeable, and unrational method unless there is an associated iron deficiency which is unusual. Hydrochloric acid in most cases can be dispensed with. Vitamin B. is of questionable but probable advantage. Naturally a patient on this regime must be given a well balanced dietary such as a normal individual would receive. In other words, one is dealing with a deficiency disease, and the one problem is to correct the deficiency by adequate replacement therapy. Adequate rest is important.

RESULTS OF MANAGEMENT

What may one expect to happen to the various symptoms and manifestations on such a regime? The answer to this question may throw some light upon the relationship of system abnormalities.

One of the first as well as one of the most striking effects of adequate therapy is the evidence of a return to normal function of the bone marrow. This is manifested by the remarkable increase in the number of reticulocytes in the blood, sometimes a rise of from one percent to 12 percent or 15 percent within a week, and a slower but notable increase in the hemoglobin readings and in the red cell count. As the last two approach normal, the reticulocyte count also approaches normal, that is it rapidly falls to a normal one or two percent. At the same time there will be noted a reduction in the number of macrocytes, poikilocytes and microcytes—the entire blood picture approaches normal. If therapy be discontinued the blood picture will again become abnormal.

This seems to establish definitely the fact that the liver extract contains a substance needed for the proper maturing of the red blood cells in the bone marrow. It has been reported that extracts from the liver of an adequately treated case of pernicious anemia, will produce a reticulocyte response in cases of pernicious anemia, while extracts from livers of untreated cases will not produce such a response, thereby increasing the evidence that E. M. F. is stored in the liver.

Equally as prompt as the improvement in the blood picture is that of the sore tongue and mouth when present. One has seen patients who were complaining bitterly of pain in the tongue greatly relieved after one or two large doses of liver extract intramuscularly. One of the most gratifying results of this form of therapy is the prompt relief of this, one of the most annoying symptoms of the disease. Not infrequently the mouth and tongue are completely relieved within ten days from the first dose of liver. But if therapy be discontinued the relapse is prompt. Again, a direct etiological relationship is suggested between the deficiency in Erythrocyte maturing Factor, or at least, between Intrinsic Factor deficiency and the pathology of tongue and mouth.

The results of therapy have not been nearly so striking or satisfactory in the cases of pernicious anemia with subacute combined degeneration of the cord. Much larger dosage is required, and a much longer period of time elapses before the benefits are obvious. There is also a great variation in the responses of various cases; as would be expected, those with milder symptoms, of shorter duration respond much more readily than the more severe cases and those of longer duration. But persistence in treatment with large doses of liver will greatly benefit a very large percentage of even those with high grade disability. One can give a favorable prognosis in the severe cases of short duration, but must be conservative about those of several years' standing.

Practically every case of pernicious anemia is troubled with paresthesias. Some of these undoubtedly are associated with sub-

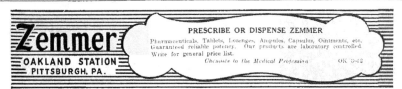

acute combined degeneration; others probably are not on this basis. The latter usually disappear promptly with adequate liver therapy; the former are likely to persist for a long time and may not disappear at all.

Loss of vibratory sense is one of the most constant of neurological findings in pernicious anemia. With adequate therapy at least a partial recovery can be expected in many cases, even with severe degenerative lesions. The same is true of sense of position, astereognosis and superficial sensation. A large percentage of patients with disturbances of gait show marked improvement, some are completely relieved. In those who remain handicapped re-education of muscles has been a most satisfying adjunct to liver therapy.

In like manner persistent adequate therapy has had a very satisfactory effect upon the lateral column symptoms in that deep and superficial reflexes have been at least partially restored to normal, and spasticity relieved. Even those with bladder and

bowel involvement have been greatly benefited, in some, normal function has been restored.

It has been suggested, and it has been my observation that in cases with neurological symptoms refractory to liver therapy improvement has been enhanced by the administration of preparations of gastric mucosa, such as ventriculin. Here, I believe, is the chief indication for any mixed therapy in pernicious anemia.

SUMMARY

1. The history of the development of our knowledge and present conceptions of Pernicious Anemia has been sketched briefly.

2. Symptoms and findings associated with Digestive, Blood and Neurological systems have been enumerated.

3. The relationship of disturbances in these systems to each other has been suggested.

4. Adequate management has been very briefly outlined and results that may be expected have been mentioned.

The Present Status of Vitamins in Neurology and Psychiatry

JAMES ASA WILLIE, M.D.

OKLAHOMA CITY, OKLAHOMA

The vast, increasing literature on vitamins, the high pressure advertising of pharmaceutical firms, and the public curiosity and "vitamin consciousness," which has been aroused by the press and radio, have all combined to make the physician more interested in vitamins. But the busy physician who attempts to bring himself up to date on this subject finds himself confronted with thousands of articles; with a confusing terminology; and an array of claims and counter-claims by different workers. At least the writer had that experience and decided therefore to try and pick out the new, essential and verified facts about vitamins, especially those facts which relate to the fields of Neurology and Psychiatry. Much of our present knowledge was learned from animal experiments and later was confirmed by similar clinical observations on humans. But the results in animals do not always coincide with those in man. A number of vitamins, for example, whose deficiency in animals causes certain deficiency syndromes, have as yet no clinical application in humans. Many complexities and unknowns face us. For instance, certain work shows that heredity plays a certain role. Further the *exact* daily reqirement of any vitamin is still un

known. This is understandable when we consider the influences of absorption, storage, and destruction, not to mention the marked variability in the minimal and optimal vitamin requirements for any particular individual. Also our problem is further complicated because single vitamin deficiencies seldom exist. Apparently too, certain safety factors operate to prevent the development of a deficiency state: (1) there is quite a margin of safety between the beginning of a deficiency disease and death; (2) there is a certain amount of storage of vitamins, especially of A and D, and (3) the body excretes less vitamin when a deficiency in that vitamin exists. In America gross deficiency states are uncommon and usually recognized. But the subclinical and latent deficiency states are very common and usually unrecognized by the physician. Four sets of factors operate to produce deficiency states: (1) an inadequate intake of the vitamin; (2) an increased need for that vitamin; (3) diminished absorption or utilization of that vitamin by the body; and (4) increased destruction or excretion of the vitamin. We shall be interested in the nature, sources, requirement, action and function, clinical features, and therapy in the case of each vitamin. For the sake of brevity the word "vitamin" will be left out as much as possible and designations such as "A," etc., will be used instead.

VITAMIN A

A is related to *carotene*, the latter being a yellow substance in certain plants. That is, A begins as carotene; the carotene is converted by a liver enzyme into A, and the liver is a storage depot for carotene. A is found abundantly in fish liver oils, egg yolks, butter and cream. A is a catalyst, which is essential in maintaining the normal state of epithelial tissues. It is in the other words a so-called epithelial protective vitamin, and is necessary for the continued health of all tissues of epiblastic origin. Thus, the brain and central nervous system, the retina, the skin and its glands and mucous membranes require A for their normal function. Where A is deficient the epithelial tissues show thickening or keratinization, followed by secondary infection and destruction. A is also a precursor of visual purple, which is the photosensitive substance in the dark retina. Deficiency of A thus causes difficulty in dark adaptation or night blindness, which can be determined quantitatively by the ophthalmologist with his biophotometer. Apparently 2,000 to 6,000 units of A represent the daily requirement.

The grosser manifestations of A deficiency are often picked up by the physician. But recent studies of large groups have demonstrated that many cases of mild to moderate A deficiency go unrecognized and that the individual himself may be unaware of its manifestations. Many people because they work under excessive light, eg., actresses, beauty operators, etc., develop early signs of A deficiency.

OCULAR SYMPTOMS—The A deficiency state begins with burning, itching, and dryness of eyes; photophobia; difficulty in reading over 10 to 15 minutes, especially at night; momentary attacks of blurring of vision at end of day; difficulty when viewing movies; dizziness; or even complete night blindness. Difficulty in driving at night may be responsible for auto accidents. The medico-legal aspects of this condition have not been realized. No such test is yet required of auto drivers or of aviators. The A deficiency state may progress to granulation and redness of the conjunctiva, softening of the cornea and blindness. In other types the skin especially over the extensor surfaces of the forearms, legs and thighs, shows keratinization of a hard, papular character that resembles goose-skin. There is some evidence that keratinization of the epithelium of the renal pelvis leading to urinary calculi may occur. Deficiency "A" also may lead to dental caries. As therapy,

A or carotene in oil or oleum percomorphum is used; giving 10,000 to 50,000 units daily.

B COMPLEX

This complex contains at least 12 fractions, four of which are now available for clinical use, namely: (1) B_1 or thiamin chloride; (2) B_2, G, or Riboflavin; (3) Nicotinic acid or the P.-P., factor and (4) Pantothenic acid. Two other less well understoood B fractions are (5) Pyroxodin and (6) Yeast Adenylic Acid.

(1) B_1 OR THIAMIN CHLORIDE

B_1 is found in yeast, milk, egg yolk, pork, etc. The daily requirement is about one to two mg. The kidney, liver and heart have a low storage capacity for B_1. B is a catalyst essential in the metabolism of carbohydrates, thus playing a part in the oxidation of lactic and pyruvic acids. Thus in B_1 deficiency we have abnormalities in pyruvic acid metabolism which is partly responsible for the disturbances of the central nervous system, and for the degeneration of the peripheral nerves. Clinically the gross B_1 deficiency states such as Beriberi with its symmetrical peripheral neuropathy and characteristic cardiovascular disturbances are familiar to the physician. Whereas, the milder and partial deficiency states often escape recognition until a severe state has blossomed out. Therefore, it behooves the physician to be on the lookout for these milder states. The milder states begin either with neurological manifestations or with a neurasthenic-like picture. Jolliffe classifies the neurological manifestations into the (1) suggestive, (2) mild, (3) moderate and (4) severe stages. In the suggestive stage the patient complains of anorexia, fatigue, heaviness of the legs, calf muscle cramps, and paresthesias in the toes and fingers. Objectively we find: calf muscle tenderness, plantar hyperesthesia and loss of vibratory sensation in the toes. The mild stage is characterized by absent ankle jerks. The moderate stage is marked by an advance in the sensory and motor changes; loss of the knee jerks; impaired position sense in the toes; atrophy of calf muscles and foot-drops. In the severe stage, we find involvement of the upper extremities; of the spinal cord; or of the cranial nerves. Certain sub-clinical B_1 deficiency states may simulate a neurotic or psychotic picture and lead to a mistaken diagnosis of a neurosis or psychosis. Here occur such symptoms as: a loss of weight and strength, indigestion and dyspepsia, epigastric burning, constipation, diarrhea, abdominal cramps, irritability, apprehension, depression, crying spells, flight of ideas, mental confusion, etc. The simulated neurotic and psychotic pictures are characteristic of thiamin, riboflavin, or nicotinic acid deficiency states, or of a combination of all three of them. Therefore, it is wise to give all three vitamins in such cases. As therapy in the B_1 deficiency states children receive five mg. thiamin intravenously or intramuscularly daily, plus ten mg. by mouth. For adults 20 to 100 mg. doses may be necessary. Such conditions as tinnitus, tabetic pains, the cerebral complications following recovery from infectious diseases, and the withdrawal symptoms that occur in the treatment of alcoholic and morphine addicts have all apparently been benefited by B_1 therapy. But large doses may cause herpes zoster. If any intense burning pain develops in any part of the body during thiamin therapy, then B_1 must be discontinued immediately. Apparently, suprarenal cortex given in conjunction enhances the effects of B_1.

(2) B_2, G, OR RIBOFLAVIN

The requirement is probably about two to five mg. daily. B_2 is essential in the oxidation processes of the cells. B_2 deficiency usually begins with "Cheilosis," ie. a pallor of mucosa of lips in the angles of the mouth, followed by superficial transverse fissures and reddened, macerated areas in the angles of the mouth; and a greasy desquamation in the nasolabial folds, in the alae nasi, in the vestibule of the nose, and on the nose. Ocular symptoms where they occur include: itching and burning of the eyes, photophobia, excessive dryness of the conjunctiva or excessive lacrimation, keratitis, vascularization and opacities of the cornea, and abnormal pigmentation of the iris, failing vision, etc. These ocular symptoms wax and wane and are worse in summer and winter. As therapy three to five mg. Riboflavin orally or intravenously in four to six doses; plus 50 to 75 gm. of brewer's yeast is sufficient.

(3) NICOTINIC ACID

A gross deficiency of nicotinic acid seemingly leads to Pellagra with its well known oral lesions, gastro-intestinal disturbances and mental aberrations. Not so well known, however, is the fact that each of these three characteristic symptom complexes, may occur alone or in any possible combination and therefore, the basic condition may easily be overlooked by the physician. When mental aberrations occur singly, many such patients are labeled neurotic, etc. Recently an "encephalopathic syndrome" due to nicotinic acid deficiency has been described. This syndrome shows the following symptoms: (1) clouding of consciousness, (2) cog-wheel rigidities of the extremities, (3) uncontrollable grasping and sucking reflexes; (4) cerebellar symptoms and (5) catatonia. Therapeutically 500 to 1,000 mg. of nicotinic acid daily or 50 to 80 mg. of it intravenously daily in 10 to 15 mg. doses, dissolved in sterile

physiologic saline solution is indicated. Also apparently the addition of nicotinic acid or of the amide to the diet produces a much larger food intake and better weight for any individual.

(4) PANTOTHENIC ACID

Is little understood yet.

(5) B_6 OR PYRODOXIN

Is still in the experimental stage. There is some evidence that it benefits cases of muscular dystrophy and lessens the muscular rigidity and weakness in cases of paralysis agitans. It is also claimed that extreme nervousness, insomnia, irritability and stomach cramps respond to it. As therapy 50 mg. of pyrodoxin in sterile physiologic saline solution is given daily.

(6) YEAST ADENYLIC ACID

This is another factor about which little is yet known. It is said to clear up intense burning of the oral mucous membrane with malnutrition, in a patient showing no evidence of pellagra. The dose is 200 mg. by mouth. Also this factor seems to increase the effectiveness of nicotinic acid in treating pellagra.

C OR ASCORBIC ACID

Occurs principally in milk, parsley, peppers, raw liver and watercress. C is a powerful reducing substance, essential in the formation and maintenance of the intercellular substance especially that of the blood vessels, dental forming organs and connective tissues. C also plays some indefinite role in respiratory function. At least 0.8 mg. of Ascorbic acid for each kilogram of body weight is used daily by healthy subjects. C seems to be stored in the adrenal cortex. The gross C deficiency state is Scurvy, with which the physician is familiar. The pathologic change here is in the intercellular substance. Especially in that of the blood vessels and bones, with softening which leads to hemorrhages into the subcutaneous, subperiosteal, gingival and other tissues. But subacute scurvy is generally unrecognized as the cause of a low state of health with fatigue, sallow complexion, and fleeting pains in the bones. Dental caries is thought to be one of the earliest signs of latent scurvy. C is essential also for the functional activities of certain cells necessary for the formation of the teeth. C deficiency also has some relationship to certain states of hemorrhagic diathesis and to certain states of macrocytic anemia.

VITAMIN D

D is found principally in liver oils of fish, egg yolks, butter, milk, and cream. D plays a part in the metabolism of calcium and phosphorus, having to do with the retention of calcium and phosphorus in the bones. Normal hepatic function seems to be necessary to insure the proper metabolism of Vitamin D. Clinical D deficiency states show up principally in the form of rickets, tetany, dental caries, and possibly osteomalacia. In regard to therapy at present massive doses of D are given. Usually as much as 500,000 international units of D_2 (calciferol) are given weekly by mouth in an oily solution with milk. One-half the dose is given on the third day and the other one-half on the seventh day of each week. In giving massive doses of D there is some danger of causing hypervitaminosis D. Symptoms of this condition are as follows: First, there is cell injury, followed by excessive deposition of calcium, but the process is reversible and reparable if the administration of vitamin is discontinued immediately. Any evidence of renal impairment or of ateriosclerosis should be a definite contraindication against excessive doses of D. Symptoms of toxicity include anorexia, and gastro-intestinal and urinary irritability. One case recently died presumably of D hypervitaminosis.

VITAMIN E

E is found principally in wheat germ oil, in lettuce, spinach, and cabbage. Recently synthetic concentrates of the alpha and beta-tocopherol forms of E have been put on the market. A lack of E in the male is thought to cause destruction of the germinative cells.

And its lack in the female is thought to be connected with spontaneous abortions and sterility. At any rate there appears to be some relationship between E and the ovarian hormone. Apparently anterior pituitary substance can be substituted for E. There is possibly a definite relationship between the inadequate intake of E and the normality of the cross-striated musculature of the body. In recent months for instance Wechsler, Stone and other workers reported remarkable cures and improvement in cases of amyotrophic lateral sclerosis, and in progressive muscular dystrophy by giving vitamin E. But other workers have gotten no results. The writer has had the opportunity of following a large series of both types of cases for the last nine months, and so far feels rather pessimistic as regards any beneficial results to be obtained by vitamin E in the above mentioned conditions. As therapy wheat germ oil is given in any amount from one dram t.i.d., upward. Ephynal or synthetic tocopherol is given daily in doses of 30 to 50 mg. either orally or intravenously. In addition foods rich in E like spinach, cabbage, lettuce etc., are given. And finally two 5 grain pills of bile salts are also given daily.

VITAMIN K

Is only being mentioned as its uses lie outside the fields of neurology and psychiatry.

Tularemia: A Report of Ten Cases*

E. H. WERLING, M.D.
Whitaker Hospital

PRYOR, OKLAHOMA

The importance of tularemia to the general practitioner is recognized by the ever increasing reports of cases occurring in the United States and many foregin countries. The recent observation of several cases prompted this report and I believe it would be well to review briefly some of the more pertinent aspects of the disease and the recent literature concerning it.

Historically, the disease was first described in 1910 by Dr. George McCoy of the Public Health Service in reporting a "plague like" outbreak among ground squirrels in Tulare county, California. McCoy and Chapin discovered and described the causative organisms in 1912, calling it Bacterium tularense after Tulare county where the disease was first observed. Dr. Edward Francis also of the Public Health Service, showed

*Read before the Section on Medicine, Annual Session, Oklahoma State Medical Association, May 21, 1941, in Oklahoma City.

in 1919 that humans acquired the disease from infected animals and called it tularemia.

The Oklahoma State Health Department reports four cases in 1936, ten in 1937, 50 in 1938, 54 in 1939, 62 in 1940. The total number of deaths was 25 or approximately 14 percent. Apparently many of the milder cases were not reported. It should be noted that the number of wild rabbits has increased markedly in the past few years in this region. For the country as a whole, 2,200 cases were reported in 1939 with 140 deaths or approximately seven percent.

The commonest source of infection is skinning infected rabbits with bare hands, or handling their pelts, and this accounts for over 90 percent of human cases in the United States. Many other animals contract the disease and are potential sources of infection. Tick bites, of the wood tick principally, rank second as the infective source. Eating insufficiently cooked wild rabbit meat has been reported as a cause of numerous cases in the United States which resulted in an exceptionally high mortality. This appears to be the source of many cases falling in the typhoid class.

Francis recognized four clinical types of the disease and this classification is still in use today.

1. Ulcero-glandular. The primary lesion is a papule of the skin, commonly on the fingers, which later becomes an ulcer accompanied by enlargement of the regional lymph nodes. Visible lymphangitis is strikingly absent and when present is due to secondary infection. The majority of human infections are contracted as the result of the organisms entering through a skin wound, inflicted at the time of infection or shortly before or shortly after the germs get on the skin. Sometimes the infection penetrates the apparently unbroken skin of the hands, but usually there is a minute cut or scratch through which the germs enter the body.

2. Oculo-glandular. The primary lesion is a conjunctivitis with enlargement of the regional lymph nodes, chiefly the preauricular and retromaxillary glands. Presumably the infection is conveyed to the eyes by fingers soiled by rabbit blood.

3. Glandular. R e g i o n a l lymphadenopathy alone occurs in this type, no primary lesion being demonstrable. It is probable that the primary lesion healed early in these cases or that it was so small that it made no impression on the patient. Patients should be questioned closely on this point as many of them do not present themselves until the second or third week of the disease, frequently long after the primary lesion has healed.

4. Typhoid type. In this type there is neither glandular enlargement nor primary ulceration. Septicemia dominates the picture, pneumonia is more frequent, and the mortality is highest. This form is common among laboratory workers who have performed necropsies on infected animals or handled infected ticks.

Most cases can be placed in one of these four groups, however the disease assumes such bizarre forms at times that accurate classification is difficult.

DIAGNOSIS

The diagnosis of tularemia is not always made easily or with certainty. This is particularly true of the typhoid type which may exist as a blood stream infection without regional lymphadenopathy or local lesions. Patients presenting atypical pneumonias, unexplained pleural effusions, unexplained toxic rashes or prolonged fever should be investigated with the diagonsis of

tularemia in mind. The great majority of cases, however, fall into the ulcero-glandular group and the diagnosis should be easy if its presence is suspected. The laboratory is frequently called upon to make the diagnosis in obscure cases and to confirm a clinical diagnosis in obvious cases. The agglutination test for the detection of agglutinins in the blood is the most widely employed of the diagnostic tests and is highly reliable. It is useless, however, in the early stages of the infection, for agglutinins are never demonstrable during the first week and occasionally may not appear until the third week. Usually a titer of about 1:640 or above is reached by the third week and this persists for years afterwards. Foshay reports a case showing a strongly positive test 33 years after recovery. On the other hand, Moss and Weilbaecher have observed an absence of agglutinin titer in severe cases. They report six fatal cases in which the diagnosis was established only at necropsy.

Foshay has introduced the intradermal test reaction as an aid in early diagnosis. This is done by injecting intradermally .05 cc of a specially prepared B. tularense suspension. A positive reaction has the appearance of a positive tuberculin test and like the latter usually requires 48 hours for its development. The chief advance claimed for the skin test is that it will confirm the diagnosis during the first week of the disease when serum agglutinins are always absent.

Moss and Weilbaecher have employed animal inoculation as a means of diagnosis in obscure cases. These investigators have found the method useful in septicemia and in severe fulminating cases, in which agglutinins may be late in appearing or may be absent throughout the illness. They also report lung puncture as a satisfactory method of obtaining material for animal inoculation in cases of atypical pneumonia in which tularemia with pneumonic involvement is suspected. Animal inoculation and culture of the organism are too technical for the average physician but they should be kept in mind as useful methods of diagnosis in obscure cases.

Of most importance is the suspicion that the disease is present. Most patients do not mention the primary lesion nor do they volunteer information regarding the recent handling of rabbits or removing a tick from any part of the body. Many are unfamiliar with such sources. Repetition of the agglutination test at weekly intervals or oftener will frequently be repaid by a positive test and indicate the correct diagnosis. A titer of 1:80 is usually considered diagnostic and a rising titer, even if low in the beginning, is also diagnostic.

TREATMENT

A great many cases are of such a mild nature that symptomatic and supportive treatment alone is adequate. Many different drugs have been utilized in the therapy of tularemia with considerable success, including neoarsphenamine, mercurochrome, iodides, quinine, acriflavine and metaphen to mention just a few. This is probably accounted for by the fact that tularemia is a disease of low mortality, about five percent, and high morbidity. There are undoubtedly many cases that recover spontaneously without ever having the correct diagnosis established. Many mild cases never consult a physician.

Lee Foshay of Cincinnati has developed specific serum therapy which is probably the most scientific advance in treating tularemia. He has studied the effect of serum on both mortality and morbidity with adequate controls. He reports a mortality rate of six percent in 518 unselected untreated cases, used as controls, while in 600 unselected treated cases the rate was 2.2 percent. The morbidity was likewise appreciably reduced.

Several observers have used sulphanilamide without influencing the course of the disease. Moss and Weilbaecher have recently reported striking improvement following the administration of sulphathiazole. It is hoped that this drug will influence tularemia in much the same way as it has pneumonia, and if these observations can be confirmed it will simplify the treatment so that it will be readily available to all. They administered two grams of the drug every three hours for the first two or three doses and then maintained a high blood level by giving one gram every three hours thereafter.

At the present time the early administration of adequate doses of antitularense serum appears to be the best form of treatment. This is especially true in the typhoid type and tularemic pneumonia in which the highest mortality occurs. The usual dose is 30-60 cc given intravenously and repeated in 72 hours if necessary. Serum sickness is very common, about 50 percent, and according to Foshay, severe in 16 percent.

A simple antiseptic dressing, such as four percent xeroform ointment, should be applied to the primary lesion and otherwise left alone. It should never be incised. Injudicious treatment of this nature may precipitate fatal septicemia. Suppurative lymphadenopathies should be incised and drained when softening has occurred, not before. Most cases show rapid improvement when this happens.

The present report covers ten cases, nine of the ulcero-glandular, and one typhoid type, observed between June, 1937 and November, 1940. All recovered. One case followed tick bite, eight handled wild rabbits, and one had no definite source. Nine had a primary lesion at the time of treatment or gave such a history. The diagnosis was confirmed in each instance by positive agglutination tests made after the first week of illness. Intradermal tests were not used. Two patients had developed large pleural effusions when first seen, but pneumonia was not observed. The first complained of fever, cough, shortness of breath and loss of weight of three weeks duration and came for examination to confirm a previous impression of tuberculosis. When his chest was bared for examination an ulcer about .5 cm in diameter was noted in the right axillary region. The lymph nodes were enlarged and tender. When questioned about this he stated that three weeks previously he had removed a wood tick from that region but had not associated it with his pulmonary complaints. The agglutination test was strongly positive. All symptoms cleared completely under symptomatic treatment. The second came because of shortness of breath which had been present about two weeks. Examination revealed a massive effusion in the left pleural cavity. The fluid was clear, amber colored and contained no cells. She volunteered the information that a week before respiratory difficulty appeared, she had had sores on both thumbs and admitted skinning wild rabbits a few days before the primary lesion was noticed. She likewise made a complete recovery under symptomatic treatment.

The diagnosis was made in one case of fever by means of the agglutination test. Recovery was prolonged and tedious. This case was placed in the typhoid group.

Six of the ten cases received .6 gm neoarsphenamine at weekly intervals with good results in five. An average of five doses was given. Two cases received sulphanilimide without any apparent benefit. One patient did not respond to neo-arsphenamine or sulphanilimide but continued on a low grade febrile course for over six months, this in spite of the fact that the regional lymph nodes suppurated, were incised and drained, and healing had occurred rather early. Apparently a transition from the ulcero-glandular to the typhoid type occurred. This patient would probably have received benefit from serum. One patient came for drainage of an axillary abscess. The primary lesion had since healed and forgotten about. The agglutination test was reported positive in all dilutions. The administration of serum as well as neo-arsphenamine must be early in the disease to derive the greatest benefit.

CONCLUSIONS

1. Tularemia is a wide spread disease showing a recent increase in reported cases.

This increase is noted along with a recent increase in the number of wild rabbits in this region.

2. Tularemia assumes bizarre characteristics at times but the majority fall into the ulcero-glandular class.

3. Tularemia should be kept in mind in obscure fevers and unexplained pneumonias. The diagnostic tests are discussed and the importance of obtaining a reliable history to exposure emphasized.

4. Specific antiserum seems to be the best method of treatment especially in the severe cases. Chemotherapy has not had adequate trial. The first reports are very encouraging regarding sulphathiazole and discouraging regarding sulphanilimide.

5. Ten cases are reported of which six received neo-arsphenamine with good results in five.

REFERENCES

1. Lee Foshay: Tularemia. Medicine, Feb. 1940. Vol. 19 No. 1.
2. Emma S. Moss and J. O. Weilbacher, Jr.: Recent Advances in the Diagnosis and Treatment of Tularemia. Southern Medical Journal, May 1941, Vol. 34, No. 5.
3. Public Health Reports, April, 1940 Vol. 55 No. 16.
4. Cecil: Textbook of Medicine.

The Diagnosis and Control of Brucellosis[*]

I: FOREST HUDDLESON, PH.D.
*Department of Bacteriology
Michigan State College*

LANSING, MICHIGAN

Brucellosis is an infection having no pathognomonic symptoms or signs. Moreover, patients in the United States rarely appear dangerously ill; hence the taking of a detailed history and the performance of a complete physical examination are readily neglected. In addition, many practitioners have not been familiar with the nature of this infection, nor are they accustomed to consider it in differential diagnosis. It is for these reasons that admittedly erroneous diagnoses have been made in so many cases. It has been gratifying, however, to see the accuracy with which brucellosis was diagnosed once the physician had seen cases or had familiarized himself with the clinical characteristics of the disease.

When the disease has been running for weeks and a temperature chart is available, the diagnosis is easy if the possibility of brucellosis is kept in mind. It is in the first weeks that difficulties arise. A list of the diseases for which brucellosis has been mistaken would include practically all the affections accompanied by a rise of temperature. The clinical symptoms, although suggestive, can never be conclusive.

The importance of laboratory tests in diagnosis has been stated repeatedly. The laboratory procedures which are of value in diagnosis are the agglutination test, the Brucellergen intradermal test, cultural studies, white blood cell and differential counts, and opsonocytophagic tests. The two of the greatest value in differential diagnosis are the intradermal and the agglutination tests. They are usually readily available, often without cost to the patient or physician. It

may be urged, therefore, that these should be more frequently used in the investigation of febrile illnesses. Agglutinins can usually be demonstrated when the patient first applies for medical advice in infections with an insidious onset, while in those with sudden onset they may not appear until the end of the second week or, according to Simpson occasionally not until the fourth week. Apparently it is true of brucellosis as of typhoid that infrequently the serum of an infected individual may persistently fail to show any agglutinins. It must always be remembered also that a positive agglutination test may be related to the past or subclinical infection and not the present ailment of the patient. Blood, urine, and stool cultures are all valuable in the study of suspected cases of brucellosis, but these are practical in diagnosis only when the patient is within easy reach of a laboratory. Any culture study in this infection will consume at least one week, and a negative report on a blood culture cannot be made reliable until the end of the third or fourth week. Moreover, negative cultural findings on one examination can scarcely be given any weight. Cultural studies are, therefore, limited in their applicability as a diagnostic test.

The white blood cell findings in brucellosis are in no way peculiar to this infection; still a leucopenia with a relative lymphocytosis will serve to rule out all but a few conditions with which this disease may be confused.

The agglutination and complement-fixation tests in their applications to *Brucella* infections have been exhaustively studied by many investigators in Europe and North America. Their value and limitations are now well established. The complement-fixation test as a routine procedure in detecting

*Read before the Public Health Meeting, Annual Session, Oklahoma State Medical Association, May 20, 1941, in Oklahoma City.

TABLE I.

The Comparative Results of Diagnostic Tests on 100 Unselected Cases of Human Brucellosis

Total No. Cases	AGGLUTINATION TITER		OPSONIC TEST		BRUCELLERGEN TEST	
	No. 1:50 or Above	No. 1:25 or Negative	No. Positive	No. Negative	No. Positive	No. Negative
100	25	75	94	6	98	2

Brucella infection has fallen into disuse because of the time and attention that are required for its operation and because it does not furnish more information than the agglutination test, which is simpler to perform and gives results just as dependable.

Two methods of performing the agglutination test to detect *Brucella* infection in human beings and animals are available: the test-tube method and the rapid method. Both have been studied critically by many workers and found satisfactory.

Brucella agglutinins as a rule do not appear in the blood until ten days after the onset of the disease. Occasionally they cannot be detected during the course of the disease. This is especially true of the chronic form. It has been the author's observation, from a comparative study of the disease on the Island of Malta and in the United States, that agglutinins are found more often in the *Br. Melitensis* type of infection than in the *Br. abortus* type. Very few, if any, *Br. melitensis* cases fail to show agglutinins during the course of the disease.

A serum agglutination titer of 1:50 or higher, obtained on a patient showing clinical evidence of infection, should be considered as presumptive evidence of active *Brucella* infection. One should rely as much on the history of the case and other confirmatory tests as on the agglutination test in detecting active *Brucella* infection in human beings.

If the serum agglutination titer of an individual, following the disappearance of all clinical symptoms and signs of the disease, is found to be slowly decreasing as shown by a repetition of tests at 30 to 60 day intervals, it is evidence of recovery from infection.

The agglutination test, which has played such an important role in the diagnosis of animal infections, is of limited value in the chronic form of human brucellosis. The writer and his associates have had the opportunity to study the value of the various diagnostic tests on 150 brucellosis patients a year for the past three years that were sent to the laboratory by physicians. Most of the cases were of the chronic form. The agglutination test was of a sufficient titer in only 25 percent of those examined to indicate active infection (see Table I).

The results of the agglutination test may also be misleading because individuals are often found to have *Brucella* agglutinins in their blood serum when they show no symptoms of *Brucella* infection. These are chiefly laboratory workers, practicing veterinarians, farmers, and packing-house employees. By way of illustration let us consider the status of veterinarians with respect to the disease. Those who are engaged in cattle practice come in contact with *Br. abortus* to a greater extent than any other single group of people. It has already been shown by serological tests made on veterinarians in Europe and this country that a considerable percentage have *Brucella* agglutinins in varying degrees in their blood. While very few of them give a history of having a clinical course of the disease, many report the occurrence of skin eruptions and malaise after removing retained placentae from aborting cows. The malaise is usually characterized by dullness, headache, sweating and aching in the muscles and joints. There may occur an elevation of the temperature. These symptoms may occur from contact with the diseased tissues or from the ingestion or inhalation of the organism alive or dead, or from the ingestion of sterile broth filtrates on which the organism has grown. It is necessary, of course, that the specific allergen pass through the epithelium of the skin, the respiratory tract or the digestive tract. Individuals in the general population as well as those in particular groups may show the symptoms just mentioned when exposed to *Brucella*.

Cross agglutination between *Brucella* antigen and those for other disease has been the subject of many papers, but only in the case of tularemia is there likely to arise confusion as to the interpretation of the test. Francis and Evans have observed that cases of tularemia may show agglutinins in a low titer for *Brucella*. In personal communications the author has been informed of two other cases of tularemia in which the blood serum showed agglutinins for *Brucella* as well as *Pasteurella tularensis*. Both cases gave a negative skin reaction.

Since the widespread occurrence of undulant fever in man in the United States was established, considerable attention has been given to the diagnosis of the disease by

TABLE II.

Comparison of the Results of the Agglutination Test with Results of Other Laboratory
Tests on 41 Clinical and 49 Subclinical Cases of Brucellosis

Total No.	Clinical Cases 41				Sub-clinical Cases 49			
	Neg.	1:25	1:50	1:100 or Higher	Neg.	1:25	1:50	1:100 or Higher
Maximum Agglutination								
Titers, No.	4	12	7	18	26	8	6	9
Blood Culture, Positive	3	12	7	13	1	0	1	1
Brucellergen Test, Negative	0	0	0	0	1	1	1	0
Brucellergen Test, Positive	4	12	7	18	25	7	5	9
Phagocytosis, Low or Moderate	3	10	6	14	16	6	4	7
Phagocytosis, Marked	1	2	1	4	0	1	1	2
Phagocytosis, Negative	0	6	0	0	10	1	1	0

allergic methods. Data have accumulated which show that this method when used alone will only detect Brucella allergy. It will not differentiate between post and active infection.

Many physicians often observe the occurrence of a symptom complex in patients not unlike that of acute or chronic undulant fever, but are confused in making a diagnosis because the serum reaction to an agglutination test for *Brucella* infection is negative. If in addition to the agglutination test an intradermal test is performed with a suitable agent and a positive reaction is obtained, this evidence alone is not sufficient to warrant a diagnosis of undulant fever, because all individuals who have been infected with *Brucella* in the past as well as those who are actively infected will show a skin reaction to a satisfactory *Brucella* allergen.

While making a study of methods for interpreting a positive Brucellergen test obtained in humans, the author and his associates discovered that the neutrophilic leucocytes in whole citrated blood of human beings who had recovered from brucellosis phagocytized *Brucella* cells in large numbers in a proper phagocytic system. It was also observed that the same type of leucocytes in whole blood from actively infected cases showed a lower degree of phagocytic activity than that seen in individuals after recovery and in the case of those who presented no past or present history of infection, little if any degree of phagocytosis was observed. The first two groups show a positive skin test, while the third group does not.

It has been the observation of the author that if a positive skin reaction is obtained in doubtful cases of brucellosis, the positive reaction does not have specific significance until a determination of the opsonocytophagic power of the whole blood is made.

The latter test should be made at the same time or within several days after the skin test is performed, because the allergen may cause an agglutinin and opsonin response.

The procedure in performing the *Brucella* opsonic test and the system of interpreting the results may be found elsewhere.

During an epidemic of melitensis brucellosis a short time ago, an opportunity was presented for making a comparative study of four diagnostic tests on 41 clinical cases, and 49 classified as subclinical. The results of this study are set forth in Table II.

The results of the blood cultures, the skin test, and phagocytosis test on each case are grouped together according to their maximum agglutination titers. Of the four clinical cases whose blood sera were negative to the agglutination test, three showed a positive blood culture on the same date. The blood examinations in two of the four cases were made ten days and seven days after onset and in one, three days before the onset. The blood culture was positive in 12 other clinical cases which at the time showed a maximum agglutination titer of 1:25. Data showing the interval between the date of onset and the date the agglutination test was made and titer obtained are set forth in Table III. The intervals varied from one to 80 days. There does not appear to be any relationship between the strength of the titer and the time the test was made after onset.

The Brucellergen skin test was positive in all clinical cases. The size of the local reaction varied from two to six cm. The results of the phagocytosis test were confusing in eight of the 41 clinical cases in that the phagocytic picture was similar to that observed in immune individuals. These results agree in many respects with the results of the phagocytic tests conducted on *Brucella melitensis* infected individuals on the Island of Malta. In many cases of *Brucella melitensis* infection, most of the leukocytes in the patients' blood in a phagocytic system showed a marked phagocytosis of *Brucella* cells. It is obvious from the results of each of the laboratory tests, that one cannot place too much reliance on any one test to confirm the early diagnosis of clinical bru-

TABLE III.

The Results of the Agglutination Test And Blood Culture on 41 Clinical Cases Of Brucellosis

Case No.	Date of Onset	Date of Tests	Blood Culture	Maximum Agglutination Titer
1	12-10-38	12-20-38	+	negative
2	12-19-38	1-30-39	+	+1:25
3	12-26-38	3-17-39	not taken	+1:500
4	12-27-38	1-7-39	+	+1:200
5	12-27-38	2-1-39	+	+1:50
6	12-28-38	1-13-39	+	+1:500
7	12-28-38	1-17-39	+	+1:50
8	12-28-38	1-27-39	—	+1:500
9	12-28-38	1-17-39	+	+1:50
10	12-28-38	1-12-39	—	+1:100
11	1-5-39	1-13-39	+	+1:50
12	1-5-39	1-23-39	+	+1:100
13	1-5-39	1-24-39	+	+1:500
14	1-6-39	1-28-39	+	+1:200
15	1-6-39	1-13-39	+	negative
16	1-6-39	1-12-39	+	+1:25
17	1-6-39	1-14-39	+	+1:100
18	1-6-39	1-9-39	+	+1:50
19	1-7-39	1-12-39	+	+1:25
20	1-7-39	1-23-39	+	+1:500
21	1-8-39	2-1-39	+	+1:500
22	1-9-39	1-13-39	+	+1:25
23	1-10-39	2-14-39	+	+1:100
24	1-10-39	1-19-39	+	+1:25
25	1-12-39	1-14-39	+	+1:25
26	1-13-39	1-14-39	+	+1:25
27	1-13-39	1-20-39	+	+1:25
28	1-13-39	1-24-39	+	+1:50
29	1-15-39	1-19-39	+	+1:50
30	1-16-39	1-19-39	+	+1:25
31	1-19-39	1-24-39	+	negative
32	1-20-39	1-24-39	+	+1:25
33	1-20-39	1-25-39	+	+1:50
34	1-23-39	1-24-39	+	+1:100
35	1-25-39	2-9-39	—	+1:500
36	1-30-39	1-27-39	—	negative
37	2-1-39	2-18-39	+	+1:200
38	2-3-39	2-1-39	+	+1:500
39	2-5-39	2-1-39	+	+1:25
40	2-7-39	2-6-39	—	+1:100
41	2-10-39	2-13-39	+	+1:25

+ = complete agglutination or positive blood culture

— = no agglutination

cellosis. The results of all the available tests taken together must be carefully analyzed in arriving at a positive diagnosis.

In considering the results on the group classified as subclinical cases, one must take into consideration the possibility that many of them may have been exposed to infection several months or years before the study was made. The results of laboratory tests conducted on groups of people during the past several years reveal that from 10 to 15 percent may have at one time been infected with *Brucella*. The results of the phagocytic test, however, in which only four of the subclinical group show a high phagocytosis, would indicate that most of them were exposed to infective material on or near the same date as the clinical cases.

It is interesting to note that a positive blood culture was obtained from each of three of the case which failed to show the slightest symptoms of the disease before or after culturing. The three cases in question showed a positive skin test and moderate degree of phagocytosis at the time the blood cultures were taken. The skin test was negative in three of the subclinical cases. Two of these showed specific agglutinins at the time of the skin test.

The data set forth in Table II show conclusively that it is possible to demonstrate active infection long after exposure to infective material in individuals who never develop clinical manifestations of brucellosis. In other words, active infection in the case of brucellosis does not necessarily imply clinical infection.

Clinical laboratories and investigators have encountered cases in which the leucocytes in whole blood were found to show a considerable degree of phagocytic activity, but at the same time the Brucellergen test was negative. Two such cases have been brought to the attention of the author.

There are two possible causes to which one can attribute the absence of Brucellergen skin allergy in a patient whose blood shows a high degree of opsonic activity for *Brucella*. One is the presence of opsonins in the blood for *Brucella* in those who have recovered from or are actively infected with *B. tularensis*. Two such cases have been brought to the attention of the author. The other is due to the failure of a small percentage of patients infected with *Brucella* to develop skin allergy and show a positive reaction to Brucellergen or other *Brucella* allergic agents.

CONTROL OF BRUCELLOSIS

A paradoxical situation exists at the present time in the control of brucellosis in that there is sufficient knowledge available on the nature of brucellosis effectively to suppress its spread in animals, and from animals to man. The important hosts of *Brucella* are known, the routes through which the organism is eliminated from the hosts have been determined, and the diagnostic procedures have been perfected to a high degree of accuracy. But despite all this usable knowledge the number of reported human cases continues to increase. The sanitarian is confronted with a perplexing problem of applying control measures effectively without affecting too seriously the economic interests involved.

Since brucellosis is primarily an animal borne disease it is exiomatic that the reduction of its incidence in man can only be brought about by either suppressing the disease in animals or by effectively breaking the infectious chains between animals and man.

Before effective control measures can be considered and put into practice in a given region, it is essential to know (1) the animal hosts, (2) the species of *Brucella* involved, (3) the means by which the organism is conveyed from animals to man. (See Table IV).

If the incidence of brucellosis is found to be high in more than one species of animal, and more than one species of *Brucella* is involved, considerable difficulty will be encountered in formulating control measures that will be applicable to all animals alike. The task becomes complex when attempts are made to prevent the transmission of the disease from one species of animal to another and from more than one animal host to humans.

If only one species of *Brucella* is found present in a given region, the problem of control is greatly simplified, but if more than one is implicated, those measures taken to suppress the dissemination of one species of *Brucella* may be unworkable for another species.

The three control measures that have been advocated and used in animal brucellosis are: (1) slaughter of infected animals, (2) segregation of infected animals from the non-infected on separate farms, (3) immunization of calves under eight months of age.

The slaughter plan for removing infected animals with the expectation of eliminating brucellosis in cattle has been in operation in certain states for 15 years, and on an extensive scale under federal supervision in most of the states for the past six years. The plan was placed in operation with a great deal of enthusiasm and has received the support of the veterinary profession and breeders' organizations. The slaughter plan was instituted in the face of the fact that previous preliminary surveys had indicated the

TABLE IV.

Viability of *Brucella* Outside the Animal Body

Material	Length of Life
Gastric juice	2 hours
Hog Cholera virus	5 months
Infected bovine fetus	7 months
Infective milk (cow)	10 days
Ice cream	30 days
Butter	142 days
Roquefort cheese	2 months
Urine (bovine)	4 days
Hog spleen (-10°F)	30 days
Hog spleen (in brine)	40 days
Mosquitoes (exposed)	48 hours
Flies (exposed)	120 hours
Soil (dry)	27 days
Soil (moist)	37 days
Tap water (25°C)	77 days
Tap water (-40°C)	114 days
Sunlight	4½ hours

incidence of infection in cattle would average 15 percent and with the knowledge that the cow is not the only host for *Brucella*. The failure of several enthusiastic advocates of the plan to give any consideration whatsoever to sources of infection other than the infected cow, and the incubation period in the disease has accounted for its failure in many instances and caused much disappointment in those directly concerned.

An unbiased analysis of the records of the cooperative federal-state Bang's disease program shows that considerable progress has been made in reducing the percentage of infected cattle and, further, the disease has been eliminated in a large number of herds. The success of the slaughter plan in eliminating the disease from infected herds appears to be inversely proportional to the size of the herd. Difficulty has been encountered in eliminating the disease from herds of a considerable size and preventing reinfections in many smaller ones. The failures in most instances cannot be attributed to laxity in sanitary practices or inadequate supervision. It is possible that when more information is available concerning the incubation period of the disease in the cow and more consideration is given to other hosts of *Brucella,* less difficulty will be met in the elimination of brucellosis from large herds.

In certain regions the milch goat or the hog is the chief reservoir for the source of the disease in man. It follows that the elimination of the disease in the cow may have little, if any effect on the lowering of the incidence of brucellosis in humans. The effectiveness of the slaughter method in infected goats and hogs is yet to be determined.

Control of the disease in cattle by means of calf vaccination is worthy of trial. Experimental data in support of vaccination of calves with a live culture of low virulence was first presented by Cotton and Buck and Smith in 1934. Since 1934, a considerable amount of data have been collected under experimental and natural conditions by several investigators which support the original findings. A high degree of protection against infection appears to be obtained in 70 percent of the vaccinated calves. The immunity appears to persist for one or more years. There have been no data obtained which indicate that the live bacteria in the vaccine is infectious for the calf under eight months of age. Vaccination of calves would in time result in the rearing of herds of cattle free from brucellosis.

There is another simple and inexpensive measure which could be taken in to prevent the spread of the disease in animals and thereby aid in keeping it under control. It is the requirement of a negative blood tes. on animals sold for breeding or for dairy purposes. If the sale of infected animals from one farm to another, or from stockyard to farm is prevented, the spread of the disease to farms where infection does not exist can be minimized. Such a measure should not be too great a burden for the farmer to bear. It would be to his interest to support and to cooperate in making the plan a success.

There still seems to exist much confusion and guessing regarding the necessary hygienic and sanitary measures that should be taken to prevent the transmission of brucellosis to humans. Today there is as much knowledge, available on the habits of *Brucella*, the channels through which they are eliminated from hosts and the means of conveyance to humans as any other pathogenic bacteria.

The incidence of the disease in humans could quickly be reduced to a minimum if the owners of livestock were taught to use more caution in the handling of infected animals, their excreta and secretions; and by the proper pasteurization of all milk from infected animals used for human consumption.

When the present knowledge is made use of to the fullest extent by sanitarians and those intrusted with the guarding of human health, brucellosis in man will be a disease of the past instead of a disease of the future.

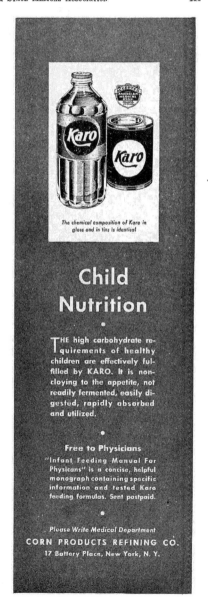

• THE PRESIDENT'S PAGE •

American Medicine scores again. "The Medical Corps at Pearl Harbor was ready" on December seventh and the story of how well those who were wounded in that dastardly assault were cared for and the results of treatment will be one of the shining examples of what true preparedness means.

Almost a year ago when most everyone thought Hawaii safe and that extensive preparations were foolish, Colonel E. S. King, Surgeon in charge of Hawaiian Army Medical Forces, organized all Army, Navy and Civilian Medical Forces so that possible disaster might be met.

Most remarkable of all results is the report that no amputations have been necessary on account of infection, and in compound fractures and flesh wounds less than four percent became infected and not a single massive infection was found ten days after the injuries.

Medical preparedness made this possible.

President.

• EDITORIALS •

PROGRAM FOR THE STATE MEETING

Elsewhere in the Journal you will find a complete outline of the program to be presented at the 50th Annual Meeting of the Oklahoma State Medical Association.

To some of you, the departure from the conventional type of program presented in the past will be a welcome change. To others, it will appear as though the activities of the various sections which make up the scientific program have been deliberately and maliciously curtailed. To still others, the idea may seem a novel experiment worthy of trial and consideration for future meetings.

Since its inception, the Scientific Work Committee has had but one aim and one goal. This is to present a high type of scientific program which will be interesting and valuable to the entire membership. Following the requests of the various sections, we have provided guest speakers for each section again this year as was done last year. The Committee felt, furthermore, that the membership should be taken into consideration in choosing subjects and material for presentation. As a result, a questionnaire was sent to each member, and we are incorporating those subjects in the program which received the largest number of requests. We extend a hearty vote of thanks to the individuals who responded to our questionnaire.

Your committee has been faced with a difficult task this year in providing guest speakers. We have also been confronted with the problem of providing a meeting place where nine sections could meet at the same time. We must admit there is no hotel or available building in Oklahoma large enough to accomodate a meeting of this size. We have made no deliberate attempt to curtail the activity of the respective sections, but it is a physical impossibility to provide each one with a suitable meeting place without subjecting the Association to the prohibitive expense of building section rooms on the floor of the Coliseum. This is the reason we have adopted the program as presented herewith.

The round-table discussion of Sulfanilamide Therapy to be participated in by all of the guest speakers, as well as the audience, is an innovation this year, and it is hoped that it will be a very valuable and instructive presentation.

Whether or not you agree with the arrangement of the program, we request your indulgence and cooperation. If there ever was a time in the history of our profession when it is essential for us, as individuals, to get behind and support organized medicine to the fullest extent, that time is now. American medicine will necessarily have to assume world leadership at the termination of the war. It behooves all of us, therefore, to become actively interested and lend full support to the component units of organized medicine which are the County and State Medical Societies. We urge you to attend this meeting, and we are confident that you will find something of interest and value in the papers presented by our essayists.— C. R. R.

MEDICINE PLUS

In this hour of trouble, embracing a worldwide war of unprecedented gravity, every good doctor must not only preserve his own equanimity, but with incredible self-control, he must pass mental poise to those who are less stable. Calm courageous attitudes while in action or in time of suspense, must become universal, if we want to win the war and preserve our democratic way of life. Otherwise, the psychologically unstable will become incapable of making constructive contributions toward the solution of our national problems. Failing in this, they not only retard progress by their own impotency, but they become a burden upon those who must carry on in spite of all obstacles.

In the history of mankind, there has never been a time when the penalties of war descended upon society in such a deadly, comprehensive fashion. Modern warfare spares no human being, not even the prenatal. Lying-in hospitals have been bombed; the sanctity of home has no security; the accumulated treasures of art are being ground into dust.

Our men on the far-flung battle front must not only meet their foes face to face, but they must fight with the deadly fear that their loved ones at home may be the innocent victims of unannounced bombing or barbarous invasion. Though our men stand at the front, they too must await news of the war. This brief comment shows what an important bearing modern warfare has upon mass psychology. Never before has there been such valid reason for universal mental strain. Already 50 percent of the hospital beds in this country are occupied by mental cases, and psychiatric deficiencies stand fifth as a cause for rejection of registrants. But doctors know it is doubtful if this high incidence of nervous and mental disease really represents a genuine decline in mental stability. It seems more reasonable to attribute the increasing prevalence of psychiatric difficulties to the trying task of adjustment in a swiftly moving, ever-changing new way of life. Unfortunately this adjustment had to be integrated with our recovery from the strain of the last world war, with its untold heroisms and self-sacrifices which, "for the safety of democracy," poured out the blood of ten million people.

If, perchance, we wonder what a doctor can do to help win a sacred cause in a world of strife and confusion, let us remember that his first duty is to keep his head clear and his hands ready for the immediate task. In so doing, he can help stabilize mass psychology and possibly stave off the evil effects of widespread hysteria, which would inevitably lead to certain defeat.

With the above in mind, doctors must help people realize that it is not necessary to draw a fine line between normal and abnormal behavior, but that it is essential for each individual to become a living example for those about him. This is no time to ask, "am I my brother's keeper?" There is both sanity and safety in service. We must do what we can to make society fool-proof. Concerted effort in this direction will do more for the fearful, wavering mind than all the medicine in the world.

Our hospitals for nervous and mental diseases are full, doctors are being called into government service, and those who remain at home are over-worked. But this is no time for us to sink into the "slough of despond." On the contrary, our fortitude and composure must serve as an antidote for those who have an idiosyncrasy toward calamity. While threatened with a lethal dose of melancholy or fear, they will need our sympathy and support. The survival of democracy will depend upon our composite response to the great emergency now claiming our attention. This emergency can be met successfully only through the elevation of our national zeal to a high average of stability and continuity. —L. J. M.

Dr. Vernon Speaks at Arkansas Meeting

Dr. W. C. Vernon of Okmulgee was guest speaker at the meeting of the Sebastian County Medical society of Arkansas, February 19, in Fort Smith, Ark.

Doctor Vernon chose "The Injection Treatment of Hemorrhoids" as the subject of his talk.

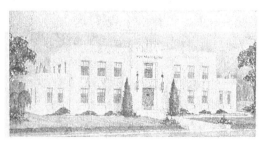

Welcome To.....

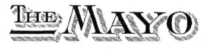

TULSA

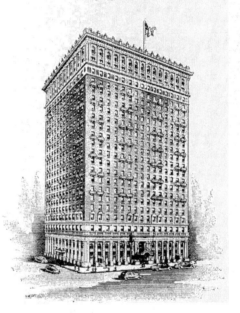

Official Headquarters

Oklahoma State Medical Association
1942 Annual Meeting

FRANK R. BENTLEY, Assistant Manager

PROGRAM

Fiftieth Annual Session of the Oklahoma State Medical Association
Tulsa, April 22, 23, 24, 1942

GREETINGS FROM THE TULSA COUNTY SOCIETY

Every other year the Tulsa County Medical Society shares honors with the Oklahoma County Society in acting as host society to the annual meeting of the Oklahoma State Medical Association. This year the Tulsa Society automatically becomes host on April 22, 23 and 24.

The Tulsa Society is alert and fully aware of its obligations when it accepts the honor as host. It shall be our duty to see that every detail is carried out in the execution of the main purpose of the meeting—the scientific program. The entertainment and side lights incident to the program shall be our responsibility to the extent that everyone in attendance will feel fully compensated for whatever sacrifice he may have made to be our guest.

In order that all events as planned shall be carried out on schedule and without detraction by holding two events at the same time, the Tulsa County Society has arranged for a special Buffet Supper at the Mayo Hotel at 6:30 p.m. on Tuesday evening, April 21. Every member of the State Medical Society is cordially invited to this affair, as guests of the local society. The supper is to be followed by two interesting speakers on medico-legal problems. If you find it possible to attend this supper, the Tulsa County Executive Secretary would appreciate a post card to that effect.

The Women's Auxiliary of our local society has made plans for entertainment of the women and they join in this formal invitation to Tulsa. Make your plans to bring your wife with you.

We shall look for you on Tuesday evening, April 21. The Buffet Supper will be a stag affair.

H. B. Stewart, M.D., President,
Tulsa County Medical Society.

General Information

HEADQUARTERS
Coliseum, Tulsa

REGISTRATION
Coliseum

All physicians except those from outside the state, visiting guests, and those on military assignment, must have membership cards for 1942 before registering. Dues will not be accepted at the registration desk except from County Secretaries.

GENERAL SESSIONS AND SECTION MEETINGS

All meetings will be held in the main foyer of the Coliseum. Section meetings will start at 9:00 A. M., and the General Sessions at 2:30 P. M.

GUEST SPEAKERS

Charles C. Dennie, M.D., Professor of Clinical Dermatology, University of Kansas School of Medicine, Kansas City, Mo.

George Herrmann, M.D., Professor of Clinical Medicine, University of Texas School of Medicine, Galveston, Tex.

John C. Burch, M.D., Associate Professor of Obstetrics and Gynecology, Vanderbilt University, School of Medicine, Nashville, Tenn.

T. Leon Howard, M.D., Associate Professor of Surgery (Urol.), University of Colorado School of Medicine, Denver, Colo.

Titus H. Harris, M.D., Professor of Neurology and Psychiatry, University of Texas School of Medicine, Galveston, Tex.

M. Edward Davis, M.D., Associate Professor of Obstetrics and Gynecology, University of Chicago, the School of Medicine, Chicago, Ill.

A. B. Reese, M.D., Assistant Clinical Professor of Ophthalmology, Columbia University College of Physicians and Surgeons, New York City, N. Y.

Robert L. Sanders, M.D., Associate Professor of Surgery, University of Tennessee College of Medicine, Memphis, Tenn.

Hugh L. Dwyer, M D., Professor of Clinical Pediatrics, University of Kansas School of Medicine, Kansas City, Mo.

HOUSE OF DELEGATES

The House of Delegates will meet Wednesday at 8.00 P. M. and at 8.00 A. M., Thursday, in the Ivory Room, at the Mayo Hotel.

COUNCIL

The Council will meet Tuesday evening, April 21, immediately following the Buffet Supper of the Tulsa County Medical Society, in the French Room, Mezzanine floor, Mayo Hotel, and thereafter on the call of the President.

SCIENTIFIC ROUNDTABLE ON SULFONAMIDE THERAPY

An innovation for the Fiftieth Annual Meeting will be the conducting of a Scientific Roundtable on Sulfonamide Therapy, in which all of the guest speakers will participate. The Roundtable will be held in the Crystal Ballroom of the Mayo Hotel, Wednesday evening, at 8:00 o'clock. An opportunity will be afforded the audience to ask questions of the guest speakers.

WOMEN'S AUXILIARY

Registration will be in the lobby of the Mayo Hotel. The complete Program will be found on this page.

TECHNICAL AND SCIENTIFIC EXHIBITS

The exhibits will be displayed in the main foyer of the Coliseum.

RESOLUTIONS

Resolutions for the consideration of the House of Delegates should be prepared and submitted at the first meeting of the House of Delegates.

TULSA COUNTY MEDICAL SOCIETY BUFFET SUPPER

The Buffet Supper will be held Tuesday evening, April 21, in the Ivory Room of the Mayo Hotel at 7:00 P. M. All members of the Association and guests of the Association are to be the guests of the Tulsa County Medical Society. An attractive program on Medico-Legal and Economic subjects has been arranged.

OKLAHOMA UNIVERSITY MEDICAL ALUMNI LUNCHEON

The Luncheon will be held at 12:00, Thursday, April 23, at the Tulsa Club.

TEA FOR DOCTORS AND WIVES

The Tea will be held from 6 30 to 7.30, Thursday evening, April 23, in the Junior Ballroom, Mayo Hotel. Everyone is cordially invited.

PRESIDENT'S INAUGURAL DINNER DANCE

The Dinner Dance will immediately follow the Tea and will be held in the Crystal Ballroom, 16th floor, Mayo Hotel. Dr. Morris Fishbein, Editor of the Journal of the American Medical Association, will be the guest speaker.

GOLF TOURNAMENT

The Golf Tournament will be held at the Tulsa Country Club and will be Medal Play over 18 holes. Those wishing to compete in the Tournament may play any time during the Meeting. Green fee will be $1.00 Carl Simpson, M.D., Tulsa, is Chairman of the Tournament.

Women's Auxiliary Program

State Auxiliary Officers

President	Secretary
Mrs. E. D. Greenberger	Mrs. E. H. Shuller
McAlester	McAlester
President-Elect	Treasurer
Mrs. Frank L. Flack	Mrs. L. S. Willour
Tulsa	McAlester
Vice-President	Historian
Mrs. Rush Wright	Mrs. A. R. Sugg
Poteau	Ada

Parliamentarian
Mrs. W. A. Fowler
Norman

CONVENTION PROGRAM

Mrs. J. W. Childs
Convention Chairman

Wednesday, April 22, 1942

9.00 A. M.—Registration   Lobby, Mayo Hotel
7:30 P. M.—Pre-convention Executive Board Meeting, in the home of Mrs. J. W. Childs, 1616 South Madison, Tulsa.

Thursday, April 23, 1942

8 30 A. M.—Registration   Mezzanine, Mayo Hotel
10.00 A. M.—Annual Meeting   Parlor, Mezzanine, Mayo Hotel
1·00 P. M.—Luncheon   Marine Room, Mayo Hotel, $1.00
            All visiting ladies invited. Tickets may be secured at the registration desk.
3.00 P. M.—Post-convention Executive Board Meeting, Parlor, Mezzanine, Mayo Hotel.

GUEST SPEAKERS
Annual Session, Oklahoma State Medical Association

Section on Dermatology and Radiology

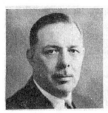

Charles C. Dennie, M.D., Professor of Clinical Dermatology, University of Kansas School of Medicine, Kansas City, Mo.

Section on Medicine

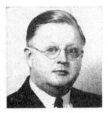

George Herrmann, M D, Professor of Clinical Medicine, University of Texas School of Medicine, Galveston, Texas.

Section on Obstetrics and Gynecology

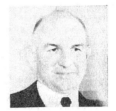

John C. Burch, M D., Associate Professor of Obstetrics and Gynecology, Vanderbilt University School of Medicine, Nashville, Tenn.

Section on Urology and Syphilology

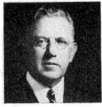

T. Leon Howard, M D., Assistant Professor of Surgery (Urol.), University of Colorado School of Medicine, Denver, Colo.

Section on Public Health

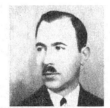

M. Edward Davis, M D., Associate Professor of Obstetrics and Gynecology, University of Chicago, the School of Medicine, Chicago, Ill.

Section on Eye, Ear Nose and Throat

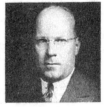

A. B Reese, M.D., Assistant Clinical Professor of Ophthalmology, Columbia University College of Physicians and Surgeons, New York City, N. Y.

Section on General Surgery

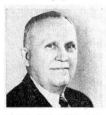

Robert L. Sanders, M.D., Associate Professor of Surgery, University of Tennessee College of Medicine, Memphis, Tenn.

Section on Neurology, Psychiatry and Endocrinology

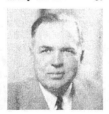

Titus H Harris, M D., Professor of Neurology and Psychiatry, University of Texas School of Medicine, Galveston, Tex.

Section on Pediatrics

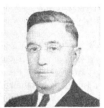

Hugh L. Dwyer, M.D., Professor of Clinical Pediatrics, University of Kansas School of Medicine, Kansas City, Mo.

Scientific Program

Oklahoma State Medical Association
April 22, 23, 24, 1942
Coliseum, Tulsa

All Sections and Sessions will meet in the General Assembly Hall in the main foyer of the Coliseum.

Wednesday, April 22
General Chairman, C. R. Rountree, M.D., Oklahoma City

9:00 A. M.
SECTION ON DERMATOLOGY AND RADIOLOGY
Onis G. Hazel, M.D., Chairman

9:00 "Sarcoid of Boeck"—Onis G. Hazel, M.D., Oklahoma City, and Wayne M. Hull, M.D., Oklahoma City.
9:20 Discussion—John H. Lamb, M.D., Oklahoma City.
9:30 "Eczema—Modern Concepts of Treatment"—Harry Green, M.D., Tulsa.
9:50 Discussion—James Stevenson, M.D., Tulsa.
10:00 "The Treatment of Pregnant Syphilitic Women and the Results of Treatment"— .
Charles C. Dennie, M.D., Kansas City, Mo.

10:30 A. M.
SECTION ON GENERAL MEDICINE
W. W. Rucks, Jr., M.D., Chairman

10:30 "Hygiene in the Tropics"—Walker Morledge, M.D., Oklahoma City.
10:50 Discussion—Carroll M. Pounders, M.D., Oklahoma City.
11:00 "Atypical Pneumonia"—Samuel Goodman, M.D., Tulsa.
11:20 Discussion—Paul B. Cameron, M.D., Pryor.
11:30 "Exigencies of Cardiological Practice"—George Herrmann, M.D., Galveston, Tex.

12:00 Noon

1:00 P. M.
SECTION ON EYE, EAR, NOSE AND THROAT
F. Maxey Cooper, M.D., Chairman

1:00 "Relation of the Eye, Ear, Nose and Throat Specialist to the General Practitioner"—Marvin D. Henley, M.D., Tulsa.
1:20 Discussion—J. F. Gorrell, M.D., Tulsa.
1:30 "Causes of Blindness in Oklahoma"—Tullos O. Coston, M.D., Oklahoma City.
1:50 Discussion—J. A. Morrow, M.D., Oklahoma City.
2:00 "Office Therapeutics"—A. B. Reese, M.D., New York City, N. Y.

General Sessions

Chairman, Finis W. Ewing, M.D., President, Oklahoma State Medical Association

2:30 P. M.
OBSTETRICS AND GYNECOLOGY
2:30 "Physiological Approach to Gynecology"—John C. Burch, M.D., Nashville, Tenn.

3:15 P. M.
DERMATOLOGY AND RADIOLOGY
3:15 "Congenital Syphilis of the Bones and Joints of Infants"—Charles C. Dennie, M.D., Kansas City, Mo.

4:00 P. M.
PEDIATRICS
4:00 "Protection of Children Against Tuberculosis"—Hugh L. Dwyer, M.D., Kansas City, Mo.

Scientific Program

Thursday, April 23

General Chairman, T. H. McCarley, M.D., McAlester

All Sections and Sessions will meet in the General Assembly Hall in the main foyer of the Coliseum.

9:00 A. M.
SECTION ON OBSTETRICS AND GYNECOLOGY

Charles Ed White, M.D., Chairman

9:00 "Obstetrical Psychosis"—Bruce R. Hinson, M.D., Enid.
9:20 Discussion—Coyne Campbell, M.D., Oklahoma City.
9:30 "Delivering the Sick Woman"—E. P. Allen, M.D., Oklahoma City.
9:50 Discussion—J. B. Eskridge, Jr., M.D., Oklahoma City.
10:00 "The Etiology of Menstrual Disturbances"—John C. Burch, M.D., Nashville, Tenn.

10:30 A. M.
SECTION ON GENERAL SURGERY

A. Ray Wiley, M.D., Chairman

10:30 "Goiter"—C. C. Hoke, M.D., Tulsa.
10.50 Discussion—
11:00 "Treatment of Varicose Veins"—R. Q. Atchley, M.D., Tulsa.
11:20 Discussion—Carl J. Hotz, M.D., Tulsa.
11:30 "Carcinoma of the Colon: Lantern Slides"—Robert L. Sanders, M.D., Memphis, Tenn.

12:00 Noon

1:00 P. M.
SECTION ON PEDIATRICS

David J. Underwood, M.D., Chairman

1:00 "Scarlet Fever Immunization"—Hugh C. Graham, M.D., Tulsa.
1:20 Discussion—J. T. Bell, M.D., Oklahoma City.
1:30 "Problems of Behavior in Child Guidance"—Harold J. Binder, M.D., Oklahoma City.
1:50 Discussion—Carroll M. Pounders, M.D., Oklahoma City.
2:00 "Emergencies of the New-born Period"—Hugh L. Dwyer, M.D., Kansas City, Mo.

General Sessions

Chairman, C. R. Rountree, M.D., Oklahoma City

2:30 P. M.
General Medicine

2:30 "Functional Heart Disorders Including the Soldier's Heart"—George Herrmann, M.D., Galveston, Tex.

3:15 P. M.
Public Health

3:15 "The Endocrines in Obstetrics and Gynecology"—M. Edward Davis, M.D., Chicago, Ill.

4:00 P. M.
Eye, Ear, Nose and Throat

4:00 "Exophthalmos Associated With Thyroid Disease"—A. B. Reese, M.D., New York City, N. Y.

Scientific Program

Friday, April 24

General Chairman, R. C. Pigford, M.D., Tulsa

All Sections and Sessions will meet in the General Assembly Hall in the main foyer of the Coliseum.

9:00 A. M.
SECTION ON NEUROLOGY, PSYCHIATRY AND ENDOCRINOLOGY
Felix M. Adams, M.D., Chairman

9:00   "Recent Advances in Psychosomatic Medicine"—Charles E. Leonard, M.D., Oklahoma City.

9:20   Discussion—F. M. Adams, M.D., Vinita.

9:30   "Neuropsychiatric Aspects of Carbon Disulphide Poisoning with Report of Two Cases Occurring in Oklahoma"—M. D. Spottswood, M.D., Tulsa.

9:50   Discussion—James A. Willie, M.D., Oklahoma City.

10:00   "Complications Following the Use of Dilantin"—Titus H. Harris, M.D., Galveston, Tex.

10:30 A. M.
SECTION ON UROLOGY AND SYPHILOLOGY
Robert H. Akin, M.D., Chairman

10:30   "Urinary Lithiasis"—J. W. Rogers, M.D., Tulsa.

10:50   Discussion—Harry H. Hudson, M.D., Enid.

11:00   "Prostatic Resection and the Result Expected"—E. Halsell Fite, M.D., Muskogee.

11:20   Discussion—Robert H. Akin, M.D., Oklahoma City.

11:30   "Malignancy of the Bladder and Prostate with Reference to New Methods of Treatment"—T. Leon Howard, M.D., Denver, Colo.

12:00 Noon

1:00 P. M.
SECTION ON PUBLIC HEALTH
John A. Morrow, M.D., Chairman

1:00   "Ideals in Rural Obstetrics"—Isadore Dyer, M.D., Tahlequah.

1:20   Discussion—Edward N. Smith, M.D., Oklahoma City, and E. R. Muntz, M.D., Ada.

1:30   "Fluoroscopic Survey of Postnatal Syphilis in a Health Department Clinic—A Preliminary Report"—David V. Hudson, M.D., Tulsa, and S. C. Venable, M.D., Tulsa.

1:50   Discussion—E. A. Gillis, M.D., Oklahoma City.

2:00   "Practical Problems in Maternal and Child Health"—M. Edward Davis, M.D., Chicago, Ill.

General Sessions

Chairman, J. D. Osborn, M.D., Frederick

2:00 P. M.
Urology and Syphilology

2:30   "The Symptoms, the Diagnosis and the Treatment of Nephroptosis"—T. Leon Howard, M.D., Denver, Colo.

3:15 P. M.
Neurology, Psychiatry and Endocrinology

3:15   "Discussion of the Depressions as Seen in the General Practice of Medicine"—Titus H. Harris, M.D., Galveston, Tex.

4:00 P. M.
General Surgery

4:00   "Complications of Duodenal Ulcers; Their Surgical Management: Lantern Slides"—Robert L. Sanders, M.D., Memphis, Tenn.

ASSOCIATION ACTIVITIES

Association Takes Over Malpractice Insurance With London and Lancashire

The Tulsa County Medical society, which two years ago caused a drastic reduction in malpractice insurance rates for the doctors of Oklahoma by working out a group policy first with the Houston Fire and Casualty company and later with London and Lancashire, requested on February 10 that the State Association become the sole holder of the Master Policy and that all future control of the policy rest with the Association.

This action by Tulsa county was promptly accepted by the Council, and a new Master Policy has been issued in favor of the Association.

The work of the Tulsa County Medical society in bringing this saving on malpractice insurance to the entire membership of the Association has been one of the finest contributions to the Association that has ever been accomplished. On the basis of an average premium of thirty-five dollars, members of the Association have been saved approximately $17,500.00 a year.

Every member of the Association who carries malpractice insurance should cooperate in this program by carrying his insurance with London and Lancashire. Details concerning the policy may be obtained by writing the office of the Association.

Councilor District 10 Holds First Annual Meeting

The First Annual Meeting of members of the Tenth Councilor District of the Association was held on the evening of February 23, at Rock Gables near Hugo, with 24 members in attendance.

The meeting was called to order by Dr. Fred Switzer, Hugo, of the Choctaw County Medical society, and was then turned over to Dr. J. S. Fulton, Atoka, Councilor for the District. Doctor Fulton complimented the group on their attendance, and stated that such meetings should be continued in the future.

Dr. Finis W. Ewing, Muskogee, President of the Association, was introduced, and then he addressed the group on the subject of "Medicine and War." Doctor Ewing also spoke on the activities of the Association.

Major Louis H. Ritzhaupt, State Medical Officer, discussed "Selective Service and the Rehabilitation Program for Rejectees." After adjournment to hear President Roosevelt's radio address, the group heard a talk on "Procurement and Assignment" by R. H. Graham, Executive Secretary of the Association.

Delegates and Alternates to Annual Meeting Are Announced

In compliance with the by-laws of the Oklahoma State Medical Association, the delegates and alternates of the county societies who have been certified to the office by the local county societies are hereby announced.

All delegates and alternates will be seated in accordance with the membership certified as of March 22.

COUNTY	DELEGATE	ALTERNATE
Alfalfa	H. E. Huston, Cherokee	
Atoka-Coal	J. C. Canada, Atoka	W. W. Cotton, Atoka
	J. B. Clark, Coalgate	R. C. Henry, Coalgate
Beckham	H. K. Speed, Sayre	E. S. Kilpatrick, Elk City
Blaine	Virginia Olson Curtin, Watonga	L. R. Kirby, Okeene
Bryan	J. T. Colwick, Durant	J. A. Haynie, Durant
Caddo	E. W. Hawkins, Carnegie	G. E. Haslam, Anadarko
Canadian	J. T. Phelps, El Reno	M. E. Phelps, El Reno
Carter	G. E. Johnson, Ardmore	F. W. Boadway, Ardmore
	J. L. Cox, Ardmore	Walter Hardy, Ardmore
Cherokee	Robert K. McIntosh, Jr., Tahlequah	Isadore Dyer, Tahlequah
	Warren Beasley, Stilwell	
	William Newlin, Sallisaw	
Choctaw	E. O. Johnson, Hugo	O. R. Gregg, Hugo
Cleveland	F. C. Buffington, Norman	O. E. Howell, Norman
	Phil Haddock, Norman	W. B. Carroll, Norman
Comanche	O. L. Parsons, Lawton	Howard Angus, Lawton
Cotton	George A. Tallant, Walters	A .B. Holsted, Temple
Craig	F. M. Adams, Vinita	Lloyd H. McPike, Vinita
Creek	C. R. McDonald, Mannford	Charles Schrader, Bristow
Custer	McLain Rogers, Clinton	Gordon Williams, Weatherford
	Ellis Lamb, Clinton	Ross Deputy, Clinton
Garfield	V. R. Hamble, Enid	
	W. P. Neilson, Enid	
Garvin	Galvin L. Johnson, Pauls Valley	
Grady	W. H. Cook, Chickasha	
Grant	E. E. Lawson, Medford	
Greer	L. E. Pearson, Mangum	J. B. Hollis, Mangum
Harmon	W. G. Husband, Hollis	Russell Lynch, Hollis
Haskell	J. C. Rumley, Stigler	William S. Carson, Keota
Hughes	W. L. Taylor, Holdenville	
Jackson	E. S. Crow, Olustee	E. W. Mabry, Altus
Jefferson	L. L. Wade, Ryan	
Kay	J. C. Wagner, Ponca City	L. I. Wright, Blackwell
	Dewey Mathews, Tonkawa	G. S. Kreger, Tonkawa

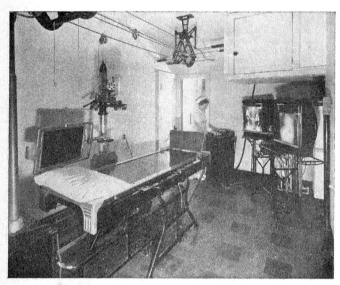

Kingfisher	F. C. Lattimore, Kingfisher	John R. Taylor, Kingfisher
Kiowa	J. M. Bonham, Hobart	
LeFlore	F. P. Baker, Talihina	
Lincoln	Ned Burleson, Prague	Carl Bailey, Stroud
Logan	L. A. Hahn, Guthrie	J. L. LeHew, Jr., Guthrie
Marshall	J. L. Holland, Madill	O. A. Cook, Madill
Mayes	Carl Puckett, Oklahoma City	V. D. Herrington, Pryor
McClain	O. O. Dawson, Wayne	G. S. Barger, Purcell
McCurtain	R. B. Oliver, Idabel	W. W. Williams, Idabel
McIntosh	Wm. A. Tolleson, Eufaula	D. E. Little, Eufaula
Murray	W. D. DeLay, Sulphur	F. E. Sadler, Sulphur
Muskogee	C. E. White, Muskogee	I. B. Oldham, Jr., Muskogee
	J. H. White, Muskogee	L. S. McAlister, Muskogee
Noble	A. M. Evans, Perry	T. F. Renfrow, Billings
Okfuskee	C. M. Cochran, Okemah	M. L. Whitney, Okemah
Oklahoma	W. F. Keller, Okla. City	W. W. Rucks, Jr., Okla. City
	Onis G. Hazel, Okla. City	Neil Woodward, Okla. City
	Walker Morledge, Okla. City	R. H. Akin, Okla. City
	L. C. McHenry, Okla. City	W. E. Eastland, Okla. City
	C. R. Rountree, Okla. City	M. F. Jacobs, Okla. City
	O. A. Watson, Okla. City	R. L. Murdoch, Okla. City
	J. B. Snow, Okla. City	R. L. Noell, Okla. City
	D. H. O'Donoghue, Okla. City	W. K. West, Okla. City
	C. M. Pounders, Okla. City	Harper Wright, Okla. City
	George Garrison, Okla. City	R. Q. Goodwin, Okla. City
	Allen Gibbs, Okla. City	George Kimball, Okla. City
Okmulgee	I. W. Bollinger, Henryetta	J. C. Matheney, Okmulgee
Osage	G. I. Walker, Hominy	Roscoe Walker, Pawhuska
Ottawa	M. A. Connell, Picher	M. M. DeArman, Miami
	Walker B. Sanger, Picher	F. L. Wormington, Miami
Pawnee	J. L. LeHew, Pawnee	R. E. Jones, Pawnee
Payne	A. B. Smith, Stillwater	R. E. Waggoner, Stillwater
Pittsburg	T. H. McCarley, McAlester	W. C. Wait, McAlester
	L. S. Willour, McAlester	Frank Baum, McAlester
Pontotoc	Ollie McBride, Ada	Sam A. McKeel, Ada
Pottawatomie	G. S. Baxter, Shawnee	E. E. Rice, Shawnee
	W. M. Gallaher, Shawnee	R. M. Anderson, Shawnee
Pushmataha	P. B. Rice, Antlers	E. S. Patterson, Antlers
Rogers	R. C. Meloy, Claremore	
Seminole	Claude S. Chambers, Seminole	Mack I. Shanholtz Wewoka
Stephens	C. N. Talley, Marlow	Claude B. Waters, Duncan
Texas	Johnny A. Blue, Guymon	Morris Smith, Guymon
Tillman	T. F. Spurgeon, Frederick	J. E. Childers, Tipton
Tulsa	R. A. McGill, Tulsa	E. Rankin Denny, Tulsa
	George Osborn, Tulsa	T. J. Hardman, Tulsa
	W. A. Showman, Tulsa	Eugene Wolff, Tulsa
	M. J. Searle, Tulsa	Carl Simpson, Tulsa
	Marvin D. Henley, Tulsa	W. A. Walker, Tulsa
	W. Albert Cook, Tulsa	W. R. Turnbow, Tulsa
	R. C. Pigford, Tulsa	M. D. Spottswood, Tulsa
	W. S. Larrabee, Tulsa	
Wagoner	H. K. Riddle, Coweta	J. H. Plunkett, Wagoner
Washington-Nowata	S. A. Lang, Nowata	K. D. Davis, Nowata
	L. D. Hudson, Dewey	J. P. Vansant, Dewey
	H. C. Weber, Bartlesville	E. E. Beechwood, Bartlesville
Washita	A. H. Bungardt, Cordell	James F. McMurry, Sentinel
Woods	D. B. Ensor, Hopeton	C. A. Traverse, Alva
Woodward	Joe L. Duer, Woodward	
	H. Walker, Buffalo	
	O. C. Newman, Shattuck	

Honorary Membership

In accordance with the provisions of the By-Laws of the Oklahoma State Medical Association, the following names of members in good standing of the Association, which have been placed on file in the office of the Association to be acted upon for honorary membership, are hereby published:

R. M. C. Hill, McLoud

Daniel F. Stough, Sr., Geary

S. P. Ross, Ada

J. C. Duncan, Forgan

Physicians Casualty Association Rates.
Policies Unchanged by Emergency

"In these days when we are all confronted with a question of shortages in various commodities and an increase in the price of those obtainable, we are happy to announce that not only will we continue to carry our policyholders at no increase in the cost of their accident and health insurance but we adopted a resolution to the effect that there shall be no restriction under our policies by reason of Army, Navy or Marine Service and this is irrespective of where such Service may take the policyholder."—Physicians Casualty Association.

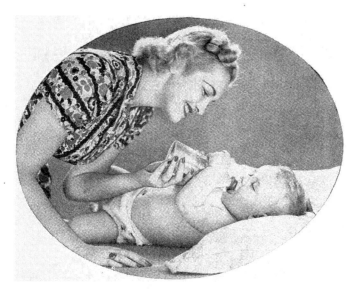

BIOLAC is complete and replete...

...because there is no lack in Biolac, except for vitamin C. Biolac feeding provides amply for all other nutritional requirements of the normal young infant, and no additional formula ingredients or supplements are necessary. It's an improved evaporated-type infant food with breast-like nutritional and digestional advantages. It is a complete formula, replete with nutritional values. Biolac is prepared from whole milk, skim milk, lactose, vitamin B_1, concentrates of vitamins A and D from cod liver oil, and ferric citrate.

Why BIOLAC is an ideal infant formula food:

- Ample provision for high protein needs of early months
- Reduced fat level for greater ease in digestion
- Enriched with vitamins A, B_1, D and iron
- All needed carbohydrate in the form of Lactose
- Sterilized for formula safety
- Homogenized to improve digestibility
- Easy to prescribe
- Convenient for mothers to use
- Economical: nothing need be added

Prescribe Biolac in your next feeding case. Professional literature on request. Write Borden's Prescription Products Division, 350 Madison Ave., New York, N.Y.

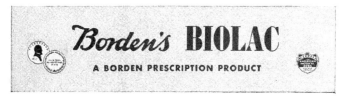

Mail to I. A. Nelson, M.D., Chairman Scientific Exhibits,
210 Plaza Court, Oklahoma City.

Application for Space in the Scientific Exhibit
of the
Oklahoma State Medical Association

Application is hereby made to the Committee on Scientific Exhibits for space at the Annual Session, Tulsa, Oklahoma

(1) ....
  (State exact title of exhibit for the program and the Journal announcement).

(2) Brief description of exhibit ....
....
....
....

(3) Exhibit will consist of the following: (check which)

  charts and posters........................... photographs...........................

  photomicrographs........................... drawings...........................

  roentgenograms........................... specimens...........................

  other material ....

(4) The following equipment will be used: (check which)

  cabinets........................... view boxes...........................

  microscopes........................... other equipment...........................

....

(5) Booth requirements:

  Length of back wall desired...........................

  Minimum requirement...........................

(6) Description of booth: The side walls are five feet, the back walls five feet or in multiples thereof, and a shelf twelve inches wide two and one-half feet from the floor will be provided. The back wall of each booth is of veneer which will permit the use of thumb tacks, etc.

  Signed: ...., M.D.

  ....
  City

Applications for Exhibit Space Cannot Be Considered After April 1

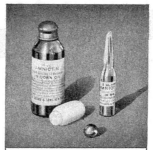

MEDICAL PREPAREDNESS

Procurement and Assignment Survey Being Made

The State Procurement and Assignment committee on March 5 mailed to the district chairmen questionnaires on all physicians of the counties in their respective districts.

In turn, the district chairmen are mailing the questionnaires to the Medical Preparedness chairmen of the county societies, asking that they immediately complete the request for the information contained therein, in order that the State Committee may have the necessary information on all physicians of the state when called upon by the Procurement and Assignment committee of the Federal government.

Every physician should bear in mind that this request is placing a tremendous responsibility on the County Medical Preparedness representative and that it is a responsibility that he did not ask for. The representatives were selected by the county societies themselves and with a full understanding that the representative and his committee might be called upon to act for the Office of Procurement and Assignment in evaluating the medical personnel of the county in relation to civilian medical care and military service.

World War II has made it necessary for an all-out effort on the part of every business and profession. Obviously, there will be instances where unanimous agreement cannot be obtained on either the method of procedure or the end result. Certainly no one can believe that any group or committee could better decide the needs of a county or community than those living and practicing there.

The procedure being followed is the democratic way. Give your support to the program and back the decision of your county society all the way.

Let us win this war.

State Committee on Procurement And Assignment Meets

The State Committee on Procurement and Assignment met February 8, at the Skirvin hotel, Oklahoma City, to discuss the work of the committee in the present emergency.

After hearing a discussion of the requests of the Office of Procurement and Assignment, as given by the chairman, Dr. Henry H. Turner, it was voted to utilize the chairmen of the Medical Preparedness committees in the counties of the state for the purpose of securing the necessary information on state doctors. The list of these chairmen appeared in the January issue of the Journal.

Each committee chairman has been sent a list of the doctors in his county and will be asked to determine the minimum number necessary for the protection of the health of the civilian population.

A similar survey was made in 1941, but cannot now be used as the basis of determining the medical personnel situation in the counties, as, since its completion, there have been changes brought about by death, removal and doctors being called into the armed forces.

The survey, when completed, will be utilized in advising the Office of Procurement and Assignment as to whether a doctor is available for military service. This method of procedure will obviously give the local doctors the opportunity of determining their local needs.

State Medical Preparedness Committee Changes Name

The Office of Procurement and Assignment, Washington, D. C., has requested of all State Medical associations that their committees on Medical Preparedness become the State Committees on Procurement and Assignment.

This request was immediately acted upon by Dr. Finis W. Ewing, President of the Oklahoma State Medical Association, and the Medical Preparedness committee will now be known as the State Committee on Procurement and Assignment.

The State Committee will continue to function through the County Medical Preparedness representatives, but the county committees will not be renamed.

One More State Doctor Called to Service

One more state doctor has been called to service by the Commanding General, Eighth Corps Area, according to the Journal of the American Medical Association.

Ordered to active duty is Dr. Lee Roy Wilhite of Perkins, who will be stationed as a Colonel at the U. S. Army Recruiting Station in Houston, Tex.

Three other state doctors whose orders to the service were revoked are:

Kinsinger, Ralph R., 1st Lieut., Blackwell

McCurdy, William C., Jr., 1st Lieut., Purcell

Preston, Thomas K., 1st Lieut., Muskogee.

Oklahoma Doctors Promoted in Navy

It has been reported to the office of the Association that Dr. Alton C. Abernethy, formerly of Altus, and Dr. M. P. Hoot, formerly of Ponca City, have been promoted to the rank of Lieutenant Commander in the naval service.

"Is This Product Council-Accepted"

This is the first question many physicians ask the detail man, when a new product is presented.

If the detail man answers, "No," the doctor saves time by saying, "Come around again when the Council accepts your product."

If the detail man answers, "Yes," the doctor knows that the composition of the product has been carefully verified, and that members of the Council have scrutinized the label, weighed the evidence, checked the claims, and agreed that the product merits the confidence of the physicians. The doctor can ask his own questions, and make his own decision about using the product, but not only has he saved himself a vast amount of time but he has derived the benefit of a fearless, expert, fact-finding body whose sole function is to protect him and his patient.

No one physician, even if he were qualified, could afford to devote so much time and study to every new product. His Council renders this service for him, freely. Nowhere else in the world is there a group that performs the functions so ably served by the Council on Pharmacy and Chemistry and the Council on Foods.

Mead Johnson and Company cooperates with both Councils, not because we have to but because we want to. Our detail men can always answer you, "Yes, this Mead Product *is* Council-accepted."

These are the Reasons why we say "Try S·M·A"

 Physicians will find that S-M-A* is not a "compromise formula." It is a complete milk formula for infants deprived of human milk.

 Cows' milk fat is replaced with the unique S-M-A fat for easy digestion and adequate nutrition. It compares physically, chemically and biologically with the fat in human milk.

 The carbohydrates in S-M-A and human milk are identical.

 With the exception of vitamin C, the vitamins essential to normal growth and development (B_1, D, and A) are included in adequate proportion in S-M-A ready to feed.

 Furthermore, iron (so difficult to provide for the bottle-fed infant) is included in S-M-A. When prepared each quart provides 10 mg. iron and ammonium citrate.

* * * * *

Excellent results with hundreds of thousands of infants is reason enough why S-M-A is the choice of a steadily increasing number of physicians.

Try S-M-A. Results tell the true story more aptly than words and pictures.

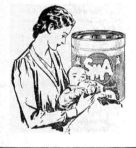

NEWS FROM THE COUNTY SOCIETIES

Dr. Richard L. Sutton, Jr., Kansas City, Mo., was guest speaker at the meeting of the Osage County Medical society, March 11, in Pawhuska. Before members of the society and guests from the Kay and Washington-Nowata County societies, Doctor Sutton discussed "Common Dermatoses."

About 12 members were present at the meeting of the Osage society, February 9, in Pawhuska. Guest speaker, Dr. Fred Glass of Tulsa, discussed "The Treatment of Burns" at this meeting.

"Diseases of the Rectum" was the topic of the talk which Dr. R. L. Murdoch, Oklahoma City, gave before the meeting of the Woodward County Medical society, March 12, in Woodward.

The society will meet April 9 in Shattuck, with Dr. Paul C. Colonna of Oklahoma City, and Dr. Paul H. Dube as speakers. Topic for discussion will be "The Diagnosis and Treatment of Fractures."

General discussion of "Congenital Dislocation of the Hip" and "The Selection of the Sulfonamide Drugs" followed the talk given on these topics by Dr. E. M. Gullatt of Ada at the meeting of the Pontotoc County Medical society, February 4 in Ada. About 13 members were in attendance.

Dr. E. A. Canada of Ada discussed "Meckel's Diverticulum" at the meeting of the Pontotoc society, February 18, in Ada.

Members of the Tulsa County Medical society are busy with arrangements for playing hosts to the Association's Annual Meeting in April.

The Tulsa county society met February 9 at the Mayo Hotel, with about 70 members in attendance. Major Louis H. Ritzhaupt, State Director of Selective Service, addressed the meeting on "Tulsa's Part in the Selective Service Program."

"The Use of Sulfonamide Drugs" was the subject of Dr. Charles M. O'Leary's discussion as guest speaker before the meeting of the Creek County Medical society, February 10, in Bristow. Doctor O'Leary discussed the treatment of peritonitis by the use of sulfanilamide and sulfathiazole in the peritoneal cavity, and the subcutaneous use of sodium sulfapyridine.

Dr. Frank Baum, McAlester, was presented with a silver plaque marking his fiftieth anniversary in the actual practice of medicine, at the Annual Inaugural Party of the Pittsburg County Medical society, January 28, in McAlester.

Dr. T. H. McCarley made the presentation of the plaque, and Dr. L. S. Willour presided as toast master for the party. Following the installation of new officers, Dr. Samuel Braden, pastor of the First Presbyterian church of McAlester, addressed the meeting.

A Symposium on Biliary Diseases was held at the meeting of the society, February 20, in McAlester. Doctor McCarley and Dr. C. E. Lively were in charge of this discussion.

Dr. Edward N. Smith of Oklahoma City was guest speaker for the meeting of the Cleveland county society, February 12, in Norman. Doctor Smith chose "Hemorrhage and Shock" as the subject for his talk.

About 20 members were present.

"Farm Security" was discussed by Dr. Charles M. Pearce before the meeting, March 11, of the Harmon county society, in Hollis.

Five members were present at the February meeting for an informal round table discussion of general problems.

A Symposium on "Lung Abscess," led by Dr. Walker Morledge and Dr. Charles M. O'Leary, was held at the meeting of the Oklahoma County Medical society, January 27, in Oklahoma City. About 75 members were in attendance.

Formal discussion of the topic was held by Dr. P. M. McNeill and Dr. J. H. Robinson.

Speakers for the program of the Oklahoma County Medical society meeting, February 24, in Oklahoma City, included Dr. L. J. Starry, Dr. N. Price Eley, Dr. L. C. McHenry and Dr. Henry H. Turner, all of Oklahoma City.

Doctor Starry discussed "Tumors of the Right Colon," and Doctor Eley led the discussion. Doctor McHenry discussed "Emergency Medical Service," and Doctor Turner gave a brief discussion of "Procurement and Assignment."

About 18 members attended the meeting of the Washington-Nowata county society, February 11, in Bartlesville, with Dr. S. A. Lang discussing "Allergy in Children" for the group.

The society is planning on presenting motion pictures, on the American Society of Clinical Pathologists and on Syphilis at a future meeting.

Dr. Henry H. Turner, Chairman of Procurement and Assignment, and R. H. Graham, Executive Secretary of the Association, both of Oklahoma City, were guest speakers at a meeting of the Seminole county society, January 14, in Seminole.

Doctor Turner discussed "Procurement of Medical Personnel for the Services," and Mr. Graham talked on "The Medical Profession's Part in Civilian Defense."

At the February 9 meeting of the Jefferson county society, a resolution was passed that the society instruct its delegate to the Annual Meeting to reduce the dues for the State Medical Association.

The society also passed a resolution that the Jefferson county society go on record as stating that participation in the County Health Unit will be discontinued as of July 1, 1942.

"Differential Diagnosis of Pulmonary Tuberculosis" was the title of the talk given by Dr. R. M. Alley of Shawnee, guest speaker for a meeting of the Garvin County Medical society, February 18, in Pauls Valley. About ten members were in attendance at the meeting.

Following Doctor Alley's talk, Dr. R. M. Anderson of Shawnee held an informal discussion. The Garvin county society will hold its March meeting at Pauls Valley, March 18, when a motion picture on Syphilis, sponsored by the Division of Veneral Diseases, U. S. Public Health Service, will be shown.

"Malpractice Insurance" was discussed by R. H. Graham, Executive Secretary of the Association, Oklahoma City, at the February meeting of the Kay County Medical society. The meeting was held February 19, in Tonkawa.

Dr. W. F. Bohlman outlined the work of the Committee on Emergency Medical and Hospital Care for members of the Blaine County Medical society at a meeting, February 19, in Watonga.

Members of the society will hear a refresher lecture on "Syphilis" sponsored by the State Health Department at their meeting March 19, in Watonga.

Plans are being made by the Pottawatomie County society for the Annual Spring Clinic. Serving on the committee in charge of preparations for this meeting are Dr. E. Eugene Rice, Dr. H. E. Hughes and Dr. Paul Gallaher.

The society met February 21, in Shawnee, with about 18 members attending the meeting. Dr. W. B. Mullins read a paper on "Recent Advances in the Treatment of Meningitis," and Dr. H. E. Hughes showed movies on "Appendicitis" and "Breast Tumors." The movies were shown through the courtesy of the Davis and Geck company.

Washington Birthday Clinic Attended by 77 Doctors

The Fourth Annual Washington's Birthday Clinic, sponsored by the Oklahoma City Internist Association, was held February 23, in Oklahoma City, with a record attendance of 77 doctors. Forty-five of the attending physicians were from over the state.

The success of the meeting was largely due to the organization work done by Dr. Mary V. Sheppard and Dr. Elmer Musick. Those appearing on the scientific program included Dr. P. M. McNeill, Dr. Bert F. Keltz, Dr. W. W. Rucks, Jr., Dr. Floyd Moorman, Dr. Wann Langston and Dr. William K. Ishmael. Those appearing on the Forum were Dr. A. W. White, Dr. L. J. Moorman, Dr. George A. LaMotte and Dr. Lea A. Riely.

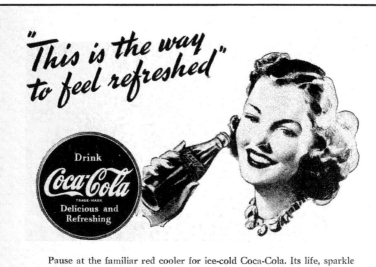

• OBITUARIES •

Dr. F. P. von Keller
1860-1942

Dr. Frederick P. von Keller, well-known pioneer Ardmore physician who was eminent in state medical circles for his outstanding work, died February 13 in the hospital which he founded and which bears his name.

Doctor von Keller was born, January 10, 1860, at Strasbourg, Alsace-Lorraine, France, of German-French parentage. Following his graduation from the the medical school of Heidelberg university in Germany, he came to the United States, where for a time he was medical examiner at Ward's Island, N. Y. Later he located in Galveston Tex., where he married Arkie Clay of Little Rock, Ark.

From Galveston, he moved to Chillicothe, Tex., in 1890, and four year later, he moved to Ardmore. Mrs. Arkie Clay von Keller passed away in 1936.

Doctor von Keller was a life member of the American Medical Association, a member of the Association of Military Surgeons of the United States, and served as president of the medical advisory board of Carter and Love counties, Oklahoma district No. 24, during the first World War. He was honored for his services in the United States Civil legion.

He was an associate professor of surgery in the College of Physicians, Dallas, from 1906 to 1907, and he was regarded as one of the best diagnosticians in the state.

He was also a member of the Beta class, the second consistory reunion held at the Scottish Rite consistory at McAlester, a member of the York Rite bodies, and a member of the Ardmore Masonic lodge No. 31.

In 1940, he married Mollie Dishman of Ardmore, who survives him. Other survivors include a daughter, Mrs. Donald M. Bretch of Oklahoma City; three granddaughters, Mrs. J. Samuel Binkley, New York City, Mrs. Donald Stuart Will, Champaign, Ill., and Mrs. Richard Gruner, St. Louis, Mo.; two great grandchildren, Donald James Frederick Binkley, New York City, and Gretchen Gruner, St. Louis; and two brothers, G. A. von Keller and L. V. von Keller, Greensburg, Kan.

Dr. John Frederick Kuhn
1872-1942

Dr. John Frederick Kuhn, another of Oklahoma City's Pioneer Doctors, has passed away. Time only will draw the curtain on the remaining few. A noble physician, a skillful surgeon, an honored gentleman and a faithful friend has died and thousands mourn his death.

Dr. Kuhn came to Oklahoma City in 1903, after finishing his residency at the Emergency hospital and at the Columbia Hospital for Women in Washington, D. C., where he trained under two great surgeons and gynecologists, Dr. J. Wesley Bovee and Dr. I. S. Stone. A few months after he established his office in Oklahoma City, where the Tradesman's National bank is now located, he married Miss Sadie Minker, of Norristown, Pennsylvania, who was a nurse he had met during his services at the Women's hosptal. Dr. and Mrs. Kuhn reared and educated their fine family in Oklahoma City. Dr. Kuhn saw our City grow to its present size. He was a loyal, progressive citizen, and possessed the qualities necessary for the expansion and culture of our beautiful City.

Dr. Kuhn was a busy doctor. His first many years, of course, were in the horse and buggy days. He was active in the promotion of good surgery in this locality and gave unselfishly his efforts to uphold the principles for its progress.

His ability was definitely recognized and no one ever questioned his loyalty and sincerity. His judgment was respected and his council secured in many of the diffi-

cult problems encountered by his colleagues. He was ready to help and give his assistance regardless of existing circumstances.

In 1912 he was appointed Instructor of Surgery in the Oklahoma School of Medicine and soon after became an Associate Professor in that Department. In 1925 he became Professor of Gynecology, which position he retained until a short time ago, when he was honored with the Emeritus Professorship. His department of Gynecology was his special pride and I believe it can be truthfully said that no one man's influence has meant more to the young doctors who have graduated from this school than that of Dr. John Frederick Kuhn's. His teaching and research activities and the countless hours given to this work were his contributions to the advancement of medical science. His desire to graduate good doctors was his daily ambition. He sacrificed the possibility of personal gain through the loyalty to the school and towards the progress of what he called the "boys."

In the passing of Dr. Kuhn, February 14, 1942, we lost a friend, a wonderful teacher, and one of Oklahoma City's greatest physicians. His devotion to his family was most beautiful. The hours spent with his students were innumerable. His interest in his private practice can be ascertained by his thousands of faithful friends and patients. His entire lfe was founded on the principles of being a "good man."—Joseph W. Kelso.

Psychiatric Institute Announced

Announcement has been made by the American Psychiatric Association of its forthcoming Fifth Postgraduate Institute for State Hospital men and other physicians interested in Psychiatry.

The Institute will open March 23 and will continue through April 3. It will be held at the Missouri State hospital, St. Joseph, Mo.

Auxiliary News

Haddon Hall will be the headquarters for the Annual Meeting of the Women's Auxiliary to the American Medical Association, which will be held at Atlantic City, New Jersey, June 8-12, 1942. Requests for reservations should be sent immediately to Haddon Hall, Atlantic City, New Jersey.

The Pittsburg County auxiliary met on February 3 at the home of Mrs. T. J. Baum, with Mrs. L. C. Kurykendall as co-hostess, for luncheon. Thirteen of the 14 members of this group were present. During the business session the following questions were discussed and action taken thereon: (1) $25.00 was sent to the Red Cross, (2) A $100.00 Defense Bond was purchased, (3) Twelve books were given to "Books for Victory." Three Red Cross Home Nursing classes are being taught. One class has been graduated. This auxiliary has also bought "Home Nursing Books" to lend to those persons who are unable to buy their own. The Pittsburg auxiliary is assisting with the feeding and clothing of a rural negro school.

On January 8 at 7:30 P.M. the Women's Auxiliary to the Cleveland County Medical Society met at the Central State Hospital, headed by Mrs. Jim L. Haddock, president. Eight of the 29 members were present. At this meeting the annual election of officers took place as follows: President, Mrs. Moorman Prosser; Vice-President, Mrs. W. B. Carroll; Secretary, Mrs. Curtis Berry; Treasurer, Mrs. W. H. Atkins. These members will take office as of September, 1942. Plans were also made at this meeting for a nurses' training course.

The Pottawatomie County auxiliary has a membership of 18 this year and meets in the homes of members. This group is headed by Mrs. Frank Keen, president. The Pottawatomie auxiliary has taken the following action during the year: $10.00 was given to Hygia; $12.00 was given to the Federal Nursing School and $10.00 was given for papers on "Tuberculosis Prevention" by seventh and eighth grade students. This auxiliary also has sent letters of thanks to Radio Stations WKY and KVOO in appreciation of the program "Doctors at Work."

Sulfadiazine Abstract Booklet A
Convenience to Physicians

With the usefulness of Sulfadiazine growing rapidly, it was felt that a booklet containing abstracts of significant recent articles would be of real convenience to physicians and others working with this important Sulfa drug. Accordingly, Lederle Laboratories, Inc., New York, N.Y. have recently made available a 64-page booklet, "Abstracts Selected from Published Articles on Sulfadiazine."

In order to compress significant material into a booklet of this size, every article on the subject appearing up to December 1, 1941, has been examined. Articles which contained only minor evidence as well as those which overlapped or reworked prior authorities have been eliminated. At the same time, no attempt was made to select the most favorable articles. The result is a terse, but authoritative review of material on Sulfadiazine, arranged topically for convenient reference. In most instances selected articles have been condensed to one page or less. In every case, bibliographies are supplied for those wishing to study the articles in full. This new booklet is available through Lederle representatives, or on request from Lederle Laboratories, Inc., 30 Rockefeller Plaza, New York, N.Y.

Pneumonia deaths will continue to decrease
steadily with this most promising Sulfonamide...

SULFADIAZINE
Lederle

THE VALUE OF SULFAPYRIDINE AND SULFATHIAZOLE in the treatment of pneumococcal pneumonias has been impressively demonstrated by extensive clinical use. Sulfadiazine, the newest of the famous sulfonamide family, shows even greater promise. The ideal sulfonamide would be flexible in its method of administration, nontoxic to the host, devoid of sensitivity effects and would be therapeutically active against a wide range of common infecting agents. Although a perfect sulfonamide is unlikely of attainment, it is believed that sulfadiazine possesses distinct advantages in the treatment of certain conditions. CECIL[1] has expressed the opinion that clinically sulfadiazine is the best of the antipneumococcal drugs.

Recently clinical workers[2] have confirmed the results of earlier investigators[3] that sulfadiazine is equal in therapeutic efficiency to sulfapyridine or sulfathiazole in the treatment of pneumococcal pneumonia; is rapidly absorbed from the gastro-intestinal tract; the blood levels obtained are usually higher than with comparable doses of sulfapyridine and sulfathiazole; and excretion takes place slowly. All these factors coupled with the *infrequency of nausea and vomiting* tend to reassure both patient and physician.

Experimentally[4] sulfadiazine has been shown to compare favorably with sulfanilamide in its action against streptococci. The excellent therapeutic activity of the drug against experimental[5] hemolytic streptococcal and Friedlander's bacillus Type B infections has encouraged the clinical trial of sulfadiazine in these infections.

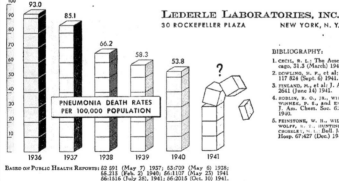

PNEUMONIA DEATH RATES PER 100,000 POPULATION

93.0 | 85.1 | 66.2 | 58.3 | 53.8 | ?
1936 | 1937 | 1938 | 1939 | 1940 | 1941

BASED ON PUBLIC HEALTH REPORTS: 52 591 (May 7) 1937; 53:709 (May 6) 1938; 55.215 (Feb. 2) 1940; 56:1107 (May 23) 1941 56:1516 (July 25), 1941; 56:2015 (Oct. 10) 1941.

BIBLIOGRAPHY:

1. CECIL, R. L.: The Aesculapian, Chicago, 31.3 (March) 1941.
2. DOWLING, H. F., et al: J. A. M. A. 117 824 (Sept. 6) 1941.
3. FINLAND, M., et al: J. A. M. A. 116: 2641 (June 14) 1941.
4. ROBLIN, R. O., JR., WILLIAMS, J. H., WINNEK, P. S., and ENGLISH, J. P.: J. Am. Chem. Soc. 62.2002 (Aug.) 1940.
5. FEINSTONE, W. H., WILLIAMS, R. D., WOLFF, R. T., HUNTINGTON, E. and CROSSLEY, M. L.: Bull. Johns Hopkins Hosp. 67:427 (Dec.) 1940.

OFFICERS OF COUNTY SOCIETIES, 1942

COUNTY	PRESIDENT	SECRETARY	MEETING TIME
Alfalfa	Jack F. Parsons, Cherokee	L. T. Lancaster, Cherokee	Last Tues. Each 2nd Mo.
Atoka-Coal	J. B. Clark, Coalgate	J. S. Fulton, Atoka	
Beckham	H. K. Speed, Sayre	E. S. Kilpatrick, Elk City	Second Tues. eve.
Blaine	Virginia Olson Curtin, Watonga	W. F. Griffin, Watonga	
Bryan	A. J. Wells, Calera	W. K. Haynie, Durant	Second Tues. eve.
Caddo	Fred L. Patterson, Carnegie	C. B. Sullivan, Carnegie	
Canadian	P. F. Herod, El Reno	A. L. Johnson, El Reno	Subject to call
Carter	Walter Hardy, Ardmore	H. A. Higgins, Ardmore	
Cherokee	Park H. Medearis, Tahlequah	Isadore Dyer, Tahlequah	
Choctaw	C. H. Hale, Boswell	Fred D. Switzer, Hugo	
Cleveland	F. C. Buffington, Norman	Phil Haddock, Norman	Thursday nights
Comanche	George S. Barber, Lawton		
Cotton	George W. Baker, Walters	Mollie F. Scism, Walters	Third Friday
Craig	W. R. Marks, Vinita	J. M. McMillan, Vinita	
Creek	Frank Sisler, Bristow	O. H. Cowart, Bristow	
Custer	Richard M. Burke, Clinton	W. C. Tisdal, Clinton	Third Thursday
Garfield	D. S. Harris, Drummond	John R. Walker, Enid	Fourth Thursday
Garvin	T. F. Gross, Lindsay	John R. Callaway, Pauls Valley	Wed before 3rd Thurs.
Grady	D. S. Downey, Chickasha	Frank T. Joyce, Chickasha	3rd Thursday
Grant	I. V. Hardy, Medford	E. E. Lawson, Medford	
Greer	G. F. Border, Mangum	J. B. Hollis, Mangum	
Harmon	S. W. Hopkins, Hollis	W. M. Yeargan, Hollis	First Wednesday
Haskell	William Carson, Keota	N. K. Williams, McCurtain	
Hughes	Wm. L. Taylor, Holdenville	Imogene Mayfield, Holdenville	First Friday
Jackson	J. M. Allgood, Altus	Willard D. Holt, Altus	Last Monday
Jefferson	W. M. Browning, Waurika	J. I. Hollingsworth, Waurika	Second Monday
Kay	J. C. Wagner, Ponca City	J. Holland Howe, Ponca City	Third Thurs.
Kingfisher	C. M. Hodgson, Kingfisher	John R. Taylor, Kingfisher	
Kiowa	J. M. Bonham, Hobart	B. H. Watkins, Hobart	
LeFlore	G. R. Booth, LeFlore	Rush L. Wright, Poteau	
Lincoln	E. F. Hurlbut, Meeker	C. W. Robertson, Chandler	First Wednesday
Logan	William C. Miller, Guthrie	J. L. LeHew, Jr., Guthrie	Last Tuesday evening
Marshall	J. L. Holland, Madill	O. A. Cook, Madill	
Mayes	L. C. White, Adair	V. D. Herrington, Pryor	
McClain	B. W. Slover, Blanchard	R. L. Royster, Purcell	
McCurtain	R. D. Williams, Idabel	R. H. Sherrill, Broken Bow	Fourth Tues. eve.
McIntosh	F. R. First, Checotah	William A. Tolleson, Eufaula	Second Tuesday
Murray	P. V. Annadown, Sulphur	F. E. Sadler, Sulphur	
Muskogee	Shade D. Neely, Muskogee	J. T. McInnis, Muskogee	First & Third Mon.
Noble	J. W. Francis, Perry	C. H. Cooke, Perry	
Okfuskee	J. M. Pemberton, Okemah	L. J. Spickard, Okemah	Second Monday
Oklahoma	R. Q. Goodwin, Okla. City	Wm. E. Eastland, Okla. City	Fourth Tuesday
Okmulgee	J. G. Edwards, Okmulgee	John R. Cotteral, Henryetta	Second Monday
Osage	C. R. Weirich, Pawhuska	George K. Hemphill, Pawhuska	Second Monday
Ottawa	J. B. Hampton, Commerce	Walter Sanger, Picher	Third Thursday
Pawnee	E. T. Robinson, Cleveland	Robert L. Browning, Pawnee	
Payne	John W. Martin, Cushing	James D. Martin, Cushing	Third Thursday
Pittsburg	Austin R. Stough, McAlester	Edw. D. Greenberger, McAlester	Third Friday
Pontotoc	R. E. Cowling, Ada	E. R. Muntz, Ada	First Wednesday
Pottawatomie	John Carson, Shawnee	Clinton Gallaher, Shawnee	First & Third Sat.
Pushmataha	P. B. Rice, Antlers	John S. Lawson, Clayton	
Rogers	W. A. Howard, Chelsea	P. S. Anderson, Claremore	First Monday
Seminole	H. M. Reeder, Konawa	Mack I. Shanholtz, Wewoka	
Stephens	E. C. Lindley, Duncan	A. J. Weedn, Duncan	
Texas	L. G. Blackmer, Hooker	Johnuy A. Blue, Guymon	
Tillman	C. C. Allen, Frederick	O. G. Bacon, Frederick	
Tulsa	H. B. Stewart, Tulsa	E. O. Johnson, Tulsa	Second & Fourth Mon. eve.
Wagoner	J. H. Plunkett, Wagoner	H. K. Riddle, Coweta	
Washington-Nowata	R. W. Rucker, Bartlesville	J. V. Athey, Bartlesville	Second Wednesday
Washita	A. S. Neal, Cordell	James F. McMurry, Sentinel	
Woods	W. F. LaFon, Waynoka	O. E. Templin, Alva	Last Wednesday
Woodward	M. H. Newman, Shattuck	C. W. Tedrowe, Woodward	

THE JOURNAL

OF THE

OKLAHOMA STATE MEDICAL ASSOCIATION

| VOLUME XXXV | OKLAHOMA CITY, OKLAHOMA, APRIL, 1942 | NUMBER 4 |

Fever Therapy*

PATRICK S. NAGLE, M.D.

OKLAHOMA CITY, OKLAHOMA

Fever therapy is a therapeutic modality of definitely established effectiveness. Its effectiveness varies from increasing the tempo of healing in self-limited diseases to arrestation of progress of incurable chronic disorders, and sometimes complete elimination or "cure" of certain diseases which lend themselves to no other manner of treatment.

Proper appreciation of it is slowly but definitely developing in the general ranks of medicine. This slowness could be discussed at length but such discussion is irrelevant. Much debate, usually burdened by rationalization and casuistry, is prevalent today as to "which" is the "best" manner of inducing artificial fever. I shall not indulge in this today.

Suffice to say, the particular technique that I shall talk about is the one with which I have had experience. By restricting my statements to data and opinions arising directly out of my immediate experience, it is hoped that the presentation will be positive and not negative, affirmative and not disputative.

In the Department of Fever Therapy at St. Anthony hospital, and in the Coyne Campbell sanitarium, fever is induced in the patient by electrical inductance. Elaborate discussion of the technicalities of this does not seem appropriate at this time. Most significantly it may be said, that by the employment of ultra short wave radio waves the fever induced in the subject is completely controlled. The temperature may be taken to any heighth deemed appropriate by the referring physician and maintained at any level for any length of time that the nature of the disease and the condition of the patient permits. The continuance and the progress of the fever may be stopped at any moment. In the experience of this writer, this is a matter of no trivial importance.

*Read before the Section on Psychiatry, Neurology, and Endocrinology, Annual Session, Oklahoma State Medical Association, May 20, 1941, in Oklahoma City.

For here, as in other radical and vigorous therapeutic procedures, the mortality of the treatment as well as the mortality of the disease must be given recognition.

Fever therapy is no novelty, although it has been exploited as such by some. It is no recent innovation in medicine and it has very definite and specific applications and appropriate uses. It is not a cure-all.

I shall list a few situations in which it is outstandingly the therapy of choice. Too frequently in these cases, it is the therapy of ultimate choice rather than first choice. I urge its earlier use.

The first condition I wish to mention is syphilis of the central nervous system. Asymptomatic sero-positive neurosyphilis may most effectively be treated by controllable artificial fever therapy in repeated courses of ten weekly treatments over a period of years. Paresis and taboparesis are ameliorated in their progress and frequently arrested by adequate fever therapy. Occasionally we see a reversal of the serology. Tabes dorsalis gives us the most dramatic proof of the effectiveness of this modality in disorders of syphilitic etiology. Here it has been observed that a patient in unremitting gastric crisis requiring hospitalization, heavy morphine sedation, and intravenous fluids, is completely relieved of symptoms after the third fever seance.

The next condition is chronic gonorrhea and its complications, gonorrheal arthritis, prostatitis, epididymitis, etc. We see these cases only after they have had vaccines and vitamines, milk shots, and typhoid injections and sulfanilamide. These people are of the group that we feel reasonably certain adequate fever completely cures.

The next category which is definitely benefited is inflammatory conditions of the eye. Iritis, corneal ulcer, certain types of conjunctivitis, and keratitis. These conditions are treated entirely upon the recommendation of the referring eye specialist, who remains in immediate responsibility and contact with the patient throughout the course of treatment.

A typical case example of the dramatic effectiveness of controllable fever therapy in inflammatory eye conditions is a case currently under treatment at St. Anthony Hospital, which is quite fresh in my mind. This 36-year-old boy is under treatment for a second attack of iritis. He has been thoroughly studied from the standpoint of focal infection and none has been established. He has been competently treated for over three weeks by one of the better eye men. The classical treatment of atropin, sterile milk, foreign protein therapy, and typhoid shots have not improved the patient. He is seen at St. Anthony's with unremitting pain in the inflamed eye. The atropin, which has been taken every few hours in the eye for relief of pain, is discontinued and the first fever treatment started. When this man's temperature reached 103 degrees, the pain in his eye was relieved. Subsequent developments established that the pain never returned. It was never again necessary to give him atropin for relief. After two bouts of fever of 105 degrees, axillary, for over two hours and each ranging to a peak of 107.4 by rectum, it is considered that the course of the iritis was interrupted. A third additional treatment is given and the patient returned home within a week after his first treatment.

Here is striking proof that all the fever producing modalities that medicine has been using and abandoning over the last 20 years have a common denominator; this is fever production. Milk shots and so-called foreign protein therapy benefit the individual who reacts to them with sufficient fever. Typhoid shots benefit the individual who reacts to them with sufficient fever.

Conditions which classically have been treated successfully by milk shots and typhoid shots are now the better and more quickly treated by the more direct and immediate application of the essential therapeutic agency, namely, increased body temperature.

Another category of diseases that we are tentatively employing fever in is "virus encephalopathies," chorea-like encephalopathies and in conjunction with intravenous vitamine B-6 occasional test cases of frank Parkinson's disease. Theoretical justification may be rationalized for use of fever in all of these situations. Empirical and practical justification is apparent in some of these conditions, chiefly chorea. Benefit is here proven.

In our experience of ten cases of chorea

for the past year and a-half, fever therapy and vitamin B-1 have relieved all cases but one. From our experience with these cases, we are realizing that chorea is a disorder with many aspects and not a clear cut and simply defined problem. One is impressed by the prominence of hysterical material encountered in these cases. Certainly a complete and competent insight into the etiology of chorea is lacking. Following is a chart of cases for the past year, treated by artificial fever therapy, indicating the type of case, the treatment, and the results.

FEVER THERAPY CASES
ST. ANTHONY HOSPITAL

DIAGNOSIS	CASES	RESULTS
Acute Iridocylitis	3	All definitely improved
Infectious Arthritis	2	Both definitely improved
Arthritis non-specific	2	Both unimproved
Sydenham's chorea	2	Both improved
Encephalitis	2	Both improved
Lung abscess	1	Unimproved
Mycosis Fungoides	1	Unimproved
Parkinson's Disease	1	Slight improvement
Neuro-Syphilis	1	Greatly improved—Serology reversed
Tabes Dorsalis	1	Treatment discontinued
Transverse Myelitis	1	Unimproved
Tabo-paresis	1	Improved
Undulant Fever	1	Improved

FEVER THERAPY CASES
COYNE CAMPBELL SANITARIUM

DIAGNOSIS	CASES	RESULTS
Encephalitis	6	5 improved
Sydenham's chorea	5	4 Improved
Paresis	6	3 Improved
Meningio Vascular Syphilis	1	Improved
Parkinson's Disease	1	Unimproved

In the control and arrestation of central nervous system syphilis it is not truly known whether high fever is spirochetocidal or not. Many workers think that they have proved that temperature of 105 is spirochetocidal. This point is of only academic importance, however, when it is so easily shown that the gross clinical aspects of a seriously disabling disease is favorably modified by six to a dozen bouts of hyperpyrexia. When the paretic can write his name again and the tabetic is free of his painful gastric crisis, the lay relatives do not ask you academic questions.

The serology of these cases is tricky and difficult to evaluate. Negative spinal fluids follow positive spinal fluids and in turn are followed by negative tests. Dependence may not be placed on a single or a few spinal fluid examinations. It is necessary for the physician to rest his judgment on a careful study and conscientious appraisal of the patient and the general clinical manifestations. Occasionally we see a reversal of the serology after treatment has been stopped for six months.

Certainly the luetic patient is never encouraged to believe he will be cured but an effort is made to instruct him to realize that his condition must and may be controlled. Although we have only been at this a few years, it is our sincere belief that those cases in which the circumstances are fortuitous, (continuous observations by the physician of the course of the patient's disease), adequate repeated courses of fever therapy will arrest the onslaught of the disease indefinitely.

PHYSIOLOGICAL ASPECTS

The alterations in the metabolism and physiology of the patient under hyperpyrexia is an extremely interesting and instructive problem. These artificially induced departures from the normal status are numerous, delicate, and little understood. These subtle chemo-physical changes are of great importance.

The totality of knowledge of human physiology has barely been tapped. It follows that many changes occurring under fever escape our appreciation. Hence our judgment of the efficiency of this treatment is, in all honesty, empirical. An increasingly accurate knowledge of the physiological chemistry of human hyperpyrexia and its effect upon parasitic organisms and non-symbiotic viruses may better be comprehended if an ecologic perspective is maintained in relation to the total process. I have little patience with the glib and over-simplified explanations imposed upon the laity and even upon the profession by some highly articulate and yet unscientific writers. Much has been written on this subject, some very little of it is worth reading. (I commend to you an article by C. F. Finney, M.D., printed in the Annals of Internal Medicine in October, 1932.)

The best work done on the chemistry of hyperthermia has been done by Danielson, Stecher, Muntwyler and Myers of the Western Reserve university in 1938. In a summary way the conclusions are as follows:

"The acid-base balance of the blood serum has been studied in a series of patients who were subjected to artificial fever. Certain of the patients were permitted to drink a chilled 0.6 percent sodium chloride solution during the treatment while others were allowed to drink iced distilled water only.

"The results of the studies which were made at the end of the period necessary to raise the body temperature from normal to the fabrile level leave little doubt that hyperventilation plays the major role in causing the initial disturbances of the acid-base balance of the blood in artificial fever.

"In patients who were permitted to drink water only, the following blood changes were encountered at the end of either two or four hours of fever: an elevated pHs, a decreased pCO2 and decreases of the (NAHCO3)s, (NACl)2, inorganic phosphorus and the serum total base concentration. The total measured acid concentration was also decreased while the undetermined acid fraction was increased. The same changes were encountered when the patients were permitted to drink the dilute saline solution with the exception that the (NACl)s was maintained slightly above the pre-fever level.

"These observations as well as the more favorable clinical conditions of the patient following fever therapy when salt is contained in the drinking water are discussed briefly."

With the rise in temperature there occurs an increase in pulse rate. This increase is found to be generally proportional to the temperature elevation. This pulse rate increase is found to be specifically in relation to the skin temperature elevation. It is this factor that makes the introduction of heat internally superior to the introduction of heat externally. Hot baths and hot steam raise the body temperature only after elevating the skin temperature, disproportionately.

The velocity of the blood flow is accelerated and no problem results as long as the blood volume is maintained. The blood velocity is reduced, however, after the patient is permitted to sweat himself out and hemoconcentration supervenes. In cases that go bad under high fever and develop heat exhaustion, the blood will sometimes be so black and thick that it is difficult to aspirate it with a needle. This perversion of physiology represents the greatest threat under treatment. Proper insight prevents its occurrence and proper treatment is always one thing, namely, intravenous sodium chloride in quantities sufficient. By sufficient I mean adequate to excessive. In one 240 pound, 15-year-old boy with chorea, it was necessary to give him, through large gauge needles in both arms, 4,500 cc's of normal saline in the course of two hours. I cite this extreme case as a matter of emphasis.

The blood pressure is usually elevated in the systolic reading a few points and almost always reduced in the diastolic reading. I have observed the diastolic reading to be zero in any number of cases. In patients that flush under treatment and sweat freely, the systolic pressure will be reduced, particularly near the end of the treatment, but unless the pulse is fast, no anxiety over shock need be entertained. In hypertensive patients, the blood pressure is always reduced under treatment and in several cases this reduction has remained permanent to date.

In conclusion, it is reiterated that controllable, artificial, electrically induced hyperpyrexia has been, in our hands and under our observation, a definitely effective therapeutic agent. In a number of disorders it is the only effective therapy available. Chief of these is general paresis. Thus far we have been fortunate in escaping all mortality.

Inflammatory conditions of the eye lend themselves most satisfactorily to this therapy.

Late and complicated cases of gonorrhea are resistant to all other forms of therapy and are readily and certainly relieved by adequate fever therapy.

Laboratory Findings in Pneumonia and Bronchitis

Report on 100 cases.

WILLIAM H. BAILEY, M.D.*

OKLAHOMA CITY, OKLAHOMA

Pneumonia, and particularly lobar pneumonia, has always been a dramatic as well as a very fatal disease. What could be more striking than the sudden onset, the chill, the high temperature, the positive signs of consolidation in the lungs, all within a period of a few hours. What more thrilling experience than to have seen the rapid change in the clinical picture of a case of pneumonia just after the crisis had occurred. Although, perhaps at the present time, much of the glamour has been taken out of this disease because of the introduction of sulfapyridine and similar drugs and the use of specific type anti-serum, this very fact has stimulated a new interest in it. It still is thrilling to see the temperature in these cases drop to nearly normal in 18 to 24 hours after sulfapyridine has been started.

In only a very few diseases will the laboratory findings remain practically the same throughout the whole course of the illness. The usual routine is that at different stages in the disease the laboratory findings will be quite different. One cannot say, dogmatically, that typhoid fever gives a positive Widal, because for the first week of the disease it is most unusual for the Widal to be positive, while the blood culture which is most often positive in the first stages of typhoid is usually negative in the latter part of the disease or soon after the Widal becomes positive.

So, also, laboratory findings are affected and changed by the treatment administered. This is brought about in two ways, first by the effect the drug has on changing the pathology and symptoms of the disease and second by the direct effect it has on the tissue or system closely associated with the test being performed. The blood culture in a case of streptococcic septecemia which has been positive is often rendered negative within a few hours after sulfanilamide has been administered.

A third factor that has its effect on the laboratory findings is that we may expect a change from the routine findings for that particular stage of the disease when some complication as a re-infection, a superimposed condition or an extension of the original pathology occurs.

All these various changes in the physical signs and symptoms of a disease are what we expect to find at different stages so why not look for changes also in the laboratory findings, for they are simply additional signs and symptoms elicited by certain specialized methods of examination.

Because of the present interest in pneumonia and because of the help given by the Pneumonia Control Program of the State Board of Health, started about a year ago, we have been able to obtain more complete laboratory data than is usually requested in the average private case. We wish to acknowledge our appreciation to the Commissioner of Health, Dr. Grady Mathews, and his assistants for this help.

All of these cases, except a very few, were admitted as patients at Wesley Hospital during the calendar year of 1940. We wish to thank the attending physicians for their cooperation in this study and for the privilege of reviewing the records of their cases.

*Doctor Bailey is now a Colonel in the army stationed at the Station Hospital, Fort Sill, Oklahoma

In most of the cases in the series the request for the sputum typing, the initial blood and urine examinations and the blood culture was received early in the disease before any chemotherapy had been started. During the first half of the year the sputum in those cases which could not be typed direct were sent direct to Mrs. Lucile Wallace of the Bacteriology department at the University of Oklahoma Medical school, who did the mouse inoculations and typing. We wish to thank Mrs. Wallace and Dr. H. D. Moor, head of the department for this valuable assistance. During the last half of the series most of the mouse inoculations have been done in the laboratory at Wesley hospital.

In a few cases, as in infants and young children, and in very old patients, a satisfactory sputum specimen could not be obtained. In these cases a specimen for culture was obtained either on a swab passed over the pharynx or a small catheter passed through the nose to the back of the throat and a small amount of mucus collected by suction with a syringe. This was incubated in a liquid culture media for eight to 12 hours and inoculated into a mouse.

1. The slide method used for the typing of the pneumococcus was the Neufeld Method which makes use of the reaction of the swelling of the capsule of the organism when brought into contact with its specific antiserum.

2. The clinical diagnoses of the 100 cases were, 59 cases of lobar pneumonia, 27 cases of bronchopneumonia and 14 cases of bronchitis.

3. Requests were received for typing 98 of these cases. Of the two cases in which no request was received, one was in an elderly woman, who had fractured her hip some three weeks before. She developed symptoms of a bronchopneumonia one day and died the next. The other case was in a man 68 years old, who had a very severe lobar pneumonia from which he died on the eighth or ninth day. We felt that in this case the attending man did not request sputum typing because of economic reasons. This in a way was unnecessary because at that time the service of the State Pneumonia Control program was available in Oklahoma county, as it is at the present time, and all of these laboratory tests could have been obtained free of charge to the patient. This service is intended for those patients in the low income group the same as it is for the indigent.

Of these 98 cases in which typing was requested we reported type pneumococci in 71 cases, streptococci in three cases, staphylococci in one and a small Gram-negative bacillus similar to the influenza bacillus in one case. In the remainder we were unable

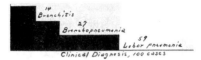

Clinical Diagnosis, 100 cases

to determine any particular organism that we thought predominated. Although not scientifically conclusive, yet for ordinary clinical purposes in cases of this nature it is customary to accept the predominating organism as the infective agent in the etiology of such a condition.

Of the 71 cases showing type pneumococci the clinical diagnoses were 52 cases of lobar pneumonia, 18 cases of bronchopneumonia and one case of bronchitis.

Of the 27 cases not typing, five were lobar pneumonia, nine bronchopneumonia and 13 bronchitis.

4. In the initial red cell counts 87 cases gave a count of over four million. Of these, 16 were over five million and 71 between four and five million. Only 13 were below four million.

5. The initial hemoglobin tests gave 90 with over 70 percent, 46 over 90 percent, with several over 100 percent and 44 between 70 and 90 percent while only ten were below 70 percent.

6. Hemoglobin estimations were taken at 48 hour and 96 hour periods for the purpose of indicating the toxic effect of sulfapyridine. In 48 hours 14 had a higher hemoglobin while 24 showed a lower percent. In 96 hours 63 showed a higher percent while 15 gave a lower reading.

7. The initial white cell count gave 15 above 25,000, 53 between 10,000 and 25,000 and 32 below 10,000.

8. In the initial counts the polymophonuclears gave 94 with polys over 70 percent, of these 33 were over 90 percent and 61 between 90 and 70 percent. Only six were below 70 percent.

9. White counts were taken at 48 hour and 96 hour periods to show the toxic effect of the drug. In 48 hours seven showed a higher white count, 33 about the same and 60 gave a lower count. In 96 hours 11 were higher, 26 the same and 63 lower.

10. The urine was tested at these same intervals. During the whole course of the disease only 18 showed albumin, 11 had a few red cells and in three we found sulfapyridine crystals.

11. Although sulfapyridine crystals are fairly typical they are rather difficult to recognize unless they are present in large numbers.

The blood cultures were positive in only two cases.

12. The specific types of pneumococci in the different pneumococcic cases found and the number of cases of each type were as follows:

Type I—4	Type XVIII—5
Type II—4	Type XIX—4
Type III—7	Type XX—0
Type IV—4	Type XXI—0
Type V—6	Type XXII—1
Type VI—7	Type XXIII—2
Type VII—4	Type XXIV—0
Type VIII—4	Type XXV—1
Type IX—1	Type XXVI—0
Type X—1	Type XXVII—0
Type XI—2	Type XXVIII—0
Type XII—3	Type XXIX—3
Type XIII—1	Type XXX—0
Type XIV—2	Type XXXI—0
Type XV—2	Type XXXII—0
Type XVI—1	Type XXXIII—1
Type XVII—0	

There were nine deaths in the whole series. One was a type II, one a type V, one a type VII, two were type XXIX, two streptococcic, and two were the two cases in which no requests for typing were received. The age incident of the deaths in this series showed all but one were over 40 years of age. The patient under 40 years who died was 30 years old and he was one of the streptococcic cases.

Considering only the proven pneumococcic cases the mortality was five in 71 cases or 7.2 percent. Cecil gives 8-12 percent in his series of over 1,000 cases before the introduction of the new chemotherapy.

Summary: In so far as this small series is concerned and from the experience we have gained we feel that we may draw the following conclusions. It will of course be realized that only 100 cases is much too small a number from which to obtain very definite information.

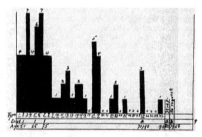

1. We consider the Neufeld method of typing pneumococci as a rapid, efficient and very satisfactory method for clinical use.

2. The borderline cases in which it is difficult for the physician to diagnose pneumonia clinically are also the ones in which it is difficult to type the sputum.

3. The most characteristic blood finding is a high polymophonuclear leukocytosis.

4. Fatal cases may have either a high or only a moderate leukocytosis.

5. Only about two percent of the cases will have a positive blood culture in the initial stage.

6. Unless satisfactory sputum specimens can be secured before chemotherapy is started the typing is very unsatisfactory.

7. Pneumococci will occasionally appear in the sputum as chains and all such specimens should be tested for typing.

8. At times the sputum, even from frank pneumonia cases, will show too few pneumococci to type direct and all such specimens should be inoculated into a mouse and typed.

9. The mortality in pneumococci pneumonia in this series was around 7.2 percent, with the most deaths occurring in patients past 50 years of age.

10. Streptococcic pneumonia is much more fatal than pneumococci pneumonia.

Obstetrical Shock

BRUNEL D. FARIS, M.D.

OKLAHOMA CITY, OKLAHOMA

Shock after delivery, unless associated with hemorrhage, rupture of the uterus, or inversion, is rare, but I have seen two cases followed by simply attempting the Crede too forcefully. Such a nervous shock sometimes follows the removal of gauze packing or any minor obstetrical procedure where an anesthetic has not been used.

Obstetrical shock is a very rare complica-tion of pregnancy, but when seen necessitates rapid and accurate treatment if the patient's life is to be saved.

It is interesting to note that one of the first manifestations of this condition is a change in the character and the rate of the pulse, followed quickly by a death-like palor, and cold, clammy skin.

De Lee states that Obstetrical shock or

nervous shock of labor may terminate fatally and many cases are cited in the literature of sudden shock in labor followed by death. There is no apparent explanation for a profound collapse of the patient and the most careful examination both at the bedside and at the autospy may not reveal the slightest abnormality. Some call this an acapnia and others peritoneal shock.

Pituitrin sometimes cause pain simulating that of a coronary occlusion, followed by symptoms of shock. Some say that Obstetrical shock is due to traumatism to the pancreas during prolonged bearing down effects—same causing insulin shock or hyperinsulinemia. The shock may resemble a form of anaphylaxis. Still others say that the vagosympathetic system is effected due to the rapid emptying of the uterus. Audeburt in 1921 collected 12 cases—of shock in labor. (Labor was spontaneous in three of them). Three he stated were due to the paralsis of the stomach, and three to the action of chloroform, and the other causes not determined. Williams suggested that arterio duodenal occlusion following acute elimination of the bulk of the abdominal contents incident to a sudden decrease in the size of the uterus might be the cause. Several cases were thought to be due to acute dilation of the stomach. There was dark fluid vomitus and death soon followed.

Crushing of the pelvic floor may cause surgical shock, similar to that following crushing of the leg. We must remember that traumatism to the abdomen may cause shock. Glotz states that striking a frog's abdomen will stop his heart. Other conditions seen complicating pregnancy which may cause shock, are heart disease, rupture of the intestines, gallbladder, pulmonary embolism and so forth.

The treatment depends on a hurried diagnosis—the foot of the bed should be elevated, one-half amp of adrenalin and one-fourth gr. morphine given, warmth to the feet, and glucose—especially for edema of the lungs or possibly embolism. (30 to 100 cc of 50 percent glucose). If we are able to rule out a pulmonary or cardiac embolism, 500 cc of ten percent glucose intravenously is used instead of the 50 percent. One thousand cc of Normal Saline is usually given at once, subcutaneously, into the thigh. Oxygen should be given. Digitalis intramuscularly is a questionable treatment that may be given, if there is reason to suspect the heart. The efficacy of coramine is questionable. The ideal treatment would be blood plasma if it could be easily obtained. Williams claims the stomach should be emptied and the patient should be treated according to the exigencies. Too often we do not recognize the so-called exigencies. Many use 10 cc of five percent calcium chloride intravenously for vascular collapse.

Anuria Following the Administration of Sulfadiazine and Sulfapyridine: Case Reports*

W. TURNER BYNUM, M.D.
FRANK T. JOYCE, M.D.
OSCAR S. PYLE, M.D.

CHICKASHA, OKLAHOMA

We wish to present two cases of unusual reactions to the sulfonamide compounds:

CASE REPORTS

Case 1, J. W., a 13-year-old white boy weighing 85 pounds was admitted to the hospital on September 27, 1941 for treatment of a six inch laceration of the left leg. The injury was caused by being run over by a wagon. The wound was cleaned and sutured and the boy was given 1,500 units of tetanus antitoxin: 48 hours later his temperature rose to 100.6 F. and a bubbling seropurulent discharge was oozing from the wound. There was a marked lymphangitis of the left leg and thigh and a left inguinal lymphadenitis. No crepitation was felt in the tissues but

gas gangrene was suspected. The wound was opened, hot packs started, and 2,000 units of combined tetanus-gas gangrene antitoxin was given for prophylaxis.

Sulfadiazine was started; the initial dose was 2.5 grams followed in fours hours by 1.5 grams and then 1.0 gram every four hours. This dosage was continued for the following 84 hours when a total of 24 grams of sulfadiazine had been given. The patient tolerated the drug well for 66 hours when 19 grams had been given. At that time he complained of aching pain in both kidney areas and cramping abdominal pains. Unfortunately, the drug was continued for five more 1.0 gram doses and during the time of those 20 hours the pain became worse and severe nausea and vomiting developed. The

*Read before the Oklahoma State Internists society, Chickasha, Oklahoma, December 4, 1941.

last voided urine specimen, which amounted to 60 cc. of grossly bloody urine, was obtained only seven hours after the patient first complained of pain in the kidney areas.

After anuria had persisted for 42 hours (Oct. 5, 1941), cystoscopy was done but ureteral catheters could not be passed higher than one-half inch because of obstruction in both ureters. The boy was returned from surgery and was given an intravenous injection of 1,000 cc. of ten percent glucose in saline. Immediately following this preparation a nephrostomy was done on the left kidney. After delivery of the kidney from the incision it was found to be swollen to about three times its normal size. Much to our surprise the renal pelvis was not greatly dilated but was tense and about 15 cc. of bloody urine was aspirated. Innumerable fan-shaped crystals were seen on microscopic examination of this urine. Fluids were given by the intravenous route and the pyelostomy drained well.

On October 9, 1941, about 36 hours following the pyelostomy on the left kidney, cystoscopy was performed again and a catheter was passed into the pelvis of the right kidney. After irrigating the pelvis urine began to flow from the catheter. The catheter was left in for two days. Within 24 hours after its removal there was a recurrence of pain in right kidney area and a decreasing urinary output so that on October 11, 1941, the catheter was replaced in the right kidney pelvis. The catheter was left in again for two days with a recession of the pain.

The patient's course was satisfactory for almost two weeks when on October 26, 1941, pain in the region of the right kidney recurred and was accompanied by a fever of 104 F. The pain and fever persisted and on October 29, 1941, the right ureter was again catheterized and urine containing four plus pus was obtained. The catheter was left in for two days and was removed because there had not been any relief of the symptoms. A perinephric abscess was suspected and proven by needling the right flank and on November 3, 1941, the abscess was drained. Fever and pain promptly subsided.

Urine has continued to drain profusely from the left pyelostomy except for a few days after October 31, 1941, when drainage through the left ureter was re-established after a successful ureteral catheterization on that date. Prior to that date it had been impossible to pass a ureteral catheter up to the left renal pelvis although this procedure had been attempted every time the patient was cystoscoped for ureteral catheterization on the right side.

For 17 days following the drainage of the perinephric abscess on the right his course was quite satisfactory. On November 20,

1941, there occurred a profuse hemorrhage from the draining sinus which subsided spontaneously. At the same time he began to pass blood and blood clots from the bladder in large quantities. The hemorrhage from the sinus occurred several times daily and it became necessary to give him 2,500 cc of blood in a period of two days. In spite of the transfusions the hemorrhages persisted and a nephrectomy on the right was done in order to control the bleeding. Because of the previous abscess it was very difficult to free the kidney and the source of the preoperative bleeding was never determined. Since then there has been no bleeding and he has not had any fever since December 5, 1941.

It has been assumed that some urine was draining from the left ureter following the catheterization of that ureter on October 31, 1941, however, since the right kidney was removed there has been no voided urine. Further attempts to catheterize the left ureter have been postponed in view of his previous trouble.

Microscopical sections of the right kidney: Section through the kidney shows diffuse suppurative infiltration of all portions of the kidney. The cortex shows many tubules filled with masses of pus. There is also a mass of infected thrombus along one edge. No sulfadiazine crystals are found in the tubules. There is rather an extensive tubular degeneration and interstitial edema. Diagnosis: Acute diffuse suppurate nephritis.

Case 2, C. W., a 48-year-old male weighing 202 pounds entered the hospital on January 6, 1941, complaining of pain in both sides of the chest, coughing, and fever. He stated that he had had "flu" for five days prior to his entrance into the hospital. Examination showed a temperature 102 F., respirations 32 per minute, and pulse 120. Except for the chest the remainder of the physical examination was normal. The lungs contained numerous rales, vocal fremitus was increased but there were no definite areas of dullness. Breath sounds were bronchovesicular in type throughout. The sputum was bloody and contained numerous pneumococci and micrococcus catarrhalis. The white blood count was 15,700. A diagnosis of bronchopneumonia was made and sulfapyridine was started. The initial dose was two grams followed in two hours with two grams and then one gram every four hours. Ten grains of sodium bicarbonate was given with each dose of sulfapyridine. About 36 hours after the drug was started and he had taken only a total of 12 grams he complained of severe cramping pain in the abdomen. He had not complained of nausea until the occurrence of the abdominal pain, but from that time on vomiting became severe. He was given two more doses of one gram each of sulfapyridine. Four hours after the appearance of the abdominal pain he complained of being unable to void. He was catheterized and one ounce of bloody urine was obtained.

Within an hour 1,000 cc. ten percent dextrose in normal saline was started intravenously but did not produce any urine in the bladder. Six hours after the anuria was discovered he was cystoscoped and crystals were seen to bulge from each ureteral orifice. With considerable difficulty ureteral catheters were pushed up into each kidney pelvis and irrigations with normal saline were carried out. The ureteral catheters were left in place and urine drained from each rather promptly. The catheters were removed 24 hours later, however, the urine was grossly bloody for another 24 hours. The patient's fever subsided and he made an uneventful recovery from both the pulmonary infection and the ureteral obstruction.

DISCUSSION

Sulfadiazine was used in the case reported above in accordance with a report by Long[1] of satisfactory results in the treatment of Cl. Welchii and Vibrion septique infections in vitro; gas gangrene was suspected in this case. Most of the literature[1,2,3,4,6,7] on this subject has stressed the low toxicity and the therapeutic advantages of sulfadiazine. In over 1,000 cases reported in the literature there have been only two previously reported cases of anuria[2,3] from the clinical use of this drug.

Sadusk and Tredway[4] in a rather thorough article on the absorption, excretion, diffusion and acetylation of sulfadiazine in man go so far as to predict that because of the great solubility of the acetylated derivative of sulfadiazine in urine that this drug would probably not produce calculi in the urinary tract of man. Contrary to this however, Lehr and Antopol[5] in a study of the toxicity of sulfadiazine in rats found that all animals that developed anuria did so because of a nephrotic type of kidney damage due to precipitation of the free drug in the renal tubules. In their study it was shown that symptoms of toxemia and death did not occur during the time of maximum concentration of the drug in the blood stream; i.e., there was no relation between blood level and precipitation of the free drug in the renal tubules. In the case of anuria from sulfadiazine reported by Thompson, Herrell and Brown[3] the blood levels were only 11.4 mgm. per 100 cc of blood at the onset of anuria. We have recently observed a patient with blood stream concentrations of sulfadiazine as high as 29 mgm. percent with no hematuria.

Lehr and Antopol as well as Thompson and associates have stressed the lessened gastrointestinal and other subjective manifestations of toxicity with the use of sulfadiazine prior to the onset of anuria and azotemia. Long[6] as well as Thompson et al have emphasized the fact that alkalinazation is of no advantage in the prevention of these kidney complications.

Anuria following sulfapyridine adminstration was first reported by Southworth and Cook[8], and later many reports appeared in the literature. We feel that our case here reported is worthy of note primarily because of the small amount of drug administered and the rapidity of the onset of anuria.

We believe that blood counts and the determination of blood levels of the particular drug given are important adjuncts to proper therapy in the administration of the pyridine, thiazole and the diazine derivatives of sulfanilamide; however, high blood levels or the total amount of the drug given give no indication of the onset or impending danger of the most dramatic and dangerous complication in the administration of these valuable drugs, i.e., anuria. It is our opinion that the only means of avoiding this occurrence is by close attention to the urinary output, i.e., keeping the 24 hour output in the neighborhood of 1,000 to 1,500 cc or above for adults and proportionally smaller amount for children, and watching closely for the occurrence of microscopic hematuria, discontinuing the drug at its first appearance, and forcing fluids.

CONCLUSIONS

In order to avoid the occurrence of anuria and its subsequent dangers in patients who are taking sulfonamide drugs it is imperative that each patient maintain a urinary output of at least 1,000 cc. daily for adults, and a correspondingly smaller amount for children. Anuria may occur if this is not observed, regardless of the amount of drug absorbed, the blood level of the drug, or whether the urine is alkaline.

BIBLIOGRAPHY

1. Long, P. H.: Sulfadiazine: The 2-Sulfanilamido-pyrimidine Analogue of Sulfanilamide, J.A.M.A., 116:2399 (May 24) 1941.
2. Finland, M., Strauss, E., Peterson, O. L.: Sulfadiazine; Therapeutic Evaluation and Toxic Effects on Four Hundred and Forty-Six Patients, J.A.M.A., 116:2641 (June 14) 1941.
3. Thompson, G. J., Herrell, W. E., Brown, A E.: Anuria after Sulfadiazine Therapy, Pro. Staff Meetings Mayo Clinic, 16:609 (Sept. 24) 1941.
4. Sadusk, J. F., Jr., Treadway, J. B.: Observations on the Absorption, Excretion, Diffusion, and Acetylation of Sulfadiazine in Man, Yale Jour, of Biology and Medicine 13:539 (March) 1941.
5. Lehr, David, and Antopol, W.: Toxicity of Sulfadiazine and Acetylsulfadiazine in Albino Rats with Special Reference to Renal Lesions and Their Significance, Urologic and Cutaneous Rev., 45:545 (Sept.) 1941.
6. Long, P. H.: Clinical Use of Sulfonamide Compounds in Prophylaxis and Treatment of Infections, Northwest Med. 40:811 (Sept.) 1941.
7. Flippin, H. F., Rose, S. B., Swartz, L., and Domm, A. H.: Sulfadiazine and Sulfathiazole in the Treatment of Pneumococcic Pneumonia, Am. Jour. of Med. Sc., 201:585 (April) 1941.
8. Southworth, H., Cooke, C.: Hematuria, Abdominal pain and Nitrogen Retention, J.A M.A. 112:1820 (May) 1939.

An Unusual Case History for Diagnosis*

D. J. UNDERWOOD, M.D.

TULSA, OKLAHOMA

Infant was a full term normal birth. Weighed 8½ lbs., delivered at St. Johns hospital and discharged on the tenth day.

Patient was re-admitted on twenty-first day, after having spent 11 days at home, with a history of coughing and choking spells which became progressively worse and became so severe that infant would not breathe for three to four minutes and would become extremely cyanotic.

Physical examinaton revealed a very sick infant—cyanotic, irregular respiration, temperature 100.8°, pulse 130, respiration 48.

Head—Nostrils filled with a yellow-gray mucous discharge.
Pharynx injected.
Ears—Drum membrane normal in appearance with light reflex present.
Neck—No pathology.
Chest—Lungs show evidence of an early pneumonia over the right side with coarse rales and increased breath sounds.
Cardio vascular—No pathology.
Abdomen—Soft, no masses or distention.
Genito urinary—Negative.
Skin—Very cyanotic during choking spells.
Extremities—Negative.

On February 18, 1941, the day of admittance, a direct smear of the throat revealed a few bacilli strongly suspicious of Diphtheria and culture revealed many diphtheroids and an occasional diphtheria bacillus. 20,000 units of Diphtheria Antitoxin was given intramuscularly.

Blood Count—Hemoglobin 85%; R.B.C. 4,240,000; W.B.C. 14,800; Neutrophiles 64; Myelocytes 0; Juveniles 0; Band 30; Segmented 34; Mononuclears 5; Kline and Kahn negative.

Urine—Acid; albumin negative; sugar one plus, ten pus cells per L.P.F. X-ray of the chest revealed a large thymic shadow with markedly involved peribronchial infiltration in all portions of lungs except a small portion of the right base.

Rx—X-ray treatment of thymus.
Sulfathiazole Gr. II every four hours.
Oxygen—Nasal catheter.
Steam inhalations.

*Read before the Section on Pediatrics, Annual Session, Oklahoma State Medical Association, May 20, 1941.

Coramine ½ ampoule.

Suction of mucous from nose and throat.

February 20, 1941—Patient still having choking spells with severe cyanosis. Unable to take fluids by mouth because of choking so 125 cc of Hartmans solution given by Hyperdermoclysis and repeated six hours later. Cevitamic acid, 25 mgm. given.

February 21, 1941—X-ray reveals a marked decrease in the size of thymus and lung fields show marked bronchitis with sufficient evidence to make it very suggestive of Bronchial pneumonia. Sulfapyradine Gr. II given every four hours. Alpa Lobelin given intramuscularly. Hartmans solution, 150 cc given and repeated in six hours by 125 cc. Spasmodic movements of eyes and lips with edema of eyes and face and extreme difficulty in swallowing. Adrenalin in oil, ¾ M given with no response. Necessary to give artificial respiration on repeated occasions—as long as 25 minutes.

Blood Count—Hemoglobin 80 percent; R.B.C. 4,000,000; W.B.C. 39,450; Neutrophiles 48; Band 14; Segmented 34; Lymphocytes 52.

February 23, 1941—Calcium gluconate Gr-V intramuscularly.

Magnesium sulphate 25 percent, 2 cc, given intramuscularly and repeated in six hours.

Gr. III Sulfapyradine in 40 cc distilled water given subcutaneous.

Hartmans 125 cc given subcutaneous.

Convulsions seemed to be controlled.

February 25, 1941—40 cc citrated whole blood IV.

Sulfathiazole Gr. II every four hours.

Hartmans solution with gavage.

Vitamin K M X.

February 27, 1941—Patient appears improved but lungs do not clear up. X-ray report shows numerous small patchy areas of density of the entire lung fields, having the characteristics of a broncho pneumonia.

Sulfathiazole Gr. III given in formula. Calciden Gr. ½, given by gavage. Continuous oxygen.

March 1, 1941—Breathing improved—Fewer attacks of coughing and choking. W.B.C. 31,650; Neuthrophiles 59; Juveniles 5, Band 27; Segmented 13; Lymphocytes 35; Eosinophiles 6.

March 2, 1941—Hemoglobin 60 percent; W.B.C. 51,450; Neutrophiles 41; Myelocytes 5; Juveniles 13; Band 10; Segmented 13; Lymphocytes 54; Mononuclears 2; Basophiles 3.

Continuous oxygen.

Vitamin K M V.

Vitamin C 25 mgm.

Sulfathiazole discontinued.

March 6, 1941—Formula by gavage. Temperature higher. Negative urine.

Sulfapyradine Gr. III every four hours subcutaneous.

March 9, 1941—Patient had repeated convulsions and appears to be in peripheral vascular collapse. Adrenaline 1—1,000 ¼ ampoule. No improvement.

Calcium gluconate Gr. V intramuscularly.

Sodium luminal Gr. ¼ hypodermically.

March 11, 1941—Twitching of mouth, right hand and foot. Spinal puncture and 25 cc removed. Clear—slight trace of Globulin. No W.B.C.

125 cc whole citrated blood intravenously.

X-ray shows a marked increase in density in the upper left lobe. Marked increase of cardiac shadow which is very suggestive of pericarditis with effusion.

March 15, 1941—Cough Plate—no pertussis bacilli. Many staph. Few gram negative bacilli.

X-ray shows a marked decrease in size of cardiac shadow both to left and right.

March 20, 1941—Cough Plate—Negative for pertussis bacilli.

Sulfathiazole Gr. I every four hours.

Oleum percomorphum M V

Vitamin K, M VIII

Cevitamic acid 50 mgm. daily.

March 24, 1941—Culture shows gram negative club shaped bacilli, cultural characteristics presumably pertussis bacilli.

March 26, 1941—Patient expired.

March 27, 1941—Pathological report: The body is that of a somewhat emaciated white male infant about two and one-half months old showing on external examination no anomalies, scars, nor lesions.

The body is opened by the usual midline incision from the sternal notch to the symphysis pubis. The chest shows a consolidation of all the lobes in both lungs with one small nodule on the left lung suggesting a tubercle. The trachea and bronchi show mucus secretion. There seems to be some infarction at the midaxillary portion of the left lower lobe. Several portions of both lungs are cut and dipped into water, most of them will not float; there is a fibrous induration in several portions. The thymus is small and the pleurae are smooth. The heart shows marked dilatation of the right side and there is a small grayish area of degeneration on the anterior surface of the right ventricle. The liver is smooth, edges somewhat rounded. On cutting the inferior vena cava and vessels from the liver a definite swelling of the liver was quite perceptible indicating a rather marked passive congestion on the right side of the heart. The spleen is fairly small. The pancreas, adrenals, stomach and small intestines show no pathology (they are examined insitu without excessive dissection).

Summary of Gross Anatomic Findings:
1. Bilateral unresolved pneumonia.
2. Pulmonitis.
3. Toxic myocarditis.
4. Cardiac failure, right side.

Microscopic Examination

Lungs: Unresolved bronchopneumonia.
Heart: Toxis myocarditis.
Liver: Moderate passive congestion.

DISCUSSION

J. B. SNOW, M.D.
OKLAHOMA CITY, OKLAHOMA

The presence of an occasional diphtheria bacilli in a culture from a patient who does not show a visible membrane in the nose or throat probably does not justify the diagnosis of diphtheria. However, I think you are always justified in giving diphtheria antitoxin when in doubt or have such a laboratory report. If diphtheria were present, it could have contributed to the lung pathology by producing weakness of the muscles of the soft palate which are usually the first to be involved, and may be affected as early as the fifth or sixth day. I doubt if an enlarged thymus produced any of the symptoms in this patient. I wonder if whooping cough was prevalent in Tulsa at this time, and whether this patient had come in contact with a case. I think two of the blood counts were rather typical of whooping cough, and late in the course, a culture showed an organism which had cultural characteristics of the pertussis bacillus. The choking spells, periods of asphyxia and the convulsions could be explained by a severe bronchitis and broncho-pneumonia complicating pertussis in a young infant. The failure of the pneumonia to respond to chemo-therapy was probably due to the organism being the pertussis or influenza bacilli instead of the penumococcus. The enlarged cardiac shadow may have been due to a terminal acute dilitation of the heart.

• *THE PRESIDENT'S PAGE* •

The Annual Meeting, April 22nd to 24th, which will commemorate the Fiftieth Anniversary of Organized Medicine in Oklahoma, should be the best attended meeting ever held in the State. A glance at the program carried in the March issue of the Journal shows a change in the general plan and guarantees everyone the opportunity to participate in the entire program.

It is my desire to use this page in this, my last opportunity to sincerely and earnestly thank the membership of the Oklahoma State Medical Association for their loyal support and cooperation throughout the year. I want to thank the office force in the Oklahoma City office for their loyal and enthusiastic aid; the members of the various committees who have given much of their time and have made many personal sacrifices for the good of medicine, and last I want to say to the Council, that their wholesome and kindly advice and wholehearted cooperation has made what otherwise might have been an onerous task the most pleasant year of my life.

It is now my desire to surrender the duties as President and commend to you, your new President and to assure him that he will have the privilege of leading the finest and most loyal group ever given any man.

Whatever success has been accomplished during the year just passed is due to the intelligent, loyal and untiring efforts of the office force, the Standing and Special Committees and the Council. Whatever errors or mistakes made must be laid at the door of your President, to each and everyone I plead that they were mistakes of the head and not of the heart.

President.

28% LESS NICOTINE IN THE SMOKE—BUT NO REDUCTION IN SMOKING PLEASURE

WHEN improving a patient's smoking hygiene, many a physician simplifies his program by advising the regular use of Camel cigarettes—the slower-burning brand. Medical-research authorities* state, and Camel's scientific tests on hundreds of samples** confirm, that a slower-burning cigarette produces less nicotine *in the smoke*.

Nicotine, as the body of scientific research agrees, is by far the leading component of tobacco smoke having systemic potentials.

Slower-burning Camels not only offer a reduction of nicotine in the smoke but assure your patients of more mildness, coolness, and flavor. Naturally, your recommendation of Camel cigarettes helps to promote patients' cooperation.

*J.A.M.A., 93:1110 — October 12, 1929
Brückner, H—Die Biochemie des Tabaks, 1936

**The Military Surgeon, Vol. 89, No. 1, p. 7, July, 1941

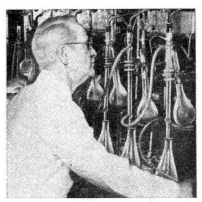

● In recent laboratory tests, Camels showed 28% less nicotine *in the smoke itself* than the average of the 4 other largest-selling brands tested—less than in the smoke of any of them. In the same tests, Camel burned 25% SLOWER than the average of the 4 other largest-selling brands tested— slower than any of them.

CAMEL

THE CIGARETTE OF COSTLIER TOBACCOS

• EDITORIALS •

FIFTY YEARS, AN EON IN MEDICAL PROGRESS

The story of the practice of medicine in Oklahoma would make one of the most interesting chapters in the history of medicine. Nowhere in the United States has there been such revolutionary progress as in this section of the short grass country.

There are doctors now living in Oklahoma who came in the early days when the practice of physic blended with the poetry of unplowed prairies and clashed with the primtive methods of the plains Indians which approached those of the Pre-Hippocratic period. The Indians lived under the fear of the supernatural and the mysterious manifestations of nature, and the Medicine Man often combined his priestly functions with the power of magic and the crude application of medicinal remedies. Oklahoma doctors who came in contact with the Indians had to contend with many of the superstitions and evil practices which confronted the father of medicine in the 5th Century, B.C. Not infrequently they found traces of primitive medicine among the white homesteaders.

Many of the white people who moved into this environment were very poor. Some of them holed in with the prairie dogs, rattle snakes, and burrowing owls, others lived above ground but in sod houses, and those who could afford a modest investment freighted in sufficient rough lumber to build small box houses. The country doctor, with horse and buggy, made the rounds day and night, tending the sick in these strange domiciles and following the stork from one homestead to another. There were no nurses, no hospitals, no clinics, no public health agencies, but the pioneer woman, calm, capable and courageous, mothered her family, shepherded her farm, nursed her neighbors and served as the doctor's aid. In those days on the plains the word neighbor meant more than Noah Webster, the pioneer in good American words, ever imagined.

Towns and cities sprang into being with facilities for growth and development which, in half a century, enabled them to stand abreast of those boasting three hundred years of traditional development. Such phenomenal progress has not been experienced in any other section of the country.

Because this was a land of opportunity, many well-educated, ambitious young doctors came here to seek their fortunes and, in spite of the fact that we had a few undesirable, early-day registrants, we started with a relatively high average of well qualified, progressive young men in the profession. Though the outside world knew and cared little about medicine in Oklahoma, the members of the local profession not only were giving the best individual medical care any pioneering people ever received, but they were keenly aware of, and actively engaged in, the most phenomenal period of medical progress the world has ever known.

Thus, they were laying the foundation for our present high position in the field of medicine. Through the development of the University of Oklahoma School of Medicine, the gradual evolution of hospital facilities, the postgraduate courses for country doctors, the development of public health services, the doctors of Oklahoma have forged an ever lengthening chain of professional achievements.

While we pause to give credit for fifty years of work well done, we should gather strength for the tasks before us. The young doctor, now standing upon the foundation which has been established through the untiring efforts of pioneering souls, should be inspired by the security which has come to him through the doctors of the "old school." Having been freed from the hardships and the time-consuming tasks of the old, he should pursue the new with a consuming desire to forge additional links in the chain which will ultimately place the medicine of the plains on a level with that in all the high places of the world.

Only through the young doctor of today can the pioneer doctor of yesterday receive his just reward. As he throws the torch to us let us say of him what the poet William E. Henley said of Lord Lister:

"We hold him for another Herakles,
Battling with custom, prejudice, disease,
As once the son of Zeus with Death and Hell."—L. J. M.

ORGANIZED MEDICINE AND PUBLIC WEAL

In this issue of the Journal Dr. Basil A. Hayes has given a concise history of the development of organized medicine in Oklahoma. Since the approaching annual meeting in Tulsa represents the 50th anniversary of the Oklahoma State Medical Association,

Dr. Hayes' historical sketch serves as a fitting contribution at this time and constitutes a valuable record.

But we must not let this half century mark pass without calling attention to the high purposes of organized medicine in Oklahoma. A careful perusal of the editorials, presidential addresses, published resolutions and committee reports in the Journal for the duration reveals one continuous unwavering theme, namely community welfare as expressed through education, sanitation and public health.

The persistent, unfaltering drive in this direction, often in the face of public indifference and political interference, is amazing. This shining record of unselfish striving for the sake of humanity serves as a well merited tribute to the worthy progenitors of our present enviable position in this field of endeavor.

We should find a way to let the people know that their safety and happiness depend largely upon the progress of medical science and its unselfish application to their daily needs. If they knew what organized medicine has done for them they would take the profession under their wings and exclaim with Socrates, "We owe a cock to Aesculapius."

The present response of our younger men to the call of our country indicates that the spirit of service abides with us.—L. J. M.

EIGHTEEN AND EIGHTY-NINE

In 1889 medicine was crossing the border, staking new claims and preparing to turn virgin soil.

The discovery of the causative agents of infectious diseases was bringing about a revolution in medical thought. Medicine was approaching the end of one of the most wonderful decades in the world's history. In this country we were entering upon a period of phenomenal scientific development.

In May, 1889, Johns Hopkins Hospital was opened. William H. Welch, William Osler, Halsted and Kelly were beginning their exceptional careers, each a pioneer in his own field. Every well-informed doctor knows much about the influence of these men upon medical education, and the development of medical science and public health. Osler was contemplating the preparation of his textbook, "The Principles and Practice of Medicine." It is said that this book, falling into the hands of one of Rockefeller's advisors led to his interest in medicine and ultimately the development of the Rockefeller Institute for Medical Research.

In 1889 Walter Reed was sent to Johns Hopkins by the Surgeon General of the United States, who instructed him to attend the clinics of Osler, Halsted and Kelley, and to stay away from the laboratory. Reed could not resist the influence of Welch. Soon Carroll came and together under Welch they laid the foundation for the ultimate control of yellow fever, an accomplishment which ranks with Jenner's discovery of vaccination against smallpox. Simon Flexner was working with Welch at this time in preparation for his work with the Rockefeller Institute. Councilman Barker and others who have occupied high places in medicine were there during the latter part of that wonderful decade.

In 1889, William Crawford Gorgas, who later collaborated with Reed and Carroll in their efforts to free the world from yellow fever, was walking the streets of Oklahoma City. He was then a young physician in military service and was attached to the army post adjacent to Oklahoma City at the time of the opening. Fifteen years later, Walter Reed wrote Gorgas, "The news from Havana is simply delightful. It shows that your acquaintance with the local conditions was much better than mine. That you have succeeded in throttling the epidemic appears beyond question and it is to your everlasting credit. A man of less discretion, enthusiasm and energy would have made a fiasco of it. Whereas you, my dear Gorgas, availing yourself of the results of the work at Camp Lazear, have rid that pest hole, Havana, of her yellow plague. All honour to you, my dear boy!"

Gorgas' work in the Panama Canal zone is well known. After thousands had died in the attempt to build the canal, Gorgas made the adventure relatively safe.

It is interesting to note that a Baltimore barefoot boy, an Oklahoma City Eighty-niner, should render such a great service to humanity and at last receive the plaudets of the whole world while he slept under the stars and stripes at St. Pauls in London, and later in Washington, where his body lay in state four days before it was conveyed to its beautiful resting place in Arlington.—L. J. M.

Noted Vitamin Scientist on Borden Staff

The Borden Vitamin Company, which has been bringing into its fold a number of research and production leaders in that field, announces that Dr. Hugh H. Darby, distinguished Columbia scientist and author of many authoritative works, has joined its staff for research and development in the production and application of vitamins and hormones.

Doctor Darby, who has been with the Department of Biochemistry of the College of Physicians and Surgeons for the past seven years as research associate, is a specialist there on vitamins and hormones, achieving wide attention for his work on the extraction and physiology of sex hormones.

THE BEGINNING OF ORGANIZED MEDICINE IN OKLAHOMA

Basil A. Hayes, M.D.

Oklahoma City, Oklahoma

The first medical meeting ever held in what is now the State of Oklahoma was on a spring afternoon 61 years ago. It was on April 18, 1881, and was in Muskogee, Indian Territory. In the minutes of the meeting, the town's name was spelled M-u-s-c-o-g-e-e, and they read in part as follows:

"At 2:00 P. M. a number of medical gentlemen met, pursuant to a previously circulated call for a mass convention for the purpose of medical organization. The convention was called to order by Dr. B. F. Fortner, who nominated Dr. G. W. Cummings to the chairmanship of the convention, which was unanimously confirmed. The organization was completed by the election of Dr. Cutler, vice-president, and Drs. Fortner and C. Harris as secretaries. The chair proceeded to state the object of the meeting by reading the original call and address appended. The chair proceeded to appoint a committee on Constitution and By-Laws, consisting of B. F. Fortner, M.D., and Felix McNair, M.D. Several communications from gentlemen professionally detained at home were read, prominently among which was one from Dr. L. M. Cravens of the Cherokee Nation, for which the convention returned a vote of thanks. Convention adjourned until 9:00 A. M. tomorrow."

The next day the organization was completed by electing Dr. B. F. Fortner, of Claremore, President. Dr. G. W. Cummings, of Muskogee, was made first Vice-President, and Dr. Felix McNair, of Locust Grove, second Vice-President. Dr. M. F. Williams, also of Muskogee, was elected Secretary; and Dr. R. B. Howard, of Fort Gibson, Treasurer. Dr. E. P. Harris, address not given, was elected Librarian. A Board of Censors was named consisting of C. Harris, E. P. Harris, J. R. Cutler, W. T. Adair, and W. H. Bailey. Other members were S. F. Moore, of Webbers Falls; A. W. Foreman, of Vinita; A. Y. Lane, of Claremore; L. M. Cravens, of Tahlequah; W. T. Adair, of Tahlequah; H. Lindsey, of Eufaula, and R. O. Trent, address unknown. They also voted in an honorary member, Dr. Clegg, of Siloam Springs, Arkansas, who was present and read a paper on "The Use of Calomel in Malarial Diseases."

It was the intention of this group to meet every six months, and it assembled again at Muskogee on September 14, of that same year. Five men had been assigned subjects upon which they were to read papers, but not one was ready, so the first day's activity consisted only of a business meeting. On the following day, Dr. Fortner presented a case of "fracture of the cranium with remarks:" Dr. C. Harris reported a case of gelsemium poisoning, giving in detail his treatment. Dr. Bailey reported a case of typho-malarial fever, treatment consisting mainly of carbolic acid. A case of heart disease was presented by Dr. Fortner and discussed by various members of the Society. Also at this meeting, the usual discussion regarding incompetent practitioners was brought up, and "it was moved that the secretary draw up resolutions expressive of our views in relation to the practice of medicine by others and those newly qualified and educated for that purpose." The resolution requested "the Chief of the Cherokee Nation cooperate with us and see that the law is enforced." It was decided that the next meeting would be held at Eufaula on February 22, 1882, and the Society adjourned.

No further minutes are available, yet the pages of the book are intact. One must assume, therefore, that this Society died for want of support and was not resurrected until seven and one-half years later. This time, again, the meeting was called in Muskogee. The date was June 28, 1889, and the minutes read as follows:

"Pursuant to a previously circulated call, a number of physicians met in the Southern Methodist Church in the City of Muskogee on the morning of June 28, 1889,

for the purpose of medical organization. The meeting was called to order by Dr. Callahan, after religious services conducted by Reverend J. Y. Bryce. Dr. R. A. Burr was called to the Chair and Dr. Bagby elected temporary secretary. The object of the meeting was then stated, and in a few appropriate words Drs. Harris and Burr welcomed the visiting gentlemen. Dr. Fortner then read the names and credentials of twenty-two applicants. The Chair appointed Drs. Fortner and Callahan a Committee on Credentials, who after consultation made the following report:

"We, the Committee on Credentials for the convention, beg to report that we have in our hands twenty-two applications for membership, all claiming, as we believe justly, graduation from colleges of medicine recognized by the American Association of Medical Colleges of the United States, and your committee recommends that the convention proceed to organize a medical association in pursuance of its original purpose with the following members: A. W. Foreman, Vinita; M. F. Williams, Muskogee; J. R. Brewer, Muskogee; J. O. Callahan, Muskogee; Charles Harris, Muskogee; R. A. Burr, Choteau; C. A. Pennington, Choteau; R. L. Fite, Tahlequah; F. B. Fite, Tahlequah; E. N. Allen, McAlester; G. R. Rucker, Eufaula; D. Dunn, Bartlesville; C. P. Linn, Claremore; A. J. Lour, Oowala; J. C. Blaud, Red Fork; G. W. Cleveland, Wagoner; G. A. McBride, Fort Gibson; W. J. Adair, J. T. Jones, Tulsa; Oliver Bagby, Vinita; B. F. Fortner, Vinita; J. S. Lankford, Atoka; E. P. Harris, Savanna."

After this second beginning, the Indian Territory Medical Association met regularly every six months. Meetings were held in Fort Gibson, South McAlester, Muskogee, Vinita, Wagoner, Atoka, and Claremore. After the third year, the program was broken into three groups, consisting of the Practice of Medicine, Obstetrics and Gynecology, and Surgery. Each years its membership grew in numbers and strength, until it attracted men even from Arkansas, Texas, and Kansas. Among others, Jabez Jackson of Kansas City attended regularly and contributed many papers and discussions to its programs. Finally, in 1906 it gave up its identity by merging with another association which had been formed in the unsettled land then known as Oklahoma Territory.

This country had been opened to settlement April 21, 1889, and along with the settlers came doctors of various kinds. About one year later a meeting was held in Guthrie for the purpose of organizing a Territorial Medical Association. The effort was unsuccessful and another was held in Edmond for the same purpose, but it likewise failed. Meanwhile, three local societies had been organized and were functioning, one in Guthrie, one in Oklahoma City, and one in El Reno. Notwithstanding this, the Oklahoma Medical Journal was begun in January, 1893, at Guthrie by Drs. E. O. Barker, H. P. Halsted, and Joseph Pinquard. In March of that year, it published the following editorial:

"Is it not about time for the doctors of this Territory to organize a Territorial Medical Society? Every state and territory except Oklahoma has a successful medical society, and Oklahoma with three hundred or more physicians without a territorial society is behind the times. We as practitioners, if we hope to keep to the front and alive to the advance of medical science, must have a place where we can meet and exchange ideas and form more friendly and closer relations.

"The Journal wishes to propound the following questions, and upon the answers will depend the organization of a Territorial Medical Society.

Question 1. Doctor, are you willing to lend your presence and what other assistance you can to the organization of a Territorial Medical Society?

Question 2. What place, in your opinion, would be the most satisfactory for the physicians to meet for organization?

Question 3. In your opinion, what date would be most acceptable to the profession?

"If sufficient answers are received, showing a desire on the part of the doctors of the Territory for an organization, we will issue a call through the Journal at a time and place indicated by the answers to the foregoing questions.

"We hope that each doctor will take sufficient interest to drop us a card immediately."

Evidently the appeal was successful and aroused a good response for the next issue we find the following:

"Territorial Call of Physicians"

"The physicians of Oklahoma Territory will meet in Oklahoma City, on May 9, 1893, for the purpose of organizing a Territorial Medical Society. The answers to the questions in the last month's Journal in reference to a territorial organization have been sufficient in number to make it advisable; a large number of physicians having responded with their approval of such a movement.

"From the answers received, we find that the most suitable place is Oklahoma City, and the time May 9th.

"In order to expedite business when we do met, we will make the hour 3:30 P.M. at the Grand Avenue Hotel."

Accordingly, on the date specified, a group of doctors met in the commercial clubrooms of the Grand Avenue Hotel and organized themselves into the Oklahoma Territorial Medical Association. The meeting was called to order by Dr. W. R. Thompson, of Oklahoma City, and Dr. E. O. Barker, of Guthrie, was elected temporary Chairman. A committee of five on permanent organization was appointed by the Chair, consisting of Dr. C. A. Cravens, of Oklahoma City; Dr. J. A. Overstreet, of Kingfisher; Dr. W. B. Camp, of Tecumseh; Dr. N. W. Mayginnes, of Stillwater; and Dr. H. P. Halsted, of Guthrie.

Dr. DeLos Walker, of Oklahoma City, was elected president of the new association. The Committee on Constitution and By-Laws recommended the adoption of the constitution and by-laws of the Indian Territory Medical Society, except that the dues were to be one dollar per year instead of two dollars per year. A scientific program was then heard and the meeting adjourned to convene again November 2nd and 3rd, 1893, at El Reno. Meetings were then held semi-annually in Oklahoma City, Guthrie, El Reno, Norman, and Shawnee, until 1904, at which time the association was reorganized along the lines laid down by the American Medical Association; and six months later it was decided to dispense with the fall meeting and merely have one annual meeting in the month of May. The following men were the charter members:

W. H. Clutter, Oklahoma City; J. M. Carson, El Reno; W. H. Snow, Norman; E. J. Trader, Council Grove; N. W. Mayginnes, Stillwater; DeLos Walker, Oklahoma City; J. R. McElvain, Oklahoma City; T. A. Cravens, Oklahoma City; J. A. Hatchett, El Reno; H. P. Halsted, Guthrie; B. L. Applewhite, Tecumseh; S. M. Barnes, Stillwater; W. McKay Dougan, Perry; A. A. Davis, El Reno; J. A. Overstreet, Kingfisher; J. E. Fenlon, Norman; J. M. Still, Noble; C. D. Arnold, El Reno; A. H. Jackson, El Reno; C. B. Bradford, Oklahoma City; J. A. Ryan, Oklahoma City; E. O. Barker, Guthrie.

This association continued to meet regularly until the year 1906, at which time it merged with the Indian Territory Medical Association to make the present Oklahoma State Medical Association.

War or No War—

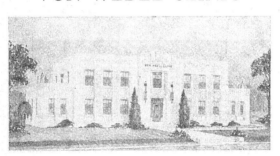

COMMITTEE REPORTS

Committee Reports To Be Made
Before House of Delegates

The following committees of the Association have elected to make verbal reports to the House of Delegates. The reports will be made at the first meeting of the House of Delegates, and in the regular order of business.

The committees are: Committee on Conservation of Hearing; Committee on Crippled Children; Committee on Study and Control of Venereal Diseases; Committee on Benevolent Fund; Committee on Credentials; Committee on Annual Session; Committee on Scientific Work; Committee on Medical Education and Hospitals; Committee on Publicity; and the Committee on Public Policy.

ANNUAL REPORT OF DISTRICT NO. 5

To the President and House of Delegates
Of the Oklahoma State Medical Association
Gentlemen:

In reporting the activities of the Councilor of the Fifth District, I hope you will consider the frailties of the flesh, for at times the heart is willing where the flesh is weak.

The Fifth District consists of nine counties with a membership of 119 members: Caddo with 22 members, Carter 26, Comanche 15, Cotton 7, Grady 19, Jefferson 10, Murray 8, Stephens 13, and Love with two or three belonging to Carter county. Of these the larger counties have very active societies, while the smaller do not have enough members to meet regularly.

Most of the counties with the exception of my own have doctors who are not members of the Association.

Your Councilor visited only one society during the year, with the exception of a Councilor District meeting held at Ardmore, January 12, which was attended by about half of the membership of the district. Ardmore was a delightful host to this meeting and all those who did not attend it certainly missed a treat both up and down stairs. The meeting was held at the Ardmore Hotel, beginning with a supper, or rather a "get-to-gether" upstairs which inspired everyone present.

The Speakers for the evening were Dr. Finis W. Ewing, President of the Association; Dr. Lewis H. Ritz-haupt, State Medical Officer; and Mr. Graham, Executive Secretary of the Association. Several guests from Oklahoma City were present.

My program for the coming year will consist of about four meetings of this type, which I believe are of more benefit than just visiting the county societies. There has been no trouble or discord in our District during the year.

Respectfully submitted
J. I. Hollingsworth, M.D.
Councilor District No. 5

ANNUAL REPORT OF DISTRICT NO. 8

To the President and House of Delegates,
Oklahoma State Medical Association
Gentlemen:

I will be frank and admit that during the past year very little has been accomplished in the 8th Councilor district so far as new constructive work is concerned.

The following County Medical Societies are active and, I believe, have held regular meetings during this period: Okmulgee, Ottawa, Muskogee, Craig and Cherokee.

I am not thoroughly acquainted with Mayes, Delaware, Adair, Sequoyah and Wagoner. Mayes and Wagoner are organized but have not functioned with regular meetings.

Delaware, Adair and Sequoyah have no organization as very few physicians live in these counties and some hold their membership in adjoining County Societies.

Okmulgee, Cherokee, Craig and Ottawa have had some

very interesting programs which has stimulated interest in these County Medical Societies.

The Muskogee County Medical Society has cut its regular meeting from two per month to one per month, this due to the increased work the membership has at this time.

Wagoner and Sequoyah have combined with Muskogee to form the Muskogee-Sequoyah-Wagoner County Medical Society. We are hoping in this way to create more interest in this section. This has not been approved as yet by the Council but I am taking the liberty of reporting this without the approval of the Council as these three County Medical Societies have voted for amalgamation.

Respectfully submitted,
SHADE D. NEELY, M.D.
Councilor District No. 8

ANNUAL REPORT OF DISTRICT NO. 9

To the President and House of Delegates of the
Oklahoma State Medical Association
Gentlemen:

I herewith tender you my report for the year 1941-42 for the Judical District No. 9, Oklahoma State Medical Association.

I have visited each of the County Societies comprising this district and wish to report to you they are in a healthy condition, are active and meeting regularly with good programs being presented to the membership.

While McIntosh County has a very small membership, the Society is meeting regularly and has in Doctors Little and Tolleson two enthusiastic officers, who at all times are working for the furtherance of orthodox medicine in Oklahoma. I have visited them several times and assisted in every way called upon in their problems presented.

LeFlore County Medical Society has only recently resumed regular meetings, having suspended meetings for a few months during the winter season. They have a healthy membership and I predict for them a good year. At the meeting on March 12, two pioneers in Organized Medicine in eastern Oklahoma were presented tokens of esteem by the Society for having been in the practice of medicine for 40 years. These two pioneers are Doctors E. L. Collins and S. C. Dean of Panama and Howe, respectively. Also as a token of their good wishes in his new location and as an appreciation for the good work done in the LeFlore County Medical Society, a token was presented to Doctor W. L. Shippey. Doctor Shippey has just recently re-moved to Fort Smith.

Pittsburg County has been active, meeting regularly with good programs being presented at each meeting. Doctor E. D. Greenberger, the Secretary, has been very energetic in obtaining membership in the County Society of practically every doctor in Pittsburg County who is eligible to membership.

Latimer County does not have a Medical Society and does not at the present time have sufficient doctors in the county to justify the organization of a society. The same is also true of Haskell County. The doctors of Latimer County belong to either Pittsburg or LeFlore County Medical Societies.

It is my suggestion that Latimer County join with LeFlore County Medical Society forming the LeFlore-Latimer Medical Society. And that Haskell County join with McIntosh County forming the McIntosh-Haskell Medical Society.

Respectfully submitted,

L. C. KUYKENDALL, M.D.
Councilor District No. 9

Report of the Committee on Necrology

The Committee on Necrology submits the following report to the House of Delegates:

Medicine's duty to humanity in the present world emergency will find physicians on all fronts. Their duty will be to save rather than to take life. Many will pay the supreme sacrifice on the battle front, many will do likewise on the home front.

As the years go on through war and peace, the physician will continue to give of himself without thought of himself. To those who no longer will hear the roll of battle drums in the call of duty, all homage is paid. Theirs has been a battle fought and won. We must carry on.

In honor of those members of the Association who have passed away during the last year, the Necrology committee submits the following resolution for adoption by the House of Delegates:

WHEREAS: Thirty-nine of our members have passed to the Great Beyond since the 1941 report of the Necrology committee of the Association, be it

RESOLVED: That the House of Delegates of the Oklahoma State Medical Association recognize the demise of these former fellow members and instruct the Secretary-Treasurer to inscribe with honor and regret the following names upon the records of the Association:

George W. Sisler	Tulsa	March 23, 1941
A. T. Hill	Stigler	April 21, 1941
*Calbert Harvey Beach	Glencoe	May 15, 1941
Peter Cope White	Tulsa	May 26, 1941
*J. E. Jones	Hollis	May 23, 1941
S. N. Mayberry	Enid	June 22, 1941
Charles D. Johnson	Tulsa	June 22, 1941
Edmund S. Ferguson	Oklahoma City	June 28, 1941
*Charles R. Silverthorne	Woodward	July 27, 1941
J. R. Holliday	Oklahoma City	August 7, 1941
*A. J. Welch	McAlester	Sept. 7, 1941
Allen G. Flythe	Durant	Sept. 21, 1941
J. C. Warmack	Oklahoma City	Sept. 26, 1941
*McClellan Wilson	McAlester	Oct. 15, 1941
C. T. Arrington	Oklahoma City	Oct. 18, 1841
C. J. Forney	Woodward	Oct. 24, 1941
*T. M. Boyd	Norman	Oct. 29, 1941
J. A. Rutledge	Ada	Nov. 2, 1941
C. K. Logan	Hominy	Nov. 14, 1941
Ruth B. Jones	Seminole	Nov. 29, 1941
Dick Lowry	Oklahoma City	Dec. 2, 1941
Jesse Bird	Oklahoma City	Dec. 9, 1941
J. B. Hix	Altus	Dec. 13, 1941
J. L. Adams	Hobart	Dec. 31, 1941
O. N. Windle	Sayre	Jan. 3, 1942
*J. W. Browning	Geary	Jan. 9, 1942
I. B. Oldham, Sr.	Muskogee	Jan. 15, 1942
*C. S. Boho	Norman	Feb. 3, 1942
John Kuhn, Sr.	Oklahoma City	Feb. 13, 1942
F. P. Von Keller	Ardmore	Feb. 13, 1942
G. D. Funk	El Reno	Feb. 26, 1942
Thomas R. Lutner	Lawton	March 7, 1942
*A. M. Young, Jr.	Oklahoma City	March 18, 1942
D. B. Stough	Vinita	March 19, 1942
A. C. Jenner	Durant	March 19, 1942
*Edward M. Harris	Cushing	
William C. Sain	Ardmore	March 7, 1942
G. R. Norman	Tulsa	Jan. 21, 1942
John Davis	Seminole	

Requiescat in Pace!

*Honorary

Respectfully submitted
R. M. Anderson, M.D., Chairman
John A. Haynie, M.D.
W. H. Livermore, M.D.

Report of the Committee on Judicial And Professional Relations

The Committee on Judicial and Professional Relations submits the following report to the House of Delegates:
Your Committee on Judicial and Professional Relations established under the new constitution and by-laws has not been presented with any questions coming under its jurisdiction concerning compensation for injuries said to have resulted from malpractice other than those cases which have been brought to the attention of the committee by requests for assistance from the Medical Defense fund.

During the 1941-42 period, five requests for assistance from the fund have been received and the assistance granted. Of these cases, one has been settled by a verdict in favor of the defendant, one in favor of the plaintiff, one dismissed, and the other two are awaiting disposition. The committee desires to express its appreciation for the manner in which cooperation has been received from those members requesting assistance and respectfully desires to reaffirm the splendid place this fund takes in the affairs of the Association.

On April 1 in addition to bonds held to the account of the Medical Defense fund as reported in the audit of the Association, there is on hand in cash the sum of $1,438.34.

Respectfully submitted
A. S. Risser, M.D.
L. C. Kuyrkendall, M.D.
J. M. Bonham, M.D.

Report of the Committee On Postgraduate Medical Teaching

The Committee on Postgraduate Medical Teaching submits the following report to the House of Delegates.

The postgraduate program in pediatrics conducted by James G. Hughes, M.D., of Memphis, Tennessee, which ended January 31, 1942, was a success from every viewpoint. The course was offered in 45 teaching centers. Additional instruction was given in Oklahoma City and Tulsa for the benefit of colored physicians. Total registration numbered 782. Doctor Hughes held 979 consultation with physicians, and spoke before a total of 6,239 citizens in his lay talks. The first circuit only, in northeastern Oklahoma, was given by Drs. Wayne A. Rupe, Peter G. Danis, and Stanley Harrison, all of St. Louis, Missouri.

The attendance throughout the state was excellent, in view of the severe epidemic of influenza which occurred during the first winter, and the call to military duty of so many of our physicians who have participated in these courses. Registration fees were refunded to those who were called to active duty between the date they enrolled and the date instruction began in their community.

Receipts from all sources amounted to $31,038.91. Total disbursements were $24,851.55. Balance at the close of the program was $6,187.36, which amount was prorated back to the contributing agencies. Bound copies of the instructor's lectures were distributed to all physicians enrolled, and a total of 600 Certificates of Attendance were issued to those whose attendance averaged 70 percent, or more.

The Committee desires to thank The Commonwealth Fund of New York, the Oklahoma State Health Department, the U. S. Children's Bureau, and the Oklahoma State Medical Association for their financial assistance, and further recommends that the House of Delegates, by resolution, express its appreciation to these contributing agencies.

We are also pleased to report that a two-year program in internal medicine is now in progress. L. W. Hunt, M.D., Assistant Professor of Medicine, University of Chicago, began instruction in northeastern Oklahoma, March 9. The teaching centers for the first circuit are Miami, Vinita, Pryor, Claremore and Bartlesville. Over 80 percent of the physicians practicing in this section of the state have enrolled, and during the first two weeks Doctor Hunt has held 48 consultations.

Further information regarding this course may be obtained at the Postgraduate Booth during the State

Medical Meeting at Tulsa, or by writing the Postgraduate Committee, Oklahoma State Medical Association, 210 Plaza Court, Oklahoma City.

Respectfully,

Henry H. Turner, M.D., Chairman,
M. J. Searle, M.D.
H. C. Weber, M.D.

Report of the Committee on the Study And Control of Cancer

The Committee on the Study and Control of Cancer submits the following report to the House of Delegates:

The Cancer Committee during the past year has devoted its work to the assistance of the program of the Women's Field Army of the American Society for the Control of Cancer.

The Women's Field Army annually sponsors an educational program on early diagnosis and treatment of cancer through the Federation of Women's Clubs of the state. During the months of April and May, their enrollment drive is made, and it is from this money that the program is financed.

In the past, the Cancer committee has annually asked for an appropriation of $750.00 from the Association to assist the work of the Committee and the Women's Field Army. However, the work accomplished for the Committee since the establishment of a full-time office for the Association no longer makes it necessary to ask for this appropriation.

Committee work during the coming two months will be heavy, since these are the months of the educational program of the Women's Field Army. Each County Medical society will be asked by the local county Captain of the Field Army to assist in the drive, in so far as it pertains to the educational feature. Doctors will not be asked to solicit enrollments.

Your Committee urges every county society to assist the women in their educational work and to enrol personally, if you feel able.

Your Committee commends and endorses the work being done by the Women's Field Army.

Your Committee also strongly recommends to the county societies that they take the initiative in sponsoring cancer education in the highschools and colleges of the state, and that through the Chairman of the Cancer committee at least one program on this second highest cause of death be made available annually to the schools.

Respectfully submitted
C. P. Bondurant, M.D., Chairman
W. S. Larrabee, M.D.
Paul B. Champlin, M.D.

Report of Committee on Medical Economics

The Committee on Medical Economics submits the following report to the House of Delegates:

Your Committee at the 1941 session of the House of Delegates reported its recommendations on the important problem of assisting the Department of Public Welfare in its Aid to Dependent Children Fund. It is now further gratifying to be able to report that upon the adoption of the report by the House of Delegates, the President at the request of the Council immediately contacted the Director of the Department of Public Welfare, and from that meeting, a committee composed of C. R. Rountree, Chairman, F. Redding Hood, R. M. Shepard, Clinton Gallaher and A. R. Sugg was appointed to give advice and aid on medical matters concerning the operation of the fund.

Since this Committee will report in detail, no further comment will be made except to commend the Council upon its outstanding accomplishments.

During the past year, the Committee has had occasion to study the problem of organized medicine and its place in the program of the Farm Security Administration's health projects for its clients.

The Committee, before meeting with representatives of the F.S.A., took a survey of the past and present programs of this type in operation in the state, and the conclusions drawn from this survey could not be made definite. In the main, the reports from the different societies were to the effect that the programs were not satisfactory for reasons of administration, inequalities and low fee payments for services rendered.

Upon meeting with F.S.A. representatives concerning this program, certain objectionable features seemed to have been eliminated, but your Committee at this time cannot report further upon the attitudes of the county societies concerning the operations of the plans under the revised system.

Your Committee recommends that no endorsement of the Farm Security Administration plans be made by the House of Delegates, but that the cooperation of organized medicine be left to the discretion of the local county societies after careful and complete study.

Your Committee further recommends that the study of its relations to the voluntary feature of medicine in medical economics by the State Association be given every impetus possible by the House of Delegates and that the Council keep constant vigil on this important phase of medicine as it pertains to world conditions and its relations to the voluntary feature of medicine in America today.

Respectfully submitted
Horace Reed, M.D., Chairman
W. A. Howard, M.D.
McLain Rogers, M.D.

Report of Committee on Industrial and Traumatic Surgery

The Committee on Industrial and Traumatic Surgery submits the following report to the House of Delegates:

Your Committee met on March 15, in Tulsa, with the Industrial committee chairmen of 22 County Medical societies of the Association, and after a discussion of the problems of medicine in industry, has the following recommendations to make to the House of Delegates:

1. That a series of programs on Industrial Medicine and Surgery be held in connection with either County Medical societies or councilor district meetings, and that speakers for these meetings be arranged for through either the State Association or the American Medical Association.
2. That the scientific program of the State Association have included in its program papers on Industrial Medicine and Surgery.
3. That the Editorial Board be requested to devote part of the Scientific section of the Journal to problems of industrial medicine.

Your Committee is further of the opinion that the war effort of the United States will rapidly develop and enlarge the field of Industrial Medicine and Surgery, and that every effort should be made by organized medicine to meet these needs. It is the opinion of the Committee that the above recommendations if adopted will materially assist to that end.

Respectfully submitted.
I. W. Bollinger, M.D., Chairman
O. S. Somerville, M.D.
W. G. Chestnut, M.D.

Report of Committee on Public Health

The Committee on Public Health submits the following report to the House of Delegates:

During the past year, your Committee has advised and cooperated with the Department of Health in its program of child immunization.

The recommendations of the Committee were transmitted to the Council, and the Council acted upon these in the affirmative.

This program is now in operation in the state and since each County society has been advised of its scope, it will not be repeated in this report.

Your Committee wishes to commend to the House of Delegates the work of the Department of Health and particularly the Commissioner, Dr. Grady Mathews, for the efforts made by his department in the field of public health and the cooperation given organized medicine.

It is the feeling of your Committee that preventive medicine will be expanded during the time necessary for the winning of the war and that organized medicine should give and expend its entire facilities and energies to accomplish this important defense measure.

Respectfully submitted

Carroll M. Pounders, M.D., Chairman

G. S. Baxter, M.D.

H. K. Riddle, M.D.

Report of the Committee on Maternity and Infancy

The Committee on Maternity and Infancy submits the following report to the House of Delegates:

NEW MATERNAL MORTALITY FORMS READY

Two Dollars Paid for Completion and Return

As soon as the exact causes of death and their modifying factors are definitely known, instead of being hidden by the present brief and obscure "death certificate," a substantial reduction in Oklahoma's maternal mortality rate is certain to occur.

The House of Delegates voted to conduct a maternal mortality survey at the last meeting of the Oklahoma State Medical Association. During the past year, this has been carried on through the Committee on Maternity on Infancy, and the plan adopted is a composite of several plans which have been brilliantly successful in other localities. Many of these have served to reduce maternity and infancy mortality rates by a spectacular decline. Sample questionnaires were obtained from these localities, and from these a form more suitable for Oklahoma was composed.

The new form was put into trial use on several instances in order to "iron out the kinks," and has recently been made available for state-wide use.

Speed Is Essential

Other states have found that the greatest single factor in making these forms effective was their prompt completion by the physician who had signed the death certificate. For this reason, a fee of two dollars will be paid the physician who completes and forwards this form promptly. The questionnaire is based on a chronological history of the patient's pregnancy and is therefore easily completed.

Causes of Death Exposed

The present form of death certificate leaves much to be desired when attempting to analyze and correct causes of obstetrical death. The present certificate may list, for instance, "death from hemorrhage," and this may be correct, but it fails to state that the patient lived twenty miles over sandy roads, or that she refused the doctor's advice until it was too late, or that no donors were available.

It is now universally recognized that eclampsia is preventable, but eclampsia can be prevented only when the patient consults the physician early enough, and then follows the doctor's orders. All such information is missing on the present death certificate, and for many years Oklahoma physicians have labored under the stigma of a high maternal mortality rate, which may or may not have been ascribable to them. The present survey will not only clarify these factors, but will also, if followed through, attack each cause of death as a separate problem.

In the City of Philadelphia, the maternal mortality rate was stationary for many years. Within a short time after the individual deaths were analyzed, the death rate was reduced by one-half. A similar detailed study in Oklahoma is certain to bear valuable fruit.

Method of Survey

When an "obstetrical death" occurs, the Bureau of Vital Statistics will fill out the first page of the new questionnaire, subsequently forwarding it to the doctor signing the death certificate.

The remaining questions follow in easy sequence, and serve to paint the complete picture of that patient's death.

It is to be emphasized that there is no effort being made to fix blame or pin responsibility. The results will be forever anonymous, and the sincere purpose is not to accuse the doctor, but to prevent another patient from dying. The Committee sincerely hopes you will never be called upon to fill out this form, but if you are, please do so promptly, cheerfully, and accurately. You will be paid for your effort.

Respectfully submitted,

Charles Ed White, M.D., Chairman

J. B. Eskridge, M.D.

J. H. Veazey, M.D.

Edward N. Smith, M.D.

J. T. Bell, M.D.

Report of the Committee on Conservation of Vision

The Committee on Conservation of Vision submits the following report to the House of Delegates:

Your Committee on the Conservation of Vision wishes to report that, after due consideration and deliberation, world events made it inadvisable to attempt to function at the present time.

The State of Oklahoma is very backward in handling its visual conservation setup. The dread disease of Tracoma has passed out of the picture. However, the numerous blind pensioners continue to have their ranks filled because of ignorance both within the medical profession and the laity.

The need of Oklahoma is:

1. Education of the physicians.
2. Education of the teachers.
3. An improvement in the handling of the defective eyes during the school age.

Your Committee endeavored to start such a program throughout Oklahoma, but due to the increased amount of work incurred by the draft, deemed it best not to attempt to function at a necessarily inadequate program.

Your Committee recommends that when the emergency has disappeared the State Medical Association make as one of its major projects the sadly deficient Ophthalmological setup in Oklahoma.

C. H. Haralson, M.D., Chairman

E. H. Coachman, M.D.

F. Maxey Cooper, M.D.

Report of Committee on Study and Control Of Tuberculosis

The Committee on Study and Control of Tuberculosis submits the following report to the House of Delegates:

The State of Oklahoma has a large incidence of tuberculosis which is not being lowered. In fact, it is increasing. This is not occurring in other states where proper measures are taken.

There is not proper supervision of tuberculosis patients in the state who are not hospitalized in one of the state sanatoria. Some counties have efficient State Health organizations which are doing good work, but there are far too many who are not supervised by these units.

Our sanatoria are only able to hospitalize about one-half of the patients who apply, and while we believe these organizations are doing excellent work, we believe there should be definite organizations for the control and treatment of tuberculosis in the state of Oklahoma, the organizations to be intelligently handled and have definite functions.

The bed space should be increased in the two state sanatoria and appropriations substantially increased to take care of these patients. The patients who can obtain competent medical supervision at home, and proper supervision from a public health standpoint, or where they are financially able to seek competent private care, should be advised to do so.

Therefore, we believe the following resolutions and recommendations are in order:

1. Be it resolved that this committee go on record as recommending a unified control of tuberculosis as to survey, care and treatment, and that a budget be prepared that will allow enough money to care for these patients and provide and equip the present sanatoria with increased bed capacity.

2. Furthermore, be it resolved that some attempt be made to secure federal funds to aid in hospitalization and care of the tuberculous. Since our country is in total war and the care of the citizens and soldiers' dependents is very vital to the nation's defense, we believe that some federal funds should be allotted in each state for the purpose of care and supervision of people suffering from tuberculosis of the lungs.

Respectfully submitted
F. P. Baker, M.D., Chairman
R. M. Shepard, M.D.
Carl Puckett, M.D.

Supplementary Report

In support of the report by the Committee on Study and Control of Tuberculosis, prepared by Dr. F. P.

Baker, Chairman, I submit the following supplementary report to emphasize the first recommendation, and which may be classed as a minority report. I am "all out" for the chairman in his attempt to bring order out of the present chaos:

Unified control of tuberculosis will be well under way when the supervision of the tuberculosis sanatoria is placed under the State Health Department, where they were from the time of establishment until 1937 when transferred to the State Board of Public Affairs. Tuberculosis is a communicable disease and its supervision and control therefore belongs to the Health Department, and the santoria are a part of the State system of tuberculosis control.

Every physician should lend his influence at the ballot box for making this legal change back to the Health Department at the next session of the Legislature. Other necessary improvements may then be made within this properly coordinated set-up.

Respectfully submitted
Carl Puckett, M.D.

ANNUAL AUDIT REPORT

Mr. R. H. Graham, Executive Secretary
Oklahoma State Medical Association
210 Plaza Court
Oklahoma City, Oklahoma

Dear Sir:

We have completed the audit of the financial records of

THE OKLAHOMA STATE MEDICAL ASSOCIATION
Oklahoma City, Oklahoma

for the period from January 1, 1941, to December 31, 1941, and submit herewith the following Exhibits:

EXHIBIT "1"—BALANCE SHEET
EXHIBIT "2"—STATEMENT OF CASH RECEIPTS AND DISBURSEMENTS
EXHIBIT "3"—OPERATING STATEMENT
EXHIBIT "4"—BANK RECONCILIATION

EXPLANATION

Since the Association operates on a Cash Receipts and Disbursements basis, the disbursements for December, which are paid in January, are included in the report for the following year.

We wish to thank you for this audit, and if we can be of further service, please feel free to call upon us.

Respectfully submitted,

H. E. COLE COMPANY

OKLAHOMA STATE MEDICAL ASSOCIATION
Oklahoma City, Oklahoma

Exhibit I

BALANCE SHEET
Dec. 31, 1941

ASSETS

	Total	Membership Fund	Journal Fund	Medical Defense Fund	Annual Meeting
Petty Cash	$ 14.94	$ 14.94	$	$	$ ....
Bank	3,930.30	2,126.54	834.42	309.34	660.00
U. S. Treasury Bonds	6,178.88	1,235.78	....	4,943.10	....
National Defense Bonds	2,220.00	....	....	2,220.00	....
TOTAL ASSETS	$12,344.12	$ 3,377.26	$ 834.42	$ 7,472.44	$ 660.00

LIABILITIES & RESERVES

	Total	Membership Fund	Journal Fund	Medical Defense Fund	Annual Meeting
1942 Membership Dues	$ 10.00	$ 9.00	$	$ 1.00	$ ....
Operating Reserve	12,334.12	3,368.26	834.42	7,471.44	660.00
TOTAL LIABILITIES & RESERVES	$12,344.12	$ 3,377.26	$ 834.42	$ 7,472.44	$ 660.00

OKLAHOMA STATE MEDICAL ASSOCIATION
Oklahoma City, Oklahoma
Exhibit 2

STATEMENT OF CASH RECEIPTS & DISBURSEMENTS
January 1, 1941 to December 31, 1941

	Total	Membership Fund	Journal Fund	Medical Defense Fund	Annual Meeting
Cash Balance—January 1, 1941	$ 3,136.55	$ 660.68	$ 1,442.53	$ 993.34	$ 40.00
Petty Cash Balance—January 1, 1941	10.00		10.00		
RECEIPTS:					
1941 Membership Dues	13,989.15	12,562.15		1,427.00	
1942 Membership Dues	10.00	9.00		1.00	
Journal Advertising & Subscriptions	7,213.01		7,213.01		
U. S. Government Bond Interest	135.00	27.00		108.00	
Annual Meeting	2,410.40				2,410.40
TOTAL CASH TO BE ACCOUNTED FOR	$26,904.11	$13,258.83	$ 8,665.54	$ 2,529.34	$ 2,450.40
DISBURSEMENTS:					
1940 Social Security Paid	$ 18.45	$ 18.45	$	$	$
National Defense Bonds Purchased	2,220.00			2,220.00	
Expenses for 1941	20,720.42	11,098.90	7,831.12		1,790.40
TOTAL DISBURSEMENTS	$22,958.87	$11,117.35	$ 7,831.12	$ 2,220.00	$ 1,790.40
Bank Balance—December 31, 1941	$ 3,930.30	$ 2,126.54	$ 834.42	$ 309.34	$ 660.00
Petty Cash Balance	14.94	14.94			
	$ 3,945.24	$ 2,141.48	$ 834.42	$309.34	$ 660.00

OKLAHOMA STATE MEDICAL ASSOCIATION
Oklahoma City, Oklahoma
Exhibit 3

OPERATING STATEMENT
1941

REVENUE

	Total	Membership Fund	Journal Fund	Medical Defense Fund	Annual Meeting
1941 Membership Dues	$13,989.15	$12,562.15	$	$ 1,427.00	$
Journal Advertising & Subscriptions	7,213.01		7,213.01		
U. S. Government Bond Interest	135.00	27.00		108.00	
Annual Meeting	2,410.40				2,410.40
TOTAL REVENUE	$23,747.56	$12,589.15	$ 7,213.01	$ 1,535.00	$ 2,410.40
EXPENSES					
Salaries	$ 7,166.82	$ 3,886.82	$ 3,280.00	$	$
Journal Printing & Mailing	3,834.29		3,834.29		
Press Clipping Service	36.00		36.00		
Journal Engraving	167.95		167.95		
Telephone & Telegraph	478.32	475.34	2.98		
Postage	626.12	560.97	65.15		
Office Rent	305.00	175.00	130.00		
Printing & Stationary	332.27	332.27			
Office Supplies	427.33	427.33			
Traveling Expense	1,029.12	842.02	187.10		
Council & Delegates Expense	574.86	574.86			
Social Security Tax	51.82	38.22	13.60		
Post Graduate Committee	2,000.00	2,000.00			
Office Equipment	175.24	175.24			
Annual Meeting	2,113.88	323.48			1,790.40
Returned Checks	1.50		1.50		
Certificate Frames	35.10	35.10			
Sundry	234.82	197.27	37.55		
Secretary's Conference	128.30	128.30			
Dr. Willour's Refund on Salary Overpayment	288.75	288.75			
Entertainment	246.87	246.87			
Dr. Long's Plaque & Picture	203.56	203.56			
Auditing & Legal	212.50	137.50	75.00		
Chamber of Commerce Dues	50.00	50.00			
TOTAL EXPENSES	20,720.42	11,098.90	7,831.12		1,790.40
Revenue over Expenses	$ 3,027.14	$ 1,490.25	—$618.11	$ 1,535.00	$ 620.00

OKLAHOMA STATE MEDICAL ASSOCIATION
Oklahoma City, Oklahoma

Exhibit 4

BANK RECONCILIATION
December 31, 1941

MEMBERSHIP FUND—Liberty National Bank
Balance per Bank Statment.. $2,498.74
Outstanding Checks:
    Voucher No. 705—Richard H. Graham............................$ 150.00
    Voucher No. 706—Dr. Finis Ewing.................................   17.52
    Voucher No. 712—Skirvin Hotel.....................................   132.50
    Voucher No. 715—Postmaster...   72.18   372.20

    Balance per Books... $2,126.54

JOURNAL FUND—Liberty National Bank
Balance per Bank Statement.. $ 886.27
Outstanding Checks:
    Voucher No. 707—Dr. L. S. Willour...............................$ 50.00
    Voucher No. 708—Dr. L. S. Willour...............................   1.85   51.85

                                                                                         $ 834.42

MEDICAL DEFENSE FUND—Liberty National Bank
Balance per Books & Bank Statement................................ $ 309.34
ANNUAL MEETING FUND—Liberty National Bank
Balance per Books & Statements.. $ 660.00

    TOTAL MONEY ON DEPOSIT....................................... $3,930.30

New Treatment of Diarrhea in Babies

Before the advent of Mead's Pectin-Agar in Dextri-Maltose, there were two methods of treating diarrhea in infants: (1) the "starvation" or "rest" method, consisting of withholding food during the duration of the diarrhea, offering the baby water and carbohydrate solutions. While this succeeded in preventing extreme dehydration, the child received practically no food to maintain nutrition, so that, when long continued, his resistance was greatly impaired. (2) the "Finkelstein method," based on the theory that some carbohydrates are especially likely to cause fermentation and prolong diarrhea. His method consisted of high protein feedings in the form of protein milk, sometimes with added carbohydrate, and continues to have many advocates, especially in breast-fed infants. One of the successful modifications has been Casec (calcium caseinate), which can be used for both breast-fed and bottle-fed infants.

In recent years, the use of raw apple and weak tea for treating diarrhea has had various proponents. The literature contains reports by Birnberg, Reglien, Kaliski, Giblin and Lischner, McCaslan, Tompkins, Borovsky, Stein, and Hunt. Smith and Fried believe that any beneficial effects from scraped raw apple are due to the partial starvation effected by the regimen. The success of apple and tea therapy has stimulated hypotheses as to the effective agent. Moro attributed its value to tannic acid. Heisler would also give credit to malic acid and to the mechanical cleansing of the intestines, while Scheer places most emphasis on indigestible bulk. Malyoth believes pectin and cellulose are the active agents.

Based on their experience with apple, Winters and Tompkins devised a mixture of pectin, agar and Dextri-Maltose which was more successful. Others have privately confirmed their finding that a mixture of this nature is of value in diarrhea. Kutscher and Blumberg studied the use of the pectin-agar mixture with and without carbohydrate. They concluded that the addition of Dextri-Maltose to the other constituents was a definite advantage. Various reasons for the effectiveness of both pectin and agar have been advanced but none has a background of experimental proof. It has been claimed that pectin is bactericidal, that its constituent galacturonic acid functions as a detoxifying agent, that it absorbs toxins and enmeshes bacteria, that its hydrophilic nature prevents dehydration, and that it is soothing to an inflamed gastrointestinal tract. Bulk is the only valuable characteristic advanced for the use of agar.

In practice, the application of this method differs from the starvation method in that full caloric feedings are immediately instituted and maintained.

The new method differs from protein milk therapy in that a diet high in carbohydrate is fed. It also has the advantage of palatability, particularly important with older children.—Mead Johnson & Company, Evansville, Ind., U.S.A.

Opportunities for Practice

Opportunity for Practice

An opportunity for practice is open in the town of Hunter, in northeastern Garfield county. For more information, any physician interested in this opportunity should contact the office of the Association, 210 Plaza Court, Oklahoma City.

What <u>better</u> proof
of
Philip Morris superiority:−

EVEN *more* conclusive than the obvious improvement in patients' conditions* on changing to PHILIP MORRIS cigarettes is this:

ON CHANGING BACK TO OTHER CIGARETTES, CONGESTION RETURNED IN 80% OF THE CASES.**

PHILIP MORRIS

PHILIP MORRIS & CO., LTD., INC.

119 FIFTH AVENUE, NEW YORK, N. Y.

* *Irritation of the nose and throat due to smoking.*
** *Laryngoscope, Feb. 1935, Vol. XLV, No. 2, 149-154.*

ASSOCIATION ACTIVITIES

450 Hear Dr. Mayo at Annual LeRoy Long Memorial Lecture

With approximately 450 people in attendance and with Dr. Charles W. Mayo of the Mayo Foundation, Rochester, Minn., as guest lecturer, the third LeRoy Long Memorial Lecture was held March 13, in the Auditorium of the Oklahoma University School of Medicine, Oklahoma City.

The lecture, which is conducted under the auspices of the Phi Beta Pi fraternity of the medical school, is an annual event. For the subject of his lecture, Doctor Mayo chose "Principles of Surgery of the Colon." He also exhibited a motion picture of a surgical operation.

General Robert U. Patterson, Dean of the medical school, opened the program with an introduction of Dr. R. M. Howard, Professor of Surgery at the medical school, who in turn introduced Doctor Mayo.

Oklahoma Pediatric Society Announces Program

Dr. Hugh L. Dwyer, Professor of Clinical Pediatrics, University of Kansas School of Medicine, Kansas City, Mo., and a guest speaker for the Annual Meeting, will appear on the Program of the Oklahoma Pediatric Society, Wednesday noon, April 22, at the Mayo Hotel, Tulsa.

Doctor Dwyer will speak to the Society on "Jaundice and Anemia of the New Born."

The Society will convene at 12:15 Noon, for a luncheon, business meeting and Doctor Dwyer's address.

Program for Medical School Alumni Meeting Is Announced

The following program for the Annual Meeting of the Oklahoma University Medical School Association, to be held at 12:00 noon, April 23, at the Tulsa club in Tulsa, has been announced. Dr. Ralph A. McGill is in charge of the program committee and the arrangements for the banquet meeting.

ANNUAL SPRING MEETING OF THE OKLAHOMA UNIVERSITY MEDICAL SCHOOL ASSOCIATION
April 23, 1942
Tulsa Club
PROGRAM
12:15   Honor Classes, 1912, 1922, 1932, 1942
        Special Tables
        Central Tables, Alumni and Guests
        BUSINESS
12:45   Prefactory Remarks, Ray M. Balyeat
12:55   Secretary's Report, Wayne M. Hull
 1:05   Committee Reports
        Miscellaneous Business
        ENTERTAINMENT
Honorary Toastmaster, Wm. F. Taylor, Emeritus
   Professor Pediatrics, Oklahoma University
   School of Medicine
 1:15   Toastmaster's Remarks
        Assisting Toastmaster, Ralph A. McGill
 1:20   Echoes, Class of 1912, Pauline Barker
 1:25   Echoes, Class of 1922, Marvin D. Henley
 1:30   Echoes, Class of 1932, John H. Lamb
 1:35   Echoes, Class of 1942, Mr. Allen Greer, President,
        Senior Class
        ADDRESS
 1:40   Wann Langston
 1:55   Adjournment

Internists to Honor Dr. Herrmann

Members of the Oklahoma State Internists Association will be hosts at a dinner honoring Dr. George Herrmann, Galveston, Tex., Wednesday, April 22, at 5:30, at the Annual Meeting of the Oklahoma State Medical Association, in Tulsa. Doctor Herrmann is guest speaker for the Section on General Medicine.

The Internists Association met December 14 as guests of the Chickasha Hospital, Chickasha, with Dr. Turner Bynum in charge of the program. It is planned to make this meeting in Chickasha an annual event.

Federal Income Tax on Accounts Receivable

In The Journal of the American Medical Association, January 10, 1942, page 149, reference was made to the fact that under section 42 of the Internal Revenue Code, accounts outstanding on the books of a taxpayer may have theretofore been on a cash receipts and disbursements basis.

It was pointed out in The Journal that this method of computing income artificially builds up the income of the taxpayer for the year of death, subjecting it to higher surtax rates and in many instances imposing a considerable hardship on the estate of the taxpayer to raise necessary funds to pay the tax. Please refer to the statement in The Journal for a detailed discussion of this matter.

On March 3, representatives of the Treasury Department appeared before the House Committee on Ways and Means which is now holding hearings on the new tax law and submitted a number of recommendations for changes in the existing law. The Tax Advisor to the Secretary of the Treasury, Randolph Paul, submitted the following Treasury Department recommendation, among others:

"Under present provisions income accrued to the date of the decedent's death must be included in the return for his last income tax period. The "bunching up" of income that may occur under this provision can work a severe hardship, as the income of the decedent may in effect be artificially raised to a much higher surtax bracket. The Supreme Court has indicated that under this provision a lawyer's share of the fees from cases pending at his death is includible in the income tax return for the year in which his death occurs even though such fees may not be collectible until years later. The same result may follow with respect to the commissions of insurance agents, executors and trustees, and the fees of doctors and other professional men. To avoid this hardship, it is suggested that the present method of treating such income be eliminated in favor of a method that taxes the income to the persons who actually receive it. Thus, the income would be made taxable to the estate or to the heir or legatee as the case may be. It is also suggested that this change be made retroactive to all open years under proper safeguards insuring payment of the tax by the recipients of income in such years."

The House Committee on Ways and Means has as yet taken no action with respect to the foregoing recommendation of the Treasury Department. I send you this information so that you may know that there is in the offing a possibility of relief from the inequities created by the present method of arriving at the income of a taxpayer for the year of death.

Sincerely yours,
J. W. Holloway, Jr.,
Bureau of Legal Medicine and Legislation,
American Medical Association

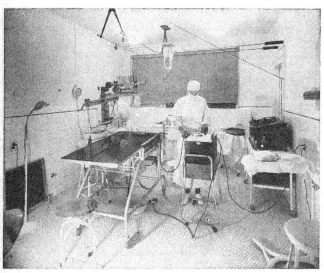

MEDICAL PREPAREDNESS

WAIVER OF PHYSICAL DEFECTS FOR LIMITED SERVICE OFFICERS

On January 30 the following communication was sent to surgeons in all corps areas and departments except the Philippine Department and to the commanding officers of all general hospitals except Sternberg General Hospital in Manila.

1. In order that the provisions of AG 210. 31 (12-19-41) RP-A, Jan. 7, 1942, subject: Waiving of physical defects for limited service officers of the supply arms and services may be carried out in a uniform manner, the following policies of this office concerning recommendations for waiver for limited service are announced:

(a) Considered acceptable for limited service:

(1) Overweight to 25 percent above average weight for age and height, and underweight to 15 percent below ideal weight, provided chest x-ray examination is n e g a t i v e for pulmonary pathologic change and other chronic disease is carefully excluded.

(2) Vision 20/400, in each eye corrected with glasses in possession of the examinee to 20/20 in one eye to at least 20/40 in the other, provided no organic disease of either eye exists.

(3) Blindness, or vision below 20/400, in one eye with vision 20/100 corrected with glasses in possession of the examinee to 20/20 in the other, provided there is no organic disease in the better eye and no history of cataract or other disease in the more defective eye which might be expected to involve the better one, and provided that, in case of ophthalmosteresis, the individual is fitted with a satisfactory prosthesis.

(4) Complete color blindness.

(5) Hearing 5/20 in each ear for low conversational voice, or complete deafness in one ear with hearing 10/20 or better in the other, provided the defect is not due to active inflammatory disease and is stationary in character.

(6) Chronic otitis media, inactive, with perforation of membrana tympani, provided there is a trustworthy history of freedom from activity for the preceding five years.

(7) Old fracture of the spine or pelvic bones which has healed without marked deformity, provided there is a trustworthy history of freedom from symptoms during the preceding two years.

(8) Loss of one hand, forearm, or lower extremity below junction of the middle and lower thirds of the thigh, provided the lost member is replaced with a satisfactory prosthesis.

(9) Pes planus, pes cavus, or talipes equinus, provided the condition is asymptomatic and does not interfere with normal locomotion.

(10) History of osteomyelitis following fracture, provided x-ray examination indicates complete healing and the condition has been asymptomatic for the preceding five years.

(11) Joints fixed or limited in motion, provided the condition is the result of injury and is nonsymptomatic.

(12) History of excision of torn or detached semilunar cartilage of knee joint, provided there is normal stability of the joint and a period of one year with complete freedom from symptoms has elapsed since the operation.

(13) Residuals of anterior poliomyelitis, without marked deformity or loss of function, originating two years or more prior to examination.

(14) V a r i c o s e veins, moderate, without edema or discoloration of skin.

(15) History of gastric or duodenal ulcer, provided there is a trustworthy history of freedom from activity during the preceding five years and provided a gastrointestinal roentgenogram at the time of examination is negative.

(16) Incomplete inguinal hernia.

(17) Small asymptomatic congenital umbilical hernia.

(18) Absence of one kidney, provided its removal has been necessitated by other than tuberculosis or malignancy and the other kidney is normal.

(b) Considered unacceptable for any service:

(1) History of malignant disease within preceding five years.

(2) Active tuberculosis of any organ and inactive pulmonary tuberculosis except as described in paragraph 2a.

(3) Syphilis, except adequately treated syphilis as described in paragraph 2b.

(4) Old fracture of the skull with bony defect greater than 2 cm. in longest diameter or with history of accompanying mental or neurologic complications.

(5) Instability of any of the major joints.

(6) History of metastatic osteomyelitis with prolonged or recurrent drainage, regardless of duration.

(7) Arthritis of the atrophic (rheumatoid) type.

(8) Any cardiovascular condition which disqualifies for general military service.

(9) History of gastroenterostomy, gastric resection, or intestinal anastomosis or operation for intestinal obstruction.

PROCUREMENT AND ASSIGNMENT SERVICE FOR PHYSICIANS. DENTISTS AND VETERINARIANS

Information from Major Sam F. Seeley, Executive Officer of the Procurement and Assignment Service for Physicians, Dentists and Veterinarians, 601 Pennsylvania Avenue, Washington D. C., states that a request has just been received by that office from the Army Air Force for two thousand five hundred physicians to be commissioned by July 1 and for six hundred physicians to be commissioned each month thereafter for the period of 1942. The total is six thousand one hundred physicians needed this year to provide adequate medical care for the Air Force. The place of the Air Force in the winning of the War is already apparent to every one.

QUALIFICATIONS

Eighty percent of the physicians to be commissioned must be under 37 years of age. The remaining 20 percent may be between the ages of 37 and 45 years. Those in the older age group must be qualified by certification as specialists preferably in the fields of surgery, ophthalmology and neuropsychiatry.

The letter of application should state the age of the applicant and the school of graduation and should indicate that he believes himself qualified physically and professionally for a commission.

All names are cleared through the Procurement and Assignment Service.

The letter, requesting application forms, should be sent to the Air Surgeon, Army Air Force, Washington, D. C.

(10) History of prostatectomy or transurethral resection of the prostate, or of prostatic hypertrophy of any degree.

(11) Chronic endocrine disease except mild hypothyroidism or mild Froehlich's syndrome.

(12) Diabetes mellitus of any degree or renal glycosuria.

(13) History of any psychosis.

(14) History of severe psychoneurosis at any time, or psychoneurosis of any degree if it has been recurrent or has shown symptoms within the preceding five years.

2. The following may be recommended for general military service with waiver:

(a) Individuals with minimal inactive lesions of primary or reinfection type pulmonary tuberculosis. These lesions may consist of:

(1) Calcified residues of lesions of the intrathoracic lymph nodes, provided none of these exceed an arbitrary limit of 1.5 cm. in diameter and the total number does not exceed five.

(2) Calcified lesions of the pulmonary parenchyma, provided the total number does not exceed ten, one of which may equal but not exceed 1 cm. in diameter, but none of the remainder may exceed 0.5 cm. in diameter.

(Note—The lesions described in (1) and (2) should appear sharply circumscribed, homogeneous and dense. Measurements refer to standard 14 by 17 inch direct project roentgenograms.)

(3) Small fibrotic parenchymal lesions represented in the roentgenogram as sharply demarcated strandlike or well defined small nodular shadows not exceeding a total area of 5 sq. cm., provided acceptance is deferred until subsequent examination demonstrates that the lesions are stationary and are not likely to be reactivated. The minimum period of time to determine this is six months. It must be recognized that either progression or regression of the lesions indicates activity.

(b) Individuals with confirmed positive serologic tests for syphilis with no clinical evidence of the disease, with convincing histories of a trustworthy diagnosis of syphilis, or with reliable histories of treatment for the disease on serologic or clinical grounds; provided:

(1) That a negative spinal fluid since infection and treatment has been reported from a trustworthy source;

(2) That, in infections estimated to be of less than four years' duration, at least 30 to 40 arsenical and 40 to 60 insoluble bismuth injections or their equivalent, with a minimum total of 75 injections, have been given, with approximate continuity (no rest periods or lapses) during the first 30 weeks of treatment; and

(3) That, except as further qualified, in infections estimated to be over four years' duration, at least 20 arsenical injections and 40 to 60 insoluble bismuth injections or their equivalent, with a minimum total of 60 injections, have been given in alternating courses; rest periods between consecutive courses not exceeding eight weeks being allowable.

In infections of unknown duration, it shall be presumed for classification purposes that those of individuals under 26 years of age are of less than four years' duration, and over 26 years, of more than four years' duration.

(Note—For the determination of treatment, the signed statement of acceptable treatment sources administering it, with total number of doses of each drug and approximate calendar dates of administration and available laboratory and clinical data, shall be required as evidence).

(c) Overweight to 20 percent above average weight for age and height, and underweight to 12.5 percent below ideal weight, provided a chest roentgenogram is negative for pulmonary pathologic changes and other chronic disease is carefully excluded.

(d) Insufficient incisor or masticating teeth, provided the mouth is free from extensive infectious processes and the examinee is wearing satisfactory dentures.

(e) Pilonidal cyst or sinus, provided there is no palpable tumor mass, no evidence of purulent or serous discharge, and no history of previous discharge or inflammation.

(f) History of healed fracture with bone plates, screws or wires used for fixation of fragments still in situ, provided x-ray examination shows no evidence of osteomyelitis and no rarefaction of bone contiguous to the fixative materials; that such fixative materials are not so located that they will be subjected to pressure from military clothing or equipment, and that one year has elapsed since their application.

(g) History of operation or of injection treatment for inguinal or small ventral hernia, provided examination three months or more following operation, or following the last injection, shows a satisfactory result.

(h) History of unilateral renal calculus, provided the condition has been asymptomatic for the preceding three years, urine examination is negative, and roentgenologic examination (flat plate) of both kidneys is negative.

(i) Absence of the spleen, provided its removal has been necessitated by a crushing injury.

(j) History of cholecystectomy, provided the condition has been asymptomatic for the preceding two years.

3. The action of the reviewing medical authority should indicate on the Report of Physical Examination, W. D., A. G. O. Form No. 63, that cognizance has been taken of any defects which do not meet the standards set forth in AR 40-105, but for which waiver is recommended by a notation as follows:

"Recommend acceptance for general military service with waiver of (here record the defect or defects)," or "Recommend acceptance for limited service only with waiver of (here record the defect or defects)."

By order of the Surgeon General:

John A. Rogers,
Lieutenant Colonel, Medical Corps,
Executive Officer.

American Board Obstetrics, Gynecology Examination Dates Set

The general oral and pathological examinations (Part II) for all candidates (Group A and B) will be conducted at Atlantic City, N. J., by the entire Board from Thursday, June 4, through Tuesday, June 9, 1942, prior to the opening of the annual meeting of the American Medical Association.

Group A, Part II, candidates will be scheduled for examination the first part of the examination period, and Group B, Part II, the latter half. Formal notice of the time and place of these examinations will be sent each candidate several weeks in advance of the examination dates.

Candidates for *reexamination* in Part II must make written application to the Secretary's Office before April 15, 1942.

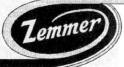

NEWS FROM THE COUNTY SOCIETIES

Members of the Creek County society met March 10 in Sapulpa to hear a program presented by guest speakers, Dr. James Stevenson and Dr. John Edwards of Tulsa, and Fletcher Johnson, attorney from Bristow.

Dr. L. C. Northrup, Ponca City, presented a two-hour moving picture and talk on Colombia and Ecuador for members of the Kay County Medical society, March 19, in Ponca City.

Members of the society have begun plans for the District Meeting in May.

A discussion of the new Postgraduate teaching course in Internal Medicine was given by L. W. Kibler, Oklahoma City, for members of the Ottawa County society at a meeting in Miami, March 19.

Dr. Clarence W. Erickson of Pittsburgh addressed the meeting on "Early Heart Failure." About 18 members of the society were present.

To honor the President of the Associatin, Dr. Finis W. Ewing, and two pioneer physicians of LeFlore county, members of the LeFlore county society met March 12 in Poteau for dinner and a scientific program. The pioneer physicians honored were Dr. E. L. Collins, Panama, and Dr. S. C. Dean, Howe. Gifts were presented to these doctors and to Dr. W. L. Shippey, who recently moved to Fort Smith, Ark.

Doctor Ewing discussed "Medical Preparedness." Dr. Shade D. Neely of Muskogee discussed "Syphilis," and Dr. L. S. McAlister, Muskogee, discussed "Malignancy." Other guests were Dr. L. C. Kuyrkendall of McAlester who discussed the work of the Council of the Association, and Dr. William H. Kaeiser, of McAlester.

The Custer County society and the Southwestern Oklahoma Medical Association met together, March 18, in Clinton, to hear three speakers present a scientific program.

Dr. Wann Langston, Oklahoma City, talked on "Circulatory Emergencies." Dr. J. William Finch of Hobart discussed "Nausea and Vomiting Following Administration of Stilbesterol," and Dr. Paul B. Lingenfelter of Clinton spoke on "Foreign Bodies of Lung and Trachea."

About 16 members of the Seminole County society met February 24, in Wewoka to hear Dr. Eugene Gillis of the State Health Department discuss "Syphilis." Doctor Gillis illustrated his talk with a motion picture.

"Phlebitis" was the topic for discussion at the meeting, March 10, of the society.

Dr. F. Redding Hood spoke on "Treatment of the Decompensated Heart" at the meeting of the Oklahoma county society, March 24, in Oklahoma City. Discussion of the paper was given by Dr. L. H. Charney and Dr. George H. Garrison, both of Oklahoma City.

The regular monthly meeting of the Cherokee County society was held on Tuesday, March 10, following a dinner at the W. W. Hastings hospital in Tahlequah.

The program, symposium on gynecological endocrinology, was presented by the following speakers: Dr. L. H. Bally, Professor of Biology, Northeastern State college, who spoke on "The Physiology of the Pituitary Gland," and Dr. Isadore Dyer, Tahlequah, who spoke on "The Definition and Role of the Female Sex Hormone in Treatment of Gynecological Conditions."

Members of the Beckham county society are making plans for a joint meeting of the physicians, dentists and lawyers of the county for the near future.

At the meeting of the society, April 14, in Sayre, Dr. P. J. Devanney read a paper on "Shock," and Dr. Hugh H. Shannon discussed his work out of the State Health department.

A motion picture on "Syphilis" was shown to members at the meeting, March 3, in Elk City.

"Certain Medical-Legal Problems in the Treatment of Fractures" was the topic of the talk given by Dr. D. H. O'Donoghue of Oklahoma City before members of the Muskogee county society, March 2, in Muskogee. Doctor O'Donoghue used x-ray films to illustrate his talk.

Others on the program were Dr. H. L. Word, Muskogee, who reviewed "Recent Advances in Treatment of Burns;" Dr. I. B. Oldham, Jr., Muskogee, who discussed "Lymphatic Leukemia," and Dr. Marvin Elkins of Muskogee,. who talked on "Emergency Surgery."

A case of Sarcoma of the Cord was discussed by members of the Carter county society at the meeting, March 20, in the Hardy sanitarium in Ardmore. The meeting followed a dinner served by Mrs. Hardy to the staff of the sanitarium and members of the society. Other discussions centered on the part of medicine in the present emergency.

Another county society to see the motion picture and hear the talk given by Dr. Eugene Gillis on "Shypilis" is the Garvin county society. Members saw the picture at their March meeting in Pauls Valley.

At this meeting, the society also joined in agreement with the U. S. F. S. A. for the care of members under the F. S. A. by members and other regularly licensed physicians of the county.

The program of the Craig County society's meeting, March 10, centered on the examination of draftees. Following this, members heard Dr. L. W. Hunt, speaker for the Postgraduate course in Internal Medicine, discuss "Arthritis," and clinics on the subject were presented.

On March 17, members met to hear Doctor Hunt's lecture on "Gastro-Intestinal Diseases."

Dr. John W. Martin, Cushing, read a paper on "Gastric Disorders" at the meeting of the Payne County society, March 10, in Stillwater, and Dr. A. B. Smith and Dr. L. A. Mitchell presented ten-minute discussions of the paper. About 17 members of the society were in attendance.

Dr. E. Goldfain, Dr. Charles R. Rountree, and R. H. Graham, all of Oklahoma City, were guest speakers at the meeting of the Alfalfa County Medical society, March 31, in Alva.

The program followed a dinner for the doctors, their wives, and guests, and a short business session. Doctor Goldfain spoke on "Neuritis, Arthritis, and Rheumatism, Diagnosis and Treatment," and Doctor Rountree discussed "Arthritis and Neuritis From an Orthopedic Standpoint." Mr. Graham then spoke on "Procurement and Assignment."

Auxiliary News

A few more months and the members of the Women's Auxiliary of the American Medical Association will be arriving in Atlantic City, New Jersey, for their Annual Convention, June 8-12.

Have you made your reservations? If not, send your request *at once* to Haddon Hall, Atlantic City, New Jersey.

On March 3, 1942, the Pittsburg auxiliary met at the Hotel Crutcher in McAlester for a meeting and luncheon. Mrs. E. H. Shuller was in charge of the meeting, due to the absence of Mrs. Pemberton, on account of serious illness. Twelve of the 15 members were present. Last year this group adopted a British child, however, they decided not to adopt a child this year but to redouble their Red Cross production. Other projects include the furnishing of cod liver oil and completion of 32 scrap books for tuberculosis children at Talihina.

The Tulsa Auxiliary met at the Chamber of Commerce Building in Tulsa on Monday, March 2. This meeting was in the form of a Health Forum, which was open to the public. Questions on health were asked from the floor and answered by the following doctors: Dr. Ralph McGill, Dr. D. L. Garrett, Dr. George Osborn, Dr. Maurice Searle and Dr. Margaret Hudson. Exhibits of Hygeia and other health charts were on display.

The Oklahoma County auxiliary met on February 25 at the Y.W.C.A. in Oklahoma City. The Scrap Book Committee, under the guidance of Mrs. Tom L. Wainwright, has completed 30 books. These have been given to the Crippled Children's hospital. Mrs. Walker Morledge, as chairman of the Social Service committee, reports completion of 12 layettes. The layettes are donated to four hospitals of the City. Mrs. Wm. K. Ishmael, Chairman of the Calling committee, has completed a list of the doctors' wives who are graduate nurses or who have nurses' training. This information has been turned to the Red Cross and the O.C.D. Bureau. The Oklahoma County auxiliary is under the guidance of Mrs. Neil Woodward and has a membership of 140. Along with Mrs. Woodward's medical auxiliary work, she is a First Aid instructor for the Red Cross and has started a class which is composed of doctors' wives.

March 5, 1942, Capping exercises were held in the auditorium of the School of Medicine building for 25 student nurses who completed their probational training.

Miss Gladys Hall, Educational Director of the American Dietetic Association inspected the school for the training of student dietitians, Thursday, March 5.

Dr. Helen S. Mitchell, Chief Nutritionist of the Defense Health and Welfare Service, Federal Security Agency, talked to dietitian students, nurses, and students and members of the faculty of the University of Oklahoma School of Medicine, on Friday, March 6, 1942.

At 4:00 P. M. on Friday, March 13, 1942, Dr. Finis Ewing, President of the State Medical Association, gave a lecture to junior and senior students on "The Future of Medicine in America," in the auditorium of the School of Medicine building.

At 8:00 P.M. on Friday, March 13, 1942, Dr. C. W. Mayo of the Mayo Clinic, Rochester, Minn., gave the third annual LeRoy Long Memorial Lecture. He spoke on the subject: "Principles of Surgery of the Colon." The talk was illustrated by means of colored pictures.

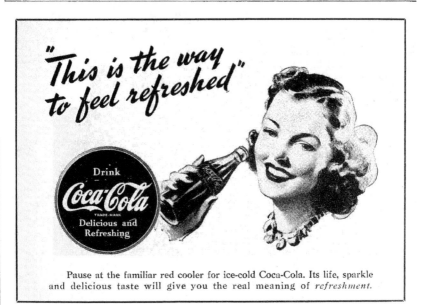

News From The State Health Department

A better organized, more effective venereal disease control program is expected for the state health department, now that a Works Project administration assistance organization is working.

Under the assistance program, a central registry for venereal disease cases and contacts has been located at the state health department. It will serve as a clearing house for all agencies treating or investigating venereal disease cases or suspected cases.

The objectives of the program are: to improve case finding, particularly among contacts who infect men in the armed forces, defense industrial workers and selectees; to work for more complete venereal disease morbidity reporting by the private physicians, and to evaluate the different techniques in venereal disease case finding.

In addition the project provides for an emphasized health education program on venereal disease, intended to give the public authentic information on the dangers of syphilis and gonorrhea and the importance of early treatment.

Clinic, nursing and laboratory assistance is also offered under the plan. Dr. E. A. Gillis, director of venereal disease control for the State Health department, Neill Sanborn, WPA supervisor of the project, and J. F. Donohue, public health service statistician, are responsible for direction of the program.

Group Hospital Service News

BLUE CROSS NEWS

In all American History there has never been a movement that has enlisted the popular support that has been given to the "Blue Cross Plans" for hospital care. From slightly over one-half million subscribers on January 1, 1937, enrollment has grown to 8,465,000 subscribers on January 1, 1942. Comparison has been made with gains in the armed forces of the Nation, and it has been found that the total induction in army, navy and marines is less than the "Blue Cross" figure. Without compulsion, appealing purely on the basis on their non-profit protection and gaining greatly from word-of-mouth publicity, which was prompted by the excellence of service rendered in the hospitals of America, the plans have accelerated their rate of growth to its highest peak. More than 1,000,000 people voluntarily enrolled in the last three months of 1941.

The proportion of persons hospitalized through "Blue Cross Plans" during the month of December increased only slightly over the previous month, which was the low point of the year. Nevertheless, approximately 62,000 subscribers were admitted to hospitals during December, and the total for the year reached 750,000 hospital patients who had the foresight to enroll in the non-profit hospital service plans.

The speed with which Americans are embracing this National Health Agency makes every million mark a milestone. An even great significance attaches to this huge volume of enrollment when the health values of the movement are realized. The enrollment of eight and one-half million persons means that in 1942 at least one million persons will be hospitalized without fear of hospital bills, and in the language of large numbers, one thousand gross of babies will be delivered in hospitals prepaid.

• OBITUARIES •

Dr. A. M. Young, Jr.
1886-1942

Another one of our older members of the medical profession in Oklahoma City passed away on March 18, 1942, at Kerrville, Tex., where he had gone to the Soldier's Hospital for treatment some two months ago.

Andrew Merriman Young, II, was born in Nashville, Tenn., on August 16, 1886. He received his preliminary education at the Battleground Academy at Franklin, Tenn., and then graduated from the Medical Department of Vanderbilt University, Nashville.

He came to Oklahoma City and was associated with the late Dr. Millington Smith, where he enjoyed a general practice. In 1924, however, he decided to become a genito-urinary specialist, so took a post-graduate course at Tulane University, New Olreans, La. He then became associated with the late Dr. W. J. Wallace in urology, later moving to an office by himself. From 1912-1917 he was a surgeon for the Frisco Railroad in Oklahoma City.

He entered the United States Army Medical corps in 1917 as a first lieutenant, and served over seas with the 36th Division, and later served as surgeon for the 131st Machine Gun Battalion. In 1918 he was promoted to the rank of Captain, in the medical corps, and saw service in Champaign and Meusse-Argonne sectors. He was discharged from Camp Dix in 1919.

At one time Dr. Young served as Assistant Surgeon in the United States Public Health Service and was a former director of the state venereal disease bureau.

He was a member of the Alpha Tau Omega social fraternity, and the Alpha Kappa Kappa medical fraternity. He belonged to our County and State Medical Societies, the American Medical Association, and was a former member of the Civitan Club.

He married Miss Morree Oswald of Nashville, Tenn., on May 6, 1912, and to this union four children were born. Dr. A. M. Young, III, has continued in his father's office, and also carries on a general practice. Millington Young is now a student in the University of Oklahoma School of Medicine. His wife, two daughters, Margaret Ann and Rose Marie, and three brothers survive.

Dr. Young had been in ill heath for some time and was forced to give up his practice and retire to his home in November, 1938. He recently went to the Soldier's Hospital at Kerrville, Tex., where he remained until his demise on March 18, 1942.—Lea A. Riley.

Dr. Thomas R. Lutner
1886-1942

Dr. Thomas R. Lutner, a practicing physician in Comanche county since 1919, died of a heart ailment, March 7, in an Oklahoma City hospital.

Recognized as one of the leading physicians of Lawton, Doctor Lutner had recently been elected Secretary of the Comanche County Medical society for 1942. He had been active in county and state medical organizations since May of 1919, when he moved to Lawton from Cameron, Tex. Doctor Lutner was an eye, ear, nose and throat specialist.

Graduated from Texas university, the Dr. John Sealy school of Galveston and Chicago university, Doctor Lutner began his practice in Cameron. When he moved to Lawton, he married Miss Sallie Draughn of Lawton.

He was active, also, in the Baptist church, the Masonic lodge and the Kiwanis club.

Survivors include his wife and a daughter, Lurleen, of the home address; a son, Thomas, a student at Kemper Military academy; and a daughter, Kathleen, a student at Baylor university, Waco, Tex.

Dr. George R. Norman
1885-1942

Dr. George Robert Norman, 56, for many years active in Tulsa county medical affairs died January 21 after a brief illness. Funeral services for the veteran eye, ear, nose and throat specialist were held at Memorial Christian church.

A resident of Tulsa for 16 years, Doctor Norman was a graduate of the University of Alabama medical school at Tuscaloosa. During the last World War, he served in the United States Army Medical Corps, and was a member of the Joe Carson post of the American Legion.

Resolution

WHEREAS, George Robert Norman has for the past sixteen years labored in Tulsa and vicinity as an active and interested member of the Tulsa County Medical Society, and

WHEREAS, during all this period he has practiced the healing art in a manner to reflect credit both upon himself and his profession, and

WHEREAS, he served with honor in the Medical Department of the armed forces of the United States in the World War I; was later identified with the Joe Carson Post of the American Legion, and a valued member of the Petroleum Lodge of the Masonic order, and

WHEREAS, the said George Robert Norman has been called to his reward by the Great Physician, and, in order that the Tulsa County Medical Society may appropriately record his useful career among us,

NOW, THEREFORE, BE IT RESOLVED by the Tulsa County Medical Society, in regular meeting assembled this 26th day of January, 1942, that the absence of Dr. Norman from our ranks will be keenly felt by us and the various organizations, of which he was an active and faithful member.

BE IT FURTHER RESOLVED that the Tulsa County Medical Society, by this means expresses its sympathy to the family of the deceased and our appreciation of his worth to his confreres in both City and State.

BE IT FURTHER RESOLVED that a copy of this Resolution be spread upon the minutes of our Society and that copy of same be transmitted by our Secretary to the bereaved family.

Roy Dunlap, M.D., Chairman,
R. G. Ray, M.D.,
S. C. Venable, M.D.,
Committee.

Dr. G. D. Funk
1905-1942

Dr. Gustavus D. Funk, El Reno physician, serving as a captain in the Medical Corps of the U. S. Army, died unexpectedly from a heart attack about 8:15 A.M. February 26, at his home in El Reno, 414 South Williams Avenue.

Arriving home Tuesday to spend a brief leave here he suffered a heart attack about 7:30 A.M. and died less than half an hour later.

Doctor Funk came to El Reno as a boy three years of age from Maryville, Mo. He was born there on May 8, 1905. He attended school here and was a star basketball player and captain on the El Reno High School teams. Following his graduation in 1923 he attended Washington and Lee at Lexington, Va., for two years and then completed his course at the University of Oklahoma, Norman.

Following his graduation he was united in marriage to Miss Rose Aderhold, daughter of Dr. T. M. Aderhold of El Reno. After two years Dr. Funk decided to change from a business career and enter the medical profession. He accordingly returned to the University of Oklahoma and in 1933 received his M.D. degree.

Doctor Funk practiced medicine in El Reno from the time of his graduation from the University of Oklahoma school of medicine in 1933, until he was called to the Army in October, 1940. Commissioned as a lieutenant when called to active duty, he later was made a captain and at the time of his death, was serving at Lubbock, Tex. He was also owner and manager of the El Reno Sanitarium. He was a member of Phi Gamma Delta social fraternity at Norman, and the Elks lodge and Rotary club in El Reno.

Survivors include his wife, his daughter, Jean, both of the home address; his mother, Mrs. John L. Funk, of El Reno; and a brother, William L. Funk, County Attorney, of El Reno.

Dr. Daniel B. Stough
1861-1942

Dr. Daniel B. Stough, pioneer physician of Vinita and Craig county, died at his home in Vinita, March 19, after an illness of several months.

Doctor Stough came to Vinita in 1907, and established a practice. He became prominent in medical circles, and held the position of county physician for years. He was a graduate of the Kentucky School of Medicine, Louisville, Ky.

Besides his activities in connection with his profession, Doctor Stough was active in the First Methodist church and the Masonic lodge.

He is survived by two daughters, Mrs. L. R. Herndon, Seminole, and Mrs. B. K. Chowning, Okemah; two sons, Dr. Daniel B. Stough, Jr., Hot Springs, Ark., and Tommie E. Stough, Baltimore Md.; and three grandchildren and one great-grandchild.

J. E. Hanger, Inc. Are New Advertisers

This issue of the Journal carries the first advertisement of J. E. Hanger, Inc., of St. Louis, Mo., manufacturers of artificial limbs.

The Oklahoma City office of J. E. Hanger, Inc. is located at 612 N. Hudson, and Mr. L. T. Lewis serves the company as Oklahoma City representative.

BOOK REVIEWS

"The chief glory of every people arises from its authors."—Dr. Samuel Johnson.

"FUNCTIONAL PATHOLOGY." Leopold Lichtwitz, M.D., Chief of the Medical Division of the Montefiore Hospital, Clinical Professor of Medicine, Columbia University, New York. 567 Pages. Grune and Stratton, New York City, 1941.

"Functional Pathology is the science which analyzes the mechanism of symptoms and disease. It can also be defined as the science of pathological manifestations during life." Hence this book takes up the age old argument about the relationship between cellular and functional pathology. The more we study the relationship between "mind" and "matter," and accept the evident liason between them, the more we will be able to accept the contents of this book for its "creative thought." Certainly the hypothalmus and pituitary cannot always verify at autopsy what was diagnosed by clinical symptoms. Example: "hypoprotamaenia and edema (hypothalmic edema) possibly also hypercholesterolemia and albumunuria point to the hypothalmus as the area of origin of the nephritic syndrome. There is of course no anatomic proof."

The hypothalmus does not make any protest to the incrimination. Its title may just as properly be called the Physiology of the Hypothalmus*, due to the pontifical position he gives that organ, as the regulator and correlator of the various organs as subject to the autonomic nervous system, which causes automatic changes in the blood supply, secretion, muscular tone, and bodily functions, either in a normal or pathological manner. He especially notes the "urinary system which consists of the renal parenchyma proper, and the vascular supply and the nerve connections from the hypothalmus down to the last nerve ending." In addition, a number of endocrine glands act on the widespread components of this system. By cooperation of the circulatory nervous and endocrine elements, with the renal parenchyma of the activity of the system is automatically integrated with that of the entire organism. One of the most interesting 40 pages is taken up with the mechanisms of kidney secretion in the normal and pathological kidneys. It shows he has put much time on this phase of medicine, and giving a very rational explanation to various points. These he tries to interpret, by bedside and laboratory methods as a clinical observer, both on the Continent and in this country. His most impressionable years were in Europe, when interest in the hypothalmus was beginning to manifest itself as a physiological entity in relation to the autonomic nervous system and endocrine glands. Even at this date, many mooted points are still under discussion, and you may not always agree with his deductions, but ever thus it has been since Claude Benard made the first piqure and made a diabetic response which he styled "internal environment."

"The anatomical relationship between hypothalmus and pituitary gland, as evidenced by their embryonic development, their spatial intimacy, and their numerous connecting nervous pathways and vascular channels, is paralleled by functional cooperation." Heat production or control, sweating, are all controlled by this hypothalmic-pituitary action on the autonomic nerves. Basal metabolism rate is altered by hypothalmic lesions. Body water is controlled by insulin, thyroxin, pitressin, hyperpathyroidism. The denervated muscle loses water and is unable to absorb it. Hence, nervous hormonal and ionial influences are responsible for the quantity of, and degrees of water fixation.

A disorder of the hypothalmic pituitary system produces Diabetes Insipidus. This same system disturbs sugar metabolism, as shown in acromegaly, hypersensitivity to insulin, after diminished function of the pituitary gland. Many now think Diabetes is an adrenal, thyroid, pituitary, liver and pancreatic maladjustment, and not that of the Iletin glands alone. These doubters have plenty of argument for their dissension to the view generally held. Posterior pituitary gland substance, or pitressin in oil, as insulin in protamine zinc solution, acts specifically on their respective troubles, but are alike diminished in specificness by emotional states.

Lesions in the hypothalmic area render the responses to the thyroid, either in an extreme sensitiveness (as in the migraine patient) to an extreme tolerance. The adrenal glands also aggrevate all thyroid symptoms. The thyroid gland is discussed in a very full text. Especial attention to the relationship of carbohydrate metabolism is given.

The novel explanations of these many clinical phenomena, with the vast amount of bibliography (mostly French and German), in its 567 pages, makes it a very interesting book to study, and gives you plenty of food for thought and invokes discussion. It Oslerizes in point of brevity the therapeutic advice, but philosophizes in a Baconian manner on the Why of symptoms and pathology. Dr. Alexis Carrel, in one of his books, sharply criticizes modern physiological investigation for far too closely confining itself to the body, merely as a machine without any adequate consideration of the driving force that animated the machine.—Lea A. Riely.

*(In 1940 a symposium on the anatomy, physiology and clinical significance of the hypothalmus included 42 investigators and the published Proceedings, containing 34 chapters, runs to 971 pages, and includes a bibliography of more than one thousand titles.)

"SYNOPSIS OF GENITOURINARY DISEASES." Austin I. Dodson, M.D., F.A.C.S., Richmond, Va. Third Edition, C. V. Mosby and Co., St. Louis.

As the author indicates in a foreword, this book is designed for medical students and as a quick reference book for the general practitioner, making no claim for technical or operative procedures. Chapters are devoted to:

Methods of diagnosis; Instruments and minor urologic procedures; Anomalies; Nontuberculous infections of the urinary tract; Urethral infections; Infections of the male genital tract and disturbances of function; Tuberculosis; Injuries; Calculous disease; Hydronephrosis; Prostatic obstruction; Neurogenic dysfunction of the bladder; Pathology in the scrotum; Tumors.

In such a limited space naturally no detailed instructions can be given, but the proportions devoted to each subject are well balanced, especially from the standpoint of practicability and general usage. Almost all conditions are mentioned and the most common are taken up in greater length. Indications for advanced urological study are given as are those for surgery without attempting to describe the procedure. The illustrations and diagrams are well chosen and helpful, not being too complicated or detailed.

The chapter on nontuberculous infections is good and is up to date. Dietary treatments are mentioned and charts given, but such subjects require more space to be properly presented. Medical management and choice of drugs in different infections is well covered. Tuberculosis and calculous disease are covered and the management of each is adequately presented.

On the whole the book is well adapted to the purpose for which is was designed. Medical students and interns may find much of value here and the general practitioner as well will find it useful to freshen his approach to genitourinary problems.—Jim M. Taylor.

The Middle Way

· · · · · · · · · · · · · IN BISMUTH THERAPY

BISMUTH ETHYLCAMPHORATE

After the intramuscular injection of 2 cc. of Bismuth Ethylcamphorate, a treponemicidal level is ordinarily reached in forty-eight to seventy-two hours. This speed of effectiveness lies between that of water-soluble bismuth salts, which are faster, and oil suspensions of bismuth salts, which are slower. Since this promptness of therapeutic action is coupled with good duration of effectiveness, Bismuth Ethylcamphorate possesses the advantages of the "middle way."

Sterile Solution Bismuth Ethylcamphorate is the bismuth salt of ethyl camphoric acid dissolved in sweet almond oil. It is available in boxes of six and twenty-five 1 cc. ampoules, and in 30 cc. vials.

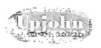

Fine Pharmaceuticals Since 1886

REVIEWS and CORRESPONDENCE

SURGERY AND GYNECOLOGY

Abstracts, Reviews and Comments From
LeRoy Long Clinic
714 Medical Arts Building, Oklahoma City

"CORTICAL EXTRACT IN THE TREATMENT OF SHOCK." Loring S. Helfrich, M.D., William H. Cassels, M.D., and Warren H. Cole, M.D.; The American Journal of Surgery, February 1942, Vol. LV, No. 2, Page 410.

In an effort to determine the efficacy of cortical extract in the prophylaxis and the treatment of shock, the extract was given to animals subjected to shocking procedures and to human beings having major operations of a magnitude apt to produce shock. In animals, shock was produced by hemorrhage and by massage of the intestine with the animal under ether anesthesia. In experimental shock produced by hemorrhage cortical extract exerted a definite but slight tendency to decrease the severity of shock, particularly when the extract was given with fluids (glucose and electrolytes). Fluids alone, i.e., without cortical extract, did not significantly prevent the fall in blood pressure although the actual survival time following hemorrhage was increased.

When cortical extract was given an hour or two before institution of intestinal massage (to produce shock), the average drop in systolic blood pressure after 40 minutes of massage was only 19.5 mm., contracted with 35.3 mm. in animals not receiving extract prophylactically. Moreover, when hemorrhage of a constant rate was instituted 90 minutes after intestinal massage was begun, there was a survival time of 36 and five-tenths minutes in animals receiving cortical extract, contrasted with a survival time of only 21 minutes in animals not receiving cortical extract. When glucose and electrolytes were given in addition to extract, the effect was still more prominent, there being no drop in blood pressure after 40 minutes of massage and an average of only 7.5 mm. after 55 minutes of massage. In other words, the beneficial effect of cortical extract and fluids (glucose and electrolytes) in prevention of shock was comparable to that which might be expected from plasma. When extract was given after shock had already been produced in animals very little beneficial effect could be demonstrated; there was little or no rise in blood pressure although further drop was slightly delayed.

Falling drop determinations showed an increase in specific gravity of blood in shock, and a decrease after hemorrhage as reported by others. Cortical extract showed a definite but slight tendency to counteract the increase in specific gravity produced by shock.

In human beings the use of cortical extract in the presence of shock was limited to a few cases due to the relative infrequency of shock, but in every instance the effect appeared to be beneficial.

In order to determine whether or not cortical extract would exert a favorable influence in prevention of shock, the average pulse rate and blood pressure was computed in a series of 15 patients receiving cortical extract prophylactically, and upon whom major operations of unusual duration and severity were performed. From the hospital records an equal number of cases (in which no cortical extract was given), with equal number of types and duration, were obtained and the average pulse rate and blood pressure likewise determined. In the patients receiving cortical extract prophylactically, the pulse rate averaged eight beats per minute slower, and the systolic blood pressure 12 mm. higher than in the patients not receiving extract. This suggests that the cortical extract tends to minimize the changes which might be interpreted as being changes preliminary to the development of shock.

Observations on animals as well as patients showed that the extract was much more effective when given prophylactically, than when given after shock was already produced.—LeRoy D. Long.

"PERITONITIS — STUDIES IN PERITONEAL PROTECTION WITH PARTICULAR REFERENCE TO ACTION OF SULFONAMIDE DRUGS IN EXPERIMENTAL PERITONITIS." H. D. Harvey, M.D., F. L. Meleney, M.D., and J. W. R. Rennie, M.D., New York, N. Y.; Surgery, February 1942, Vol. 11, No. 2, Page 244.

Acute gangrenous perforated appendicitis was produced in dogs, which resulted apparently uniformly in generalized peritonitis.

Eighty-seven and one-half percent of the untreated controls died of peritonitis.

Preoperative peritoneal protection afforded by bactragen, E. coli vaccine or E. coli bacteriophage did not lower the mortality or significantly prolong life.

Sulfathiazole placed in the peritoneal cavity in the vicinity of the appendix was of little apparent benefit; sulfanilamide similarly used seemed to have some value in lowering the mortality and in prolonging life.

Enteral administration of sulfapyridine, sulfathiazole and, less definitely, of sulfanilamide, was followed by a striking lowering of mortality. In the case of sulfathiazole, the mortality fell to 8.3 percent, compared to 87.5 percent for the controls. The mortality with sulfapyridine was 37.5 percent, with sulfanilamide 50 percent.

The peritonitis in each case cultured was found to be due to a mixture of organisms, among which the varieties commonly found in human peritonitis were predominant; that is, E. coli, enterococci, Cl. welchii.

The authors, in experiments with mice and guinea pigs, attempted to render the peritoneal cavity immune to infection by the organisms that commonly cause peritonitis in man. They found that several substances injected intraperitoneally 24 hours before the organisms would afford limited immunity. They then took what seemed to be the best of these substances and compared their effect upon peritonitis in dogs with the effect of some of the sulfonamide drugs. The lesion produced in the dogs resembled that encountered in human beings, in that it was a peritonitis caused by a mixed growth of intestinal organisms emanating from a focus of gangrenous cecal appendage. It seems significant that preoperative immunization of the peritoneum had little effect upon this type of lesion. The authors say that they cannot express the degree of effectiveness of the sulfonamides in terms of minimal lethal doses but that they believe their experiments justify further trial as preventive and curative agents for peritonitis in man. They fail to demonstrate any advantage in intraperitoneal use of the crystals of these drugs, as opposed to administration by other routes. They, however, make the statement that in their opinion these experiments should not be taken literally and that the problems of route of administration and even of the type of sulfonamide drug should be solved clinically.

They believe that their experiments have shown that there is strong evidence that the sulfonamide drugs, properly selected and administered, will be of use in lowering the death rate from peritonitis. They also think their experiments show that there was slight evidence of benefit from preoperative injection of substances into the peritoneal cavity in the effort to produce peritoneal immunity, but that the benefit was slight and definitely less than that afforded by the sulfonamide drugs. It appeared that there is no benefit to be derived from preoperative injections that cannot be better obtained from the sulfonamides.

Their conclusions were as follows:

"1. Various substances injected into the peritoneal cavity of mice or guinea pigs will produce an immunity to peritonitis caused by subsequent intraperitoneal injection of intestinal organisms.

2. The immunity appears to be nonspecific in nature.

3. The degree of immunity against organisms as obtained from the intestinal tract or from pus in the peritoneal cavity is usually of the order of ten minimal lethal doses. Only against strains of E. coli, whose virulence had been artifically enhanced, did the immunity rise to the order of 1,000 minimal lethal doses.

4. In experiments involving over 7,000 animals, no protecting substance of unique value was found. The best protecting agents were the irritative ones, such as the vaccines, potent sera, bactragen, or aleuronat and starch mixture.

5. In dogs with generalized peritonitis following artifically produced acute gangrenous perforated appendicitis, the immunity afforded by preoperative intraperitoneal injections of the best of the protecting agents was not sufficient to lower the mortality.

6. In a parallel series of dogs, however, postoperative enteral administration of the sulfonamide drugs, especially sulfathiazole, was followed by a striking lowering of mortality. Intraperitoneal use of these drugs was less effective.

7. On the basis of this evidence we recommend the use of the sulfonamides clinically but do not recommend the use of preoperative injections."—LeRoy D. Long.

"THE USE OF ESTROGENS IN THE TREATMENT OF DYSURIA AND INCONTINENCE IN POSTMENOPAUSAL WOMEN." Udall J. Salmon, M.D., Robert I. Walter, M.D., and Samuel H. Geist, M.D., New York, N. Y.; American Journal of Obstetrics and Gynecology. November 1941. Vol. 42, No. 5, Page 845.

"1. Sixteen postmenopausal women with urinary symptoms (urinary frequency, urgency, and incontinence), which were refractory to orthodox treatment, were found to have an estrogen deficiency.

2. Acting on the assumption that the urinary symptoms were related to the estrogen deficiency, these patients were treated with estrogens.

3. Relief of symptoms was achieved in all but three cases.

4. Relief of symptoms ran parallel with evidence of estrogenic effect in the vaginal smears.

5. Symptoms recurred gradually after the discontinuation of therapy, coincident with the re-appearance of signs of estrogen deficiency in the smears.

6. Patients could be kept symptom-free on a maintenance dose of estrogens.

7. One the basis of the observations reported here, it is concluded that: (a) a syndrome consisting of urinary frequency, dysuria, and incontinence in elderly women can be caused by a long-standing estrogen deficiency; (b) in advanced stages, the estrogen deficiency leads to atrophic erosions of the mucous membrane of the urethral meatus similar in appearance to the erosions in "senile vaginitis;" this "senile urethritis and periurethritis" causes urgency, painful micturition, and frequency; (c) the estrogen deficiency also leads to impairment of the bladder sphincter function which results in incontinence.

8. It is suggested, on the basis of these observations, that postmenopausal women, upon whom vagino- or urethroplasty is contemplated for the relief of incontinence, whether or not a cystocele or urethocele is present, be examined for evidence of estrogen deficiency, and, if such a deficiency is found, that they be given a full course of estrogens as a therapeutic trial."

COMMENT: This is a well conducted study on a small group of patients with a fairly common and usually discouraging group of symptoms. Their results have been excellent. Though I have undertaken this form of treatment for this particular group of symptoms in only a few patients recently, I have observed improvement in urinary incontinence, urgency, and frequency, in a fairly large group of women who have been treated for senile vaginitis by the use of estrogens.—Wendell Long.

"ECTOPIC PREGNANCY." Goodrick C. Schauffler, M.D., and Frederick O. Wynia, M.D., Portland, Oregon; American Journal of Obstetrics and Gynecology; November 1941. Vol. 42, No. 5. Page 786.

"1. Sixty-five cases with the pathologic diagnosis of ectopic pregnancy are reviewed. For the report some general considerations are omitted in favor of the more pertinent and timely aspect of the problem.

2. The impression that previous operations, abortions, and pelvic infection contribute to the incidence of ectopic pregnancy is supported by our findings.

3. Hematology and blood pressure observations support generally accepted conclusions. Our experience with transfusion parallels that of most other observers. Autohemoclysis, as an emergency measure, has been used with consistent benefit, where more suitable blood is not available.

4. In 28 cases surgery other than removal of the ectopic pregnancy was performed but not in the presence of infection or free bleeding. Those patients did exactly as well as the rest of the group. It is thought that this surgical attention may account for the fact that no second ectopics are recorded (28 percent sterilized). Other reported incidence is 3.6 to 22 percent.

5. Our mortality rate is three percent. Diagnosis was 80 percent correct. The routine use of the Friedman test has improved our percentage of correct diagnoses.

6. Seventeen endometriums were available for pathologic examination. Had these tissues been obtained by curettage, diagnosis would have been assisted in only six out of the 17 and definitely confused in the remainder.

7. Microscopic examination of the tubes and other tissues indicates some further basis for the hypothesis of ectopic placentation in areas of ectopic endometrium or decidua.

8. Cul-de-sac puncture has been harmless and exceedingly valuable in diagnosis. The peritoneoscope has been used. Its status is discussed.

9. Three unusual cases are reported and illustrated."

COMMENT: This article is abstracted not because of any unusual features but because it is a comprehensive and clear review of the unselected group of patients with ectopic pregnancy. Though a relatively infrequent disease, ectopic pregnancy is an important one from a practical diagnostic point of view because this diagnosis must be considered in the differential diagnosis of a great many very common pelvic conditions.—Wendell Long.

"PELVIC PAIN." Robert D. Mussey, M.D., and Robert B. Wilson, M.D., Rochester, Minnesota; American Journal of Obstetrics and Gynecology, November 1941. Vol. 42, No. 5. Page 759.

"This follow-up study of pelvic pain was attempted with the full realization that pain is not a diagnostic entity and that treatment or operation is ordinarily carried out for the relief of any one symptom, such as pain. However, it seemed to be desirable to know the percentage probability of relief of pain associated with various pelvic disorders."

Four or more years following examination of them in 1936, questionnaires were sent to 500 patients included in a previous study of pelvic pain. ·Each patient was asked whether the pain was completely relieved, partly relieved, or not relieved. Replies of 310 of the 500 questionnaires form the basis of this report.

Of the 310 patients, 193 complained primarily of lower abdominal pain while the remaining 37.7 percent complained of backache or menstrual pain, or they made multiple complaints.

Of the 310 patients, 131 were subjected to surgical operation with complete or partial relief of the pain in 104 or 79 percent.

The remaining 179 were treated by non-surgical medical measures with complete or partial relief of the pain in about 66 percent.

''When a reasonably accurate diagnosis is made of pelvic lesions which cause pain and which are amenable to surgical measures complete or partial relief of pain may be expected in 79 percent of cases, depending on the condition and the nature of the operation.

Nonsurgical lesions or pain for which organic cause is not found, may be relieved in not more than 66 percent of cases; in this group fall a considerable number of patients, about a fourth of all patients who complain of pelvic pain, who have no demonstrable organic lesion or who suffer from varying degrees of chronic nervous exhaustion. The scientific integrity of the physician is best maintained by his explaining to this type of patient, who is difficult to satisfy and reassure, the physiologic basis of her pain.''

It is interesting to note that of the 54 patients complaining of backache, only six were subjected to surgical operation. This correctly reflects the present attitude about backache and its relatively infrequent cause by surgical disease of the pelvic genitalia.

COMMENT: This is a valuable contribution from a practical point of view. While it is true that pain is not a diagnostic entity, pain is a symptom for which many women seek relief and it requires the most meticulous care of the physician to obtain an accurate interpretation of the pain and after this is done, it demands sound judgment to advise and administer the proper treatment whether it be surgical or nonsurgical.

This review demonstrates that such care in interpretation and such judgment in treatment was employed. In addition, it sets forth the results of such careful interpretation and treatment. Despite the fact that this study represents only 310 of the 500 patients to whom questionnaires were sent, it is reasonably accurate and demonstrates the caution with which the treatment of pain in the pelvis must be undertaken.—Wendell Long.

EYE, EAR, NOSE AND THROAT
Edited by Marvin D. Henley, M. D.
911 Medical Arts Building, Tulsa

"THE RELATIONSHIP BETWEEN DISEASES OF THE UPPER RESPIRATORY PASSAGES AND THE SURGERY OF THE CHEST." F. C. Ormerod. London. The Journal of Laryngology and Otology, August, 1941.

According to the author the relation between abscess of the lung and operations on the tonsils has been a matter of knowledge and discussion for the past 30 years.

Richardson in 1912-1913 was the first to discuss lung abscess as a sequalae of tonsillectomy.

Chevalier and Chevalier Lawrence Jackson in 1933 expressed the opinion that the postoperative lung infection was embolic or pyaemic in origin and never due to aspiration.

Myerson in 1922 reported the results from 100 cases of bronchoscopic examination immediately following a

tonsillectomy. Blood was found in the trachea in 76 cases.

Iglauer in 1928 found blood in the trachea after tonsillectomy in 40 percent of the cases after general anaesthetic and in 38 percent of the cases after local anaesthetic.

Ochsner and Nesbit in 1927 showed that the lymphatics draining the tonsillar region empty directly into the venous system at the junction of the internal jugular and subclavian veins and therefore infection could not pass directly to the lungs by the lymph stream.

The author names the four obvious tracts for connection between the upper and lower respiratory: 1. Aspiration. 2. Lymph stream. 3. Blood stream. 4. Direct continuity. He says that on the whole the aspiration theory seems to be the most obvious, the blood stream or embolic route being responsible possibly for a number of cases. The lymphatic route may account for an occasional case. Broncho-sinusitis disease and its sequalae may explain many cases of bronchiectasis though probably not abscess in the lung.

"BLINDNESS, AS RECORDED IN THE NATIONAL HEALTH SURVEY." Amount, Causes and Relation to Certain Social Factors. Rollo H. Britten, senior statistician. U. S. Public Health Service. Public Health Reports, vol. 56, No. 46, page 2191-2215, November 14, 1941.

In the National Health Survey, special consideration was given to the subject of blindness. The National Health Survey was a house-to-house canvass of many urban families in 18 states. The analysis is confined to 2,498,180 white and colored persons in surveyed urban areas. The extent of this survey lends particular value to the findings on blindness. From the nature of the survey and its methods it may be assumed that the cases of blindness recorded represent persons who were totally blind or had vision sufficient merely to distinguish between light and dark.

The number of persons per 100,000 recorded as being blind in both eyes was 83, the number of blind in one eye only 326, and the number blind in one or both eyes 409. The prevalence of blindness was greater among males than among females, the difference being particularly marked for blindness in one eye only. More than one-fourth of all the blind were over 75 years of age; two-thirds were over 55 years of age. Practically all were past or within the working ages. Among children the rate was 12 per 100,000 for blindness in both eyes and 86 per 100,000 for blindness in one or both eyes. In each succeeding age group there was found a marked increase in the rate, which reached the extreme figure of 2,918 (both eyes) and 6,630 (one or both eyes) among persons 85 or more years of age. According to the statistics there is an estimated annual incidence of new cases of blindness (both eyes) of 6.6 per 100,000 population. The males showed a higher annual incidence of new cases in both eyes up to about 70 years of age; above that age the incidence was greater among females.

Accident was recorded as the cause of blindness in one-sixth of the cases of blindness in both eyes and in one-half of the cases of blindness in one eye only. The remainder may perhaps be ascribed to disease and to congenital causes or causes associated with early infancy. Cataract, glaucoma, or other diseases of the eye were recorded as the cause in more than half of the cases of blindness reported as due to disease. Degenerative disease was the major cause for diseases which did not originate in the eye. Syphilis and gonorrhea did not appear in the list of causes on account of the public nature of the survey.

Further analysis of blindness by accident showed that more than a third of the cases were results of occupational accidents. A fourth of all cases of blindness in both eyes and a third of all cases in one eye only which were caused by accidents were due to home accidents. As a cause of blindness in both eyes, cataract ranks first, whereas for blindness in one eye only, occupational accidents ranks first; second position is held by degenerative diseases and home accidents, respectively; third position by glaucoma and cataract, respectively. For blindness in both eyes, falls, motor vehicles, burns, and firearms and fireworks were the principal means of injury; for blindness in one eye only cutting and piercing instruments were by far the most important means. It was found that the higher rate of blindness in males is due to the greater frequency of accidents among them. The prevalence of blindness due to accident was about five times as great among males as among females. It was also proved that accidents are more frequent causes of blindness in the younger ages and diseases in the older ages. Sixteen percent of the cases of blindness in both eyes were due to accident; for blindness in one or both eyes the percentage was 42.

Blindness was much more prevalent in the colored than in the white populations, the rates being respectively 146 and 76 per 100,000 for blindness in both eyes. Blindness had a higher incidence rate in cities under 100,000 population than in larger cities. Two-thirds of the blind were in families with annual incomes under $1,000. Ten percent of the blind were reported as being employed. The prevalence of blindness (both eyes) was relatively low among the employed workers, a large proportion of the blind being in the "unemployable" group. Nearly two percent of the "unemployable" males, aged 15-64, were blind in both eyes.

"CARDIOSPASM; OBSERVATIONS ON THE USE OF PROSTIGMINE;" a clinical and experimental report. Jacob Meyer and H. Necheles, Chicago. The Journal of Laboratory and Clinical Medicine, volume 27, Number 2, page 162-168, November 1941.

The accepted therapy for cardiospasm in the past has been (a) gastric lavage; (b) dilation of the cardia; (c) the use of antispasmodics. Psychotherapy, diathermy, and vitamin B1 have been reported to be of value. These measures have been effective to a degree in relieving the patient of discomfort and in improving his general nutrition. The esophagus has in most instances remained the same size, and patients have had recurrent symptoms but with a minimum of discomfort despite a large esophagus.

Much evidence has accumulated recently to show that cardiospasm is often related to damage to vagus fibers or to damage and loss of ganglion cells of the myenteric plexus of the esophagus at the cardia. In accordance with this theory, recently, intractable cardiospasm has been relieved successfully by bilateral cervicothoracic sympathetic ganglionectomy. This may be considered as proof of sympathetic "achalasia."

On the basis of the same theory, assuming that achalasia or cardiospasm is a condition in which degenerative changes have taken place in the myenteric plexus of the lower esophagus, through which the parasympathetic nerves effect normal peristalsis, drug therapy for achalasia and megaesophagus can be elaborated. Drugs that affect the parasympathetic system may be used to produce increased tonus and peristalsis of the esophagus. In the present experiments, eserine and prostigmine were employed, the latter being the drug of choice because it lacks the disagreeable by-effects of the former.

The authors observed a 21 years' old female patient with cardiospasm for over two years. During this time, prostigmine was administered for a period of time, and again withheld. When the prostigmine was withheld, the patient would return with more complaints and ask that the drug be continued. This was true even though she had had periodic dilatation of the cardia. The patient had been dilated previously at other institutions, but she had not experienced the same degree of improvement as from prostigmine and dilatation. She had also undergone an extensive course of psychotherapeutic treatment at another institution with no apparent improvement.

To the same patient, under fluoroscopic observation a barium meal was administered and one mg of prostigmine was injected intramuscularly. Fifteen minutes later, increased peristalsis and tonus were observed. The increased contractions of the esophagus were particularly marked above the cardia, and the barium meal was emptied rapidly into the stomach. Injection of ergotamine into another patient likewise revealed increased tonus and peristaltic rate of the esophagus.

Experiments on anesthetized dogs confirmed the observations made on the patients and further reveal that the prostigmine acts not only through stimulation of the parasympathetic innervation of the esophagus, but also through a direct effect on its musculature.

It seems therefore logical to give prostigmine or ergotamine for the treatment of cardiospasm. It is a promising method of treatment of this condition. The prostigmine may be given in doses of 15 mg three times daily for several weeks. It can be given intermittently for several years. The method is best combined with local dilatation of the cardia.

"THE GENERAL PRACTITIONER'S PART IN THE CAMPAIGN FOR THE PREVENTION OF BLINDNESS FROM GLAUCOMA." Mark J. Schoenberg, New York, New York State Journal of Medicine, volume 41, Number 22, page 2216-2219, November 15, 1941.

Out of hundreds of thousands of ambulatory patients daily consulting medical practitioners throughout this land, at least 30 percent are 40 years of age or more. It is within this age group of patients that one has to look for the present and future glaucoma victims. Patients afflicted with glaucoma are potentially victims of partial or total loss of sight. It is estimated that there are approximately 200,000 blind persons in this country, of whom over 20,000 are blind from glaucoma. The general practitioner is the first usually to have an opportunity of detecting or at least suspecting the presence of glaucoma at an early stage. Suspecting the glaucoma, the general practitioner is in the position to direct his patient as soon as possible to ophthalmologists or eye clinics for checkups.

The author gives six points the investigation of which frequently suffices to obtain enough evidence to detect or suspect the existence of glaucoma:

1. Measure the acuity of vision. The cause of subnormal vision of one or both eyes must always be investigated.

2. Examine the size of the pupils and their reaction to light. Inequality of pupils or poor reaction to light is not to be ignored.

3. Feel with the fingers whether the eyes are normally soft or hard. One can acquire this "feel" by instruction and practice.

4. Examine each eye with the ophthalmoscope and find out whether the optic disks are pale or excavated.

5. Ask the patient about the occurrence of occasional blurring or clouding of vision, seeing rainbow rings around a distant light, one-sided headaches, discomfort in or around the eyes after movies, excitement, and worry. Inquire whether the patient experiences difficulty in reading in spite of recently prescribed glasses.

6. Ask whether there is a case of glaucoma in the family.

The glaucoma problem is one of growing importance, for it is probable that its incidence is rapidly increasing. In great part this is due to the rise in the population age group of those over 40 and to the strain and worry to which a large part of the adult population has been subjected in recent years. It is of the utmost importance to make a concerted move to attack this problem. To do this it is essential to get the cooperation of all physicians practicing medicine in adults.

There is for instance the acute glaucoma, which has a stormy beginning and runs a stormier and exciting course. It is characterized by excruciating pain in and around the eye, almost complete loss of vision, one-sided headaches, nausea, vomiting, dilatation of the pupil, and cloudy cornea. Occasionally, the inexperienced physician may think he is dealing with a gastric upset or iritis. And yet, the diagnosis is simple; loss of vision, hardening of the eyeball, congestion, and cloudy cornea are parthognomonic of acute glaucoma. Immediate action can save the eye from blindness. The diagnosis of chronic glaucoma, particularly the noncongestive type, offers many difficulties to the general practitioner. Relatively few cases can be uncovered by him in the earlier stages. However, if he becomes conscious of the frequency of glaucoma and knows its symptoms, great progress can be made in diagnosing many cases before too much irreparable damage has been done.

"THE PROBLEM OF TRACHEOTOMY IN LARYNGEAL SUFFOCATION IN CHILDHOOD." Rene Mayoux. Le Journal de Medicine de Lyon. volume 22. Number 522. page 421-423. October 1941.

Laryngeal suffocation which is not the result of diphtheria is the most frequently due to subglottic edema. In France, it is the general practice that the physician waits with the tracheotomy until there is an urgent need for it, when the dyspnea is great and when pulmonary complications can be still prevented. In America, tracheotomy is done at a much earlier stage of the disease, and its purpose is not only to make the glottis permeable by a metallic tube but also to render the aspiration of secretion from the bronchi possible. According to Chevalier Jackson, aspiration of the secretion which obstructs the bronchi is an indispensable complement of any tracheotomy. Le Mee also recommends bronchial injection of a sodium borate solution in order to stimulate the work of the ciliated epithelium of the bronchi. Thus, in the American practice, tracheotomy is not a palliative operation performed in emergency cases, but a truly curative therapeutic measure that may prevent the pulmonary complications in cases of suffocating laryngitis.

Formerly it was thought that such children die from bronchopneumonia. In fact, there is rarely a bronchopneumonia; the physical signs are caused by atelectasia of the lungs, which is a result of bronchial obstruction by accumulated secretion. Formerly, physicians even thought that tracheotomy may cause pulmonary complications. Now, we know that the contrary is true: by early tracheotomy, it is possible to prevent the development of pulmonary complications.

Considering the French view and the American view, one wonders which to accept. The author reports several cases which are evidently opposite to the American doctrine on tracheotomy and its therapeutical effects. There were five children: two recovered, and three died. The autopsy found no secretion in the trachea or the bronchi. In one of the fatal cases, repeated attempts were made to aspirate bronchial secretion through the tracheotomy tube, but only a small quantity of mucus was removed, without any improvement in the patient's dyspneic condition. It is also true that in none of the fatal cases was bronchopneumonia found, and the histological examination showed leukocytes and fibrine in the alveoli, and pus in the smaller bronchi. It almost seems that the tracheotomy and the endobronchial medication in the three fatal cases aggravated the pulmonary lesions.

The truth is that there are different types of suffocating laryngitis. The types may vary according to the nature of the epidemic and, even according to geopathological factors. There is the disease described by Chevalier Jackson and others under the term of tracheobronchitis fulgurants. Though the dyspnea is the same as in suffocating laryngitis, and the clinical aspect of the disease is only slightly different, the tracheobronchitis is entirely different from suffocating laryngitis. It is characterized by the presence of abundant exudates and edema in the trachea and the large bronchi—but this is not a laryngitis. Here, the only effective treatment is tracheotomy followed by aspiration. And an early tra-

cheotomy is imperative. The recognition of this new disease, and the existence of an effective therapeutic measure for it makes it necessary to examine the larynx with direct laryngoscopy in all cases of suffocating laryngitis: detection of abundant secretions, with congestion or edema of the tracheal mucosa indicate an immediate tracheotomy. The disease is rare in France.

The types of suffocating laryngitis observed in France, and occuring in the course of measles, grippe, or spontaneously, are two. In one type, the laryngeal lesion and the subglottic edema constitute the entire disease. This type is easily cured, and tracheotomy is rarely if ever necessary.

But, beside this purely local form, there is also a rather severe type of suffocating laryngitis. There are two essential factors in death from suffocating laryngitis: the intensity of the toxi-infection, and the bronchopneumonia. The pulmonary changes are usually not secondary to the laryngitis: they develop simultaneously with the laryngitis as seen in the "grippe" of the entire respiratory tract. In this type, the role of bronchial obstruction, and of atelectasis is of little significance, and patients with this type of suffocating laryngitis cannot be saved by tracheotomy.

PLASTIC SURGERY
Edited by George H. Kimball, M. D., F. A. C. S.
912 Medical Arts Building, Oklahoma City

"HUMAN BITES OF THE HAND." Harry Miller. M.D.. and James M. Winfield. M.D. Surgery. Gynecology and Obstetrics, Vol. 74. Feb. 1, 1942, No. 2.

Experience in many communities has yielded abundant proof of the danger which attends neglect of wounds contaminated with human mouth organisms. As the concomitant sequelae and resultant functional disturbances are often of a most serious nature, the importance of the correct management of the early and late human bite lesions cannot be over-emphasized. There is a definite tendency for these infections, when once established, to extend and to invade into deeper and more vital structures, the lesions rapidly becoming foul smelling, necrotizing, and resistant.

The organisms implanted in the tissues of the hand are often most virulent. The part played by such anaerobes as the fusiform bacillus and the spirochete of Vincent has been repeatedly pointed out. Although these organisms are not always demonstrable in cultures and smears from human bite wounds, dark field examination of fresh wet smears will demonstrate their presence in a higher percentage of instances. Anaerobic cultures observed over a period of seven to ten days will often yield much information. Streptococci and staphylococci alone and in symbiosis, as well as other contaminants such as the colon bacillus, various fungi, and occasionally the Spirocheta pallida play an important role in producing and prolonging these necrotizing infections.

In order to gain a lucid concept of the problems involved in the prophylaxis and treatment of these lesions one must appreciate the anatomic complexity of the tissues which predisposes to extension of infection rather than to localization, particularly under conditions of neglect, as well as the low resistance of fibrous connective tissue and cartilage, to infection.

A knowledge of the mechanism of production, the usual sites of injury, the extent and depth of the lesion, and the possible course of extension of the infection is of considerable aid in the intelligent management of these cases.

Human bite injuries usually occur during the course of fist fights or drunken biting brawls. Consequently, the lesions range from actual bites of the phalanges and hand to puncture wounds and lacerations produced by a fist striking exposed teeth. When the closed fist is used in striking a blow the knuckles of the second and third metacarpals receive the major force of the impact. This is primarily due to the fact that these bones are longer and stronger than the other metacarpals and, furthermore, they are more immobile. In this position the dorsal ligaments, extensor tendons, and skin are tightly stretched across the metacarpal, and will easily cause a sharp, resisting surface to penetrate the joint cavity or to damage underlying structures.

A more rare mechanism, that of the sucking of hangnails or of clean lacerated wounds by the patient or a concerned bystander, will account for contamination with mouth organisms in a small number of cases. One of the patients included in our group of late infected cases acquired a severe infection following the biting of a hangnail.

In regard to the extent and depth of the lesion, the injury may present itself as: (1) a simple abrasion over the phalanges, knuckles, or palmar surface of the hand or wrist, involving only the epidermis; (2) a complete avulsion of segments of skin, subcutaneous structures and occasionally of bone; (3) a penetrating laceration either partially or completely severing the extensor tendon; (4) a wound which may have opened into the dorsal subcutaneous space, subtendinous bursa, dorsal subaponeurotic space, or the joint cavity.

In 1930, Mason and Koch published a paper on human bite infections of the hand in which they demonstrated experimentally the lines of spread of infectious agents from the region of the metacarpophalangeal joint. This paper has been unsurpassed in the presentation of essentials and remains the outstanding contribution on this subject.

Obviously, abrasions and avulsion lacerations offer little opportunity for the establishment of an anaerobic infection. Lacerations, however, which have penetrated the subcutaneous layers and opened into the subtendinous tissues and joints, present ideal conditions for the production of fetid, necrotizing infections because of the relatively anaerobic conditions, the low resistance of fibrous tissue and synovial membranes, the anatomic complexity of structures favoring the spread of infection, and the presence of traumatized tissue. Consequently, the infections occurring on the dorsal aspect of the hand in and about the metacarpophalangeal joint potentially and actually carry the graver prognosis. Because of the shift of tissues particularly about the knuckles, infection may be carried from an original point of entrance to a relatively distant area.

Infection occurring from an injury over the proximal phalanx may extend both superficial and deep to the expansion of the extensor tendon. From this position it may extend along the lumbrical and interosseous tendons to involve the lumbrical space.

Laceration of the extensor tendon with the implantation of infection but without penetration into the joint may occur. Here the extension of infection will be extracapsular and subtendinous, the subtendinous bursa and subaponeurotic space becoming contaminated. Should the joint be infected infection may penetrate into the subtendinous bursa and subaponeurotic space as well as under the expansion of the extensor tendon over the perimal phalanx from which point infection will travel, as described, namely, to the lumbrical canal and large fascial spaces in the palm of the hand.

The dorsal subcutaneous space is usually involved early. This follows subcutaneous penetration with or without laceration or displacement of the tendon or extension into the joint.

The flexor tendons and their synovial sheaths are rarely invaded from behind. A dense fibrous sheath and the accessory volar ligament serve as an adequate barrier. Late in the course of infection, especially in neglected cases, the flexor tendon sheaths may be invaded.

Believing the results obtained by those surgeons using chemical and electrocautery methods in the primary treatment of early human contaminated wounds are not entirely satisfactory, we have followed in our clinic the suggestion made by Mason and Koch in 1930 of cleansing the wound with soap and water combined with gentle debridement. The recognition of early human bites as such is often quite difficult. Falsification of history is common especially in the white patient, and often results in contraindicated primary suture. A definite and comprehensive regimen has been developed, comprising a searching history, complete examination, and treatment.

The routine treatment employed is as follows: The area about the wound is gently washed with soap and water for five minutes following which the wound itself is thoroughly washed with soap and water and irrigated with saline for a further period of ten minutes. Following this procedure, the edges are gently retracted and the lesion examined, in order to determine the extent of injury if possible. These wounds are not probed since the information obtained is meager and the danger of carrying infectious agents more deeply into the tissues is great. Following mechanical cleansing and a very limited debridement, wet dressings are applied. No attempts are made to repair the rent in the joint capsule. Hands are splinted in the position of function. Lacerations are never sutured nor are injuries to deeper structures repaired. The major catastrophes in our series have occurred in those cases in which wounds were primarily sutured. Patients return daily for examination and if there is joint involvement, are usually hospitalized. In certain of the initial cases in this series patients were observed and treated in conjunction with Dr. R. E. Speirs who has reported these previously. A total number of 61 early human bites of the hand have been given prophylactic treatment during the past three years. All patients seen within four hours after the occurrence of injury were considered early cases. Friedrich has pointed out that a lag phase of six hours exists before organisms contaminating a wound become acclimated to the human tissues. This lag phase in the case of organisms transfered from the human mouth is greatly shortened and there may be only a brief interval before the organisms are accustomed to their new environment. Those cases already presenting swelling and evidence of infectious extension were not included in this series of early cases even if patients were seen within the four hour period and were considered as late cases.

The accompanying table illustrates an interesting grouping of these injuries. It will be noted that 34 lesions involved the fingers while 18 occurred in the region of the knuckle. Of the total number of cases, five showed mild inflammatory reaction characterized by swelling and tenderness without suppuration and only one gave evidence of gross infection. Two of the knuckle injuries exhibiting inflammation had been sutured primarily due to falsification of history but the sutures were removed almost immediately and the wound treated as a human bite. One of the compound fractures with the tip of the terminal phalanx completely bitten off showed mild inflammation. The compound fractures were usually hospitalized for a short period. The case referred to in the footnote was a most extensive injury, the fifth finger having been almost completely bitten off at the base of the proximal phalanx, tooth injuries of the third and fourth metacarpophalangeal joints and three lacerations over the dorsum of the hand. It was necessary to remove the fifth finger. The third and fourth metacarpophalangeal joints became stiff and the dorsal skin sloughed requiring a subsequent graft. Obviously, gross suppuration occurred in this hand, but we were able to save the major portion of the hand and to obtain a fair functional result. In none of the early cases, except the last mentioned, was it necessary to resort to amputation.

A more complete analysis has been made of the last 27 cases. In this group ten were knuckle injuries, five of these occurring on the third right knuckle and one on the third left knuckle. Two occurred on the second right knuckle. Of the 17 finger injuries, the first, second, and fifth right fingers were most commonly involved. There were ten extensor tendon lacerations and one flexor tendon laceration. The metacarpophalangeal joint was known to be entered in three instances, but no doubt lacerations involving the joint were more frequent than this, as the positive determination of the extent of the injury in this region is often difficult to ascertain.

Over 60 percent of the cases were between the ages of 15 and 25 years, 18 being males, nine females: 19 were colored, and eight white. Of 22 cases the functional result in 20 was excellent, good in one, and poor in one (cases described previously).

The average wound healing time for the whole series of 61 cases was 8.5 days and for the group of 27 cases 9.9 days.

The after-care consisted essentially of splinting and the application of continuous saline, boric acid, or magnesium sulphate soaks for a period of 48 hours. The wet dressings were discontinued at this time if the wounds remained clean. Splinting was continued to complete healing.

This relatively simple course of management of early human bite injuries has given results which have been most gratifying. Unfortunately, the patient, when first seen often has a fully established infection, and regardless of the adequacy of treatment, frequently is condemned to a prolonged illness which may result in loss of parts and occasionally in loss of life.

In marked contrast to the prophylactic treatment and management of the early human bite injuries, is the therapeutic problem presented by the late infected human bites. These wounds are already in serious conditions, and sometimes extensively infected. As in other infections of this type, adequate surgery is essential with emphasis on somewhat earlier and more radical drainage. In general, the basic principles enunciated by Kanavel, Koch, Mason, and others relative to the treatment of established hand infections should be adhered to scrupulously. It should be unnecessary and is obviously impractical to outline the treatment in the most minute detail. Suffice it to say, that under general anesthesia, and in a bloodless field, the hand is throughly cleansed with soap and water. Then an extremely careful, meticulous debridement is performed, with removal of as much infected, gangrenous sloughing tissue as possible, and in addition with adequate drainage for all areas of infection. Definite mention should be made regarding metacarpophalangeal joint infections. The joint capsule should be opened transversely by one to a 1.5 centimeter incision which usually gives sufficient drainage. As has been pointed out earlier in the paper, infections of this type when implanted in certain regions may characteristically spread along certain lines to involve adjacent or deeper structures. The deepest anatomic plane involved should be inspected, as the infection may spread along the lowermost plane. Infection of the joint, if adequately drained, does not always result in a completely ankylosed joint as in many instances excellent function is obtained. An understanding of the pathogenesis of the advance of infection is essential to the correct surgical management of these severe infections, since it is only by locating those areas of greatest potential danger and recognizing the presence of infection that the lesion can be intelligently and satisfactorily managed. One should be slow to amputate extensively infected fingers but extensive drainage of the soft parts is essential. Often a useful part may be preserved or if amputation later becomes necessary, more of the extremity may be saved. Amputation should be avoided in the presence of an acute infection.

The wounds are then loosely packed with vaseline gauze and usually massive wet dressings are applied. A considerable variety of antiseptic solutions have been employed. In addition to saline, boric acid, and magnesium sulphate solutions, we have utilized and rather favor the use of Dakin's solution; it being our impres-

sion that the wounds remained cleaner and that sloughs separated more readily with consequently better drainage when the latter solution was used. Hydrogen peroxide, potassium permanganate, and chromic acid solutions also were used without notable success. Zinc peroxide, arsenicals, and sulfanilamide did not produce strikingly favorable results. The fingers, hand, and arm are then splinted and put at rest in the position of function and whenever possible arranged so that the position will favor dependent drainage. It is our belief that practically without exception cases of this type should be hospitalized. A Wassermann should be done in all patients presenting human contaminated lesions.

As has been stated, the initial injuries in the late infected cases occurring in the region of the knuckle outnumbered those of the finger. In 34 of the 54 patients the knuckles were involved, 15 occurring over the third metacarpophalangeal joint, the others scattered and of the group of 34 cases, the joint cavity itself was infected in 19 instances. There were 19 cases with lesions of the fingers 16 injuries being on the dorsal surface, and three on the volar surface. In six cases the middle interphalangeal joint was involved. As might be expected, partial or complete laceration of extensor tendons occurred in 18 cases and in only six were the flexor tendons partially severed. There was one case presenting a laceration of dorsum of the hand alone.

In several cases there was multiple involvement of joints, fascial spaces, and tendon sheaths. However, in 12 cases infection was confined to the dorsal subcutaneous space and in 21 cases both the dorsal subcutaneous and the dorsal subaponeurotic space was infected. Infection of the midpalmar space was present in three cases and this seems significant in that this space is not commonly involved in the usual hand infection. In one case infection extended from an involvement of the index flexor tendon and its sheath to the thenar space. In another case the ulnar, radial bursa, retroflexor space, and bones of the wrist and hand became so severely infected from a knuckle lesion that amputation through the forearm was required. From an original focus at the metacarpophalangeal joint, infection spread to the lumbrical spaces in nine cases. Thirteen cases of a total 48 developed stiff fingers and five cases amputation of parts was required, in one of which it was necessary to perform amputation through the forearm.

In spite of the severity of these infections, the average length of healing was 34 days and 9.4 was the average number of hospital days. No fatalities occurred in this group of cases.

As has been noted in the literature, these infections are prone to recurrence and frequent exacerbations. In our series there were three such instances, one in three weeks, one in two months, and one in three years' time.

Since instituting the described management of early human bite lesions, the number of late cases admitted to the hospital have been definitely fewer in number. For a short interval during a change in the resident staff, the late infected cases increased, and it was found that the treatment of the early cases was not being carried out as outlined.

The careful evaluation of results in the treatment of human bite infections is difficult because of the variations in the virulence of the contaminating organisms and the resistance of tissue. The criterion of the length of stay in the hospital is not a good index to the extent or severity of the infection. These studies have convinced us that good results in the treatment of human bite infections of the hands can be obtained only by attention to details and adherence to surgical principles. Careful cleansing and gentle handling of tissues have reduced our incidence of severe infections and adequate drainage, fixation of parts and irrigation are fundamental necessities in the treatment of the late infections.

Summary

1. The prophylactic treatment of early "human bite" injuries handled under the regimen of soap and

water cleansing, limited debridement, wet dressings, and splinting is simple and effective, the results obtained being superior or equal to those attained when actual or chemical cauterization was utilized.

2. The correct management of the "early human bite" cases has reduced the number of late infected cases and we feel that prompt and intelligent treatment of the infected cases has been disabling and deforming sequelae.

3. In dealing with the late infected cases a clear understanding of the mechanism, depth of penetration, and degree of injury in relation to the spread of established infection is essential for adequate and correct surgical treatment.

Comment: Anyone who has treated cases of human bites of the hand will appreciate this fine article. The results speak very favorably for the treatment rendered. I believe every surgeon will find this abstract useful.

CARDIOLOGY

Edited by F. Redding Hood, M. D.
1200 North Walker, Oklahoma City

"INTERPRETATION OF BLOOD PRESSURE BEHAVIOR DURING PREGNANCY AND THE PUERPERIUM." R. A. Bartholomew and E. D. Colvin. (Condensed from American Journal of Obstetrics and Gynecology, 41: 646, 1941.)

The observation that hypertension complicates pregnancy, either early or late in gestation, is rightfully regarded as of serious significance. "Since it may indicate either vascular disease or true toxemia, differentiation of these conditions assumes much importance, not only in the management of the pregnancy, but in the final classification and ultimate prognosis of the disorder.

"It is our purpose to point out certain observations during pregnancy and the puerperium, which not only aid in interpreting the behavior of the blood pressure, but which will enable one to predict that a moderate rise in blood pressure will probably occur in the latter part of pregnancy. It is desired to emphasize, particularly, the value of retinal examination in the differentiation and management of true toxemia and vascular disease, and the importance and examination of the formalin-fixed placenta in the final classification of the disorder."

"Hypertension, present early in pregnancy or arising later in pregnancy, is interpreted on the basis of vascular disease or true toxemia according to the following behavior and characteristics:

1. If, on retinal examination early in pregnancy, there is evident disturbance in the A-V ratio (ratio of diameter of arteries to veins), varying from 1 to 2 to 2 to 3, or 1 to 2 up to 1 to 3, 1 to 4 or more, it is evident that the pregnancy is complicated by vascular disease. The more marked the disturbance in A-V ratio, the earlier the onset of hypertension in pregnancy and the more marked the increase in light reflex and A-V compressions. Hemorrhages and exudates are usually not seen unless the disturbance is severe and of long standing, with associated kidney involvement. Localized arterial spasms are not seen unless there is a superimposed toxemia.

"Hypertension due to true toxemia rarely occurs as early as the fifth month but becomes increasingly frequent after the seventh month. The A-V ratio is normal and the arterial spasms, at first sharply localized, become spindle-shaped and elongated with the increasing hypertension until, in severe cases, there is generalized constriction and the A-V ratio becomes much disturbed. Since the disturbed ratio is due to spasm rather than sclerosis, there is no corresponding increase in light reflex or A-V compressions, which helps to rule out vascular disease.

2. Edema, headache and albuminuria are much less pronounced in vascular disease than in true toxemia with a comparable elevation of blood pressure.

3. Following the initial rise in blood pressure and appearance of albumin, subsequent observations at weekly intervals show very gradual increases in hypertension as compared to true toxemia. Superimposed true toxemia causes rapid increase in edema, headache, hypertension, albuminuria, and the appearance of acute placental infarcts.

4. The more severe cases of vascular disease, which occur much more frequently among colored than white women, usually show a striking and unexplainable response to rest in bed. One frequently observes a blood pressure of 180/100 return nearly to normal after several days' rest in bed. An immediate return to the former high level is noted when the patient again resumes the upright position, even though she carries on no physical exertion. These cases also show marked fluctuation in blood pressures from day to day for no apparent reason.

"In contrast to this behavior, hypertension due to true toxemia is not much influenced by rest in bed or indeed by any other measures. It remains persistently elevated and tends to increase. Edema may lessen with rest in bed but headache and albuminuria increase. Arterial spasms, at first sharply localized, become spindle-shaped, elongated, and finally produce generalized constriction. Hemorrhages in the retina may occur. Finally, examination of the formalin-fixed placenta shows the acute types of toxic infarcts.

5. The concentration test on the urine and the blood chemistry values are seldom affected in either vascular disease or toxemia of pregnancy, unless advanced cardiorenal disease or severe toxemia have seriously affected the kidneys. However, the uric acid value, which is usually normal in vascular disease, is definitely increased in toxemia, due probably to increased liver damage in the latter.

6. Hypertension and retinal changes due to vascular disease persist throughout the puerperium and show a gradual tendency to increase. This is likewise true of toxemia, if expectant treatment is followed, induction of labor delayed, and the patient subjected to long continued harmful effects on her vascular system and liver. In such cases, hypertension and albuminuria usually persist and subsequent observations show that the patient has acquired vascular disease. However, it is well recognized that marked hypertension due to fulminating toxemia, subsides quickly after spontaneous or induced labor, apparently leaves the patient none the worse for the experience.

7. Finally, examination of the formalin-fixed placenta from cases of hypertension due to vascular disease, shows no infarcts of the toxic types, namely the 'C', 'D', 'E' and possibly the 'B' types. If infarcts of these types are present, they are proof of the toxic origin of the hypertension."

Hence, in the examination of the retina and the formalin-fixed placenta, more accurate diagnosis and classification of cases of hypertension during pregnancy are made possible. When a distinct disturbance in A-V ratio is seen early in pregnancy, a warning is given of the probability of hypertension occurring in the latter part. "The extent of the increase and the stage of pregnancy at which it will appear are directly proportionate to the degree of disturbance in the A-V ratio. Examination of the formalin-fixed placenta serves as a check in the final classification of the nature of the hypertension. Type 'A' infarct (White) is nontoxic; Type 'B' (yellow) is usually associated with slight hypertension and albuminurial Type 'C' (brown yellow) is associated with moderate toxemia; Type 'D' (brown) is associated with severe toxemia and type 'E' (black) is associated with acute or fulminating toxemia. It must be remembered that true toxemia may be so mild that except for a slightly greater degree of albuminuria and edema, it may simulate the picture above described as due to vascular disease with slight disturbance in A-V ratio."

The authors predict that when the types and significance of placental infarcts are more generally recognized, and the value of retinal examination in pregnancy is appreciated, there will result not only more uniform statistics concerning pregnancy complicated by toxemia and vascular disease, but more rational management of pregnancy when complicated by these conditions.

ORTHOPAEDIC SURGERY
Edited by Earl D. McBride, M. D., F. A. C. S.
605 N. W. 10th, Oklahoma City

"INSUFFICIENCY FRACTURE OF THE TIBIA RESEMBLING OSTEOGENIC SARCOMA." George E. Pfahler. The Amer. Jr. of Roentgenology and Radium Therapy. XLV, 209, 1941.

The author first reviews the literature and known facts concerning this type of fracture. He describes it as an incomplete fracture of the cortex of the bone, resulting from excessive strain and affecting just one side of the bone. In most cases the fracture line is not discernible in the roentgenogram until after a month or more. The first symptom is pain on exertion at the site of the lesion, often with early swelling due to edema, and with a later swelling caused by callous formation. The process is similar to that seen in the so-called "march fracture" of the metatarsals.

Since the pain and swelling with new-bone formation are often seen without the fracture line being visible, a diagnosis of osteogenic sarcoma is a natural mistake, and one which the author emphasizes as being a tragic one. Cessation of activity and weight-bearing will result in complete cure.

A case report with roentgenograms is also given.

"COXA PLANA, WITH SPECIAL REFERENCE TO ITS PATHOLOGY AND KINSHIP." H. Jackson Burrows. The British Jr. of Surg., XXIX, 23, July, 1941.

"1. Coxa plana proves histologically to be a condition of necrosis of bone followed by repair.

2. The necrosis differs from ordinary aseptic necrosis in showing lysis of trabeculae.

3. Infection cannot be excluded as a cause of the lysis, but is highly improbable.

4. The results of animal experiments suggest that the lysis is not due to arterial anaemia occurring in the special anatomical circumstances of the presence of bone in an envelope of cartilage.

5. A possible cause is some form of vascular disturbance other than arterial anaemia,—either venous obstruction or haematoma; the anatomical circumstances are such that either of these events might have profound results.

6. Recognition of the special pathological changes assists the accurate definition of 'osteochondritis juvenilis' occurring at sites other than the hip and the rejection of alleged examples which lack the essential criteria which might properly justify an analogy with coxa plana.

7. Recognition of histological criteria that the following are akin to coxa plana: osteochondritis of the tarsal scaphoid bone (Kohler's disease), of the metatarsal head (Freidberg's disease or Kohler's disease), and of the semilunar bone (Kienbock's disease).

8. On grounds of critical radiology, without histological information, it is probable that osteochondritis of the vertebral body in infants (Calve's disease) and osteochondritis juvenilis of the capitellum (Panner's disease) are further examples.

9. Other alleged examples of osteochondritis juvenilis, with one or two possible exceptions, probably belong to unallied conditions and are not analogous to coxa plana.

10. In assessing these conclusions, only the weight it deserves should be accorded to evidence based on identity of histological appearances or the results of animal experiments.''

INTERNAL MEDICINE
Edited by Hugh Jeter, M. D., F. A. C. P., A. S. C. P.
1200 North Walker, Oklahoma City

"METABOLISM AND DIABETES"—Review of certain recent contributions. Edward H. Rynearson and Alice G. Hildebrand, Rochester, Minn. Archives of Internal Medicine, 68:134-75, July, 1941.

A summary of 128 published reports over the past year dealing with glycogen and carbohydrate metabolism, diabetes mellitus, Insulin and its modifications, hyperinsulinism, the pituitary gland, obesity and various subdivisions.

The mortality rate of diabetes in the United States has resumed an upward trend. There are probably 500,-000 to 600,000 cases, and it appears that at the end of the present decade the figure will reach 1,000,000. The general conclusion has been that there is no evidence of trauma itself causing diabetes, although it may cause latent diabetes to be manifest. There is now considerable evidence that pregnant diabetic patients may have hormonal imbalance, and that toxemia may be prevented by replacement therapy . . . although diabetic children may have a disturbance of some other endocrine system, the only real facts available indicate that the only acknowledged deficiency is that of Insulin, and that many of the other changes are secondary. As yet there is no conclusive evidence that any one type of diet is suitable for every physician to prescribe. However, the majority of internists are prescribing diets which are higher in carbohydrates and lower in fat than those which were used previously.

There is unanimity of opinion that Protamine Zinc Insulin has a definite role in treatment, but little evidence that Crystalline Insulin has a much different effect than the unmodified type of Insulin used in past years.

There is increasing insistence that the term "hyperinsulinism" be reserved for those cases in which there is proof that the symptoms are caused by excessive production of endogenous insulin. Recent work on the pituitary indicates that affording the pancreas the benefit of physiologic rest improves diabetes by reducing strain on the remaining island cells, and also permitting restoration to function of some of the exhausted cells. If Insulin is given during the period of overwork diabetes may often be prevented.

The current literature on obesity is concerned chiefly with the extremely controversial subject of pathogenesis. It is considered to be either exogenous or endogenous. Supporters of the latter theory are not at all in agreement as to the site of disturbance.

"THE PATHOLOGY OF DIABETES MELLITUS." Shields Warren, Boston, Mass. New York State Journal of Medicine, 41:2432-36, December 15, 1941.

The pathology of diabetes mellitus is partly well understood and partly still confused. The lesions of the islands of Langerhans, particularly hyalinization and fibrosis, are adequate to explain some cases of the disease. Their experimental production in dogs and cats by anterior pituitary extract, apparently following the occurrence of hydropic degeneration of the insular cells, suggests the reality of the assumed relationship between the pituitary gland and the pancreas. Yet, the mechanism of production of hyalinization of the islands is still unknown. The occurrence of amyloid and paraamyloid reactions may be significant. Thus far, the significance of rather striking hyaline deposition in some functioning adenomas and carcinomas of the islands has not been determined.

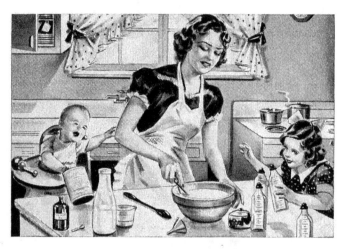

Why let a busy mother
upset your formula balance?

THE OPTIMAL NUTRITION which your baby feeding prescriptions provide... may be lost through errors in formula preparation.

For even the best-intentioned mothers may make mistakes in measuring. Or leave out important supplements. Or fail to follow instructions completely.

Biolac makes such formula errors all but impossible, because:

1. Formulas are made by simply diluting Biolac with water.

2. Biolac provides completely for *all* the nutritional requirements of early infancy except for vitamin C.

3. No supplementary formula ingredients are necessary.

4. The adequate carbohydrate content of Biolac is processed in the milk, is in equilibrium and is sterile.

5. The nutritional completeness of Biolac is guaranteed by strict laboratory control of manufacturing operations and assays of product composition which are recognized in its A.M.A. Council acceptance.

Thus in prescribing Biolac you have these extra assurances that your babies will actually receive in their formulas the optimal nutrition you prescribe.

Biolac nutritional values equal or exceed recognized standards. For complete information, write Borden's Prescription Products Division, 350 Madison Ave., New York, N.Y.

Biolac is prepared from whole milk, skim milk, lactose, vitamin B_1, concentrate of vitamins A and D from cod liver oil, and ferric citrate. It is evaporated, homogenized, and sterilized.

Visit our Booth No. 50 at the Tulsa meeting

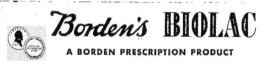

Borden's **BIOLAC**

A BORDEN PRESCRIPTION PRODUCT

OFFICERS OF COUNTY SOCIETIES, 1942

COUNTY	PRESIDENT	SECRETARY	MEETING TIME
Alfalfa	Jack F. Parsons, Cherokee	L. T. Lancaster, Cherokee	Last Tues. Each 2nd Mo.
Atoka-Coal	J. B. Clark, Coalgate	J. S. Fulton, Atoka	
Beckham	H. K. Speed, Sayre	E. S. Kilpatrick, Elk City	Second Tues. eve.
Blaine	Virginia Olson Curtin, Watonga	W. F. Griffin, Watonga	
Bryan	A. J. Wells, Calera	W. K. Haynie, Durant	Second Tues. eve.
Caddo	Fred L. Patterson, Carnegie	C. B. Sullivan, Carnegie	
Canadian	P. F. Herod, El Reno	A. L. Johnson, El Reno	Subject to call
Carter	Walter Hardy, Ardmore	H. A. Higgins, Ardmore	
Cherokee	Park H. Medearis, Tahlequah	Isadore Dyer, Tahlequah	
Choctaw	C. H. Hale, Boswell	Fred D. Switzer, Hugo	
Cleveland	F. C. Buffington, Norman	Phil Haddock, Norman	Thursday nights
Comanche	George S. Barber, Lawton		
Cotton	George W. Baker, Walters	Mollie F. Scism, Walters	Third Friday
Craig	W. R. Marks, Vinita	J. M. McMillan, Vinita	
Creek	Frank Sisler, Bristow	O. H. Cowart, Bristow	
Custer	Richard M. Burke, Clinton	W. C. Tisdal, Clinton	Third Thursday
Garfield	D. S. Harris, Drummond	John R. Walker, Enid	Fourth Thursday
Garvin	T. F. Gross, Lindsay	John R. Callaway, Pauls Valley	Wed before 3rd Thurs.
Grady	D. S. Downey, Chickasha	Frank T. Joyce, Chickasha	3rd Thursday
Grant	I. V. Hardy, Medford	E. E. Lawson, Medford	
Greer	G. F. Border, Mangum	J. B. Hollis, Mangum	
Harmon	S. W. Hopkins, Hollis	W. M. Yeargan, Hollis	First Wednesday
Haskell	William Carson, Keota	N. K. Williams, McCurtain	
Hughes	Wm. L. Taylor, Holdenville	Imogene Mayfield, Holdenville	First Friday
Jackson	J. M. Allgood, Altus	Willard D. Holt, Altus	Last Monday
Jefferson	W. M. Browning, Waurika	J. I. Hollingsworth, Waurika	Second Monday
Kay	J. C. Wagner, Ponca City	J. Holland Howe, Ponca City	Third Thurs.
Kingfisher	C. M. Hodgson, Kingfisher	John R. Taylor, Kingfisher	
Kiowa	J. M. Bonham, Hobart	B. H. Watkins, Hobart	
LeFlore	G. R. Booth, LeFlore	Rush L. Wright, Poteau	
Lincoln	E. F. Hurlbut, Meeker	C. W. Robertson, Chandler	First Wednesday
Logan	William C. Miller, Guthrie	J. L. LeHew, Jr., Guthrie	Last Tuesday evening
Marshall	J. L. Holland, Madill	O. A. Cook, Madill	
Mayes	L. C. White, Adair	V. D. Herrington, Pryor	
McClain	B. W. Slover, Blanchard	R. L. Royster, Purcell	
McCurtain	R. D. Williams, Idabel	R. H. Sherrill, Broken Bow	Fourth Tues. eve.
McIntosh	F. R. First, Checotah	William A. Tolleson, Eufaula	Second Tuesday
Murray	P. V. Annadown, Sulphur	F. E. Sadler, Sulphur	
Muskogee	Shade D. Neely, Muskogee	J. T. McInnis, Muskogee	First & Third Mon.
Noble	J. W. Francis, Perry	C. H. Cooke, Perry	
Okfuskee	J. M. Pemberton, Okemah	L. J. Spickard, Okemah	Second Monday
Oklahoma	R. Q. Goodwin, Okla. City	Wm. E. Eastland, Okla. City	Fourth Tuesday
Okmulgee	J. G. Edwards, Okmulgee	John R. Cotteral, Henryetta	Second Monday
Osage	C. R. Weirich, Pawhuska	George K. Hemphill, Pawhuska	Second Monday
Ottawa	J. R. Hampton, Commerce	Walter Sanger, Picher	Third Thursday
Pawnee	E. T. Robinson, Cleveland	Robert L. Browning, Pawnee	
Payne	John W. Martin, Cushing	James D. Martin, Cushing	Third Thursday
Pittsburg	Austin R. Stough, McAlester	Edw. D. Greenberger, McAlester	Third Friday
Pontotoc	R. E. Cowling, Ada	E. R. Muntz, Ada	First Wednesday
Pottawatomie	John Carson, Shawnee	Clinton Gallaher, Shawnee	First & Third Sat.
Pushmataha	P. B. Rice, Antlers	John S. Lawson, Clayton	
Rogers	W. A. Howard, Chelsea	P. S. Anderson, Claremore	First Monday
Seminole	H. M. Reeder, Konawa	Mack I. Shanholtz ,Wewoka	
Stephens	E. C. Lindley, Duncan	A. J. Weedn, Duncan	
Texas	L. G. Blackmer, Hooker	Johnny A. Blue, Guymon	
Tillman	C. C. Allen, Frederick	O. G. Bacon, Frederick	
Tulsa	H. B. Stewart, Tulsa	E. O. Johnson, Tulsa	Second & Fourth Mon. eve.
Wagoner	J. H. Plunkett, Wagoner	H. K. Riddle, Coweta	
Washington-Nowata	R. W. Rucker, Bartlesville	J. V. Athey, Bartlesville	Second Wednesday
Washita	A. S. Neal, Cordell	James F. McMurry, Sentinel	
Woods	W. F. LaFon, Waynoka	O. E. Templin, Alva	Last Wednesday
Woodward	M. H. Newman, Shattuck	C. W. Tedrowe, Woodward	

THE JOURNAL

OF THE

OKLAHOMA STATE MEDICAL ASSOCIATION

| VOLUME XXXV | OKLAHOMA CITY, OKLAHOMA, MAY, 1942 | NUMBER 5 |

The Physiological Approach to Gynecology[*]

JOHN C. BURCH, M.D.
CHARLES A. MELLA, JR., M.D.

NASHVILLE, TENNESSEE

During the last ten years, a foundation has been laid for the application of the physiological concept of disease to the subject of gynecology. In seeking a topic for today's discussion, one useful to the clinician at the bedside, nothing seemed more appropriate than the physiological approach of gynecology. The basis of this physiological approach is a realization of the importance of the various activities of the sexual organs in the normal life of women.

Physiological consideration of any gynecological problem involves an appraisal of the patient's functional needs, of the extent of the functional disturbances, and of the effect of treatment on genital function. The *choice* of treatment is dictated by the type of pathology present, and the functional requirements of the individual.

As examples of this physiological approach, let us consider briefly some phases of the problems of discharge and of menstrual disorders.

In the juvenile form of vulvovaginitis, especially that due to gonorrhea, physiology has provided the answer. The child's thin vaginal mucous membrane becomes excoriated and the subepithelial tissues infected. Administration of estrogen causes a proliferation of the mucous membrane with healing of the infected areas. The proliferated epithelium becomes resistant to the disease.

TeLinde[1] recommends the use of vaginal suppositories and reports 175 cures in as many patients. He inserts an estrogen suppository of 1,000 I.U. nightly, and continues this for two weeks after the first negative smear. Russ and Collins,[2] in 25 cases, used 1 mg. of stilbestrol orally t.i.d. for seven days and obtained 100 percent cures.

In senile vulvovaginitis, continued estrogenic treatment is likewise of advantage in overcoming atrophy. A return to the mature type of epithelium is accompanied by a disappearance of symptoms.

Touching briefly on cervical disease, we believe that infection has been overemphasized and functional hypersecretion overlooked. In this connection the recent contributions of Wollner,[3] and of Bourne and Bond[4] are highly pertinent. While these authors make a strong case for a functional leukorrhea, the subject needs further study. At present, we are investigating some aspects of this problem.

In treating discharge it is well to be on the lookout for functional leukorrhea. It results from an endocrine hypertrophy and hyperplasia of the endocervix with an accompanying outpouring of an alkaline mucoid secretion. This is a factor in the development of erosions, and the production of suitable environment for the trichomonas vaginalis vaginitis. Unless the excess cervical secretion is eliminated, cure of the erosion or of the trichomonas vaginitis is impossible. Treatment can be directed at the underlying endocrinopathy or at the overactive endocervix. While endocrine therapy of functional leukorrhea is still in an embryonic stage, there are many methods for the elimination of an overactive endocervix. Among these are the scalpel, the actual cautery, conization, and electro-coagulation. Each must be used with careful discretion. No one method is suitable for all cases.

In approaching the subject of menstrual disorders, it is well to remember that the first principle in the therapy of any condition is an accurate diagnosis. For some years our group has been engaged in studies relating to the diagnosis of the disorders of menstruation. A detailed exposition of the

*Read before the General Session, Annual Session, Oklahoma State Medical Association, April 22, 1942, in Tulsa.

experiemental evidence which we have obtained can be found in previous publications.[5-6-7] On the basis of this evidence we have formulated a working concept which may be stated as follows: "A functional menstrual disorder can result from a lesion in any of the endocrine glands or from some general constitutional condition secondarily affecting the endocrine system. Whatever the primary disease conditions, it operates by producing a disturbance of the endocrine activity of the ovary, and this in turn gives rise to abnormal conditions in the lower genital tract. The endometrium indicates roughly the degree of ovarian involvement. There is no constant correlation between the primary lesion, the endometrial changes, and the type of menstrual disturbance."

From this it follows that ovarian, pituitary or thyroid disease and other types of endocrine or nonendocrine disease may give rise to endometrial changes and menstrual disorders of identical types, and each, on the other hand, may cause endometrial changes and menstrual disorders of quite different types. In other words, a menstrual disorder is not a disease but a symptom, referable to a variety of conditions. These disorders are not local disturbances; they are expressions of constitutional abnormalities and must be considered from the general, rather than the local standpoint.

The first step is to rule out organic pelvic disease, such as abortion, fibromyoma, carcinoma and so forth. Occasionally, this is difficult. A common error is to treat symptoms resulting from a small submucous fibroid by endocrine means. Conversely, other fibroids may be removed and an associated endocrine lesion overlooked. Diagnostic procedures such as the uterosalpingogram and the endometrial biopsy deserve mention here.

Having eliminated organic lesions, we must next determine the endocrine gland primarily affected and the presence and nature of contributory conditions, if any. For this, a thorough history and general examination are a requisite, with special attention to the constitutional status. It should never be forgotten that the elimination of the contributory disease and the proper and intelligent application of general medical measures directed at building up the general health of the patient are the keystones on which successful endocrine treatment rests.

With respect to endocrine diagnosis our knowledge is admittedly incomplete but sufficiently accurate to be of clinical value. Hormone assays and extensive laboratory tests are not necessary. The only essential special studies include endometrial biopsy, a few simple physical measurements, sugar tolerance tests (by oral galactose method or

the usual glucose tolerance curve) and basal metabolism determinations. Goldzieher's[8] specific dynamic action test may be of value in conjunction with the B.M.R. These studies can be carried out efficiently in the office as well as the hospital.

A working knowledge of the endocrine states supplemented by any of the standard texts on endocrine diagnosis will give the information necessary for interpreting the data obtained from history, physical examination and special studies. Evaluation of the data will usually lead to a working appraisal of the situation which will be found to correspond with the final diagnosis in a satisfactory percentage of the cases. After the tentative diagnosis is made, one is in a position to select the proper methods, endocrine and otherwise, indicated in a specific case.

The physiologically-minded gynecologist, in his attack on the problem of functional menstrual disturbances, has, as his objective, the return to the normal cyclic variations. This cannot be done in every case, and in such instances he approximates the norm as best he can, under the existing circumstances. Reorganization and restitution of the patient's genital interrelationships with an eye to her total structure, her future needs, her psyche and her sex life, he keeps in mind constantly. Resort to surgery he holds in abeyance. He has at his command a number of endocrine preparations, one or a combination of several of which may enable him to restore useful function to the patient. The products include the gonadotropes, the sex sterols and thyroid.

Gonadotropes are of three kinds: (1) chorionic; (2) pituitary; and (3) equine.

The chorionic gonadotrope, formerly referred to as the anterior pituitary-like hormone (A.P.L.) is derived from pregnancy urine or placenta. Many excellent preparations are available. In intact animals, they produce ovulation and corpus luteum formation, but in hypophysectomized animals they produce only theca luteinization. These extracts have been widely used clinically, more frequently formerly than at present, with varying degrees of success. Some investigators continue to obtain exceptional results, while others, notably Hamblen,[9] doubt their therapeutic worth. The excretion of an increased amount of pregnandiol follows their use; however, it seems definitely proved they do not produce ovulation or structural changes in the mature human ovary or endometrium.[10] Their most reliable action is a gonad-maturing one, best seen in male cryptorchidism and indicated in young girls with primary ovarian failure. In elderly women with primary ovarian failure they are apt to be worthless. They are useful in secondary ovarian failure for their stimulative action during the time one is waiting for more specific measures to take effect. On the whole, too much has been claimed for these preparations, which, however, are useful when used according to their indications.

The pituitary gonadotropes are derived from the gland itself and consist of two fractions: follicle stimulating and luteinizing. Ovulation is dependent upon a proper combination of the two fractions. Unfortunately these extracts with their wide potentialities for stimulation and restoration of normal function, have not been produced in a sufficiently stable form to render them useful clinically until quite recently. They are now in the process of clinical evaluation.

In the last year, work has been done on a preparation which combines chorionic gonadotropin and the pituitary synergist. This product, termed Synapoidin (Parke-Davis) has been reported to produce increase in ovarian size and follicle growth with luteinization.[10] Untoward effects such as overstimulation, hemorrhage into follicles, and cyst formation are seen from overdosage.[11] We have observed comparable effects at laparotomy in cases to whom this preparation was given pre-operatively.

Equine gonadotropes are derived from the serum of the pregnant mare. The use of this substance, P.M.S., has been reported to produce startling results by Davis and Koff,[12] Siegler[13] and others. We have not been impressed by its efficacy in producing ovulation in the woman with subthreshold ovarian activity, but have noted that supernumerary ovulation can be produced in the normally-ovulating woman. These preparations may have some value perhaps in the treatment of first-degree ovarian failure due to pituitary disease. Although the substance is said to be practically protein-free, one must test by intradermal and conjunctival tests for sensititvity before administration.

Some investigators have reported encouraging results from treatment with a combination of equine and chorionic gonadotropic preparations. [10-14-15] Greenblatt and Pund[16] state that bleeding induced with this combination occurs almost always from an estrogenic endometrium; no pregnant responses were obtained as regards menstrual cycles or ensuing pregnancies.

Sex sterols include the estrogens, progesterone and male hormone preparations. The estrogens are the most important of the group and are used by practically all practitioners. Their action is: (1) stimulative upon the luteinizing activity of the pituitary;[16] (2) sedative upon the nervous system;[17] (3) tropic upon the genital tract.[18]

Their use is indicated in pituitary failure because of the stimulative action on the pituitary, and because they substitute for the secondary deficiency in estrogen. In these cases it is usually advisable to use them in conjunction with thyroid, because of the action of this hormone on the pituitary and because of the secondary thyroid deficiency which often exists.

With regard to the second use, that on the nervous system, they are of value for the treatment of ovarian failure at or near the menopause or following operation. On account of this, they have been used extensively in menopausal conditions, although the observations of Pratt and Thomas[19] perhaps indicate that their effect has been overestimated. In my own practice, I have found them highly satisfactory.

As concerns the third use, action on the lower genital tract, the estrogens are extremely useful in the treatment of vulvovaginitis of infancy[20-19-21] and atrophic disturbances of the menopause.[22-23-24]

Hamblen[25] has reported excellent results from the treatment of menometrorrhagia by the cyclic employment of 10,000 I.U. of estrogen daily for 21 days followed by five mg. of progesterone daily for five days. Most of the patients treated obtained regular cycles and some continued to menstruate regularly after cessation of treatment. This form of therapy is rational when applied to the pituitary and Ovarian groups. If used in thyroid cases, supplemental therapy with thyroid will be required.

In pituitary cases, dosages of the estrogens range from 1,000 to 10,000 I.U. per day (in the case of tablets orally) or from one to three teaspoonfuls per day of the preparation known as emmenin. For the vulvovaginitis of infancy, the dosage should be 1,000 I.U. daily in the form of a vaginal suppository. The amount necessary to control menopausal symptoms will vary according to the amount of estrogen produced by the patient's own ovaries. The average dosage ranges from 6,000 to 60,000 I.U. weekly. In some instance, larger amounts will be needed.

The practical value of the estrogens has been somewhat limited due to the expense and the intramuscular mode of administration. These disadvantages have led investigators to seek other substances with estrogenic activity and a number of these have been synthesized. Stilbestrol, recently released for general consumption, is the most important. This substance, obtained from stilbene, differs chemically from the natural estrogens, but has all their biologic properties. It is relatively nontoxic, effective orally, and much cheaper than the natural estrogens. By various methods of comparison, different authorities give various value for the relative potency of one mg. of stilbestrol, compared with international units of estrone as follows: subcutaneously, one mg, equals 10,000 to 50,000 I.U.;[26-27-28-29-31] orally, one mg. equals 40,000 to 50,000 I.U.[27-28-29-30]

I have been fortunate in having had at my disposal a generous supply of this material which I have used in a large series of cases. A number of these patients had severe amenorrhea and were refractory to other forms of treatment. One milligram of stilbestrol daily for 25 days produced a menstrual flow in a high percentage of these difficult cases. Mild toxic reactions, chiefly nausea and vomiting have been observed. No serious reactions have been noticed. Reactions can be avoided somewhat by administering the drug at bedtime and combining it with small doses of phenobarbital.

Karnaky[32] reports successful results with the use of stilbestrol in stopping excessive uterine bleeding due to functional causes. Five to 25 mg. of stilbestrol in oil, according to the amount of bleeding, are given into the anterior lip of the cervix with a long needle and syringe. The patients can be kept from bleeding indefinitely. If the condition is not alarming and the bleeding mild, stilbestrol orally in five mg. doses daily can be used to control bleeding. Recently, I have had some success with this method.

Progesterone, the hormone of the corpus luteum, is now available commercially and has been used in a variety of conditions. In my own experience and that of others, it has proved to be of some value in cases of threatened abortion or functional uterine bleeding. Albright[33] states he has been using daily doses of five mg. for five consecutive days for the prolonged bleeding of glandular cystic hyperplasia. His objective is the production of endometrial regression. Zondek[34] reports he is using progesterone in a simplified treatment for amenorrhea. Fifty mg. of progesterone hypodermically or 300 mg. of pregneninolone orally over a two to five-day period are followed by bleeding.

The male hormone (testosterone propionate) has been the subject of intensive investigation regarding its action on the pituitary and on the female genital tract.[35-36-37-38] Its chief use in gynecology is for the control of uterine bleeding. Clinical reports indicate that daily doses of 25 mg. every other day for three or four days will usually control for the moment the severest forms of menorrhagia. Fairly complete control can be obtained by a monthly dose of 125 to 250 mg. If given in larger amounts, signs of masculinization may appear, as noted by Greenhill and Freed.[39] These are transitory and regress, for the most part, in a period of several months' time.

Thyroid is perhaps the most useful of all the hormones in the treatment of gynecological conditions. Its use is indicated in primary hypothyroidism and in hypothyroidism secondary to pituitary disease. In either condition the drug is given in doses sufficient to raise the basal metabolic rate to normal or until it produces symptoms. It is best always to start with a small dose, such as one-half grain each day, and to continue this dosage for a period of six weeks, at which time the metabolism is determined and the dosage increased by one-fourth to one-half grain. After another six weeks, the dosage is again increased by small amounts only. If symptoms appear before the metabolism reaches normal, the dosage should be reduced a little for a period of six to eight weeks and then increased again. It is almost impossible to find a patient who will not tolerate thyroid if given in this manner. Two points should be stressed. In the first place, there is frequently a paradoxical fall in the basal metabolic rate in spite of marked clinical improvement. Youmans and Riven[40] consider this a sign confirming the diagnosis and indicating good results. In the second place, in most cases of true primary hypothyroidism, the drug, once started, must be continued indefinitely. If it is discontinued, these patients return to their former disagreeable status and treatment has to be carried out all over again.

Radiation and surgery still occupy a prominent place in the treatment of menstrual disorders. Radiation may be depressive and destructive, or stimulative, as some term low-voltage dosage radiation. This latter has produced good results in the hands of Mazer[41] and others, and the dosage recommended apparently can do harm. However, there is still much to be learned concerning this form of treatment. Destructive radiation of the type employed near the menopause, (1,600 to 2,000 r) will, of course, stop bleeding and make the ovarian failure complete. In a carefully selected group of cases, this is the method of choice, but it should not be used in the younger age groups or in the cases in which the well-known contraindications exist. In the young patient extreme complications arise, frequently throwing her life out of balance; sexual, reproductive, and menstrual functions are lost; the major portion of the endocrine function disappears. Here, above all, preservation of useful function is mandatory.

In the consideration of surgery, we find curettage an excellent method to check bleeding temporarily and to allow time for specific measures to take effect. The endometrium thus obtained is valuable for ruling out carcinoma, and acting as an "indicator" tissue to determine the degree of ovarian involvement. In certain cases, hysterectomy associated with postoperative endocrine therapy is the most satisfactory means of treatment. I find myself frequently resorting to vaginal hysterectomy in those cases where there are associated pelvic lesions such as prolapse or cystocele; of course, as stated previously, an intensive investigation with the evaluation of the need for the menstrual and reproductive functions is considered for each individual; the preservation of useful function and the destruction of harmful disease is practiced with every patient to the fullest extent.

Fibroid tumors are a frequent cause for pelvic surgery. It has been shown by Nelson[42] (previously postulated by Witherspoon)[43] that these tumors have an endocrine significance. Not infrequently the tumors and ovaries are removed and an associated endocrine imbalance completely overlooked. In this connection, therefore, it is well to remember that surgery or destructive radiological procedures do not cure an endocrinopathy, but merely remove the symptoms and may exaggerate the underlying endocrine process. The endocrine status of these patients should be determined and they should be treated accordingly.

In conclusion let us again point out that the physiological approach invokes an appraisal of the patient's functional needs, of the functional disturbance, and of the physiological effect of treatment. Its watchwo. is the maintenance of useful function.

BIBLIOGRAPHY

1. TeLinde, R. W. Treatment of gonococcic vaginitis with estrogenic hormone: Further studies. J.A.M.A. 1938, 110:1683.
2. Russ, J. D. and O. G. Collins. The treatment of prepuberal vulvovaginitis with a new synthetic estrogen. J.A.M.A. 1940, 114:2446.
3. Wollner, A. A preliminary study of the cyclic histologic changes of the human cervical mucosa in the intermenstrual period. Amer. Jour. Obs. and Gyn. 1936, 32:365.
The physiology of the human cervical mucosa. Surg Gyn. and Obst. 1937, 64:758.
The histologic correlationship of endometrial and cervical biopsies. Amer. Jour. Obs. and Gyn. 1938, 36:10.
The etiology and treatment of endocervicitis and cervical erosions. Amer. Jour. Obs. and Gyn. 1939, 37:947.
4. Bourne, A. and L. T. Bond. Discussion on the pathology of cervicitis. Proc. Royal Soc. Med. 1940, 33:787.
5. Burch, J. C., G. S. McClellan et al. The diagnosis and classification of menstrual disorders. J.A.M.A. 1937, 108:96-101.
6. Idem: The menstrual problem. Southern M.J. 1938, 31:80-83.
7. Burch, J. C. The general significance of the disorders of menstrual interval and flow. International Clinics, 1937, 4:65-70.
8. Goldzieher, M. A. Relation of the anterior lobe to the specific dynamic action of protein. Association Research in Nervous and Mental Disease, Research Publications, 1938, 17: 536-546.

9. Hamblen, E. C. The clinical evaluation of ovarian responses to gonadotropic therapy. Endocrinology, 1939, 24: 848-866.
10. Greenblatt, R. R. and E. R. Pund. The gonadotropins: A clinical and experimental study. Southern Med Jour. 1941, 34:780-741.
11. Buxton, C. L. Certain gonadotropic extracts: Effects on anovulatory cycles and amenorrhea. Amer. Jour. Obst. and Gyn. 1941, 42:226.
12. Davis, M. E. and A. K. Koff. The experimental production of ovulation in the human subject. Amer. Jour. Obst. and Gyn. 1938, 36:188-199.
13. Siegler, S. L. Further experiences with the hormone of pregnant mare serum. Endocrinology, 1940, 27:387.
14. Hamblen, E. C. Endocrine therapy of functional menometrorrhagia and ovarian sterility. Jour. of Clin. Endocrinology. 1941, 1:211-221.
15. Rydberg, E. and E. Ostergaard. The effect of gonadotropic hormone treatment in amenorrhea. Acta Obst. et Gynec. Scandinav. 1939, 19:222-246.
16. Ellison, E. T. and J. C. Burch. The effect of estrogenic substances on the pituitary, adrenals and ovaries. Endocrinology, 1936, 20:746-752.
17. Sevringhaus, E. L. The relief of menopausal symptoms by estrogenic substances. J.A.M.A. 1935, 104:624-628.
18. Papanicolau, G. N. and E. Shorr. The action of ovarian follicular hormone in the menopause. Amer. Jour. Obst. and Gyn 1936, 31:806-831.
19. Pratt, J. P. and W. L. Thomas. The endocrine treatment of menopausal phenomena. J.A.M.A. 1937, 109:1875-1877.
20. Lewis, R. M. and E. L. Adler. Endocrine treatment of vaginitis of children and of women after the menopause. J.A.M.A. 1937, 109:1872-1875.
21. TeLinde, R. W. The treatment of gonococcic vaginitis with estrogenic hormone. J.A.M.A. 1938, 110:1633-1638.
22. Hawkinson, L. F. The menopause syndrome: Estrogen. J.A.M. 1936, 111:390.
23. Mazer, C. and S. L. Israel. The symptoms and treatment of the menopause. Med. Clinics of N.A. 1935, 19:205-226.
24. Wiesbader, H. and R. Jurzrok. The menopause. Endocrinology, 1938, 23:32-38.
25. Hamblen, E. C. Therapeutic use of the sex sterols in functional menometrorrhagia. Endocrinology, 1939, 24:13.
26. Dodds, E. C., W. Lawson and R. L. Noble. Lancet, 1938, 1:1389.
27. Emmens, C. W. Journal Physiology, 1939, 95:379.
28. Kreitmair, H. and Sieckmann, W. Klin. Wchnschr. 1939, 18:156.
29. Mazer, C., S. L. Israel and E. Ravetz. J.A.M.A. 1941, 116:675.
30. Leighty, J. A. and H. J. Wick. Endocrinology, 1939, 25:597.
31. Frank, R. T., M. A. Goldberger and G. Felshin. Endocrinology, 1940, 27:381.
32. Karnaky, K. J. Personal communication. Am. Jour. Obst. and Gyn. 1942, 43:385.
33. Albright, F. A.O.A. Lecture, Vanderbilt Medical School, March 19, 1942.
34. Zondek. B. Simplified hormonal treatment of amenorrhea. J.A.M.A. 1942, 118:765.
35. Freed, S. C., J. P. Greenhill and S. Soskin. Biphasic effect of male sex hormone on the pituitary. Proc. Soc. Exp. Biol. and Med. 1938, 59:440-442.
36. Gaines, J. A., U. J. Salmon and S H. Geist. Effect of testosterone propionate upon the endometrial cycle. Proc. Soc. Exp. Biol. and Med. 1938, 38:779-783.
37. Mazer, M. and C Mazer. The effect of prolonged testosterone propionate administration. Endocrinology, 1939, 24: 175-181.
38. Williams, C., D. Phelps and J. C. Burch. The effect of testosterone on experimentally produced endometrial hyperplasia in the guinea pig. Endocrinology, 1939, 25: 312-317.
39. Greenhill, J. P. and S C. Freed. Virilism in women. J.A.M.A. 1939, 112:1373-1574.
40. Youmans, J. B. and S. S. Riven. Hypothyroidism without myxedema. Annals of Internal Med. 1932, 5:1497.
41. Mazer, C. and G. Baer. The therapeutic value of low-dosage irradiation of the Pituitary gland and ovaries in functional menstrual disorders. Amer. Jour. Obst. and Gyn. 1939, 37:1015-1034.
42. Nelson, W. O. Endometrial and myometrial changes induced in the uterus of the guinea pig by the prolonged administration of estrogenic hormone. Anat. Rec. 1937, 68:99-102.
43. Witherspoon, J. T. Interrelationship between ovarian follicle cysts, hyperplasia of the endometrium and fibromyomata. Surg. Obst. and Gyn. 1933, 58:1026.

Obstetrical Psychosis*

BRUCE R. HINSON, M.D.

ENID, OKLAHOMA

All of us who care for women during gestation are more or less aware of and familiar with the physiological adjustments that must be made during this period, and in many instances we can take steps to relieve many of their discomforts. We also readily admit that these women are subject to unusual emotional stress, but all too few of us take adequate steps to help the patients to obtain a better emotional equilibrium. I feel that sometimes the emotional discomforts and anxieties that these women feel far outweigh any physiological adjustments that must be dealt with. By heeding such symptoms as unusual irritability, persistent insomnia, and feeling of confusion we might do a great deal to prevent the development of a serious psychosis, or deepseated neurosis that would result in invalidism.

Approximately nine percent of all females committed to institutions for the mentally ill date their illness from a pregnancy. About 75 such women are committed to Oklahoma State mental hospitals each year. Formerly when certain mental symptoms appeared in pregnant women, doctors referred to these symptoms as a psychosis of pregnancy, considering this condition a clinical entity, but at present it is the concensus of opinion of psychiatrists that the psychoses appearing during or following pregnancy do not differ from the psychoses appearing in non-pregnant women. Any strain comparable to a pregnancy might precipitate the same mental difficulty. There are many instances in which women who have had preceding psychotic episodes develop very similar psychotic findings with pregnancy. The psychosis of pregnancy is not an uncommon occurrence, but appears less often than some sequelae. It is estimated that a psychosis appears about once in every 400 to 500 deliveries. This has been borne out by my personal experiences.

We classify the psychoses of pregnant women not only as to the type of psychosis, such as toxic-exhaustive, manic-depressive, or schizophrenic, but as to the time of its occurrence, whether during pregnancy, the puerperium, or lactation period. Any one of these three types of psychosis may appear in any one of the three stages mentioned; however, we usually see the toxic-exhaustive type in the latter weeks of pregnancy or late in the lactation period.

The toxic-exhaustive falls into a class of its own because as a rule it is obviously the result of a definite organic disturbance, such as puerperal sepsis, toxemia of late pregnancy, post-partum hemorrhage, prolonged nursing of the baby, or general debility. The psychosis usually disappears when the organic disturbance has been relieved. Atkin, 1938, reported acute delirium and prolonged confusion in the puerperium as the result of severe secondary anemia, and all patients were completely relieved by restoring the blood picture to normal by use of various iron compounds and liver concentrates. The toxic-exhaustive psychosis is the usual type that results from prolonged lactation, and is found more commonly in multiparous women who are malnourished, overburdened with the care of their other children, and who nurse their babies well into the second year. The condition is usually relieved by weaning the baby, taking away part of the mother's burdens or responsibilities, and initiating steps to help her regain a physiological equilibrium. She should also be placed under the care of a competent psychiatrist.

This type of psychosis is characterized by acute delirium and confusion arising from profound toxemia or exhaustion, and is not necessarily dependent upon previous emotional instability. The severity of the psychosis has a definite relation to the severity of the toxemia, and the psychosis is usually relieved when the toxin is removed. Individuals developing this toxic-exhaustive type, and who also have a neuropathic taint as a rule make a slower recovery and are given a poorer prognosis even though the toxin is removed. This group, as a rule, carries a high mortality, not because of the psychosis, but because of the underlying pathology. It takes a fairly normal physical constitution to withstand successfully a psychosis. According to F. M. Adams of the Eastern Oklahoma Hospital, individuals suffering from this type of psychosis give a much graver prognosis than do the manic-depressive and schizophrenic types. Of their admissions in the past five years, they have had an 80 percent mortality from this type of psychosis,

*Read before the Section on Obstetrics and Gynecology, Annual Session, Oklahoma State Medical Association, April 23, 1942, in Tulsa.

with almost the reverse being true of the manic-depressive and dementia-praecox types.

The psychoses appearing during gestation most commonly occur in the last trimester, and the vast majority are in women with a definite neuropathic or psychopathic taint. Many of them, have had previous definite mental illnesses. The majority of them will be found to have been emotionally unstable, queer, and anti-social. Piker, 1938, found, in reviewing 946 cases of psychoses of pregnancy, that 24 percent of them occurred during pregnancy, and 76 percent occurred postpartum. The common types of psychoses developing during gestation are schizophrenia and the depressed phase of manic-depressive, although we do see some acute confusion and delirium in the latter months as a result of concurrent toxemia.

Quoting from McGeorge, 1938, *Mental Disorder and Childbirth,* "Pregnancy indirectly may give rise to a variety of conditions. For example, the fear of what should be a natural physiological process, engendered by reports of the maternal death rate, may result in an hysterical reaction. Pregnancy may be a period of mental stress to a perfectly healthy woman to which its associated pain and danger makes it an ordeal. It is even more so to one who is psychologically unstable. The presence of bodily disease and toxemia increases the danger of the development of psychopathic symptoms; for the toxemia alone is sufficient for this. . . . All authorities agree that revulsion to husband and child is a common feature of this form of mental disorder. The patient becomes very suspicious, depressed, and jealous, and suicidal tendencies are often evident."

Termination of the pregnancy because of the appearance of a psychosis does not alter the course of the psychotic process, unless it is due purely to an acute toxemia. Termination of the pregnancy might have a deleterious psychological effect in itself. Abortions, whether accidental or induced, may result in a depressive or confusional state because of disappointment or self-reproach.

I recall that during my internship I delivered a woman of her third child, all three of her children having been delivered in the sanitarium. The patient was admitted each time one month preceding delivery with an acute depression and marked suicidal tendencies, and each time, within two month following delivery, was discharged and remained well until her next pregnancy.

The onset of the purely functional type may be quite insidious, being preceded for several weeks by the patient complaining of sleeplessness, anxiety, indifference, and depression; or the onset may be very sudden, and the psychosis appear complete, the patient being almost uncontrollable within a period of a few hours.

My records show one patient, aged 26, primipara, having a perfectly normal prenatal course, with no evidence of toxemia until one month before delivery, when suddenly in the middle of the night, she awoke hallucinating, was disoriented, had bizarre delusions and hallucinations. She was given constant attendance the following month and subsequently delivered, without difficulty, normal full-term twins. Following delivery there was an increase in her psychotic symptoms, and she was transferred to a mental hospital. Six weeks later she was successful in a suicide attempt.

According to most authorities, psychoses developing in the latter weeks of pregnancy give a better prognosis than those appearing in the very early months, but this has not been my experience.

If the obstetrician is to serve his patient well he must have knowledge of the patient's previous emotional stability. Inquiry should certainly be made into previous nervous conditions and information obtained as to the emotional stability of the patient's immediate family. With this knowledge the doctor will be forewarned if the patient has apparent pre-psychotic symptoms. By taking adequate steps to combat insomnia, increasing irritabiltiy, and moodiness he may be able to forestall a serious mental breakdown. If necessary, an attempt should be made to lessen the family difficulties and responsibilities of the patient. Adequate sleep is an absolute requirement, and sedatives should be given in sufficient quantity to obtain rest. The usual barbiturates will suffice.

Seventy-five percent of the women developing psychotic symptoms do not do so until after delivery. The time of onset varies from one week post-partum to 14 or 16 months. In this group we find many cases that are due purely to toxemia and have no hereditary taint as a foundation for their illness. This toxic type is usually violent, appears suddenly, and as a rule runs a relatively short course, either to recovery or fatality. Many of these die, not as a result of their psychosis but, as I have pointed out elsewhere, as a result of their underlying sepsis or toxemia. With immediate and proper care for the toxemia, some of these women will make an uneventful and complete recovery from their psychotic symptoms. Those that die of their psychoses usually are suicides. Individuals that carry the unfavorable prognosis and have the longest recovery time are those that have had previous mental illnesses or have a definitely bad heredity.

The care of these people after delivery should be in the hands of a competent psychiatrist. Those presenting depressed symptoms of a manic-depressive psychosis can be given a fairly good prognosis for that particular phase, but no assurance can be given as to the possibility of recurrence; however, the probability is that with each subsequent pregnancy there will be a return of the psychosis. The advisability of further pregnancies depends entirely upon each individual case, and the patient should rely on the judgment of the psychiatrist.

Probably the most serious type of psychosis is a schizophrenia developing in the early weeks following delivery. The onset is usually slow, appearing in individuals who have had definite schizoid personalities. They have always been more or less seclusive, solitary, and sensitive, and given to day-dreaming. With the onset of their illness they ordinarily become indifferent, caring little about their personal appearance, their social obligations, and their usual work. This indifference occasionally extends to actual neglect of the new baby. Many cases of infanticide are the direct result of an unrecognized schizophrenia. All of these individuals are institutional cases. It is impossible to predict what they might do next. They do not show the marked suicidal tendencies of the depressed manic-depressive. They commit suicide usually by accident rather than by design.

Before the advent of various types of shock treatment for schizophrenia, this type of psychosis, appearing post-partum, was given a very grave prognosis. It still carries a more serious outlook than does the manic-depressive type. Since the introduction of the insulin, the metrozol, and electric shock treatments, the outlook for the schizophrenic patient is much brighter. As a rule they have a longer recovery time and their recovery is less complete than the other forms of psychosis. Few psychiatrists will trust the recovery to the extent that they will advise subsequent pregnancies.

At present I have a patient with a schizophrenic remission of one year's standing. Very suddenly she developed a hebophrenic phase of schizophrenia about six weeks post-partum. She had a very definite neurotic history, but had delivered one normal, full-term child two years previously without any mental difficulty. She became fairly well stabilized after about 35 shock treatments, and four months confinement in a mental hospital. At present she is at home doing very well, but under reduced responsibilities.

SUMMARY

1. There is no true psychosis of pregnancy. The pregnancy merely acts as the precipitating cause, similar to any other stresses that bring on a psychosis.

2. The obstetrician may do his patient a great service by properly evaluating her emotional stability.

3. Active treatment of the prodromal symptoms may avoid the precipitation of a psychosis.

4. The new advances in psychiatric treatment have given these patients a much better prognosis.

5. The advice of a psychiatrist should be sought, and his recommendations followed from the earliest development of serious symptoms.

REFERENCES

McGeorge, John: Mental Disorder and Childbirth, Medical Journal of Australia, 11:671 (October 22) 1938.
Piker, Phillip: Psychoses complicating childbearing, American Journal of Obstetrics and Gynecology, 35:901 (May) 1938.
Atkin, I.: Post-partum Macrocytic Anaemia Associated with Confusional States, Lancet, 234:434 (February 19) 1938.
Titus: 2nd Edition, Management of Obstetric Difficulties; Chapter 35, Complications of Puerperium.

DISCUSSION

COYNE H. CAMPBELL, M.D.
OKLAHOMA CITY, OKLAHOMA

This has been an excellent presentation of a very important clinical problem. Dr. Hinson has given an accurate summary of available information and has correlated this with his own experiences. There is really very little to add and the discussion can best be directed toward emphasis upon certain facts.

Although a psychosis appears only about once in every 400 to 500 deliveries; it should be mentioned that borderline psychotic states and distressing neurotic symptoms complicate the gestation and post partum periods with at least an equal if not a greater frequency than the occurrence of psychoses.

A study of the personality background of the pregnant woman is very important. If the individual develops emotional instability in relationship to pregnancy, and if a careful study reveals no evidence of previous similar distress; a toxemia arising out of some definitely discernible organic pathology should be assumed.

The toxic-exhaustive psychoses are perhaps more specific than other types, and constitute a very serious problem, with a high mortality rate.

It has been correctly pointed out that there is no such thing as a psychosis of pregnancy. This may be said in relationship to all of the so-called "functional" psychoses, because as yet nothing is really known regarding a specific etiology of these disorders. Even such assumed clinical entities as dementia-praecox, involutional psychoses and manic depressive psychoses so overlap in their manifestations that the diagnosis of either one is a mere name for something about which very little is understood.

It is likely that the content of delusions are largely conditioned by current problems of the individual. The frequent occurrence of, and fears of impulses in the mother, that she may injure, or even murder the infant, would be replaced by some other type of impulse under different conditions of stress. The above symptomatology constitutes, however, the only specificity with reference to the psychoses of pregnancy.

A careful study of 50 consecutive cases who have come under personal observation reveals that those who develop psychotic symptoms early in pregnancy have the most unfavorable prognosis. Those who develop symptoms insidiously after three or more months following delivery also offer a serious prognosis. The patients who develop psychoses immediately following delivery or acutely in the late gestation period have shown a more favorable recovery rate.

The symptoms of anxiety, insomnia, obsessions, fears, and depression that occur during pregnancy and following delivery should be treated by correction of any physical complications, suggestive therapy reassurance, and sedation. Sodium amytal has proven to be the drug of choice. If adequate response to this treatment does not occur, the physician should suspect the possibility of a malignant psychiatric disorder.

A careful inventory of the personality background in every obstetrical case should be made by the physician. Certainly a history of prevoius nervous breakdown or severe emotional instability should place the physician on guard as to the probability of a potential psychosis. Psychiatric consultation is necessary in circumstances under which malignant symptoms such as hallucinations and extreme depression become manifest, and in those instances when the more minor symptoms do not respond to ordinary therapy.

A careful investigation as to the existence of organic toxic disturbances should of course first be made. As Doctor Hinson has pointed out, advising relatives to whether the patient should become pregnant again is an individual matter, but as a rule it is well to advise sterilization at an appropriate time following recovery from the psychosis in those with a history of inadequate personality structure prior to pregnancy.

Shock therapy cannot be used during pregnancy but has been given without complications as early as one week following delivery. It is certainly the treatment of choice in the depressions with suicidal tendencies. Electric and metrazol shock are used in these cases. Perhaps insulin treatment is preferable in the schizophrenic psychoses that come on insidiously. Electric and metrazol are used with fair results in the acute schizophrenic disorders. The toxic exhaustive psychoses are treated by an attempted removal of the cause for the toxemia, adequate food and fluid intake, proper elimination, supportive measures of various types, hydrotherapy, vitamin therapy, and in selected cases, electro-shock may be tried.

Early treatment of the beginning symptoms as emphasized by Doctor Hinson is most important and undoubtedly is preventive of later serious complications.

Hygiene in the Tropics[*]

WALKER MORLEDGE, M.D.
OKLAHOMA CITY, OKLAHOMA

This paper is the result of a request by some of the younger physicians in Oklahoma City for a statement about life in the tropics. These young men believe that some of them might be called upon to live or do medical service in a tropical climate. The basis of my knowledge of life in a hot climate is seven years spent in Zululand, South Africa. A part of this time was devoted to medical mission work and a part to service for the South African government.

Life in the tropics differs from life in Oklahoma in the following ways: (1) excessive heat; (2) excessive moisture; (3) the presence of numerous insects with the prevalence of insect-born diseases; (4) poor hygienic standards of tropical people; (5) danger of moral and physical degeneration due to the above factors.

HEAT

Anyone who has spent a summer in Oklahoma can appreciate what prolonged and excessive heat can do to one's energy and initiative. In the tropics the excessive heat is continuous, and causes profuse perspiration. In many tropical climates there is excessive moisture in the atmosphere which interferes with the evaporation of perspiration. This causes clothing to feel sticky and clammy

*Read before the Section on General Medicine, Annual Session, Oklahoma State Medical Association, April 22, 1942, in Tulsa.

and the individual is not cooled as he is in a dry climate. Increase in perspiration leads to a decreased urinary output and easy fatigueability. With hot nights one does not awaken rested and refreshed in the morning. Food spoils easily. Frequently, owing to the retarded state of civilization, ice is not available nor is electricity for the preservation of food. This means that in many places in the tropics canned foods, including milk, and hot drinks, must replace fresh foods and iced drinks. Moreover, fresh vegetables which have been raised under proper conditions of sanitation frequently are not available. Respiratory diseases, scarlet fever, and acute rheumatism are much less frequent in the tropics, but there are many more cases of gastro-intestinal infections and insect-born diseases, such as malaria, dengue fever, yellow fever, sleeping sickness, etc.

MOISTURE

Excessive moisture in the atmosphere is depressing, even in a temperate zone. An excessive moisture with a temperature in the 90's or above saps one's energy and initative. His clothing is damp, mildew gathers on clothes, leather goods, and on walls. To prevent mildew leather goods and clothes must be dried and sunned. If electricity is absent, fans are not available. During my stay in the tropics, air conditioning was unknown.

THE PRESENCE OF INSECTS

Life is a constant battle against insects. One must always be on his guard against mosquito bites. The battle to prevent mosquitoes from breeding and multiplying is unceasing. Houses must be screened and the screen doors kept closed. The screen must be of mesh small enough to exclude the fly and mosquito. Even in a screened house it is safer to sleep under a mosquito net, but that does not add to the person's comfort. The prudent householder in the tropics makes at least one weekly inspection of his premises to see that there are no stagnant pools of water. No tin cans or old glass should be allowed around the premises, for if they contain water, they are potenial breeding places for mosquitoes. No roof gutter pipe can be allowed to become obstructed; no mud puddle can be tolerated; even the palm trees must be inspected to be sure that no water collects between the branches and the trunk. Irrigation trenches have to be kept clean. In other words, every breeding place of the mosquito must be eliminated if at all possible.

During my stay in Africa a severe epidemic of malaria was spread by sugar cane. This cane was cut in areas where mosquitoes were infected, then transported some miles by rail. It was noted when the cane was unloaded that many mosquitoes flew out from the cane, and a very severe epidemic

followed in this community. An infected mosquito can be carried by automobile, rail, or airplane, thus spreading either malaria, dengue, or yellow fever through distant communities.

The British in North Africa have lessened the instances of gastro-intestinal infection at least 50 percent by a constant battle against flies. This was accomplished by destroying refuse in which flies breed, by screening cooking quarters and by supplementing these methods of extermination by swatting, traps, and other means. When one remembers that in the Boor War and the Spanish-American War that more men died by gastro-intestinal causes than were killed by guns, the importance of the relationship between food and flies is at once apparent. Tropical ants are large and often vicious. They crawl into one's clothes if one lies on the ground. Their bite is agonizing and may result in severe infection.

POOR LOCAL HYGIENE

In most localities civilization is not far advanced. To date the white man with his advanced civilization has been kept from the hot climates partly by malaria and partly because he prefers the temperate zone. The other races which live in the tropics are not so energetic, they have low standards of morals, and usually are ignorant and superstitious. Intestinal disease and intestinal parasites abound. It is most difficult for a physician to instill into the minds of ignorant people who have no conception of bacteria, ideas of modern sanitation. If the native African believes that disease comes as a curse or as the result of evil spirits, it is hard for him to become enthusiastic about the destruction of mosquitoes and the draining of swamps. In the same way, it is hard to impress upon the tropical cook boy the need for sanitary measures in the preparation of food. The heat and moisture of the tropics affect the native, and thus help conduce his ignorance and indolence. The white man in the tropics is likely to suffer from ennui, and to relax his own physical and moral standards. Because of the lack of suitable amusement and activities, some white men have immoral association with native girls, many of whom have syphilis. Some drink excessively to relieve the monotony of life, hence the white man in the tropics needs to be warned of these dangers.

CLOTHING

For protection of the head the old sun helmet has proved its worth, but many helmets are hot and uncomfortable. A light double felt hat with some air spaces between the two hats is more satisfactory. The danger of sun stroke is always present. During the hot hours of the day one should, if possible, try to be in the shade. Though sunstroke may occur, it is not common. Most cases so reported are tropical malaria. If one is not exposed to direct sunshine, shorts, and shirts with short sleeves, open at the neck are preferable. To keep up one's morale, he should shave and dress for dinner.

FOOD

In the preparation of food it is most important to have intelligent and well-trained servants, if possible, servants who know something about hygiene and are intelligent enough to appreciate its value. One should never overeat or overdrink. As mentioned above, electricity and ice may not be available, and this rules out fresh meat, with the exception of chicken. The banana with its thick skin is rarely contaminated by dis ease. Vegetables should be washed very thoroughly, for they might have been raised in unhygienic surroundings.

WATER

Unless one is certain about the water supply, it is best to drink hot tea. This usually causes perspiration and thus helps to cool the body. Or, boiled water can be put in a porous earthen jar and hung where the breeze can strike it. The water slowly seeping to the surface, leads to rapid evaporation and cools the jar. Such water will be many degrees cooler in temperature than the surrounding air.

SLEEPING QUARTERS

As mentioned above, the sleeping room must be carefully screened and in every malaria-infected district it is wise to have in addition a mosquito net on a frame to drop over one's bed. Before turning out the light, the net should be lowered down over the bed, tucked in around the mattress, and the space underneath the net carefully inspected to be sure no mosquito is imprisoned. The net adds very little to the heat, but it certainly gives the sleeper a feeling of security. If one has to sleep in the open, he should have a net by all means. Smoke from fires and tobacco may help to drive away mosquitoes. The mosquito repellants such as oil of citronella or cod liver oil rubbed on the exposed surfaces helps somewhat to prevent mosquito bites.

MALARIA

Malaria has been the chief factor in keeping the white man out of the tropics. It may have been malaria which defeated Hannibal in the plains of Italy before he met the armies of Rome. Malaria may have been one of the causes for the overthrow of ancient Greece. Repeated military campaigns with resultant neglect of farm land and the development of swamps would result in malarial increases. It is known that some of the Grecian people lost their vigor and initiative

and developed large spleens. The same might be said of the ancient Romans. It was malaria which prevented the French from building the Panama Canal. The malaria mosquito bites usually just before and after sunrise and just before and after sunset. If one can avoid being out at these hours, he may escape malarial infection. The question of atabrine and quinine for malarial prophylaxis is still debatable. However, if one has but a short period of duty in malaria-infected country and must be out at all hours, I believe it is wise to take at least ten grains of quinine daily to prevent the development of the infection.

In bathing, especially on the east coast of Africa, in Egypt, southern India, and Maylaia, one must remember the danger of bilharzia. This is contracted by bathing or washing in infected water, as well as drinking it. The disease is characterized by passing blood in the urine or bloody stools. It is so common in Egypt that no British soldier has been allowed to bathe or wade in the Nile or its tributaries. The organism cannot live in salt water. In salt water bathing, however, one must always remember the presence of sharks. These are supposed not to swim in active breakers.

SKIN INFECTIONS

Due to heat and moisture, skin infections are more prevalent and more difficult to heal than in other climates. Small abrasions and mosquito bites need to be sterilized and carefully protected so that infection will not develop. The treatment of snake bite is too long to be discussed in this paper.

The British have had more experience in tropical life than almost any other white people. In more than half of their cases where civil servants are sent home because of ill health, the etiology has been found to be nervous breakdowns and neurosthenia. The children of white parents in tropical climates tend to grow tall and gangling with a mild anemia. To some extent this tendency can be obviated by having the children spend the hottest part of the year in the mountains. If one is stationed in a tropical climate, he should ask the advice of either native residents or servants about the prevalence of malaria, intestinal disease, etc., about the danger of local bathing, and then take proper steps to protect his own health.

In this paper malaria has been mentioned repeatedly. It is a most serious disease and in tropical countries often it is deadly. The newcomer in the tropics must treat it with the utmost respect and do his best to avoid contracting the disease. If malaria and intestinal parasites can be avoided, a sojourn in the tropics should prove to be interesting and instructive without serious effect on subsequent health.

Coronary Thrombosis

FLOYD MOORMAN, M.D.

OKLAHOMA CITY, OKLAHOMA

The circulation of the heart is not only of immense importance, but it is peculiar in that it constitutes the blood supply to a muscle, which is maintained by that muscle's own contraction.

In 1708 Thebesius, followed later by Haller, Morgagni and Senac, by careful dissections, came to the conclusion that anastomoses exist between both coronary arteries. Haller stated that these were quite rich and occurred with frequency at the root of the pulmonary artery, in the posterior sulcus longitudinalis, in the right ventricle, at the apex of the heart, on the surface of the ventricles and through the vasa vasorum of the great vessels.

1799 Parry and Jenner first interpreted the clinical syndrome known as angina pectoris as due to calcification of the coronary arteries and the autopsy findings on John Hunter's heart, after Jenner had diagnosed his condition, corroborated this view.

Many other investigators made reports pro and con as to anastomoses between the coronary arteries.

In 1880 Langor showed that anastomoses exist between the coronary arteries and those of the pericardium, and through these, with the internal mammary artery. He showed further that by means of the vasa vasorum of the pulmonary artery, connection also takes place with the bronchial arteries and through branches from the auricles, with the diaphragm.

In 1907 Spalteholz employed a chrome-yellow suspension in gelatine for injections with subsequent dehydration and clearing in benzol and carbon disulphide. By this method he was able to obtain a reconstruction of the cardiac circulation which was vastly superior to anything hitherto obtained. His conclusions were as follows:

(a) No end arteries exist in the heart.
(b) Rich anastomoses occur in all layers of the heart and, through the vasa vasorum, on the great vessels.
(c) In the thick muscle of the left ventricle, perpendicular vessels penetrate to anastomoses under the endocardium.
(d) The papillary muscles are particularly rich in anastomoses.
(e) With growth, the appearance of the vessels on the surface shows a typical alteration.

In 1921 Gross[1] published his classic mono-him to the opinion that anastomoses exist and that the condition of the heart musculature and potency of the vessels played an important part in determining the degree of compensation which can take place after obliteration. He suggested that the vessels of Thebesius might serve as accessory nutritive channels in such cases.

In 1921 Gross[1] published his classic monograph "The Blood Supply to the Heart." His work consists of the study of 100 hearts at different age periods in which he injected barium sulfate suspension in gelatine. After injection, the hearts were x-rayed stereoscopically, cleared and then dissected and sectioned. His conclusions were as follows:

(a) Anastomoses exist between the right and left coronary arteries both in their capillary as well as precapillary distribution.
(b) Anastomoses exist between the branches of each coronary artery.
(c) Anastomoses in the heart are universal and abundant.

He also states that there is still no accurate knowledge of the exact nature as well as architectural arrangement of these anastomoses and that after a very careful study of this question he came to the conclusion that the heart is perhaps the richest organ in the body as regards capillary and precapillary anastomoses between branches of the same coronary artery as well as between branches from both coronaries.

The older the individual the more free and patent are the anastomoses. An old heart, is therefore much more prepared to receive with relatively little or no damage, the brunt of a sudden obliteration of a nutrient vessel.

Herrick[2] stated that a gradual obliteration of a vessel allows time for the existing anastomoses to widen and compensation to take place. Here Gross has shown that the arteriae telae adiposae are of considerable importance. These are what may be called fat branches. They are seen in greatest number in the fat under the pericardium, namely, in the grooves between the chambers and over the sites of the main coronary branches, where they exist as delicate parallel accompanying vessels whose distance from the main branches varies directly with the amount of fat present. They also form a rich network of interanastomosing delicate vessels upon the outer coats of the root of the aorta and the pulmonary artery. These fat vessels arise largely from the first portions of the right and left circumflex arteries.

According to Wearn and his collaborators there exist in addition to anastomoses between branches of the coronary system, anastomoses between branches of the coronaries and those branches of the aorta which supply the pericardium. There are also arterioluminal vessels which connect the coronaries directly with the ventricular cavities, arteriosinusiodal vessels also connecting the coronaries with the ventricular cavities through myocardial sinusoids, and the Thebesian veins. Flow in these vessels increases when the coronaries are gradually blocked and then it may proceed in the reverse of the normal direction. The passage of dyes into the heart wall from the coronary sinus has also been described after experimental occlusion of the coronaries. It is possible that in early diastole the pressure in the right auricle may be adequate to move blood along in the reverse direction through Thebesian veins into the ventricle. The possibility that the heart obtains enough oxygen for light work, even from venous blood, is great, in view of its capacity to utilize the whole of the oxygen carried.

Clinical and experimental studies have demonstrated that there is often an extensive anastomosis between the right and left coronary arteries and between the branches of these arteries. This anastomosis exists chiefly between the smaller arterioles and probably, in the capillary bed. At times, the heart is capable of withstanding even extensive interference of the blood supply through the development of an effective collateral circulation. Instances are not infrequently encountered at necropsy in which the heart has recovered in a surprising fashion from the occlusion of one of the main branches of the coronary arteries. Smith[3] observed a case in which the descending branch of the left coronary artery was ligated in the repair of a stab wound of the heart, and following recovery from the operation, there was no apparent impairment in the cardiac function.

The first case of coronary occlusion correctly diagnosed during life was reported by Dr. Adam Hammer of St. Louis. He saw the patient in consultation on May 4, 1876 and gave a masterly description of the history and physical findings, part of which I will here repeat. "The percussion of the cardiac area showed no abnormal dullness, the heart could be outlined on the chest without great difficulty and as far as position and size were concerned must be considered as normal. Percussion of the lungs also showed no dullness, so that one was justified in excluding a

pleuritic effusion as well as pneumonia or any other infiltration. Auscultation of the lungs showed everywhere normal respiratory sounds, only here and there were a few fine rales, such as commonly occur in marked hyperemia of the lungs.

"The auscultation of the heart however, showed some remarkable findings. The heart beat was weak, one every eight seconds. Upon the sound of each systole and diastole which although weak could be clearly made out and were without any murmur, there followed immediately a clonic spasm of the heart, which beat forcibly upon the applied ear with a sort of rustling, lasted exactly five seconds with the same intensity and then ceased as if cut off. I can compare these rapid successive twitchings of the heart muscle with nothing better than with the marked tremor of the hand of a man who is suffering from delirium tremens.

"What impressed me particularly about this case and attracted my attention in the highest degree, was the sudden appearance and the steadily progressive course of the collapse. I thought that only a sudden, progressively increasing disturbance in the nutrition of the heart itself such as a cutting off of the supply of nourishment could produce such changes as this case showed, and that such an obstruction could be produced only by a thrombotic occlusion of at least one of the coronary arteries. From lack of ground for any other satisfactory explanation, I was carried away by this thought. I mentioned my conviction to my colleague at the bedside. He, however, had a nonplussed expression and burst out 'I have never heard of such a diagnosis in my whole life' and I answered 'nor I also.' "

Permission for an autopsy was obtained from the relatives. The autopsy findings confirmed the diagnosis. Hammer remarks that obtaining of an autopsy in America is attended by great difficulties and goes on to say, "How often have I purchased this permission by giving up my fee for professional services and in certain cases I have had to pay money out of my pocket in order to succeed."

Doctor Hammer returned to Europe in 1877 and this case was reported in Vienna in 1878.

In 1896 George Dock published the first account of a case of coronary thrombosis in America diagnosed during life and confirmed by autopsy findings.

During the years that it has been my privilege to practice medicine no condition has interested me more than coronary thrombosis. Thirty years ago very little was known about the clinical manifestations of acute obstruction of the coronary arteries. Herrick in 1912 gave one of the earliest clinical descriptions and emphasized the fact that the condition need not be fatal.

ETIOLOGY

Heredity seems to play an important part. In the majority of cases atheroma is to blame; this consists of senile softening with yellowish fatty areas in the endarterium. Thickening and calcification ensue and the arteries may become brittle. The frequency of coronary disease in myxedema supports the idea of a factor of disturbed metabolism.

Syphilis, rheumatic disease and diabetes have seemed to be an etiological factor in some cases. Congenital abnormalities of the coronary arteries may rarely be a cause.

Many other factors such as tobacco, alcohol, high protein diet, overwork, infection and faulty metabolism have been mentioned, but none have been proved or consistently found. Hypertension is frequently followed by general arteriosclerosis, including sclerosis of the coronary arteries.

Coronary disease predominates in males, various studies giving ratios ranging from 4:1 to 7:1.

Leary in 1934, after detailed microscopic study in a large group of cases of coronary sclerosis thought that the changes represented a disturbance in the lipoid metabolism of the body.

Willius[4] made a study of the plasma lipoids in coronary disease and in normal persons as controls. The patients comprised those of the fourth to the eighth decades inclusive. The lipoids studies included cholesterol, cholesterol esters, lecithin, fatty acids and total lipoids. This study consisted of 107 cases of coronary sclerosis and 200 cases in the control series. The results were rather striking in that he found a significant increase in all the lipoids in the patients with coronary sclerosis.

Some interesting speculations may be introduced as a result of these studies. For instance, man is the only known creature that dies relatively young from coronary disease and if he attains an advanced age, atherosclerosis universally develops. Furthermore, man is the only known creature who, from soon after birth to old age partakes of a diet relatively high in fat, including such foods as milk, cream, butter, eggs and animal fats. Atherosclerotic lesions closly resembling those of man have been experimentally produced in herbivorous animals, notably in rabbits, by the feeding of diets rich in cholesterol. It thus seems probable that some relationship between hyperlipemia and atherosclerosis exists.

Willius goes on to say that the lipoid hypothesis of coronary disease, becomes of special interest for it offers the only tenable explanation to date of the discrepancy in incidence, according to sex. It is acknowledged that, during pregnancy, the storage of lipoid in the body is greatly increased as part of a physiologic reaction for the nutrition of the developing fetus. It, therefore, appears logical to suggest that women are endowed with a more active and perhaps more perfect metabolism, which permits them to utilize completely the recurrent excesses of stored lipoid and to accomplish this without incurring arterial deposition. Men, apparently, are not endowed with such an active and perfect lipoid metabolism.

During recent years there has been some differences of opinion as to the part that unusual exertion or emotion might play in precipitating a coronary accident. Paterson[5] states that actually there is definite evidence to prove that hours or even days elapse between the time of the inception of the thrombus and the moment when occlusion, with its resulting cardiac pain, occurs. He reports two cases that came to necropsy and in which the pathologic study revealed that formation of a thrombus was a gradual and not a rapid process and says that in order to eliminate physical exertion or emotion as a precipitating factor in coronary thrombosis, the activities of the patient should be investigated not only for the few hours prior to the attack but for many days previously. He gives two principal factors which appear to be involved in the mechanism of capillary rupture: (1) softening, by atheroma, of the tissues surrounding and supporting the capillary wall, (2) high intracapillary blood pressure.

The age incidence of coronary thrombosis and intimal hemorrhage corresponds roughly with that in which atheroma usually develops, i.e. late middle life. Intimal capillaries, because they arise directly from the main coronary lumen, are exposed constantly to a relatively high blood pressure and because of their peculiar position, will be sensitive to sudden increases in the coronary blood pressure and should this occur, these capillaries will be in imminent danger of dilatation and rupture, particularly if the surrounding tissues are in a state of laxity from atheromatous degeneration.

James B. Herrick[6] presents a number of conditions which he has seen mistaken for coronary thrombosis and which should be mentioned in this discussion. Angina pectoris and coronary thrombosis are closely related pathologically. Thrombosis may be an incident in the history of frequently recurring angina of effort. From the standpoint of prognosis and treatment, it is worth while to distinguish, if possible, between the pain brought on by effort, which disappears after rest and use of nitrates, and the more enduring pain which may come on without provocative effort and is accompanied by shock, dyspnea, arrhythmia, fever, leukocytosis, and altered electrocardiogram. The one condition speaks for a temporary relative ischemia of the cardiac muscle, the other for a more permanent ischemia. It should be remembered also that in some cases recurring attacks of angina are the sequelae of thrombosis and that angina of effort may cease after a coronary occlusion has converted the area of muscle that previously caused the pain into a scarred area, practically dead, inert and painless.

Arrhythmias: Cardiac irregularities not dependent on a coronary lesion may stimulate acute coronary obstruction, particularly if they occur in suddenly developing paroxysms—extrasystoles, auricular fibrillation or flutter. All the classical signs and symptoms of coronary occlusion (precordial pain, fever, leukocytosis, feeble pulse, low blood pressure and inversion of the T wave in the various leads of the electrocardiogram) may frequently occur at the onset of paroxysmal auricular tachycardia. It has also been pointed out that the coronary T wave of the electrocardiogram may occur in pericarditis with effusion.

Frank cases of neurocirculatory asthenia may usually be easily recognized. On the other hand, this condition may present a difficult puzzle.

The pain and distressed breathing, together with changes in cardiac action due to syphilitic aortitis, with or without definite aneurism, may be misinterpreted. So may the sudden severe pain of a dissecting aneurism—which occurs usually in a non-syphilitic individual with hypertension, with its shock and frequently altered heart rate and rhythm. Rupture of the aorta into the pericardial sac, a not uncommon termination of dissecting aneurism, may resemble acute coronary thrombosis.

Cases of pleurisy, pneumonia, carcinoma of the bronchus and massive collapse of the lung have been mistaken for acute coronary obstruction.

Acute spontaneous pneumothorax has been the cause of the error. An embolus, perhaps a thrombus, in the pulmonary artery, unless the embolus is small, may cause symptoms that mimic those seen in the fulminant type of acute coronary obstruction. Herpes Zoster may be a source of diagnostic error, at least until the skin lesion appears and is recognized.

Symptoms caused by abdominal conditions may simulate those of a cardiac accident. To remember this possibility and to exclude these causes first is usually all that is necessary.

Coronary thrombi are not unusual in diabetics, who are prone to have arteriosclerosis. Oncoming coma may simulate a coronary attack. On the other hand, one must not too hastily diagnose chronic unrecognized diabetes in a patient who has an acute thrombosis, for sugar in the urine is not unusual in patients suffering from this accident.

THE CLINICAL PICTURE

As a general rule the patient is suddenly seized with a severe substernal or precordial pain. The pain may be referred into the shoulders, the upper midback, the arms or the neck. In some instances the pain may be in the upper abdomen and simulate some acute surgical condition. In the more severe cases the pain is followed by shock, (weak, thready pulse, pale cold clammy skin covered with perspiration, low blood pressure). The facial expression is usually one of apprehension and the breathing may be rapid and difficult. He is usually found propped up in bed or sitting up in bed or in a chair as this position is more comfortable and these individuals are often kept in this position in contra-distinction to the treatment of shock from other causes in which the foot of the bed is usually elevated. Cases of coronary thrombosis without pain have been reported and undoubtedly do occur. Cardiac irregularities, particularly auricular fibrillation may be observed especially in patients with posterior infarction. In anterior infarction a pericardial friction rub may be heard after 12 to 48 hours. Fever and leucocytosis occurs usually on the second day following the accident. Levine[7] brought out an important fact in that fever is often overlooked if the temperature is taken by mouth as these patients are in shock and the periphery of the body may be actually cold in the presence of a true fever. This error will be avoided if rectal temperature is taken.

The development of mural thrombi often results in embolic phenomena and is always a dreaded and serious complication. In one of my patients this occurred on the third day with what appeared clinically to be emboli in the abdominal viscera, producing severe upper abdominal pain that could not be relieved by frequent doses of opiates, death occurring on the fourth day following occlusion. In another case of a man who developed pulmonary emboli with bloody sputum and numerous rales in the chest, recovery took place. If emboli come from the left ventricle, hemiplegia, renal, splenic or mesenteric infarcts may result or gangrene of one of its extremities. If they originate in the right ventricle pulmonary embolism or infarction occurs.

Nausea and vomiting may often be a distressing symptom and result from the disease or from the administration of opiates. There is often a sensation of discomfort in the epigastrium which usually comes on several days after the acute episode, and in some instances it is difficult to convince the patient that he does not have stomach trouble.

The heart sounds are usually muffled and different types of arrhythmias may occur. Rales are often present particularly in the base of the lungs and in cases accompanied by acute pulmonary edema, bubbling and sonorous rales are heard throughout the chest.

Pardee first established the fact during the early hours or days after attack, the ventricular complex may take on a peculiar form. This consisted of a high take-off of the T wave from the Q-R-S complex before the latter reaches the iso-electric line in one or another of the customary three leads. The T waves become rounded and dipped and finally peculiarly inverted.

Electrocardiography has not only been valuable in diagnosis, but has enabled us to predict in many cases the exact location of the area of infarction. Injuries to the anterior part of the heart generally occurring in the lower lateral portion of the left ventricle near the apex and resulting from a thrombosis of the descending branch of the left coronary artery are associated with one type of electrocardiogram. Similar injury to the posterior part of the ventricle, either resulting from a thrombosis of the circumflex branch of the left artery or of the right coronary artery, produce a different set of changes. In the former the high take-off of the T. wave with subsequent inversion of the T wave and the appearance of a Q wave in lead one. In the latter type these similar changes occur in lead three. Wilson has shown that while the changes in the T wave are often transient with even complete restoration of the normal appearing upright T wave, the changes in the initial ventricular complexes, notably the Q wave, are apt to be permanent. In this way one may be enabled to suspect months or years after an attack, that one previously had taken place. The recent introduction of the fourth or chest lead by Wilson, Wolferth and Wood has further increased the usefulness of electrocardiography.

TREATMENT

The first consideration is to relieve pain and combat shock. Morphine in $\frac{1}{4}$ grain doses repeated every 30 minutes if necessary, is used to relieve pain. Larger doses, even as much as one grain of morphine is advocated by some, but in my experience such dosage has been unnecessary and is not without danger. Pantopon and Dilaudid in 1/6 and 1/20 grain doses may be better tolerated than morphine in some instances. The use of oxygen by nasal catheter or the tent is often a life saving measure. Shock is combated by the use of heat and stimulants, such as coramine and caffeine sodium benzoate. In my experience, coramine has been a valuable drug in the treatment of shock. These patients are more comfortable with the head of the bed elevated 30 to 45 degrees. Complete physical and mental rest is of the utmost importance. Digitalis is recommended if signs of congestive heart failure develop and in cases of persistent auricular fibrillation. If paroxysmal ventricular tachycardia complicates coronary occlusion quinidine may be given three or four times daily, in three grain doses, as long as the tendency persists. If syncope occurs in the presence of a slow pulse in cases of auriculoventricular heart block, $\frac{1}{2}$ or one cc. of 1:1000 adrenalin should be given subcutaneously, but if unconsciousness and ventricular asystole are present intracardial administration is indicated. In less severe cases of heart block, ephedrine by mouth will be sufficient.

The administration of glucose intravenously, 50 to 100 cc. of a 50 percent solution, after the acute symptoms have subsided is highly recommended by some cardiologists. I usually give strained honey or Dexin a pure form of sugar, in fruit juices several times daily. Normal saline should be given subcutaneously if dehydration develops. The bowels should be disregarded for the first few days. If necessary an enema may be given on the fourth or fifth day. The use of a bed pan is desirable.

Diet during the early days should be confined to liquids, gradually returning to a normal diet in small amounts.

A dry, slightly bitter wine such as sherry may be given before meals for anorexia. The judicious use of alcohol is thought by some to be of real therapeutic value in coronary disease. Tobacco is thought to be harmful and should be either entirely eliminated or firmly moderated.

In nervous patients a sedative, such as one of the bromides or barbiturates may be given as indicated.

The services of a nurse when this can be afforded by the patients is desirable at least for the first week or two.

Rest in bed for six or eight weeks, and in some cases longer, should be carried out. Then the patient may be permitted to be up in a chair and gradually increase his activities. It is desirable to limit his activities permanently to some extent. Periodic examinations every two or three months, should be encouraged. Ordinary physical examination may reveal no significant findings, while fluoroscopic and electrocardiographic examinations often offer much valuable information.

BIBLIOGRAPHY

1. Gross, Louis—The Blood Supply to the Heart—Paul B. Hoeber 1921.

2. Herrick, J. B.—"Clinical Features of Sudden Obstruction of the Coronary Arteries," Journal A.M.A. 1912, 59, 2015.

3. Smith, Fred M.—Cyclopedia of Medicine, Vol. III. F. A. Davis Co. Philadelphia.

4. Willius, F. A.—Staff Meetings of the Mayo Clinic, November 22, 1939.

5. Paterson, J. C.—Journal A.M.A. 112:895 (March 11) 1939.

6. Herrick, James B.—Ann. Int. Medicine 11:2079—2084, June 1938.

7. Levine, Samuel A.—Clinical Heart Disease, W. B. Saunders Co. 1936.

Squibb Now Packages Diphtheria Toxoids According to New Recommended Dosages

Following the recommendation of the Committee on Administrative Practice of the American Public Health Association of two doses of diphtheria toxoid alum precipitated, or three doses of diphtheria toxoid, for immunization against diphtheria, E. R. Squibb and Sons, New York, are now supplying Diphtheria Toxoid Alum Precipitated Squibb in two-dose packages and Diphtheria Toxoid (Ramon) Squibb in three-dose packages.

The new recommended dosages are the outgrowth of comprehensive studies which have shown conclusively that a higher percentage of children receiving 2 x 1 cc. doses of diphtheria toxoid alum precipitated, or three doses of diphtheria toxoid, will be subsequently Shick-negative, than those children to whom only 1 cc. of diphtheria toxoid alum precipitated or 2 x 1 cc. of diphtheria toxoid—the heretofore commonly used dosages—is administered.

Squibb diphtheria toxoids are now packaged as follows:

Diphtheria Toxoid Squibb (Anatoxin Ramon):
  3 x 1 cc. vials,—(one complete immunization)
  30 cc. vial —(ten complete immunizations)
  1 cc. vial for reaction test.
Diphtheria Toxoid Alum Precipitated Refined Squibb:
  2 x 1 cc. vials,—(one complete immunization)
  2 x ½ cc. vials,—(one complete immunization)
  10 cc. vial —(five complete immunizations)
  5 cc. vial —(five complete immunizations)

Opportunities for Practice

Announcement has been made of two vacancies in a hospital association in Arkansas, one for a general practitioner, and the other for a physical examiner and relief doctor. Both positions include salary, office supplies, and mileage allowances.

Any physician who desires more information should contact the Executive office, 210 Plaza Court, Oklahoma City.

An opportunity is open in a town of 1,000 population, with a large, surrounding trade territory of 2,000 population. Any physician who is interested in this opportunity may inquire for further information at the Executive Office of the Association, 210 Plaza Court, Oklahoma City.

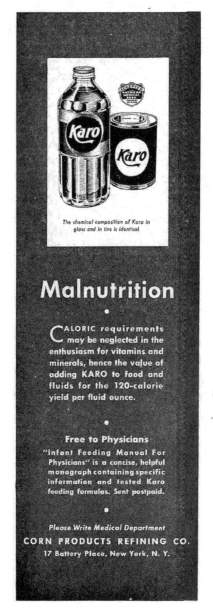

· THE PRESIDENT'S PAGE ·

"The President's Page" was created primarily to provide the members of the Oklahoma State Medical Association a monthly report from their president. The writer now finds himself serving in a "dual capacity," president of the Association, and secretary of the Oklahoma State Board of Medical Examiners.

At this writing there is a very important matter that will confront the members of the medical profession, and it is the opinion of the writer that this page could not be put to better use at this time, than to call to the attention of the members that on June 1, and not later than June 10, they will be required to renew their licenses to practice medicine in this State.

The law does not make provisions for extension of time, neither does it provide that you be notified. Failure to comply with this law could subject you to prosecution, and the Board of Medical Examiners could suspend or revoke your license.

If you secured a permit last year, simply send in the $3.00 fee, and request a permit for this fiscal year. Be sure to sign your name in full. If this is your first registration, write for application and when you return the application, remit the fee.

Those of you who are members of your county medical society can do your fellow doctors, who are not members of their county society, a great favor by calling their attention to this law, and they will appreciate your effort in helping them.

James D Osborn

President.

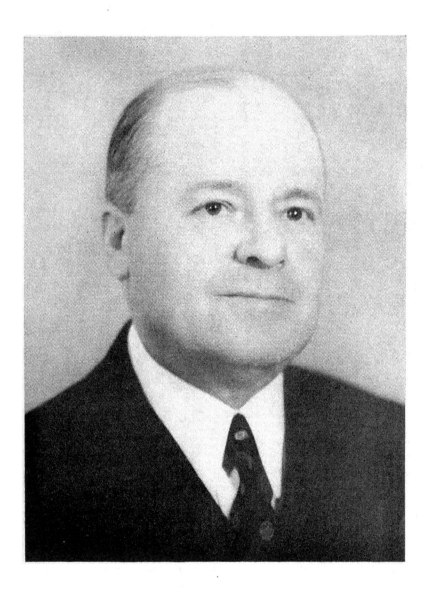

• EDITORIALS •

THE STATE MEETING

The Fiftieth Anniversary meeting of the Oklahoma State Medical Association has passed into the realm of creditable history. Every member of the State Association is indebted to the retiring president for earnest and efficient administrative service; to the council for its fine spirit of cooperation and unselfish devotion in all of its deliberations; to the Scientific Work Committee for untiring persistence in building a splendid program, in spite of many obstacles; to the Tulsa group for their part in making the meeting a success. In this connection, the pre-convention buffet supper, presided over by Tulsa County's genial president, deserves special mention. Finally, the executive secretary and his efficient staff merit the highest praise.

As highlights of the meeting, history will hold that the scientific roundtable was an outstanding event. This is attested by the record attendance and the profound interest displayed throughout this special session, and made more obvious by the general manifestation of reluctance when the expiration of time made it necessary to close the conference.

Of equal historical moment was the president's inaugural dinner, characterized by the absence of the usual long inaugural address, and the presence of the versatile editor of the Journal of the American Medical Association. Those who heard Dr. Morris Fishbein will agree that in the course of 250 years, old Pepys has lost none of his erudition.

The performance of the guest speakers, bringing to us the best from the various special fields, deserves the highest commendation.

The plan of the Scientific Work Committee, which brought the total membership together in one group for the purpose of all out acquisition of general medical knowledge, including that coming from the highly specialized groups, was considered most helpful. At this time, when total warfare is smashing many barriers, especially in civilian practice, and making it necessary for doctors, as far as possible, to broaden their skills and enlarge their scope of activities, the plan seemed to be particularly fitting.

Obviously, the best specialists should be good, all-round doctors, because they have learned to look upon the patient as a composite whole in need of both physical and psychological consideration. Such a specialist, in case of emergency, can honorably return to the humble art of caring for the sick. Many modern doctors who view the problems of the patient with a level vision are inclined to approve the Scientific Work Committee's plan for the State Medical Association Programs in order that all may learn more about every phase of medicine.

It is generally admitted that the members of highly specialized groups in section meetings at state medical associations, usually spend their valuable time telling each other what they already know. In national association meetings, the highly specialized groups have the opportunity to learn what is new in the particular speciality of their choice, by calling attention to progress in widely separated sections of the country, but this does not relieve them of the responsibility of knowing something about the art and science of medicine as a whole.

Finally, the members of the State Association are indebted to the Federal Government for the informative and helpful discussions of "The Medical Doctor in Selective Service," by Major Robert A. Bier, and "The Procurement and Assignment Service" by Thomas A. Hendricks. The two addresses were so well received and they proved to be so helpful to many of those present, it would appear that the Program Committee should bear this in mind when the next annual meeting approaches. Even when the war passes, there will be many allied interests deserving our serious consideration and possibly a place on the program.

The occasion for these serious addresses warrants much concern and causes us to wonder what may be said of Oklahoma medicine in 1942-43 when our successors celebrate the one-hundredth anniversary of the State Medical Association. Let us strive to give it the luster of unfaltering devotion.

OLD AGE AND TRANSFUSIONS

In the light of present developments, it is interesting to note that James Mackenzie in his book, "The History of Health and the Art of Preserving It," printed by William Gordon in 1758, says that "care is due with regard to health, namely, in childhood, youth, manhood and old age." Significantly, he adds, "Of these four periods, the Gerocomice or care of old age, is the only one (so far as I know) taken notice of before Pythagoras."

Among the intriguing methods employed to sustain vigor and bring about rejuvenation, he refers to Ulysses' advice to his father, Laeretes, "in the last book of the Odyssey, line 258:

Warm baths, good food, soft sleep, and generous wine,

These are the right of age, and should be thine.

"On this passage Galen remarks that 'the poet's rule was excellent; which directed an old man, after bathing and refreshing himself with food, to take some rest; for old age being naturally cold and dry, those things which moisten and warm, as bathing, eating, and sleeping, are the most proper for it.'"

After a long, interesting discussion, Mackenzie closes by referring to the history of transfusion and its early purposes:

"About a hundred years ago, a new and gallant effort was made to mend distempered constitutions, and consequently to prolong life, by supplying the human body with young and healthy blood from other animals.

"The first hint of this great attempt was given at Oxford, anno 1658, by Dr. Christopher Wren, Savilian Professor of Astronomy there, who proposed to the honourable Mr. Boyle, a method of transfusing liquors in to the veins of living animals.

"In 1666 his hint was farther improved, at the same perennial source of ingenuity and learning, by Dr. Richard Lower, who invented the method of transfusing blood out of one animal into another.

"He was followed by several ingenious men at London, and particularly by Dr. Edmund King, who rendered Lower's method of transfusion still more easy and commodious. And as it was intended by the royal society that those trials should be prosecuted to the utmost variety which the subject would bear, by exchanging the blood of old and young, sick and healthy, fierce and timid animals; various experiments were accordingly made with surprising effects upon lambs, sheep, dogs, calves and horses.

"From England this invention passed into France and Italy, where after old, decrepid and deaf animals had their hearing and the agility of their limbs, restored by the transfusion of young and healthy blood into their veins, and other wonderful cures had been achieved, J. Denis, doctor of physics at Paris, with the assistance of Mr. Emerez, ventured to perform the operation on men in that city: And Johann Gulielm. Riva, a surgeon of good reputation, made the same experiments at Rome."

After some over enthusiasm with reference to transfusions from animals to human beings, deaths occurred and the practice fell into disrepute and was prohibited by the Pope in Italy and the king in France.

The author closes the book with these significant remarks:

"Thus was defeated a noble essay, begun with prudence in England, but rashly pursued in foreign countries, which, had the first trials on the human species been conducted with care and caution, might in time have produced most useful and surprising effects.

"But after all, I am of opinion, that the greatest efforts of the human mind to extend a vigorous longevity much beyond fourscore, will generally prove ineffectual; and that neither the total alteration and discharge of old distempered humours, by a course of resolvent medicine, nor the substitution of fresh vital juices in their room, prescribed by the great lord Verulam and Boerhaave; nor the transfusion of young blood into our veins, tho' performed with the utmost precaution and dexterity, will ever avail to bestow strength and vigour on the bulk of mankind, for any great number of years, beyond the limits marked out by the Psalmist, and much less to produce rejuvenescency. Tho' I am persuaded, at the same time, that these methods prosecuted to accuracy, and reduced, if possible, to a general and easy practice, would make the life of man hold out, free from the usual complaints of decrepitude, longer than it does at present, since we see every day, that an extraordinary strength of constitution, managed with common prudence, often exceeds an hundred years."

Judging from this account the old boys from Homer and Pythagoras down, including Pliny Galen, Paulus Aegineta, and Boerhave anticipated our old age problem and wanted to do something about it. Also it is interesting to note Mackenzie's reluctance to give up his glimmering persuasion that the transfusion of blood possessed certain virtues that were being abandoned for want of accuracy and ease of practice. He was seeing the transfusion of blood "through a glass darkly," while we see it "face to face."

Vice-President of Upjohn Firm Dies

Malcolm Galbraith, vice-president and director of sales of the Upjohn company, died Friday morning, April 10, in Kansas City.

Mr. Galbraith was born in Bowmanville, Ontario, Canada, October 23, 1876. He received his bachelor of pharmacy degree at Ontario College of Pharmacy in 1898, entering the drug business in Ontario the same year. He later became a naturalized citizen of the United States. In 1909, he left the H. K. Mulford company of Philadelphia to join the Upjohn company. In October 1929, he was elected to the board of directors and named director of sales. He was made vice-president of the company in May, 1936.

ASSOCIATION ACTIVITIES

50th Anniversary Meeting Held In Tulsa, April 22, 23, 24

The Fiftieth Annual Meeting of the Association, held in Tulsa, April 22, 23 and 24, was highlighted by two new features—the Scientific Roundtable on Sulfonamide Therapy participated in by all guest speakers, and the substitution of a president's guest speaker for the Annual Inaugural Address given by the incoming President. Morris Fishbein, M.D., Editor of the Journal of the American Medical Association, Chicago, was the guest speaker at the Inaugural dinner and spoke to on overflow crowd on "American Medicine in the War."

From the response given these two new features, there is little doubt that they will be retained by the Annual Meeting committee and the Council of the Association as permanent additions to the program.

Annual Election of Officers

New officers and members of the Council were elected Thursday morning, April 23, at the last meeting of the House of Delegates. Those elected to serve with the new president, J. D. Osborn, M.D., of Frederick, are James Stevenson, M.D., President-Elect, Tulsa; Galvin L. Johnson, M.D., Vice-President, Pauls Valley; George H. Garrison, M.D., Speaker of the House of Delegates, Oklahoma City, and H. K. Speed, M.D., Vice-Speaker of the House of Delegates, Sayre. W. A. Howard, M.D., Chelsea, was reelected as delegate to the American Medical Association, and Finis W. Ewing, M.D., Muskogee, the outgoing president, was elected as alternate.

New Members Elected to Council

New councilors were elected for Districts No. 6 and No. 7, J. V. Athey, M.D., Bartlesville, being elected to succeed James Stevenson, M.D., Tulsa, the President-Elect, in District No. 6, and Clinton Gallaher, M.D., Shawnee, to succeed J. A. Walker, M.D., of Shawnee, in District No. 7. All other members of the Council were reelected to succeed themselves.

Auxiliary Officers for 1942-43

The Woman's Auxiliary of the Association at its business luncheon, Thursday noon, held its annual election of officers, and the following members will direct the activities of the Auxiliary for the coming year; Mrs. Frank L. Flack, President, Tulsa; Mrs. F. Maxey Cooper, President-Elect, Oklahoma City; Mrs. J. L. Haddock, Vice-President, Norman; Mrs. James Stevenson, Recording Secretary, Tulsa; Mrs. H. Lee Farris, Treasurer, Tulsa; Mrs. Clinton Gallaher, Historian, Shawnee, and Mrs. E. D. Greenberger, Parliamentarian, McAlester. Mrs. Joseph Kelso, Oklahoma City, was elected delegate to the Annual Meeting of the Woman's Auxiliary to the American Medical Association.

105 members of the Auxiliary registered for the meeting, and out-of-state guests were registered from Chicago, Greenville, S. C., and Independence, Kan.

Nine Guest Speakers Presented

The Scientific Program of the meeting of the Association had as guest speakers: Charles C. Dennie, M.D., Professor of Clinical Dermatology, University of Kansas School of Medicine, Kansas City, Mo.; George Herrmann, Professor of Clinical Medicine, University of Texas School of Medicine, Galveston, Tex.; John C. Burch, M.D., Associate Professor of Obstetrics and Gynecology, Vanderbilt University School of Medicine, Nashville Tenn.; T. Leon Howard, M.D., Associate Professor of Surgery (Urol.), University of Colorado School of Medicine, Denver, Colo.; Titus H. Harris, M.D., Professor of Neurology and Psychiatry, University of Texas School of Medicine, Galveston, Tex.; M. Edward Davis, M.D., Associate Professor of Obstetrics and Gynecology,

University of Chicago, the School of Medicine, Chicago; A. B. Reese, M.D., Assistant Clinical Professor of Ophthalmology, Columbia College of Physicians and Surgeons, New York City; Robert L. Sanders, M.D., Associate Professor of Surgery, University of Tennessee College of Medicine, Memphis, Tenn.; and Hugh L. Dwyer, M.D., Professor of Clinical Pediatrics, University of Kansas School of Medicine, Kansas City, Mo.

The Scientific Program was changed from the custom of past years in that all programs were conducted in the General Assembly Hall and followed each other consecutively. This allowed all doctors in attendance to hear the entire program. Whether this plan will be continued in the future will be determined by a survey to be taken among the members of the Association who registered at the meeting.

In addition to the guest speakers on the Scientific Program, the General Assembly was addressed by Major Robert A. Bier, Assistant Medical Director of Selective Service, Washington, D. C., who spoke on "The Medical Doctor in Selective Service," and Thomas A. Hendricks, personal representative of Frank Lahey, M.D., President of the American Medical Association, in the Office of Procurement and Assignment, who discussed the part physicians will play in national defense through the work of the Office of Procurement and Assignment and the State and County Medical associations.

House of Delegates

The House of Delegates completed its work in two meetings. Resolutions were adopted in behalf of the University of Oklahoma School of Medicine; endorsing the compulsory vaccination for smallpox and diphtheria program; expressing the opinion that the necessity under present state laws of placing on birth certificates the words "illegitimate" or "born out of wedlock" is to the detriment of the individuals concerned; expressing appreciation for the financial assistance given by the State Health Department, through the Children's Bureau, and the Commonwealth Fund to the Postgraduate Committee's program, and gratefully acknowledging to the Tulsa County Medical society the appreciation of the Association for the society's efforts in bringing about the present Group Malpractice insurance coverage for members of the Association through the London and Lancashire Indemnity company of New York.

In addition to these resolutions, the House of Delegates instructed the President to appoint special committees to study, for the best interests of the public, radio advertising of worthless nostrums and other forms of medication, and the rendering of expert testimony by physicians who are not qualified. The delegates to the American Medical Association were instructed to oppose any change in the rules of ethics of the American Medical Association which would make it not unethical for ophthalmologists to give lectures to and consult with opticians and optometrists.

Amendments

Two amendments to the Constitution were introduced, one concerning the time at which delegates to the American Medical Association would assume office, and the other defining the succession of the Vice-Speaker of the House of Delegates to the Speakership.

Amendments to the By-Laws were also introduced and passed. These amendments were: a provision for Associate membership in the Association; a provision for physicians to belong to adjoining county societies when permission is received from the society of the county of their residence; a provision for the revocation of honorary and associate membership; the creation of a standing committee on Prepaid Medical and Surgical Plans; a

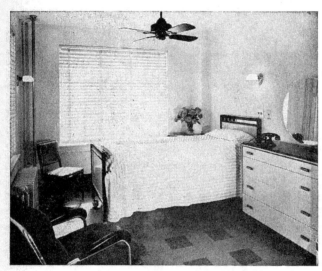

provision to allow honorary members to be counted as fully paid members in the consideration of the number of delegates a county society is entitled to send to the House of Delegates; a provision changing the duty of the selection of the Editor-in-Chief of the Journal from the Editorial Board to the Council; and a provision changing the manner in which the Scientific Program shall be arranged by placing the responsibility on the Scientific Work committee.

The House of Delegates also elected the following physicians to honorary membership: R. M. C. Hill., McLoud; Daniel F. Stough, Sr., Geary; S. P. Ross, Ada, and J. C. Duncan, Forgan.

The complete transcript of the proceedings of the House of Delegates along with the Council and Committee reports will be published in the June issue of the Journal.

Golf Tournament

The Golf Tournament which was held at the Tulsa Country club as a running tournament for the three days of the meeting found C. H. Cooke, M.D., Perry, winner of the Low Medal championship trophy, and Frank Stuart, M.D., Tulsa, the winner of the Lev Prichard runner-up cup.

In the Handicap flight, J. C. Peden, M.D., Tulsa, was first place winner and received the Nestle's Milk award, and Roy Emanuel, M.D., Chickasha, won the Industrial Printing company trophy as runnerup. Other physicians receiving awards were Charles Eads, M.D., Silas Murray, M.D., Paul Grosshart, M.D., Philip M. Schreck, M.D., and Jeff Billington, M.D., all of Tulsa; William P. Longmire, M.D., Sapulpa, and Paul Champlin, M.D., Enid.

Frisco Rates and Time Schedules For A.M.A. in Atlantic City

The following is a time schedule and rate list of the Frisco Railroad lines to Atlantic City, N. J., where the Annual Session of the American Medical Association will be held June 8-12, 1942.

These fares and the time schedule are given as of April 15, and are subject to change.

Rates

	FROM	
	Okla. City	Tulsa
Round trip first class fare to Atlantic City, good for 30 days	$80.80	$77.95
Federal tax	4.04	3.90
Round trip first class fare to Atlantic City, good for 30 days, in one direction via New York City	86.10	83.20
Federal tax	4.31	4.16
Lower to Philadelphia (one-way)	12.50	11.90
Federal tax	.63	.60
Seat in parlor car, Philadelphia to Atlantic City	65c	
Federal tax	3c	

Schedule

Lv. Okla. City	Frisco "Meteor"	5:25 PM Daily.
Lv. Tulsa	'' ''	8:25 PM Daily.
Ar. St. Louis	'' ''	8:10 AM Next day.

	Pennsylvania RR	Baltimore & Ohio
Lv. St. Louis	9:12 AM	12:00 (noon) 9:30 AM Daily.
Ar. Philadelphia	5:51 AM	7:26 AM 10:30 AM Next day.

Via Pennsylvania Reading Seashore Line

Lv. Philadelphia	8:20 AM Daily	11:30 A M Daily.
Ar. Atlantic City	9:45 AM Next day	12:40 PM Same day.

State Board of Medical Examiners Hires Attorney

J. D. Osborn, M.D., Secretary of the Oklahoma State Board of Medical Examiners, Frederick, has announced that the Board has retained the services of Mr. L. L. Corn, 908 Perrine Bldg., Oklahoma City, as Attorney for the Board.

The position of Attorney was created by the enactment by the last legislature of the Annual Registration Act for doctors of medicine.

Mr. Corn will be the investigating officer in all cases of alleged violations of the medical practice act, and every member of the association should give every assistance possible to help Mr. Corn and the Board in the enforcement of the laws governing the practice of medicine.

All physicians should bear in mind that under the Annual Registration Act they must register annually with the State Board of Medical Examiners. The registration fee is $3.00 and must be paid on or before June 10 of each year. If the fee is paid by check, the Annual Registration card will not be issued until the check has cleared. All checks or money orders should be made payable to the Oklahoma State Board of Medical Examiners and should be sent to J. D. Osborn, M.D., Secretary, Frederick, Okla.

Pottawatomie County Society Holds Spring Conference

Dr. A. C. Ivy, Professor of Physiology in Northwestern University School of Medicine, Chicago, Ill., and Dr. A. E. Hertzler, Professor of Surgery in the University of Kansas Medical School, Halstead, Kans.; were guest speakers for the Annual Spring Clinical Conference of the Pottawatomie County Medical society, March 28, in the Aldridge hotel, Shawnee.

About 75 doctors, including guests from Muskogee, Chickasha, Holdenville and Oklahoma City, attended the Conference. The afternoon program centered around gall bladder conditions, with Doctor Ivy speaking on "The Physiology of the Gall Bladder," and Doctor Hertzler discussing "The Surgical Aspects of the Acute Gall Bladder."

The subject for the evening program was thyroid conditions. Doctor Hertzler spoke on "The End Results of Total Thyroidectomy," and Doctor Ivy on "The Physiology of the Thyroid Gland."

Dr. Paul C. Gallaher of Shawnee, Committee Chairman, was in charge of the program.

Dr. Clifford C. Fulton, a member of the Association from Oklahoma City, has been placed in charge of a new naval organization school for enlisted men.

Doctor Fulton, a Lieutenant Commander in the naval services, is stationed at the U. S. Naval hospital, in Corpus Christi, Tex., where he was head of a Surgical ward before his promotion to head of the school.

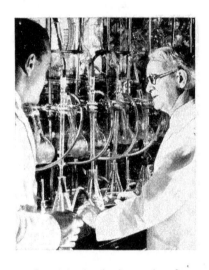

OF LESS NICOTINE SMOKE

Is a reduction of nicotine *in the smoke itself* of real physiologic importance to a regular Camel smoker?

A prominent physician states in an important article** on smoking, that when injections of nicotine were increased by only 25%, profound changes in blood pressure occurred.

The "Pleasure Factor"

In addition to a desirable reduction in nicotine intake, Camel offers another big advantage—a bid for patients' cooperation in a program of smoking modification. Camel is the slower-burning cigarette for more mildness, coolness, flavor!

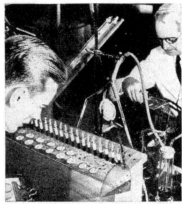

In the same tests, Camel burned SLOWER than any of the 4 other largest-selling brands tested.

* J.A.M.A., 93:1110 — October 12, 1929
Brückner, H—Die Biochemie des Tabaks, 1936
**The Military Surgeon, Vol. 89, No. 1, p. 7, July, 1941

SEND FOR REPRINT of an important contribution to medical literature—"The Cigarette, The Soldier, and The Physician," *The Military Surgeon,* July, 1941. This significant analysis reveals many new angles about smoking that should be valuable to you when modifying patients' smoking without disturbing their smoking enjoyment. Write to Camel Cigarettes, Medical Relations Division, 1 Pershing Square, New York City.

Name_____

Street_____

City_____ State_____

MEDICAL PREPAREDNESS

War Session on Medical, Hospital Problems May 28 in Oklahoma City

The American College of Surgeons announces the scheduling of a "War Session" on May 28 in Oklahoma City, with headquarters at the Biltmore hotel. Invited to participate are all physicians, medical students, and representatives of hospitals in the states of Oklahoma and Kansas. The object of the meeting is to bring to them authoritative information on meeting the problems of wartime medicine, and outstanding speakers on the program will be representatives of the Surgeon Generals' offices of the United States Army and the United States Navy, and of the Office of Civilian Defense and the Procurement and Assignment Service.

The Oklahoma City meeting will be the last of a series of 27 meetings being held under the sponsorship of the American College of Surgeons in which participation has been provided for members of the medical and hospital profession in every state in the Union and the District of Columbia.

The meeting will open at 9:00 o'clock in two sections —one for the medical profession and the other for hospital representatives. Panel discussions on treatment of war injuries to the chest and on prevention and treatment of shock will occupy the first group. A forum on civilian defense as related to hospitals will be held by the second group.

At 10:45 a joint meeting for physicians, surgeons and hospital representatives will be conducted. A joint luncheon will follow with the Procurement and Assignment Service as the subject of discussion.

Separate sessions will again be held in the afternoon. For the medical group there will be panel discussions on treatment of wounds of soft parts and on fractures. For the hospital group has been arranged a panel discussion on special problems incident to the war as affecting hospitals.

The evening program will commence with dinner at 6:00 o'clock followed by panel discussions on treatment of burns and of war injuries to the skull and face. The medical and hospital groups will participate jointly in the dinner and evening programs.

The "War Sessions" supplant the usual Sectional Meetings of the American College of Surgeons. The large attendance which they have attracted in all of the cities in which they have so far been held shows the great interest of medical and hospital people in obtaining information on how they can best serve the nation to bring about a speedy victory.

150 Association Members Are in Active Service

The following members and former members of the Association have been reported to the Office of the Association as serving with the armed forces of the nation. The list, which contains the names of 150 physicians, includes their home addresses and addresses in the services when the latter addresses are known, and gives each physician's name by the county of his residence before he was called into service.

ALFALFA
DUNNINGTON, W. G., Cherokee, 189th F. A., Camp Barkeley, Abilene, Tex.
ATOKA
COTTON, W. W., Atoka————
BECKHAM
TRACY, G. W., Erick, 120th Med. Regt., Camp Barkeley.
BLAINE
CLARK, BEN P., Okeene————
COX, A. K., Watonga, Camp Bowie, Tex.

BRYAN
BAKER, A. T., Durant, Camp Barkeley.
COKER, B. B., Durant, 3449 Lover's Lane, Dallas, Tex.
DUEWALL, R. H., Durant, Camp Wolters, Tex.
PAUL, WM. G., Durant, 107 E. Artillery Post, Fort Sam Houston, Tex.
CADDO
ANDERSON, P. H., Anadarko, Dallas, Tex.
COOK, EDWARD T., JR., Anadarko, 368th Inf., Ft. Huachuca, Ariz.
MILES, JOHN B., Anadarko, Station Hospital, Camp Barkeley.
CANADIAN
CRADEN, PAUL, El Reno————
CARTER
CARLOCK, J. HOYLE, Ardmore, Fort Sam Houston, Tex.
PERRY, FRED T., Healdton, Camp Barkeley.
SMITH, JAMES, Ardmore, Wm. Beaumont General Hospital, El Paso, Tex.
STONE, S. N., Ardmore, Naval Hospital, San Diego, Cal.
CHOCTAW
WATERS, FLOYD L., Hugo, Camp Wolters, Mineral Wells, Tex.
CLEVELAND
BEELER, T. T., Norman, Fort Knox, Ky.
COOLEY, BEN., Norman, Fort Bliss, El Paso, Tex.
HOOD, J. O., Norman, 179th Infantry, Fort Sill.
WILLARD, D. G., Norman, Naval Hospital, San Diego, Cal.
COTTON
VAN MATRE, REBER M., Walters, San Antonio, Tex.
CREEK
MOTE, PAUL, Sapulpa, U. S. Receiving Station, San Diego, Cal.
SISLER, FRANK H., JR., Bristow————
ZAMPETTI, H. A., Drumright, Fort Logan, Colo.
CUSTER
BULLOCK, BERNARD, Clinton, Fort Sam Houston, Tex.
HINSHAW, J. R., Butler————
KENNEDY, LOUIS, Clinton————
PAULSON, ALVIN W., Clinton, Randolph Field, Tex.
GARFIELD
BAKER, R. C., Enid, 189th F.A., Camp Barkeley.
BOND, IRA T., Enid, Special Troops, 45th Division, Camp Barkeley.
JACOBS, R. G., Enid, Naval Hospital, San Diego, Cal.
ROBERTS, C. J., Enid, Station Hospital, Camp Wolters, Mineral Wells, Tex.
ROSS, GEORGE, Enid————
GRADY
BAZE, ROY E., Chickasha————
OHL, C. W., Chickasha, 189th F. A., Camp Barkeley.
HARPER
PIERSON, DWIGHT, Buffalo————
HUGHES
DAVENPORT, JOHN, Holdenville, 1323 Fulton Ave., Fort Sam Houston, Tex.
JOHNSTON, L. A. S., Holdenville————
KERNEK, CLYDE, Holdenville————
JACKSON
ENSEY, J. E., Altus, 120th Quartermaster Regt., Fort Sill.
STARKEY, W. A., Altus, Camp Barkeley.
JOHNSTON
SCOTT, GEORGE W., Tishomingo, Station Hospital, Fort Sill.

KAY
KENNEDY, VIRGIL N., Newkirk———
MOHLER, E. C., Blackwell, 26th General Hospital, Fort Sill.
RISSER, PHILIP, Blackwell, Navy Hospital, San Diego, Cal.
LeFLORE
BRADLEY, FRANK, Talihina, Camp Wolters, Mineral Wells, Tex.
LOWREY R. W., Poteau, Fort Sam Houston, Tex.
ROGERS, G. A., Talihina, Weatherford, Tex.
LOGAN
RITZHAUPT, LOUIS H., Guthrie, State Selective Service Headquarters, Oklahoma City.
LOVE
LAWSON, PATRICK, Marietta, 179th Inf., Fort Sill.
MARSHALL
RAFF, J. G., Madill, 158th Infantry, Camp Barkeley.
MURRAY
FOWLER, ARTHUR, Sulphur, 158th F. A., Camp Barkeley.
PRATHER, FRANK W., Sulphur———
MUSKOGEE
ATKINS, PAUL N., JR., Muskogee, Station Hospital, Fort Sill.
DOYLE, W. H., Muskogee, 622 First Court, Clayton, Mo.
HOLCOMBE, R. N., Muskogee, 180th Infantry, Fort Sill.
KAISER, G. L., Muskogee, 180th Infantry, Camp Barkeley.
OGLESBEE, C. L., Muskogee, 180th Infantry, Fort Sill.
REYNOLDS, JOHN H., Muskogee, Station Hospital, Fort Sill.
WEAVER, W. N., Muskogee, 1804 Tenth Street, Brownwood, Tex.
WOLFE, I. C., Muskogee, 180th Infantry, Fort Sill.
OKFUSKEE
BLOSS, C. M., JR., Okemah, Camp Grant, Rockford, Ill.
OKLAHOMA
BAILEY, W. H., Oklahoma City, Station Hospital, Fort Sill.
BEATY, C. SAM, Oklahoma City, 320 Spafford Ave., San Antonio, Tex.
BOLEND, REX G., Oklahoma City, 45th Division, Fort Devens, Mass.
BRANHAM, D. W., Oklahoma City———
BROWN, GERSTER W., Oklahoma City, Naval Hospital, Charleston, S. C.
CLARK, JOHN V., Oklahoma City, Camp Barkeley.
COLEY, JOE H., Oklahoma City, Naval Hospital, San Diego, Cal.
DeVANNEY, LOUIS R., Oklahoma City, Marine Recruiting Station, Oklahoma City.
DRUMMOND, N. ROBERT, Oklahoma City, Randolph Field, Tex.
EMENHISER, LEE K., Oklahoma City, San Antonio, Tex.
FOERSTER, HERVEY A., Oklahoma City, Camp Barkeley.
FULTON, CLIFFORD C., Oklahoma City, U. S. Naval Hospital, Corpus Christi, Tex.
HAZEL, ONIS G., Oklahoma City———
HOLLINGSWORTH, C. EDWARD, Oklahoma City, Fort Richardson, Anchorage, Alaska.
HOWARD, ROBERT B., Oklahoma City, LaGarde General Hospital, New Orleans, La.
HUBBARD, RALPH W., Oklahoma City—(foreign service).
HYROOP GILBERT L., Oklahoma City, Los Angeles, Cal.
KURZNER, MEYER, Oklahoma City, Naval Air Station, San Diego, Cal.
LINDSTROM, W. C., Oklahoma City, 82nd Inf. Div., Camp Claiborne, La.
MARIL, JOSEPH J., Oklahoma City, Post Hospital, Fort Sill.
MARTIN, H. C., Oklahoma City, Station Hospital, Fort Sill.
McCLURE, WILLIAM C., Oklahoma City, Long Beach Naval Dispensary, Long Beach, Cal.

MELVIN, JAMES H., Oklahoma City, 1614 D Ave., Brownwood, Tex.
MILES, W. H., Oklahoma City, 120th Med. Regt., Camp Barkeley.
MILLER, NESBITT L., Oklahoma City, Camp Barkeley.
RECORDS, JOHN W., Oklahoma City, Fort Bliss, El Paso, Tex.
RICKS, J. R., Oklahoma City, Camp Chorrea, Balboa, Canal Zone.
SADLER, LeROY H., Oklahoma City, Camp Bowie, Brownwood, Tex.
SANGER, F. A., Oklahoma City, 120th Med. Regt., Camp Barkeley.
SANGER, W. W., Oklahoma City, Station Hospital, Fort Sill.
SEWELL, DAN E., Oklahoma City, Station Hospital, Army Air Base, Albuquerque, N. M.
SHORBE, HOWARD B., Oklahoma City, Station Hospital, Fort Sill.
SMITH, CHARLES A., Oklahoma City, Fort Huachuca, Ariz.
STRECKER, WM. E., Oklahoma City, Station Hospital, Camp Wolters, Mineral Wells, Tex.
TACKETT, O. H., Oklahoma City, Panama Canal Zone.
WATSON, I. N., Edmond, Sheppard Field, Wichita Falls, Tex.
WILDMAN, S. F., Oklahoma City, Recruit Reception Center, Camp Wolters, Tex.
OKMULGEE
SMITH, C. E., Henryetta, Quarters 31, Fort Logan, Colo.
OSAGE
DALY, JOHN F., Pawhuska, 21st and Walnut, Philadelphia, Pa.
HEMPHILL, PAUL H., Pawhuska, 120th Medical Regt., Camp Barkeley.
RAGAN, TILLMAN, Fairfax, Med. Corps, Ft. Ringgold, Rio Grande City, Tex.
OTTAWA
AISENSTADT, E. ALBERT, Picher, Office of Surgeon, Ft. Jay, Governor's Island, N. Y.
BISHOP, CALMES, Picher, Palacias, Tex.
PAWNEE
LE HEW, E. W., Pawnee, 179th Infantry, Fort Sill.
PAYNE
DAVIDSON, W. N., Cushing, Station Hospital, Camp Barkeley.
PERRY, DANIEL L., Cushing, 120th Med. Regt., Camp Barkeley.
WALTRIP, J. R., Yale, 158th F. A., Camp Barkeley.
WILHITE, L. R., Perkins, 210 Plaza Court, Oklahoma City.
WRIGHT, J. W., Stillwater———
PITTSBURG
KLOTZ, WM. F., McAlester, Ft. Richardson, Anchorage, Alaska.
PONTOTOC
BIGLER, IVAN E., Ada, Lou Foote Flying Service, Stamford, Tex.
CHEATWOOD, W. R., Ada, Camp Wallace, Tex.
McDONALD, GLEN W., Ada, 120th Med. Regt., Camp Barkeley.
MURRAY, E. C., Ada, Ft. D. A. Russell, Marfa, Tex.
WEBSTER, W. H., Ada, 120th Med. Regt., Camp Barkeley.
ROGERS
ANDERSON, P. S., Claremore, Miami, Fla.
ANDERSON, W. D., Claremore, Victoria, Tex.
BIGLER, E. E., Claremore, Station Hospital, Fort Sill.
NELSON, D. C., Claremore, Fitzsimmon, Denver, Colo.
SEMINOLE
DEATON, A. N., Wewoka, 160th F. A., Camp Barkeley.
LYONS, D. J., Seminole, Camp Barkeley.
TERRY, JOHN B., Wewoka, Kelly Field, Tex.
STEPHENS
KING, E. C., Duncan, Australia.
SMITH, LESTER P., Marlow, 179th Infantry, Fort Sill.
TEXAS
BLUE, JOHNNY A., Guymon, Naval Recruiting Station, Oklahoma City.

TILLMAN
FISHER, ROY L., Frederick, Randolph Field, Tex.
FRY, F. P., Frederick, Co. B., 2nd Medical Bureau, Ft. Sam Houston, Tex.
TULSA
AKINS, JACK ODIE, Tulsa————.
DAVIS, T. H., Tulsa, Carlisle Barracks, Carlisle, Pa.
DENNY, E. RANKIN, Tulsa, La Garde General Hospital, New Orleans, La.
EWELL, W. C., Tulsa, Fort Sam Houston, Tex.
FORD, R. B., Tulsa, U. S. Naval Station, Corpus Christi, Tex.
HAMMOND, JAMES H., Tulsa, 120th Med. Regt., Camp Barkeley.
PITTMAN, COLE D., Tulsa, Chanute Field, Rantoul, Ill.
POLLOCK, SIMON, Tulsa, Camp Hulen, Tex.
SMITH, ROY L., Tulsa, Naval Training School, College Station, Tex.
TURNBOW, W. R., Tulsa————
YANDELL, HAYES R., Tulsa————
WASHITA
DARNELL, E. E., Sentinel, Enemy Alien Internment Camp, Stringtown.
LIVINGSTON, L. G., Cordell————
STOWERS, AUBREY E., Sentinel, Camp Barkeley.
WASHINGTON
COLLETTE, E. L., JR., Dewey, Camp Grant, Rockford, Ill.
ETTER, F. S., Bartlesville————
WORD, LEE B., Bartlesville————
WOODS
SIMON, JOHN, Alva, Reception Center, Fort Sill.
WOODWARD
ENGLAND, MYRON C., Woodward, Camp Hulen, Palacias, Tex.

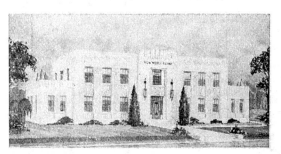

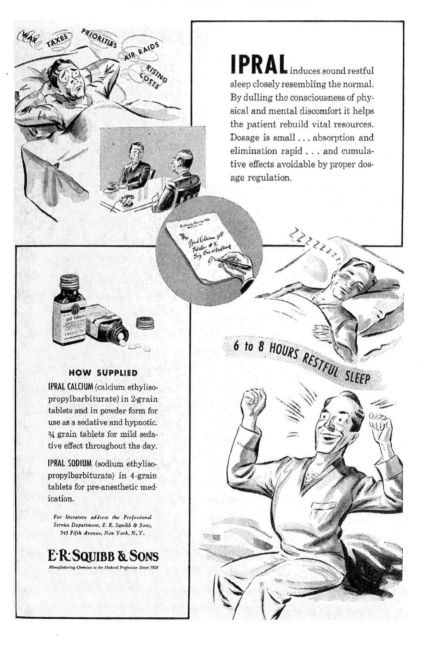

IPRAL induces sound restful sleep closely resembling the normal. By dulling the consciousness of physical and mental discomfort it helps the patient rebuild vital resources. Dosage is small . . . absorption and elimination rapid . . . and cumulative effects avoidable by proper dosage regulation.

6 to 8 HOURS RESTFUL SLEEP

HOW SUPPLIED

IPRAL CALCIUM (calcium ethylisopropylbarbiturate) in 2-grain tablets and in powder form for use as a sedative and hypnotic. ¾ grain tablets for mild sedative effect throughout the day.

IPRAL SODIUM (sodium ethylisopropylbarbiturate) in 4-grain tablets for pre-anesthetic medication.

For literature address the Professional Service Department, E. R. Squibb & Sons, 745 Fifth Avenue, New York, N. Y.

E·R·SQUIBB & SONS

Manufacturing Chemists to the Medical Profession Since 1858

NEWS FROM THE COUNTY SOCIETIES

A Farm Security Administration plan for Cherokee county was discussed by Dr. Charles M. Pearce, Dallas, Regional Medical Director, at the meeting of the Cherokee County Medical society, April 14, in Tahlequah. About 12 members were in attendance.

Dr. Isadore Dyer, Tahlequah, discussed important notes taken at the Second American Congress on Obstetrics and Gynecology.

The Cherokee county society will have as its guests at its May meeting a medical group from Tulsa, who will participate in the program of the meeting.

The Washington-Nowata County society has adjourned its meetings until the completion of the Postgraduate course in Internal Medicine being conducted in that section of the state by Dr. L. W. Hunt. The Washington-Nowata society plans to resume its meetings late in May.

A Symposium on Pneumonia highlighted the meeting of the Pittsburg County society, April 14, at the St. Mary's hospital in McAlester. Twenty members were present to participate in the discussion.

Dr. E. H. Shuller, chairman, read a short paper and discussions of diagnosis, medical management, surgical complications, differential diagnoses including multiple x-rays of pneumonias and allied conditions, were held by the doctors present.

A Symposium on Fractures will be the feature of the next meeting to be held May 28 in Antlers with members of the Southeastern Oklahoma Medical association. Dr. James S. Speed of the Willis Campbell clinic in Memphis, Tenn., will be the guest speaker for this meeting.

"Some Observations of a Medical Officer in the Philippine Islands" was the topic of the talk given by Dr. G. E. Johnson of Ardmore at the meeting of the Garvin County Medical society, April 15, in Pauls Valley.

An informal discussion of Doctor Johnson's talk was held by the 12 members in attendance, and the meeting was adjourned.

The next meeting will be held May 20 in Pauls Valley.

At the buffet dinner meeting of the Oklahoma County Medical association, April 28, in Oklahoma City, Dr. Joseph W. Kelso discussed "Repair of the Perineum."

About 145 members were present at the association's March meeting when Dr. F. Redding Hood and Dr. Henry H. Turner were speakers. Doctor Hood spoke on "Treatment of the Decompensated Heart," and Dr. Lou H. Charney and Dr. George H. Garrison led discussion on this talk. Doctor Turner gave a brief talk on Procurement and Assignment.

"The Present Status of Endocrinology in General Practice" was the subject of the talk given by Dr. Henry H. Turner of Oklahoma City at a meeting of the Muskogee County society, April 6, in Muskogee.

About 16 members of the society were present.

Dr. J. B. Morey, Dr. Forrest Dean and Dr. John A. Wrenn were speakers at the Pontotoc County society meeting, April 1, in Ada. Twelve members of the society were present.

Doctor Morey spoke on "Tularemia," and Doctor Dean on "Coronary Heart Disease." Doctor Wrenn reported on a recent meeting of the State Committee on Industrial and Traumatic Surgery.

Nine doctors and their wives were guests of the Woodward County Medical society at a meeting in Shattuck,

April 9. About 18 members of the Woodward County society and their wives attended the meeting.

"Fractures" was the topic for discussion on the scientific program, and Dr. C. R. Rountree of Oklahoma City and Dr. Paul Dube of Shattuck were the speakers.

"Sulfonamides" is the topic for the program planned for the May 14 meeting of the society, with Dr. V. M. Rutherford as speaker.

Dr. Wann Langston of Oklahoma City and Dr. F. P. Baker of Talihina were guest speakers at a meeting of the Kay County Medical society, April 16, in Blackwell. Thirteen members of the society attended the meeting.

Following a discussion of the immunization program, Doctor Langston spoke on "Cardiac Emergencies," and Doctor Baker on "Pulmonary Tuberculosis, Diagnosis and Treatment."

Dr. Eugene A. Gillis of the State Health Department will be the society's chief speaker at a meeting, May 21, in Tonkawa, when he will discuss "Syphilis in All Its Phases." The society also is making plans for the District meeting to be held in June, at Ponca City.

Dr. Charles M. Pearce of Dallas presented a discussion of the FSA plan for medical care at the meeting of the Pottawatomie County society, April 18, in Shawnee. About 18 members were present.

"Tumors of the Uterus" was the topic of Dr. John Carson's talk on the scientific program for the evening.

Dr. Charles W. Haygood was appointed chairman for the P. T. A. Summer "Round-Up" of Pre-School Children.

New officers were elected at the meeting of the Stephens County Medical society, April 28, at the Wade hotel, in Duncan.

Dr. A. J. Weedn of Duncan was elected president, and the following other officers were elected to serve with him: Dr. E. H. Lindley, Duncan, Vice-President; Dr. W. K. Walker, Secretary-Treasurer; Dr. C. N. Talley, Marlow, delegate; Dr. J. L. Patterson, Duncan, alternate; and Dr. C. N. Talley, Marlow, and Dr. W. S. Ivy and Dr. S. S. Garrett, both of Duncan, censors.

Doctor Ivy and Doctor Patterson will serve on the Program committee, and Doctor Lindley, Doctor Talley and Doctor Patterson on the Tuberculosis committee. Those who will serve on the Cancer committee are Doctor Ivy, Dr. A. M. McMahan of Duncan, and Doctor Patterson.

Following the business session, two guest speakers from Oklahoma City presented a scientific program. Dr. B. F. Burton spoke on "Surgery of Melanotic Moles," and Dr. C. L. Brundage on "Skin Diseases (Dermatitis Contact)."

The Tri-County Medical Society, which is composed of members from the Caddo, Grady and Stephens County Medical societies met March 19, in Chickasha, with about 25 members attending the meeting.

Guest speakers were Dr. Wendell Long and Dr. Wann Langston, both of Oklahoma City. Doctor Long presented a paper on "Functional Uterine Bleeding," and Dr. Wann Langston presented a paper on "Cardiac Emergencies."

Dr. Finch Elected to College of Physicians

Dr. J. William Finch of Hobart has been elected a Fellow of the American College of Physicians.

Doctor Finch attended the Annual Meeting of the College at St. Paul, Minn., April 20-24, at which time he was inducted into the College.

Group Hospital Service News

Prepaid Hospital Care for Rural Areas

As though in answer to the Federal inference that voluntary hospitalization plans have not penetrated to all economic and vocational strata, Oklahoma's own Blue Cross Plan has just achieved signal success in rural enrollment.

Whether the population in and surrounding the city of Alva constitutes rural, or only semi-rural residents, does not make the recent campaign less noteworthy. The fact is, only one place of business has a sizeable payroll: 33 employees, of which perhaps only 17 work six days a week. A half-dozen other firms employ between 12 and 15 each.

As of March 15, 1942, Group Hospital Service more than doubled the number of Alva subscribers formerly enrolled. The names of approximately 750 Alva men, women, and children are now registered under the Blue Cross. The ineligibility of persons over 65 to enroll reduced the whole from which the Blue Cross drew its members.

Civic interest in the work of the non-profit plan devised a convenient method for payment of subscribers' monthly dues when the city council instructed the city clerk to post hospitalization dues on the water bill. This unique procedure is, to our knowledge, without precedent and may be the solution to the collection problem among rural groups in Oklahoma and elsewhere.

As a late payment of a water bill carries the penalty of discontinuation of supply, very few residents delay payment. It is presumed that the identification of "water" with "hospitalization" will effect the same promptness in Blue Cross payments.

The Alva General Hospital, city owned, helped materially during the campaign. Several new rooms have recently been made available. Front page publicity was given the drive by the Review-Courier, and the Blue Cross movie, "Worries Away," was shown four nights in local theatres without charge to the plan or the city. The beginning of the campaign was announced from many of Alva's church pulpits. Mr. Tom Greene, Regional Director, who co-ordinated the drive, spoke at the Rotary, Kiwanis, and Professional and Business Women's luncheons. Blue Cross posters were displayed around town and a special folder was distributed.

Backbone of the campaign was a staff of eight Alva women, who, after being instructed in the Plan, visited every residence (in districts), answering questions and accepting applications.

The importance of everyone of these forces of education and solicitation moves us to judge that without them, the Blue Cross Plan would have entered into "Individual enrollment" with its attendant poor selection.

To assure sound procedure, no applications were accepted after March 15, 1942, nor will they be accepted until that time next year.

No—the deterrent to voluntary hospitalization plans is not financial brackets, nor means of livelihood, nor geography. It is the *confusion* that exists in the minds of those who would choose prepaid care. On one hand is the non-profit plan; on the other, commercial insurance which in turn is broken down into perhaps three types and 15 underwriters.

Hospital care is as important to community health as police protection is to community welfare. Imagine the duplication, the fiasco, that would result, if eight distinct police organizations patrolled a community's streets!

We think we know which hospitalization system will best suit most people, and with more Alva-like cooperation from employers and municipalities the answer will be apparent to everyone.

Experience on the Alva procedure will be watched and studied carefully. If satisfactory in every way, the same plan will be offered to other communities that are interested. While the procedure used is experimental in some phases and not intended to be employed in all Oklahoma communities at once, it does have a bearing in determining future activity.

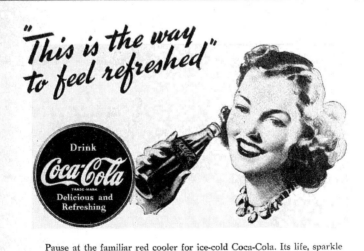

Pause at the familiar red cooler for ice-cold Coca-Cola. Its life, sparkle and delicious taste will give you the real meaning of *refreshment.*

BOOK REVIEWS

"The chief glory of every people arises from its authors."—Dr. Samuel Johnson.

"THE BLOOD BANK AND THE TECHNIQUE AND THERAPEUTICS OF TRANSFUSIONS." Kilduffe and DeBakey. The C. V. Mosby Company, St. Louis, Mo.

This book represents a clear and concise reference source for most problems relating to the important therapeutic procedure of transfusions.

It relates most interestingly the historical background of blood transfusion, relating its place as a therapeutic agent.

In discussing the rational indications and contraindications of blood transfusion, the book outlines and explains in detail the six fundamental physiologic principles which are essential in its consideration. These are: (1) increase in fluid bulk or volume of circulating blood, (2) immediate increase in the oxygen-carrying capacity of the blood, (3) increase in protein concentration of blood, (4) increase in the coagulability of the blood, (5) possible stimulation of hematopoiesis, and (6) addition of immunologic factors.

Under indications for blood transfusion the authors enumerate: (1) Hemorrhage, (2) peripheral circulatory failure, (3) pre-operative and post-operative therapy, (4) hypoprotonemia, (5) blood dyscrasias, (6) infections, (7) intoxications and poisonings, (8) debility.

The chapter dealing with the technique of blood typing and compatability tests is complete in detail, clear in description, and illustrated very graphically by cuts and photographs.

The blood bank, its operation, and changes which occur in stored blood, are explained in detail in four chapters with beautiful illustrations of technique.

Kilduffe and DeBakey devote several chapters to the transfusion of Plasma, both citrated and dried; the various methods employed to collect and administer plasma, the indications and techniques for its use. They made the statement that "the blood bank of the present may be in large measure replaced by the plasma bank of the future."

In view of the increasing interest in "blood banks," and plasma transfusions, and the important role that these therapeutic measures will play in Military Medicine this book is most timely, most interesting, and deserves a prominent place on the library shelf of most every physician.—Tom Lowry.

―――――

"INTRODUCTION TO DERMATOLOGY." Sutton and Sutton. Fourth Edition, cloth, $9.00. 904 pp., 723 illustrations. C. V. Mosby Company, St. Louis, Mo.

"Introduction to Dermatology," by Sutton and Sutton is the answer to the many requests from medical students and general practitioners for a more condensed edition of Sutton's "Diseases of the Skin" which has been so popular as an elaborate authority on dermatology for more than 20 years. Now the fourth revision of "Introduction to Dermatology" has appeared with numerous new and clear illustrations of various skin diseases, as well as many more pages of discussion of later thought originating largely from recent research and clinical experience. The addition of 35 pages of bibliography in the back of the book, which addition contributed so much to the popularity of the original Sutton's "Diseases of the Skin," has advanced this text into a class of its own.

This book discloses the same alertness and discrimination of the authors and publishers in their endeavor to give physicians and students the very best in the fewest pages, and should meet with the same gracious popularity as their previous editions.—Everett S. Lain.

"SURGERY OF THE AMBULATORY PATIENT." L. Kraeer Ferguson, A.B., M.D., F.A.C.S. 645 Illustrations. Philadelphia: J. B. Lippincott Company, 1942. $10.00. A Section on Fractures by Louis Kaplan, A.B., M.D., F.A.C.S.

From the inside front covers, which are occupied by illuminating instructive charts, to the index this book is filled with practical instructive items for the use of the young surgeon and the general practitioner; not the specialist. Therein lies its appeal. Finally, a book has been written and published which fills the great void which has heretofore existed between the medical school and the finished surgeon. For all this Dr. Ferguson and his collaborator Dr. Louis Kaplan, who has written the section on Fractures, will be thanked by the inarticulate thousands who have longed for just such a volume.

The book is very profusely illustrated with photographs and explanatory diagrams. It is divided into three sections: 1. Surgical Principles and Lesions, 2. Regional Surgery, and 3. The Musculoskeletal System. In the first section anesthesia, preparation for operation, post-operative care, infections and specific surgical lesions are discussed in considerable detail. In the second section, the various surgical lesions which might be classified as non-confining from the scalp to the foot are considered from the standpoint of region involved, anatomical considerations, etiology and most particularly treatment. The final section considers fractures and dislocations generally and then passes on to a consideration of the common fractures of both upper and lower extremities. Many reproductions of the X-ray films are included in the section with detailed explanation of the various maneuvers used in orthopedic treatment.

The book is large. It must be so since it is so comprehensive. It is also stoutly bound which again is essential since the binding will be greatly strained from frequent use in the hands of those for whom it is especially written.—L. J. Starry.

―――――

"EFFECTIVE LIVING." C. E. Turner, A.M., Sc.D., Dr. P.H., and Elizabeth McHose, B.S., M.A. C. V. Mosby Company, 1941.

It is difficult to discuss Effective Living in an effective way, but the authors of this book have presented many helpful facts in a clear-cut, straightforward manner, and it is to be hoped that they may reach many of the young people who are facing a new way of life with many difficult problems ahead.

In this volume, Effective Living is discussed under three main heads: "1. Effective Living for the Individual; 2. Effective Living in the Family; and 3. Effective Living in the Community." These are vital subjects which when properly understood, should help every youth reach his full capacity as an individual, as a unit in his family, and as a member of society. This is a high and holy purpose which should interest every good citizen.

The discussion proceeds in an orderly and interesting fashion. The text is supplemented by 164 attractive and instructive illustrations.

This is a book doctors may recommend to patients, to mothers and fathers, and to teachers and pupils. Each page is followed by a series of self-teaching questions and at the end of the text there is a page of source materials; also, Appendix A, which deals with the Control of Communicable Diseases, and Appendix B, which gives a plain and effective coordination. In addition, there is a glossary and a comprehensive Index.—L. J. Moorman.

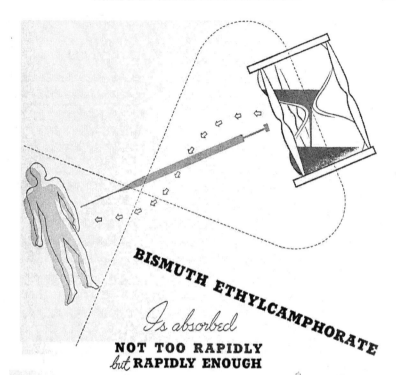

BISMUTH ETHYLCAMPHORATE

Is absorbed

NOT TOO RAPIDLY
but RAPIDLY ENOUGH

Because the effectiveness of Bismuth Ethylcamphorate (injected intramuscularly) endures a longer time than does that of water solutions of bismuth salts, it makes possible a more convenient (weekly) visit interval for the patient. On the other hand, since it is more rapidly and completely absorbed than are oil suspensions of insoluble bismuth compounds, less material in terms of metallic bismuth is needed to maintain a therapeutic level, and danger of toxicity is minimized.

Sterile Solution Bismuth Ethylcamphorate is the bismuth salt of ethyl camphoric acid dissolved in sweet almond oil. It is available in boxes of six and twenty-five 1 cc. ampoules, and in 30 cc. vials.

Fine Pharmaceuticals Since 1886

REVIEWS and CORRESPONDENCE

SURGERY AND GYNECOLOGY

Abstracts, Reviews and Comments From
LeRoy Long Clinic
714 Medical Arts Building, Oklahoma City

"THE END RESULTS OF THE SIMPSON OPERATION IN SIXTY-ONE PATIENTS DELIVERED AT TERM." American Journal of Obstetrics and Gynecology. April 1942, Page 690. **Brooke M. Anspach and John B. Montgomery. Philadelphia, Pa.**

The authors emphasize the fact that retroflexion and retroversion of the uterus do not necessarily produce symptoms and that uterine suspension should be undertaken only after all other possibilities of origin of symptoms have been carefully explored.

On the other hand there are patients who have symptoms produced by a retroversion retroflexion of the uterus and require uterine suspension. "During the childbearing age, treatment of retroflexioversion of the uterus may be required: (a) to promote conception, (b) to favor the normal course of pregnancy, (c) to relieve various symptoms, the most frequent of which are low abdominal distress and backache, worse in the erect posture and upon exertion, better when lying down."

They discuss the natural requisite of a suspension operation during the reproductive years. It entails no disadvantage during a subsequent pregnancy and labor and the uterus must remain in good position.

It is felt that this requisite makes it desirable to use the inner parts of the round ligaments which are stronger, more muscular, and participate more in the involution of the uterus.

They consequently prefer in average patients the Simpson operation which has the advantage that the modified Gilliam operation is carried out extra-peritoneal. The operative technique is briefly discussed.

From 1921 to 1941 a total of 500 Simpson operations were performed. Fifty-eight of these patients were sterilized by ligation or excision of the tubes and of the remainder, many women used contraceptive measures and many were nearing the menopause.

There were 76 patients pregnant after the Simpson operation.

Fifty-six of these delivered at term by natural passages and five had Caesarean section at term for other indications than suspension. Abortion occurred in 11 patients. Two of these were induced.

"Bearing in mind the statement of Litzenberg, who reviewed the literature, that 'the proportion of one abortion to five viable births is supported by authorities from many countries,' we may conclude that the altered anatomic relations brought about by the operation did not predispose to abortion. On the contrary we have a definite number of patients in whom the performance of the Simpson operation after failure of postural and pessary treatment put an end to a repetition of abortion in early pregnancy."

Of the 61 patients delivered at term, 58 maintained a cure with the uterus in a normal position after delivery.

COMMENT: Most patients with retroversion and retroflexion of the uterus are suffering no symptoms from this condition and do not require an operation for its correction. The cause of symptoms can usually be found by a more careful and painstaking investigation and when any type of uterine suspension is undertaken in patients where such careful investigation does not precede operation, many patients will have the same symptoms which they had before.

However, there are selected patients who do require uterine suspension during the reproductive years and this paper is important because it deals with the effect of the uterine suspension upon pregnancy and also the effect of pregnancy upon the uterine suspension.

For the past 14 years I have employed the Simpson operation in the great majority of those patients upon whom I have performed a uterine suspension and I can unreservedly endorse the statement of these authors about the wisdom of employing the inner portions of the round ligaments and the very satisfactory results from operation.

I can also endorse the almost uniformly satisfactory results of patients who have delivered after operation.

It can likewise be said that this type of suspension does not interfere with the normal course of the pregnancy.

It may be added, in concurrence with the opinion of Doctors Anspach and Montgomery, that this type of suspension has never in my experience interfered with conception.

It is consequently to be recommended that patients who have been carefully selected for uterine suspension have a modified Gilliam type suspension. It is my preference to perform the Simpson operation because the round ligament is drawn through the extraperitoneal space entirely. The Crossen operation satisfies the criteria for the suspension but there is a potential opening in the side of the pelvis that has to be closed separately from the principal portion of the operation and it is for this reason that my preference lies in the Simpson operation.—Wendell Long.

"A COMPARATIVE STUDY OF TUBAL INSUFFLATION AND LIPIODOL INJECTION IN STERILITY." David Feiner, Brooklyn, N. Y. American Journal of Obstetrics and Gynecology. April 1942, Vol. 43, Page 639.

There is a very comprehensive study based on the results of investigation of tubal patency in 706 consecutive cases.

831 insufflations were given to 541 patients. There was one death with the pathological diagnosis "Rupture of a coronary vein, hemopericardium, pulmonary thrombosis, and chronic myocarditis."

Uterosalpingorrhaphy with lipiodol was performed on 337 patients. A total of 84 patients conceived tubal insufflation and a total of 58 patients conceived within one year following uterosalpingorrhaphy.

Six patients showed gross' morbidity following uterosalingorrhaphy and there was one case of mortality from peritonitis.

There were 20 patients who showed patency to lipiodol visualization after a negative insufflation. It was thought that this was probably due to isthmospasm.

"The relative merits of carbon dioxide insufflation and lipiodol injection are considered. The view is expressed that carbon dioxide insufflation should always precede the use of lipiodol. However, lipiodol may be information in the majority of cases without some of the drawbacks of lipiodol. The use of lipiodol should be reserved in the main for those cases of nonpatency in which accurate localization of the obstruction is desired.

"The therapeutic value of uterotubal insufflation is seen in many ways in cases of partial obstruction; a greater or more normal degree of patency may be established in certain cases showing a complete obstruction. Tubal patency may be re-established by the breaking down of adhesions, the expulsion of a plug of mucus or the straightening of the kinks. Dysmenorrhea is sometimes relieved; pregnancy follows insufflation in a certain proportion of cases.

"My personal experience and the review of literature indicates that routine lipiodol injections are not harmless and that as a diagnostic method lipiodol injections carry a morbidity and mortality even though small. In sterility cases in which one tube is occluded, or both tubes show partial obstruction as demonstrated by air insufflation, lipiodol injection should be used cautiously, as complete occlusion may result and thus defeat the primary objective."

COMMENT: Both of these procedures are now well established and of tremendous assistance in the investigation and correction of sterility.

There would seem little doubt but that most would agree that carbon dioxide insufflation should always precede the use of lipiodol. However, lipiodol may be very useful, particularly in those patients in which accurate localization of the obstruction is desired when some surgical interference is contemplated.—Wendell Long.

"CRITERIA OF AN ACCEPTABLE OPERATION FOR ULCER. The importance of the acid factor." Owen H. Wangensteen, M.D., and B. Lannin, M.D.; Archives of Surgery, March 1942, Page 489.

The authors believe that the empiric surgical approach to the ulcer problem has come to an end. In the past 50 years of accumulated experience a mass of conflicting data has accumulated with reference to the accomplishment of operation in the management of ulcers without a clearcut definition of the criteria of an acceptable operation. It now appears that the cause of this confusion is not difficult to detect. There having been no general agreement among clinicians or investigators concerning the cause of ulcer, the surgeon knew only that the objective of his craftmanship was to prevent recurrence of ulcers; in determining how to attain that end, he had little or no help to guide him. It was not surprising, therefore, that the surgeon groped about aimlessly for procedures which he hoped might accomplish his objectives of obviating recurrence of ulcer since he did not know how ulcer came about, what was demanded of a satisfactory operation, or how his handicraft mediated its influence.

The authors believe that all this has now changed. They think that accumulating evidence indicates clearly that acid is the important factor in the genesis of ulcer. They admit that it is not known what are the factors that condition the capacity of the gastric mechanism to secrete acid or what other factors may thwart or favor digestion of tissue by acid. However, they believe that unneutralized hydrochloric acid secreted by the stomach may bring about the formation of ulcer in every instance.

It has been found that, by stimulating the intrinsic gastric secretory mechanism with histamine in beeswax, from which histamine is liberated slowly, ulcer may be produced in a large number of laboratory and domestic animals.

In their series of patients, they report upon seven types of gastric operations and they recommend as satisfactory only two types of operations out of the total number of seven types.

It is their conviction that, in their hands, the following two kinds of operations alone are satisfactory.

(a) Three-quarter resection, including the pylorus and antrum with Hofmeister retrocolic anastomosis.

(b) Finsterer exclusion operation with excision of the remnant of the antral mucosa.

Their patients who have undergone the Three-quarter gastric resection may eat anything; the imposition of dietary restrictions is unnecessary. Within four months after operation, usually, the gastric capacity of the majority of these patients has returned to normal, so that they can eat a full sized holiday meal without distress. They point out that the thin walled fundus is the most dilatable portion of the stomach. Most of these patients hold their weight satisfactorily. A number gain weight. They have found no evidence of anemia or dietary deficiency in patients upon whom the Three-quarter gastric resection has been performed. They believe that inasmuch as Castle found that the fundus of the human stomach contains the intrinsic anti-anemic factor in abundance, it is not likely that anemia will follow such operation. They are uncertain as to whether such patients will need particular notice with regard to iron and calcium requirements in the future.

Their clinical experience suggests that the operative risk of the Three-quarter resection for ulcer is between two and three percent—a mortality rate no greater apparently than that reported by other investigators employing the small antral resection, or the operation of small gastric excision with Polya anastomosis.

In the surgical management of ulcer, it is to be remembered that the ulcer itself is not the disease but that it is only the end effect of unneutralized hydrochloric acid digesting away the wall of the stomach or the duodenum. It is the active gastric secretory mechanism which is responsible for the ulcer diathesis. Failure of operation to depress gastric secretion effectually compromises seriously the likelihood of the success of the procedure. There would appear to be some room for discriminating and effective choice among operations for ulcer, but there is little option between an acceptable operation and one which fails to meet the requirements of a satisfactory operation.

By far the most important criterion of an acceptable operation for ulcer is that it reduce gastric acidity effectually.

In their experience the two operations mentioned above (out of the total number of operations tried) appear to meet the requirements of a satisfactory operation.

Their objectives of an acceptable operation are, first, that it relieve the patient subjectively and remove the ulcer diathesis; second, that it prevent recurrent ulcer; third, that it do not compromise the future of the patient.

It appears that extensive removal of gastric tissue (Three-quarter resection) is necessary to insure achlorhydria and to give assurance of meeting the first two requirements of an acceptable operation. Their observation suggests that the achlorhydria of the Three-quarter resection so desirable to protect against recurrence of ulcer, meets adequately the third requirement of an acceptable operation, in that these patients lead active useful lives without any evidence of deficiency disorder.

The only known manner in which the secretion of acid may be depressed effectually is by sacrificing a liberal portion of the gastric mucosa.

In order to insure achlorhydria, excision of the antral mucosa is mandatory. They suggest that the antral mucosa may contain a harmonal stimulant of gastric secretion other than histamine.

COMMENT: Dr. Wangensteen's preference for Three-quarter resection is well known. In view of his unsatisfactory result with less radical operation, one is inclined to agree with him that Three-quarter resection is necessary to accomplish desired achlorhydria.

However there are other well known surgeons who are not yet convinced of the absolute necessity for Three-quarter resection.—LeRoy D. Long.

"WAR SURGERY AND TRAUMATIC LESIONS."

This excellent symposium includes three papers of importance with the following titles:

1. Early Diagnosis of Craniocerebral Injuries
2. Stab Wounds of Chest Wall and Lungs
3. Diagnosis in Abdominal Trauma

The symposium appears in April 1942 issue of the American Journal of Surgery. Early Diagnosis of Craniocerebral Injury: Donald Monroe, M.D., American Journal of Surgery, April 1942, Page 3.

An appreciation of diagnostic fundamentals is of more than usual importance in dealing with head injuries. "Brain surgeons" who have been trained in the more leisurely schools of neurology and tumor neurology are frequently at a loss in the hurly-burly of craniocerebral injuries in which decisions have to be made rapidly and without benefit of the detailed meticulous study that tradition has decreed must precede the diagnosis of intracranial disease. Moreover, the clouding of the picture by associated injuries, rapid intracerebral changes that may not only vitiate otherwise reliable signs but actually apparently reverse their significance, and the complications such as surgical shock and dehydration lead to profound diagnostic errors, ill-conceived therapy and higher mortality. There is a great need for sanity and objectivity in the diagnosing of the intracranial pathological conditions that result from acute craniocerebral injury.

A prerequisite of any acute craniocerebral injury, except perforating wounds of the skull, is the demonstration of the fact that there has actually been an injury to the patient's head and that he has been knocked unconscious as the direct result of that injury.

Accurate diagnoses of uncomplicated non-operable craniocerebral injuries are dependent, first, upon the history and then upon a study of the make-up and pressure of the cerebrospinal fluid. Diagnoses made without these data are inferential rather than factual.

Accurate diagnoses of uncomplicated, operable craniocerebral injuries will always include a word picture of the associated non-operable cerebral condition. In addition, certain data that are obtainable only by special x-ray examination, palpation through a scalp wound, a detailed history of the development of symptoms after the accident, and the use of an exploratory trephination whenever the patient's progress does not coincide with the diagnosis already made, are necessary.

More attention should be paid to the possibility of significant complications of acute craniocerebral injury. This is particularly true in regard to surgical shock, toxic-dehydration and acidosis.

Accurate diagnoses of common complications of acute craniocerebral injury will depend upon the knowledge of the cerebral pathological condition that has been produced by the head injury, a study of the pulse pressure, a study of the patient's history in relation to exposure to heat, fluid intake and limitation, the administration of dehydrants and the level of the intracranial pressure.

"STAB WOUNDS OF THE CHEST WALL AND LUNGS."
Alex Steward. M.D., American Journal of Surgery, April 1942. Page 15.

No class of wounds, unless it be in a few centers of the brain, involves the essential physiologic processes of the body more rapidly than wounds of the chest. In addition to the rapid physiological changes which must be met, many pathologic sequelae may be expected. No class of wounds requires more accurate judgment at onset or more persistent care during its course.

Injuries and wounds of the chest have been classified in various ways. Lilienthal divides them into superficial, penetrating and perforating, the last two classes being differentiated only by degree. Cole divides them into external and internal chest injuries. Bigger calls them

perforating and non-perforating. A similarly explicit description may be made of superficial wounds which involve layers of the thoracic wall to the parietal pleura, and deep wounds which extend through the parietal pleura to varying depths.

Peculiarly, very few bayonet wounds of the chest were seen in the hospitals during World War I. The reasons given for this are: first, that the wounds were so severe that the victim failed to survive the trip, second, that the armies were taught to lunge for the abdomen so that the bayonet would not be caught in the ribs and, third, in case the bayonet was difficult to withdraw, to shoot it loose.

CONCLUSIONS: 1. Care must be taken in examining and repairing superficial chest wounds.

2. The immediate closure of deep chest wounds should be done and aspiration or valve control or internal pressure should be used.

3. The mistaking of systemic shock for right heart embarrassment and the danger in using intravenous solutions in the presence of increased intrapleural pressure is emphasized.

4. There is a difference in treatment and results of wounds involving the pulmonary and those involving the bronchial vessels.

"DIAGNOSIS IN ABDOMINAL TRAUMA." Ambrose H. Storck. M.D., American Journal of Surgery. April 1942. Page 21.

When a traumatic lesion of the abdomen, due either to penetration or blunt violence, is suspected or known to exist, diagnosis embraces more than the mere determination of whether peritoneal perforation has occurred, and even more than estimation of the probable existence and extent of visceral injury. Upon a complete determination of the patient's status in respect to shock, hemorrhage, and associated injuries, depend both the selection and the timing of the therapeutic measures which are discussed. In addition to immediate or pre-operative studies, observations at the time of operation, and recognition of the late complications which follow traumatic lesions of the abdomen, are still other important phases of diagnosis.

An account of the circumstances under which the injury was incurred, as well as a description of the mechanism of the injury, often furnish valuable information. For example, in considering the possible damage done by a blunt force or by a projectile following a known course, if the urinary bladder was recently emptied it may escape injury; while if distended at the time the wound was sustained, the bladder may not only have been struck but is likely to have been extensively lacerated as a result of the explosive force exerted by its noncompressible fluid contents. Likewise, evacuation of the bowel shortly before injury favorably influences the amount of spillage of intestinal contents. The physical attitude of the patient when wounded may greatly influence the course of a projectile, and in the instance of subcutaneous wounds, the type and direction of the blunt force often suggests the probable location of visceral lesions. Information concerning the period of time elapsed since the injury was sustained, and the character of first aid or other previous treatment is also of value in planning the management of patients with abdominal injuries.

Prompt determination of the existence of abdominal visceral injury, extensive hemorrhage, shock, or associated chest as well as craniocerebral injury is especially necessary when patients are to be transferred in airplanes flying at high altitudes. Lovelace has reported on the deleterious effects caused by reducing atmospheric pressure in the presence of any of these conditions, and has also drawn attention to the increased outpouring of stomach and intestinal contents caused by expansion of gas in these viscera when atmospheric pressure is lowered. Therefore, only those ambulance air transports which have cabins that can be sealed to permit maintenance of barometric pressure near that at ground level are safe conveyances for seriously wounded patients.

Even in obscure cases with either penetrating wounds or visceral injuries caused by blunt force, diagnosis is usually possible before shock and hemorrhage, or extravasation of gastro-intestinal content, have been fatally prolonged or extended.

The clinical manifestations as well as the findings obtained by clinical laboratory, x-ray and endoscopic methods of study, which permit early diagnosis and serve as a guide to therapy, are presented.

The indications for and method for exploring the abdominal wall wound as well as peritoneal cavity, are detailed.

Criteria for the selection of cases requiring operative treatment, and for the timing for surgical intervention, are given.

Methods of determining the presence and extent of hidden lesions at the time of operation, are discussed. The complications which frequently follow abdominal injuries are considered in respect to the importance of their early recognition.—LeRoy D. Long, M.D.

EYE, EAR, NOSE AND THROAT
Edited by Marvin D. Henley, M. D.
911 Medical Arts Building, Tulsa

"USE OF NONSPECIFIC BACTERIAL VACCINE IN CHRONIC COUGHS AND THE COMMON COLD OF CHILDREN." H. Goldstein. Archives of Pediatrics. vol. 59, p. 50-56, January. 1942.

The cause of the common cold is believed to be a filtrable virus, and, as far as known, there is no specific available. Various polyvalent catarrhal and cold vaccines of stock bacterial combinations are being used with varying results. These are being used with the hope that secondary invaders may be prevented from causing infections of a serious nature of the nose, throat and respiratory tract. Some of the vaccines are effective to a partial extent; others not at all.

The author used many stock vaccines with unreliable effect. Some would act better than others in certain patients. In a number of children the commonly used cold vaccines failed to work, whether given during an attack of a common cold in order to abort or benefit it, or before one gets a cold in order to prevent it.

This lack of having any specific vaccine or other means of therapy to apply for relief of the suffering patients during attacks of common cold and chronic coughs led the author to seek a remedy for them to ameliorate their attacks. After several clinical trials, he found that bacterial vaccine of B.tyhposus containing 1,000 million organisms per cc achieved startling results.

The new method of vaccine therapy was used on 380 children, who have been suffering either from distressing coughs or repeated attacks of acute common cold. Many of them had a muco-purulent discharge in the nasopharynx, an angry red granular appearing pharyngeal wall, enlarged lingual tonsil, and running nose. Some complained of a clogged feeling in the nose and head, and a few gave a history of having sinus congestion and defective nasal breathing. Several of them showed bronchitis and rarely wheezing.

The dosage of B.typhosus vaccine was as follows: initial dose of 0.1 cc, two days later 0.2 cc intradermally, then subcutaneous injections were given every third day increasing in dose by 0.1 cc until 0.5 cc were given. In some instances the optimum dose reached was 0.7 cc to 1.0 cc depending on the local and general reactions of the child. Most of the children were relieved from their coughing spells after the first or second injection, and the coughing stopped after the third or fourth treatment. In children who came down with an acute head cold

the first or the second injection brought complete relief. In a number of the children, prophylactic intradermal injections of 0.2 cc every two or three months for a period of one to two years prevented further attacks of colds.

It seems that this treatment changes the vulnerability of the upper respiratory tract and its mucous membrane, making it more resistant to the existing infection, and preventing the progress of the attack of colds. All in all, complete relief was brought to 90 percent of the children.

The B.typhosus vaccine has nonspecific antigenic properties also, which stimulate antibody formation, such as opsonins or similar substances, having certain effects that weaken or prepare the bacteria, making them attractive for phagocytic activity.

The author found that the smaller doses gave the best therapeutic results. In one instance a child of three years was coughing for over a period of several months. He had a congested nasopharynx, and rough breathing sounds. 0.1 cc B.typhosus vaccine was injected parenterally, and three days later 0.2 cc vaccine was additionally given. Since then, the child has been well and free from cough and nasopharyngeal infection. Such phenomenal results have been observed in the great majority of the cases treated.

"THE BLOCKED EAR OF THE CAISSON WORKER." A. Almour. Laryngoscope. vol. 52, p. 75-81, January 1942.

The "blocked ear" is an expression used by the caisson worker, or sandhog, to denote some disturbance to the drum, tympanic cavity, or both, which has resulted from a failure to equalize the intra- and extratympanic air pressure. This can occur during compression or decompression. The most important predisposing factor of blocking the ear is some degree of tubal occlusion, and the majority of blocked ears occur in workers who do not stay away from their work during an attack of common cold, or who still did not recover from an attack of cold.

The caisson worker, upon being locked in the compression apparatus is able to equalize at all times the pressure of the air in the middle ear with the changing pressure in the air lock. He is taught to do this by learning how to inflate his middle ears by swallowing repeatedly while he is in the lock. Where, however, a tubal obstruction is present, the ability to auto-inflate is lost.

The immediate symptoms of blocked ear is severe, stabbing pain in the affected ear and a sensation of extreme fullness. Speech is heard with no difficulty, but sounds hollow and muffled. Otoscopic examination enables one to classify cases; the second degree cases may be further subdivided into mild, moderate and severe forms.

In the first degree of blocked ear there is a marked retraction of the drum, with hyperemia of its blood vessels. The upper portion of the drum is hyperemic chiefly, while the lower half of the pars tensa of the drum approximates the normal color. Otalgia disappears quickly.

In the mild forms of second degree blocked ear, one or more hemorrhages are found in the tympanic membrane. They appear as purplish spots. A solitary hemorrhage is chiefly in the posterosuperior quadrant. The hemorrhages do not form bullae, and can never be confused with the hemorrhagic blebs of a grippe otitis.

In the moderate form of second degree blocked ear, one finds an intratympanic hemorrhage, with or without hemorrhage into the drum itself. The tympanis membrane is retracted and the bony landmarks accentuated, and it presents a diffuse purplish color. In the severe form, it is possible to visualize the incudostapedial articulation. The pressure of this joint against the membrane may result in a perforation. Such perforations may occur anywhere, and they may be of any size and number. The posterosuperior quadrant is affected most often. Free bleeding may or may not accompany this type of blocked ear. Thus, bleeding from the ear is not an evidence of an injury to the internal ear.

In the vast majority of cases of blocked ear wherein no perforation has occurred the hearing returns to within normal limits after measures have been instituted to re-establish the patency of the Eustachian tube. Heat, in the form of diathermy, has aided in hastening the absorption of hemorrhages. The average time for accomplishing this has been 16 days. Where a perforation of the drum has occurred, the hearing loss may be anything from a few decibels to 30 decibels.

There may be some difficulty in evaluating the permanent disability of caisson workers due to blocked ear. There is no definite characteristic of a hearing loss due to a blocked ear. There is no pre-employment examination; moreover, there is no reliable audiometer on the market to test hearing acuity in a standardized form.

"EXOPHTHALMOS." A. D. Ruedemann. The Annals of Otology, Rhinology & Laryngology, vol. 50, p. 1164-1171, December 1941.

The patient with a protruding eye always presents a difficult problem for the diagnostician. There are usually several possible diagnoses, and the final decision as to the nature of affection can be made only after an operation on the orbit.

Exophthalmos is either bilateral or unilateral. The bilateral type is limited to general disease. The unilateral type is the one which causes the trouble. Congenital orbital defects and congenital eyeball defects must be differentiated. One orbit may be shallowed out and the globe pushed forward.

Cases of exophthalmos due to trauma are now seen more frequently. The history and roentgen examination will reveal the change in the size of the orbit. Protrusion of the eye may be produced either by compression of the orbital cavity by extraorbital lesions, or the orbital content may be increased by local tissue reaction or by new growth.

It is important to remember that the orbit is completely occupied at all times by the eyeball, muscles, fat, nerves, vessels, blood volume, and a certain amount of lymph. The eyeball cannot be pushed back into the orbit; the only direction the eyeball can go is forward. A considerable amount of new orbital tissue is required to move the eyeball forward one millimeter. The volume increase of the orbit must be about 1,600 cubic millimeter in order to push the eyeball outwards by one millimeter. This must be borne in mind when dealing with orbital tumors or lesions, as physicians are frequently surprised by the size of the abscess or the size of the local growth in the presence of only a small amount of exophthalmus.

Intracranial lesion itself does not, as a rule, change the position of the eyeball except in very rare cases. When changes in the position of the eyeball do occur with increased intracranial pressure, the diagnosis is so obvious that differentiation is not necessary.

In children, certain sinuses are absent up to seven and eight years of age. Therefore, unilateral exophthalmos is rarely due to sinus disease in a child. Exophthalmos in children should be divided into two groups: (1) the inflammatory group, and (2) the non-inflammatory group. If it is inflammatory, the sinuses must be excluded immediately or the possibility of an orbital cellulitis or abscess secondary to some general condition. Any precious constitutional disease may produce or lead to an orbital abscess. Yet, surgical measures to aid in diagnosis should not be undertaken unless all other measures have been tried.

An inflamed prominent eye in a young child always leads to some trouble posterior to the eye, but does not always mean that the orbit must be entered in order to make a diagnosis or give treatment. This is especially true in the cases of orbital edema with some stasis of the blood due to involvement of the ethmoid or the antrum in which poor drainage from the nose is present. In these cases, especially if a diagnosis of sinus disease could be made, the patient should be put to bed and given supportive measures, such as frequent applications of heat to the face, drops to the nose, and suction to establish drainage through the nose. The eyeball will go back into position without the disfiguring scar from an orbital operation.

In the noninflammatory groups in children, an intermittent exophthalmos may be present due to a vascular tumor of the orbit, to encephalocele, dermoid cysts, or occasional sarcoma. Every possible diagnostic point must be investigated in order to determine the etiological factor in unilateral exophthalmos.

The position of the eyes aids in the differential diagnosis. Lesions invading the orbit from without or surrounding areas, usually push the eyeball into position opposite to the invaded area. This is not always exactly correct, however.

Unilateral exophthalmos occurring in adults requires considerable study before a definite diagnosis can be established. Spontaneous exophthalmos may follow a strong sneeze if there is a dehiscence of the orbital wall on the nasal side. This is a type of emphysema, and one may feel the air moving under the palpating finger. A light blow upon the orbit may produce sufficient injury to the nasal bony wall of the orbit to cause such a dehiscence.

Sudden exophthalmos may follow the washing out of the maxillary sinus under pressure. This is not a serious accident, unless pus is pushed into the orbit.

It is important to remember that acute and noninflammatory orbital edema is associated with angioneurotic edema and other allergic factors, and also is associated with the early stages of trichinosis. New growths appearing in the orbit of an adult may be inflammatory or noninflammatory. The sarcomas are usually noninflammatory and usually come down into the orbit from above or occur in at least 75 percent in the superior half of the orbit.

Most metastases in the orbit have been secondary to carcinoma, these arising elsewhere in the body. Orbital carcinoma are usually infiltrating new growth, produce pain, are inflammatory, and tend to early fixation of the eyeball. They usually come from the antrum or the nasal side of the orbit, and are unilateral as a rule.

Cases of pulsating exophthalmos are not rare. The history is not always definite and the expected bruit is not always present. It may be transitory, both to the patient and to the examiner. Until the automobile era, most cases of pulsating exophthalmos were secondary to spontaneous rupture of a vessel within the orbit, trauma playing a very minor role. The cases now are usually traumatic in origin, being due to automobile injuries. Every case of exophthalmos should be listened to with a stethoscope for a diagnostic bruit.

Pseudotumors of the orbit in adults are not uncommon, arising usually from a posterior ethmoid cell. The entire orbit is invaded by low grade granulation tissue which usually is painful, inflamed and insidious in growth.

Panophthalmia is another inflammatory process occurring in the orbit. It arises from the anterior portion of the socket and is usually so obvious that diagnosis is immediate. All in all, the diagnosis of exophthalmos is made by exclusion only. It requires painstaking study in every instance, and examination of the nose and throat is always necessary in a patient with a protruding eye. Roentgenograms are of great help but are not to be relied upon entirely.

"TRACHEOBRONCHIAL VARICES AND HEMORRHAGIC TRACHEOBRONCHITIS; ITS ENDOSCOPIC RECOGNITION." J. M. Remolar, and L. A. Samengo. Archivos argentinos de enfermedades del aparato respiratorio y tuberculosis, vol. 9, p. 312-319, November 1941.

Formerly, bronchoscopic examination was restricted to a few indications, and the use of the bronchoscope was thought to be an instance of malpractice in cases of hemoptysis. Now, recurrent hemoptysis is one of the chief indications for bronchoscopic examination. It is the only means to detect the primary source of bronchial bleeding, whether the blood originates from tumors, varices, ulcers or hemorrhagic inflammations.

Varices in the tracheobronchial tree are rather frequent according to the published medical literature, but they are often mistaken for tuberculosis, or bronchial dilatation or for other sources of hemorrhage. Their pathogenesis and etiology is unknown, since there have been no biopsies and no autopsies made in such cases. It is told that such varices show the lability of the venous system, which itself is a non-committal statement.

One should distinguish isolated tracheobronchial varices, varices resulting from general systemic disease, and hemorrhagic tracheitis. Tracheobronchial varices may occur in liver cirrhosis, leukemia, hemophilia, purpura, severe jaundice, etc. They may also develop in chronic industrial poisoning, in workers who are exposed to irritating gases, war gases, or to lead and arsenic. Cases of hemorrhagic tracheobronchitis are mostly due to infection. Syphilis has also been incriminated as a factor in producing tracheobronchial manifestations with hemorrhage. Of course, tuberculosis is the most frequent cause of hemorrhagic tracheobronchitis. Rosenthal proved that the Pfeiffer bacillus may also provoke acute tracheobronchial inflammations with bleeding.

The clinical picture is characterized by bloody sputum without exact pulmonary signs, discrete retrosternal pain, and general malaise. The clinical course is favorable and spontaneous healing will occur within from ten to 15 days. This is true for most cases of grippe tracheobronchitis.

Another factor in bronchial bleeding is bronchomycosis and bronchospirochaetosis. The latter is caused by Castellani's spirochaete, and is manifested in the form of chronic tracheitis. Recently, Collet stated that deficiency of vitamin C may also be a predisposing factor in the pathogenesis of varices or hemorrhagic tracheitis. In the present author's clinical material the lack of vitamin C proved to be of importance in the maintenance of hemoptysis, and administration of this vitamin was an excellent adjuvant.

The endoscopic exploration of the tracheobronchial tree is the only procedure that may ascertain a correct diagnosis. The bronchoscopic aspect varies. One may find a few varices, which are mostly on the posterior wall of the trachea over or below the glottis. Or, there may be diffuse lesions over a red, congested mucosa, of different color and size; this is the more common type of varicous lesions. In hemorrhagic tracheobroncitis there is intensive hyperemia of the mucous membrane with numerous small and large varicosities; the mucosa is covered with pseudomembranes and blood coagula.

The only available and successful treatment of these conditions is by means of the bronchoscope. The varices are cauterized with 10 percent of silver nitrate. Lesions in the second stage can still be cured easily, but in more advanced cases repeated bronchoscopic treatment will be needed. In general, one or two treatments are sufficient for the cure of tracheobronchial varices.

CARDIOLOGY
Edited by F. Redding Hood, M. D.
1200 North Walker, Oklahoma City

"TREATMENT OF CONGESTIVE HEART FAILURE."

In a lecture before the New York Academy of Medicine, Paul D. White (Bull. New York Acad. Med. 18:18, 1942) presents some pertinent remarks concerning treatment of congestive failure.

"Digitalis, in any one of numerous effective forms, still remains the drug par excellence for myocardial failure, no matter what the heart rhythm," says White, "although the results are more spectacular in the presence of auricular fibrillation with rapid heart rate."

One should be certain that dyspnea or edema is of cardiac origin and not a result of pulmonary disease or local stasis before digitalis is administered. Nor is digitalis of value when congestion is the result of chronic constrictive pericarditis unless auricular fibrillation has occurred as a complication to speed up the heart rate, in which circumstance it does help a lot.

It is important to avoid giving digitalis in doses sufficient to upset the patient inasmuch as the drug will probably be needed during the rest of his life and should not be made excessively distasteful. White points out that so-called sensitiveness or idiosyncrasy to digitalis is usually a result of physical or mental repugnance to previous toxic dosage. He states that he has never encountered an instance of true allergy to digitalis.

Three other observations concerning digitalis should be emphasized. The first concerns occasional drug intoxication immediately following vigorous mercurial diuresis, which may be wrongly attributed to the diuretic. In these patients, a good deal of digitalis as well as water may be released suddenly from the tissues and produce a toxic saturation of digitalis.

The second point concerns the different strengths of digitalis preparations. Many have been increased in strength to accord with the international standard of the U. S. Pharmacopeia. Others have retained their old strength on which most physicians have based routine digitalis dosage for years.

White states: "Since the new potency is from 30 to 50 percent stronger than the old, it behooves us always carefully to note the statements on the labels of the preparations we are using to avoid the possibility of disagreeable or even dangerous digitalis intoxication which I have found to have become, quite abruptly, increasingly frequent throughout the country in the last few years because of the general lack of appreciation of this important fact."

The third point "concerns the use of digitalis in modest dosage, say at the rate of one or one-half the usual daily ration without digitalization first, in cases of considerable myocardial strain and enlargement before the muscle fails, in order to prevent congestive failure. Dr. Henry Christian advised this some years ago and I believe it is a wise move, despite the difficulty of proof of its efficiency."

Mercurials given intravenously have assumed an important and useful role as diuretics in congestive failure, but there is some neglect of milder diuretics that may be taken by mouth and suffice as adjuvants to rest and digitalis.

ORTHOPAEDIC SURGERY
Edited by Earl D. McBride, M. D., F. A. C. S.
605 N. W. 10th, Oklahoma City

"MUSCLE BEHAVIOR FOLLOWING INFANTILE PA-
RALYSIS." Herbert E. Hipps. The American Journal
of Surgery, LIII, 314, 1941.

The author reports a study of a series of cases of
infantile paralysis in which he attempted to determine
whether or not a paralyzed muscle tries to recover when
placed at rest in a relaxed position. He did not use
transplanted muscles in the study or muscles which were
hard to demonstrate, such as the quadratus lumborum.
The only patients used were those receiving physiotherapy and brace treatment, or rest and braces. The
grading system used was as follows: zero, trace, poor,
fair, good, normal.
The results in the three age groups studied were:
(1) Six months to six years—37.3 percent improvement;
(2) Six years to 15 years—44.7 percent improvement;
(3) Sixteen years and over—27.3 percent improvement.
Two hundred and eighty-seven muscles, graded poor
plus, fair, or good, showed much improvement in 87
percent of the cases; 276 muscles graded zero, trace,
or poor showed slight or no improvement in 90 percent.
Thus, he concludes that muscles which have been
paralyzed a long time, and grade only zero to trace or
poor, will not benefit by prolonged rest or physiotherapy,
while those which grade poor plus, fair, or good can
be expected to improve with physiotherapy.
He makes the unanalyzed statement that 25 miscellaneous patients who received adequate treatment made an
average improvement of 47.5 percent; 21 patients who
received inadequate treatment made an average improvement of 20.6 percent.
Twenty-three cases were studied to determine the
relative efficiency of early treatment, beginning immediately after the temperature subsided, with the following results:
(1) Early complete rest with splinting—23.8 percent.
(2) Early physiotherapy—68.5 percent.
(3) No treatment(small number of patients)—31.1
percent.

"END RESULTS OF SYNOVECTOMY OF THE KNEE
JOINT." Ralph K. Ghormley and David M. Cameron.
The Amer. Jr. of Surg. LIII, 455, 1941.

The authors review Swett's original paper in which
were stated the three theoretical considerations on which
to base operation for this condition.
1. With foci removed, the inflammatory process in
the joints subsiding, and the usual means of absorption
of the inflammatory exudate having failed, manual removal of the exudate might promote the resumption of
joint function.
2. Such operations might be helpful, not alone by
the mechanical improvement, but by removal of organisms capable of continuing the process.
3. Stimulation of metabolism, by prompt restoration
of function in atrophic disused joints and muscles, might
occur.
The authors state that synovectomy may be employed
in a joint in which extensive induration and fibrosis of
the capsule, enlargement of the synovial villi, and persistent increase of joint fluid are present. The causes
of such conditions may be as follows: chronic atrophic
arthritis, traumatic arthritis, benign tumors, osteochondromatosis, syphilitic arthritis, intermittent hydrarthrosis,
synovitis ossificans, hypertrophic arthritis, synovial tuberculosis, synovitis caused by a foreign body.
Their results indicate that synovectomy is most useful
in traumatic arthritis, synovial osteochondromatosis, and

xanthoma or benign tumors. It is of less value, although
indicated, in some cases of chronic infectious arthritis.
It is of value in chronic synovitis, but the prognosis
should be guarded; this holds true also in intermittent
hydrarthrosis.

"FRESH COMPOUND FRACTURES. TREATMENT BY
SULFONAMIDES AND BY INTERNAL FIXATION IN
SELECTED CASES." Willis C. Campbell and Hugh
Smith. Jr. A.M.A. CXVII, 672, 1941.

The authors' report is based on three years of experience in this method of treatment, and includes a
series of 50 private patients treated under optimum
surgical conditions, with adequate postoperative care and
follow-up, and 93 patients of the municipal hospital
treated under less favorable conditions. Sulfonamides
were used in the entire series; metallic, internal fixation
in 42 of the cases; and primary closure of wounds in
the majority. No set routine was followed for all
compound fractures, but in general the treatment consisted in adequate debridement, copious irrigation with
normal saline, and implantation of five to 20 grams of
sulfanilamide crystals in the wound, metallic fixation
when indicated—using vitallium stainless steel—followed
by primary closure in all cases except those of more
than 12 hours' duration, those with soft tissues so extensively mangled that closure of the skin was impossible,
or those in which complete debridement was impossible,
as in shotgun wounds of a fleshy part.
In comparing this entire group with a group of 75
compound fractures in which neither internal fixation nor
the sulfonamides were used, it was found that the percentage of union and non-union, and the average time
required for union in the two groups, was approximately
the same.
Primary closure, in conjunction with sulfonamide
therapy, did not increase the incidence of gas gangrene,
nor was there a sufficiently striking decrease in its
incidence to indicate a particularly beneficial effect of
the sulfonamides on the gas-producing organism. The
incidence of infection was reduced from 33.3 to 18.1
percent; only two of 143 patients wro received sulfonamide died from infection, as compared with three in
the control series.
In a comparison of the 40 patients in whom internal
fixation was used, with the 52 in whom no internal
fixation was used, it was found that there were 14
infections and 11 non-unions in the former group, and
11 infections with three non-unions in the latter. There
was little difference in the average period required for
union between those with and those without internal
fixation. The high incidence of infection and non-union
in the group with internal fixation, is partially explained
by the fact that it was used in those with severe fractures in whom a higher percentage of infection and
non-union could be expected. The authors feel that
their results have been materially improved by these
measures, and do not hesitate to use internal fixations
when indicated.

"CALCIUM DEPOSITS IN THE SHOULDER AND SUB-
ACROMIAL BURSITIS." A Survey of 12,122 Should-
ers. Boardman Marsh Bosworth. The Jr. of A.M.A.,
CXVI, 2477, 1941.

The author examined, clinically and by roentgenograms, the shoulders of 6,061 unselected persons, and
found 165, or 2.7 percent, of the group had calcium deposits about the shoulder. Of the total group, 5,061
were followed over a three-year period. During this
time 70 patients had symptoms of pain in the shoulder.
The cases appeared more frequently in males below the
age of 50, and especially in patients whose work required long periods of use of the arms in abduction.
The author feels that there is a definite occupational
factor in the formation of these deposits. A few deposits were found to occur in as short a time as two
months, but it was felt that the majority developed
slowly over a number of months.

In diagnosing these cases, the author advocates the use of a fluoroscopic and spot-film roentgenographic technique to prevent the overlooking of otherwise obscure calcium deposits.

In treating these cases, it must be remembered that some will heal spontaneously. Others may be improved or cured by such means as heat (infra-red diathermy) or irrigation methods. The author, however, prefers surgical excision of the deposits as being the surest means of complete relief. After such a procedure, the patient may expect to return to work, without symptoms, in about three weeks.

INTERNAL MEDICINE

Edited by Hugh Jeter, M. D., F. A. C. P., A. S. C. P.
1200 North Walker, Oklahoma City

"INFECTIOUS MONONUCLEOSIS." Diseases of the Blood, Second Edition, Roy R. Kracke. Infectious Mononucleosis. A. Bernstein. Med. 19:85, 1940.

The following is a summary of the subject of Infectious Mononucleosis taken largely from the above.

(Benign Lymphadenosis) (Glandular Fever) (Acute Benign Lymphoblastosis) (Acute Benign Leukemia) (Acute Lymphadenosis) (Monocytic Angina) (Lymphocytosis of Infection)

All of these names have been assigned to the disease from time to time and by different authors and are given you because collectively they convey the nature of the disease.

History

The disease seems to have been first recorded in 1885 by Filatow in Russia, who called it an idiopathic lymphadenopathy of children. An epidemic involving 96 children in Ohio was reported by West in 1896. Terfinger in 1908 reported an epidemic of 150 cases occurring in adults. Sprunt and Evans in 1920 introduced the name infectious mononucleosis, and following this many reports have been made. The last and perhaps the most important contribution to literature is a monograph by Bernstein.

Etiology

The disease has been reported from all parts of the world. Kracke believes it is probably non-existent in negroes. It is more prevalent in children and young adults, but old individuals have been known to be affected. Infants under the age of six months are considered to be immune. More cases of males than females have been reported. No seasonal or occupational incident of importance has been reported. The disease may be epidemic or sporatic. Epidemics seem to be more likely among children and sporatic cases the rule for adults. Incubation period varies from five to 15 days and it is assumed that the infection is transmitted by fairly close contact, although it is unusual for more than one child in a family to become infected.

Considerable investigation has been done in connection with the search for a specific etiological agent, both in the human and in animals, without success.

Symptoms

The onset is gradual, the patient has fatigue, dull headache, general malaise, sore throat, lymphadenopathy and after about six days becomes febrile. The cervical (posterior auricular usually not involved), axillary and inguinal glands usually become considerably enlarged and moderately tender and at the end of about the first ten day period the patient complains of moderate sore throat.

Symptoms as summarized by Isaacs and his associates are as follows: "Headache, general malaise, sore throat, tenderness of the glands, backache, chilliness, anorexis, coryza, sweating, weakness, cough, dizziness, sore bleeding gums, nausea, stiff neck, epistaxis, stomatitis, abdominal pain, rash, photophobia and conjunctivitis. The temperature ranges from 102° to 105°, enlargement of the glands is practically 100 percent and suppuration of glands has seldom been observed. The spleen is palpable in about 40 percent of the cases but never extremely large.''

Like most acute infectious diseases, there is considerable variation in the severity and, likewise, the symptoms. As a rule no complications occur and the disease runs a course of 20 to 30 days.

Diagnosis

Although the disease presents a fairly characteristic clinical syndrome, certain laboratory procedures are of definitely specific value.

The macrolymphocytosis is an outstanding feature. The term macrolymphocytosis is preferable to the term mononucleosis, because the cells which predominate during the course of this disease are not always the classical large mononuclear cells. Regardless of this technicality, a persistent finding in these cases is that of a high percentage, 40 to 90, of lymphocytes which are larger than normal, and whether they are to be called large mononuclears or immature lymphocytes is only a technicality. The total number of myeloid cells or neutrophils is ordinarily decreased, which makes neutropenia a conspicuous finding from the very onset and of the neutrophils present, most are immature in form.

We may say then, in brief, that the blood picture is that of leucocytosis, neutropenia and macrolymphocytosis.

Anemia is against the rule and thrombocytes are ordinarily average or slightly decreased in number and normal in quality. Bleeding time may be slightly prolonged, but is ordinarily within normal limits and the clotting time is universally normal. There has been no consistant relation to any blood group. Blood chemistry is normal.

For some strange reason the serological tests for syphilis have been falsely positive in 18 percent (Bernstein). The Widal Agglutination Test has also been reported positive in an occasional case.

The Heterophile Antibody Test

Heterophile simply means that antibodies are present which cause a reaction such as agglutination or hemolysis with antigens other than those involved in their production. In this instance the antigen involved in the production of the disease of infectious mononucleosis is not known but the serum containing antibodies is found to agglutinate and occasionally hemolyze the red cells of the sheep, the goat and the ox. In other words, the reaction toward cells or antigens other than those which cause the disease, hetero- meaning other and -phile meaning affinity. The heterophile antibody or Paul-Bunnell Test, therefore, amounts to a simple test in which the serum in different dilutions is added to sheep cells in suspension. Agglutination is easily observed.

Normal blood may contain sheep cell agglutins up to a titer of 1:80. In infectious mononucleosis the dilution ranges much higher, from 1:160 to as high as 1:40,000, and in one case 1:160,000 was reported. The test becomes positive four or five days after the onset of the disease and remains positive in relatively high dilutions for six to 12 months. Serum which has been kept in the ice box for as long as three years has been found to give a strong positive reaction. The age of the sheep cells, the concentration of the sheep cells and the length of incubation may be factors in connection with the titer of the serum, but the test is invariably strongly positive and a matter of dilution has no clinical significance. Ordinarily two hours incubation is allowed. Bunnell ran tests for heterophile antibodies in over 2,000 patients representing 76 clinical entities and none showed a titer higher than 1:32, while the cases of infectious mononucleosis ranged from 1:62 to 1:4096. Therefore, the presence of a definitely positive heterophile antibody test is practically absolute assurance that the patient is suffering from infectious mononucleosis. Cases of serum sickness may likewise give a positive in high dilutions.

The biopsies of lymph nodes have shown diffuse hyperplasia with no absolutely characteristic histopathological pattern. The abnormal lymphocytes that appear in the blood stream may be recognized in large numbers in the lymph nodes.

No valuable information has been obtained from autopsies. This is as might be expected because death has rarely occurred.

Differential Diagnosis

Leukemia, agranulocytosis, Vincent's angina, diphtheria, tonsillitis, syphilis, Hodgkin's disease, tuberculosis and occasionally some other similar type disease may at the onset present a similar picture.

Acute lymphatic leukemia offers the greatest difficulty in differentiation in so far as the laboratory findings are concerned. Leukemoid states simulating leukemia or simulating infectious mononucleosis may occur. However, neither true lymphatic leukemia nor leukemoid states give a positive heterophile antibody test.

Treatment

There is no specific treatment. Isolation and symptomatic therapy are adequate. Serums, sulfanols, x-ray and other agents have been used without satisfactory results. Bed rest during the febrile period and modified ambulatory activities for a week to ten days following cessation of fever is recommended.

UROLOGY

Edited by D. W. Branham, M. D.
502 Medical Arts Building, Oklahoma City

"INFLUENCE OF TEMPERATURE ON SULFATHIAZOLE THERAPY OF GONOCOCCAL INFECTIONS." Frederick B. Bang, Nashville, Tenn. Journal of Urology, March, 1942.

The use of the chick embryo as an experimental host for gonococci allows an in vivo study of chemotherapy at different temperatures. It is noteworthy that not only is therapy more effective at temperatures above 37° C., but it is less effective below.

A small series of hospitalized male patients with acute gonorrheal urethritis was treated for five days with the usual dose of sulfathiazole combined with moderate hyperpyrexia. The results of such treatment were favorable and the authors thought that the addition of hyperpyrexia was an enhancing addition to the successful treatment of gonorrhea.

"DISTURBANCES OF THE ACID-BASE BALANCE OF THE BLOOD: THEIR SIGNIFICANCE AND INFLUENCE ON PROGNOSIS IN ELDERLY PATIENTS." H. S. Rupert, Greely, Colo. Journal of Urology, Mar. 1942.

The kidneys' ability to maintain the acid-base balance of the blood is an important element of renal function and is not given the attention it deserves. Neglect of this function probably accounts for a few instances of mortality when surgery is performed. The author suggests that the CO_2 combining power of the blood be determined and if it be low, steps are to be taken to counteract this. They suggest the intravenous administration of sodium lactate, 1/6 molar solution or blood transfusion as the best procedure to control acidosis.

"PROSTATIC OBSTRUCTION IN YOUNG ADULTS." REPORT OF FIVE CASES. H. A. Fowler, Washington, D. C. Journal of Urology, Jan. 1942.

The authors report five instances of true prostatic hypertrophy occurring in young individuals, the youngest 19 years and the oldest 26 years. They discuss the etiology of prostatic hypertrophy in the light of its occurrence in young individuals. They feel that to account for such cases one must assume some factor or factors other than changes incident to the male climacteric as the cause of hormonal imbalance; one that may become operative at any age, possibly of congenital origin.

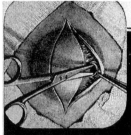

Time-tested dependable

LOCAL ANESTHETIC

LOCAL anesthesia with Novocain has been induced for countless numbers of major and minor operations. Novocain has stood the test of time, having clearly demonstrated its efficiency and relatively high safety.

The strength of solutions required for various types of injections has been standardized by extensive experience as follows: for infiltration, 0.5 per cent solution; for blocking nerve trunks 1 per cent solution; for spinal anesthesia a total dose of from 50 mg. to 200 mg. (or the equivalent 10 per cent solution, further diluted with spinal fluid).

Novocain is available, with and without Suprarenin*, in various sized ampules containing several concentrations and in tablets of different formulas. Few preparations are supplied in such a large variety of convenient, ready-to-use forms.

*Suprarenin (trademark), brand of synthetic epinephrine.

Write for copy of "Novocain—Its Use as a Local Anesthetic for General Surgery" which describes numerous procedures of local anesthesia, profusely illustrated with drawings made in the clinic by a physician artist.

NOVOCAIN
Reg. U. S. Pat. Off. & Canada

Brand of PROCAINE HYDROCHLORIDE

•

Pharmaceuticals of merit for the physician

NEW YORK, N. Y.   **WINDSOR, ONT.**

OFFICERS OF COUNTY SOCIETIES, 1942

COUNTY	PRESIDENT	SECRETARY	MEETING TIME
Alfalfa	Jack F. Parsons, Cherokee	L. T. Lancaster, Cherokee	Last Tues. Each 2nd Mo.
Atoka-Coal	J. B. Clark, Coalgate	J. S. Fulton, Atoka	
Beckham	H. K. Speed, Sayre	E. S. Kilpatrick, Elk City	Second Tues. eve.
Blaine	Virginia Olson Curtin, Watonga	W. F. Griffin, Watonga	
Bryan	A. J. Wells, Calera	W. K. Haynie, Durant	Second Tues. eve.
Caddo	Fred L. Patterson, Carnegie	C. B. Sullivan, Carnegie	
Canadian	P. F. Herod, El Reno	A. L. Johnson, El Reno	Subject to call
Carter	Walter Hardy, Ardmore	H. A. Higgins, Ardmore	
Cherokee	Park H. Medearis, Tahlequah	Isadore Dyer, Tahlequah	
Choctaw	C. H. Hale, Boswell	Fred D. Switzer, Hugo	
Cleveland	F. C. Buffington, Norman	Phil Haddock, Norman	Thursday nights
Comanche	George S. Barber, Lawton	W. F. Lewis, Lawton	
Cotton	George W. Baker, Walters	Mollie F. Scism, Walters	Third Friday
Craig	W. R. Marks, Vinita	J. M. McMillan, Vinita	
Creek	Frank Sisler, Bristow	O. H. Cowart, Bristow	
Custer	Richard M. Burke, Clinton	W. C. Tisdal, Clinton	Third Thursday
Garfield	D. S. Harris, Drummond	John R. Walker, Enid	Fourth Thursday
Garvin	T. F. Gross, Lindsay	John R. Callaway, Pauls Valley	Wed before 3rd Thurs.
Grady	D. S. Downey, Chickasha	Frank T. Joyce, Chickasha	3rd Thursday
Grant	I. V. Hardy, Medford	E. E. Lawson, Medford	
Greer	G. F. Border, Mangum	J. B. Hollis, Mangum	
Harmon	S. W. Hopkins, Hollis	W. M. Yeargan, Hollis	First Wednesday
Haskell	William Carson, Keota	N. K. Williams, McCurtain	
Hughes	Wm. L. Taylor, Holdenville	Imogene Mayfield, Holdenville	First Friday
Jackson	J. M. Allgood, Altus	Willard D. Holt, Altus	Last Monday
Jefferson	W. M. Browning, Waurika	J. I. Hollingsworth, Waurika	Second Monday
Kay	J. C. Wagner, Ponca City	J. Holland Howe, Ponca City	Third Thurs.
Kingfisher	C. M. Hodgson, Kingfisher	John R. Taylor, Kingfisher	
Kiowa	J. M. Bonham, Hobart	B. H. Watkins, Hobart	
LeFlore	G. R. Booth, LeFlore	Rush L. Wright, Poteau	
Lincoln	E. F. Hurlbut, Meeker	C. W. Robertson, Chandler	First Wednesday
Logan	William C. Miller, Guthrie	J. L. LeHew, Jr., Guthrie	Last Tuesday evening
Marshall	J. L. Holland, Madill	O. A. Cook, Madill	
Mayes	L. C. White, Adair	V. D. Herrington, Pryor	
McClain	B. W. Slover, Blanchard	R. L. Royster, Purcell	
McCurtain	R. D. Williams, Idabel	R. H. Sherrill, Broken Bow	Fourth Tues. eve.
McIntosh	F. R. First, Checotah	William A. Tolleson, Eufaula	Second Tuesday
Murray	P. V. Annadown, Sulphur	F. E. Sadler, Sulphur	
Muskogee	Shade D. Neely, Muskogee	J. T. McInnis, Muskogee	First & Third Mon.
Noble	J. W. Francis, Perry	C. H. Cooke, Perry	
Okfuskee	J. M. Pemberton, Okemah	L. J. Spickard, Okemah	Second Monday
Oklahoma	R. Q. Goodwin, Okla. City	Wm. E. Eastland, Okla. City	Fourth Tuesday
Okmulgee	J. G. Edwards, Okmulgee	John R. Cotteral, Henryetta	Second Monday
Osage	C. R. Weirich, Pawhuska	George K. Hemphill, Pawhuska	Second Monday
Ottawa	J. B. Hampton, Commerce	Walter Sanger, Picher	Third Thursday
Pawnee	E. T. Robinson, Cleveland	Robert L. Browning, Pawnee	
Payne	John W. Martin, Cushing	James D. Martin, Cushing	Third Thursday
Pittsburg	Austin R. Stough, McAlester	Edw. D. Greenberger, McAlester	Third Friday
Pontotoc	R. E. Cowling, Ada	E. R. Muntz, Ada	First Wednesday
Pottawatomie	John Carson, Shawnee	Clinton Gallaher, Shawnee	First & Third Sat.
Pushmataha	P. B. Rice, Antlers	John S. Lawson, Clayton	
Rogers	W. A. Howard, Chelsea	George D. Waller, Claremore	First Monday
Seminole	H. M. Reeder, Konawa	Mack I. Shanholtz, Wewoka	
Stephens	A. J. Weedn, Duncan	W. K. Walker, Marlow	
Texas	L. G. Blackmer, Hooker	Johnny A. Blue, Guymon	
Tillman	C. C. Allen, Frederick	O. G. Bacon, Frederick	
Tulsa	H. B. Stewart, Tulsa	E. O. Johnson, Tulsa	Second & Fourth Mon. eve.
Wagoner	J. H. Plunkett, Wagoner	H. K. Riddle, Coweta	
Washington-Nowata	R. W. Rucker, Bartlesville	J. V. Athey, Bartlesville	Second Wednesday
Washita	A. S. Neal, Cordell	James F. McMurry, Sentinel	
Woods	W. F. LaFon, Waynoka	O. E. Templin, Alva	Last Wednesday
Woodward	M. H. Newman, Shattuck	C. W. Tedrowe, Woodward	

THE JOURNAL
OF THE
OKLAHOMA STATE MEDICAL ASSOCIATION

| VOLUME XXXV | OKLAHOMA CITY, OKLAHOMA, JUNE, 1942 | NUMBER 6 |

The Management of Depressions As Seen in General Practice

TITUS H. HARRIS, M.D.

GALVESTON, TEXAS

When a psychiatrist is asked to present a paper before a group of medical men whose interest lies principally in the field of general medicine he is confronted with the problem of selecting a subject for discussion which is of practical value and yet one about which he, as a psychiatrist, is qualified to speak. There are many subjects that would fall into this category because psychiatry is no longer a narrow field of medicine confining itself to the management of chronic psychotic patients. On the contrary, psychiatry permeates every field of medicine. The surgeon, for example, appreciates the need for caution in making the decision to operate a neurotic patient; yet at times these patients develop surgical conditions. He should also realize the importance of proper management of such a patient in order to avoid post-operative complaints. The dermatologist certainly realizes the relationship between emotional tension and anxiety and certain of the urticarias. The internist has his spastic colon patients, and he, too, knows that treatment confined strictly to the colon keeps them living in terms of diet and elimination, all of which does little for the patient. I could go on mentioning every specialty in medicine, showing that after all, we are dealing with people who are sick and not individual organs or systems, and we must realize that people are struggling to achieve the most in life and in so doing they worry and they suffer defeats, which in turn influence the behavior or function of that person to an extent where one might develop a pain, or a skin lesion, or an eye complaint, or a spastic colon, depending on the total life experience of that particular individual.

Medical schools have realized that psychiatry is fundamental in medical education during the past ten or fifteen years, and so much so that this subject is taught throughout the four years of the curriculum. The study of a normal person his origin and function, is presented in the freshman year along with anatomy and physiology. In the second year pathological behavior or psychopathology is presented along with organ pathology. Then in the last two years clinical psychiatry is taught, not so much in the psychopathic hospital as in the medical and surgical wards of the general hospital and in the general hospital out-clinic.

So when the psychiatrist is selecting a subject of general medical interest he has a wide range from which to choose. For example, he might talk about the psychiatric management of essential hypertension, or the treatment of the irritable colon; or an especially good subject would be the management of the menopause situation. But at this time I have selected the subject—"The Management of Depressions as Seen in General Practice"—because I can think of no other subject fulfilling the requirements outlined above more completely than does a discussion of the depressive reactions.

I refer particularly to the mild depressed states that are so close to the borderline of health and illness that the patients are often thought not to be ill at all, and are subjected to rebuke for their complaints instead of the sympathetic consideration which they deserve. This disease is among the most common in medicine and, I am sure, one of the greatest burdens to the physician. It has been said by a well known psychiatrist that next to the common cold the simple depression is the most common disease seen by physicians. These conditions are important because, with proper management, the recovery rate is practically 100 percent, and recovery is complete in every respect, and also because 95 percent of the suicides occur among these patients. Since they are recoverable, they should receive just as much skilled care as we give pneumonia or any other acute disease.

The frank or major depressions are easily recognized. There is much agitation in the involutional type, and usually their delusional expressions of a self-accusatory type make one immediately put them in the class of the mentally sick. These patients generally express a need of punishment for some imaginary sin or criminal act. Such patients may believe that they are to be arrested and put in the penitentiary, or are doomed to suffer unto eternity and burn in hellfire. With such a disturbance of the mental content they are promptly considered psychotic, and institutional treatment is advised. Suicide is frequent among this group, but occurs less often because that tendency is recognized early in the illness and prevented by appropriate hospital care.

The severe depressions of the manic-depressive type, too, are easily recognized with the usual slowing up of mental and physical activity and the history of a previous attack of despondency or excitement which required hospital care.

In contrast, the very common simple depressions are not easily recognized unless one understands the clinical picture. They are most often thought of as a psychoneurosis or a simple unnecessary worry syndrome. In describing the simple depression, it is necessary to compare the symptoms with those of a psychoneurosis and to discuss the difference between the two conditions since at times they are very much alike and difficult to differentiate from each other. A psychoneurosis implies a disease state or symptom which, while disordered function is present, is not caused by pathological tissue change. It represents a reactive state, that is, the symptom is motivated by some situation that is unsatisfactory to the patient and is actively going on at the moment, and, therefore, will continue until the situation ceases to exist, or at least ceases to be distasteful. Thus treatment (in the form of psychotherapeutic measures) must be active and directed toward removing the cause.

These characteristics are not true of a depression. A depression represents an episode of illness in a previously healthy person, and the basis for the symptoms comes from within as a result of illness, and not in any sense are they due to external factors, situations, conflicts, and sources of worry. On the contrary, the depressive illness will create a situation which might appear to be the actual source of worry.

For example, a young woman decided she had made a mistake by marriage and attempted suicide rather than suffer the unhappiness caused by her supposed mistake. Yet after recovery she was quite happy to remain in the married state.

Another patient, a physician who had always been happy and successful in his work, decided that the town in which he lived was the reason for his miserable plight, and firmness and much persuasion were necessary to prevent his moving to another community. This attitude, too, disappeared with recovery from the depression.

I mention these two examples to illustrate how an apparently logical source of worry is really created by the illness and represents a symptom of it.

A psychoneurosis will promptly respond when the cause has been corrected. It will respond to suggestion and to persuasion and encouragement, but a depression, again, represents an episode of fixed illness in the same sense that fever is fixed, and will not immediately respond to anything that is done. Often economic reverses are the primary cause of worry; yet restoration of satisfactory economic conditions will not influence the course of the illness. Again, a psychoneurosis may have existed for many months or years, while the simple depression usually lasts only a few months. A psychoneurosis is usually preceded by months or years of an unhappy existence, while a depression may occur without even a precipitating cause and usually develops in previously well adjusted, happy people. A phychoneurosis more often presents physical complaints, while the depression's symptoms are concerned largely with a general feeling of sadness. A psychoneurosis is continuous and usually without a history of a previous attack, while in the case of depressions we may be able to obtain a history of a previous episode many years before or even an attack of mild elation or excitement, which may have gone unnoticed at the time.

I draw the distinction between a psychoneurosis and a depression so sharply because the two are so different in the mechanism of production, in the prognosis, and in treatment. The common names by which the depression is known are many. A few may be mentioned — nervous exhaustion, neuro-exhaustion, chronic nervous exhaustion, neurasthenia, or a chronic nerve fatigue —all implying an exhausted or weakened state of the nervous system, and none implying a true episode of illness affecting the emotional function of the individual. And all too often, when this condition occurs in women around middle life, it is thought of as a menopause state. The symptoms of this condition are so classical that one can make the diagnosis by the complaints offered by the relative or the patient. Such statements as the following are common:

"He is all washed up. He worries all the time over nothing. He has nothing to worry him, yet he worries all the time. He can't sleep. He doesn't want to do anything but sit around and brood. Doctor, I am afraid sometimes that he might do something desperate, the way he talks." Or the patient may say, "I have no energy. I can't enjoy anything any more."

Questioning then will bring out the following symptoms: He has lost interest in everything. Things he formerly enjoyed he no longer likes. He has to drive himself to do everything. It takes him longer to do simple tasks. He is weak and easily exhausted. He has no appetite and can't sleep. He is constantly preoccupied with what is happening to himself and can't divert his attention to anything else. He feels that life is a burden and not worth living, and careful questioning nearly always brings out thoughts of suicide. Many physical symptoms may be present—a hot burning scalp, indigestion, constipation, and, in women, an absence of menstruation.

A young lady, described by the father as having always been bright and cheerful, returned home for the holidays and seemed listless and cared nothing about social activities, which formerly had interested her very much. She did not complain much to her parents, but seemed let down, and they thought she had had some trouble in school. When she left home to return to her school, she left a note expressing sorrow for the disappointment she had caused her parents, and directed them how to dispose of certain of her things. When brought to the office this girl came in bright and smiling, and it was hard to realize that she was sick; yet questioning brought out the fact that she was tired, could not do her work well, felt hopeless about the future, could not apply herself, and actively contemplated suicide. Further questioning showed that she had had an episode five years before, with similar symptoms, and later a period during which she was gayer and happier than she had ever been before.

A physician seen some time ago stated that he felt so miserable that his wish would be fulfilled if he could have a fatal automobile accident. He stated that he knew he was losing his practice and that every time he saw a patient he knew the patient would not return, none of which was true. In spite of urgent demands to his relatives that he be put in a hospital for protection, he was permitted to continue his work. He committed suicide by jumping from a tenth floor window. This patient was one of the most highly respected physicians in the state, and had carried on a most commendable work. He had a history of a brief, previous episode of depression fifteen years before.

What is the nature and the cause of this condition? Perhaps it will seem unusual for a psychiatrist to attempt to explain depressions on a physiological basis; yet certain evidence seems to support such a conception —the suddenness of onset and equal suddenness of remission in many of them, and then the almost dramatic response to the recently discovered shock therapy. Physiologists and anatomists have fairly definitely established an emotional center in the brain. We know, too, that one important function of the individual or personality is to feel or express emotion or affect. The depression, then, may be thought of as a disease of the emotional mechanism. Therefore, the symptoms would primarily result from disturbed feeling function, and secondarily, the disease would influence thinking in a depressive way, and also influence the function of certain organs or systems through the effect of tension on the vegetative nervous system. We might compare the development of a depression to the development of fever following exposure to extreme heat. The heat regulating mechanism is upset, and fever occurs as a result of over-production of heat and inadequate elimination. So with a depressive reaction, the individual is subjected to so much tension that finally the emotional mechanism is upset, and there is produced from within the patient a disturbance of feeling with the development of depressive symptoms. A very large group of individuals have a sensitive emotional mechanism, and, therefore, develop a disease of this function more easily than others, in the same sense that certain people develop tuberculosis or an allergic state more easily than do others. The threshold of resistance varies. In those with a low threshold very little in the way of psychic trauma or anxiety or tension is necessary to produce a depressed state. Thus we see many recurrences of this disease, while in others there is a high threshold, and we see depressions occur only after severe external tension and few or widely separated recurrences. Thinking of the depressions in this way it is easy to understand the symptoms and offer a prognosis both as to recurrence and outcome.

This illness, the depression, is often thought to be due to endocrine imbalance, especially when the disease occurs in women around the mid-period of life. But even here, it is our opinion that there is no causative relationship, and if endocrine symptoms occur, they are secondary to the depressed state, and not in any sense a cause. Many of you no doubt have treated such patients with ovarian hormones, and have seen them recover, but we must not forget that we are dealing with a disease which recovers spontaneously, and will recover with any form of treatment as long as the patient is adequately supported and does not fall a victim of suicide.

As to prognosis, we can always predict a favorable outcome for the particular episode. The average duration is a few months. Recovery will be complete, and the individual will be just as capable as before the illness, and if there is no history of a previous attack we need not expect recurrences. If there is a history of repeated attacks, we may expect recurrences to occur, although this is not always the case. Statistics indicate that 50% of the manic-depressive type do not recur, and the probability is less in the other types of depression. An opinion seems to be present among the medical profession that the outlook for the depressive patient is bad with regard to recurrences, and advice is frequently offered with regard to future occupation on this basis. For example, a patient under observation is an aviator, and because of a single attack his wife was advised that he should never attempt to fly again. The implication, on the part of the physician, is that he may not recover and that recurrence is likely. In this instance I would not advise a change in occupation. On occasions patients are discharged from jobs carrying responsibility because of a single attack of depression. It is our responsibility to correct such mis-information through educational measures.

In considering the treatment of the depressions it is most important to discuss the question of suicide. As has been indicated, 95 percent of all suicides occur in this group of conditions. Every depression must be considered a potential suicide. After the diagnosis has been established an effort should be made to evaluate the possibility of suicide. This can be done by keeping in mind certain facts to be discussed. In the first place, it is incorrect to assume that a person who talks of suicide will not commit the act. Yet this is a view which seems to be very prevalent. I believe that all patients with a suicidal tendency will talk about it if given an opportunity to do so by a sympathetic listener. Many will have expressed a wish to die. Once an attempt has been made and it is felt to be genuine, no further chance should be taken, and such a patient should be hospitalized immediately. If a patient shows agitation or if he expresses guilt feelings or expresses a need to be punished for supposed sins or criminal acts, he should be considered suicidal. Of particular importance is the patient who feels that he is a burden to his family and that they would be better off if he were out of the way. Patients often commit suicide in order for their family to obtain life insurance. We should be on our guard, too, when a depression suddenly improves. This often means that a decision to commit suicide has been reached, and with the issue settled, the tension lessens. Such guides are valuable, but of more importance is that most of these patients, if talked to frankly and questioned in an understanding way, will admit suicidal thoughts and desires, and the tendency can be adequately evaluated. If it can be determined that suicide is a probability, then hospitalization for protection is absolutely necessary, because certainly the patient can be watched more closely in a hospital than he can at home, regardless of what precautions are utilized.

If it is determined that suicide is not a danger, and since the illness is self-limited and recovery is spontaneous, then treatment amounts to supporting the patient and seeing that he gets adequate nutrition and rest. Encouragement and sympathy are important. An explanation as to the nature of the illness will help, and if a patient is told that he will, with certainty, recover, and if the physician explains his limitations in the matter of actual treatment, then confidence is established, and the patient will not go from physicians to physician looking for help. I believe it is helpful, too, to carefully explain to the patient that he is sick and that the control of his symptoms is beyond any effort that he himself can make. I often compare the illness to typhoid fever and mention to the patient that he is just as helpless to help himself get well as the typhoid patient is to throw off his fever.

It is very important to explain this situation to relatives of patients because the unfortunate patient is usually derided and nagged because he won't quit his "silly worrying." We must not expect any treatment we offer to alter the course of the illness. If we are certain of the diagnosis, we need not worry about the patient's recovery. If you can understand such a patient in this way, the patient will not be the burden that he often seems to be. Some tonic medication, in the form of injections that can be given at the office, will keep the patient under supervision, where encouragement can be offered and his physical health improved. Sleep is always an important question and can best be handled by the barbiturate group of drugs. These drugs are not harmful if taken only for sleep, and can be given safely over a long period of time. It is best not to use bromide because of the danger of intoxication and delirium in this type of patient. Diversion of any kind is helpful; however, since these patients have to drive themselves they will not take part in any activity unless forced to or led by a suitable companion or relative, and often this is such a burden that it accomplishes nothing. Nor can psychotherapy in the strict sense be utilized in the depressions. We should, of course, encourage, try to understand, sympathize, and influence the patient to accept treatment, and we should establish a deep feeling of confidence on the part of such a patient—all of which is a part of psychotherapy, but we do not think it helpful to try to discover hidden conflicts and try to establish a relationship between these and the disease, in such a patient. This, of course, is not true of a psychoneurosis. In the case of a psychoneurosis, trying to alter the relationship between the patient and his situation is the chief approach to therapy. But in the case of the depressions we are concerned with an episode of illness which recovers spontaneously, with the patient returning to his normal way of feeling and thinking.

In outlining the treatment of depressions one must mention the remarkable results being achieved now with shock therapy. Statistically eighty to eighty-five percent of these patients recover in a very short time with this plan of treatment; yet we do not want to subject a patient to this drastic plan of treatment if it can be safely avoided. I will try to mention what I consider to be the indications for shock treatment. I believe that those who have had experience in treating depressions feel that the electro-shock method is best. It seems to be less hazardous, and certainly is more agreeable to the patient and probably gets better results than does either metrazol or insulin. Shock therapy is a specialized type of treatment and should be used only by one who is experienced in this method.

I would think of the following circumstances as indicating a need for this form of treatment:

First, in the presence of suicidal tendencies such a patient cannot be adequately and completely protected even in a psychiatric hospital, so shock therapy is much less a danger and should be used. Many times thoughts of suicide will disappear even after the first few treatments.

For example, one patient had already spent three months in one hospital and was advised to take a trip south during the winter. He became worse and attempted suicide. A constant attendant was necessary even after reaching the hospital; yet with electro-shock therapy he was completely well in one month and returned home.

We find certain depressions that linger on for months or even a year or two. This would seem to be an indication for shock treatment. A recent patient had a depression of a very mild degree for three years. Only two treatments were necessary to interrupt the condition in this case, and he was in the hospital for only one week.

In the presence of extreme agitation, where the question of management is doubtful, shock therapy should be used.

And then in the case of involutional depression where the prognosis is never very good with the ordinary methods of treatment, shock therapy should be used because a very high percentage of this type of patient quickly recovers with shock therapy.

Again, we frequently find patients who for various reasons need to be hospitalized, but because of economic factors, it is necessary to get the patient well as quickly as possible. I believe shock therapy is indicated in that sort of situation.

The hospital management of depressions has been completely changed with the advent of the shock program. We no longer need to think of these patients having to remain in hospitals for an indefinite period of time at a great expense. We can now think of weeks of treatment instead of months, and we have reached the point of thinking of these patients almost as we would acute infections. It is a fact now that even a severe depressive illness can be carried to recovery within as short a period of time and with no more expense that the average uncomplicated operation.

But I don't want to imply by this that all cases suffering from depressions should be hospitalized, nor do I wish to convey the impression that shock therapy is the treatment of choice. As has been stated, the mild depressions, which by far make up the majority, recover regardless of what we do or fail to do, and the important thing is to understand the type of illness we are treating and not be annoyed by the failure of our treatment to influence the course of the disease, and yet to be able to assure the patient and the family that recovery will take place, watch for evidence of suicidal thoughts, and above all, appreciate the fact that we are treating an episode type of disorder, and that having had such an illness a person is just as able to carry on in his life work as before.

The Diagnosis and Treatment of Goiter

Clarence C. Hoke, M.D.

TULSA, OKLAHOMA

The fact that we have a national and an international society for the study of a particular gland—the thyroid—indicates the importance of that organ. We know that, in health, the thyroid gland performs certain definite functions especially in connection with the control of the rate of oxidation in the tissues (metabolism) and, also perhaps with the storage of glycogen especially in the liver.

In the diseased states which we recognize as toxic nodular and toxic diffuse goiter the gland produces a secretion which is abnormal not only in quantity but also in character Hertzler has tritely stated that after we reach adult life we know not whether the thyroid be friend or foe.

Clinicians and surgeons alike with the widest experience in the management of thyrotoxicosis agree that the proper treatment of this condition is resection of the diseased thyroid gland.

We are concerned chiefly with two types of goiter—the adenomatous or nodular and the diffuse parenchymatous or so-called exophthalmic goiter. There is perhaps a third type representing a combination of these two or adenomatous goiter with hyperplasia.

The patient with adenomatous goiter may go along for many years without symptoms referable to the thyroid gland. In other cases symptoms may be produced in a relatively short time. In the earlier stages of this type the patient may consult the physician or surgeon because of the deformity resulting from the presence of one or more nodular areas in the thyroid gland.

A little later this same patient may seek relief because of pressure symptoms resulting from tracheal compression. Often this type of goiter is partially and at time wholly substernal. These goiters often go untreated for as long as twenty or thirty or even forty years and then the patient comes in complaining of not only deformity and pressure symptoms but also of dyspnoea, palpitation, tachycardia, weakness, weight loss and nervousness—the result of cardiac damage and of general visceral involvement by the toxins elaborated in the degenerated adenomatous tissue of the thyroid. It is known that thyrotoxicosis is associated with varying degrees of liver damage.

On Physical examination these patients exhibit varying degrees of deformity of the neck due to one or more lumps in the thyroid gland. If the goiter is large or partly or wholly substernal there may be marked dyspnoea or hoarseness or both and the patient may be obliged to avoid the recumbent position because of these pressure symptoms. There is practically always an associated hypertension and tachycardia and there is usually a certain degree of cardiac arythmia. In cases of long standing and marked toxicity there may be complete cardiac decompensation with signs or severe liver damage. Unexplained persistent tachycardia or other signs of cardiac abnormality should always at least make us think of the possibility of thyrotoxicosis. Especially in those of middle age or beyond this is frequently due to toxic substernal adenomatous goiter. Marked engorgement of the veins of the neck may result from pressure of a large goiter of any type. A careful fleuroscopic examination of the chest will usually reveal a substernal goiter if present.

The B. M. R. is usually elevated in toxic nodular goiter but not with the uniformity or degree observed in toxic diffuse goiter.

About ninety-five percent of the cases of thyroid malignancy occur in this adenomatous type of goiter.

Surgery in this type of goiter is indicated chiefly for the relief or prevention of the following conditions — deformity — pressure — cardiac and visceral damage and malignancy.

The diffuse parenchymatous, hyperplastic or so-called exophthalmic goiter occurs usually in youth or middle age and ordinarily gives us a pretty sick patient in a matter of months as a result of hyperthyroidism whereas the adenomatous goiter frequently requires years to produce a comparable degree of toxicity.

The chief symptoms in a typical case of hyperthyroidism are restlessness—nervousness—palpitation—weakness—heat intolerance—excessive appetite. Nausea—emesis and diarrhoea are not infrequent. Crises and remissions occur spontaneously.

The chief physical findings are varying degrees of diffuse enlargement of the thyroid gland with signs of increased vascularity and probably with bruit and thrill over the thyroid arteries. The gland is fairly smooth but firm and granular. Exophthalmos and other eye signs may or may not be present. There is a definite persistent tachycardia and often fibrillation or other types of arythmia. The systolic blood pressure at least is elevated and the pulse pressure in the typical case seventy or more. The skin is moist and there is a fine tremor of the fingers. The patient is restless, nervous and apprehensive. There is evidence of definite and often marked weight loss and of marked muscular weakness especially in the lower extremities. The B. M. R. is uniformly elevated.

In this second type of toxic goiter surgery is indicated for the control of these numerous symptoms and signs of hyperthyroidism.

The preoperative treatment is the most important step in the management of thyrotoxicosis. The time element is of the greatest importance. Adequate preoperative preparation is especially important in the patient with hyperthyroidism and in this connection I would like to emphasize the well known but of't neglected fact that Lugol's solution need not and should not be given except as part of the preoperative and postoperative treatment of patients with toxic goiter.

A careful history and physical examination and a B. M. R. should always be done. At this time it is well to summarize the findings and to estimate the probable surgical risk before any treatment is started. The patient is then put to bed. Visitors are excluded—all stimulants are withheld—sedatives and hypnotics are used as necessary. A high caloric high carbohydrate diet is given and an ice cap is placed over the precordium.

After a variable period of from one to three weeks or longer on this regime there is a definite decrease in all the symptoms and a corresponding improvement in the patient's general condition. When it is apparent that no further improvement is to be expected from these measures then and not until then is iodine given. Time is a factor of the greatest importance.

A good method is to give ten drops of Lugol's solution in a glass of orange juice three times daily for a period of ten to fourteen days or sometimes a little longer. In this time the maximum benefit from iodine is, in the average case, obtained. During this period of iodine administration it is neither necessary nor desirable to keep the patient in bed constantly. In fact these patients come to operation in better condition if during this latter period they are allowed to be up and walking about to some extent.

In very toxic goiters it may be well to supplement the diet for several days before operation by the use of intravenous glucose.

Light gas anesthesia, especially during the more difficult stages of the operation, using an intratracheal tube and with or without novocaine infiltration or block will probably be the anesthetic of choice in the average case of toxic goiter.

The exposure must be adequate, hemostasis complete and all manipulations as careful and gentle as possible. The suture material whether silk or catgut should be as light and as small in amount as is consistent with good surgery. Drainage will probably be advisable in the average case. Both drainage material and skin sutures can usually be out in forty-eight hours or sooner.

After operation the patient will be more comfortable if placed in a half sitting position (about forty-five degrees) with the head propped well forward. Sufficient morphine is used to control pain and restlessness but not enough to abolish the cough reflex. The administration of adequate amounts of glucose and Lugol's solution intravenously during the first few postoperative days helps to maintain satisfactory control of toxic symptoms as well as to supply the patient with the necessary fluid and nutritional requirements.

In the postoperative care of toxic goiter patients medicated steam appears to be of considerable value in relieving the discomfort associated with the accumulation of tenacious mucus in the trachea and bronchial tree.

The postoperative use of oxygen helps to control toxic symptoms and to prevent or relieve the accumulation of excessive secretions in the trachea and bronchial tree.

The average patient can be up in a chair about the third or fourth postoperative day and home by the fifth or seventh day—depending upon the circumstances of the particular case, freedom from complications et cetera.

About ten drops of Lugol's solution daily may be given for a period of a few weeks to several months—or longer depending upon the condition of the patient and the attitude of the surgeon. Some experienced surgeons think that the use of Lugol's solution postoperatively is not necessary.

Regardless of the claim of some surgeons that they are doing total thyroidectomies in practically all their toxic goiters it is evident that most experienced surgeons will continue to do a reasonably radical subtotal resection rather than a so-called total removal—for obvious reasons.

There is still a definite indication for a graded operative procedure in certain very toxic goiters or in those in which resection is technically difficult and in which there is a grave surgical risk.

Ideals In Rural Obstetrics*

ISADORE DYER, B.S., M.D.**

TAHLEQUAH, OKLAHOMA

The practice of obstetrics varies so greatly when a comparison is made between large urban areas and rural areas, that the methods pertaining to maternal care are related only in principle. The type of patient, the travel, the facilities for delivery, and the fee involved, could be listed as the more important factors that tend to make the comparison interesting. Before ideals can be discussed, an appreciation of the problem involved should be attempted.

Babies are delivered by three types of individuals: obstetricians, general practitioners, and midwives. Since Oklahoma has no midwife registration, the last category can include anyone from a relative to a poorly experience self-styled midwife, and this includes the so-called "neighbor woman." The national figures available to support this statement are significant. Each year over 2,000,000 live births occur, or one birth every 14 seconds. There are an additional 75,000 stillbirths and an undetermined number o abortions. Of the live births, 250,000 have no medical attendant, 200,000 are delivered by physicians trained as obstetricians[1], and 250,000 are delivered by students, internes and residents. Eighty-five percent of the specialists practice in cities of more than 100,000 population, but less than one percent in rural areas of 10,000 or less population. This leaves 1,500,000 women or about two-thirds of the total to be delivered by general practitioners. More than one-half of the live births occur in rural areas and of these, 84% in the home. In the State of Oklahoma in 1939, 32% or 13,833 live births occured in hospitals, and 29,638 in the home, of which 27,845 were delivered by physicians. Therefore it would seem logical to turn attention to that group who have as their lot, the responsibility, as well as the criticism, in supplying the bulk of live babies to the nation.

In evaluating the capability of the average physician for this task, it is alarming to note that during his medical school training he delivered less than 10 women, and about the same number during his internship.[1] Many internships have no training in home delivery. Eventually, he finds himself in a rural community in a practice wherein obstetrics is essential and necessary, working under the poorest of conditions, usually alone and unassisted. In his hands and judgment rests the Herculean task of producing live, healthy offspring and maintaining the life of the mother.

There is a marked difference between the practice of the specialist in the large city and the general practitioner in the rural area. The former significantly attends a patient, who, because of her environment, is better informed in the matter of maternal care. The matter of travel is rarely a problem, hence frequent visits during the prenatal period are possible. The delivery is usually accomplished in a well equipped hospital with adequate assistance and facilities for anasthesia. Birth rooms are arranged in such a manner that members of the family offer no added hazard or interference since no admittance is allowed to them. The more famous or popular the specialist, the more attention is afforded him, and in many instances he has the added assistance of a well trained resident or assistant to watch the patient and call him when his services are most needed. Medical and obstetrical consultants are as close to him as the telephone and a well equipped laboratory and X-ray is readily available. Delivery is accomplished in a well lighted room with up-to-date delivery equipment. Nursery facilities are available for the new-born baby under rigid regieme and supervision. Postpartum care is administered according to accepted principles and the fees are remunerative.

The picture changes remarkably in the experience of the rural practitioner in a rural area. The rural patient has not had the advantages of her urban sister. She relies upon her mother and older relatives for advice, the substance of which often is related to well known superstitions. Due to lack of education along the newer modes of maternal care, she is unaware of the importance of securing prenatal care and unless taught, does not present herself to the physician until late in the third trimester of pregnancy. Travel is an acute problem, and often only done when the desire for proper care overcomes the many difficulties and obstacles in securing transportation. Only by constant urging and commendation will a patient secure prenatal care regularly. The delivery itself has many variations. Perhaps one of the most important factors lies in the

*Read before the Section on Public Health, Oklahoma State Medical Association, Tulsa, Oklahoma, April 24, 1942.
**Consultant Obstetrician, Cooperative Health Unit, District No. 1, Oklahoma State Health Department, Tahlequah, Oklahoma.

home itself. The variations on this theme are countless. It can safely be said that rural homes can vary between one room shacks with little or no furniture, poor heat and leaky roofs to well furnished, well built, modest farm homes. The water supply may vary from a spring to a properly protected well. Sewerage disposal can vary from just a quick throw out of the back door to approved privies. Still, there is universally poor lighting, and lack of assistance, and equipment comparable to the city hospital and consultation. In addition, a delivery in the home, like a wake or a wedding, is the community signal for all curious and interested persons to gather around. At best, the rural practitioner is surrounded by the able assistance and advice of at least two mothers-in-law, two fathers-in-law, a husband, and at least a neighbor and a "widow woman" or two. The time spent traveling to the delivery bed, as well as the time spent in the home, often consumes the better part of a day or night, and after the delivery is done, the patient and baby are left to the mercy of home remedies and community lore. Significant enough is the fact that the fee involved is usually one-tenth to one-fourth of that obtained by the fraternal collegue in the large city. Post-partum care is only administered if the physician takes the time to insist upon examining the patient six weeks after delivery and if this examination is included in the delivery fee.

In evaluating ideals in rural obstetrics one must not loose sight of the fact that the same problems complicating the pregnancy, the delivery and the puerperal period will present themselves in both urban and rural women. In the latter, additional problems of edemic disease and diet will add complications. It then becomes the sacred duty of each and every rural practitioner who accepts the responsibility of maternal care, to detect and treat these complications to the best of his ability. Much can be gained in both successful outcome of mother and baby if efforts have been made to guard against known obstetric conditions which would make a home delivery hazardous.

Complete co-operation from the patient is necessary. This involves painstaking minutes of teaching and education, and in no other field of medicine can the patient-physician relationship be more satisfying or appreciated. The following program is suggested and although time does not permit of detailed discussion of each point, the practice of these principles would help to improve and simplify the rural obstetrical problem.

1. Urge early supervision and prenatal care by popularizing the practice of having the expectant mother visit the attending physicians office at least once a month. If pre- natal, delivery and postpartum care is included in *one* fee, the patient soon learns that she is missing care which could have been obtained for the same fee.

2. At the first visit the doctor should make a complete physical examination and evaluate the effect the pregnancy could have on the given patient. This would necessarily include an evaluation of the bony pelvis. It would be better for all concerned if a pelvic disproportion were detected early, and a hospital delivery planned, than to diagnose this condition later on in the home during labor.

3. Emphasis must be placed upon the importance of searching for syphilis by doing a blood test. If syphilis is found it must be treated.

4. Watch for toxemias. Twenty-four percent of maternal deaths are due to toxemias. Remember that when the patient herself is mindful of some complication in this regard, the toxemia is usually advanced and has been present for some time. It takes little effort to examine the urine, to weigh the patient and take the blood pressure. Return visits will be made if the patient finds that her physician actually is in search of complicating factors. If early toxemia is detected, it should be treated and the patient closely observed with a view of escaping the hazards of eclampsia with convulsions.

5. Follow some accepted plan for control of weight as well as proper diet practices. This would include the administration of vitamin K during the last two weeks of pregnancy. Printed diet instruction will usually be followed more readily than oral instruction and are far more impressive to the patient. If efforts are made to maintain gain in weight of not more than twenty-five pounds, the delivery will usually be less troublesome.

6. Instruct the patient to prepare the home for delivery. Again, printed instructions for supplies needed for home care, as well as the actual preparation of the delivery bed are indispensable. These instructions should also include notes describing danger signals concerned with bleeding and signs of impending toxemia. They should include detailed information in regard to when the doctor is to be summoned for delivery. The last will often eliminate unnecessary trips made before progress would warrant the presence of a physician.

7. If there exists a health department in the vicinity, enlist the services of a public health nurse to aid in the education of the patient and in the preparation of the home. Literature will also be available to the patient from the local or central health offices, by merely filing a card and directing it to the proper office.

8. Plan and follow a well organized technique for delivery, and practice it uniformly. It does not matter whether a wet or dry technique is used, as long as it is simple enough to employ under any condition. Remember that 42 percent of maternal deaths are the result of infections. Make efforts to prevent these by properly preparing the patient and by using every means to prevent contamination. Do as few pelvic examinations as possible and if these are done, take steps to use an aseptic technique. DO NOT INTERFERE WITH THE NORMAL PROGRESS OF LABOR. A perfectly normal labor can easily become complicated by the unwarranted meddling of an over-anxious physician. Pituitrin given indiscriminately will, in the long run, do more harm than good to the patient. Its use certainly endangers the life of the baby. By producing tonic and convulsive uterine contractions the forceps are directed to the fetal head. Rapid delivery brought about by the use of pituitrin endangers the soft parts of the mother and increases the danger of hemorrhage from a cervical laceration. It would be better to diagnose the cause for the long labor and attempt correction, than to admit defeat or ignorance and blast the baby into the world with pituitrin. Learn the simple procedure of passing a tracheal catheter. This will save many a baby's life. Secure good light if you have to carry a torch. Do not be reluctant to seek help and assistance if a situation arises wherein you feel unable to properly manage the difficulty. It is far better to have a live mother and be humble than to loose a mother and maintain false pride. Again printed instructions for immediate post-partum care and baby care are of greater value to the patient than trying to instruct her or a member of the family at a time when their emotions would affect their memory. If possible, clear the home of all but necessary help.

9. Ideally, the assistance of a nurse in attendance is most helpful. Either train one locally who will be available at all times, or prevail upon local officials and the health department to establish nurses for delivery. This one aid, to properly prepare the patient, to give anasthesia and care for the baby would make the problem of home delivery 50 percent less troublesome. If there is any doubt of this statement, inquire as to its value of any physician living in an area where nurses are available for delivery calls 24 hours per day.

10. Be prepared for any emergency. Hemorrhage, trauma and shock account for 23 percent of maternal death. One of the best aids available today are the ergonovine preparations. Don't hesitate to administer these intravenously if necessary. Every woman who is to be left in the home should receive ergonovine by mouth for at least 24 hours. This will lessen the danger of late uterine relaxations and hemorrhage that might be fatal. Carry a uterine pack to be used in extreme emergencies. Learn to properly pack a uterus when the rare necessity arises. Carry intravenous solutions, at least one each of 25 percent glucose in distilled water for eclampsias, 5 percent glucose in normal saline for shock, and 10 percent glucose for toxemias in shock. The administration of such solutions is simple and the equipment required is not difficult to carry. Be prepared to administer transfusions in the home. The technique for typing and collecting blood is not difficult and the margin of safety well warrants the effort.

11. Visit the patient at least once during her postpartum period. This will serve to emphasize the important stay in bed, and check on the manner in which the instructions are being carried out.

12. Examine the patient at the sixth post-partum week. Observe the effects of childbirth on the reproductive system. Correct childbirth injuries. Treat erosions of the cervix and uterine displacements. Do not discharge the patient until she has returned to normal.

There are many rare complications of pregnancy that might not be covered in the twelve points given, still the three prominent causes of maternal deaths can be remarkably lowered by adopting the principles outlined. *Toxemias* can be detected and remember that. Fifty percent of all deaths from toxemias are in patients not receiving prenatal care. *Infection* and *hemorrhage* can be prevented or treated, and the lowering of the mortality rate from these three prominent causes of death would affect 89 percent of the 9,000 odd women who die each year. For the 11 percent of deaths due to other varied complications, the rural practitioner needs the help and assistance of a trained specialist and is not to be condemned for failure in management.

Perhaps the day will come when every rural practitioner will be afforded adequate consultation facilities, to assist him when he most needs that help. Delivering babies in rural homes at best is no easy procedure, but adhering to good ideals can and will make the ultimate outcome a pleasant one for the mother, baby and physician.

BIBLIOGRAPHY
1. Daily, E. F.: Problems of Obstetrics Practice in Rural Areas of the United States. Conn. State Medical Journal, 4:2, February, 1940.

DISCUSSION
E. R. MUNTZ, M.D.
ADA, OKLAHOMA

Doctor Dyer's discussion of the difficulties

encountered in rural obstetrics reveal his actual experience in the field tempered with study and good judgment. He should be complimented for again directing the attention of the profession in general to the problems of rural obstetrics which he has so clearly defined. The program suggested by Doctor Dyer includes fundamental principles of Modern Obstetrics which have been proven time and again to be absolutely essential to satisfactory results. I simply wish to add a loud "Amen."

In regard to the future I think we can justifiably be optimistic. Improvement in obstetrical care in general has been apparent in this country in the past few years, and I feel certain that these trends will continue at even a more rapid rate in the next few years. Physicians are giving more serious thought and study to Obstetrics, as a result of the efforts of our teaching profession to improve obstetrical care. Medical schools, which in the past gave little time to obstetrics, are now alloting more time to this field of study in their curriculums. I also believe that Medical educators are realizing the great value of properly conducted home delivery services in teaching practical Obstetrics to medical students. Post-graduate study and "refresher courses" are becoming more popular and avilable to the practicing physician and, although this effort to improve the practice of obstetrics is still in its infancy, definite progress is being made as all of us in Oklahoma are aware. It is my hope that our Medical schools will enlarge this program in the future.

Doctor Dyer has briefly mentioned the frequent inadequacy of rural obstetrical fees, a fact with which most of us present to-day are cognizant. It seems to me that some readjustment of the remuneration to the physician for modern obstetrical care in rural areas is definitely in order if we are to finally reach our ideal objectives. Popular fees for obstetrical care in many rural areas with which I am acquainted simply will not purchase the type of care which Doctor Dyer has outlined. Even in this phase of the problem, however, I believe that some progress is evident, as the public comes to more fully appreciate what modern obstetrical care should include. In speaking of this matter, I am not disregarding the necessity for charity and semi-charity service in obstetrics as in all other branches of medicine whether in urban or rural practice, and I am sure that the American physician will continue to give freely of his services to those in need as he has done in the past.

A Review of War Surgery

GREGORY E. STANBRO, M.D.

OKLAHOMA CITY, OKLAHOMA

In ancient times surgeons built up their experience in the work shops of war. History reveals that wars are always a stimulus to great surgical advance. Increase in knowledge and improvement of principles is progressive, but in war, by necessity, there is an acceleration of interest and opportunity augments advance. Many methods developed in the World War are no longer new and as much is learned, likewise men become great. Practically all of our knowledge concerning amputations is a result of war experience. Chest surgery was only a name until the radical changes and progress initiated during the World War by Duval and others. Neurosurgery was in its swaddling clothes before 1914 and the pioneering by Cushing and others. The understanding of shock by the shock commission, in the late World War, gave us great help. Fracture principles of today such as skeletal traction, the walking caliper, local anesthesia, the Orr treatment, the maggott treatment, etc. all are the outcome of the World War. Therefore many surgical principles layed down as a result of the last war have stood the test of time and augmented by knowledge during the late automobile era are the sheet anchors of present principles and procedures. Debridement and excision of war wounds are in reality a fulfillment of principles laid down in 1897 by the German surgeon Friedreich but not accepted until the World War.

The present war is distinctly different from previous wars. It is different in its conception of attack and defense, as well as the vulnerability of the civilian population. The enemy is exposed from above as well as on the ground. This war is being called the war of the "crouching man" for on hearing a noise, man, civilian or military, crouches and the posterior body is exposed to injury.

Methods of inflicting wounds change as rapidly as methods of treatment, and proper care of wounds and the management of the wounded, necessitates some understanding of ballistics, the science of the motions "of projectiles." In this war the rifle bullet is sharper and changed in contour. It travels 1 7/8 to 2 1/4 miles. The muzzel velocity of the German rifle bullet is 2800 feet per second and at the end of 600 yards its velocity is still 1100 feet per second or the velocity of sound. The trajectory of a bullet follows a great curve, governed by the pull of gravity. The bullet rotates on its own axis and it oscillates or travels crosswise of its course even turning base foremost, at times. This oscillation or wobble beings early in its course, under 600 yards and has a terrific explosive effect on wounds. Later in its course the missile meets less resistance, has less wobble, and therefore less explosive effect. At the end of its course there again is a wobble and the bullets lodge in the body as they become spent.

High explosive shells are in casings filled with highly explosive trinitrotoluene. They are still fired by the artillery and trench mortars and burst by means of a detonatory which comes into action by contact. The fragments contained are 600 to 1500 in number and vary from a millet seed in size to jagged masses of iron many pounds in weight. The fragments are irregular in shape, create the worst wounds, are very destructive of tissue, and bury foreign bodies, clothing, etc. in the body.

Grenades and bombs encased in iron are segmented, contain fragments, and also scatter stone and earth adding to their severity and becoming secondary projectiles themselves.

While in the World War only 2 to 18 percent of wounds were from bombs and grenades in this war there is an enormous increase, by reason of the aerial bombs and torpedoes. The surface wounds may be small but the underlying injury is terrific. The high explosive shell, by necessity, has a strong casing where as the aerial bomb is only dropped and therefore has only a thin casing and is filled to the maximum with high explosive. It breaks into millions of fragments which travel 4000 feet per second and cause a devastating effect on the tissues.

The high explosive force of these bombs and their resultant phenomenon have come to be known as blast injuries. A bomb was originally defined as "a ball of fire" and air bombing has been developed by the Germans until 50 to 500 kgm. aerial bombs are used which are incredibly destructive and may destroy a city block. The aerial bomb is fired by combustion or detonation and chemical action takes place with terrific velocity. High explosives are violent, detonating at the rate of several miles per second, the blast resulting in supreme compression followed by a suction wave. At every point in the immediate vicinity there occurs a momentous wave of high pressure and then a negative suction pressure wave due to the reduced density of the air behind the compression wave. Although each lasts but a fraction of a second, the negative suction

pressure lasts longer than the positive compression. Therefore bombs dropped in the streets of Spain and England pulled out the metal shutters on the stores and the walls of the buildings fell or were pulled into the street. The bomb which drops inside a house pulls the walls in upon the victims instead of forcing the walls outward as would be expected. On account of this force and the suddenness of the blast, the effect on the human body is as though the body was struck by a solid object. Men are picked up with no mark of injury and only blood trickling from their noses, who at autopsy show numerous hemorrhages of their brains, lungs, ruptured viscera, retroperitoneal hemorrhages etc. Thus all types of injuries from minor to the most severe may result with no external evidence of injury. Taking a group in which there is one blast case, there are undoubtedly others which will be overlooked unless one understands blast results. A severe compression under positive and negative pressure has occurred. The patients should be treated for shock. They may bleed from the lungs for 48 hours. The lesions may be symmetrical or otherwise, pulmonary lesions predominating. The pulmonary lesions are caused by lowering of the alveolar pressure by the negative suction waves with rupture of the alveolar capillaries, or distention of the lungs with air by the high pressure of compression. Pulmonary damage may also be caused by the impact of the pressure waves against the chest wall. Blast injuries may damage the brain, the chest, the abdomen, or the spinal cord. They should be recognized as among the severest of injuries and treated for shock out of all proportion to the apparent severity of the injury.

With reference to head wounds four principles of treatment are cited and these are not new principles. Remove ineffective material and dead brain tissue, remove blood clot, extra dural or sub-dural, and consider whether retained foreign bodies should be removed. There is definite evidence that sulfanilamides tend not only to localize the infection but to delay the necessity for operation. This is a definite hint toward conservatism.

The outstanding fact to be established is: Has the dura been penetrated? Every means should be employed to determine this fact. If and when the dura is open, damage to nerve paths, avenues of infection etc. may result. The dural wound should not be opened unless the surgeon is prepared to go ahead, and complete the surgery indicated.

Chest wounds like wounds of the abdomen are of high mortality, a large percent never reaching the base hospital. Operative procedure for hemorrhage is of primary importance. Open pneumothorax is the bugbear of the sucking wounds and must be stopped at once, by packing the wound with vaseline gauze taped tightly. Aspiration of hemothorax is indicated and may be life saving. Hemorrhage in the lung may cause pulmonary collapse, and, or coughing up of clot, inspiration into the other lung complicating the picture by pneumonia and later abscess, gangrene, and circulatory failure, following in succession. Debridement of the wound and resection of ribs may be necessary. The mortality is 30 to 40 percent in the best hands. In France before the British left Dunkirk there were 2000 patients in the British general hospitals. Less than a dozen of these were chest cases which, in itself, is evidence of the gravity of chest injuries. They usually do not reach the hospitals.

In the South African War of 1900 McCormac's aphorism was "A man wounded in the abdomen dies if he is operated upon and remains alive if he is left in peace." This same policy was carried out in the Russo-Japanese War and until 1915 in the World War. Ten percent of 1,185,000 killed outright in the World War died of shock and hemorrhage of penetrating wounds of the abdomen. In this war the great increase in use of H.E.S., aerial bombs, etc. has increased the mortality of the abdominal wounds by their multiplicity and wide range of destructive action and complications.

In 1915-1918 and 1936 the "look and see policy" was used and found to save most lives. Blast injuries and the low velocity projectiles of modern warfare, increased difficulties of collection, transportation, and treatment have almost counteracted the advances in methods of treating these cases. Forty-seven percent of 500 cases were inoperable. The early operation has become almost routine even though the mortality is terrific. The patient is treated for shock while being prepared otherwise for surgery. He is operated promptly if his condition permits, as the high percentage of hemorrhage deaths in abdominal wounds demand prompt surgery. Surgery and transfusion during the operation offers the best chance in the hemorrhagin or perforation type of case. Local patching of wounds of the intestines is preferred to resection but when resection is mandatory, end to end anastamosis is the method of choice. There are a greater number of wounds of the ileum because of the multiplicity of the coils. Wounds of the jejunum are apt to remain circumscribed and everted due to the thickness of the wall while those of the ileum are ragged and explosive permitting rapid escape of the contents and the early development of peritonitis. Meticulous control of the bleeding, cleansing the peritoneal cavity and drainage (rarely) are the custom. Abdominal injuries on account of the destructive and complicated character have the gravest prognosis and an appalling mortality. Excision of wounds of the entrance and exit, should be carried out *after* the laparotomy.

Wound excision replaces all attempts at local disinfection. Having made an elliptical incision, the skin is undermined, the edges retracted and the tract is excised in one piece down to the peritenoneum, never allow the knife to enter the tract. If this does occur one should change gloves and instruments. If and when satisfied that the wound is clean and hemostatic a contaminated wound is thereby converted into a clean one. Close the wound in layers without drainage. The destructiveness of these wounds is incompatible with life and the problem of today has become one of prevention and prophylaxis. Armor is being recommended. Steel helmets met adverse criticism in the last war for some time but were eventually accepted, and some form of body armor may be the answer here.

Wounds of war are being treated as in the World War, by excision. The best results are being obtained when they can be treated within four to eight hours, which also was proven in the World War. Incidentally, Lister stated that after six hours his treatment was of no value. Amputation is unusual unless the injuries are grave, the wounds multiple, or the main blood vessels destroyed. "No matter how severe the destruction of skin, the comminution of bone, or the contamination of tissues, if the main blood vessels are not destroyed the limb can usually be saved." The blood vessels being intact, bone fragments are removed with extreme conservatism, infection is treated by adequate drainage, immobilization and chemotherapy. Skin destruction is later covered by grafting, and non-union overcome by continuous prolonged fixation in plaster. Stiffness and disuse of joints is conquered by early active exercise. If amputation is mandatory the conical or short flap operation is replacing the guillotine. The conical amputation can be done at the site of election as quickly and does not necessitate re-amputation. It shortens the suffering, reduces the morbidity and lowers the mortality. The short flap operation, though taking slightly longer is also being done rather than the hurried unsatisfactory guillotine. Always obtain a second expert opinion before amputating! If it is necessary, operate through the wound even though it is the site of election. When this is necessary traction sutures are applied and the stump is left open, to overcome soft tissue retraction and permit drainage.

Advances in fracture treatment have always come about during wars. Only in war do all the problems involved present themselves for study. Epocal progress resulted during the World War. Again, the war in Spain added improved principles and substantiated methods of previous probable value. During the interval between wars the great number of automobile era road accidents has kept up interest and progress.

Fractures in war are caused by bullets from rifles, grenades, high explosive shells, bombs, etc. Aerial bombs, as has been mentioned, are most destructive. It has finally been appreciated that a traumatized bone should not be treated as a separate and distinct entity but as an organic tissue which reacts similarly to other tissue. Therefore, the treatment of fracture wounds has two motives, first, the avoidance or over coming of infection and second, an attempt to obtain the best reduction and by immobilization secure consolidation of the fracture without disability.

In 1897 Friedreich advocated wound excision as if they were neoplasms but it was not until the World War that this principle was finally appreciated and accepted. Vital tissues are not easily infected and removal of devitalized tissue deprived of circulation is the first step toward infection prevention. In war wounds, excision is therefore the first step, for soft tissue infection is primary and the bone involvement is secondary. The skin edges are excised, the devitalized tissue removed, including the whole muscle if the nutrient artery is gone. Muscle spaces should be cultured. As during the World War, results are based on the time, following the trauma, the wounded was received and the hour the devitalized tissue was excised. If sutures will produce the slightest tension do not suture. Do not suture if there is any doubt about tissue vitality. The wound having been excised, a plaster non-padded cast is applied. Truetta, in Spain, used plain gauze between muscle layers for drains before the plaster application. Rigorous immobilization is the best means of preventing and combating infection. (Rigorous means prevention of muscular movement and plaster casts are the answer.) The only disadvantage of plaster is the inability to inspect the wounded limb at intervals. A window neutralizes all the other advantages of the cast. Window oedema developes. It permits the curious to change the dressing, and allows movement of the muscles.

Traumatic, surgical or secondary shock in varying and severe degrees is the handmaiden to any trauma, burn, blast, and crushing injury. There is no new information on the problem but there is a fuller appreciation of certain phases since the World War. Santy, on the battle fields of France in the World War, observed that the early wounded were calm and collected. The pulse was slow and full. The skin was dry. However, treatment for secondary shock was mandatory because as Santy said, "The wounded was not shocked yet." Waiting for the established picture of shock, means waiting for tissue asphyxia, peripheral circulatory collapse and death.

Shock is the process of loss of blood volume, brought about through tissue asphyxia which results from inadequate blood flow. Given inadequate circulation and we have shock. It is caused by hemorrhage, dehydration, pain, cold, fear, asphyxia and exhaustion. It should be prevented by transfusion of plasma or blood, by fluids, morphine, warmth, reassurance, oxygen, rest, psychological and physical.

Traumatic or wound shock means the loss of blood or plasma or both. It may be local, general or both. As a consequence of the reduction in blood volume there is an inadequate venous return to the right heart, a decline in the cardiac output, fall in blood pressure, stagnant anoxia, peripheral circulatory failure and death. The treatment ideal is the replacement of fluid at the earliest possible moment in the form in which it has been lost, for only when the flow of blood to the tissues has been re-established has the treatment of shock become effective.

Great progress has been made in the methods of obtaining, preserving, transporting and administering blood or substitutes for blood. Salt solution or glucose (isotonic) are better for prevention, as dehydration is one of contributing cause of shock, and these isotonic solutions replace the deficit in the extra cellular fluids. However, where there is gross damage to the capillary bed these solutions are valueless or even harmful as they wash protein out of the blood stream and accentuate the hypoproteinemia. Hypertonic solution may be even worse. Therefore solutions of crystalloids are not satisfactory and acceptable blood substitutes in the treatment of shock. Whole blood, fresh or preserved, is a satisfactory fluid for intravenous induction in the treatment of shock. It restores the red blood cells and augments plasma protein concentration. Loss of whole blood is tolerated better than loss of plasma. Only whole blood or plasma may safely, effectively, and permanently restore the volume of the circulation. Of these plasma is preferable, for, volume for volume, plasma supplies twice as much osmotically active protein as whole blood and it is nutritionally more effective. It need not be typed, is easily administered, and finally is readily preserved as a dry powder or in liquid state for as long as desired. Therefore; Treat shock early, give morphine, apply heat, furnish liquids, demand rest, give plasma, administer oxygen (90%). Cortin or other suprarenal extracts may be used.

It is obvious that the problem of burns is titanic in total war. The internal combustion engine, the incendiary bomb, the flame projectors, flame throwing tanks and the flash from high explosive shells all do their part to create the enormous number of burn casualties which are admitted to the hospital. The blowing up of oil tanks both on land and on the sea also produce great numbers of burns, not to mention the burns resulting from phosgene and mustard gases which go to complete the total.

Primarily, burns should be treated for shock before treating the burn itself. A burn is a particular type of wound and the only wound which is primarily sterile. The surface area of a burn governs its gravity rather than the depth. The character of the shock associated with the burn is identical in all respects with the traumatic or secondary shock of other wounds. However, the added loss of the serum protein of the burn surface to the plasma protein loss add to the severity of the shock. They are shock casualties and hecome shock deaths. The shock having been adequately treated, there is still no agreement as to the ideal treatment of the burn surface. It is agreed that the burn surface area should be thoroughly cleansed under an anesthetic if necessary and one of several procedures carried out. Tannic acid 5% may be applied except on the face and hands, one percent aqueous solution of gentian violet is preferred by some and triple aniline dye by others. (1:400 gentian violet, 1:400 brilliant green, 1:400 flavine. Follow by spraying with 5% tannic acid.) Tannic acid and silver nitrate are a popular principle of treatment. The Bunyan envelope method, a rather new development, may become popular. It consists of daily applications of electrolytic sodium hypochlorite solution applied inside large sealed oil skin or tissue envelopes. The saline bath has its advocates. Again, tannic acid is applied by other men, removed on the fifth to eighth day and continuous Dakin's solution packs applied.

Anesthesia is mentioned only to state that the use of intravenous Pentothal sodium and Evipal stand out favorably in the present war literature. Local anesthesia is almost uniformly condemned. Gas-oxygen is being used and of course drop ether is being administered to some extent.

In conclusion, it is obvious that the man who first cares for the wounded is supreme in importance. His judgment and care governs and determines the recognition and treatment of shock. The original handling of the wound, the control of the sucking wounds of the chest, the determination of sacrificing or saving a traumatized limb, etc. etc. is in his hands.

To date the outstanding war advances in surgical principles are the use of PLASTER —PLASMA—AND CHEMOTHERAPY.

The extensive use of the non-padded plaster cast protects and immobilizes the injuried part. There is relief of pain and rapid disappearance of shock which is the best compliment to wound excision. The immobilization prevents infection and promotes healing. It prevents loss of function and promotes fracture union. It permits immediate operation followed by prompt transportation which expedites and provides for more adequate and ultimate complete care. The objections to this closed method are few. If the blood supply to the part is inadequate and gangrene results, the cast should not have been applied originally.

Plasma now obtained is prepared, stored, dried, transported and made available is the ideal treatment in shock. In itself this advance is epochal. The soldier can carry dried plasma. Before the war is much older he will be able to carry synthetic plasma protein which, when added to crystalloid solutions will be even more efficacious than true plasma.

Perhaps the most fascinating aspect of the modern treatment of war wounds is the advent of chemotherapy. Though still experimental, it is the consensus of opinion that through the use of the sulfonamides, wounds are in a healthier state and less heavily infected than in the last war. All the sulfonamides have been and are being used. Sulfathiazole is more apt to cause cold abscesses sulfanilamide is more uniformily preferred. The effects of chemotherapy are most striking ing streptococcus wounds. Fortunately B.Welchii is more susceptible to chemotherapy than the other anaerobes. It is the general belief than the sulfonamides are directly bacteriostatic.

Nothing has been said about the remarkable results of Moorhead at Pearl Harbor. The Pearl Harbor catastrophe occurred on a beautiful, warm sunshining day at one of the cleanest locations in the world. The results were remarkable but can hardly be compared with the wounded treated under usual most unsanitary war conditions.

Prostatic Resection and the Results Which May Be Expected

E. HALSELL FITE
Fite Clinic
MUSKOGEE, OKLAHOMA

During a period roughly covered by the first twenty-five years of this century, surgery of the prostate acquired a high degree of excellence. This was due to many factors but perhaps more than anything else, it was due to a better understanding of the problems presented, and in particular to an appreciation of the necessity of proper preoperative preparation.

Then a very startling chain of events began to take place. Stern developed his resectoscope and Davis began to put it to use. (And here I want to digress long enough to pay tribute to Davis, who never quite received the honor due him for his pioneer work in this field.) He was soon followed by many men doing resections in large numbers, and almost immediately what many regarded as a type of urological heresy broke out. Resectionists made the statement that they were not preparing their patients preoperatively. A large number of prostatectomists raised a tumult of objections, and the argument was on. Some of those doing hugh numbers of resections presented long series of cases apparently demonstrating beyond doubt that they were correct in stating that preoperative preparation was unnecessary in the majority of cases. This was countered by the prostatectomists' statement that in large private clinics under special conditions preoperative preparation might be unnecessary, but that this was definitely a special condition and could not be reproduced elsewhere.

I have entered into several such arguments and have made the statement that most cases if handled properly do not need preoperative care such as is mandatory for open prostatectomy. However, I had never analyzed a series of my cases. As I represent not the large clinic but the average private clinic, it occurred to me that an analysis of a series of my cases might really be of more value as a yard stick of what the average man has to face and can expect than are the reports of the huge series. This analysis was started for my own benefit, and I did not try to report any very considerable number, but starting on a given date, haphazardly selected, I decided to analyze twenty-five consecutive cases from my private practice, not including any from my work with the Veterans Bureau. I missed two in the middle of the series, which were later included for the

sake of accuracy, and thus there are twenty-seven cases analyzed.

The cases were divided into those receiving no preoperative drainage, those receiving one to four days preoperative drainage, and those receiving longer than four days preparation. The reason for the middle class was that we felt that four days did not constitute any appreciable preoperative preparation, and yet the question might be raised that they had received preoperative catheter drainage.

In class I there were eleven cases or 40 percent.

In class II there were eight cases or 30 percent.

In class III there were eight cases or 30 percent.

As we had suspected we found that class II was composed mostly of cases which for no important reason had simply been delayed in operation after entry to the hospital. Five of the eight cases definitely should have been included in class I; three might be included in class III as they were kept in the hospital for short periods of observation; one because of urinary tract infection, and two because of large residuals. This, if rearranged, left class I consisting of sixteen cases or 60 percent, and class III consisting of eleven cases or 40 percent, or if class I and II, as seems most proper, were taken together, 70 percent received immediate operation, and in 30 percent operation was delayed for preoperative drainage.

We then analyzed the cases of prostatic obstruction with a view of determining those which could be operated with relative safety without preoperative preparation. I found I was using the following five prerequisites:—

1. The patient should appear to be in pretty good physical condition as well as have a negative physical examination.

2. He should be able to void fairly well, though he may have several ounces residual urine. I have operated several cases, however, who had been catherizing themselves for long periods.

3. The blood urea and nitrogen should not be markedly raised, and the p.s.p. test should not be too much delayed. A much delayed peak of curve is evidence of serious kidney damage.

4. The internist should be able to say that the circulatory system is satisfactory and that other medical conditions, if any, are under control.

5. Bladder or kidney stones or other serious urinary pathology should not be present.

The patients, of course, have thorough clinical examination, including physical, laboratory, and X-ray examinations as indicated by their histories and other findings. Those cases not meeting the above requirements are placed on preoperative drainage and treatment. I usually use a simple small indwelling catheter, though in the cases where the physical condition is extremely poor and the renal damage severe, I prefer open suprapubic drainage, since by this method there is no chance of accidental obstruction to the drainage system since if the catheter becomes plugged for any reason, the urine can escape around it. Also, it is more comfortable for long periods of drainage, and the urethritis of long catheter drainage is avoided.

Of the eight cases properly falling in class III, six were extremely ill, and in my opinion four of them could not have been successfully treated without resection of the vesical neck. Many complicating factors existed.

Lest someone think this series is composed of selected cases, particularly of younger men, the following age figures are given:—

The average age of the whole series was 68 years.

20 were above 65 years of age.

11 were above 70, and

3 were above 80, the oldest being 86.

The post operative records are quite startling, I think. I keep all "out to town" cases in the hospital fourteen days after operation, no matter how well they are doing. Out of the twenty-seven cases there was one death. This patient died of sepsis on the second post operative day, and had been considered an excellent risk preoperatively. This makes the mortality percentage about 4%, which of course is the lowest it could be in a small series if anyone at all died. This is also much higher than my total mortality, which runs less than one percent. And, anyone operating for anything on men of this age is bound to have a mortality around one percent.

Of the twenty-six remaining cases, all but four left the hospital by the fourteenth day or sooner. Of the four who stayed longer, one was in the hospital three days over time because of an acute respiratory infection contracted the day he was supposed to go home; one was in six days over time because of minor delayed hemorrhage; and two were hospitalized for 33 and 31 days postopera-

tively because their bladders did not regain tone sooner. These cases had had 53 and 50 ounces residual when operated. Of the eight cases in class III, six were out of the hospital within the fourteen day period. The other two were the two cases of huge residual just mentioned.

CONCLUSIONS

That with due precautions and careful selection of cases, any competent resectionist can operate on a majority of his cases without prolonged preoperative preparation, and he may expect excellent results.

That the post operative recovery in these cases is unusually rapid and free from sequelae such as severe sepsis, etc., and that severe post operative reactions are rare.

That in properly performed resections, hemorrhage is most infrequent, and does not constitute a serious complication when properly managed.

That a substantial economic gain is made by omitting or limiting the period of preoperative treatment.

That even a greater economic saving is accomplished through the short post operative hospitalization and rapid convalescence.

The author recognizes that a series of twenty-five cases is rather small, but believes the above conclusions are justified, especially in the light of experience, both antidating and following the series presented.

Try Pablum On Your Vacation

Vacations are too often a vacation from protective foods. For optimum benefits a vacation should furnish optimum nutrition as well as relaxation, yet actually this is the time when many persons go on a spree of refined carbohydrates. Pablum is a food that "goes good" on camping trips and at the same time supplies an abundance of calcium, phosphorus, iron, and vitamins B. and G. It can be prepared in a minute, *without cooking*, as a breakfast dish or used as a flour to increase the mineral and vitamin values of staple recipes. Packed dry, Pablum is light to carry, requires no refrigeration. Easy-to-fix Pablum recipes and samples are available to physicians who request them from Mead Johnson and Company, Evansville, Ind.

Opportunities for Practice

Opportunity For Practice

There is an opportunity for practice in Waynoka. Anyone who is interested, can receive further information by contacting the Executive Office, 210 Plaza Court, Oklahoma City.

American Urological Association Will Meet

The Western Branch of the American Urological Association will hold its annual convention this year at Hotel Del Monte, Del Monte, California, from June 22 to June 24.

· THE PRESIDENT'S PAGE ·

On July 14th, the Democratic and Republican primaries will be held for the usual purpose of selecting the public officials that will guide the destiny of our State and Federal Governments.

Never in the history of our country has there been a greater need for calm, cool, and deliberate selection of these candidates. It is every persons obligation as a patriotic citizen, to exercise his franchise in their selection.

I urge you to contact these candidates, evaluate their qualifications, ascertain their views on matters concerning public health, and then vote for the person who, in your opinion, will best represent you.

Bear in mind that unless you do your part, you cannot criticize the selection of others.

Sincerely yours,

President.

The "troublesome weed" will soon harass
your patients with contact dermatitis—

POISON IVY EXTRACT
Lederle

THE OLD BUGABOO OF VACATIONISTS, poison ivy, will soon rear
its ugly head! In the spring and summer the plant is most
poisonous, as it is then loaded with sap and its leaves and stem
are more susceptible to injury.

The prophylactic injection of "Poison Ivy Extract *Lederle*" * can
establish a complete immunity to the usual direct contact with
Rhus toxicodendron radicans in at least a considerable proportion of
susceptible persons. Two injections, given within a two-week
interval, are sufficient to protect a large proportion of such persons against the inconvenient and distressing dermatitis resulting
from ivy poisoning. This should be of interest to farmers and military land forces at this time as well as to vacationists.

In the *treatment* of ivy poisoning, one or two injections of "Poison
Ivy Extract *Lederle*" often give marked relief within a short time.

Pain on injection is seldom experienced with the Lederle extract, which is an *acetone extract in almond oil*. Literature on the
details of this treatment available to the physician on request.

PACKAGES:
2 syringes (1 cc. each)
1 syringe (1 cc.)
*"Poison Oak Extract *Lederle*" is available for the Pacific Coast states.

LEDERLE LABORATORIES, INC.
30 ROCKEFELLER PLAZA   NEW YORK, N. Y.

Specify Lederle

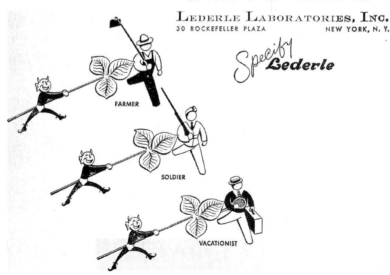

FARMER

SOLDIER

VACATIONIST

• EDITORIALS •

SUGAR

In the rationing of Sugar, the resulting psychological burden becomes a physiological boon. The overloaded liver and the hard pressed pancreas, may now find a little well earned cellular liesure.

As a result, there will be a decline in the incidence of Obesity, Diabetis and decayed teeth. It has been stated that food rationing during World War 1, also reduced the incidence of heart troubles, gallstones and constipation.

The rotund individual, who take up their belts will feel better and live longer and according to recent reports, will be less likely to die of Cancer. Dr. Albert Tannenbaum of Michael Reese Hospital, Chicago, has recently shown that people of average weight or below average, are not as susceptible to cancer as those who are overweight. In the laboratory he has shown that mice, on a low ration of starches and sugars manifest increased resistance toward the development of cancerous tumors.

Cane sugar was not available for general consumption in England, until the later part of the 16th Century. Shakespeare, Linacre and William Harvey wrought without sugar as we know it today. It is said that sugar was unknown to the Ancient Greeks. If it were possible to have Greek culture and Greek intellect with Grecian physical grace and charm sans sugar, why should we worry about rationing.

THE FERRULE OF CALAMITY

Much of the world's work and a generous share of its thinking and planning have been done by the sick. "Sickness and pain remind us of our nothingness and keep us in virtue."

In the summer of 1880 a sick, young doctor opened an office at 519 Pine Street, Philadelphia. Soon he sought admission to the United States Navy, because he was too ill to follow private practice. He passed his examination with high honors, but "his delicate constitution barred him from service." Dr. J. M. DaCosta diagnosed tuberculosis and advised that he "go west." Following this advice, he did the heath resorts from Philadelphia to Los Angeles. "Moreover, early in his travels he was convinced, from the ages of the men sleeping beneath the stones in the historic grave yards throughout the west, that the climate was of little value." Finally he completed his cure on his father's farm in the Alleghenies and in 1883 he again opened his office at 519 Pine Street. Though he had not planned to treat consumptives, they came in droves and the poor he had with him always. This young doctor was Lawrence F. Flick.

On May 7, 1942, a great throng of people from all parts of the United States gathered in a great banquet hall at the Bellevue-Stratford Hotel in Philadelphia to celebrate the 50th anniversary of the Pennsylvania Tuberculosis Society, and to pay tribute to its founder, who assembled the first group of its kind in the world for an organization meeting in his office at 519 Pine Street, April 22, 1892.

In 1891, this young physician, with prophetic vision, said:

"It is my firm conviction, after careful study of the question, that, with our present knowledge of the etiology of the disease, we have it in our power completely to wipe it out. . . . To do this would of course require well-organized boards of health, an enlightened public, and the cooperation of the entire medical profession."

Directly and indirectly Dr. Flick's influence has permeated practically every public health activity in the United States during the past fifty years. He advocated registration of the tuberculous, beds for consumptives; and free beds for the poor. He founded White Haven Sanatorium. His work and writings engaged the attention of the steel magnate Henry Phipps and led to the establishment of the Henry Phipps Institute for the Study, Treatment and Prevention of Tuberculosis.

He was instrumental in bringing about the organization of the National Tuberculosis Association in 1904, and he initiated the plans to bring the International Congress on Tuberculosis to the United States in 1908.

He was known as benefactor, teacher, organizer, author, and historian. His memberships, honors, activities and publications are too numerous for inclusion in this short notice.

OKLAHOMA IN THE UPPER THIRD

In the State Board number of the Journal of the American Medical Association, May 9, 1942, statistical columns show that the University of Oklahoma School of Medicine is one of twenty-two out of sixty with no failures before state boards. Sixty-four of Oklahoma's graduates, distributed among ten state examining boards were examined without a single failure.

This is something the University of Oklahoma should be proud of. In view of the fact that today there are not enough doctors under forty-five years of age in the United States to supply the needs of the army and navy, we take pride in the fact that Oklahoma is contributing its full quota. The Oklahoma state legislators, who have been so loath to give adequate financial support to the Medical School, should take notice. We need more doctors, the Medical School needs more money. There will be another session of the State Legislature and let us hope. a generous appropriation for medical education.

MEDICINE AND WAR

The Governments team for the recruitment of physicians is now functioning daily at Plaza Court, Oklahoma City, and for this board we bespeak the generous response, so characteristic of Oklahoma doctors.

As the young men of the Medical profession pass into the Army and Navy, it is obvious that those who are left behind must gird their loins with the sword of service and take on the knighthood of Civilian practice.

Deep in the heart of every worthy physician there is a heroism that brooks no obstacles. To meet the present emergency the average doctor will broaden his skills and enlarge his activities to include the varied needs of the Civilian population. Sickness, suffering, and death may rob him of well earned leisure and comfort, but nothing can dim his sense of professional duty or curb his mounting courage in pursuit of the same. Throughout the land, there are many physicians of the old school. In fact, there are few communities without a William MacClure to fight the drifts and ford the streams for the people of his "glen." Such professional devotion knows no reserve and withholds no kindly deed.

No doctor at the front will serve with more valour. The government and the people should see that each in his sphere, at home and abroad, has the best available chance for the greatest possible good.

"FROM EACH ACCORDING TO HIS ABILITY, TO EACH ACCORDING TO HIS DESERTS."

This motto, popular some years ago, might be a good slogan for the medical profession to adopt, at least for the duration. The present war is so vast and many sided that every qualified physician may have something to contribute for the ultimate victory of democratic principles. In our civilization,

already highly complex and made more so by the demands of total war, there is room and need for every talent and ability which physicians as a class command. As the need enlarges, an increasingly large number of our profession will be drawn into the various branches of the armed services until ultimately practically every professionally qualified and reasonably able bodied physician under forty five years of age will be enlisted. This will place a tremendous burden upon all physicians—upon those who remain as well as those who answer the call to go. And the physicians of America will not fail. However, those of our number who are called will go more gladly if they know that our armed forces are so organized that special abilities will be fully utilized in the fields wherein they have specially prepared themselves. A less efficient organization than this is unworthy of the profession, of the service arms and of the country we desire to serve and save.

We who perforce must remain at home bespeak for our colleagues who go the full opportunity to serve where they are best qualified to do so. Furthermore, those of us who are left behind must ever be considerate of the best interests of those called away. We will do well to remember that we, too, can make real contributions to national safety and victory in promoting public and industrial health, civilian defense in its many aspects, in maintaining "morale" and so continuing the high standards of our profession. For while at present the second part of the above motto is relatively unessential, it may be true that unless we help win this war for democracy, there may be for us and our people neither dinner nor desserts.—A. S. R.

WE ARE PROUD

At the annual meeting of the National Tuberculosis Association, held in Philadelphia the first week in May, Dr. Lewis J. Moorman was honored by election to the post of President-Elect of the organization.

To all who know Dr. Moorman this honor at the hands of his colleagues in his specialty comes as a well earned recognition of his secure place in the field of his chosen labors. Having demonstrated that happy combination of competent practitioner, thorough scientist and fluent and lucid writer, it is to be expected that his talents should receive from time to time such appropriate recognition as has just been conferred upon him.

Lest some might suspect he has departed from his usual modest ways, these words of commendation and recognition were not the product of his editorial pen but rather a feeble attempt on the part of his host of admirers to bring a newsworthy item to the attention of the profession in Oklahoma.—N. R. S.

ASSOCIATION ACTIVITIES

Proceedings of House of Delegates

Oklahoma State Medical Association
April 22-23, Tulsa, Oklahoma

The following transcripts of the two meetings of the House of Delegates, in Tulsa, April 22 and 23, have been edited. All actions of the House of Delegates have been included. The Council Report together with the Reports of the Councilors and Special Committees not published in the April Journal of the Association appear on the pages as noted in the transcript of the minutes.

WEDNESDAY, APRIL 22, 1942

The first session of the House of Delegates at the Fiftieth Anniversary Annual Meeting of the Oklahoma State Medical Association held April 22 to April 24, 1942, at Tulsa, was called to order in the Ivory Room of the Mayo Hotel, at 10:00 P. M., Wednesday, April 22, by the Speaker of the House, Dr. P. P. Nesbitt of Tulsa.

Following the call to order by the Speaker, the roll was called by the Chairman of the Credentials Committee, Dr. W. A. Howard of Chelsea, and the following motion made:

MOTION: Dr. W. A. Howard

"Inasmuch as a quorum is present, I move that the Speaker declare the House in session and proceed with the business that is to be transacted."

SECONDED: Dr. H. K. Speed

Motion carried.

Following the calling of the roll, the Speaker in compliance with the provisions of Chapter III, Section 4, Subsection (a), of the By-Laws, appointed the following Reference Committees: Sergeant-At-Arms—Dr. H. C. Weber, Bartlesville and Dr. Ralph A. McGill, Tulsa; Resolutions Committee—Dr. George H. Garrison, Chairman, Oklahoma City, Dr. A. H. Bungardt, Cordell and Dr. Charles Ed White, Muskogee; and Tellers and Judges of Elections—Dr. L. Chester McHenry, Chairman, Oklahoma City, Dr. S. A. Lang, Nowata and Dr. Carl Puckett, Oklahoma City.

Following the appointment of the above committees, the Chairman called for the reading of the minutes of 1941 Meeting of the House of Delegates, and it was moved

MOTION: Dr. L. S. Willour

"Inasmuch as the minutes of the preceding session were published in the Journal of the Association, I move that the reading of the same be dispensed with and that they be approved as published."

SECONDED: Dr. J. D. Osborn

Motion carried.

Immediately following the above motion and its adoption, in compliance with the provisions of Chapter VII, Section 3, of the By-Laws of the Association, the Speaker called for the reports of the Officers.

At this time, Mr. R. H. Graham, the Executive Secretary of the Association, read the Council Report. (See page 262.)

Upon completion of the reading of the Council Report by Mr. Graham, the following motion was offered:

MOTION: Dr. L. A. Hahn

"I move that the Report of the Council be accepted by the House of Delegates."

SECONDED: Dr. George Osborn

Following the motion, Dr. A. S. Risser of Blackwell was granted the permission of the floor and at which time he made the following comments: "In my opinion, this is one of the best and most widely viewing reports that this Association has ever presented. I definitely

think the Council and the Executive Secretary should be highly commended for their consideration and the views that have just been presented in the annual report of that body. A mere clapping of the hands is not sufficient. This body of men have looked forward into the future as far as possible. It is my opinion that, as individuals and as a body of scientists doing things, it will be our task to bring these many things to a conclusion. I think that this report deserves the commendation of every member in this State Association."

Dr. L. S. Willour of McAlester was granted the floor following Dr. A. S. Risser's remarks and made the following observations: "According to the report, as just read by the Executive Secretary, the setting of dues will be left in the hands of the Council—the same not to exceed $12.00 and to remain at $10.00, if possible. I am heartily in favor of this procedure. In this way, the Council will be given enough money to run the State Association from the dues of those who stay at home. I would even be in favor of the dues being raised to $15.00, if necessary, to maintain the state office."

The Speaker of the House, upon the completion of the remarks by Dr. A. S. Risser and Dr. L. S. Willour, stated the original motion and asked the pleasure of the House concerning its adoption. The motion made by Dr. L. A. Hahn that the Council Report be accepted, and duly seconded by Dr. George Osborn, was unanimously approved.

Following the Report of the Council, the Chair called for the Reports of the Councilors of the Association, and upon request by the Speaker, the following motion was offered:

MOTION: Dr. W. S. Larrabee

"I move that we properly approve the Reports of the Councilors upon their completion in the natural sequence of order."

SECONDED: Dr. W. A. Showman

Motion carried.

At this time, the Executive Secretary was granted the privilege of the floor and stated that he had the report for Councilor District No. 1, but that it had been received in the office of the Association too late for publication in the April issue of the Journal, which issue had carried other Councilor and Committee Reports that had been received in time for inclusion in that particular issue. Following this statement, Dr. O. E. Templin of Alva, the Council of District No. 1, asked that Mr. Graham read his report. (See page 266.)

Upon completion of the reading of this report, Dr. V. C. Tisdal of Elk City, the Council of District No. 2, was recognized by the Speaker and presented his report. (See page 266.)

The Councilor of District No. 3, Dr. C. W. Arrendell of Ponca City, was next granted the privilege of the floor and made his annual report (See page 266.)

Following the report of Dr. Arrendell, the Chair called for the report of the Councilor from District No. 4, Dr. Tom Lowry of Oklahoma City. (See page 267.)

Upon the completion of Dr. Lowry's report, the Speaker remarked that the report of Dr. J. I. Hollingsworth of Waurika, Councilor from District No. 5, had appeared in the April issue of the Journal of the Association. Upon call, Dr. Hollingsworth stated that he had nothing further to add.

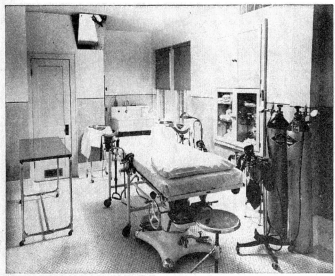

The Speaker next asked for the report of the Councilor from District No. 6, Dr. James Stevenson of Tulsa. (See page 267.)

In order, the next Councilor District was No. 7, but the Speaker stated that word had come to him that it was impossible for Dr. J. A. Walker of Shawnee to be present; therefore, no report was given.

At this time, Dr. Nesbitt, the Speaker, stated that the report for Councilor District No. 8, represented by Dr. Shade D. Neely of Muskogee, had been published in the April issue of the Journal.

Likewise, the same observation was made concerning District No. 9 with Dr. L. C. Kuyrkendall of McAlester as the Councilor.

The Speaker next called upon Dr. J. S. Fulton of Atoka, the Councilor of District No. 10, for his report. (See page 267.)

Following the report of Dr. Fulton, Dr. Shade D. Neely of Muskogee was granted the permission of the floor and made a supplementary report for Councilor District No. 8. (See page 267.)

At this time, the Speaker asked the pleasure of the House concerning the Councilor Reports, and the following motion was offered:

MOTION: Dr. L. Chester McHenry

"I move that the Reports of the Councilors be accepted."

SECONDED: Dr. Marvin D. Henley

Motion carried.

Following this action, the Speaker stated that in the absence of Dr. A. H. Bungardt of Cordell, he would appoint Dr. Ned R. Smith of Tulsa to serve on the Resolutions Committee in his place.

Following this substitute appointment, the Speaker, Dr. Nesbitt, stated that the next order of business would be the report of the Standing Committees.

The first Committee to report was the Credentials Committee and, since the report of this Committee had been published in the Journal, it stood approved.

Dr. Finis W. Ewing next gave the report of the Annual Session Committee by making the following statement: "This meeting is the answer and my report. I sincerely hope the meeting will be all you expect, and that it will be satisfactory to you. The fine cooperation given by the Tulsa County Medical Society, the work by Mr. Graham, the untiring efforts of Dr. C. R. Rountree and the other two members of the Scientific Work Committee, Dr. T. H. McCarley of McAlester and Dr. R. C. Pigford of Tulsa, and others that have been engaged in any way, is sufficient answer."

Upon motion by Dr. McLain Rogers of Clinton, seconded by Dr. F. W. Boadway of Ardmore, the report was accepted.

Following this action, the Speaker called upon Dr. C. R. Rountree of Oklahoma City, Chairman of the Scientific Work Committee, who stated that he had no further report to make at this time since the scientific program being presented was the report of the Committee.

At this time, the Speaker stated that the next Committee listed was that of Medical Education and Hospitals. Upon request, Mr. Graham was recognized and read, with the permission of Dr. Galvin L. Johnson of Pauls Valley, the Chairman, the following report:

Report of Committee on Medical Education and Hospitals

Your Committee on Medical Education and Hospitals desires to make the following recommendations to the House of Delegates concerning rules and regulations governing the licensing and operation of hospitals in the State of Oklahoma: 1. That, at the present time, there are no state statutes which set standards by which hospitals, clinics, institutions, sanitariums or infirmaries used for the treatment or care of medical and surgical elements are governed. 2. That this problem should have the attention of the State Legislature. 3. That the present laws allowing the creation of hospitals by irresponsible and uneducated layman for the purpose of promoting for gain the public without proper supervision is negligent and not to the best interest of the public and should be strictly regulated. 4. That any program licensing hospitals by state statutes should have for its minimum requirements those of either the American Hospital Association or the American College of Surgeons.

The Speaker, at this time, stated that the next report would be from the Committee on Publicity of which Dr. L. J. Starry of Oklahoma City was the Chairman but, inasmuch as Dr. Starry was not present, no report was made.

The next report to be considered in order was that of the Judicial and Professional Relations Committee, and the Speaker stated that this report had been published in the April issue of the Journal. Following this statement, Dr. A. S. Risser, Chairman of the Committee, was granted the permission of the floor, at which time he said: "Gentlemen: The work which has been done by the Tulsa County Medical Society concerning malpractice insurance stands as a monument. Observations which come from insurance men are to the effect that every suit for malpractice is founded on a misunderstanding or on remarks made by some physician in regard to certain cases. The medical profession can help in this respect by being careful about what is said. It has been proved that the better class of legal men are unwilling to take up malpractice cases. The solution of this problem lies in our hands alone."

At this time, the privilege of the floor was granted to Dr. F. W. Boadway of Ardmore, Chairman of the Public Policy Committee, by the Chair, who stated: "Gentlemen: The Public Policy Committee has had a quiet year. There has been no legislation to look after. One bill; namely, H. R. 4476 in the United States Congress which provided for the employment of osteopaths as internes in army hospitals was called to the attention of the membership. This action resulted in correspondence being sent to the proper officials in Washington. As a conclusion, next year is election year, and there will probably be lots to look after." The report of the Committee was approved.

The Speaker announced that this completed the Reports of the Standing Committees and that the next order of business would be that of the Reports of the Special Committees.

The Reports of the following Committees were published in the April Journal of the Association and were approved as published: Conservation of Vision, Industrial and Traumatic Surgery, Maternity and Infancy, Necrology, Postgraduate Medical Teaching, Study and Control of Cancer, Study and Control of Tuberculosis, Medical Economics and Public Health.

Following approval of the published Committee Reports, the Reports of the Committees on Conservation of Hearing, Study and Control of Venereal Diseases, Crippled Children, Benevolent Fund and Prepaid Medical and Surgical Service were approved as given by the Chairmen. (See page 268.)

For the next order of business, the Speaker recognized Dr. C. R. Rountree, Chairman of the Medical Advisory Committee to the Public Welfare Board, for a report to the House of Delegates on this important activity of the Association. Since the work of this Committee has been one of the progressive steps taken by the Association in the past year and since there was some discussion following the reading of the Report, the contents will be included in the minutes.

Report of Medical Advisory Committee

The Medical Advisory Committee to the State Department of Public Welfare, named by the President of the State Medical Association, and appointed by the State Director of Public Welfare, is composed of five members, one advisory member and two ex officio members, as follows: Members—Dr. C. R. Rountree, Chairman, Oklahoma City; Dr. F. Redding Hood, Vice-Chairman, Oklahoma City; Dr. Alfred R. Sugg, Ada; Dr.

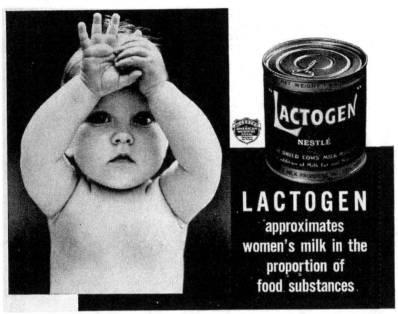
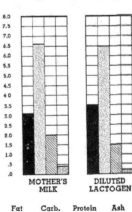

Clinton Gallaher, Shawnee, and Dr. R. M. Shepard, Tulsa; Advisory member—Dr. Mootman Prosser, Norman; Ex officio members—Dr. Finis W. Ewing, President of the Oklahoma State Medical Association, Muskogee, and Dr. Tullos O. Coston, Consulting Ophthalmologist of the State Department of Public Welfare, Oklahoma City. Miss Olivia Hemphill, Assistant Supervisor, Division of Public Assistance, represents the Department of Public Welfare at the meetings of the Medical Advisory Committee.

Meetings are held on the second Sunday in each month, eight monthly meetings having been held.

In setting up a Medical Advisory Committee, the services which the State Department of Public Welfare desired of the Committee were outlined as follows: 1. To give counsel to the agency in regard to policies, standards and procedures relating to the health of applicants for and recipients of aid of dependent children. 2. To serve in an advisory capacity to the agency in the review of reports of physicians submitted as evidence of the incapacity of the parents in establishing eligibility for aid to dependent children. 3. To advise with the agency in the development of suitable plans by which adequate medical examinations and review of such examinations by qualified medical personnel may be secured by the county departments of public welfare. 4. To advise with the State Department of Public Welfare to assure a discriminating and effective use of available facilities for health care. 5. To encourage the appointment of local medical advisory committees where they are needed, and to correlate the efforts of such committees. 6. To interpret to physicians throughout the state the purpose of the aid to dependent children program and the significance of the medical examination as a factor in determining eligibility for assistance and in planning for the welfare of the family. 7. To act as a liaison between the Department of Public Welfare and doctors over the state who examine applicants for aid to dependent children.

The Committee at first reviewed all of the reports of physicians on cases which were recommended for aid to dependent children where the incapacity of the parent was a factor in eligibility. The number of cases made it impossible for the Committee to discuss broader phases of the program, confining the discussion to specific cases involved; therefore, it was decided to divide the state into five districts, with each member responsible for studying the medical report and available social data on the cases in his particular district, prior to the regular meeting. On cases presenting no question as to whether or not an applicant is physically incapacitated, as determined by the medical report, a recommendation is made immediately to the Department of Public Welfare by the district member. When the member questions the incapacity of the parent, the medical report is held for study by all members of the committee at their regular meeting, and a recommendation is then made to the Department.

From July 1, 1941, through March 1, 1942, the Department of Public Welfare has referred 712 cases to the Committee. Recommendations have been made by the Committee on 604 of these cases, with the remaining 108 cases pending. The county recommendation was sustained on 504 of the 604 cases, but not sustained in 82 cases. The Committee found that in 81 cases there was insufficient evidence of physical incapacity, while one case recommended for denial by the county, was considered eligible from a physical standpoint by the Committee. There were 18 cases disposed of for other reasons, such as death, moved out of the State, etc.

The study of the medical reports in the individual cases consumes a great amount of the Committee's time. It is felt, however, that the Committee can be of greater service to the State Department in assisting in developing a reconstructive program for those families where physical incapacity of the parent exists. It is anticipated that as the work of the Committee progresses, it will be possible to spend more time on the development of policies and less time on the individual cases.

The Committee has studied the form which was being used by the Department for recording the findings of the examining physicians and recommended a revision of the form. While the new form is more adequate it is not proving entirely saitsfactory and it is the purpose of the Committee to work with the Department in making further revision of this form. It was found that there was a Department regulation stipulating that to be eligible for aid to dependent children because of physical incapacity, the incapacity must cover at least a twelve months' period. Consequently, examining physicians were being requested to make a definite statement as to the exact length of time an individual would be incapacitated. It was the opinion of the Committee that this regulation should be modified and a recommendation to this effect was made to the Commission. The Commission has now set a six months' period of incapacity. It is hoped that in the future this regulation may be further modified in order to make it possible for the physician to report on the present condition of the patient without considering his condition at a future specified time, thus enabling those persons who are definitely incapacitated to receive assistance for the children, and give the parent an opportunity to secure the necessary care and attention, before he becomes permanently disabled.

The Committee has also considered the advisability of paying fees to those physicians who are requested to make examinations. This question of fees was discussed in an executive session prior to our last meeting, and will be taken up with those administering the program before a definite recommendation is presented to the Commission.

It is the opinion of the Committee that giving assistance to families where the parent is incapacitated does not entirely solve the problem. Many of these incapacitated parents could be rehabilitated if proper treatment were available. It is our understanding that because of lack of funds, the Department can pay only 60 percent of the budget deficit. This means that many times the incapacitated parent is not able to follow the recommendation of his doctor, and his recovery is delayed because of insufficient food or because he attempts to augment this assistance by working when he should not. This tends to make for permanency of incapacity. The facilities for medical care, as you all know, are limited for this group of persons who are without means of support. It is the desire of the Committee to have as one of its future objectives the consideration of ways in which this group may have better medical and hospital facilities in order to rehabilitate them so that they will not remain permanently dependent.

The greatest handicap in planning a more effective aid to dependent children program is the inadequacy of funds for this group. Assistance funds provided by the Sales Tax in Oklahoma are so ear-marked that the Department of Public Welfare can pay only 60 percent of the budget deficit for children in need of assistance, while 100 percent of the budget deficit can be paid the needy aged and blind. Budgets for all these groups are determined on a very conservative basis and are not entirely adequate even when paid on a 100 percent basis, but if the funds are not ear-marked for definite groups, but paid into a general assistance fund, a more equitable distribution of the funds would be possible and as much could be done proportionately for children in their formative years as for the aged and blind. Because of insufficient funds, the Department has not been able to consider medical care in planning with families in these groups to meet their needs, other than to include actual cost of medicine and special diets where recommended by a physician. At present in the aid to dependent children program only 60 percent of the cost of medicine or special diets, included in the budget, would actually be received by the needy family.

The Committee has also given much thought to ways and means of interpreting the work of the medical profession to the Department, and the objectives of the aid to dependent children program to the medical profession. The purpose of the aid to dependent children program is to provide food, clothing and shelter to those children who meet the requirements as set by law and regulations, and physical incapacity of a parent to provide for his children is only one of several possible conditions that might render children eligible for aid to dependent children. Letters have been written to each of you and we have tried, whenever possible, to discuss this program with you individually.

The physicians of the State have given the Committee splendid cooperation, and we will need your further assistance in carrying out the Committee's work effectively.

Following the reading of the Medical Advisory Committee Report, it was moved

MOTION: Dr. McLain Rogers

"I move that the Report of the Medical Advisory Committee be accepted."

SECONDED: Dr. A. S. Risser

Preceding the adoption of the above motion, the Chair recognized Dr. F. W. Boadway of Ardmore who stated: "I was in hopes that some mention would be made about the people who don't want to get well but would rather be dependent on some organization for their day to day existence."

Following this statement, Dr. Rountree was again granted the privilege of the floor, and made the following supplementary remarks: "During the time the Medical Advisory Committee has functioned, it is estimated that approximately 12.4 percent of the cases that have been recommended for assistance by the counties have been recommended for denial by the Medical Advisory Committee. In several instances, however, some of the cases that have been denied the first time have been re-submitted to the members of the Committee and have been given approval after more information was secured."

At this time, the Speaker recognized Dr. Finis W. Ewing who stated: "This Committee, of which I am very proud, has been functioning only nine months instead of a year. As Dr. Rountree has already stated, approximately 12.4 percent of the cases that have been recommended for assistance have been recommended for denial by the Committee. The Committee has also been responsible for the stopping of an increase of applications. As you will remember, the Report of the Medical Economics Committee last year stated that the State Department of Public Welfare was very desirous that the State Medical Association appoint a Committee to counsel with them on recommended applications. In compliance with approval from the House of Delegates and in response to the appeal from the Public Welfare Department, the Committee was appointed. Again, may I say that I am indeed proud and pleased with the work accomplished by this Committee."

Following Dr. Ewing's remarks, Dr. Nesbitt requested of the House the pleasure of the motion concerning the acceptance of the Medical Advisory Committee Report, and the original motion by Dr. McLain Rogers, duly seconded by Dr. A. S. Risser, was approved unanimously.

Next, the Speaker stated that inasmuch as Dr. Clinton Gallaher of Shawnee, Chairman of the Committee on Medical Testimony, was not present at this time, the report would be called for later and that the House would proceed with the next order of business which, according to the agenda, was the invitation for the next annual session.

At this time, Dr. Tom Lowry of Oklahoma City was recognized by the Chair. "In the absence of the Chairman of the Oklahoma County Delegation, I take the privilege of representing that body and extending to the members of the Oklahoma State Medical Association an invitation to be our guests in Oklahoma City for the 1943 Annual Meeting."

Following the invitation in behalf of the Oklahoma County Delegates, the following motion was made:

MOTION: Dr. Sam A. McKeel

"I move that we accept the invitation of Oklahoma County to be their guests in 1943."

SECONDED: Dr. O. E. Templin

Motion carried.

Following this order of business, Dr. Nesbitt asked Dr. James Stevenson of Tulsa, a member of the Committee on Medical Testimony, if he would like to give the report for that Committee in the absence of the Chairman, and Dr. Stevenson stated that Dr. Gallaher was in possession of the report and that unforeseen circumstances had, no doubt, prevented his being present.

At this time, the Speaker asked the Executive Secretary to read the amendments to the Constitution and the By-Laws that had been presented for consideration. (The amendments appear in full in the proceedings of Thursday morning, April 23.) Following this action, there being no further introductions from the floor, the Chair stated that final consideration would be given to the amendments to the By-Laws the following morning and that it would be necessary for the amendments to the Constitution to lay over one year before final action could be taken.

The next order of business, according to the Speaker, was unfinished business of the preceding session, and the privilege of the floor was extended to Mr. Graham, who made the statement that the adoption of the new and official seal for the Association had been inadvertently omitted at the 1941 meeting. The following motion was made:

MOTION: Dr. L. C. Kuyrkendall

"I move that the House approve the seal."

SECONDED: Dr. J. D. Osborn

Motion carried.

There being no other old business to be considered, the next order pertained to the introduction of new business.

The Speaker recognized Mr. Graham, who read the Official Call to the Officers, Fellows and Members of the American Medical Association signed by the President, Dr. Frank H. Lahey, the Speaker of the House of Delegates, Dr. H. H. Shoulders, and the Secretary, Dr. Olin West, that had been received in the office of the Association.

The next order of business to be considered, according to the Speaker, concerned a communication petitioning for the creation of the Muskogee-Sequoyah-Wagoner County Medical Society. Mr. Graham was recognized and observed that the doctors in Sequoyah County belonged to the Cherokee Society since there were not sufficient members in that County to maintain an organization, and that although Wagoner County elected officers annually, due to the fact that there were only three members, it was impossible for them to have an active Society. Mr. Graham further observed that the request was in conformity with the provisions of the Constitution and By-Laws of the Association. He further stated that the following resolution submitted to the office of the Association by the Muskogee County Medical Society had been given Council approval at its meeting on March 29:

"That the membership of the Muskogee County Medical Society petition the Council of the Oklahoma State Medical Association for the amalgamation of the Muskogee, Sequoyah and Wagoner County Medical Societies.

"That the title of this Society then be changed to Muskogee-Sequoyah-Wagoner County Medical Society."

Following these statements, it was moved

MOTION: Dr. O. E. Templin

"I move that the House concur in the action of the Council, and that the above resolution, as read, be adopted."

SECONDED: Dr. J. D. Osborn

Motion carried.

Following the adoption of the above motion, the Chair stated that the next order of business to be considered would be the budget of the Association, and called upon Dr. L. J. Moorman of Oklahoma City, Secretary-Treasurer of the Association, to present the budget.

MOTION: Dr. Galvin L. Johnson

"I move that the budget, as read, be approved and accepted."

SECONDED: Dr. V. C. Tisdal

Motion carried.

At this time, Dr. Nesbitt stated that Dr. George H. Garrison was the Chairman of the Resolutions Committee and that he was in possession of several that had been referred to his Committee for consideration. The Speaker asked if there were other resolutions to be introduced from the floor at this time, but there was no response. (The resolutions appear in full in the proceedings of Thursday morning, April 23.)

The Speaker stated that the next order of business to be considered would be the election of Honorary Members to the Association. Mr. Graham was recognized and stated that, in accordance with the provisions of Chapter I, Section 3, Subsection (b), of the By-Laws of the Association, the four following names had been submitted to the office of the Association for election to Honorary Membership: R. M. C. Hill, McLoud; Daniel F. Stough, Sr., Geary; S. P. Ross, Ada; and J. C. Duncan, Forgan.

MOTION: Dr. W. S. Larrabee

"I move that the names, as read, be accepted for election to Honorary Membership."

SECONDED: Dr. V. C. Tisdal

Motion carried.

Following this action, Dr. Nesbitt stated that Dr. J. D. Osborn, Secretary of the State Board of Medical Examiners, would, at this time, make several pertinent remarks for the benefit of the membership pertaining to the Annual Registration Act—there following a general discussion by the Delegates.

Following this discussion, the Speaker stated that, inasmuch as he had omitted one of the items of new business on the agenda, he would recognize Dr. P. F. Herod of El Reno, Delegate from the Canadian County Medical Society, who desired to offer, in behalf of that Society, a motion concerning Affiliate Membership in the American Medical Association for Dr. T. M. Aderhold of El Reno.

MOTION: Dr. P. F. Herod

"I move that this House of Delegates instruct the Secretary to execute the necessary forms to be given to the Delegates to the American Medical Association convention to present to the proper committee requesting Affiliate Membership for Dr. Aderhold."

SECONDED: Dr. Garvin L. Johnson

Motion carried.

On motion of Dr. W. S. Larrabee, duly seconded and supported, the House adjourned at 12:00 P. M. to recess until 8:00 A. M., Thursday morning.

THURSDAY, APRIL 23, 1942

The second and final session of the House of Delegates convened at 8:50 A. M., Thursday morning, April 23, Dr. P. P. Nesbitt, the Speaker, presiding.

Following roll call by the Credentials Committee, the Committee announced a quorum present, and upon motion duly seconded, the report of the Credentials Committee was adopted.

The Speaker opened the morning session by stating that Dr. George H. Garrison was in possession of two letters he would like to read to the Delegates. Upon being granted permission of the floor, Dr. Garrison stated the letters were from Mayor R. A. Hefner and Dr. Harry H. Sorrels, Chairman of the Conventions Committee, extending a cordial invitation to the members of the Oklahoma State Medical Association to meet in Oklahoma City in 1943, and following this obversation, Dr. Garrison read the letters.

The next order of business was the reading of resolutions which had been introduced at the preceding session and referred to the Resolutions Committee. The Speaker recognized Dr. George H. Garrison, Chairman of the Committee, and all resolutions recommended by the Reference Committee were adopted. The resolutions are as follows:

University of Oklahoma School of Medicine

"Resolved by the Oklahoma State Medical Association in Annual Meeting assembled that:

This Association desires to record the interest it feels in the welfare and progress of the University of Oklahoma School of Medicine. The Association recommends that this institution receive adequate appropriations at the hands of the Legislature in order that it may advance and keep abreast of the progress in medical education, and continue to be, as it now is, a credit to the State.

Be it further resolved that a copy of this Resolution be sent on the first day of the next meeting of the State Legislature, to the Governor of the State, to the Speaker of the House, to the President Pro Tem of the Senate, to the Chairmen of the Senate and House Appropriations Committee, to the President of the University of Oklahoma, to the President of the Board of Regents of the University of Oklahoma, and to the President of the Oklahoma State Regents for Higher Education."

Rules of Ethics

"WHEREAS, There is a movement under way to request the House of Delegates of the American Medical Association at the coming 1942 meeting to rescind a rule of ethics adopted by that House of Delegates in 1935, making it unethical for ophthalmologists to give lectures to and consult with opticians and optometrists; and

WHEREAS, It is conceded that to care for the diseases and conditions of the human eye demands the unusual knowledge and skill of a graduate physician who has been especially prepared, and

WHEREAS, The eye is an integral part of the body; and

WHEREAS, No one but a physician so trained should be permitted to diagnose, treat or prescribe for eye conditions; and

WHEREAS, Lectures or other forms of instruction to opticians and optometrists by ophthalmologists is not only a breach of the principles of medical ethics, but is also to the detriment of the ocular health of the public by giving it a false sense of security; and

WHEREAS, General Health and ocular comfort depend on the best medical care,

THEREFORE, BE IT RESOLVED THAT the Oklahoma State Medical Association go on record as opposing any attempt to rescind this rule of ethics preventing ophthalmologists lecturing to or consulting with opticians and optometrists, and be it further resolved that our Delegates to the American Medical Association be advised of this action and be instructed to actively oppose any change in this rule of ethics."

Medical Testimony

"WHEREAS, expert medical testimony is a vital factor in securing just and meritorious decisions and rulings in the Courts and Commissions of the State of Oklahoma, and

WHEREAS, such testimony in this state has fallen far short of its rightful function through the failure of medical witnesses to govern their actions by the high professional canons; and

WHEREAS, the integrity and ethical standards of our profession are being jeapordized by biased and prejudiced testimony; and

WHEREAS, the professional societies and associations of other states have attempted to meet this responsibility by the formulation of plans and the appointment of commissions aimed at the enactment of rules and regulations to correct this condition; and

WHEREAS, the Minnesota State Medical Association has been singularly successful in this respect,

NOW, THEREFORE, be it resolved that the President of the Oklahoma State Medical Association appoint a committee to investigate the plan or plans of medical associations or societies of other states and submit a report of their study, with their findings and recommendations to the House of Delegates at its next annual meeting.''

Appreciation to Tulsa County Medical Society

''WHEREAS, The Tulsa County Medical Society by foresightedness and organization ability brought into being a group liability insurance policy for members of the Tulsa County Medical Society and later made it available to members of the Oklahoma State Medical Association; and

WHEREAS, Their continued interest and effort developed that group insurance to its present level of efficiency; and

WHEREAS, The development of such a plan has meant to physicians of Oklahoma an actual saving in premiums of $10,000.00 annually; and

WHEREAS, The Tulsa County Medical Society has relinquished the sponsorship of this group coverage and transferred the master policy to the Oklahoma State Medical Association,

THEREFORE, Be it resolved that the Oklahoma State Medical Association express its appreciation to the Tulsa County Medical Society for this splendid endeavor and accomplishment, and further that a copy of this resolution be sent to the Tulsa County Medical Society.''

Commonwealth Fund

''The House of Delegates in this Fiftieth Annual Session desires to express thanks and appreciation to The Commonwealth Fund of New York, for their liberal financial support in making possible the postgraduate instruction in obstetrics and pediatrics, also internal medicine for 1942 and 1943, in the State of Oklahoma.

It is the judgment of this House of Delegates, from numerous reports throughout the State, that hundreds of physicians in our medical profession have benefitted by reason of these courses.''

State Health Department

''The House of Delegates in this Fiftieth Annual Session desires to express thanks and appreciation to the Oklahoma State Health Department, and the United States Children's Bureau of Washington, D. C., for their financial support in making possible the postgraduate instruction program in pediatrics in the State of Oklahoma.

It is the judgment of this House of Delegates, from numerous reports throughout the State, that hundreds of physicians in our medical profession have benefitted by reason of the postgraduate programs in Oklahoma.

Further, that a copy of this resolution be sent to Dr. Grady F. Mathews, Commissioner, Oklahoma State Health Department; also a copy to the United States Children's Bureau, Washington, D. C.''

Compulsory Vaccination for Smallpox and Diphtheria

''WHEREAS, The health of the nation is at all times the consideration of the physician and,

WHEREAS, In the present world emergency there will be great shifts in population and resultant concentrations,

NOW THEREFORE BE IT RESOLVED that the House of Delegates endorse in principle the program of the Woman's Auxiliary of the Tulsa County Medical Society concerning compulsory vaccination for smallpox and diphtheria.''

Radio Advertising

''WHEREAS, The radio is a great and increasing means of commercial advertising, and

WHEREAS, Many nostrums and worthless forms of medication are advertised to the detriment of the public,

THEREFORE, Be it resolved that the Council and House of Delegates instruct the President to appoint a committee to function for the best interest of the public and organized medicine.''

Wording of Birth Certificates

''WHEREAS, The stigma of illegitimacy placed upon a birth certificate by the state laws of Oklahoma is unfair to the innocent child born out of wedlock and

WHEREAS, The designation of 'illegitimate' or 'born out of wedlock' on the birth certificate is injurious to the future of such a child,

NOW THEREFORE BE IT RESOLVED, that the Oklahoma State Medical Association endorse the principles embodied in the New York law, which prohibits any statement on a birth certificate concerning the marital status of the parents of the child, and issued to all children, the sense of which law is as follows:

A certification of birth shall contain only the name, sex, date of birth and place of birth of the person to whom it relates, and all other date on the original birth certificate reported by the attending physician concerning illegitimacy shall be deleted; however, a certificate copy of the original certificate of birth shall be issued upon order of a court of competent jurisdiction or upon a specific request by the person, if of age, or by a parent or other lawful representatives of the person to whom the record of birth relates if such request is to be issued for genealogical purposes.

NOW THEREFORE BE IT FURTHER RESOLVED, that a copy of this resolution be sent to the Governor of the State of Oklahoma, the Speaker of the House of Representatives and the Lieutenant Governor as the presiding officer of the Senate.''

Following the adoption of resolutions, the Speaker asked that the Vice-Speaker, Dr. H. K. Speed of Sayre, preside.

At this time, Dr. Speed recognized Mr. Graham, who read amendments to the By-Laws that had been submitted for consideration by the House of Delegates.

Chapter IX, Section 10, Subsection (a)
Re: Addition of the Name of a Committee

That Chapter IX, Section 10, Subsection (a), of the By-Laws, be amended as follows: Add to the names of committees:

''Prepaid Medical and Surgical Service.''

Chapter I, Section 3, Subsection (b)
Re: Honorary Members

Chapter I, Section 3, Subsection (b), of the By-Laws, be amended as follows: Add to the last paragraph the following sentence:

''Honorary Members shall be considered the same as fully-paid members in computing the membership of the County Societies for the purpose of determining the number of Delegates that the County Societies shall be entitled to send to the House of Delegates as provided in these By-Laws.''

Chapter I, Section 3, Subsection (d)
Re: Associate Members

Amend Chapter I, Section 3, of the By-Laws, by adding another division following Subsection (c) to be designated as Subsection (d):

''The House of Delegates may elect to Associate Membership any person who cannot qualify for either Active, Honorary or Junior Membership if, in the majority opinion of the House of Delegates, his contributions to medicine or the Association justifies the conferring of such an honor. Any County Society may place before the House of Delegates petitions for Associate Membership, after having first submitted the petition to the Council at least ninety (90) days before the Annual Meeting and receiving Council approval of the petition.

''Petitions for Associate Membership may also originate in the Council, however, in all instances, all petitions for Associate Membership must be published in the issue of the Journal published at least thirty (30) days before the Annual Session.''

Following the reading of the above amendment, the following comments were made:

Dr. John A. Haynie of Durant: 'I think the amendment is too broad reaching.''

Dr. McLain Rogers of Clinton: ''The action is still in the House of Delegates, and I see no objection.''

Dr. W. S. Larrabee of Tulsa: ''The action concerning the election of Associate Members must first be passed by the County Society, then the Council and finally the House of Delegates. I can see no objection to the adoption of this amendment.''

Dr. J. D. Osborn of Frederick: ''This particular amendment has been proposed by the Council to take care of a situation that has arisen in the State of Oklahoma concerning doctors who are practicing with the Federal Agencies, for instance, at the town of Muskogee, and in other towns. They are doctors who are not in private practice but with Governmental Agencies; therefore, are not required to take out a license to practice medicine in the State of Oklahoma. These physicians do not care to go to the trouble and expense of being licensed in Oklahoma. Some of these men would like to be members of the Association but, according to the Constitution and By-Laws, as they now stand, it is impossible. The election of certain doctors to Associate Membership would still be in the hands of the House of Delegates, and in my opinion, would be handled with perfect safety."

Dr. A. S. Risser of Blackwell: "If this had been an organization in France a good many years ago, this particular discussion would have been applicable to men like Louis Pasteur. It is my understanding that the intention is to honor men who support the cause of the profession for the general public. We are perfectly safe in adopting this amendment."

Chapter I. Section 5
Re: Revocation of Honorary and Associate Members

Amend Chapter I, of the By-Laws, by adding another division to be designated as Section 5:

"Any Honorary or Associate Membership may be revoked by a two-thirds vote of the House of Delegates when, in the opinion of the House of Delegates, the conduct or actions of the Honorary or Associate Member violates any of the principles of the code of ethics of the Association, or whose conduct or actions are not becoming to the honor conferred."

Following the reading of this amendment, Dr. P. P. Nesbitt resumed the Chairmanship.

Chapter XI. Section 3, Subsection (a 1)
Re: Membership in Adjoining Society

Amend Chapter XI, Section 3, Subsection (a), of the By-Laws, by adding another division to be designated as Subsection (a 1).

"Any physician living near a county line may hold membership in the medical society of the county adjoining his residence if it is more convenient for him to attend the meetings of the medical society of the adjoining county, but before a physician is affiliated with a medical society in a county in which he does not reside, the consent of the medical society in the county of which he does reside must be first obtained."

Chapter II. Section 5
Re: Section Sessions

Chapter II, Section 5, of the By-Laws, shall be amended to read as follows:

"The sections authorized for separate meetings and a division of the scientific work shall be determined by the Scientific Work and Annual Session Committees, with approval of the Council."

Chapter VII. Section 11
Re: Editor of the Journal

Chapter VII, Section 11, of the By-Laws, to be amended as follows: Delete the last sentence, which reads

"The Board shall organize as soon as possible and elect an Editor-in-Chief."—(Election of Editor-in-Chief provided for in Chapter VIII, Section 4, Subsection (a), of the By-Laws.)

Chapter VIII. Section 4. Subsection (a)
Re: Editor-in-Chief

Amend Chapter VIII, Section 4, Subsection (a), of the By-Laws, in the following manner: Insert before the last sentence

"The Council shall designate one of the elected board members as Editor-in-Chief, and this designation shall, at all times, be subject to change by the Council by giving thirty (30) days written notice to the Editor-in-Chief."

Dr. L. S. Willour of McAlester: "I oppose this amendment to the By-Laws."

Dr. Finis W. Ewing of Muskogee: "This amendment has been recommended to the House by the Council, and their thought when suggesting this change was that it would dispose of the fact that one of the three doctors on the Editorial Board might be more or less embarrased by having to vote for himself."

Dr. H. K. Speed of Sayre: "The Council is the safest body of this Association, and I firmly believe their judgment in passing on the members of the Editorial Board and selecting the Editor-in-Chief is safe and sound. I believe the amendment should be adopted."

Dr. L. S. Willour of McAlester: "The Journal of the Association is published under the immediate direction of the Council and under the supervision and direction of the Editorial Board. This authority is stated in the Constitution and By-Laws. The job of publishing the Journal should be given to the Editorial Board and it should then be made their responsibility. I think that the Editorial Board composed of the three members selected by the Council are more capable of electing an Editor-in-Chief than are the members of the Council."

Dr. J. D. Osborn of Frederick: "Dr. Ewing has stated one of the reasons why this amendment should be adopted. In addition, I think the Council is as competent or more so to elect an Editor-in-Chief than is the Editorial Board. In a committee of three, it would become necessary for one man to vote for himself. I also want to second what Dr. Speed has said. The Council is a group of level headed and clear-thinking men."

Following the reading of the amendments to the By-Laws, it was moved by Dr. Kuyrkendall, seconded by Dr. Galvin L. Johnson, that they be adopted, and carried unanimously.

At this time, Mr. Graham read the amendments to the Constitution that had been introduced.

Article VIII, Section 4
Re: Vacancy of the Speaker of the House

Article VIII, Section 4, of the Constitution, to be amended in the following manner:

"Vacancies created by the death, resignation, or removal of the above-named officers shall be filled by temporary appointment by the Council, such appointment being effective until the next annual meeting of the House of Delegates, which shall elect a successor to complete the unexpired term, if any, except the President, whose place shall be filled by the Vice-President, and the Speaker of the House of Delegates, whose unexpired term shall be filled by the Vice-Speaker."

Following the reading of this amendment, the Speaker stated that it would be necessary for this amendment to wait for final action until the 1943 session to comply with the provisions of Article XIII of the Constitution.

Article VIII. Section 3
Re: General Officers

Amend Article VIII, Section 3, of the Constitution, as follows:

"All of the above officers shall assume the duties of their respective offices immediately upon the close of the annual session at which they were elected to serve and shall serve until their successors have been elected and installed with the exception of the Delegates to the American Medical Association who shall take office the first of January succeeding his election."

At this time, the Speaker stated that it would also be necessary for this amendment to lay over until the 1943 session.

The next order of business was the election of officers. The Speaker announced that the first election would be that of President-Elect and recognized Dr. H. C. Weber of Bartlesville, who made the following remarks: "Mr. Chairman and Members of the House of Delegates: There are a lot of good men but some would not be able to give this office the time that is absolutely necessary and which will be essential next year. Tulsa County has a capable man, and I know he will give all the time that is necessary to such a position if he is elected. I should like to place in nomination the name of Dr. James

Stevenson, who has been a member of the American Medical Association and the Oklahoma State Medical Association for at least twenty years. Dr. Stevenson came to Tulsa from the little town of Cherokee, and I think he has done very well. In the last three years, Jim Stevenson has given the State Association more time than any other man—he was Chairman of the Committee that hired the Executive Secretary, was partially responsible for the establishment of group hospitalization in the State of Oklahoma and was President of the Tulsa County Medical Society when they had very poor attendance. By a lot of hard work, I understand Jim has been able to encourage more of the doctors here in Tulsa to attend the regular county meetings.''

Dr. Finis W. Ewing of Muskogee: "It gives me pleasure to have the opportunity to second Dr. Weber's nomination. It has been my pleasure to have been intimately associated with Dr. Stevenson, and I sincerely concur in the statement that he will make an excellent President.''

Dr. H. K. Speed of Sayre: "I move that the nominations cease and that Dr. Stevenson be elected by acclamation.''

Dr. L. S. Willour of McAlester: "A year ago, Dr. Stevenson came before the House of Delegates and said nice things about me, and I liked them. At this time, I want to reciprocate by seconding Dr. Speed's motion that he be elected by acclamation.''

The motion carried.

Following his election, Dr. Stevenson made the following remarks to the Delegates: "Mr. Speaker and Gentlemen: I should like to take this opportunity to thank Dr. Weber, Dr. Ewing and Dr. Willour for their many kind words. I only hope they are merited, and I'll certainly need the help of everyone. At this time, I pledge my very best endeavors to act as your leader.''

Following the election of President-Elect, nominations were in order for Vice-President.

The Speaker recognized Dr. F. W. Boadway of Ardmore, who remarked: "I should like to place in nomination the name of a man who has been a member of the House of Delegates for a good many years and who is a member of several committees—Dr. Galvin L. Johnson of Pauls Valley.''

Dr. G. E. Johnson of Ardmore: "Several years ago, Dr. Johnson was President of the Southeastern Medical Association which is composed of seventeen counties. Seriously, Dr. Johnson has always worked for organized medicine and the sick man, boy and girl of our State and, of course, always in an honorable way. He is a leader. I would like to second the nomination of Dr. Boadway.''

Dr. W. L. Taylor of Holdenville: "I move that Dr. Johnson be elected by acclamation.''

The motion was seconded by Dr. J. D. Osborn, and carried unanimously.

Following his election, Dr. Johnson made the following statement: "Thank you, and I'll do the best I can.''

Next, the House was in order for the election of Speaker of the House of Delegates, and Dr. Nesbitt recognized Dr. O. E. Templin of Alva: "Gentlemen: It is important that we have a good Speaker of the House just as well as a good President. Since the beginning, we have had a good Speaker. We will certainly not be letting down the standards, and I should like to place in nomination the name of a person who is well versed in parliamentary procedure, Dr. George H. Garrison of Oklahoma City.''

The motion was seconded by Dr. A. S. Risser of Blackwell, and Dr. I. W. Bollinger of Henryetta moved that Dr. Garrison be elected by acclamation, duly seconded by Dr. Templin, and carried.

At this time, Dr. Garrison made the following statement: "Thank you. I appreciate very much the recognition and the position which the Speaker of the House carries with it. I am indeed grateful to Dr. Templin for his remarks. I shall do the best I can with your help.''

In order, the next election was for Vice-Speaker of the House of Delegates. Dr. Nesbitt recognized Dr. L. S. Willour of McAlester, who placed in nomination the name of Dr. H. K. Speed of Sayre. There being no further nominations, Dr. Galvin L. Johnson moved that the nominations be closed and Dr. Speed be elected by acclamation. The nomination was properly seconded by Dr. J. D. Osborn and carried.

The Speaker next called for nominations for that of Delegates to the American Medical Association to serve for 1942-43. Dr. Marvin D. Henley of Tulsa was recognized by the Chair and made the following nomination: "I should like to place in nomination the name of a man with whom everyone is well acquainted. He is a good man and has been our Delegate to the A. M. A. for the last two years. The doctor to whom I refer is Dr. W. A. Howard of Chelsea.''

Following this nomination, Dr. H. C. Weber moved that the nominations cease and that Dr. Howard be elected by acclamation. The motion was duly seconded by Dr. Finis W. Ewing and carried.

Following the election of Dr. Howard as Delegate to the American Medical Association, Dr. Nesbitt observed that nominations were in order for Alternate Delegate to the American Medical Association, and Dr. I. W. Bollinger of Henryetta was recognized by the Chair and made the observation that he wished to place in nomination the name of Dr. Finis W. Ewing of Muskogee. Dr. Galvin L. Johnson moved that the nominations cease and that Dr. Ewing be elected by acclamation. The motion was duly seconded and carried.

At this time, Dr. Nesbitt, the Speaker, stated that there was a mistake in the years the Councilors were to serve since the provisions of the By-Laws, as adopted at the 1940 session, according to Chapter IV, Section 2, Subsection (a), had not been followed; therefore, there was only one Councilor whose term was correct as listed, this being Dr. Tom Lowry of Oklahoma City, Councilor of District No. 4. Dr. Nesbitt continued by saying that in 1940, the Councilors were to have been elected for the following terms: Districts 1, 4, 7 and 10 for one year; Districts 2, 5 and 8 for two years and Districts 3, 6 and 9 for three years. The Speaker further observed that the only way to get the term straightened out was for all of the officers to be declared for re-election except District No. 4, which was correct. Further explanation was made to the effect that to get the Councilors' terms in proper sequence at this time, Districts 3, 6 and 9 should be elected for one year; Districts 1, 7 and 10 for two years and Districts 2, 5 and 8 for three years. This opinion was concurred in by the Delegates, and the Speaker requested the Delegates to retire and prepare their nominations for Councilors from their respective districts.

Immediately following the recess of the House, Mr. David Milsten, attorney and member of the Tulsa Speaker's Bureau from the Office of Civilian Defense, was introduced by the Speaker and spoke to the Delegates on the doctor's place in the civilian defense set-up.

At this time, the Delegates from the nine named districts advised the Chair that their nominations for Councilors were in order. The first to be considered were those Councilors who would serve for one year, and Dr. A. S. Risser of Blackwell nominated Dr. C. W. Arrendell of Ponca City as Councilor from District No. 3; Dr. M. J. Searle of Tulsa nominated Dr. J. V. Athey of Bartlesville as Councilor from District No. 6; and Dr. L. S. Willour of McAlester nominated Dr. L. C. Kuyrkendall of McAlester as Councilor from District No. 9

In order, the Councilors who would serve for two years were next named, and Dr. C. R. Rountree of Oklahoma City nominated Dr. O. E. Templin of Alva as Councilor from District No. 1; Dr. W. L. Taylor of Holdenville nominated Dr. Clinton Gallaher of Shawnee as Councilor from District No. 7; and Dr. John A. Haynie of Durant nominated Dr. J. S. Fulton of Atoka as Councilor from District No. 10.

The Councilors to serve for three years were next proposed, and Dr. McLain Rogers of Clinton nominated Dr. V. C. Tisdal of Elk City as Councilor from District No. 2; Dr. G. E. Johnson of Ardmore nominated Dr. J. I. Hollingsworth of Waurika as Councilor from District No. 5; and Dr. Finis W. Ewing of Muskogee nominated Dr. Shade D. Neely of Muskogee as Councilor from District No. 8.

Following these nominations, Dr. J. D. Osborn moved the election of three physicians as Councilors. The motion was duly seconded by Dr. Finis W. Ewing and carried.

Following the election of Councilors, the Speaker requested the pleasure of the House concerning the installation of officers, and it was moved by Dr. L. S. Willour that they be automatically installed, duly seconded by Dr. W. L. Taylor and carried.

Immediately following the above motion and its adoption, it was moved by Dr. George H. Garrison of Oklahoma City that the Tulsa County Medical Society be extended a vote of appreciation in behalf of the State Medical Association for the outstanding manner in which they had entertained the members of the Association during the 1942 Annual Meeting. The motion was duly seconded by Dr. O. E. Templin and adopted.

Following this motion and its adoption, Dr. George H. Garrison moved that the House of Delegates extend a vote of thanks to the Scientific Work Committee for the remarkable program which the Association had been privileged to attend. Dr. Finis W. Ewing seconded the motion, and it was unanimously adopted.

At this time, Dr. L. S. Willour moved that the Secretary be instructed to send to Dr. J. A. Walker of Shawnee, the retiring Councilor from District No. 7, an appropriate letter in behalf of the House of Delegates of the Oklahoma State Medical Association expressing their best wishes and extending their appreciation for his faithful service in behalf of the Association. The motion was seconded by Dr. A. S. Risser and carried.

Following this action, Mr. Graham was extended the privilege of the floor and stated that the following telegram had been received by Dr. Finis W. Ewing, retiring President of the Oklahoma State Medical Association, from Captain James G. Hughes, Camp Gordon, Augusta, Georgia, who had recently completed the teaching of a postgraduate course in Pediatrics in the state: "Best wishes to all my Oklahoma friends for a successful meeting."

At this time, Dr. Nesbitt announced that the desk of the Speaker was cleared and unless there was other business to be transacted a motion for adjournment was in order. Dr. J. D. Osborn of Frederick moved the House adjourn. The motion was seconded by Dr. Finis Ewing of Muskogee and carried.

ANNUAL REPORT OF THE COUNCIL

Since the last report by the Council on its stewardship of the association, world conditions have developed to such an extent as to make the activities of organized medicine one of the first lines of defense. For this reason, if for no other, the Association must and will maintain a progressive attitude and leadership in the protection of the Public Health and the staffing of the medical corps of our military forces. Already 150 members of the Association have taken up service in the armed forces of our government and in the immediate future many others will be called.

In reporting the activities of the Association for the year 1941-42, the Council has deemed it advisable to refrain from too much elaboration on past activities, in order that a complete discussion may be had on the future courses and policies of the Association in the war years ahead.

During the past year, the financial position of the Association has remained in a sound condition, although its reserves have not been augmented by any large increase. The financial statement has been published in the Journal, and time will not be taken to review it now. The financing for 1942-1943 will be presented in a later paragraph and in more detail.

As each of you know, during the last year, the problem of medical defense brought about by the questionnaire of the American Medical Association and the program of the Office of Procurement and Assignment has been the one of paramount importance. The response of the profession through the county societies has been little short of miraculous and every chairman and member of committees participating in the work, as well as the individual members, can feel a justifiable pride in their accomplishment. The Council is also of the opinion that now as never before the necessity and value of a full-time office has been clearly pictured and justified in the work accomplished by the Office of the Association in the defense program. ·.

The Council, after hearing periodic reports from the Procurement and Assignment Committee, is fully cognizant of the fact that this voluntary effort on the part of organized medicine may in isolated instances seem to work hardships and injustices on some, but in the final analysis it is the true democratic way to accomplish the needed end result. Every delegate is urged in reporting to his county society to stress the present need for the cooperation and unity of the profession in order that the greatest service possible will be rendered to the greatest number of people.

Your Council is of the opinion that in the near future there probably will be a forced dislocation of physicians unless the medical profession can and will see that its services and abilities are made available to both urban and rural communities that are now without the services of any physician.

To this end your Council urges and requests that each and every county society survey its immediate territory and population to see that the people in the area are having care made available to them on a basis that they can afford.

The county societies are requested to consider the towns and rural population surrounding their geographic boundaries when the neighboring county is without an organized medical society.

This is a responsibility of medicine that it must assume. If this cannot be accomplished, then any alternate plan advanced by outside agencies cannot be factually criticized.

Committee activity during the past year has been most gratifying. There has not been a single committee called upon to function that has not responded in an aggressive manner.

The reports of the committees have been published in the April Journal and will not be read into the Council's report. However, the Council does wish to call special attention to the work of the Postgraduate Committee, the Advisory Committee to the Public Welfare Department, the Scientific Work Committee, and the Committee on Procurement and Assignment.

The Postgraduate Committee has again made it possible for the membership to have postgraduate work available in the local communities at a time when it is of the utmost value. The program for the coming two years is on Internal Medicine, and every member should take advantage of it. The assistance given by the Commonwealth Fund of New York and the Oklahoma State Department of Health is gratefully and sincerely acknowledged. Without their support, the programs could not be conducted. The very fact that this program is still in operation with the same contributing agencies speaks sufficiently for the splendid work of the committee.

The Scientific Work Committee this year was confronted with a most difficult task. Past actions of the House of Delegates in creating scientific sections until at the present time there are nine, plus the mushroom growth of attendance at the Annual Meeting, called for physical requirements for the holding of the Annual Meeting that were difficult to meet. The meeting that we have attended today and will attend for the next two is the result of many hours' work done by this committee. Your attention is directed to the policy of the committee in providing for the last two years guest speakers for all sections and the splendid, well-rounded program that has been developed. The Scientific Roundtable on Sulfonamide Therapy that is on the program is also the result of the creative attitude of the committee in presenting an interesting and beneficial program. It is also interesting to report that these many additions and innovations have been accomplished with little, if any, additional cost to the Association, since a vigorous campaign to obtain technical exhibitors has been successful enough to finance the new features. In this connection, the Council should like to suggest that each of us show our appreciation to these exhibitors by visiting and registering at their booths. It is only by evincing honest interest in the exhibits that their continued support can be solicited.

In a preceding paragraph, special reference was made to the work of the Advisory Committee to the Public Welfare Department. A report of the activity of the committee will be made by the Chairman that will give complete and factual information concerning its accomplishments. However, your Council cannot refrain from citing this committee for its outstanding work and for the fact that the members of the committee have seen fit to meet once each month since last July without remuneration. The Council herewith wishes to emphasize its complete endorsement of the work being done by the committee and to urge that every member give his complete cooperation.

The Procurement and Assignment Committee also has not been without its problems. Since its work affects the practice of every doctor either directly or indirectly, all of its requests to the County Societies should receive calm and deliberate consideration. Your attention is again directed to the purpose of the Committee, which is to assure adequate medical care to the civilian population and at the same time make available for military duty as many physicians as possible. Your Council is not unmindful of the magnitude of this vital factor of medical care as it pertains to all-out war and the responsibilities resting upon the County Societies and their Committees, and wishes to observe to you, as Delegates representing the County Societies, that unless medicine in this voluntary manner can meet the demands that will be placed upon it, it may be necessary for more drastic action to be put in effect to secure physicians for military duty. Your Council is firmly of the opinion that medicine will not fail in its responsibilities and desires to compliment the Committee for its efficient work. The cooperation of every physician is vital and necessary.

The special attention called to the work of the preceding four committees does not in any way reduce or minimize the work of all other committees. The Public Health Committee was extremely active in cooperating with the Public Health Department in its program of immunization, which is now in progress. The Cancer Committee is again active in its work with the Women's Field Army of the American Society for the Control of Cancer. This year's program will be an extensive one and the assistance of the profession will be requested in conducting lay lectures on the necessity for the early diagnosis and treatment of cancer. You are individually urged to give every support possible to the Women's Field Army and to enroll yourselves.

The Industrial and Traumatic Surgery Committee report speaks adequately enough for its initial work in this fast developing field. The Council heartily endorses its objectives and will give every assistance possible in promoting its work. The Economics Committee during the past year completed a thorough survey of the opinions of the county societies and their attitude toward the Health Program of the Farm Security Administration. Its report should be studied by all societies having this problem presented to them. The Council subscribes to the conclusion of this committee that no definite recommendation can be made as to whether a county society should cooperate in the program, but that the decision must rest solely with the local society after a careful study is made as to the local need for the program.

The reports of the committees call for careful study and consideration by every delegate, and criticisms and opinions should be freely expressed. It is only in this manner that the Council and committees can be guided in following the wishes of the membership.

The preceding paragraphs have expressed the report of the Council on committee work and the following paragraphs will report activities directly sponsored either by or through the Council and the executive office.

During the past year, the Tulsa County Medical Society requested that the State Association assume complete control and ownership of the Master Policy for malpractice insurance for members of the Association that had been developed by that society in cooperation with the London and Lancashire Indemnity Company of New York through Eberle and Company of Oklahoma City. This transfer has now been made, and the Master Policy changed to the State Association. This contribution by the Tulsa Society is probably the greatest that has ever been made by a county society, as through its efforts the members of the Association are now saving many thousands of dollars more annually on their insurance premiums than they are paying in dues. The Council wishes to state in this connection that the present malpractice premium is based on premium income versus the loss ratio on paid claims, and that the amount of premium that will be charged in the future will depend on the protection given every member of the Association by his conferee when he is the victim of an unwarranted suit. Every member should also in so far as is possible assist this activity by carrying his insurance with London and Lancashire.

Many of you no doubt attended the Second Annual Secretaries Conference, which was held December 14, in Oklahoma City. This meeting which was inaugurated two years ago has rapidly become one of the foremost meetings of the year. The program for last year was highlighted by the appearance as guest speaker of Sam Seeley, M.D., Executive Officer of the Office of Procurement and Assignment, Washington, D. C. The Council feels that it is justified in being proud of this innovation and urges all who can to attend this meeting when it is held.

The Council is also pleased to be able to report to the Delegates that its brief presented to the Treasury Department of the United States for an exemption from the payment of federal income tax on the basis that the Association was a non-profit, scientific and educational Association, was successful. It might be of further interest to the delegates to know that his ruling has been made to few medical organizations, and speaks well for the work of the auditors and the officers of the Association.

The Journal during the past year has been ably directed by the Editorial Board, and special attention should be called to the development of the Editorial Page. The features of interest to the profession that were started in 1940-41, including the news notes from the Medical School, Public Health Department, Group Hospital Service, and the Woman's Auxiliary, have been maintained, and the Book Review section has been expanded. Color advertising was approved, and the Journal cover converted to color. Every assistance is pledged the Editorial Board by the Council in its effort to improve at all times the Journal, both scientifically and as an economic news medium.

While each individual councilor has either reported in the Journal, or will give a verbal report of the activity in his Councilor District, it is nevertheless of interest to note the splendid acceptance of the Councilor District meetings that were held during the past year. Every effort will be made by the Council to expand this activity during the coming year, in order that the County Societies may be kept in constant touch with the affairs of the Association.

Outside of the general activities under the auspices of the Association, and yet activities in which the Association is vitally interested and in which the physician plays a prominent part, are Selective Service, the Committee on Health and Housing of the Office of Civilian

Defense and the Group Hospital Service—the Blue Cross Plan. The Council wishes to commend Major Louis H. Ritzhaupt as State Medical Officer, Dr. Grady F. Mathews as Chairman of the Health and Housing Committee, and Mr. N. D. Helland as Director of the Blue Cross Plan, for the direction and cooperation they have manifested in the execution of their positions, and to pledge full support of the Association to the aims and ideals of their undertakings.

The Council also recommends that the House of Delegates reaffirm its original position concerning the action of the Board of Medical Examiners in the ruling made by that Board concerning refugee physicians. The Council further recommends that the House of Delegates give its full support to the recently enacted Annual Registration Act and the purpose it will serve. It is understood by the Council that the Secretary of the Board of Examiners will make a report to the House on the operation of the law and its recent action in securing an attorney.

That the coming war years will be difficult ones for medicine in its organized position, as well as for the private practitioner, is an obvious assumption that probably would be concurred in by all.

As viewed by the Council, the activities of the Association and its obligation to society must be continued and even expanded, in so far as the resources of the Association can justify this continuance and expansion.

Your Council is of the opinion that the activities of the Association for the coming year should be limited to complete cooperation with the all-out effort of the United Nations to win the war and to a protection of the health of the people in whatever manner this latter problem may present itself.

Medical defense both at home and in foreign fields may tax the entire resources and abilities of the medical profession. Those who stay at home must never lose sight of the sacrifices being made by others.

January 1, 1943, will find the destinies of the State of Oklahoma in the hands of a new governor and legislature. Each and every member of the Association is urged to exercise his heritage and prerogative as an individual citizen in the selection of the public officials and legislators who will formulate the laws and conduct the business of state and local governments. Politics is no longer a game participated in by a few, for today politics is business and business is politics. Whether this is as it should be is immaterial, but it does place a greater responsibility on the electorate. As private citizens, you should interview and consult with all candidates for public office on their attitudes concerning measures that will effect the health of the public, and each of us should work diligently for the election of those officials whose concepts of the divisions between government and private initiative is to the best interests of the public at large.

Since many county societies will have their membership depleted by virture of members serving in the armed forces, it is urged that those members remaining at home be diligent in continuing the work of the local society.

Concerning the financing of the Association during the war years—your attention is directed to the provision of the By-Laws which places the amount of dues for membership as the duty of the House of Delegates, and to the problem this presents to the Council in its endeavor to anticipate the financial needs of the Association for 1943.

To present the subject properly, a brief summary will be given of the present financial condition of the

Association and the Council's interpretation of this condition as it pertains to the 1943 year of operation.

As of January 1, 1942, the Association had on hand as operating assets before the payment of any 1942 dues the sum of $2,454.75. This reserve had been accumulated on the basis of dues of $10.00 by a membership of 1,456 in 1940 and 1,430 in 1941. At the present time, the Association has 1,348 members, of which 57 have paid $4.00 dues, since they are serving in the armed forces. This leaves a total of 1,291 as full dues paying members for the year 1942. While the amount paid in by this membership plus the accumulated reserve is sufficient to operate the Association adequately for the current year, it does not take into consideration the anticipated needs for 1943, which must be dealt with at this time.

Since practically all medical students, interns and residents have already accepted commissions in the armed forces, as exemplified by the action of the students of the Oklahoma University School of Medicine where all but five out of 224 have taken commmissions, which is indeed a splendid record, it is obvious that there will be relatively few new members for the Association, as these physicians will go directly into service, immediately upon completing one year of internship.

Anticipating that the next six months will see many more members being called into military service who in turn will not be available as full dues paying members for 1943, the Council recommends to the House of Delegates that it empower the Council to set the dues for membership on or before December 1, after considering the needs of the Association for 1943 and the probable number of members who will be available at that time, and further that the Council be instructed to set the dues at $10.00 per year, unless it is absolutely impossible to operate the Association at this figure, but that under no circumstances shall the dues be raised in excess of $12.00 per year, and that after 1942 and for the duration of the war, the dues of members serving in the military forces be $4.00 annually.

The budget which will be presented by the Council has been given careful consideration and has been compiled on a conservative basis. There have been only two raises in the budget over the last year, one in the amount of postage which was raised in consideration of the coming legislative year, and the other is for secretarial work in the office which has for some time been in need of adjustment. The salary of the Executive Secretary and the Editor of the Journal have not been increased.

In consideration of this proposal, the Council pledges to the House of Delegates that in every phase of Association activity, it will practice the strictest economy and operate the Association on a sound and conservative basis.

In closing this report, each delegate is urged to speak freely concerning the proposals of the Council and its conduct of the Association's affairs during the past year.

The Resolutions Committee in its report will submit several resolutions that have had your Council's approval. The Council here again urges that each delegate express himself if he does not subscribe to the opinion of the Council.

Your Council pledges itself to give to the membership of the Association in the coming year a sincere and conservative administration. The Council solicits your cooperation, assistance, and criticism at all times, and charges you to remember that the Association belongs to the membership and not to the Council, your officers, or any individual.

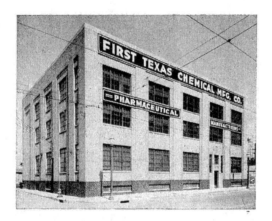

COUNCILOR DISTRICT REPORTS

In addition to the Councilor District Reports published in the April issue of the Journal of the Association, the following reports were made before the House of Delegates at the time of the 1942 Annual Meeting in Tulsa:

ANNUAL REPORT DISTRICT NO. 1

To the Officers and Members
Of the Oklahoma State Medical Association

Gentlemen:

During the past year I have cooperated as well as possible with all the activities sponsored by the State Association. I have written many letters to stimulate renewal of membership for 1942. Much time has been spent in examination of selectees for the Army. I have complied with all requests from the state office relative to procurement of Medical Officers and any other duties that have been requested of me.

I have attended at my own expense Council Meetings in Oklahoma City on the following dates: July 21, 1941; September 14, 1941; and March 29, 1942.

I have attended meetings throughout the district as follows: Cherokee, May 27, 1941; Supply, June 12, 1941; Cherokee, January 27, 1942; Woodward, March 12, 1942; Shattuck, April, 1942.

The Woodward County Society covers Woodward, Harper, and Ellis County and is well organized. Woods and Alfalfa Counties are well organized and active. Texas County is organized but inactive. Beaver and Cimarron Counties are not organized. Owing to the small number of physicians in the last three counties it is practically impossible for a society to function.

Respectfully submitted,

O. E. Templin, M.D.
Councilor District No. 1.

ANNUAL REPORT DISTRICT NO. 2

To the President, and House of Delegates
Of the Oklahoma State Medical Association

Gentlemen:

District No. 2 consisting of nine counties, Roger Mills, Beckham, Greer, Harmon, Washita, Kiowa, Custer, Jackson and Tillman, wishes to bring you the following report of the state of conditions existing among the county societies and doctors as follows:

We are pleased to report that the county societies are functioning with an increased enthusiasm, a desire for medical advancement in the way of knowledge as demonstrated by the large number in attendance at the Post Graduate Course given in Obstetrics the past fall and winter.

There is a progressive, cooperative and patriotic atmosphere as has been demonstrated by the large number of men who have entered the armed service forces. The doctors of my district are fully aware of their responsibility and are cooperating in every measure possible in national defense in a very sane and reasonable frame of mind.

The economic condition of my district has given some relief to the doctors during the past year. Cooperative medicine in my own town and the western part of the state has not as yet been satisfactorily combated. We have had nothing to offer the people to relieve the psychological effect of this new movement. We have had no way of making them believe that we were trying to offer them anything that was different from the old form and system of medicine. Personally, I do not wish to convey the idea that it is not sound, reasonable and fair; yet the psychology has been preached to them and is a deadly weapon to the regular ethical practitioner.

The economic improvement as stated above has given some relief to the old family physician, but not anything like satisfactory in its effect. It is my opinion and the opinion of many of my colleagues that something should be offered the people that is ethical and stable, giving them free choice of medical and hospital care. The speaker spent one year with a committee helping and lending all support possible to the Group Hospital Service plan. This does not meet the needs of the rural community; it has not been applied or worked in our community where, by all means, from my view point, any attempt to show the people that we are trying to offer them something different, has failed. It works well in a large industrial center, but where the rural communities are and where the poison has sprung from in the way of cooperative medicine, we have had no relief.

I should like to report to you that the Cooperative Hospital or Community Hospital in my town has done very little in the way of open, unethical advertisement during the past year. The organizer has two sons that are apparently capable and men that I like personally very much. This year it is my understanding that they are offering a medical care for $3.00 per year for a family of four to six and are collecting the regular hospital fee for hospitalized cases. I am giving you this report so that you may know something of the durability and the impression made by a new attempt to change the way of medical and surgical care.

I wish to commend the farsightedness, fidelity and untiring efforts of our State Board of Medical Examiners under the leadership of the President of the Board of Examiners, Sam McKeel and our President-elect, J. D. Osborn, Jr. Sec., and other members for their strenuous efforts to keep our state from being flooded with refugee doctors, thereby giving an immense relief to the regular men of my district. I voice the sentiment of all my colleagues in this statement. The work that has been done by the Post Graduate Committee has been appreciated and we wish to conclude our report by commending the sane, conservative and constructive course pursued by the President of our State Medical Association for the year 1941-1942.

Respectfully submitted,

V. O. Tisdal, M.D.
Councilor District No. 2.

ANNUAL REPORT DISTRICT NO. 3

Officers and Members of the House of Delegates
Of the Oklahoma State Medical Association

Gentlemen:

My one year of having served as a Councilor of District No. 3 has been of extreme pleasure. Due to inexperience, I have not been able to give very much to the Council during the past year. Personally, however, I have received a liberal education from my association with the members of the Council during the past year. It has indeed been a pleasure to serve with and under Dr. Ewing, our President, and I would also like to say that I am now able to more and more appreciate the services rendered by our Executive Secretary Mr. Graham. I have the feeling that all of the County Societies have yet to learn to know Mr. Graham and his capabilities to the best advantage. I should, however, like to bring to the attention of each of you the fact that he is able and willing to help the County Medical Societies, and I am sure the State Association will be better off if we will use him more. I should also like to say that it has been a pleasure to serve with the other members of the Council, most of whom are older and more experienced than I. I can assure you that the executive functions of the Association are in very good hands.

As to the status of District No. 3—there are seven counties in this district; namely, Kay, Grant, Garfield, Payne, Pawnee, Noble and Major, with a present total of 110 paid members. Of these counties, Kay, Garfield, and Payne are active and smoothly functioning Societies. The other four counties are small with three members in Grant, six in Noble, seven in Pawnee and four in Major. Because of the small number of doctors in some of the counties, the Societies do not meet regularly. There has, however, been some attempt made to bring about the amalgamation of Payne and Pawnee Counties, Kay and Garfield Counties, Major with Garfield, and Grant County with either Garfield or Kay.

It is now my plan to have a Councilor District meeting around June 1. I understand some of the other Districts have been having these meetings, and I think it is definitely a good thing. On the whole, District No. 3 is progressing nicely.

Respectfully submitted,
C. W. Arrendell, M.D.
Councilor District No. 3.

ANNUAL REPORT DISTRICT NO. 4

Members of the House of Delegates
Of the Oklahoma State Medical Association
Gentlemen:

District No. 4 is composed of six counties—Blaine, Kingfisher, Canadian, Logan, Oklahoma and Cleveland. Logan, Oklahoma and Cleveland Counties are functioning smoothly. There has been an attempt made to unite Blaine, Kingfisher and Canadian counties with the plan of having one meeting a month. Thus far, there has been one such meeting that Mr. Graham, the Executive Secretary, and I have attended. Most of our time has been spent with the Procurement and Assignment Committees.

To my knowledge, each County Society, on the whole, is functioning satisfactorily.

Respectfully submitted,
Tom Lowry, M.D.
Councilor District No. 4.

ANNUAL REPORT DISTRICT NO. 6

Officers and Members of the House of Delegates
Of the Oklahoma State Medical Association
Gentlemen:

There are six counties in District No. 6, but only five Societies as Washington and Nowata counties are combined into one Society. It is one of the very finest Societies in the State, holding regular meetings. In that Society, they carry out one idea which is indeed very excellent. At the beginning of the year, a Committee works out the complete program for the year, and they then assign topics to the members so that the individual doctor has time to prepare the particular subject and present a worthwhile paper.

I am also proud of the smoothly organized Rogers County Society as there are few doctors in that county. They meet regularly every month, and to my knowledge, Slim Howard is responsible. Osage County is also to be commended. It is the largest county in area in the State of Oklahoma. The meetings are held in Pawhuska, and there has been one large meeting this year, when they had a very interesting Speaker from Kansas City. The Creek Society functions smoothly with the meetings alternating between Sapulpa and Bristow.

Then there's Tulsa County—but, I'd better not elaborate here as it's my home Society. I do, however, wish to express, in behalf of the Tulsa County Medical Society, their thanks for the kind words of commenda-

tion given by the Council for offering to the State Association the group malpractice insurance policy.

Respectfully submitted,
James Stevenson, M.D.
Councilor District No. 6.

SUPPLEMENTARY REPORT OF DISTRICT NO. 8

To the House of Delegates
Of the Oklahoma State Medical Association
Gentlemen:

During the past year, our County has voted for the amalgamation of Wagoner, Sequoyah and Muskogee Counties into one Society, and this action has been approved by the Council.

Also, I should like to urge that the County Societies not elect members to the respective organization too hastily. It seems to me that it would be advisable to send the individual application for membership to the office of the Association at least sixty days before a member is voted on and accepted by the local Society. During this period, there would be sufficient time for available information to be secured concerning the particular doctor.

This procedure would allow Mr. Graham, through various channels, to make a detailed report to the Society about the doctor before he is elected to membership. It is my appeal to all County Societies that we cooperate with the Executive Secretary in getting reports concerning the applicant before he is elected a member of a society.

Respectfully submitted,
Shade D. Neely, M.D.
Councilor District No. 8.

ANNUAL REPORT DISTRICT NO. 10

Members of the House of Delegates
Of the Oklahoma State Medical Association
Gentlemen:

District No. 10 represents the tail end of the Councilor Districts, being composed of the southeast portion of the State. Several of the counties in my District have only three or four members, yet they are organized and have regular medical meetings. I always attempt to meet with them. Bryan County has a good Medical Society, and I have not missed a meeting during the year. Atoka-Coal is a small but good Society. The membership is very small, but we have not missed a meeting this year.

This year, we have had a Councilor District Meeting in the southeastern part of the State. Through the fine cooperation of the Executive Secretary, we had a meeting of all the Counties in my District at Hugo in Choctaw County. The doctors are very scarce in this particular section of the State, but there were 25 members present at the Councilor District Meeting. I think it was a very fine meeting and likewise very enjoyable, and we feel that each District would do well to have a Councilor District Meeting once a year.

Throughout the year, I have written letters to doctors who have not paid their dues. All together, however, I feel that I have not done my duty as well as I should, but I am alone in Atoka, therefore, it is inconvenient for me to get away often. It seems that I do not have the time to spend, and too, I guess I am getting stingy with the years. I feel that I should spend as much time as I can at home with my wife, but I hope that if I am re-elected Councilor for my District that I can make a better report next year.

Respectfully sumbitted,
J. S. Fulton, M.D.
Councilor District No. 10.

COMMITTEE REPORTS

The following reports of Special Committees of the Association were presented to the House of Delegates at the time of the Annual Meeting held in Tulsa, April 22, 23 and 24:

Report of Committee on Benevolent Fund

Inasmuch as one of the members of this Committee on the disposition of the Medical Defense fund is sick and unable to be here, also from the fact that there is some difference as to just exactly how it should be disposed of, we beg to let the fund stand as it is for the time being, and that those in whose hands it is being directed invest it in the very best manner possible, with a view later of converting it into some sort of a benevolent fund for the benefit of the indigent doctors.

Report of Committee on Conservation of Hearing

Your committee on the Conservation of Hearing desires to submit the following report: Feeling that it might be well to have a survey of the various sections of the state regarding their reaction toward what might be done in the conservation of hearing, the committee attempted, by a questionnaire, to sound out the opinion of the Eye, Ear, Nose and Throat men in the various sections. The results of this questionnaire, we are sorry to report, were of very little effect since only a very small number of the men responded with answers. Therefore, this report, instead of giving a cross-section of the majority of the Eye, Ear, Nose and Throat men of the state, represents a very small response. The results may be summed up in the following:

1. That any tissue or hypertrophy that causes pharyngeal congestion tends to lessen hearing.

2. That an adenoidectomy beneficially influences hearing in cases of hypertrophy.

3. That parent, though usually the first to detect any hearing loss, never do anything about it because they believe the child will "grow out of it."

4. Therefore, instructions by all medical men as to the necessity of early education about lymphatic growths in the vault of the pharynx should be stressed.

5. The audiometer test in the school room has resulted in very little improvement in the educational interest produced in the parent toward caring for any defects noted. Sometimes it seems that all such measures tend to produce in the parent a possible hope that the State or some good agency will, in time, appear to carry out and on the corrections made known by such all-inclusive and free examinations that are made.

6. In Enid, we made an audiometric examination in our public schools. The results of the examination were followed by a fairly good check on the ones who had definite decrease in hearing with the result that most of those are now waiting for somebody to come along with police powers and make them carry into effect the recommendations made.

7. While it is obvious that the teachers and doctors must cooperate as the only practical way to determine the number and degree of deafness present in our young, this does not in any way result in any effective measures being employed to care for the defects so noted. Unless the parents can be thoroughly and actively sold on the necessity for action, should any conditions be found that are injurious to the hearing, no solution will ever be worth either its trouble or expense. Most of the work that has been done in audiometric tests is of value solely because it has established a percentage knowledge that can be used by the profession and the teachers in making them more alert to help educate both the student and parent on the frequency of deafness among the children. I have seen no tangible results that could be measured of any other value it offers.

Report of the Committee on Study and Control of Venereal Disease

The physicians of the state in cooperation with the state and local Health Departments are trying to stamp out syphilis by treating all cases of infectious venereal diseases and by locating and examining their contacts which if found infectious are treated.

The committee requests that the Oklahoma State Medical Association urge all physicians to report promptly to the Health Departments all cases of Venereal Diseases coming under their care for diagnosis or treatment.

The Committee further reports that the Oklahoma Social Hygiene Association was organized February 6, 1942, to combat venereal diseases and that members of the medical profession are cooperating with this organization. The president is Mr. Lee Jones, Bell Telephone Building, 405 North Broadway, Oklahoma City.

The committee further recommends that the Oklahoma State Medical Association go on record as taking the following position concerning Venereal Disease Control in the State of Oklahoma:

First, that the control of venereal disease requires elimination or regulation of commercialized prostitution.

Second, that the medical inspection of prostitutes is untrustworthy, inefficient, gives a false sense of security, and fails to prevent the spread of infection.

Third, that the commercialized prostitution is unlawful and physicians who knowingly examine prostitutes for the purpose of providing them with medical certificates to be used in soliciting are participating in an illegal activity, and are violating the principles of professional conduct of the Oklahoma State Medical Association.

Report of Committee on Prepaid Medical and Surgical Service

Your committee appointed for the study of prepaid medical and surgical care wishes to offer the following report.

The lay public is concerned as never before about health and medical and surgical care. This concern is attracting the attention of private promotion groups, insurance companies, social reform foundations and the Federal Government. These various agencies are offering plans and advocating procedures that do not primarily consider the relation of patient and physician. We feel that if these conditions are allowed to continue that they will do so to the detriment of the medical profession.

To correct this situation, your Committee recommends the following:

1. That the State Association establish a permanent committee to handle these problems. That this committee should be composed of members whose term of membership should be staggered so as to preserve its continuity.

2. Secondly, that the State Medical Association instruct its various County Societies to establish committees for the study of prepaid medical and surgical care, and to urge them to start immediately upon the consideration of their individual local problems and, if possible, to work out a plan suitable to their locality.

3. Thirdly, that these county committees would be in close liason with the State Committee and the Council seeking advice and counsel and that before they put any local plan into action they would have the approval of the State Committee.

REPORT OF ANNUAL MEETING OF AUXILIARY

The Women's Auxiliary to the Oklahoma State Medical Association met in Tulsa with headquarters at the Mayo Hotel on April 22, 23 and 24. Mrs. L. H. Stuart reported 105 registered.

Out of state guests came from Chicago, Greenville, S. C., and Independence, Kan., and doctors' wives from the following cities attended: Seminole, Grove, Antlers, Bartlesville, Pawhuska, Anadarko, Carnegie, Poteau, Oklahoma City, McAlester, Miami, Shawnee, Norman, Ada, Sapulpa, Altus, Chickasha, Hominy, Guthrie, Depew, Coalgate, Blackwell, Durant, Ryan, El Reno and Tulsa.

The Pre-Exectuive Board meeting was held in the home of Mrs. J. W. Childs, convention chairman, on Wednesday evening April 22. There were 15 members present. Mrs. Edward D. Greenberger presided. Various matters of interest to the auxiliary were discussed. The Nominating, Tray, Budget and Auditing committees were appointed. At the close of the meeting Mrs. J. W. Rogers, assisted by Mrs. Childs, served a light lunch.

The Annual Meeting was called to order at 10:00 A. M. Thursday, April 23, in the Parlor of the Mayo hotel, by the president, Mrs. Edward D. Greenberger. Excellent reports were made by the following committees: Public Relations, Mrs. W. T. Mayfield, Norman; Program Health Education, Mrs. James Stevenson, Tulsa; Hygeia, Mrs. Frank L. Flack, Tulsa; Exhibits, Mrs. J. W. Rogers, Tulsa, and Organization and Tray, Mrs. Rush Wright, Poteau. The eight counties organized had representatives present with reports of their actvities throughout the year. Space does not permit a full report but a few highlights will prove interesting.

Muskogee County, organized during the year, won honorable mention in the A .M. A. Hygia Contest. The Public Relations and Philanthropic work of Pittsburg County (McAlester) was outstanding. Oklahoma County has the largest membership with 138 active members. They completed 12 layettes and 54 scrapbooks. With a large number of their membership studying or teaching First Aid, Nutrition, and Home Nursing, their Red Cross work warrants commendation. Pontotoc County, (Ada), sewed for the Red Cross and made dressings for the Valley View Hospital, Pottawatomie County, (Shawnee) knitted for the Red Cross, assisted with the Federal Nursery School and sponsored an Essay Contest on "Tuberculosis" in the city schools. Cleveland County, (Norman) sponsored classes in Home Nursing and sold 21 subscriptions to Hygeia. These classes were taught by three of their own members who are graduate nurses. LeFlore County reported a very active year in Red Cross, Public Relations and Philanthropic work. A great deal of interest was evidenced in a Health Forum sponsored by Tulsa County. Representatives from a large number of women's clubs were present. Tulsa gave 61 six-month Hygia subscriptions to county schools and gave the County Medical Society $75.00 for their library.

The Auxiliary went on record favoring legislation for immunization for smallpox and diphtheria. They also resolved to assist the Red Cross in every way possible. Tulsa County won the "Silver Tray Award" for the most complete program during the year.

Following the business meeting, a luncheon was served in the Marine Room of the Mayo hotel, with 108 present. Mrs. J. W. Childs, convention chairman, presided. Mrs. James Stevenson announced the program. Mrs. L. D. McClatchey, Bartlesville, State Commander of the Women's Field Army of the American Society for the Control of Cancer, gave a short talk. Miss Theressa Fro Grimes, vocalist, presented a group of songs and Mrs. F. R. Rickey whistled several solos. Mrs. Frank L. Flack, president, 1942-43, addressed the membership.

A Post-Executive Board meeting was held immediately following the luncheon. The tea and dinner dance of the Association concluded the entertainment for the Convention.

INAUGURAL ADDRESS

MRS. FRANK L. FLACK
Tulsa, Oklahoma
President 1942-43, Woman's Auxiliary

As we enter another year, we find our country facing a great national crisis. It should stimulate all of us to find in what way we can be of most value to our families, our community, our State and our Nation. While our doctors' wives are usually leaders in their community, I feel that we can accomplish still more than we have in the past. Anatole France once said: "The future is hidden from us all, even from those who make it." We can get the jitters about the fate of our country and go around in circles and accomplish very little, or we can calmly evaluate our qualifications, find the thing we are best fitted for and work at our task with enthusiasm and energy. Service should be our motto for the year. We have a grave responsibility to use our organization to the fullest extent to promote the various activities of our program.

Before completing our plan for the year, our executive board will be advised by the National Board and learn some of their ideas. I have already had some correspondence with Mrs. Frank Haggard, of San Antonio, president-elect of the Woman's Auxiliary to the American Medical Association. I feel that she will be an excellent executive and very helpful to our Oklahoma organization.

First, I urge that all counties have committees to correspond with the State committees.

I think the field of Public Relations can be enlarged to include the duties of a Health Defense committee. I would suggest that your auxiliary membership be classified as to their ability. Find out what members have been trained in nursing, clerical work, nutrition and First Aid. The information gained by such a survey will then be available to use in an emergency. I would suggest that you provide programs on health subjects to other women's organizations. A Health Forum like one held in Tulsa the past year is of great value.

One of the finest means of promoting health education is the Hygeia magazine. Essay contests in some phase of better health usually create interest. Increase your information so that when matters of health are discussed in your presence you can give the facts.

We hope to have an increase in Hygeia subscriptions the coming year. Better health would result if this magazine were placed where it likely would be read. Gather up old numbers and distribute them.

Concerning the Student Loan Fund, it is my opinion that it would be well to do something definite with it.

I would like to see more publicity in our State and National Journals.

There has been nothing to do in the matter of legislation in the past year except to keep informed concerning what is going on in other states which might be an issue in our state when legislature convenes. Your state chairman will inform you if your help is needed.

There are many more counties which should be organized. I expect to communicate with the county medical presidents and see if we cannot interest more counties in this.

I am asking for a close cooperation between the county committee chairmen and the state chairmen.

While the purely social side of our lives will be displaced this year to a large extent with war work, we must not neglect it altogether. One objective in our constitution is to promote acquaintanceship among physicians' families that fellowship may increase.

If there is any doubt in your mind about some phase of your program, always consult your County Medical society. Each county should have a Medical Advisory Council.

Make your auxiliary an outstanding organization in your county. Doctors' wives should be leaders. Aside from their qualifications in their own right, their close association with the medical profession, composed of men of the best education, the highest ethics, the most dependable, the most honorable in their community, should undoubtedly inspire them to greater heights. The ideals of the medical profession have always been of the highest. Let us assist them by continuing to make our organization one of the same caliber. If my year as your leader is to be a success, I must have your cooperation. I will try to give you my best.

Semi-Annual Meeting of Southeastern Medical Association

J. S. Speed, M.D., of the Campbell Clinic, Memphis, Tennessee, was the Guest speaker at the semi-annual meeting of the Southeastern Medical Association held in Antlers, May 28. Dr. Speed presented the subject of "Compound Fractures." Other physicians appearing on the program were J. T. Colwick, Durant; Woodrow Williams, Idabel; L. S. Willour, McAlester; and Earl Woodson, Poteau.

On Wednesday evening, May 27th, all guests of the Association attended a fish fry on the banks of the Kiamichi, sponsored by the Antlers Lion's Club and Antlers Physicians. Approximately sixty physicians were in attendance.

The Southeastern Medical Association meetings are always outstanding events and the Association is to be complimented for the part it plays in promoting scientific medicine.

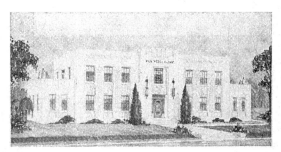

MEDICAL PREPAREDNESS

Procurement and Assignment Chairmen Meet in Omaha

All State Medical Association Procurement and Assignment Chairmen west of the Mississippi River, met with officials of the War Department, Office of Surgeon General, Selective Service, and Procurement and Assignment in Omaha, Nebraska, May 8. Also attending the meeting were the Army recruiting boards for the 22 states who are serving in their respective capacity by authority of the Surgeon General.

Dr. Henry H. Turner and Dick Graham, representing the Association, and Colonel Lee R. Wilhite and Captain Oliver H. Cornelius, the latter two of the recruiting board for Oklahoma, were present.

The meeting outlined the immediate needs of the Army for physicians which as previously reported is 16,000 by December 31, 1942, and the probable need for 32,000 during 1943, as well as the simplified method of induction which has been established by the creation of the recruiting boards.

Addressing the meeting were Col. G. E. Isaacs and General Wharton of the War Department, Col. J. R. Hudnall and Col. H. C. Gibner, Surgeon General's office, Lt. Col. Sam F. Seeley, Office of Procurement and Assignment, and Col. Richard H. Eanes of Selective Service.

Outside of the announcement of the establishing of the recruiting boards and the simplified method of commissioning of physicians, was the explanation of the cooperation to be developed between the offices of Selective Service and Procurement and Assignment. This is of particular interest to all physicians under the age of forty-six.

OCCUPATIONAL DEFERMENTS OF DOCTORS, DENTISTS AND VETERINARIANS

The following memorandum (1-420) was sent to all state directors by Lewis B. Hershey, director of the Selective Service System, Washington. D. C. This amendment involves a change from Corps Area Committee of Procurement and Assignment Service to separate state chairmen for medical doctors, dentists and doctors of veterinary medicine and also a change with respect to the consideration of dependency in classifying such registrants.

NATIONAL HEADQUARTERS
SELECTIVE SERVICE SYSTEM
21st Street and C Street, N.W.
Washington, D. C.
January 28, 1942.
Amended April 28, 1942
Memorandum to all State Directors (1-363)
Local Board Release (89)

Subject: Occupational Deferments of Medical Doctors, Dentists and Doctors of Veterinary Medicine (III).

1. Information previously distributed by this headquarters clearly indicates an overall shortage of medical doctors, dentists and doctors of veterinary medicine in the nation. Since war was declared, the shortage of these professional men has become acute. It is now manifest that every qualified doctor, dentist and veterinarian must serve where he can render the greatest professional service to the nation.

2. In order to accomplish this purpose, the President, by executive order, has formed the Procurement and Assignment Service. This service was formed primarily for the purpose of gathering and making available information with respect to the supply of qualified practitioners in the fields of medicine, dentistry and veterinary medicine, with a view of securing the most effective allocation of medical manpower as indicated by the requirements of the armed forces, civilian needs and industrial medicine.

3. To work with the headquarters of the Procurement and Assignment Service there has been appointed for each state and the District of Columbia a state chairman for medical doctors, a state chairman for dentists and a state chairman for doctors of veterinary medicine. These state chairmen will secure information concerning their respective professions and will give advice regarding the allocation of medical manpower.

4. When considering the classification of any registrant who is a qualified medical doctor, dentist or doctor of veterinary medicine, the director of Selective Service desires that local boards, through the state director, shall consult with the respective state chairman of the Procurement and Assignment Service.

5. In considering the classification of a registrant who is a qualified medical doctor, dentist or doctor of veterinary medicine, the local board may, if it finds such registrant should not be deferred for reasons other than dependency, take into consideration the pay and allowances which such registrant would receive in the event he is commissioned in the armed forces. In practically all instances the pay and allowances of such registrant, if he was commissioned as an officer, would be sufficient to eliminate the question of dependency.

In consideration of the above and since the lowest rank that can be given a physician is First Lieutenant, it is obvious that where the local Selective Service board requests information concerning qualified physicians and the rank they may secure there will be a few deferments for reasons of dependents.

Should any physician not accept a Commission when tendered, it is the duty of the State Chairman of Procurement and Assignment to forward that physicians name to the State Director of Selective Service.

ARMY RECRUITING BOARD FOR OKLAHOMA

The recruiting board for physicians, dentists and doctors, of veterinary medicine is now located at 211 Plaza Court, 10th and Walker, Oklahoma City, telephone 7-0976, and is under the direction of Colonel Lee R. Wilhite, representing the Surgeon General, and Captain Oliver H. Cornelius of the Office of the Adjutant General.

The recruiting board has full authority to order physical examinations, waive physical defects, grant commissions, and administer the oath of office.

All physicians below the age of fifty-five, desiring to obtain commissions should immediately contact the board: An appointment is not necessary.

The board is particularly anxious to interview physicians under the age of forty-five.

Waiver of Physical Defects For Limited Service Officers

The Surgeon General of the U. S. Army announced April 23 the following policies of his office concerning recommendations for waiver for limited service officers. These policies were announced in order that the provisions of AG-210.31 (12-19-41) RP-A Jan. 7, 1942, may be carried out in a uniform manner.

1. a. Considered acceptable for limited service:

(1) Overweight to 25 per cent above average weight for age and height, and even greater degrees of overweight, provided the individual is not decidedly obese and provided that because of his special training in civil life he is peculiarly fitted to fill a particular technical assignment in the Army; and underweight to 15 per cent below ideal weight, provided chest x-ray examination is negative for pulmonary pathologic conditions and other chronic disease is carefully excluded.

(2) Any degree of uncorrected vision, provided it is corrected with glasses in possession of the examinee to 20/20 in one eye and to 20/40 in the other and provided that no organic disease of either eye exists.

(3) Blindness or corrected vision below 20/40 in one eye with vision 20/200 corrected with glasses in possession of the examinee in 20/20 in the other, provided there is no organic disease in the better eye and no history of cataract or other disease in the more defective eye which might be expected to involve the better one, and provided that in case of ophthalmosteresis the individual is fitted with a satisfactory prosthesis.

(4) Complete color blindness.

(5) Hearing 5/20 in each ear for low conversational voice, or complete deafness in one ear with hearing 10/20 or better in the other, provided the defect is not due to active inflammatory disease and is stationary in character.

(6) Chronic otitis media, inactive with perforation of membrana tympani, provided there is a trustworthy history of freedom from activity for the preceding five years.

(7) Old fracture of the spine or pelvic bones which has healed without definite deformity, provided there is a trustworthy history of freedom from symptoms during the preceding two years.

(8) Loss of one hand, one forearm, or one lower extremity below the junction of the middle and lower thirds of the thigh, provided the lost member is replaced with a satisfactory prothesis.

(9) Pes planus, pes cavus or talipes equinus, provided the condition is not more than mildly symptomatic, does not interfere with normal locomotion and has not interfered with the individual's vocation in civil life.

(10) History of osteoymelitis following fracture, provided x-ray examination indicated complete healing and the condition has been asymptomatic for the preceding five years.

(11) Joints fixed or limited in motion, provided the condition is the result of injury and is nonsymptomatic.

(12) History of excision of torn or detached semilunar cartilage of knee joint, provided there is normal stability of the joint and a period of one year with complete freedom from symptoms has elapsed since the operation.

(13) Residuals of anterior poliomyelitis, without pronounced deformity or loss of function, origination two years or more prior to examination.

(14) Varicose veins, moderate, without edema or discoloration of skin.

(15) History of gastric or duodenal ulcer, provided there is a trustworthy history of freedom from activity during the preceding five years and provided that the gastrointestinal roentgenogram at the time of examination is negative.

(16) Incomplete inguinal hernia.

(17) Small asymptomatic congenital umbilical hernia.

(18) Absence of one kidney, provided its removal has been necessitated by other than tuberculosis or malignancy and the other kidney is normal.

b. Considered unacceptable for any service.

(1) History of malignant disease within preceding five years.

(2) Active tuberculosis of any organ and inactive pulmonary tuberculosis except as described in paragraph 2a.

(3) Syphilis, except adequately treated syphilis as described in paragraph 2b.

(4) Old fracture of the skull with bony defect greater than 2 cm. in longest diameter or with history of accompanying mental or neurologic complications.

(5) Instability of any of the major joints.

(6) History of metastatic osteomyelitis with prolonged or recurrent drainage, regardless of duration.

(7) Arthritis of the atrophic (rheumatoid) type.

(8) Any cardiovascular condition which disqualifies for general military service.

(9) History of gastroenterostomy, gastric resection, intestinal anastomosis or operation for intestinal obstruction.

(10) History of prostatectomy or transurethral resection of prostate or of prostatic hypertrophy of any degree.

(11) Chronic endocrine disease except mild hypothyroidism or mild Froelich's syndrome.

(12) Diabetes mellitus of any degree or renal glycosuria.

(13) History of any psychosis.

(14) History of severe psychoneurosis at any time, or psychoneurosis of any degree if it has been recurrent or has shown symptoms within the preceding five years.

2. The following may be recommended for general military service with waiver:

a. Individuals with minimal inactive lesions of primary or reinfection type pulmonary tuberculosis. These lesions may consist of:

(1) Calcified residues of lesions of the intrathoracic lymph nodes, provided none of these exceed an arbitrary limit of 1.5 cm. in diameter and the total number does not exceed five.

(2) Calcified lesions of the pulmonary parenchyma, provided the total number does not exceed ten, one of which may equal but not exceed 1 cm. in diameter, but none of the remainder may exceed 0.5 cm. in diameter.

(Note: The lesions described in (1) and (2) should appear sharply circumscribed, homogeneous and dense.

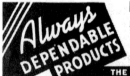

Measurements refer to standard 14 by 17 inch direct projection roentgenograms.)

(3) Small fibrotic parenchymal lesions represented in the roentgenogram as sharply demarcated strandlike or well defined small nodular shadows not exceeding a total area of 5 sy. cm., provided acceptance is deferred until subsequent examination demonstrates that the lesions are stationary and are not likely to be reactivated. The minimum period of time to determine this is six months. It must be recognized that either progression or regression of the lesions indicates activity.

b. Individuals with confirmed position serologic tests for syphilis with no clinical evidence of the disease, with convincing histories of a trustworthy diagnosis of syphilis or with reliable histories of treatment for the disease on serologic or clinical grounds, provided.

(1) That a negative spinal fluid since infection and treatment has been reported from a trustworthy source;

(2) That in infections estimated to be of less than four years' duration at least thirty to forty arsenical and forty to sixty insoluble bismuth injections or their equivalent, with a minimum total of seventy-five injections, have been given, with approximate continuity (no rest periods or lapses) during the first thirty weeks of treatment; and

(3) That, except as further qualified, in infections estimated to be over four years' duration, at least twenty arsenical injections and forty to sixty insoluble bismuth injections or their equivalent, with a minimum total of sixty injections, have been given in alternating courses; rest periods between consecutive courses not exceeding eight weeks being allowable.

In infections of unknown duration it shall be presumed for classification purposes that those of individuals under 26 years of age are of less than four years' duration and over 26 years of more than four years' duration.

(Note: For the determination of treatment, the signed statement of acceptable treatment sources administering it, with total number of doses of each drug and approximate calendar dates of administration and available laboratory and clinical data, shall be required as evidence.)

c. Overweight to 20 per cent above average weight for age and height, and underweight to 12.5 per cent below ideal weight, provided chest x-ray examination is negative for pulmonary pathologic conditions and other chronic disease is carefully excluded.

d. Insufficient incisor or masticating teeth, provided the mouth is free from extensive infections processes and the examinee is wearing satisfactory dentures.

e. Pilonidal cyst or sinus, provided there is no palpable tumor mass, no evidence of purulent or serious discharge and no history of previous discharge or inflammation.

f. History of healed fracture with bone plates, screws or wires used for fixation of fragments still in situ, provided x-ray examination shows no evidence of osteomyelitis and no rarefaction of bone contiguous to the fixation materials; that such fixative materials are not so located that they will be subjected to pressure from military clothing or equipment, and that one year has elapsed since their application.

g. History of operation or of injection treatment for inguinal or small ventral hernia, provided examination three months or more following operation, or following the last injection, shows a satisfactory result.

h. History of unilateral renal calculus, provided the condition has been asymptomatic for the preceding three years, urine examination is negative and roentgenologic examination (flat plate) of both kidneys is negative.

i. Absence of the spleen, provided its removal has been asymptomatic for the preceding two years.

j. History of Cholecystectomy, provided the condition has been asymptomatic for the preceding two years.

3. The action of the reviewing medical authority should indicate on the Report of Physical Examination, W. D., A. G. O. Form No. 63, that cognizance has been taken of any defects which do not meet the standards set forth in AR 40-105, but for which waiver is recommended by a notation as follows:

"Recommend acceptance for general military service with waiver of (here record the defect or defects)", or

"Recommend acceptance for limited service only with waiver of (here record the defect or defects)."

4. It should be understood that this communication sets forth the policy of this office with regard to recommendations, for waiver in the case of applicants for appointment and officers of the Reserve components under consideration for extended active duty. It is not intended that officers already in active service shall be recommended for appearance before retiring boards because of defects which would be considered disqualifying according to the policies set forth. The recommendations of disposition boards of general hospitals will be based on the principle that officers should be retained on active duty as long as they are capable of rendering efficient service unless they have conditions not incident to the service which are likely to progress to incapacity and eventually result in retirement in line of duty. The findings of disposition boards should clearly indicate that the officer under consideration is physically fit for limited service only when such is the case.

By order of the Surgeon General:

John A. Rogers,
Colonel, Medical Corps,
Executive Officer.

News From The State Health Department

"Thanks to the cooperation of the physicians of the state, Oklahoma is now well along in the national program to immunize all children against the common communicable diseases as a war-time measure," Dr. G. F. Mathews, commissioner of the state health department said today.

At the suggestion of President Roosevelt, physicians, civilian defense workers and public health personnel have undertaken the tremendous task of protecting all children against typhoid fever, diphtheria, smallpox, tetanus and pertussis.

In Oklahoma the President's suggestion was taken to the Oklahoma State Medical Association for the consideration of the physicians of the state. The Medical Association agreed to approve the project, and leave it up to each county society to work out the best method for doing the work.

Preliminary reports show that 40 counties are conducting a systematic, organized campaign to arouse public interest in the immunization program. Private physicians are scheduling clinics at specified places and on certain dates.

"The program is working in true democratic style, with each county making its own plans to suit each locality, and the work is being done," the commissioner said. Each county is making its own financial arrangements, with the price for immunization varying from nothing for each immunization to $1.00.

The work is being done in all but a few counties of the state, and in over 40 of the counties an organized campaign to convince the public of its value is being undertaken, he said.

The project was assigned to the civilian defense organization, which is helping the physicians make arrangements. Biologics are being furnished by the State Health Department.

"We know that this request constituted a tremendous job, to immunize all the children in the state means reaching many thousands, but we're encouraged over the start already made, and there seems little doubt that Oklahoma physicians will do this job, along with the many others given them during this emergency," he said.

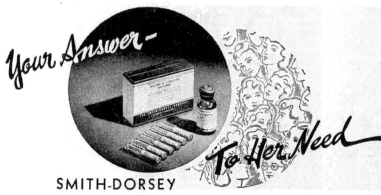

SMITH-DORSEY
Solution of Estrogenic Substances (in Peanut Oil)

Mercy walked with the discovery of the remedial action of estrogenic substances. It walks today . . . where carefully regulated laboratories produce and distribute theses products. . . . And most of all, where competent physicians — alert to symptoms — administer estrogens for these various conditions: natural and artificial menopause, gonorrheal vaginitis in children, kraurosis vulvae, pruritis vulvae. . . .

Supplied as follows by the SMITH-DORSEY LABORATORIES:

Ampoules —	1 cc. Ampoule 10,000 units per cc.
In boxes of 12, 25 and 100	10 cc. Ampoule Vials 5,000 units per cc.
1 cc. Ampoule 2,000 units per cc.	10 cc. Ampoule Vials 10,000 units per cc.
1 cc. Ampoule 5,000 units per cc.	10 cc. Ampoule Vials 20,000 units per cc,

The SMITH-DORSEY COMPANY   -   Lincoln, Nebraska

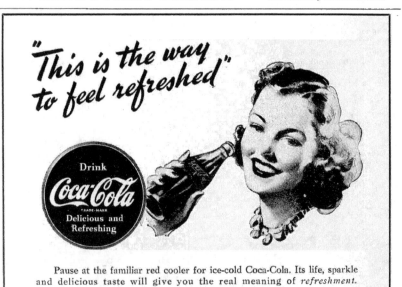

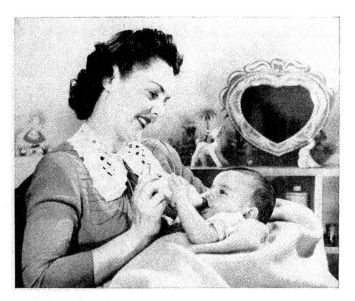

BIOLAC is complete and replete...

...because there is no lack in Biolac, except for vitamin C. Biolac feedings provide amply for all other nutritional requirements of the normal young infant, and no additional formula ingredients or supplements are necessary. It's an improved evaporated-type infant food with breast-like nutritional and digestional advantages. It is a complete formula, replete with nutritional values. Biolac is prepared from whole milk, skim milk, lactose, vitamin B_1, concentrates of vitamins A and D from cod liver oil, and ferric citrate.

Why BIOLAC is increasingly popular:
- Ample provision for high protein needs of early months
- Reduced fat for greater ease in digestion
- Enriched with vitamins A, B_1, D and iron
- All needed carbohydrate present as Lactose
- Sterilized for formula safety
- Homogenized to improve digestibility
- Easy to prescribe
- Convenient for mothers to use
- Economical: because it's complete

Prescribe Biolac in your next feeding case. Professional literature on request. Write Borden's Prescription Products Division, 350 Madison Ave., New York, N. Y.

 Borden's BIOLAC

A BORDEN PRESCRIPTION PRODUCT

OFFICERS OF COUNTY SOCIETIES, 1942

★

COUNTY	PRESIDENT	SECRETARY	MEETING TIME
Alfalfa	Jack F. Parsons, Cherokee	L. T. Lancaster, Cherokee	Last Tues. Each 2nd Mo.
Atoka-Coal	J. B. Clark, Coalgate	J. S. Fulton, Atoka	
Beckham	H. K. Speed, Sayre	E. S. Kilpatrick, Elk City	Second Tues. eve.
Blaine	Virginia Olson Curtin, Watonga	W. F. Griffin, Watonga	
Bryan	A. J. Wells, Calera	W. K. Haynie, Durant	Second Tues. eve.
Caddo	Fred L. Patterson, Carnegie	C. B. Sullivan, Carnegie	
Canadian	P. F. Herod, El Reno	A. L. Johnson, El Reno	Subject to call
Carter	Walter Hardy, Ardmore	H. A. Higgins, Ardmore	
Cherokee	Park H. Medearis, Tahlequah	Isadore Dyer, Tahlequah	
Choctaw	C. H. Hale, Boswell	Fred D. Switzer, Hugo	
Cleveland	F. C. Buffington, Norman	Phil Haddock, Norman	Thursday nights
Comanche	George S. Barber, Lawton	W. F. Lewis, Lawton	
Cotton	George W. Baker, Walters	Mollie F. Seism, Walters	Third Friday
Craig	W. R. Marks, Vinita	J. M. McMillan, Vinita	
Creek	Frank Sisler, Bristow	O. H. Cowart, Bristow	
Custer	Richard M. Burke, Clinton	W. C. Tisdal, Clinton	Third Thursday
Garfield	D. S. Harris, Drummond	John R. Walker, Enid	Fourth Thursday
Garvin	T. F. Gross, Lindsay	John R. Callaway, Pauls Valley	Wed before 3rd Thurs.
Grady	D. S. Downey, Chickasha	Frank T. Joyce, Chickasha	3rd Thursday
Grant	I. V. Hardy, Medford	E. E. Lawson, Medford	
Greer	G. F. Border, Mangum	J. B. Hollis, Mangum	
Harmon	S. W. Hopkins, Hollis	W. M. Yeargan, Hollis	First Wednesday
Haskell	William Carson, Keota	N. K. Williams, McCurtain	
Hughes	Wm. L. Taylor, Holdenville	Imogene Mayfield, Holdenville	First Friday
Jackson	J. M. Allgood, Altus	Willard D. Holt, Altus	Last Monday
Jefferson	W. M. Browning, Waurika	J. I. Hollingsworth, Waurika	Second Monday
Kay	J. C. Wagner, Ponca City	J. Holland Howe, Ponca City	Third Thurs.
Kingfisher	C. M. Hodgson, Kingfisher	John R. Taylor, Kingfisher	
Kiowa	J. M. Bonham, Hobart	B. H. Watkins, Hobart	
LeFlore	G. R. Booth, LeFlore	Rush L. Wright, Poteau	
Lincoln	E. F. Hurlbut, Meeker	C. W. Robertson, Chandler	First Wednesday
Logan	William C. Miller, Guthrie	J. L. LeHew, Jr., Guthrie	Last Tuesday evening
Marshall	J. L. Holland, Madill	O. A. Cook, Madill	
Mayes	L. C. White, Adair	V. D. Herrington, Pryor	
McClain	B. W. Slover, Blanchard	R. L. Royster, Purcell	
McCurtain	R. D. Williams, Idabel	R. H. Sherrill, Broken Bow	Fourth Tues. eve.
McIntosh	F. R. First, Checotah	William A. Tolleson, Eufaula	Second Tuesday
Murray	P. V. Annadown, Sulphur	F. E. Sadler, Sulphur	
Muskogee	Shade D. Neely, Muskogee	J. T. McInnis, Muskogee	First & Third Mon.
Noble	J. W. Francis, Perry	C. H. Cooke, Perry	
Okfuskee	J. M. Pemberton, Okemah	L. J. Spickard, Okemah	Second Monday
Oklahoma	R. Q. Goodwin, Okla. City	Wm. R. Eastland, Okla. City	Fourth Tuesday
Okmulgee	J. G. Edwards, Okmulgee	John R. Cotteral, Henryetta	Second Monday
Osage	C. R. Weirich, Pawhuska	George K. Hemphill, Pawhuska	Second Monday
Ottawa	J. B. Hampton, Commerce	Walter Sanger, Picher	Third Thursday
Pawnee	E. T. Robinson, Cleveland	Robert L. Browning, Pawnee	
Payne	John W. Martin, Cushing	James D. Martin, Cushing	Third Thursday
Pittsburg	Austin R. Stough, McAlester	Edw. D. Greenberger, McAlester	Third Friday
Pontotoc	R. E. Cowling, Ada	E. R. Muntz, Ada	First Wednesday
Pottawatomie	John Carson, Shawnee	Clinton Gallaher, Shawnee	First & Third Sat.
Pushmataha	P. B. Rice, Antlers	John S. Lawson, Clayton	
Rogers	W. A. Howard, Chelsea	George D. Waller, Claremore	First Monday
Seminole	H. M. Reeder, Konawa	Mack I. Shanholtz ,Wewoka	
Stephens	A. J. Weedn, Duncan	W. K. Walker, Marlow	
Texas	L. G. Blackmer, Hooker	Johnny A. Blue, Guymon	
Tillman	C. C. Allen, Frederick	O. G. Bacon, Frederick	
Tulsa	H. B. Stewart, Tulsa	E. O. Johnson, Tulsa	Second & Fourth Mon. eve.
Wagoner	J. H. Plunkett, Wagoner	H. K. Riddle, Coweta	
Washington-Nowata	R. W. Rucker, Bartlesville	J. V. Athey, Bartlesville	Second Wednesday
Washita	A. S. Neal, Cordell	James F. McMurry. Sentinel	
Woods	W. F. LaFon, Waynoka	O. E. Templin, Alva	Last Wednesday
Woodward	M. H. Newman, Shattuck	C. W. Tedrowe, Woodward	

THE JOURNAL
OF THE
OKLAHOMA STATE MEDICAL ASSOCIATION

VOLUME XXXV	OKLAHOMA CITY, OKLAHOMA, JULY, 1942	NUMBER 7

Military Medicine*

ROBERT U. PATTERSON, M.D.

DEAN, UNIVERSITY OF OKLAHOMA SCHOOL
OF MEDICINE

Military Medicine connotes a large group of diseases. In a strict sense, it also includes surgical conditions since they inevitably occur among troops. However, military surgery is generally considered and taught as a separate subject in those educational institutions which take cognizance of the diseases and injuries associated with wars, and in the peace time training of the military and naval forces of any country.

My remarks today, however, will be restricted to consideration of the diseases that are commonly associatde with assemblages of men composing organizations of the Army as they live in garrisons, camps, or when on active service in a theatre of operations. While there are certain conditions that are peculiar to service tboard ships of the Navy requiring special preparation and treatment, with a few particular exceptions such as those that are connected with the living conditions of the crews of submarines, the same conditions of disease that exist in Armies are also to be found among Naval forces, particularly when the Navy is engaged in operations ashore, or on duty in Navy yards, or other Naval establishments. So that military medicine has a general applicability to both the services. This includes also the special operations of military and naval *Air* Forces, and those of the Marine Corps which form a part of the Navy.

Military medicine therefore comprehends consideration of the disease entities to be found among military and naval forces wherever they may be situated. During recent years, and particularly is this true during the present war, service in the colder climates such as Labrador, Iceland, Norway, Russia, Alaska, and Siberia are calling for

*Address delivered to the students of the University of Texas School of Medicine, Galveston, Texas, June 5, 1942.

special preparations by the medical services of all the belligerents now actively engaged in operations in these areas or who anticipate the great probability that they will be. It is entirely possible that service of many elements of military and naval forces of some of the belligerents will become necessary in the *Antarctic* as well as the *Arctic* regions.

However, most commonly, and this has been the fact so far during the present great struggle, hostilities have been largely limited to the temperate and tropical zones. Therefore, so-called tropical medicine very definitely plays a most important part in any study of military medicine. Tropical medicine may be described as the study of those diseases which, though they exist often quite commonly in the temperate or cooler zones, are found to be most prevalent in tropical or sub-tropical countries, i.e., in countries or portions of them having the same isothermic temperatures as in the definite geographic tropics. Why such diseases are so prevalent there is a result of the special climate conditions in those localities. An explanation of tropical environments and why they support certain diseases seems to be indicated.

The *tropics* are generally considered or defined as those portions of the earth's surface situated between the Tropic of Cancer north of the equator, and the Tropic of Capricorn south of that defining line. This comprises a belt or area of approximately 47 degrees of latitude extending north and south. As the earth turns, the solar rays are almost constantly vertical over parts of this area. Because of variations in the orbits of the sun and earth, as the sun approaches the geographical limits of the upper areas of the tropical zone near the Tropic of Cancer, and the lower limits near the Tropic of Capricorn, there is naturally an extension over and above the defined tropical region, and north and south of it, so that their influences and conditions are often felt even as far north as the 35th degree of north latitude, and approximately to the 30th degree of south latitude.

Without other influencing factors one would expect the same temperatures in the tropical belt completely around the world. This, of course, is not so. Areas other have great differences of temperature and of what we designate as climate. This is because of many influencing phenomena, each of which has a direct bearing upon the character of the climate in any given portion of the tropics or sub-tropics. These important factors in determining climate are many, but the principal ones regulating climate may be set down as due to meteorological conditions. For example, temperature, humidity, or varying degrees of air water saturation, currents or movements of the air over the surfaces of the land and water, the distance traveled over water by prevailing winds, the effects of temperature of water surfaces due to ocean currents, and barometric pressures. Actual physical characteristics of the earth's surface have a profound effect. Mountains and high altitudes completely change temperatures and so-called climates by their presence in comparison with the conditions found at lower or tidewater levels.

One has only to mention the influence upon the climate of the British Isles and Norway of the Gulf Stream, or the effect of the Japan current upon countries whose shores are washed by it in the northeastern Pacific areas. The warmer climates have been classified variously but usually into four belts: (1) the equatorial belt, (2) the trade wind belt, (3) the monsoon belt, and (4) the mountain climates.

In the equatorial belt close to the equator, there are frequent alterations of season, that is periods of winds and periods of calm, and by reason of the phenomenon that the heated air in that region is heavy with moisture carried by the trade winds, there are varying amounts of rain and clouds. The northeast and southeast trade winds produce periods of calm and periods of maximum and minimum temperatures. There are in this belt two short wet and two short dry seasons. There is practically uniform barometric pressure in areas between the high pressure and low pressure belts of the northern and southern hemispheres producing an area known to sailors as the "doldrums". Light winds coming from first one direction and then another in these areas permit the water surfaces to become heated and this in turn affects the air lying over it which, as it warms,

rises. As this warm and vapor laden air gains sufficient elevation, it cools, and the moisture is condensed with resulting clouds and heavy rains.

In the trade wind belt, the winds have very constant qualities with daily changes in temperature. These produce rains or dry periods. A few hundred feet of altitude or obstruction of air currents by mountains or land elevations produce great changes in temperature. It is said that 300 feet of elevation will cause a lowering of temperature of one degree compared with sea level, unmodified by other influences. This is not entirely correct as temperatures at a given level depend upon the expansion of the air, air currents, the humidity, or water saturation, the kind of terrain, i.e., rocky or good soil, and the type of wind direction at a given time. India has its Simla; the Philippines has its Baquio, although at present the latter is no longer in our control.

A striking example of the effect of the factors above mentioned is illustrated in the Panama Canal region. The height of the land at no point close to the Canal is over a few hundred feet, and along the course of the Canal not more than forty or fifty feet, even in the "cuts". Yet within forty miles of the two oceans, on the Atlantic side there is an annual rainfall of more than 300 inches, while on the Pacific side only about 170. This latter figure is far in excess of anything seen in the temperate zones.

The constant warmth and moisture in the tropics provide conditions which produce vast forests and jungles, and lush growth of vines and underbushes. It favors the rapid development of many harmful forms of reptiles, insects, and pathogenic parasitic organisms and other harmful lower forms of life. Enough has been said to indicate that the vectors of many diseases flourish in the tropics and cause a large number of those which we classify as tropical. As I have already stated, in many instances such diseases are found also in the temperate zones though not to the same extent. Amebic dysentery and bacillary dysentery are not confined to those regions although much more prevalent in the tropics than elsewhere. One readily recalls the epidemic of amebic dysentery which occurred in Chicago during the last World's Fair. Amebic dysentery is found and is endemic in many parts of the south and southwest of the United States. In the Philippines and in other tropical countries, the incidence is high. Malaria is common in the United States, particularly in the southern states, including Texas and Oklahoma, but the incidence in the tropics is far in excess of anything that one ever sees in the temperate zones. Malaria in Panama and in Central and South America is the most serious cause of morbidity and mortality in those areas. All of these tropical diseases have to be considered and classed as a part of the larger division of "military medicine", so that those who teach military medicine readily understand that there will be overlapping with several other teaching departments and will require the collaboration and cooperation of those who instruct in tropical medicine, general medicine, hygiene and public health or preventive medicine, and even with the Departments of Urology and Syphilology, which concern themselves, among other things, with venereal diseases. The great protean disease, syphilis, is no respecter of climate, zone, race, or color.

I will not dwell upon the effects of all tropical climates upon the general health, or upon the energy or resistance of members of the white races who are obliged to live in the tropics without a change or return at regular intervals to temperate climates. It is well established that though tuberculosis in the United States still takes a heavy toll of life, it is without doubt the greatest cause of morbidity and death among the native inhabitants of tropical countries. The only exceptions to this would be during pandemics such as Asiatic cholera or plague. Therefore, serious consideration of tropical diseases cannot be eliminated and must be considered as a part of the programme in any course of study properly purporting to teach military medicine. At this very time we have thousands of our own troops and naval personnel stationed in the tropics, and in the Antipodes, and many more are going.

One who has had military service is fully cognizant of the fact that certain diseases common in the New England states are seldom seen or are as serious in the southern United States, and many of them are rare in the tropics. However, anyone who thinks that respiratory diseases are uncommon in the tropics is seriously in error. The constant perspiration on the slightest exertion even when wearing the lighest of clothing, plus the rapid chilling that so frequently follows in those with the lowered resistance so commonly present during a tour of tropical service by personnel of the Army or Navy, produces an astonishingly high incidence of respiratory infections. This is exclusive of tuberculosis, which I have already mentioned.

The special and changing environment of personnel who serve with the Air Forces has led to special study known as "Aviation Medicine". It is also a very definite part of "Military Medicine".

Time will not permit dwelling on the many ramifications of military medicine in one discourse, but later I will consider briefly some of the more serious diseases to be confronted whenever aggregations of troops are assembled, or among the crews of ships, or in Naval and Marine Corps shore operations either alone, in cooperation with, or in support of operations by the Army. In the Army Medical School in Washington, D. C., tropical medicine is included in and taught definitely as a part of military medicine. As a prerequisite to the study of military medicine, one should consider the general functions of the medical departments of both the services.

First, let it be said that the principal duty of the medical departments of Armies is to keep men on the firing line, i.e., fit to fight. The medical department wields an important effect upon the winning of battles if their duties are properly performed. During the first World War, the medical department of the Army returned to the firing line in the American Expeditionary Forces in France the equivalent of seven full divisions. A division at that time comprised 27,000 officers and men. We now have so-called smaller "square" divisions, and "triangular" divisions. These men were returned to duty in that war. This would not have been the case had the methods in vogue at the time of the Spanish-American War, or even as late as the Russo-Japanese War in 1904-1905 been in practice. It is essential, therefore, that in any consideration of military medicine, one should have a clear understanding of the scope of the responsibilities of medical officers.

Briefly, the medical department of the Army (and this of course applies generally to the Navy, also) has the following responsibilities:

1. To prevent the admission of the physically unfit to the services.

2. By appropriate sanitary or preventive medical measures to maintain the health of the forces.

3. To provide professional care whenever and wherever needed.

4. To provide a system of orderly and rapid evacuation in war of all sick and wounded from the field to medical department hospitals and other installations so as to relieve the fighting forces of the encumbrance of sick or wounded. This is done by medical personnel and requires the organization of a series of definite medical troop units and other institutions extending from the combat troops actually in the fighting line and in the theatre of operations, back through the various echelons of command and supply to the

zone of the interior. This latter usually is in the home territory but may be overseas.

5. When military personnel become no longer physically fit for service, to secure their prompt discharge with due regard to the interest of the government and of the individual.

Each disease which may be classed as coming under the heading of military medicine should be studied as to history, etiology, epidemiology, pathology, clinical manifestations, treatment, and prevention. Some of the more important diseases and conditions which belong definitely to military medicine are malaria, typhoid fever, typhus fever, acute respiratory infections, yellow fever, Asiatic cholera, plague, the dysenteries, measles, scarlet fever, mumps, chicken pox, beri beri, diseases due to food deprivations, the fractures and injuries common to many branches of the service as a result of extra hazards, wounds and injuries due to active hostilities, practically all of the parasitic diseases, and those of the tropics.

It is impracticable and undesirable to attempt in a discourse of this kind to do more than indicate some of the diseases belonging to certain important groups of military medicine as just mentioned, and to speak more particularly of a few of the most striking ones to serve as important examples.

YELLOW FEVER

The importance of yellow fever, both in its bearing on the military services as well as upon the civil population, has been generally recognized by the profession for many years and is quite fully appreciated by all modern students of medicine. Yellow fever was the scourge of the western hemisphere, particularly in the Caribbean area, for centuries. Its existence in the western hemisphere had a most important effect on the geographical expansion of our own country. Had it not been for yellow fever, Napoleon's troops, under his brother-in-law, General Le Clerc, after overrunning Santa Domingo would probably have, and did intend to, take over the territory comprising the Louisiana Purchase, which the United States obtained from France in 1803. From the Louisiana Purchase have been carved some 14 states of our Union.

There were a number of notable epidemics of yellow fever in our country, the best known one being that described by Benjamin Rush, which occurred in Philadelphia the latter part of the 18th Century. Yellow fever was first *officially* mentioned in the report of The Surgeon General of the Army in February, 1820. Serious epidemics occurred among troops as well as among the civilian population in Louisiana in the period between 1819 and 1824. It seriously affected the efficiency of the operation of our Army during the Mexican War when it appeared among those forces landing at Vera Cruz under General Scott, before they could reach the high, salubrious interior. Probably the year 1867 stands out as the worst epidemic of yellow fever among our military forces. It appeared at Brownsville, Texas, about October 1st of that year being introduced by Austrian troops who formerly belonged to Emperor Maximilian's Army in Mexico, but who had been disbanded. They provided the focus from which the disease spread to many of the southern states. The classical experiments of Walter Reed and his Board, consisting of Carroll, Lazear, and Agramonte, marked an epoch in preventive medicine. Reed and his co-workers proved beyond all doubt that yellow fever was conveyed from one patient to another by the bite of a mosquito, first called the Culex Fasciata, but now known as Aedes Egypti. We now are also aware that there are other vectors besides the mosquito, and that virus of yellow fever can be conveyed to other by the fresh blood of patients suffering from yellow fever even through the uncut surface of the skin, if the skin is thus contaminated, and provided also that the patients are at a proper stage of the disease.

It is well established that the endemic foci of yellow fever in Africa and Brazil are kept alive in monkeys and a number of other lower animals. Experimental studies with mice have led to the development of an immunizing means of treatment for those who have to proceed to tropical areas where yellow fever is or may be present. All Army troops at the present time who are dispatched to the tropics are given immunizing doses against yellow fever, i.e., a certain number of so-called "mouse units", just as for years we have been routinely giving typhoid prophylaxis and small pox vaccination on induction to the service.

Historically, it is well known that Dr. Carlos Finlay of Havana, Cuba, was the first person to advance the theory that yellow fever was transmitted by the bite of a mosquito. He did not prove it, but his observations were correct as was so brilliantly proven by Reed and his colleagues in Cuba in 1900 and 1901. Reed's Board demonstrated that yellow fever was only infectious if the patient suffering from that disease was bitten by a mosquito during the first three days of his illness, and that the mosquito itself could not transmit the disease to another individual until after an interval of 12 days, which permitted certain developments of the virus to take place in the body of the mosquito.

William Crawford Gorgas, afterwards Surgeon General of the Army, was Chief Health Officer of Havana, Cuba, at that time, and was the first to put to practical application the discovery of the Reed Board, and was able to free Havana of yellow fever for the first time in several centuries. Later General Gorgas, while serving as Chief Health Officer of the Panama Canal Zone during the building of the Canal, by using similar mosquito control methods as he had in Havana was able to rid the Canal Zone of yellow fever, and very largely control the incidence of malaria. Prior to the inauguration of sanitary measures in the Canal Zone by Gorgas, it had been impossible for Europeans to carry on the work of building the canal on account of the tremendous mortality. It was said that for every tie placed in the Panama Canal railroad across the isthmus, there was a death of one laborer. There is still a town on the railroad called Matachin, because so many Chinese laborers died in that locality.

It was because of the high mortality among the European laborers that the famous French engineer, Ferdinand De Lesseps, failed to build the Canal and that work was not resumed until many years afterwards the United States undertook it in the early part of the present century. The canal was finally opened to navigation in 1914. The engineering feat of building the Canal was carried out by the great Army engineer, Goethals.

While serving in the Second Occupation of Cuba, 1906-1909, I had the privilege of meeting Drs. Finlay, Guiteras, and Agramonte, all then living in Havana and constituting what was known as the Yellow Fever Board. Their function was to see and diagnose all suspected cases of yellow fever in the city of Havana and adjacent territory. As a young medical officer, I was given an opportunity by them to see a number of cases of yellow fever that were being treated in the Beneficencia Hospital in that city.

TYPHOID FEVER

Though not as spectacular as a cause of death as yellow fever, typhoid fever has played a more important part in our military history. In times past it was one of the greatest causes of morbidity and mortality among United States troops as well as among civilians.

Typhoid fever was confused with typhus fever and with malaria until 1829, when the French pathologist, Louis, gave it its name. The pathology of the disease was accurately described by Gerhard, an American student of Louis, in 1837, and it was then shown that typhoid fever was an entity, and entirely distinct from typhus fever. It then became generally recognized that these two were different diseases. The name *typhoid* was given to the disease because of resemblance to *typhus* fever in some of its clinical aspects. The first official mention of typhoid fever as a separate disease in Army records was made in the report of The Surgeon General of the Army in 1851. Typhoid fever took a tremendous toll in the Continental Army at Cambridge, Massachusetts, in 1775. It played a very serious part among our troops in the War of 1812. There were known to be more than 80,000 cases of typhoid fever in the Northern Army alone during the Civil War, and at that time the mortality was extremely high—not less than 37 percent of those who contracted typhoid fever died. Typhoid fever among military forces declined after the Civil War until the early nineties. In the Spanish-American War, thyphoid fever broke out in most of the concentration camps. It has been variously estimated that about 20 percent of the entire Army, regular and volunteer, during that war suffered from the disease, and that typhoid fever caused 86 percent of all death from disease which occurred during that war.

The work of Walter Reed, Victor C. Vaughan, and Edward Shakespeare, constituting a special board during the Spanish-American War to investigate the epidemiology of typhoid fever, indicated that the disease was carried through infection of food and or water, and in certain cases was conveyed to individuals by bacteria-laden dust, and also by flies passing from the open latrines into the unscreened mess halls and kitchens of the troops, thus contaminating the foods.

Time will not permit going into a history of the development of typhoid prophylaxis. The British attempt to do so in the Boer War by use of typhoid vaccination was not very successful, nor was it in the hands of the Germans later in West Africa. Briefly, Sir Almyroth Wright, by experiments showed that if patients were injected with killed cultures of typhoid bacilli it would produce in them immunizing bodies which would protect such individuals from infection by the typhoid bacillus just as if they had previously had an attack of the disease. Captain Frederick F. Russell (now Brigadier General, retired) made a study of the methods of typhoid vaccination used by the British and Germans among the civil population in 1908. Upon his return, a Board was appointed by The Surgeon General of the Army to consider the whole subject. The men on the Board with Captain Russell were Victor C. Vaughan, Simon Flexnar, William Councilman, John Musser, Alexander Lambert, and

William S. Thayer. These distinguished scientists served for more than a week on this Board as a patriotic duty and at considerable personal financial loss. As a result the Board was convinced that typhoid prophylaxis was practicable and safe. It was introduced first into our Army as a voluntary measure, in 1909. It was made compulsory in the fall of 1911. The American Army was the only Army fully protected by typhoid prophylaxis in the World War. The Germans, French, and British, especially the two former, lost thousands from this disease before the prophylaxis was put into practice on a large scale as in the American Army.

After typhoid prophylaxis was introduced into our service in 1909 only a few cases were reported in the Army until 1912. There were no deaths in the Army from typhoid fever from that date until 1925. During part of this period among 286,000 men who entered the Army as recruits, the absence of the disease was remarkable. In the World War there were only 546 cases of typhoid fever among the enlisted men in camps in the United States and a large proportion of those contracted the disease before reporting at the camps. The prophylactic material is made in large quantities at the Army Medical School laboratories in Washington. During the World War, to the typhoid portions of the prophylaxis was added a certain amount of paratyphoid A and paratyphoid B killed cultures. This was known as "triple typhoid vaccine". After the World War, the paratyphoid B fraction was omitted since

that form of paratyphoid is more common in Europe than in the United States. Later the paratyphoid A was also omitted. The old Rawlins "mother strain" from which typhoid prophylaxis material was made for so many years was changed about 1935 in the Army, and a new and more satisfactory culture is being used. In the World War more than four million men were mobilized and out of that great number there were only 1,529 cases admitted to sick report as a result of typhoid fever. This was actually one admission during the World War for every 382 cases of typhoid fever which occurred during the Spanish War. The latter in an Army of less than 300,000 men. This outstanding achievement in preventive medicine is a good example of what scientific medicine is able to do in these days as a result of research. A triumph of preventive medicine.

These few examples are all that can be mentioned today in the limited time. In closing, it seems justifiable to conclude that so-called military medicine, embracing as it does so many diseases usually taught in many different departments in the curricula of medical schools, merits a special place or department in any school that wishes to deal adequately with the subject. Collaboration and cooperation with the other teaching departments is essential. This plan is now being followed in a number of the more progressive schools of our country. The importance of *military medicine* cannot be overemphasized.

Protection of Children Against Tuberculosis[*]

HUGH L. DWYER, M.D.

KANSAS CITY, MISSOURI

Recent data published by the Metropolitan Life Insurance Company show that in the short space of two decades the mortality from tuberculosis has been reduced two-thirds for white persons and one-half for colored. In females the decline has been more rapid so that now they have a lower mortality than males. For example, in 1920 the rate for white females was 93.4 per 100,000 population and in 1940 it had declined to 25.3, a reduction of 73 percent. In

*Read at Annual meeting, Oklahoma State Medical Association,Tulsa, April 22, 1942.

white males the death rate declined 63 percent during these twenty years. In the white race, death from tuberculosis is becoming a problem of the aged, although in this group the decline has followed the general trend downward. In 1920 the chances of a newborn white child dying of tuberculosis was six in 100; in 1940 it was less than three in 100.

Of all the communicable diseases tuberculosis takes the greatest toll. Each year it kills 70,000 persons in the United States and it is estimated on the basis of hospital admissions that there are 400,000 persons at large who are spreaders of tubercle bacilli. It is not generally appreciated that the highest mortality in white persons is between the ages of 65 to 70 for men and 70 to 75 for women. In infants under one year, the rate is approximately 40 per 100,000. The lowest rate is seen in children between five and nine years.

In this country most authorities hold that there are at least two stages in the development of tuberculosis, primary tuberculosis or first infection type, formerly called childhood tuberculosis, and re-infection tuberculosis, formerly called adult tuberculosis. The first infection sensitizes the tissues, but seldom if ever does the child succumb to a single primary infection. The individual can resolve a primary infection to the calcified state. However he can do this only once. The next time tubercle bacilli circulate in the body the tissue change is a necrotizing process and active disease of the lung parenchyma follows.

There are no symptoms of primary tuberculosis unless the infection is extensive and in the few in which symptoms appear, they subside in a few weeks. Thereafter, throughout the remainder of the life of the patient the primary lesion produces no symptoms. After the first infection the individual will react to tuberculin in sufficient dosage but in only 20 to 25 percent can changes be detected by X-ray examination.

Consumption, therefore, does not develop as a result of first infections; such lesions as they cause uniformly resolve and calcify at any age in which they occur according to Myers and Stewart. Lincoln[1] at Bellevue Hospital, on the other hand, found that 20 percent of the children with X-ray evidence of primary tuberculosis died of the disease within one year. Consumption develops following reinfection from without or from an activation of the first infection. The lesions of primary infection appear in the middle and lower thirds of the lungs. The fact that lesions of chronic pulmonary tuberculosis develop in the upper parts of the lungs leads the Bellevue school to the belief that this is a complication of the primary infection tuberculosis rather than re-infection. They also contend that the development of chronic pulmonary tuberculosis is related to the development of sexual maturity and that the re-infection theory fails to explain the occurrence of chronic pulmonary tuberculosis so much earlier in girls.

The lesions of re-infection tuberculosis usually appear first in the subapical part of the lungs and may exist for years without symptoms, physical signs or a tendency to spread. A sub-clinical pulmonary tuberculosis occasionally is present in the early stage of the re-infection phase when a silent pulmonary lesion becomes clinically active with symptoms. This may occur in young adults, notably medical students or student nurses, who a few months previously had a negative tuberculin reaction.

To prevent tuberculosis in children it is necessary that they be kept from contact with a tuberculous adult. Once the primary infection is acquired they should be protected against re-infection. It is during the first year and again during adolescence that the disease is mostly likely to develop. Not infrequently an unsuspected active case in the home is brought to light when a positive tuberculin test discloses a primary infection in a school child.

There are students of tuberculosis who believe there is a certain degree of immunity following the first-infection and that such infections, after early infancy, are not a handicap to the child. The majority contend that only harm can come from first infections. The experience at Lymanhurst where some 2,467 children with primary infection were observed for several years prompted Stewart[2] to say, "there is no form of tuberculosis that is prevented by the first invasion of tubercle bacilli,—we believe that primary infection is the first step along the path which leads too often to all the serious reinfection varieties." At this same clinic[3] it was found that reinfection tuberculosis developed in nine times as many children with a positive tuberculin reaction as in those of the same age with a negative test. the ratio of mortality in the two groups was 38:1. Nearly 70 percent of all cases of phthisis in children has occurred in those known to have had primary infections previous to the time re-infection occurred.

There is always a danger to children from intimate association with persons about whom nothing is known regarding their freedom from tuberculosis. Parents, servants and other adults in the home have been known to infect and re-infect the child with disastrous results. Not infrequently the infection has been acquired from an elderly relative thought to have asthma or bronchitis which in reality was communicable tuberculosis. Every pediatrician who does tuberculin tests on children has experienced the discovery of active disease in a parent, when this was not suspected. Practically all childhood tuberculosis is acquired from close association with adults who have "open" tuberculosis.

Twenty years ago, Charles Hendee Smith prompted a study by the New York Tuberculosis Association of transmission of tuberculosis to children by servants. Within recent years the American Academy of Pediatrics through its Committee on Contact Infections', has stimulated interest in the danger of tuberculosis from household domestics and from teachers and other school personnel. At the time Smith attacked the problem he met a great deal of resistance to his efforts to have all servants have a clean bill of health. Since that time, public appreciation of the danger to children from this source has increased rapidly. Now the health of the school teacher is recognized as an important item in protecting the child.

Contact between children and tuberculosis nursemaids or other servants will be less frequent when parents are convinced of the necessity of employing only those who have had a recent health examination. Tuberculosis is relatively more common in the young negro women. A physical examination that does not include a good X-ray plate of the chest is of little value when one is looking for tuberculosis. If there is any place where pre-employment and subsequent periodic examinations including the roentgenogram is needed, it is among those whose work brings them intimately in contact with children. At present there is a widespread interest in blood examinations for syphilis and occasionally parents arrange for a serologic examination for those who work in their kitchens. Obviously there is comparatively little danger from the transmission of syphilis to children. In fact, there is no comparison in the health hazard to children between syphilis and tuberculosis and the prevention of the spread of tuberculosis from this source awaits only the education of the public to its need and some provision for less expensive X-ray examinations.

Ten years ago Jordon described the transmission of tuberculosis to school children in Minnesota by a teacher with far advanced, but unrecognized, tuberculosis. The teacher instructed the band and occasionally would demonstrate the use of a wind instrument by blowing into it, then handing it to the child. Sputum transferred in this manner resulted in 33.5 percent of the boys of the band giving a positive tuberculin test whereas only 15.7 percent of the remainder of the class were positive. Among the 173 teachers, janitors and other adult personnel of this school, five had re-infection type tuberculosis.

Lindberg made a tuberculosis survey in Macon County, Illinois, and found that in 705 school teachers, 315 were infected and nine actively tuberculous. Jordon, in 1936, found the sputum positive in eight of 786 teachers, and of 64 pupils exposed to a tuberculous teacher 42.6 percent were tuberculin positive while of 161 pupils of the same

school and age group only 11.2 percent were positive.

Harrington and associates in Minneapolis reported the examination of 3,600 school teachers and janitors, 68 of whom showed X-ray evidence of tuberculosis and six had positive sputum.

In 1930, Dietrich reported three families in which four children developed tuberculosis from tuberculous nurse-maids and two of the children died.

About two-thirds of the largest cities in the nation require a health certificate from teachers before appointment. The smaller the community the fewer require this. In 1934, twenty states required such an examination. In none of these compulsory examinations was a tuberculin test or an X-ray plate of the chest required. This condition is improving rapidly as a result of the educational efforts of the American Academy of Pediatrics and now several states are considering legislation to require a school employee to have periodic X-ray examinations of the chest.

The physician needs to be impressed with the need of tuberculin tests in all the children in his practice. The education of the public, school authorities and physicians alike offers a fruitful field for the County and State Medical Societies. All too often the family physician interprets the positive tuberculin reaction made in the child at school of no importance. Physicians have told parents that the positive test means only that the child has picked up the germ but that it means nothing and have not taken any steps to find the source of the infection in the home. Proper epidemiological procedures which would often find "open" tuberculosis in some member of the household, has largely been limited to families dependent upon free dispensaries, and usually municipal or university clinics have a separate department for tuberculosis.

The recently developed patch test should contribute greatly to widespread tuberculin testing in private practice. This requires only the application of adhesive tape containing tuberculin after cleansing of the skin with acetone. The area between the scapulae is chosen because the test cannot be distributed by bathing for a period of 48 hours. The patch test is proving to be as reliable as the Pirquet test in which Old Tuberculin is applied in a scratch on the skin of the forearm. The Mantoux or intradermal test with 0.1 cc. of a dilution of O. T. is most widely used. One may safely start with a 1-1000 dilution giving 0.1 mgm of tuberculin except where tuberculosis is suspected in which event a weaker dilution is advisable. Some children, relatively few, who react negatively to 0.1 mgm will be positive with 1.0 mgm.

Every physician should do some kind of a tuberculin test in the families under his care. The patch test is sufficient to make the family tuberculosis conscious. There is some objection to the use of hypodermic needles in families apparently well, and it is not always convenient for the doctor to make up dilutions to tuberculin and have a special syringe for this alone. The easily applied, harmless patch test will interest the family in X-ray examinations as well as more sensitive intradermal tests.

Stewart has demonstrated the value of testing every member of the family at intervals and states that the program of tuberculosis control will never be complete until the family physician will do tests on his patients. His patients should not have to visit another physician or health department clinic to learn whether they are free from tuberculosis. The tuberculin test is the simplest and sometimes the only way the presence of the disease can be discovered.

When Mantoux tests of the children in a family are negative, even if one or more adults have positive reactions, it can be assumed that the adult positives are not spreading tubercle bacilli and therefore X-ray examinations can be safely deferred. All households can be accredited as contagious-free units solely upon the results of the Mantoux test. Only in those homes where a child reacts positively it is imperative that all positive reacting adults have an X-ray plate of the chest made.

In schools, tuberculin testing may well be limited to two age groups, six and sixteen, or the first grader and the high school junior. Positive reactors in the kindergarten or first grade should be followed into the home to find and remove the source of infection and this is more likely of accomplishment in the younger group of positive reactors. All adolescents or high school children who react positively should have a roentgenogram annually to detect early the reinfection tuberculosis. For some unexplained reason, the development of chronic pulmonary disease is related to sex maturity and we know nothing about preventing this.

What should be done with the child who has a positive test? He should not be removed from school or home because he is not a source of damage to others. There is little to be gained by X-ray examination of positive reacting children between five and fifteen years of age. Why do tuberculin tests on private patients in this age period? The most product result of discovering positive

reactors in children in private practice will come from the follow-up work that is done, finding the source, in the home or in the school and if possible breaking the contact. If there is to be no follow-up there is little purpose in tuberculin testing any child before puberty.

The most fruitful field of case finding is among adults. The family and intimate associates of every known tuberculous patient should be investigated. The promiscous testing of school children is too costly for the number of cases of reinfection tuberculosis discovered. In a Chicago study involving 167,435 adolescents and children, it was found that the cost of discovering one tuberculous child was $450.00.

Because of the increased prevalence of tuberculosis in the negro, and the danger of the negro as a spreader of tubercle bacilli, more concerted case-finding efforts can well be devoted to this group. In our experience, the testing of all negro high school and grade school pupils has proven worth while. It is this age group who is entering that period of life when active pulmonary tuberculosis develops. The procedure of the future in case-finding would seem to be a roentgenologic survey of men and women in areas of excessive mortality, or whose work brings them in close association with children. In some surveys the miniature X-ray film has stepped into first place as a case-finding instrument. Our experience with the 35 m.m. photoflouroscopic film with several thousand adults, has not been impressive. Admittedly, it is of great educational value.

In the autumn of 1941 the Kansas City Department of Health obtained an X-ray machine for making 35 m.m. films of the chest at a cost of two or three cents each. All city employees, school teachers and other school personnel, negro maids who were registered at employment agencies supplying domestic help, and negro pupils of high schools and grade schools were invited to avail themselves of the opportunity to come in for an examination. In arranging for this survey these groups were assured that the results of the examination would be made known only to the individual and that no one would jeopardize his or her position by information revealed in this examination.

We embarked upon this survey as a case-finding project, aware of the fact that miniature films could not be relied upon in many cases to make a positive diagnosis of tuberculosis. As a result of the examinations, those X-rayed were divided into three groups; the first, those with easily recognized lesions; second, those with negative films; and third, the largest group, those with suspicious films. Those with positive films were advised to go to their personal physicians who could obtain a report of the Health Department's finding. Those with suspicious chest films were told the result of the examination warranted a more complete and a standard X-ray chest plate made by their physicians.

The cooperation on the part of the school people was exceptionally good. The survey was continued to include volunteers for civilian defense qualifying for auxiliary firemen and policemen. In high school groups, as many as 250 could be examined in one afternoon. During the first six months, more than 4,000 have been examined.

Many persons who submitted to the examination with this 35 m.m. film have gone to private physicians. A few far advanced cases of pulmonary tuberculosis were found, some whose work brought them into close association with children.

This survey, which is an inexpensive method of sifting out persons who are in need of a more complete examination, has made many people interested in tuberculosis. With the opening of the school term in September, 1942, the Board of Education will require all teachers, clerks and janitors to present evidence of a complete physical examination including a 14 x 17 X-ray plate of the chest. The examination form provided for this purpose will be reviewed by a committee of three outstanding physicians, one a radiologist with a long experience in tuberculosis. This examination will be required every three years. By this means a great advance will be made in the protection of the child at school. The educational value of chest examinations in school teachers is bound to result in an increased interest in the health of all those who might transmit tuberculosis to the child at home.

BIBLIOGRAPHY

1. J. Ped. 20:128, (Jan.) 1942.
2. Am. Jo. Dis. Child., 59:1034, (May) 1940.
3. J. A. M. A, 112:1306, 1939.
4. J. A. M. A., 113:1873, (Nov. 18) 1939.

Transfusion Accidents and Iso-immunization (Rh Factor)

F. D. SINCLAIR, M.D.
Springer Clinic

TULSA, OKLAHOMA

Less than two years ago a 32 year old multiparous housewife was admitted to a Metropolitan New York hospital with signs of a ruptured uterus at term and a dead fetus. Cesarean section delivered a ten pound, edematous infant. Because of the mothers existing anemia, a transfusion was given (donor and patient Group A (Moss II). A second transfusion was given that evening for signs suggesting shock. The next morning she was deeply jaundiced, and the hemoglobin had dropped from 60 percent to 46 percent. A third transfusions was given. Partial anuria developed. By the seventh day, hemoglobin had dropped from 46 percent to 40 percent in the absence of any bleeding. A fourth transfusion was given and for the first time was followed by signs of obvious reaction, chills and fever. The patient failed to rally and died two days later.

This case illustrates the evil possibilities in seriously ill patients requiring repeated transfusions. It is desirable to prevent such dangerous reactions. This case, focused the attention of the attending doctor on the possible common etiology of erythroblastosis fetalis, which caused the death of that baby, and transfusion accidents in pregnancy. Such transfusion accidents are not the results of errors in blood matching but are caused by the presence in the mothers blood of immune, intra-group agglutinins.

Landsteiner and Weiner (January 1940) had six months previously reported on an agglutinin which they had developed in rabbits by the injection of blood from the Macacus rhesus monkey. When tested with human bloods, this agglutinin demonstrated the presence of a new substance in the human red blood cells which they called the Rh factor (Rh from *rh*esus). Further studies on the general population have revealed that 86 percent are Rh positive and 14 percent are Rh negative. In other words, 86 percent of the random population have inherited this Rh antigen in their red blood cells and 14 percent do not have it. The antibodies which this antigen stimulates in a susceptible host are called the anti-Rh agglutinins. This Rh factor is inherited as a simple mendelian dominant much like the A & B factors which differentiate the four blood groups.

Further study on the cause of intra-group transfusion accidents associated with pregnancy has established the importance of the concept of iso-immunization of the mother by a blood factor in the fetus transmitted from the father. Iso-immunization simply means immunization by factors within a single species. This theory of iso-immunization is employed to explain the etiology of ery-throblastosis fetalis. This is a well recognized condition of newborn infants formerly described as familial hemolytic disease of the newborn. It may appear in three accepted clinic forms: hydrops fetalis, interus gravis and congenital anemia of newborn. With critical analysis of material, incidence will run as high as one in less than 200.

How does this iso-immunization of the mother occur and how is the fetus affected? The theory postulates that the father is Rh positive and because this factor is dominant, it is frequently transmitted to the fetus, which makes the fetus also Rh positive. The mother is Rh negative. The leakage of the fetal blood cells must occur through the villus into the maternal circulation. This is one particular feature which is contrary to accepted teachings. Here in the maternal circulation the Rh positive blood cells act as an antigen causing the mother to produce Anti-Rh antibodies in response to this stimulation. These agglutinins in the mothers serum are transferred back through the placenta to act on the susceptible blood of the fetus. Then the trouble starts for the developing child. The principle action of these antibodies in the test tube is agglutination of the Rh positive cells but in the living organism the end result is hemolysis and continuous destruction of the red blood cells. This originates the well known train of events—severe progressive anemia, higher percentages of circulating normoblasts and extra-medullary hematopoiesis.

Dr. Philip Levine reports in substantiating this theory a series of 153 mothers who have delivered one or more babies suffering from ery-throblastosis fetalis. Of these 153 women, 93 percent were Rh negative in contrast to the expected 14 percent of the random population. Since the incidence of Rh negative bloods is very high in these mothers, it could be anticipated on the basis of this theory that the fathers and infants are Rh positive. Of the 89 husbands tested, 89 were Rh positive (100 percent). Of the 76 infants tested, 76 were Rh positive (100 percent). The final proof of this iso-immunization theory can be supplied by the demonstration of anti-Rh agglutinins in the mothers blood. Two months post partum, approximately 50 percent of these women show the presence of anti-Rh agglutinins.

Generally speaking, the sooner after delivery this test is made, the better, for the antibodies disappear rapidly. Better still, in the future, bloods from pregnant women suspected because of previous history, should be studied during pregnancy as the titre fluctuates and apparently is not consistently present.

This iso-immunization theory has several practical applications, particularly as regards transfusions. For example, special care should be exercised in transfusing women who have recently delivered infants with erythroblastosis, unexplained dead fetuses, record of habitual aboration or a history in the past of still born fetus, neonatal deaths or transfusion reactions. Particularly in emergencies involving the recently delivered woman with dead fetus, it is far safer to use pooled plasma rather than blood transfusions, unless the donor can be thoroughly tested. It might be stated at this time that in the absence of immediately available sera for specific Rh tests, these transfusion reactions can be prevented by subjecting the cross matching to the "warm agglutinin" test. In other words, the donor's cell suspension and the patient's serum should be incubated for 30 minutes at 37 degrees C. This modification is highly essential for proper selection of completely compatible donors.

A second example of the practical application of this theory is the Rh negative patient (any Rh negative person—14 percent of population) who must receive repeated transfusions over a period of weeks or months. This patient must be protected from possible iso-immunization through receiving blood repeatedly from Rh positive donors. Any early transfusion would stimulate Anti-Rh agglutinins. These in turn would hemolize Rh positive blood cells given the patient in subsequent transfusions. It is probable that anti-Rh agglutinins are responsible for about 90 percent of all intra-group transfusion accidents, after repeated transfusions or in pregnancy at the first transfusion.

A third example is found in transfusing newborn babies with erythroblastosis fetalis or more minor degrees of congenital anemia. In these cases it is preferable to use Rh negative blood rather than Rh positive because the affected infant, it has been shown, will maintain higher levels of hemoglobin and red blood cell counts. The anti-Rh agglutinins which still might be present in the baby's serum would hemolize the Rh positive blood cells the baby received by transfusion. Certainly, these critically sick infants should not be further insulted by transfusion from the mother, whose blood undoubtedly still contains large amounts of Anti-Rh agglutinins.

How do you diagnose or test Rh positive and Rh negative bloods? One or more drops of human Anti-Rh serum are mixed in a small test tube with two drops of washed 1 percent suspension of the unknown blood. Shake and incubate at 37 degrees C. for one hour. Centrifuge at low speed for 1 minute, resuspend by shaking and read either grossly or under the microscope. Unfortunately at the present time, these potent human Anti-Rh sera are not yet available commercially. They are obtained from mothers who have recently been delivered of infants with erythroblastosis fetalis. You can appreciate the difficulties of commercial production. This fact will undoubtedly impede the progress of physicians interested in this problem and the more widespread testing of this theory.

Detection of Anti-Rh agglutinins in human sera is done as follows: Two drops of serum to be tested are added to ten tubes each containing two drops of 1 percent suspension from ten different Group A (Group IV Moss) bloods, at least one of which is Rh negative. These tubes are then incubated for one hour at 37 degrees C., centrifuged at low speed for one minute, resuspended and examined grossly or microscopically.

Dr. Philip Levine in his original work on this theory used three potent Anti-Rh sera in making the investigation of the 153 cases previously mentioned. These bloods were Group AB, A and O (Moss I, II and IV). At first the investigation moved slowly because the first potent serum was Group A (Moss II), and could not be used with all bloods to be tested because of the presence of agglutinins Anti-A and Anti-B. Later, by using Witebsky's group specific soluble substances A and B, which inhibit the action of agglutinins Anti-A and Anti-B, it was possible to test all unknown sera with the three known Anti-Rh sera in parallel. One complicating feature was that the three potent testing sera did not give entirely parallel reactions with bloods tested.

In addition there are several controversial points which become obvious in studying this question. For example, how can you explain the 7 percent Rh positive mothers who have had babies with erythroblastosis fetalis? These are explained as probably due to other and yet unknown blood factors similar to Rh. In erythrobastosis, for example, we know nothing of the circumstances which permit the immunization of an occasional Rh negative mother by an Rh positive baby and not the immunization of the vast majority of such mothers.

My interest in this Rh factor was stimulated at the second American Congress on Obstetrics and Gynecology in St. Louis early in April, 1942. Here I met Dr. Philip Levine, studied his exhibits and attended the round table discussion on this subject. My purpose in presenting this theory before the Tulsa County Medical Society is purely to arouse more widespread appreciation of this problem. Nothing original is claimed.

However, the evidence presented fairly well establishes the theory of iso-immunization as to pathogenesis of erythroblastosis fetalis. This theory also explains 90 percent of intra-group transfusion reactions. It has been a very worthwhile contribution to medical knowledge. Perhaps, it is most valuable to obstetricians and pediatricians but every physician has at times a seriously ill patient who must be repeatedly transfused. You can observe these precautions and prevent undesirable and perhaps fatal transfusion reactions.

BIBLIOGRAPHY

Levine, Philip: Amer. J. Obst. & Gynec., 42:165, 1941.
Levine, Katzen, Burnham: J. A. M. A., 116:825, 1941.
Wolfe and Neigus: Amer. J. Obst. & Gynec., 40:31, 1940.
Lyman Burnham: Amer. J. Obst. & Gynec., 42:389, 1942.
Levine, Burnham, Katzin and Vogel: Amer. J. Obst. & Gynec., 42:925, 1941.

Injection of Varicose Veins

R. Q. ATCHLEY, M.D.

TULSA, OKLAHOMA

Much thought and discussion and many original ideas and solutions and many sure shot methods have been introduced into the literature since Hippocrates (500 B.C.) wrote his shrewd observation about varicosities and their treatment. From this maze of ideas, propounded solutions and discussion has come a steady but slow improvement in treatment of vascular varicosities and their sequellae. It would be interesting but valuable time wasted to incorporate in an article of this kind a lengthy narration of the detailed history of how the treatment of varicose veins has been brought up to its present status. It is probably needless to say that failures, disappointments and even deaths have been the reward for those who have unraveled the vascular puzzle for us thus far. The why of varicose veins, ulcers and eczema stimulates our imagination sufficiently to seek a classification.

CLASSIFICATION OF VARICOSE VEINS

Four groups of varicose veins are recognized by Bernsten.

1. The uniformally dilated vein with one segment markedly dilated.
2. The common type encountered in which the veins are tortuous, nodular and not uniform in caliber.
3. The high type of varicosity reaching from the sapheno-femoral opening to the middle of the leg.
4. The sunburst or the spider burst branching superficial type.

The much discussed and debatable subject of hemostatic pressure comes in for consideration. It seems that back flow or back pressure is a great contributory factor especially so when the valves are incompetent. It is not entirely nonexistant by any means when competency exists as the elasticity of the valves allow some considerable sagging so to speak contributing to it. It is found that varicosities exist with competent valves thus supporting the above assertion.

It has been demonstrated by Adams that venous pressures as great as 260 mm. of mercury do exist in veins of the leg. Posture and straining greatly affects pressures in the two saphenous systems.

Family characteristics enter into the causative factors in that the stability of the venous system of the lower extremities especially, may vary as any family physique may vary. The veins may have weak walls and valves and the venous map may not be the same and anastomosing angles may be such that upright pressures may be increased.

Pregnancy is a recognized and obvious factor and will not be discussed further.

Occupations that require long strenous stress and strain on the lower extremities increasing the abdominal pressures are great contributory factors.

Abdominal tumors produce a similar effect as pregnancy.

Flat feet are found in many cases of varicose veins and considered by some a contributing factor but is probably a coexisting tissue dyscrasia. According to DeTakats and Quint fifty-eight percent are associated with varicose veins.

Another factor not much discussed, is the quality or firmness of the supporting structures in which the veins run, or the vein bed so to speak. It is a common observation in our clinic that soft fat in the legs carry large varicose veins and the walls seem to be consistently thin thus contributing to

tortuosity and large varicosities and the sequellae.

Phelgmas alba dolens will be mentioned just to say that it may cause large varicose veins in the superficial system as a compensatory factor.

Some recognize an endocrine factor with good supporting evidence.

In conclusion to this section of this paper it may be mentioned that varicose veins practically are nonexistant in quadrupeds supporting the haemostatic pressure theory.

INDICATIONS FOR TREATMENT

Regardless of what the etiological factors may be in a given case, with few exceptions, injection treatment will help the condition and many times bring about a cure. This does not mean that the etiological factor should be disregarded and not remedied when possible. It is my experience however that eliminating the predisposing cause is very difficult in a great majority of cases and frequently impossible.

The topic of saphenous ligations provokes discussions for and against but in reviewing the literature and from experience one can glean the conclusive thought that in selected cases it is indicated but it is not such a simple procedure as some would have us think DeTakats states that saphenous pressure returned to former levels soon after ligations. Adams also states that the varicose state rapidly progresses after ligation in a great number of cases.

A conclusive thought would be that recanalization is not so frequent after ligations as before.

PATENCY TESTS

Patency tests as Trendelenburg, Perthes, comparative tourniquet test, and compression tourniquet test of Morhorner and Ochsner, and percussion test of Schwartz are all important, but the fact that there are so many tests provokes the thought that maybe there are inaccuracies in interpretation and actual guiding aid in them, when used. The principal good to be derived from them is whether or not the deep return circulation is adequate to carry on if the superficial system is obliterated. It seems that the great majority are difficult to interpret. The question should be put to the patient whether or not has had a milk leg. If he has had one he will surely know what the term is and if he hasn't he will likely *not* know what the term is. If there is little swelling, induration or discoloration of the leg especially below the knee cautious injection is pretty safe. After some experience is gained in observing the leg one can sense so to speak the average condition of the deep circulation. It might be said that the patient wants relief and that can acutally be given by an intelligent scrutiny and selected treatment. In our clinic, few patency tests are done. This, I know is not according to the usual teaching but we believe that with extreme caution, and that is strenuously followed, the thrombotic index can be determined and success accomplished. By the thrombotic index we mean that reaction the veins show by the initial injection or in other words the sensitiveness the patient shows to the drug given. Incorporated in this index goes the allergic principle that the patient might show. We have, by this caution process injected numerous cases that have had milk legs of various severity. Great grief is born of over zealousness to effect a cure rapidly.

SOLUTIONS

Schlerosing solutions have been a great problem but through the years of disappointment and failure some good safe solutions have been worked out. I think most medical men know what is desired in a good sclerosing solution. Probably the most popular solution just now is Sodium Morrhuate 5 percent and Dextrose and Sodium Chloride probably runs next. They are safe with average caution and a small spill will not be a terrifying situation. An *old solution* must not be neglected and is 30 percent Sodium Chloride. It is a very painful one but really does a good sclerosing job. It has the great advantage of being extremly physiological when diluted by the blood. There are more recent ones on the market but I have had too little experience with them. The average dose of 5 percent Sodium Morrhuate runs from 2 cc. to 4 cc. but occasionally in large veins the amount can be increased, but cautiously. The average dose for Dextrose and Sodium Chloride is about 10 cc. and likewise can be increased in large veins.

TECHNIQUE

The technique of injection is by far the most essential of all procedures. A poor technique means poor, and a great many times disastrous results.

The ordinary office operating table can be used by allowing the patient to stand at its foot with the lower section turned down. A small foot stool should be placed so the patient can stand on it and sit upon the table with ease when the injection is to be made, thus allowing the emptying, to a certain extent, of the distended veins and in turn get a maximum intravenous concentration of the solution. The skin should be cleansed with alcohol and not a colored solution. McPheters and Rice and others, having proven by fleuroscopic demonstrations that usually the flow of blood in varicose veins is caudad and not cephalad, the site of injection should

be selected at a high point so the solution will gravitate downward, thus obliterating as much vein as possible. When the needle is inserted and blood is freely aspirated, the patient is allowed to sit down and if the veins are not sufficiently collasped the lower section of the table can be raised, very carefull, placing the limb in a horizontal position.

If a careful technique is followed many times the veins can be evacuated by stripping and blocking by the fingers of an assistant. Extreme care should be exercised that the puncture site be not disturbed, lest the posterior wall of the vein be punctured, the wall be torn or the needle slip from it. The solution should be injected slowly, occasionally aspirating blood into the syringe. The rate of injection should be about 1 cc. per fifteen seconds for the average solution. Faster than this gives more cramp like pain and movement of the patient and probably a spill into the tissues. As the veins become thrombosed, the sites of injection can be brought downward, leaving the veins around the ankles last because frequently when reached they are already thrombosed. Four to six inches and sometimes more can be well thrombosed with the average injection. If pressure seems to retard the process of the syringe plunger, too much force should not be exerted as the vein might burst or get a spill back through the needle puncture. The injection should be about every five to six days as the thrombotic index indicates. After injection a small compression pad of gauze is placed over the puncture wound and held tightly by a strip of adhesive for twenty-four hours. Some wear spiral elastic bandages during the course of treatment.

The greatest pitfall of a poor technique is a spill with a resulting slough, which takes from one to three months to heal, but, needless to say, the vein at that particular point is destroyed. Normal saline injected around a spill will minimize the slough. In indurated legs the veins if found are frequently felt as grooves and give a sense of fluctuation to the palpating finger. It seems that most veins of this type have thin walls and are the treacherous ones to inject, they tear easily and are sensitive to the solution. Small injections are usually the best as severe reactions usually follow. It is needless to say a dull needle would tear the vein and cause a spill. In the aged, doses should be reduced from the average as it seems their tolerance is poor.

A tourniquet helps to identify small and deep veins but usually a varicose vein can be found if the legs are pendant and the veins sufficiently large to give trouble. Injections should not be given near an ulcer if the veins can be identified away from it because additional sloughing is not likely to occur. Some operators never inject the internal saphenous above the knee but others do so with caution. It seems that if the injection is done slowly blocking off the vein by pressure with the finger there is little danger.

LIGATIONS

Ligations of the internal saphenous vein combined with injections give the greatest percentage of permanent cures.

To do ligations an accurate knowledge of the patency of the deep veins should be had. There is some controversy, however, relative to the advantage of ligation and injections over injections alone. Ochsner and Mohorner state that fifteen percent recur by the combination technique compared to sixty percent recurrences when injections alone are done. Any ligation proceedure brings with it a mortality rate since a great many of the patients are old or have some surgical contra-indication, saying nothing of their predisposition to respiratory complications. Recurrences after the injection treatment are always more amendable to subsequent treatment and they carry a very low mortality rate according to DeTakats seven deaths in 53,000.

THE ULCER

The varicose ulcer is the greatest problem of the entire varicose vein situation, especially in the aged and neglected cases.

They must be differentiated from ulcers of luetic, diabetic, traumatic, post operative, tuberculous and chemical orgin. The cardiac and deficiency ulcer must not be overlooked. In a few ulcer cases we find two or more factors are operating to cause the ulcer. Constricting bands as garters tend to accelerate the stasis with its accompaning anoxemia, increased carbon dioxide content and N.P.N. of the blood. It is probably needless to say stagnation with varicosities produces the above conditions in the majority of cases. The skin resistance to trauma and infection is greatly reduced causing eczema and sloughing followed by infection. The skin in the area below the mid portion of the lower leg is usually edematous and indurated. It may be smooth and pit on pressure. The veins are difficult to find in this hard edematous tissue but if they can be found they will frequently appear as grooves. If they can not be found some varicosities above the induration can be easily found and injected. Injections near an ulcer should be avoided because the increased pressure in already damaged tissue may cause sloughing.

A comparatively safe distance from the ulcer for injection is three-fourth to one inch. When injection is made near an ulcer great care must be taken to avoid injury to the vein wall by pressure. The dose should be cut in half because as above stated excessive intra tissue may produce a slough. This type of slough heals slowly. Many of these ulcers especially in the clinic cases have had every conceivable method of treatment, often resulting in secondary infections that preclude any type of injection until the infection is cleared up. Rest, hot saline packs, sulfa compounds by mouth and local antiseptics should quickly overcome the infection. It is surprising how promptly an ulcer may heal when the stagnation begins to subside. Iodine painted in the crater of the ulcer followed by balsam peru ointment 10 percent stimulates granulation. Metuvit ointment is highly lauded by Schmier of Brooklyn in an article written in 1934. Vitamin deficiencies should be discovered and properly treated. This was worked out in the University Hospital at Oklahoma City in 1941. Kreig suggested Vitamin B for relief of pain in infected ulcers (10 mg. three times daily at first). This should be decreased to 5 mgm. daily when the pain subsides. The soft rubber sponge called the venous heart by DeTakats is an aid and has the advantage of cleanliness. It is applied to the ulcer over vaseline gauze and secured by an elastic spiral bandage. The unna boot has great merit in this condition. It has the advantage of fitting the leg and distributing the pressure equally thus giving uniform support. It can be removed as frequently as necessary as it becomes quite aromatic if the ulcer produces much discharge. Spiral elastic bandages are beneficial especially where large varicosities exist and as stated above they hold the rubber sponge in place.

ECZEMA

Eczema is a complication equally as important and difficult to combat as the varicose ulcer. It usually is of the moist type involving the lower half to two-thirds of the tibio fibular region corresponding to the ulcer area. The hearty cooperation of a dermatologist is essential along with the various other procedures.

COMMENT

Injections of varicose veins in pregnancy can safely be done with the average precautions. The doseage should be smaller and for obvious reasons a quinine drug should never be employed.

Injection of varicosele is very difficult and unless there is some contra indications it should be treated surgically.

Varicosities of the vulva can be much more easily injected than varicocele but the dose should be exceedingly small. Sodium Morrhuate 5 percent (5 to 10 mm.) should be used and at much longer intervals between injections.

• THE PRESIDENT'S PAGE •

The Medical Profession has faced and conquered many scientific problems. American physicians have given the people of this country the greatest life expectancy of any nation on earth. Medicine in gaining its stature has always led rather than followed.

Today our way of life is being challenged by a disease that cannot be conquered in the test tube or on the surgical table. It is a disease that can only be stamped out by the might of armies and materials.

Medicine's problem today is to give to the military forces of our country the finest medical care that can be rendered.

That this will call for personal sacrifice, there is no doubt. But the loss of business as usual is a small price to pay for the priviledge of living in a free America.

At the present time through Procurement and Assignment Service, Medical manpower is being assembled. Your country needs physicians. It needs and will get the young and well-trained physicians. Every medical man under forty-five years of age should determine whether he is physically fit to have the honor of serving his country.*

Now is the time to face the facts and win this war.

Don't wait for John. Ask yourself the question—What am I doing commensurate with my ability and training to sustain for myself and family the American way of life?

"If it's worth having, it's worth fighting for."

*Authority for Physical Examination may be received by contacting Colonel Lee R. Wilhite, Medical Recruiting Board for Oklahoma, 211 Plaza Court, Oklahoma City, Oklahoma.

Sincerely yours,

James D Osborn

President.

• EDITORIALS •

OKLAHOMA MUST NOT FAIL

In this issue of the Journal there is a news story about Oklahoma's response to the needs of Procurement and Assignment. Every doctor of military age should read that story and make his decision. In this section of the country, where true Americanism is undiluted, doctors will not stand by and let the young men go to battle unattended. They must go with the assurance that their health will be safeguarded, their wounds promptly cared for and their suffering aleviated.

The following is a quotation from a letter written by one of America's most eminent physicians. "All the young men are keen to get into service, and this is as it should be. Those who do not go into army or navy active service, if they are fit and of proper age, will, I am sure, miss a very valuable experience and probably regret it in after years. I wish I were not too old."

If you are a young doctor, think it over, and make your decision before the candle burns out. Be sure you do not permit procrastination to slay the flickering flame within, which fortifies you against outer darkness, and the hideous dreads which hound the souls indecision. This tiny light, so mortal warm and brave may be calling you to your life's greatest achievement. There is something more than a mere crescendo of high sounding words in Thomas Mordaunt's:

"One crowded hour of glorious life,
Is worth an age without a name."

TUBERCULOSIS AND WAR

The continuous war on our ancient adversary, tuberculosis, was going well until the nations of the world entered into war with each other.

In this country during the past 50 years the subtle evasive, ubiquitous tubercle bacillus has been forced to gradually retreat. But every inch of ground gained has exacted its price in the skillful application of the accepted methods of control, plus eternal vigilence. In spite of this gain the remaining reservoir of infection is sufficient to break through our lines of defense and rapidly regain lost domain, the moment our offensive and defensive measures slacken. Such measures are so varied and so dependent upon settled social and economic factors it is impossible to avoid serious alterations and dislocations in time of war.

Tuberculosis agencies and public health workers cannot wholly overcome the breaks in our defensive lines occasioned by the exigences of war, such as mental anxiety, neutritional deficiencies, over work, and often the indiscrete expenditure of mounting wages in diversions which deplete physical energy. Of equal importance is the shifting of large groups of population with concentrations in industrial centers, upsetting and over-taxing existing public health services. The latter includes the problems of adequate housing, sanitary engineering, educational and recreational facilities.

Already the centers of urban population are feeling the strain. It is reported that of the seven cities with more than 100,000 population in New York State, five showed an increase of the tuberculosis death rate for 1941. The city of Buffalo, over run with war industry, had an advance in the death rate from 46.0 in 1940 to 54.2 in 1941.

Wichita, Kansas, supplies a good example of an urban population with high ideals and adequate budgeting for public health, educational, cultural and recreational facilities, suddenly faced with the necessity of taking care of more than 12,000 additional families. Certain cities in Oklahoma are facing similar problems. It is impossible to make the necessary adjustments without seriously upsetting many of the important defensive measures now employed against tuberculosis.

Fortunately we know, better than ever before, that early diagnosis and adequate control constitute the greatest safeguard against the rapid spread of the disease. We know that the x-ray will discover many early cases that might otherwise escape the most thorough examination. Though universal x-raying at great expense would represent good economy, it must be accepted as an impossible undertaking at the present time. Fortunately the United States, Canada and Great Britain require an x-ray of the chest in every man considered for military service. By the end of 1942 approximately five million chest x-rays will have been made by the U. S. induction boards. This will give us infinately greater protection than we had during the last world war. No doubt the saving in pensions will greatly exceed the cost of x-ray service.

Most of the young men rejected because of x-ray findings will have minimal disease. They should be informed of the true significance of these findings and urged to have the most approved management. Also it is to be hoped the government after having used the best known screen against tuberculosis, will re-x-ray those accepted for service every six to twelve months to determine the subsequent development of tuberculosis in the millions of screened subjects. This is important in order that early cases may be discovered and given adequate management and that others may be protected against otherwise undiscovered contact with the disease. In addition the accumulation data over a period of years will be of great value in the development of diagnostic and preventive measures.

Routine x-rays of the chest should be required among employees in all war industries with the same end in view. In fact industry as a whole is practicing false economy when it omits the x-ray of the chest in routine employment examinations.

It is estimated that six million young women will be engaged in industry if the war continues. Not one of these should be permitted to work without first having a chest x-ray. In this country young women are more susceptable to tuberculosis than men in the same age group and these young women are going into industry at the most susceptable age and they will be required to take on the mental and physical strains for which they have not been prepared, thus making it doubly important to exercise added vigilence against the development of tuberculosis.

In addition to our obligations in the special fields noted above, we must follow the usual maticulous preventive measures which have robbed tuberculosis of its high place in statistical columns.

EXCEPT A GRAIN OF WHEAT FALL IN THE GROUND

Now that the world is being cracked up because we have broken the commandments, it may be well to heed some of the precepts in the Book. This is not a sermon but a plea for the art of medicine which is so badly needed when the anchor is slipping. Regardless of the doctors creed, he must admit our cherished way of life is truly an interpretation of the ten commandments and the sermon on the mount.

In this time of turmoil, the doctor should strive to become his patient's mentor. It is doubtful if the people of America were ever so in need of the art of medicine. Science and reason are essential in medical progress, but in time of trouble the spirit seeks sympathy and understanding, even beyond the point of reason and logical analysis. In the hour of darkness, the doctor must find the light; in the day of confusion, he must be calm; in case of want, he must share his patient's penury; in the time of dire disaster, he must stand firm. Not only must he attend birth; sustain life, relieve suffering, dissipate fear and inspire confidence, but if need be, he must witness the separation of soul and body, and strive to comfort those who are stricken and bewildered by the last great mystery of life's incomprehensible cycle. Always he must seek to bring about the best possible spiritual and physical adjustments, regardless of social, moral and financial conditions. In spite of war, social, political and financial upheavals, medicine must hold fast the golden thread of truth and follow its traditional devotion to the welfare of society through the care of the sick and the prevention of disease. The doctors reward is in his work. If his task is well performed, ultimately social and political justice must accord his profession the position it deserves.

The above principles apply to the humblest member of the profession. This is a time when little men in their souls and their decisions may become great. There is nothing so elevating as unstinted, sacrificial service. Today, doctors small and great, at home and at war, cannot escape the opportunity to glorify their profession through the personification of all that is great and good. Fearless and defiant, without regard for his own safety, the doctor whether on the foreign line or on the civilian front, shall stand or fall in line of duty. "Except a grain of Wheat fall in the ground and die, it abideth alone; but if it die, it bringeth forth much fruit."

Without the fruits of the art and the science of medicine we will not only lose the war but our American way of life.

WHEN MEDICINE FAILS THE PEOPLE PERISH

Disease has liquidated many a golden age. The plague laid a hand on Pericles and the Roman Empire was shaken from its foundation by chills and fever.

American Medicine nursed the American Colonies through a calamitous era and suffered with Washington at Valley Forge to help achieve our National identity. It helped hold soul and body together in the early days when the Doctor was both preacher and practitioner. It then participated in the unprecedented progress of Medical science which reached a peak in the eighteen-eighties and ultimately safeguarded our National health by the advancement of public health and sanitary engineering. Without this protection for rapidly growing urban populations and to meet the health hazards occasioned by the intermingling of all Nations through modern transportation, disease would not only have impeded National progress but it would have decimated the population. At this time the Nation could not carry on thirty days without the protection Medicine affords.

Yet, the accrued benefits are so obscured by our self complacency, the Medical profession receives little intelligent thought and less merited credit. It is natural that the average Citizen should accept the evolution of National health protection as a matter of fact but it is astonishing that the spectacular control of infectious diseases leaves him unmoved. American Medicine has not only given protection against cholera, yellow fever, small pox, malaria and typhoid, but it cleaned up Havana and moved on to build the Panama Canal and to prove that the whole world may become habitable under modern preventive measures.

The high level of Army health today compared to that of a few decades ago is unbelievable. The brilliant execution of American Military medicine at Pearl Harbor writes a new chapter in the field of Scientific accomplishments. The Medical profession now has sufficient knowledge to carry on the present war virtually without loss of life from disease, even in the equatorial zone, if adequate supplies are always available.

A free Medical profession on a small average income, grateful for the privilege of working seven days a week, with unlimited hours, has achieved for this country the highest health level and, the lowest morbidity and mortality rates existing today among all the comparable nations of the world.

If the government would consider this record and devote more attention to the pro-vision of facilities for continued Medical progress and materials for Medical service and less attention to anticipated regimentation and the consequent annulment of personal initiative, National medical progress would be promoted.

Throughout the land many members of the Medical profession are serving their communities and the nation without remuneration in order to help meet the exegencies of war. Many more are leaving their home and their established practice without assurance of patronage when they return, in order to serve their country. This unselfish action should be compared with the present demands of labor and industry.

The government representative who delivered the ultimatum at the Atlantic City meeting of The American Medical Association, recently hobnobbed with labor at a great meeting in Pittsburg and in spite of sufficient previous provocation on the part of labor unions to arouse the ire of all good Americans, this spokesman for the government, expressed his hearty commendation with never a "Must or Else".

It should be remembered that Doctors are numbered in the thousands while labor runs into the millions, consequently doctors "Must or Else", *while labor must be let alone, "or else."* Political expediency thou art a jewel.

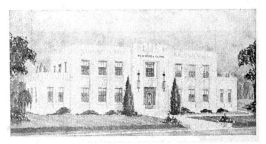

ROSTER
Oklahoma State Medical Association
1942

(Members are listed according to the county of their residence).

(*Indicates the member is serving in the armed forces).

ADAIR
BEASLEY, WARREN A. ....*Stilwell*
(member Cherokee Co. Medical Society)

ALFALFA
DOUGAN, A. L. ....*Carmen*
(member Woods Co. Medical Society)
HARRIS, G. G. ....*Helena*
HUSTON, H. E. ....*Cherokee*
LANCASTER, L. T. ....*Cherokee*
PARSONS, JACK F. ....*Cherokee*
STEPHENSON, Walter L. ....*Aline*
(member Woods Co. Medical Society)
WEBER, A. G. ....*Goltry*

ATOKA
BRIGGS, T. H. ....*Atoka*
*COTTON, W. W. ....*Atoka*
DALE, CHARLES D. ....*Atoka*
FULTON, J. S. ....*Atoka*
HUNTLEY, H. C. ....*Atoka*

BEAVER
BENJEGERDES, THEODORE D. ....*Beaver*
(member Woods Co. Medical Society)
DUNCAN, J. C. (honorary) ....*Forgan*
(member Woodward Co. Medical Society)
McGREW, EDWIN A. ....*Beaver*
(member Woods Co. Medical Society)

BECKHAM
BAKER, L. V. ....*Elk City*
DENBY, J. M. ....*Carter*
DeVANNEY, P. J. ....*Sayre*
JONES, C. F. ....*Erick*
KILPATRICK, E. S. ....*Elk City*
LEVICK, J. E. ....*Elk City*
McCREERY, R. C. ....*Erick*
McGRATH, T. J. ....*Sayre*
PHILLIPS, G. W. ....*Sayre*
SLABAUGH, R. M. ....*Sayre*
SPEED, H. K. ....*Sayre*
SPENCE, W. P. ....*Sayre*
STAGNER, G. H. ....*Erick*
STANDIFER, O. C. ....*Elk City*
TISDAL, V. C. ....*Elk City*

BLAINE
BOHLMANN, W. F. ....*Watonga*
BUCHANAN, F. R. ....*Canton*
CURTIN, VIRGINIA OLSON ....*Watonga*
GRIFFIN, W. F. ....*Watonga*
KIRBY, L. R. ....*Okeene*
MILLIGAN, E. F. ....*Geary*
STOUGH, D. F., JR. ....*Geary*
STOUGH, D. F., SR., (honorary) ....*Geary*
(member Canadian Co. Medical Society)

BRYAN
*BAKER, ALFRED T. ....*Camp Barkeley, Abilene, Texas*
BLOUNT, W. T. ....*Durant*
CAIN, P. L. (honorary) ....*Albany*
COCHRAN, R. L. ....*Caddo*
*COKER, B. B. ....*Dallas, Texas*
COLWICK, J. T. ....*Durant*
COLWICK, O. J. ....*Durant*
DICKEY, R. P. ....*Caddo*

HAYNIE, JOHN A. ....*Durant*
HAYNIE, W. KEILLER ....*Durant*
McCALIB, D. C. ....*Colbert*
MOORE, CHARLES F. ....*Durant*
MOORE, W. L. ....*Bokchito*
NICHOLS, JONAH ....*Durant*
PRICE, CHARLES G. ....*Durant*
RUSHING, G. M. ....*Durant*
SAWYER, R. E. ....*Durant*
SIZEMORE, PAUL ....*Durant*
TONEY, S. M. ....*Bennington*
WANN, C. E. (honorary) ....*Albany*
WELLS, A. J. ....*Calera*
WHARTON, J. T. ....*Durant*

CADDO
BENWARD, JOHN H. ....*Children's Hospital, St. Louis, Mo.*
CAMPBELL, GEORGE C. ....*Anadarko*
DIXON, W. L. ....*Cement*
HASLAM, G. E. ....*Anadarko*
HAWKINS, E. W. ....*Carnegie*
HAWN, W. T. ....*Binger*
HENKE, J. R. ....*Hydro*
INMAN, E. L. ....*Apache*
JOHNSTON, R. E. ....*Anadarko*
KERLEY, W. W. ....*Anadarko*
LYONS, MASON R. ....*Apache*
McCLURE, P. L. ....*Fort Cobb*
McMILLAN, C. B. ....*Gracemont*
*MILES, J. B. ....*95th Station Hospital, Ft. Bliss, Texas*
PATTERSON, FRED L. ....*Carnegie*
PUTNAM, W. B. ....*Carnegie*
SULLIVAN, CLARENCE B. ....*Carnegie*
WILLIAMS, R. W. ....*Anadarko*

CANADIAN
ADERHOLD, THOMAS M. (honorary) ....*El Reno*
BROWN, HADLEY C. ....*El Reno*
CATTO, W. B. ....*El Reno*
CLARK, FRED H. ....*Calumet*
*CRADEN, PAUL J. ....*El Reno*
DEVER, HARVEY K. ....*El Reno*
**FUNK, G. D. ....*El Reno*
GOODMAN, GEORGE LEROY ....*Yukon*
HEROD, PHILIP F. ....*El Reno*
JOHNSON, ALPHA L. ....*El Reno*
LAWTON, W. P. ....*El Reno*
MILLER, W. R. ....*Cowgill, Mo.*
MYERS, PIRL B. ....*El Reno*
PHELPS, JOSEPH T. ....*El Reno*
PHELPS, MALCOM E. ....*El Reno*
RICHARDSON, D. P. ....*Union City*
RILEY, JAMES T. ....*El Reno*
WARREN, R. C. ....*Yukon*
WIGGINS, C. W. ....*Concho*
(member Custer Co. Medical Society)
**Died, February 26, 1942

CARTER
BARKER, E. R. ....*Healdton*
BOADWAY, F. W. ....*Ardmore*
CANADA, J. C. ....*Ardmore*
CANTRELL, D. E., JR. ....*Healdton*
CANTRELL, D. E., SR. ....*Healdton*

CANTRELL, EMMA JEAN ....Healdton
COX, J. L. ....Ardmore
GILLESPIE, L. D. ....Ardmore
GORDON, J. M. ....Ardmore
HARDY, WALTER ....Ardmore
HATHAWAY, W. G. ....Lone Grove
HIGGINS, H. A. ....Ardmore
JACKSON, T. J. ....Ardmore
JOHNSON, C. A. ....Wilson
JOHNSON, G. E. ....Ardmore
JOHNSON, WALTER ....Ardmore
KETCHERSID, J. W. ....Countyline
MEAD, W. W. ....Ardmore
MOTE, W. R. ....Ardmore
MOXLEY, J. N. ....Ardmore
POLLOCK, JOHN R. ....Ardmore
REID, ROGER ....Ardmore
SULLIVAN, R. C. ....Ardmore
SWINBURNE, GRACE ....333 Crystal Pulaski Heights,
                                Little Rock, Ark.
VEAZEY, J. HOBSON ....Ardmore
VEAZEY, LYMAN C. ....Ardmore

CHEROKEE

ALLISON, J. S. ....Tahlequah
BAINES, SWARTZ ....Tahlequah
*BARNES, HARRY E. ....Camp Robinson,
                                Little Rock, Ark.
DYER, ISADORE ....Tahlequah
GRAY, JAMES KARADINE ....Tahlequah
HINES, S. J. T. ....Tahlequah
MASTERS, H. A. ....Tahlequah
McINTOSH, R. K., JR. ....Tahlequah
MEDEARIS, P. H. ....Tahlequah

CHOCTAW

GREGG, O. R. ....Hugo
HALE, C. H. ....Boswell
JOHNSON, E. A. ....Hugo

CIMARRON

HALL, HARRY B. ....Boise City
        (member Texas Co. Medical Society)

CLEVELAND

ATKINS, W. H. ....Norman
BERRY, CURTIS ....Norman
BRAKE, CHARLES A. ....Norman
*BUFFINGTON, F. C. ....Norman
CARROLL, W. B. ....Norman
DAVIS, E. P. ....Norman
        (member McClain Co. Medical Society)
FOWLER, W. A. ....Norman
GASTINEAU, F. T. ....Norman
GRIFFIN, D. W. ....Norman
HADDOCK, J. L. ....Norman
*HADDOCK, PHIL ....Norman
*HOOD JAMES O. ....179th Inf., A.P.O. No. 45,
                        c/o Postmaster, New York City
HOWELL, O. E. ....Norman
LAMBERT, J. B. ....Lexington
LOY, WILLIAM A. ....Norman
MAYFIELD, W. T. ....Norman
MERRITT, IVA S. ....Norman
NIELSEN, GERTRUDE ....Norman
PROSSER, MOORMAN P. ....Norman
*RAYBURN, CHARLES R. ....Norman
*REICHERT, R. J. ....San Luis Obispo, Cal.
RIEGER, J. A. ....Norman
SCHMIDT, ELEONORA ....Norman
STEEN, C. T. ....Norman
STEPHENS, E. F. ....Norman
WICKHAM, M. M. ....Norman
WILEY, GEORGE A. ....Norman
*WILLARD, D. G. ....San Diego Base Hospital,
                                San Diego, Cal.
WOODSON, O. M. ....Norman
        (member LeFlore Co. Medical Society)

COAL

CLARK, J. B. ....Coalgate
CODY, ROBERT D. ....Centrahoma
HENRY, R. C. ....Coalgate
HIPES, J. J. ....Coalgate

COMANCHE

ANGUS, DONALD A. ....Lawton
ANGUS, HOWARD ....Lawton
ANTONY, JOSEPH T. ....Lawton
BARBER, GEORGE S. ....Lawton
BERRY, G. L. ....Lawton
DOWNING, GERALD G. ....Lawton
DUNLAP, ERNEST B. ....Lawton
FERGUSON, LAWRENCE W. ....Lawton
FOX, FRED T. ....Lawton
GOOCH, L. T. ....Lawton
HAMMOND, FRED W. ....Lawton
HATHAWAY, EUEL P. ....Lawton
JOYCE, CHARLES W. ....Fletcher
KNEE, LOREN C. ....Lawton
LEWIS, W. F. ....Lawton
MARTIN, CHESLEY M. ....Elgin
PARSONS, O. L. ....Lawton

COTTON

BAKER, G. W. ....Walters
CALVERT, HOWARD A. ....Walters
HOLSTED, A. B. ....Temple
JONES, M. A. ....Walters
SCISM, MOLLIE ....Walters
TALLANT, GEORGE A. ....Walters

CRAIG

ADAMS, F. M. ....Vinita
BAGBY, LOUIS ....Vinita
BRADSHAW, J. O. ....Welch
DARROUGH, J. B. ....Vinita
HAYS, P. L. ....Vinita
HERRON, A. W. ....Vinita
LEHMER, ELIZABETH E. ....Vinita
MARKS, W. R. ....Vinita
McMILLAN, J. M. ....Vinita
McPIKE, LLOYD H. ....Vinita
SANGER, PAUL G. ....Vinita
**STOUGH, D. B. ....Vinita
**Died, March 19, 1942.

CREEK

BISBEE, W. G. ....Bristow
COPPEDGE, O. C. ....Bristow
COPPEDGE, O. N. ....316 Walnut St.,
                                Philadelphia, Pa.
COPPEDGE, O. S. ....Depew
*COWART, O. H. ....Bristow
CROSTON, GEORGE C. ....Sapulpa
*CURRY, J. F. ....Sapulpa
HAAS, H. R. ....Sapulpa
HOLLIS, J. E. ....Bristow
JONES, ELLIS ....Sapulpa
KING, E. W. ....Bristow
LAMPTON, J. B. ....Sapulpa
LEWIS, P. K. ....Sapulpa
LONGMIRE, W. P., JR. ....Sapulpa
LONGMIRE, W. P., SR. ....Sapulpa
McDONALD, C. R. ....Mannford
*MOTE, PAUL ....U. S. Receiving Station,
                                San Diego, Cal.
OAKES, CHARLES G. ....Sapulpa
PICKHARDT, W. L. ....Sapulpa
REESE, C. B. ....Sapulpa
REYNOLDS, E. W. ....Bristow
REYNOLDS, S. W. ....Drumright
SCHRADER, CHARLES T. ....Bristow
SISLER, FRANK H. ....Bristow
*SISLER, FRANK, JR. ....Bristow
STARR, O. W. ....Drumright
WHARTON, J. L. ....Depew

CUSTER

ALEXANDER, C. J. ....Clinton
BOYD, T. A. ....Weatherford
*BULLOCK, BERNARD ....503 Hollywood Ave.,
                                San Antonio, Tex.
BURKE, RICHARD M. ....Clinton
CUNNINGHAM, C. B. ....Clinton
CUSHMAN, H. R. ....Clinton
DEPUTY, ROSS ....Clinton
DOLER, C. ....Clinton
ENGLEMAN, C. C. ....Clinton

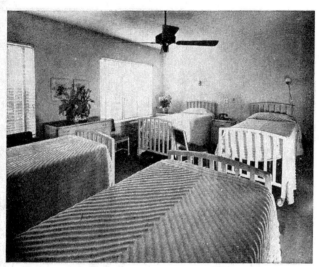

FRIZZELL, J. T. ....Clinton
GAEDE, D. ....Weatherford
GOSSOM, K. D. ....Clinton
*HINSHAW, J. R. ....Butler
*KENNEDY, LOUIS ....Clinton
LAMB, ELLIS ....Clinton
*LINGENFELTER, PAUL B. ....San Luis Obispo, Cal.
McBURNEY, C. H. ....Clinton
MILLER, E. A. ....Bagdad Copper Corp.,
                                           Hillside, Ariz.
*PAULSON, ALVIN W. ....Randolph Field, Tex.
ROGERS, McLAIN ....Clinton
RUHL, N. E. ....Weatherford
STOLL, A. A. ....Clinton
TISDAL, WILLIAM C. ....Clinton
VIEREGG, F. R. ....Clinton
*WILLIAMS, GORDON ....Army Aircraft School,
                                         Amarillo, Tex.
WOOD, J. GUILD ....Weatherford

DELAWARE

WALKER, C. F. ....Grove
    (member Craig Co. Medical Society)

DEWEY

LOYD, E. M. ....Taloga
    (member Custer Co. Medical Society)
MABRY, W. L. ....Leedey
    (member Beckham Co. Medical Society)
SEBA, W. E. ....Leedey
    (member Beckham Co. Medical Society)
VINCENT, DUKE W. Vici
    (member Woodward Co. Medical Society)

ELLIS

BEAM, J. P. ....Arnett
    (member Woodward Co. Medical Society)
DUBE, PAUL H. ....Shattuck
    (member Woodward Co. Medical Society)
*NEWMAN, FLOYD ....San Luis Obispo, Cal.
    (member Woodward Co. Medical Society)
NEWMAN, M. HASKELL ....Shattuck
    (member Woodward Co. Medical Society)
NEWMAN, O. C. ....Shattuck
    (member Woodward Co. Medical Society)
NEWMAN, ROY ....Shattuck
    (member Woodward Co. Medical Society)
SHANNON, HUGH R. ....Arnett
    (member Beckham Co. Medical Society)

GARFIELD

*BAKER, R. C. ....Camp Barkeley,
                                   Abilene, Texas
CHAMPLIN, PAUL B. ....Enid
*CORDONNIER, BYRON J. ....Enid
DUFFY, FRANCIS M. ....Enid
FEILD, JULIAN ....Enid
HAMBLE, V. R. ....Enid
HARRIS, D. S. ....Drummond
*HINSON, BRUCE R. ....Enid
HOPKINS, P. W. ....Enid
HUDSON, F. A. ....Enid
HUDSON, HARRY H. ....Enid
McEVOY, S. H. ....Enid
MERCER, WENDELL J. ....Enid
METSCHER, ALFRED J. ....Enid
*NEILSON, W. P. ....Enid
NEWELL, W. B., JR. ....Enid
NEWELL, W. B., SR. ....Enid
REMPEL, PAUL H. ....Enid
RHODES, W. H. ....Enid
ROBERTS, D. D. ....Ft. Bliss, Tex.
*ROSS, GEORGE ....Ft. Bliss, Tex.
ROSS, HOPE ....Enid
SHEETS, MARION E. ....Enid
*TALLEY, EVANS E. ....San Luis Obispo, Cal.
VANDEVER, H. F. ....Enid
WALKER, JOHN R. ....Enid
WATSON, JOHN M. ....Enid
WILKINS, A. E. ....Covington
WILSON, GEORGE S. ....Enid

GARVIN

ALEXANDER, ROBERT M. ....Paoli
CALLAWAY, JOHN R. ....Pauls Valley
GREENING, WILLIAM P. ....Pauls Valley
GROSS, T. F. ....Lindsay
JOHNSON, GALVIN L. ....Pauls Valley
*LINDSEY, RAY H. ....San Luis Obispo, Cal.
MONROE, HUGH H. ....Pauls Valley
PRATT, CHARLES M. ....Lindsay
ROBBERSON, MARVIN E. ....Wynnewood
ROBBERSON, MORTON E. ....Wynnewood
SHI, AUGUSTIN H. ....Stratford
SHIRLEY, EDWARD T. ....Pauls Valley
SULLIVAN, CLEVE L. ....Elmore City
WILSON, H. P. (honorary) ....Wynnewood

GRADY

*BAZE, ROY E. ....Chickasha
BAZE, WALTER J. ....Chickasha
BONNELL, W. L. ....Chickasha
BOON, U. C. ....Chickasha
BYNUM, W. TURNER ....Chickasha
COOK, W. H. ....Chickasha
DOWNEY, D. S. ....Chickasha
EMANUEL, LEWIS E. ....Chickasha
EMANUEL, ROY E. ....Chickasha
HENNING, A. E. ....Tuttle
JOYCE, FRANK T. ....Chickasha
LARKIN, H. W. ....Minco
    (member Logan Co. Medical Society)
LEEDS, A. B. ....Chickasha
LITTLE, AARON C. ....Minco
LIVERMORE, W. H. (honorary) ....Chickasha
MASON, REBECCA H. ....Chickasha
McCLURE, H. M. ....Chickasha
MITCHELL, C. P. ....Chickasha
PYLE, OSCAR S. ....Chickasha
RENEGAR, J. F. ....Tuttle
SCHUBERT, H. A. ....Chickasha
WOODS, LEWIS E. ....Chickasha

GRANT

HARDY, I. V. ....Medford
LAWSON, E. E. ....Medford
LIVELY, S. A. ....Wakita

GREER

CHERRY, G. P. (honorary) ....Mangum
HARP, ROBERT F. ....Mangum
HOLLIS, J. B. ....Mangum
LANSDEN, J. B. ....Granite
LEWIS, R. W. ....Granite
LOWE, J. T. ....Mangum
PEARSON, LEE E. ....Mangum
POER, E. M. ....Mangum
RUDE, JOE C. ....Duke Hospital,
                                 Durham, N. C.

HARMON

HOLLIS, L. E. ....Hollis
HOPKINS, S. W. ....Hollis
HUSBAND, W. G. ....Hollis
LYNCH, R. H. ....Hollis
RAY, W. T. (honorary) ....Gould
STREET, O. J. ....Gould
YEARGAN, W. M. ....Hollis

HARPER

CAMP, EARL (honorary) ....Buffalo
    (member Woodward Co. Medical Society)
HILL, H. K. ....Laverne
    (member Woodward Co. Medical Society)
*PIERSON, DWIGHT ....Buffalo
    (member Woodward Co. Medical Society)
WALKER, HARDIN ....Buffalo
    (member Woodward Co. Medical Society)
WINCHELL, F. Z. ....Buffalo
    (member Woodward Co. Medical Society)

HASKELL

CARSON, WILLIAM S. ....Keota
RUMLEY, J. C. ....Stigler
THOMPSON, W. A. ....Stigler
WILLIAMS, N. K. ....McCurtain

HUGHES

DAVENPORT, A. L. ....Holdenville

FLOYD, W. E. ...._Holdenville_
GEORGE, L. J. ...._Stuart_
   (member Pittsburg Co. Medical Society)
HAMILTON, S. H. ...._Non_
HICKS, C. A. ...._Holdenville_
HOWELL, H. A. ...._Holdenville_
KERNEK, PAUL ...._Holdenville_
LETT, L. M. ...._Dustin_
MAYFIELD, IMOGENE ...._Holdenville_
MUNAL, JOHN ...._Holdenville_
PRYOR, V. W. ...._Holdenville_
TAYLOR, W. L. ...._Holdenville_
WALLACE, C. S. ...._Holdenville_

JACKSON

ABERNETHY, E. A. ...._Altus_
ALLGOOD, J. M. ...._Altus_
BERRY, THOMAS M. ...._El Dorado_
CROW, E. S. ...._Olustee_
FOX, R. H. ...._Altus_
*HOLT, WILLARD D. ......_Station Hosp., Brooks Field, San Antonio, Texas_
MABRY, E. W. ...._Altus_
McCONNELL, L. H. ...._Altus_
MEREDITH, J. S. ...._Duke_
   (member Greer Co. Medical Society)
REID, JOHN R. ...._Altus_
SPEARS, C. G. ...._Altus_
STULTS, J. S. (honorary) ...._Altus_
TAYLOR, R. Z. ...._Blair_

JEFFERSON

ANDRESKOWSKI, W. T. ...._Ryan_
BOBBITT, F. S. ...._Ringling_
BROWNING, W. M. ...._Waurika_
COLLINS, D. B. ...._Waurika_
DERR, J. I. ...._Waurika_
DILLARD, J. A. ...._Waurika_
EDWARDS, F. M. ...._Ringling_
HOLLINGSWORTH, J. I. ...._Waurika_
MAUPIN, C. M. ...._Waurika_
WADE, L. L. ...._Ryan_

JOHNSTON

RAINS, S. W. ...._Wapanucka_
   (member Bryan Co. Medical Society)

KAY

ARMSTRONG, W. O. ...._Ponca City_
ARRENDELL, C. W. ...._Ponca City_
BEATTY, J. H. ...._Tonkawa_
BECKER, L. H. ...._Blackwell_
CLIFT, MERL ...._Blackwell_
CURRY, JOHN R. ...._Blackwell_
GARDNER, C. C. ...._Ponca City_
GHORMLEY, J. G. ...._Blackwell_
GIBSON, R. B. ...._Ponca City_
*GORDON, D. M. ...._Ponca City_
GOWEY, H. O. ...._Newkirk_
HARMS, EDWIN M. ...._Blackwell_
HOWE, J. H. ...._Ponca City_
KINSINGER, R. R. ...._Blackwell_
KREGER, G. S. ...._Tonkawa_
MALL, W. W. ...._Ponca City_
MATHEWS, DEWEY ...._Tonkawa_
McELROY, THOMAS ...._Ponca City_
MILLER, D. W. ...._Blackwell_
MOORE. G. C. ...._Ponca City_
MORGAN, L. S. ...._Ponca City_
NEAL, L. G. ...._Ponca City_
NIEMANN, G. H. ...._Ponca City_
NORTHCUTT, C. E. ...._Ponca City_
NUCKOLS, A. S. ...._Ponca City_
RISSER, A. S. ...._Blackwell_
VANCE, L. C. ...._Ponca City_
WAGGONER, E. E. ...._Tonkawa_
WAGNER, J. C. ...._Ponca City_
WALKER, I. D. ...._Tonkawa_
WHITE, M. S. ...._Blackwell_
WRIGHT, L. I. ...._Blackwell_
YEARY, G. H. ...._Newkirk_

KINGFISHER

ANGLIN, J. E. ...._Dover_
DIXON, A. ...._Hennessey_

GOSE, C. O. ...._Hennessey_
HODGSON, C. M. ...._Kingfisher_
*LATTIMORE, F. C. ......_Co. C, 30th Med. Tng. Bn., Camp Grant, Ill._
MEREDITH, A. O. ...._Kingfisher_
PENDLETON, JOHN W. ...._Kingfisher_
STURGEON, H. VIOLET ...._Kingfisher_
*TAYLOR, JOHN R. ......_Will Rogers Field, Oklahoma City_
TOWNSEND, B. I. ...._Hennessey_

KIOWA

BONHAM, J. M. ...._Hobart_
BRAUN, J. P. ...._Hobart_
FINCH, J. WILLIAM ...._Hobart_
HATHAWAY, A. H. ...._Mountain View_
MOORE, J. H. ...._Hobart_
WALKER, F. E. ...._Lone Wolf_
WATKINS, B. H. ...._Hobart_

LATIMER

CALLAHAN, J. S. ...._Wilburton_
   (member Pittsburg Co. Medical Society)
HARRIS, J. M. ...._Wilburton_
   (member Pittsburg Co. Medical Society)

LeFLORE

BAKER, F. P. ...._Talihina_
BEVILL, S. D. ...._Poteau_
BOOTH, G. R. ...._LeFlore_
COLLINS, E. L. ...._Panama_
DEAN, S. C. ...._Howe_
DORROUGH, J. ...._Monroe_
FAIR, E. N. ...._Heavener_
GILLIAM, WILLIAM C. ...._Spiro_
HENRY, M. L. ...._Heavener_
MINOR, R. W. ...._Spiro_
ROLLE, NEESON ...._Poteau_
SHIPPEY, W. L. ...._Fort Smith, Ark._
VAN CLEAVE, WILLIAM E. ...._Talihina_
WOODSON, E. M. ...._Poteau_
WRIGHT, R. L. ...._Poteau_

LINCOLN

ADAMS, J. W. ...._Chandler_
BAILEY, CARL H. ...._Stroud_
BROWN, F. C. ...._Sparks_
BROWN, R. A. ...._Prague_
   (member Pottawatomie Co. Medical Society)
BURLESON, NED ...._Prague_
DAVIS, W. B. ...._Stroud_
ERWIN, PARA ...._Wellston_
HURLBUT, E. F. ...._Meeker_
JENKINS, H. B. ...._Tryon_
MARSHALL, A. M. ...._Chandler_
NICKELL, U. E. ...._Davenport_
NORWOOD, F. H. ...._Prague_
ROBERTSON, C. W. ...._Chandler_
ROLLINS, J. S. ...._Prague_

LOGAN

ANDERSON, ROY W. ...._Guthrie_
BARKER, PAULINE ...._Guthrie_
CORNWELL, N. H. ...._Coyle_
GARDNER, P. B. ...._Guthrie_
GRAY, DAN ...._Guthrie_
HAHN, L. A. ...._Guthrie_
HILL, C. B. ...._Guthrie_
LEHEW, JOHN LESLIE, JR. ...._Guthrie_
MILLER, W. C. ...._Guthrie_
PETTY, C. S. ...._Guthrie_
*PETTY, JAMES S. ...._Guthrie_
RINGROSE, R. F. ...._Guthrie_
*RITZHAUPT, LOUIS H. ...._Guthrie_
ROGERS, C. L. ...._Marshall_
SOUTER, J. E. ...._Guthrie_

LOVE

LOONEY, M. D. ...._Marietta_
   (member Carter Co. Medical Society)

MAJOR

McCROSKIE, M. R. ...._Fairview_
   (member Garfield Co. Medical Society)
RYAN, ROBERT O. ...._Fairview_
   (member Garfield Co. Medical Society)

SPECHT, ELSIE ....*Fairview*
   (member Garfield Co. Medical Society)

MARSHALL

COOK, ODIS A. ....*Madill*
HOLLAND, JOHN LEE ....*Madill*
YORK, JOSEPH FERRELL ....*Madill*

MAYES

BAILEY, F. M. ....*Chouteau*
   (member Oklahoma Co. Medical Ass'n)
CAMERON, PAUL B. ....*Pryor*
HERRINGTON, V. D. ....*Pryor*
JOHNSON, WILLIAM P. ....*Pryor*
MORROW, B. L. ....*Salina*
RUTHERFORD, S. C. ....*Locust Grove*
SMITH, R. V. ....*Pryor*
WERLING, E. H. ....*Pryor*
WHITAKER, W. J. ....4057 Arts St., New Orleans, La.
WHITE, L. C. ....*Adair*

McCLAIN

BARGER, G. S. ....*Purcell*
DAVIS, S. C. ....*Blanchard*
DAWSON, O. O. ....*Wayne*
KOLB, I. N. ....*Blanchard*
McCURDY, W. C., JR. ....*Purcell*
McCURDY, W. C., SR. ....*Purcell*
ROYSTER, R. L. ....*Purcell*
SLOVER, BENJAMIN W. ....*Blanchard*
WOOD, W. M. ....*Purcell*

McCURTAIN

BARKER, N. L. ....*Broken Bow*
CLARKSON, A. W. ....*Valliant*
McCASKILL, W. B. ....*Idabel*
MORELAND, J. T. ....*Idabel*
MORELAND, W. A. ....*Idabel*
OLIVER, R. B. ....*Idabel*
SHERRILL, R. H. ....*Broken Bow*
WILLIAMS, R. D. ....*Idabel*
WILLIAMS, W. W. ....*Idabel*

McINTOSH

FIRST, F. R. ....*Checotah*
JACOBS, LUSTER I. ....*Hanna*
LITTLE, DANIEL E. ....*Eufaula*
STONER, RAYMOND W. ....*Checotah*
TOLLESON, WILLIAM A. ....*Eufaula*
WOOD, JAMES L. ....*Eufaula*

MURRAY

ANNADOWN, P. V. ....*Sulphur*
BALL, ERNEST ....*Sulphur*
BROWN, BYRON B. ....*Davis*
DeLAY, W. D. ....*Sulphur*
MORTON, RALPH ....*Sulphur*
POWELL, W. H. ....*Sulphur*
SADLER, F. E. ....*Sulphur*
SLOVER, GEORGE W. ....*Sulphur*
WRENN, JOHN ....*Sulphur*
   (member Pontotoc Co. Medical Society)

MUSKOGEE

BALLANTINE, H. T. ....*Muskogee*
BRUTON, L. D. ....*Muskogee*
COACHMAN, E. H. ....*Muskogee*
DORWART, F. G. ....*Muskogee*
EARNEST, A. N. ....*Muskogee*
ELKINS, MARVIN ....*Muskogee*
EWING, FINIS W. ....*Muskogee*
FITE, E. H. ....*Muskogee*
FITE, W. P. ....*Muskogee*
FULLENWIDER, C. M. ....*Muskogee*
HAMM, SILAS G. ....*Haskell*
*HOLCOMBE, R. N. ....64th Med. Regt.,
                    Camp Bowie, Tex.
KLASS, O. C. ....*Muskogee*
KUPKA, JOHN F. ....*Haskell*
McALISTER, L. S. ....*Muskogee*
McINNIS, J. T. ....*Muskogee*
MILLER, D. EVELYN ....*Muskogee*
MITCHELL, R. L. ....*Muskogee*
   (member Craig Co. Medical Society)
MOBLEY, A. L. ....*Albuquerque, N. M.*

MOLLICA, STEPHEN G. ....*Muskogee*
NEELY, SHADE D. ....*Muskogee*
NICHOLS, J. T. ....*Muskogee*
OLDHAM, I. R. ....*Muskogee*
RAFTER, JOHN R. ....*Muskogee*
REYNOLDS, JOHN ....*Muskogee*
*REYNOLDS, JOHN H. ....*Muskogee*
SANDERS, H. U. ....*Muskogee*
SCHNOEBELEN, RENE E. ....*Muskogee*
SCOTT, H. A. ....*Muskogee*
THOMPSON, M. K. ....*Muskogee*
WALKER, JOHN H. ....*Muskogee*
WARTERFIELD, F. E. ....*Muskogee*
WHITE, CHARLES ED ....*Muskogee*
WHITE, J. HUTCHINGS ....*Muskogee*
*WOLFE, I. C. ....180th Inf., Ft. Sill
WORD, HARLAN L. ....*Muskogee*
*WOODBURN, J. TINDER ....*Muskogee*
ZELDES, MARY ....*Muskogee*

NOBLE

COLDIRON, D. F. ....*Perry*
COOKE, C. H. ....*Perry*
DRIVER, JESSE W. ....*Perry*
EVANS, A. M. ....*Perry*
FRANCIS, J. W. ....*Perry*
HEISS, J. E. ....*Perry* .
RENFROW, T. F. ....*Billings*
WIGNER, R. H. ....*Marland*

NOWATA

DAVIS, KIEFFER D. ....*Nowata*
KURTZ, R. L. ....*Nowata*
LANG, S. A. ....*Nowata*
ROBERTS, S. P. ....*Nowata*
SCOTT, M. B. ....*Delaware*

OKFUSKEE

BOMBARGER, C. O. ....*Paden*
BRICE, M. O. ....*Okemah*
COCHRAN, C. M. ....*Okemah*
JENKINS, W. P. ....*Okemah*
LUCAS, A. C. ....*Castle*
MELTON, A. S. ....*Okemah*
PEMBERTON, J. M. ....*Okemah*
PRESTON, J. R. ....*Weleetka*
SPICKARD, L. J. ....*Okemah*
WHITNEY, M. L. ....*Okemah*

OKLAHOMA

ADAMS, ROBERT H. ....515 N. W. 11th St.
AKIN, ROBERT H. ....400 N. W. 10th St.
ALFORD, J. M. ....Medical Arts Bldg.
ALLEN, E. P. ....1200 N. Walker
ALLEN, GEORGE T. ....1200 N. Walker
ANDREWS, LEILA E. ....1200 N. Walker
APPLETON, M. M. ....400 N. W. 10th St.
*BAILEY, W. H. ....Station Hospital, Ft. Sill
BAIRD, W. D., JR. ....210½ W. Commerce St.
BAKER, MARGUERITE M. ....1104 N. E. 63rd St.
BALYEAT, RAY M. ....1200 N. Walker
BARB, T. J. ....318 S. W. 25th St.
BARKER, C. E. ....1200 N. Walker
BARRY, GEORGE N. ....Medical Arts Bldg.
BATCHELOR, JOHN J. ....Medical Arts Bldg.
BATTENFIELD, JOHN Y. ....State Health Dept.
BAUM, E. ELDON ....Perrine Bldg.
BEDNAR, GERALD ....Medical Arts Bldg.
*BELL, AUSTIN H. ....San Luis Obispo, Cal.
BELL, J. T. ....State Health Dept.
BERRY, CHARLES N. ....Medical Arts Bldg.
BINDER, HAROLD J. ....628 N. W. 21st St.
BINKLEY, J. G. ....Medical Arts Bldg.
BOATRIGHT, LLOYD C. ....Perrine Bldg.
BOGGS, NATHAN ....Perrine Bldg.
*BOLEND, REX ....24th Evacuation Unit,
                    Camp Rucker, Ala.
BONDURANT, C. P. ....Medical Arts Bldg.
BONHAM, WILLIAM L. ....Medical Arts Bldg.
BORDER, CLINTON L. ....American Nat'l Bldg.
BORDER, FOWLER ....330 N. W. 10th St.
   (member Greer Co. Medical Society)
*BORECKY, GEORGE I. ....Barksdale Field, La.
BRADLEY, H. C. ....Perrine Bldg.

*BRANHAM, D. W. .... *U. S. N. R., San Diego Base Hospital, San Diego, Cal.*
BREWER, A. M. ....*Perrine Bldg.*
*BROWN, GERSTER W. ....*Naval Hospital, Charleston, S. C.*
BRUNDAGE, C. L. ....*1200 N. Walker*
BURTON, JOHN F. ....*1200 N. Walker*
BUTLER, H. W. ....*1200 N. Walker*
CAILEY, LEO F. ....*Medical Arts Bldg.*
CAMPBELL, COYNE H. ....*131 N. E. 4th St.*
CANNON, J. M. ....*210½ W. Commerce St.*
CATES, ALBERT M. (honorary) ......*2733 N. E. 20th St.*
CAVINESS, J. J. ....*Medical Arts Bldg.*
CHAFFIN, ZALE ....*Municipal Bldg.*
*CHARNEY, L. H. ....*Medical Arts Bldg.*
CLARK, ANSON L. ....*Medical Arts Bldg.*
*CLARK, JOHN V. ....*Camp Barkeley, Abilene, Tex.*
CLARK, LeMON ....*Medical Arts Bldg.*
CLARK, RALPH O. ....*1706 S.E. 29th St.*
CLOUDMAN, H. H. ....*Medical Arts Bldg.*
CLYMER, C. E. ....*Medical Arts Bldg.*
COLEY, A. J. (honorary) ....*Hightower Bldg.*
*COLEY, JOE H. ....*4086 Jackdaw St., San Diego, Cal.*
COLLINS, H. DALE ....*Medical Arts Bldg.*
COLONNA, PAUL C. ....*800 N. E. 13th St.*
COOPER, F. MAXEY ....*Medical Arts Bldg.*
COSTON, TULLOS O. ....*Medical Arts Bldg.*
COTTEN, DAISY V. H. ....*807 N. W. 23rd St.*
**DAILY, H. J. ....*Medical Arts Bldg.*
DANIELS, HARRY A. ....*610 N. W. 9th St.*
DeMAND, F. A. ....*1200 N. Walker*
DERSCH, WALTER H. ....*Medical Arts Bldg.*
DEUPREE, HARRY L. ....*Medical Arts Bldg.*
*DEVANNEY, LOUIS R. ....*Navy Recruiting Station, Oklahoma City*
DICKSON, GREEN K. ....*1200 N. Walker*
DOUDNA, HUBERT E. ....*800 N. E. 13th St.*
DOWDY, THOMAS W. ....*Medical Arts Bldg.*
EARLY, RALPH O. ....*Medical Arts Bldg.*
EASTLAND, WILLIAM E. ....*Medical Arts Bldg.*
*EMENHISER, LEE K. ....*1004 Gorgas Circle, Ft. Sam Houston, Tex.*
ERWIN, FRANTZ B. ....*Medical Arts Bldg.*
ESKRIDGE, J. B., JR. ....*1200 N. Walker*
FAGIN, HERMAN ....*Nat'l Aid Life Bldg.*
FARIS, BRUNEL D. ....*Medical Arts Bldg.*
FARNAM, LARRY M. ....*1200 N. Walker*
FELTS, GEORGE R. ....*625 N. W. 10th St.*
FERGUSON, E. GORDON ....*Medical Arts Bldg.*
FISHMAN, C. J. ....*132 N. W. 4th St.*
FLESHER, THOMAS H. ....*Edmond*
*FOERSTER, HERVEY A. ....*349th Engineer Regt., Camp Claiborne, La.*
*FORD, HARRY C. ....*Medical Arts Bldg.*
FRIERSON, S. E. ....*Medical Arts Bldg.*
FRYER, SAM R. ....*119 N. W. 5th St.*
*FULTON, C. C. ....*Marine Camp, West of San Diego, Cal.*
FULTON, GEORGE ....*American Nat'l Bldg.*
GALBRAITH, HUGH M. ....*First Nat'l Bldg.*
GALLAGHER, C. A. ....*610 N. W. 9th St.*
GARRISON, GEORGE H. ....*1200 N. Walker*
GEE, O. J. ....*Medical Arts Bldg.*
*GIBBS, ALLEN G. ....*San Luis Obispo, Cal.*
GINGLES, R. H. ....*State Health Dept.*
GLISMANN, M. B. ....*911 N. W. 23rd St.*
GLOMSET, JOHN L. ....*1200 N. Walker*
GOLDFAIN, E. ....*228 N. W. 13th St.*
GOODWIN, R. Q. ....*Medical Arts Bldg.*
GRAHAM, A. T. ....*26 S. W. 25th St.*
HACKLER, JOHN F. ....*State Health Dept.*
HALL, CLARK H. ....*Medical Arts Bldg.*
HAMMONDS, O. O. ....*623 N. E. 18th St.*
HARBISON, FRANK ....*510 N. W. 12th St.*
HARBISON, J. E. ....*510 N. W. 12th St.*
HARRIS, HENRY W. ....*1200 N. Walker*
HASKETT, PAUL E. ....*Hales Bldg.*
HASSLER, F. R. ....*State Health Dept.*
(member Pottawatomie Co. Medical Society)
**Died, April 26, 1942.

HASSLER, GRACE C. ....*Medical Arts Bldg.*
HAYES, BASIL A. ....*625 N. W. 10th St.*
*HAZEL, ONIS G. ....*Tampa, Fla.*
HEATLEY, JOHN E. ....*Medical Arts Bldg.*
*HERRMANN, JESS D. ....*San Luis Obispo, Cal.*
HETHERINGTON, A. J. ....*2014 Gatewood*
HICKS, FRED B. ....*Medical Arts Bldg.*
HIGHLAND, J. E. ....*610 N. W. 9th St.*
HIRSHFIELD, A. C. ....*Medical Arts Bldg.*
*HOLLINGSWORTH, C. EDWARD ....*Ft. Richardson, Anchorage, Alaska*
*HOOD, F. REDDING ....*LeGarde General Hospital, New Orleans, La.*
HOWARD, R. M. ....*1200 N. Walker*
HUGGINS, J. R. ....*2225 Exchange Ave.*
HULL, WAYNE M. ....*1200 N. Walker*
HUNTER, GEORGE ....*County Court House*
HYROOP, GILBERT L. ....*Medical Arts Bldg.*
*ISHMAEL, WILLIAM K. ....*Will Rogers Field, Oklahoma City*
JACKSON, A. R. ....*2528½ S. Robinson*
JACOBS, MINARD F. ....*Medical Arts Bldg.*
JANCO, LEON ....*10 West Park*
JETER, HUGH ....*1200 N. Walker*
JOBE, VIRGIL R. ....*400 N. W. 10th St.*
JONES, HUGH ....*Medical Arts Bldg.*
KELLEAM, E. A. ....*125 S. W. 42nd St.*
(member LeFlore Co. Medical Society)
KELLER, W. F. ....*Medical Arts Bldg.*
KELSO, JOSEPH W. ....*Medical Arts Bldg.*
KELTZ, BERT F. ....*Medical Arts Bldg.*
KERNODLE, STRATTON E. ....*First Nat'l Bldg.*
*KIMBALL, GEORGE H. ....*San Luis Obispo, Cal.*
*KUHN, JOHN F., JR. ....*San Luis Obispo, Cal.*
**KUHN, JOHN F., SR. ....*Medical Arts Bldg.*
LACHMAN, ERNEST, ...*801 N. E. 13th St.*
LAIN, E. S. ....*Medical Arts Bldg.*
LAMB, JOHN H. ....*Medical Arts Bldg.*
LAMBKE, PHIL M. ....*105 N. W. 23rd St.*
LaMOTTE, GEORGE A. ....*Colcord Bldg.*
LANGSTON, WANN ....*Medical Arts Bldg.*
*LEMON, CECIL W. ....*San Luis Obispo, Cal.*
LENEY, FANNIE LOU ....*400 N. W. 10th St.*
LEONARD, C. E. ....*181 N. E. 4th St.*
LEVY, BERTHA M. ....*1200 N. Walker*
LEWIS, A. R. ....*Hightower Bldg.*
*LINDSTORM, W. C. ....*82nd Inf. Div., Camp Claiborne, La.*
LINGENFELTER, F. M. ....*1200 N. Walker*
LITTLE, JOHN R. ....*Ramsey Tower*
LONG, LeROY D. ....*Medical Arts Bldg.*
LONG, WENDELL ....*Medical Arts Bldg.*
LOVE, R. S. ....*Perrine Bldg.*
LOWRY, TOM ....*1200 N. Walker*
LOY, C. F. ....*400 N. W. 10th St.*
LUTON, JAMES P. ....*Medical Arts Bldg.*
LYON, JAMES I. ....*Edmond*
MacDONALD, J. C. ....*301 N. W. 12th St.*
MARGO, ELIAS ....*605 N. W. 10th St.*
*MARTIN, HOWARD C. ....*Station Hospital, Ft. Sill*
MARTIN, J. T. ....*1200 N. Walker*
MASTERSON, MAUDE M. ....*Medical Arts Bldg.*
MATHEWS, GRADY F. ....*State Health Dept.*
(member Cherokee Co. Medical Society)
*MATTHEWS, SANFORD ....*Army Aircraft School, Amarillo, Tex.*
McBRIDE, EARL D. ....*605 N. W. 10th St.*
*McCLURE, WILLIAM C. ....*Naval Dispensary, Long Beach, Cal.*
McGEE, J. P. ....*1200 N. Walker*
McHENRY, L. C. ....*Medical Arts Bldg.*
McKINNEY, MILAM F. ....*Medical Arts Bldg.*
McLAUCHLIN, J. R. ....*Plaza Court Bldg.*
McNEILL, P. M. ....*Medical Arts Bldg.*
MECHLING, GEORGE S. ....*1200 N. Walker*
MESSENBAUGH, J. F. ....*Colcord Bldg.*
MESSINGER, R. P. ....*807 N. W. 23rd St.*
*MILES, W. H. ....*Camp Barkeley, Abilene, Texas*
**Died, February 13, 1942.

*MILLER, NESBITT L. ...._Division Surgeon, A.P.O._
No. 45, c/o Postmaster, New York City
MILLS, R. C. ...._Hightower Bldg._
MOOR, H. D. ....800 _N. E._ 13th St.
MOORE, B. H. ...._Perrine Bldg._
MOORE, C. D. ...._Perrine Bldg._
MOORE, ELLIS ...._Medical Arts Bldg._
MOORMAN, FLOYD ....1200 _N. Walker_
MOORMAN, LEWIS J. ....1200 _N. Walker_
MORGAN, C. A. ...._First Nat'l Bldg._
MORLEDGE, WALKER ....1200 _N. Walker_
MORRISON, H. C. ....807 _N. W._ 23rd St.
MORROW, J. A. ....510½ _N. W._ 19th St.
(_member Sequoyah Co. Medical Society_)
*MULVEY, BERT E. ...._San Luis Obispo, Cal._
MURDOCH, L. H. ...._Medical Arts Bldg._
(_member Blaine Co. Medical Society_)
MURDOCH, RAYMOND L. ...._Medical Arts Bldg._
MUSICK, E. R. ...._Medical Arts Bldg._
MUSICK, V. H. ...._Medical Arts Bldg._
MUSSIL, W. M. ...._Medical Arts Bldg._
MYERS, RALPH E. ....1200 _N. Walker_
*NAGLE, PATRICK S. ...._Fitzsimmons, Denver, Colo._
*NEEL, ROY L. ...._Medical Arts Bldg._
NICHOLSON, BEN H. ....301 _N. W._ 12th St.
*NOELL, ROBERT L. ...._San Luis Obispo, Cal._
O'DONOGHUE, D. H. ...._Medical Arts Bldg._
O'LEARY, CHARLES M. ...._Medical Arts Bldg._
PARRISH, J. M., JR. ....1200 _N. Walker_
PATTERSON, ROBERT U. ....700 _N. W._ 18th St.
PAULUS, D. D. ....301 _N. W._ 12th St.
PAYTE, J. I. ....2429 _Aurora Court_
PENICK, GRIDER ...._Colcord Bldg._
PHELPS, A. S. ...._Medical Arts Bldg._
PINE, JOHN S. ...._Medical Arts Bldg._
POSTELLE, J. M. ...._Medical Arts Bldg._
POUNDERS, CARROLL M. ....1200 _N. Walker_
PRICE, JOEL S. ....1200 _N. Walker_
PUCKETT, CARL ....22 _West_ 6th St.
(_member Mayes Co. Medical Society_)
RANDEL, HARVEY O. ...._Medical Arts Bldg._
RECK, JOHN A. ...._Colcord Bldg._
*RECORDS, J. W. ...._Ft. Bliss, Tex._
REED, HORACE ....1200 _N. Walker_
REED, JAMES R. ...._Medical Arts Bldg._
REEVES, C. L. ....400 _N. W._ 10th St.
REICHMANN, RUTH S. ....124 _N. W._ 15th St.
*RICKS, J. R. ...._Camp Correa,_
Balboa, Canal Zone
RIELY, LEA A. ...._Medical Arts Bldg._
RILEY, J. W. ....119 _N. W._ 5th St.
ROBINSON, J. H. ....301 _N. W._ 12th St.
RODDY, JOHN A. ...._Ramsey Tower_
ROGERS, GERALD ....1200 _N. Walker_
ROSENBERGER, F. E. ...._Perrine Bldg._
ROUNTREE, C. R. ....1200 _N. Walker_
*RUCKS, W. W., JR. ...._San Luis Obispo, Cal._
RUCKS, W. W., SR. ....301 _N. W._ 12th St.
*SADLER, LeROY H. ...._Brownwood, Tex._
SALOMON, A. L. ....1200 _N. Walker_
*SANGER, F. A. ....64th _Med. Regt.,_
Camp Bowie, Tex.
SANGER, F. M. ...._Key Bldg._
SANGER, WINNIE M. ...._Key Bldg._
*SANGER, W. W. ...._Station Hospital, Ft. Sill_
*SEBA, CHESTER R. ...._San Luis Obispo, Cal._
SELL, L. STANLEY ...._Medical Arts Bldg._
SERWER, MILTON J. ....1200 _N. Walker_
*SEWELL, DAN R. ...._Army Air Base,_
Albuquerque, N. M.
SHACKELFORD, JOHN W............._State Health Dept._
SHAVER, S. R. ...._Medical Arts Bldg._
(_member Garfield Co. Medical Society_)
SHELTON, J. W. ...._Hightower Bldg._
SHEPPARD, MARY S. ....1200 _N. Walker_
SHIRCLIFF, E. E., JR. ....128 _N. W._ 14th St.
*SHORBE, HOWARD B. ...._Station Hospital, Ft. Sill_
*SMITH, CHARLES A. ...._Ft. Huachuca, Ariz._
SMITH, DELBERT G. ...._First Nat'l Bldg._
SMITH, EDWARD N. ....400 _N. W._ 10th St.
SMITH, RALPH A. ....443½ _N. W._ 23rd St.

SNOW, J. B. ....1200 _N. Walker_
STANBRO, GREGORY E. ...._Medical Arts Bldg._
STARK, W. W. ....829 _N. W._ 25th St.
(_member Okmulgee Co. Medical Society_)
STARRY, L. J. ....1200 _N. Walker_
STILLWELL, R. J. ...._American Nat'l Bldg._
**STONE, S. N. ...._Edmond_
STOUT, MARVIN E. ....209 _N. W._ 13th St.
*STRECKER, WILLIAM E. ...._Camp Wolters, Tex._
SULLIVAN, ELIJAH S. ...._Medical Arts Bldg._
TABOR, GEORGE R. (_honorary_) ...._First Nat'l Bldg._
TAYLOR, CHARLES B. ...._Medical Arts Bldg._
*TAYLOR, JIM M ...._San Luis Obispo, Cal._
TAYLOR, WILLIAM M. ....625 _N. W._ 10th St.
THOMPSON, WAYMAN J. ....1200 _N. Walker_
*TOOL, DONOVAN ...._Camp Gruber, Okla._
TOWNSEND, CARY W. ...._Medical Arts Bldg._
TRENT, ROBERT I. ...._Medical Arts Bldg._
TURNER, HENRY H. ....1200 _N. Walker_
*VALBERG, E. R. ...._Sheppard Field,_
Wichita Falls, Tex.
VON WEDEL, CURT ....610 _N. W._ 9th St.
WAILS, T. G. ...._Medical Arts Bldg._
*WAINWRIGHT, TOM L. ...._Medical Arts Bldg._
*WATSON, I. NEWTON ...._Sheppard Field,_
Wichita Falls, Tex.
WATSON, O. ALTON ....1200 _N. Walker_
WATSON, R. D. ...._Britton_
WEIR, MARSHALL W. ...._Ramsey Tower_
WELLS, EVA ...._Medical Arts Bldg._
WELLS, LOIS LYON ....800 _N. E._ 13th St.
WELLS, W. W. ...._Medical Arts Bldg._
WEST, W. K. ....1200 _N. Walker_
WESTFALL, L. M. ...._Medical Arts Bldg._
WHITE, ARTHUR W. ...._Medical Arts Bldg._
WHITE, OSCAR R. ....1200 _N. Walker_
WHITE, PHIL E. ...._Perrine Bldg._
*WILDMAN, S. F. ...._Camp Wolters, Tex._
WILKINS, HARRY ...._Medical Arts Bldg._
WILLIAMSON, SAM H. ...._Jones_
WILLIAMSON, W. H. ....128 _N. W._ 14th St.
WILLIE, JAMES A. ...._Medical Arts Bldg._
WILSON, KENNETH J. ...._Medical Arts Bldg._
WITTEN, HAROLD B. ...._Harrah_
*WOLFF, JOHN POWERS ...._San Luis Obispo, Cal._
WOODWARD, NEIL W. ....1200 _N. Walker_
WRIGHT, HARPER ....318 _S. W._ 25th St.
YOUNG, A. M., III ...._Medical Arts Bldg._
**_Died, April 16, 1942._

OKMULGEE

BOLLINGER, I. W. ...._Henryetta_
BOSWELL, H. D. ...._Henryetta_
CARLOSS, T. C. ...._Morris_
CARNELL, M. D. ...._Okmulgee_
COTTERAL, J. R. ...._Henryetta_
EDWARDS, J. G. ...._Okmulgee_
HOLMES, A. R. ...._Henryetta_
HUDSON, W. S. ...._Okmulgee_
KILPATRICK, G. A. ...._Henryetta_
LESLIE, S. B. ...._Okmulgee_
MABEN, CHARLES S. ...._Okmulgee_
MATHENEY, J. C. ...._Okmulgee_
McKINNEY, G. Y. ...._Henryetta_
MING, C. M. ...._Okmulgee_
MITCHENER, W. C. ...._Okmulgee_
RAINS, HUGH L. ...._Okmulgee_
RODDA, E. D. ...._Okmulgee_
SIMPSON, N. N. ...._Henryetta_
TRACEWELL, GEORGE L. ...._Okmulgee_
VERNON, W. C. ...._Okmulgee_
WATSON, F. S. ...._Okmulgee_

OSAGE

AARON, WILLIAM H. ...._Pawhuska_
ALEXANDER, E. T. ...._Barnsdall_
BAYLOR, RICHARD A. ...._Fairfax_
DOZIER, BARCLAY E. ...._Shidler_
GUILD, CARL H. ...._Shidler_
HEMPHILL, GEORGE K. ...._Pawhuska_
*HEMPHILL, PAUL H. ....120th _Med.Bn., A.P.O. No. 45,_
c/o Postmaster, New York City
KARASEK, MATTHEW ...._Shidler_

KEYES, E. C. _____Shidler
LIPE, EVERETT N. _____Fairfax
SMITH, RAYMOND O. _____Hominy
SULLIVAN, B. F. _____Barnsdall
WALKER, G. I. _____Hominy
WALKER, ROSCOE _____Pawhuska
WEIRICH, COLIN REID _____Pawhuska
WILLIAMS, CLAUDE W. _____Pawhuska
WORTEN, DIVONIS _____Pawhuska

OTTAWA

*AISENSTADT, E. ALBERT _____Ft. Jay,
Governor's Island, N. Y.
BARRY, J. R. _____Picher
*BISHOP, CALMES _____Palacias, Tex.
CANNON, R. F. _____Miami
CHESNUT, W. G. _____Miami
COLVERT, GEORGE W. _____Miami
CONNELL, M. A. _____Picher
CRAIG, J. W. _____Miami
CUNNINGHAM, P. J. _____Miami
DeARMAN, M. M. _____Miami
DeTAR, GEORGE A. _____Miami
HAMPTON, J. B. _____Commerce
HETHERINGTON, L. P. _____Miami
HUGHES, A. R. _____Miami
JACOBY, J. SHERWOOD _____Commerce
KERR, WALTER C. H. _____Picher
McNAUGHTON, G. P. _____Miami
MURRY, A. V. _____Picher
PRATT, T. W. _____Miami
RALSTON, BENJAMIN W. _____Commerce
RUSSELL, RICHARD _____Picher
SANGER, WALTER B. _____Picher
SAYLES, W. JACKSON _____Miami
SHELTON, B. WRIGHT _____Miami
SIEVER, CHARLES W. _____Picher
STAPLES, J. H. L. _____Afton
WORMINGTON, F. L. _____Miami

PAWNEE

BARBER, L. C. _____Ralston
BROWNING, R. L. _____Pawnee
HADDOX, CHARLES H. _____Pawnee
JONES, R. E. _____Pawnee
LeHEW, J. L. _____Pawnee
ROBINSON, E. T. _____Cleveland
SADDORIS, M. L. _____Cleveland
SPAULDING, H. B. _____Ralston

PAYNE

BASSETT, CLIFFORD M. _____Cushing
*DAVIDSON, W. N. _____Hdqs. 3rd Army,
San Antonio, Tex.
DAVIS, BENJAMIN _____Cushing
FRIEDEMANN, PAUL W. _____Stillwater
*FRY, POWELL E. _____Stillwater
LEATHEROCK, R. E. _____Cushing
MANNING, H. O. _____Cushing
MARTIN, E. O. _____Cushing
MARTIN, JAMES D. _____Cushing
MARTIN, JOHN F. _____Stillwater
MARTIN, JOHN W. _____Cushing
MITCHELL, L. A. _____Stillwater
MOORE, CLIFFORD W. _____Stillwater
OEHLSCHLAGER, F. KEITH _____Yale
PUCKETT, HOWARD L. _____Stillwater
RICHARDSON, P. M. _____Cushing
ROBERTS, R. E. _____Stillwater
SEXTON, C. E. (honorary) _____Stillwater
SILVERTHORN, LOUIS E. _____Stillwater
SMITH, A. B. _____Stillwater
SMITH, HASKELL _____Stillwater
THOMPSON, W. C. _____Stillwater
WAGGONER, ROY E. _____Stillwater
*WILHITE, L. R. _____Medical Recruiting Board,
Oklahoma City

PITTSBURG

BARTHELD, FLOYD T. _____McAlester
BAUM, FRANK J. _____McAlester
BUNN, A. D. _____Savanna
DORROUGH, JOE _____Haileyville
ELLIS, H. A. _____Pittsburg

GREENBERGER, EDWARD D. _____McAlester
KAEISER, WILLIAM H. _____McAlester
KILPATRICK, GEORGE A. _____McAlester
KUYRKENDALL, L. C. _____McAlester
*LEVINE, JULIUS Base Infirmary, Geiger Field, Wash.
*LIVELY, C. E. _____Station Hospital, Lincoln, Nebr.
McCARLEY, T. H. _____McAlester
MILLER, FRANK A. _____Hartshorne
MILLS, C. K. _____McAlester
MUNN, JESSE A. _____McAlester
NORRIS, T. T. _____Krebs
PARK, JOHN F. _____McAlester
PEMBERTON, R. K. _____McAlester
RAMSEY, W. G. _____McAlester
RICE, O. W. _____McAlester
SAMES, W. W. _____Hartshorne
SHULLER, E. H. _____McAlester
STOUGH, A. R. _____McAlester
WAIT, WILLIAM C. _____McAlester
WILLIAMS, C. O. _____McAlester
WILLOUR, L. S. _____McAlester
WILSON, HERBERT A. _____McAlester

PONTOTAC

BENTLEY, J. A. _____Allen
(member Hughes Co. Medical Society)
BRECO, J. G. _____Ada
BRYDIA, CATHERINE T. _____Ada
CANADA, ERNEST A. _____Ada
COWLING, ROBERT E. _____Ada
*CUNNINGHAM, JOHN A. _____Ada
CUMMINGS, I. L. _____Ada
DEAN, W. F. _____Ada
FORSYTHE, THOMAS _____Allen
(member Hughes Co. Medical Society)
GULLATT, ENNIS M. _____Ada
LANE, WILSON H. _____Ada
LEWIS, E. F. _____Ada
LEWIS, M. L. _____Ada
McBRIDE, OLLIE _____Ada
McKEEL, SAM A. _____Ada
MILLER, O. H. _____Ada
*MOREY, J. B. _____Ada
MORRIS, R. D. _____Allen
(member Hughes Co. Medical Society)
*MUNTZ, E. R. _____Ada
NEEDHAM, C. F. _____Ada
PADBERG, E. D. _____Ada
PETERSON, WILLIAM G. _____Ada
ROSS, S. P. (honorary) _____Ada
SEABORN, T. L. _____Ada
SUGG, ALFRED R. _____Ada
WEBSTER, M. M. _____Ada
WELBORN, O. E. _____Ada

POTTAMATOMIE

*ALLEY, RALPH M. _____Ft. Sam Houston, Texas
**ANDERSON, R. M. _____Shawnee
BAKER, M. A. _____Shawnee
BALL, W. A. _____Wanette
BAATER, GEORGE S. _____Shawnee
BYRUM, J. M. _____Shawnee
CAMPBELL, H. G. _____St. Louis
CARSON, F. L. _____Shawnee
CARSON, JOHN M. _____Shawnee
CORDELL, U. S. _____Macomb
CULBERTSON, R. R. _____Maud
FORTSON, J. L. _____Tecumseh
GALLAHER, CLINTON _____Shawnee
GALLAHER, PAUL C. _____Shawnee
GALLAHER, W. M. _____Shawnee
HAYGOOD, CHARLES W. _____Shawnee
HILL, R. M. C. (honorary) _____McLoud
*HUGHES, HORTON E. _____Shawnee
HUGHES, J. E. _____Shawnee
KAYLER, R. C. _____McLoud
KEEN, FRANK M. _____Shawnee
MATTHEWS, W. F. _____Tecumseh
McFARLING, A. C. _____Shawnee
McFARLING, JOHN _____Shawnee
MULLINS, WILLIAM B. _____Shawnee
NEWLIN, FRANCES P. _____Shawnee
**Deceased July 16, 1942.

PARAMORE, C. F. ....Shawnee
RICE, E. EUGENE ....Shawnee
ROWLAND, T. D. ....Shawnee
WALKER, J. A. ....Shawnee
WILLIAMS, ALPHA McADAMS ....Shawnee
YOUNG, C. C. ....Shawnee

PUSHMATAHA

CONNALLY, D. W. ....Antlers
HUCKABAY, B. M. ....Antlers
LAWSON, JOHN S. ....Clayton
PATTERSON, E. S. ....Antlers
RICE, P. B. ....Antlers

ROGER MILLS

CARY, W. S. ....Reydon
 (member Beckham Co. Medical Society)
HENRY, J. WORRALL ....Cheyenne
 (member Beckham Co. Medical Society)

ROGERS

ANDERSON, F. A. ....Claremore
*ANDERSON, P. S. ....Miami, Fla.
*ANDERSON, W. D. ....Victoria, Tex.
BESON, CLYDE W. ....Claremore
*BIGLER, E. E. ....Station Hospital, Ft. Sill
CALDWELL, C. L. ....Chelsea
COLLINS, B. F. ....Claremore
HOWARD, W. A. ....Chelsea
JENNINGS, K. D. ....Chelsea
MELINDER, ROY J. ....Claremore
MELOY, R. C. ....Claremore
WALLER, GEORGE D. ....Claremore

SEMINOLE

CHAMBERS, CLAUDE S. ....Seminole
*DEATON, A. N. ....Beaumont General Hospital,
        El Paso, Tex.
*FELTS, CLIFTON ....Camp Gruber, Okla.
GIESEN, A. F. ....Konawa
GRIMES, JOHN P. ....Wewoka
HARBER, J. N. (honorary) ....Phoenix, Ariz.
HARTSHONE, WILLIAM O. ....Cromwell
JONES, W. E. ....Seminole
KNIGHT, CLAUDE B. ....Wewoka
*LYONS, D. J. ....Australia
*LYTLE, WILLIAM R. ....Camp Gruber, Okla.
McGOVERN, J. D. ....Wewoka
MOSHER, D. D. ....Seminole
PACE, L. R. ....Seminole
REEDER, H. M. ....Konawa
RIPPY, O. M. ....Seminole
SHANHOLTZ, MACK I. ....Wewoka
STEPHENS, A. B. ....Seminole
*TERRY, J. B. ....Kelley Field, Tex.
VAN SANDT, GUY B. ....Wewoka
VAN SANDT, MAX M. ....Wewoka
WALKER, A. A. ....Wewoka
WILLIAMS, J. CLAY ....Wewoka

SEQUOYAH

NEWLIN, W. H. ....Sallisaw

STEPHENS

GARRETT, S. S. ....Duncan
IVY, WALLIS S. ....Duncan
LINDLEY, E. C. ....Duncan
LINDLEY, E. H. ....Duncan
McCLAIN, W. Z. ....Marlow
McMAHAN, A. M. ....Duncan
PATTERSON, J. L. ....Duncan
RICHARDSON, R. W. ....Duncan
SLATON, F. K. ....Comanche
 (member Alfalfa Co. Medical Society)
TALLEY, C. N. ....Marlow
THOMASSON, E. B. ....Duncan
WALKER, W. K. ....Marlow
WATERS, CLAUDE B. ....Duncan
WEEDN, ALTON J. ....Duncan

TEXAS

BLACKMER, L. G. ....Hooker
*BLUE, JOHNNY A. ....Nat'l Naval Medical Center,
        Bethesda, Md.
HAYES, R. B. ....Guymon
LEE, DANIEL S. ....Guymon
OBERMILLER, R. G. ....Texhoma
SMITH, MORRIS ....Guymon

TILLMAN

ALLEN, C. C. ....Frederick
ARRINGTON, J. E. ....Frederick
BACON, O. G. ....Frederick
*BOX, O. H., JR. ....Greenwood, Caddo Parish, La.
CHILDERS, J. E. ....Tipton
COLLIER, E. K ....Tipton
FOSHEE, W. C. ....Grandfield
FUQUA, W. A. ....Grandfield
OSBORN, J. D. ....Frederick
SPURGEON, T. F. ....Frederick

TULSA

ADAMS, R. M. ....Tulsa County Clinic
 (member Kiowa Co. Medical Society)
ALLEN, V. K. ....Medical Arts Bldg.
ARMSTRONG, O. C. ....Medical Arts Bldg.
ATCHLEY, R. Q. ....507 S. Cincinnati
ATKINS, PAUL N. ....Medical Arts Bldg.
BARHAM, J. H. ....314 Daniels Bldg.
BEESLEY, W. W. ....1733 S. Lewis St.
BEST, RALPH L. ....Medical Arts Bldg.
BEYER, J. WALTER ....McBirney Bldg.
BILLINGTON, J. JEFF ....Tulsa County Clinic
BIRNBAUM, WILLIAM ....915 S. Cincinnati
BLACK, HAROLD J. ....Medical Arts Bldg.
BOLTON, J. FRED ....Medical Arts Bldg.
BOONE, W. B. ....2112 W. 41st St.
BRADFIELD, S. J. ....Medical Arts Bldg.
BRADLEY, C. E. ....Medical Arts Bldg.
BRANLEY, B. L. ....Medical Arts Bldg.
BRASWELL, JAMES C. ....Medical Arts Bldg.
*BROCKSMITH, H. A. ....Medical Arts Bldg.
BROGDEN, J. C. ....Medical Arts Bldg.
BROOKSHIRE, J. E. (honorary) ....409 S. Boulder
BROWNE, HENRY S. ....Medical Arts Bldg.
BRYAN, W. J., JR. ....Medical Arts Bldg.
CALHOUN, C. E. ....Sand Springs
CALHOUN, W. H. ....Medical Arts Bldg.
CARNEY, A. B. ....915 S. Cincinnati
CHALMERS, J. S. ....Sand Springs
CHARBONNET, P. N. ....Medical Arts Bldg.
CHILDS, D. B. ....1226 S. Boston Place
**CHILDS, H. C. ....1226 S. Boston Place
CHILDS, J. W. ....1226 S. Boston Place
CLINTON, FRED S. (honorary) 230 E. Woodward Blvd.
CLULOW, GEORGE H. ....1307 S. Main
COHENOUR, E. L. ....Medical Arts Bldg.
COOK, W. ALBERT ....Medical Arts Bldg.
COULTER, T. B. ....Medical Arts Bldg.
CRAWFORD, WILLIAM S. ....Nat'l Bank of Tulsa Bldg.
CRONK, FRED Y. ....Medical Arts Bldg.
CULLUM, J. E. (honorary) ....1808 Eastern Court
 (member Pottawatomie Co. Medical Society)
DAILY, R. E. ....Bixby
DAVIS, A. H. ....Medical Arts Bldg.
DAVIS, GEORGE M. ....Bixby
*DAVIS, T. H. ....Hdq. Div. Arty., A.P.O. No. 45,
     c/o Postmaster, New York City
DEAN, W. A. ....Medical Arts Bldg.
*DENNY, E. RANKIN ....Camp McCoy, Wis.
DUNLAP, ROY W. ....Medical Arts Bldg.
EADS, C. H. ....Medical Arts Bldg.
EDWARDS, D. L. ....Philcade Bldg.
EDWARDS, JOHN ....Medical Arts Bldg.
ETHERTON, MONTE C. ....10½ S. Lewis
EVANS, HUGH J. ....Medical Arts Bldg.
*EWELL, W. C. ....Med. Det. 106 C. A. Bn.,
        Camp Hulen, Tex.
FARRIS, H. LEE ....Medical Arts Bldg.
FLACK, F. L. ....Nat'l Bank of Tulsa Bldg.
FLANAGAN, O. A. ....912 S. Boulder
FORD, H. W. ....Oklahoma Bldg.
*FORD, R. B. ....Corpus Christi, Tex.
FORRY, W. W. ....Bixby
FRANKLIN, ONIS ....Broken Arrow
*FRANKLIN, S. E. ....San Luis Obispo, Cal.
FULCHER, JOSEPH ....Medical Arts Bldg.
GARRETT, D. L. ....Medical Arts Bldg.
**Deceased.

GILBERT, J. B. ....Nat'l Mutual Bldg.
GLASS, FRED A. ....Medical Arts Bldg.
GODDARD, R. K. ....Skiatook
GOODMAN, SAMUEL ....Medical Arts Bldg.
GORRELL, J. F. ....Medical Arts Bldg.
GRAHAM, HUGH C. ....1307 S. Main
*GREEN, HARRY ....Medical Arts Bldg.
GROSSHART, PAUL ....Medical Arts Bldg.
HALL, G. H. ....Palace Bldg.
HARALSON, C. H. ....Medical Arts Bldg.
HARDMAN, T. J. ....Medical Arts Bldg.
HARRIS, BUNN ....Jenks
HART, MABLE M. ....2529 S. Boston Place
HART, M. O. ....1228 S. Boulder
HAYS, LUVERN ....Medical Arts Bldg.
HENDERSON, F. W. ....Medical Arts Bldg.
HENLEY, MARVIN D. ....Medical Arts Bldg.
*HENRY, G. H. ....San Diego, Cal.
HILL, O. L. ....915 S. Cincinnati
HOKE, C. C. ....Philtower Bldg.
HOTZ, CARL J. ....Springer Clinic
HOUSER, MORTIMER A. ....McBurney Bldg.
HUBER, W. A. ....Medical Arts Bldg.
HUDSON, DAVID V. ....21 N. Cincinnati
HUDSON, MARGARET G. ....Medical Arts Bldg.
HUMPHREY, B. H. ....Sperry
HUTCHISON, A. ....Bixby
HYATT, E. G. ....Springer Clinic
JOHNSON, E. O. ....Medical Arts Bldg.
JOHNSON, R. R. ....Sand Springs
JONES, WILLIAM M. ....915 S. Cincinnati
KEMMERLY, H. P. ....Medical Arts Bldg.
KORNBLEE, A. T. ....1307 S. Main
KRAMER, ALLEN C. ....Medical Arts Bldg.
LARRABEE, W. S. ....Medical Arts Bldg.
LAYTON, O. E. ....Collinsville
LEE, J. K. ....Medical Arts Bldg.
LeMASTER, D. W. ....Medical Arts Bldg.
LHEVINE, MORRIS B. ....Medical Arts Bldg.
LONEY, W. R. R. ....Medical Arts Bldg.
LOWE, J. O. ....915 S. Cincinnati
LUSK, E. M. ....915 S. Cincinnati
LYNCH, THOMAS J. ....Philcade Bldg.
MacDONALD, D. M. ....1739 S. Utica
MacKENZIE, IAN ....Medical Arts Bldg.
MARGOLIN, BERTHE ....Medical Arts Bldg.
MARKLAND, J. D. ....Medical Arts Bldg.
MATT, JOHN J. ....Medical Arts Bldg.
MAYGINNES, P. H. ....Palace Bldg.
McDONALD, J. E. ....Nat'l Mutual Bldg.
McGILL, RALPH A. ....Medical Arts Bldg.
McKELLAR, MALCOLM M. ....Springer Clinic
McQUAKER, MOLLY ....1552 E. 17th Place
MILLER, GEORGE H. ....Atlas Life Bldg.
MINER, JAMES L. ....Medical Arts Bldg.
MISHLER, D. L. ....Springer Clinic
MITCHELL, TOM HALL ....Nat'l Bank of Tulsa Bldg.
MUNDING, L. A. ....Medical Arts Bldg.
MURDOCK, H. D. ....Medical Arts Bldg.
MURRAY, P. G. ....Medical Arts Bldg.
MURRAY, SILAS ....Medical Arts Bldg.
**MYERS, F. C. ....Daniels Bldg.
NEAL, JAMES H. ....1944 N. Denver Place
NELSON, FRANK J. ....Medical Arts Bldg.
NELSON, F. L. ....Atlas Life Bldg.
NELSON, I. A. ....Medical Arts Bldg.
NELSON, IRON H. ....Medical Arts Bldg.
NELSON, M, O. ....Medical Arts Bldg.
NESBITT, E. P. ....Medical Arts Bldg.
NESBITT, P. P. ....Medical Arts Bldg.
NORTHRUP, L. C. ....1307 S. Main
OSBORN, GEORGE R. ....Medical Arts Bldg.
PAVY, C. A. ....Medical Arts Bldg.
PEDEN, JAMES C. ....Medical Arts Bldg.
*PERRY, FRED ....Will Rogers Field, Oklahoma City
PERRY, HUGH ....Atlas Life Bldg.
PERRY, JOHN O. ....Medical Arts Bldg.
PIGFORD, A. W. ....Medical Arts Bldg.
**Died June 7, 1942.

PIGFORD, R. C. ....Medical Arts Bldg.
*PITTMAN, COLE D. ....Chanute Field, Rantoul, Ill.
*POLLOCK SIMON ....Camp Hulen, Tex.
PORTER, H. H. ....Medical Arts Bldg.
PRESSON, L. C. ....1305 E. 15th St.
PRICE, H. P. ....Medical Arts Bldg.
RAMEY, CLYDE ....Palace Bldg.
RAY, R. G. ....915 S. Cincinnati
REESE, K. C. ....Medical Arts Bldg.
REYNOLDS, J. L. ....Alexander Bldg.
RHODES, R. E. L. ....Medical Arts Bldg.
RICHEY, S. M. (honorary) ....3830 W. 41st St.
ROBERTS, T. R. ....Wright Bldg.
ROGERS, J. W. ....Medical Arts Bldg.
ROTH, A. W. ....Medical Arts Bldg.
RUPRECHT, H. A. ....Springer Clinic
RUPRECHT, MARCELLA ....Springer Clinic
RUSHING, F. E. ....Medical Arts Bldg.
RUSSELL, G. R. ....Springer Clinic
SCHRECK, PHILIP M. ....Medical Arts Bldg.
*SCHWARTZ, HERBERT N. ....Will Rogers Field,
                                        Oklahoma City
SEARLE, M. J. ....Medical Arts Bldg.
SHAPIRO, DAVID ....Atlas Life Bldg.
SHEPARD, R. M. ....Medical Arts Bldg.
SHEPARD, S. C. ....Medical Arts Bldg.
SHERWOOD, R. G. ....Wright Bldg.
*SHIPP, J. D. ....Will Rogers Field,
                                        Oklahoma City
SHOWMAN, W. A. ....Medical Arts Bldg.
SIMPSON, CARL F. ....Medical Arts Bldg.
SINCLAIR, F. D. ....Springer Clinic
SIPPEL, MARY EDNA ....1542 E. 15th St.
SISLER, WADE ....Mercy Hospital
SMITH, D. O. ....Springer Clinic
SMITH, NED R. ....Medical Arts Bldg.
*SMITH, ROY L. ....Naval Training School,
                                        College Station, Tex.
SMITH, RURIC N. ....Medical Arts Bldg.
SMITH, W. O. ....Philcade Bldg.
SPANN, LOGAN A. ....Braniff Bldg.
SPOTTSWOOD, MAURICE D. ....Medical Arts Bldg.
SPRINGER, M. P. ....Springer Clinic
STALLINGS, T. W. ....724 S. Elgin St.
STANLEY, M. V. ....904 N. Denver
STEVENSON, JAMES ....Medical Arts Bldg.
STEWART, H. B. ....2500 E. 27th Place
STUART, FRANK A. ....Nat'l Mutual Bldg.
STUART, LEON B. ....Medical Arts Bldg.
SUMMERS, C. S. ....Daniels Bldg.
SWANSON, K. F. ....Springer Clinic
THOMPSON, OLIVER H. ....615 W. 14th Place
TRAINOR, W. J. ....Medical Arts Bldg.
UNDERWOOD, DAVID J. ....Medical Arts Bldg.
UNDERWOOD, F. L. ....Medical Arts Bldg.
UNGERMAN, A. H. ....Medical Arts Bldg.
VENABLE, S. C. ....Tulsa County Clinic
WALKER, WILLIAM A. ....Kennedy Bldg.
WALL, GREGORY A. (honorary) ......1159 N. Cheyenne
WALLACE, J. E. ....Medical Arts Bldg.
WARD, B. W. ....Wright Bldg.
WEST, T. H. ....Medical Arts Bldg.
WHITE, ERIC M. ....Medical Arts Bldg.
WHITE, N. S. ....Medical Arts Bldg.
WILEY, A. RAY ....Medical Arts Bldg.
WITCHER, R. B. ....Medical Arts Bldg.
WOLFF, EUGENE G. ....St. John's Hospital
WOODSON, FRED E. ....Medical Arts Bldg.
*YANDELL, HAYS R. ....Medical Arts Bldg.
ZINK, ROY ....Daniels Bldg.

WAGONER

BATES, S. R. ....Wagoner
DIVINE, D. G. ....Wagoner
    (member Muskogee Co. Medical Society)
JOBLIN, W. R. ....Porter
    (member Muskogee Co. Medical Society)
PLUNKETT, J. H. ....Wagoner
RIDDLE, H. K. ....Coweta

WASHINGTON

ATHEY, J. V. .... *Bartlesville*
BEECHWOOD, E. E. .... *Bartlesville*
CHAMBERLIN, E. M. .... *Bartlesville*
CRAWFORD, HORACE G. .... *Bartlesville*
CRAWFORD, JOHN E. .... *Bartlesville*
DORSHEIMER, GEORGE V. .... *Dewey*
*ETTER, FORREST S. .... *Bartlesville*
GENTRY, RAYMOND C. .... *Bartlesville*
GREEN, OTTO I. .... *Bartlesville*
HUDSON, LAWRENCE D. .... *Dewey*
KIMBALL, M. C. .... *Bartlesville*
　　　(*member Osage Co. Medical Society*)
KINGMAN, W. H. (*honorary*) .... *Bartlesville*
LeBLANC, WILLIAM .... *Ocheleta*
PARKS, SETH M. .... *Bartlesville*
REWERTS, FRED C. .... *Bartlesville*
RUCKER, RALPH W. .... *Bartlesville*
SHIPMAN, WILLIAM H. .... *Bartlesville*
SMITH, JOSEPH G. .... *Bartlesville*
SOMERVILLE, OKEY S. .... *Bartlesville*
STAVER, BENJAMIN F. .... *Bartlesville*
TORREY, JOHN P. .... *Bartlesville*
VANSANT, J. P. .... *Dewey*
WEBER, HENRY C. .... *Bartlesville*
WEBER, SHERWELL G. .... *Bartlesville*
WELLS, CEPHAS J. .... *Bartlesville*
WELLS, THOMAS .... *Bartlesville*
*WORD, LEE B. .... *Bartlesville*

WASHITA

ADAMS, ALLEN C. .... *Cordell*
BENNETT, D. W. .... *Sentinel*
BUNGARDT, A. H. .... *Cordell*
*DARNELL, E. E. .... *Enemy Alien Camp,*
　　　　　　　　　　　　　Stringtown, Okla.
FREEMAN W. H. (*honorary*) .... *Sentinel*
　　　(*member Kiowa Co. Medical Society*)
HARMS, J. H. (*honorary*) .... *Newton, Kan.*
JONES, J. P. (*honorary*) .... *Dill*
*LIVINGSTON, L. G. .... *Australia*
McMURRY, JAMES F. .... *Sentinel*
NEAL, A. S. .... *Cordell*
*STOWERS, AUBREY E. .... *120th Med. Bn., A.P.O.*
　　　No. 45, c/o Postmaster, New York City
TRACY, C. M. .... *Sentinel*
WEAVER, E. S. .... *Cordell*
WEBER, A. .... *Bessie*

WOODS

CLAPPER, EBENEEZER P. (*honorary*) .... *Waynoka*
ENSOR, DANIEL B. .... *Hopeton*
GRANTHAM, ELIZABETH (*honorary*) .... *Alva*
HALL, RAY LORMER .... *Alva*
HUNT, ISAAC S. (*honorary*) .... *Freedon*
LaFON, WILLIAM F. .... *Waynoka*
ROYER, CHARLES A. .... *Alva*
*SIMON, JOHN F. .... *Reception Center, Ft. Sill*
SIMON, WILLIAM E. .... *Alva*
STEPHENSON, ISHMAEL F. .... *Alva*
TEMPLIN, OSCAR E. .... *Alva*
TRAVERSE, C. A. .... *Alva*

WOODWARD

CHUMLEY, C. P. .... *Supply*
DARWIN, D. W. .... *Woodward*
DAY, JOHN I. .... *Supply*
DUER, JOE L. .... *Woodward*
*ENGLAND, MYRON .... *Camp Hulen, Tex.*
JOHNSON, H. L. .... *Supply*
KING, FRANK M. .... *Woodward*
LEACHMAN, THAD C. .... *Woodward*
MITCHELL, CLARENCE .... *Supply*
ORRICK, GEORGE W. .... *Supply*
RUTHERFORD, V. M. .... *Woodward*
TEDROWE, C. W. .... *Woodward*
TRIPLETT, T. BURKE .... *Mooreland*
WILLIAMS, C. E. .... *Woodward*

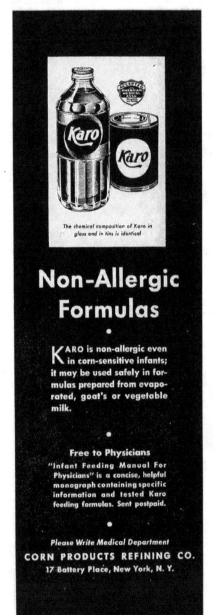

ASSOCIATION ACTIVITIES

ATLANTIC CITY MEETING AMERICAN MEDICAL ASSOCIATION

In spite of gasoline rationing on the Eastern Seaboard, 8,238 physicians registered for the Ninety-Third Annual Session of the American Medical Association, June 9, 10, 11 and 12, in Atlantic City, New Jersey.

Registration for the first three days found 34 Oklahoma physicians in attendance. Those attending from Oklahoma were: Ray M. Balyeat, Anson L. Clark, Tullos O. Coston, William Edgar Eastland, Grace Clause Hassler, Hugh Jeter, Josephine S. Kelso, Burt F. Keltz, John H. Lamb, Wendell Long, Earl D. McBride, L. Chester McHenry, J. M. Parrish, Jr., Robert U. Patterson, John W. Riley, Henry H. Turner and W. K. West, all of Oklahoma City; Victor K. Allen, H. J. Black, Walter H. Calhoun, E. O. Johnson, I. A. Nelson, A. W. Pigford, H. B. Stewart and Fred E. Woodson, all of Tulsa; Harry Lowens, Muskogee; Paul B. Champlin, Enid; H. G. Crawford, Bartlesville; Isador Dyer, Talequah; Walter A. Howard, Chelsea; J. Holland Howe, Ponca City; Paul B. Lingenfelter, Clinton; A. S. Risser, Blackwell, and Wildridge Clark Thompson, Stillwater.

The Annual Session this year was known as the Pan American Meeting, and 140 physicians from other American countries were in attendance.

The action of the House of Delegates dealt mainly with problems related to the war effort, medical service plans, and the improvement and enlargement of the functions of the American Medical Association.

The three general scientific sessions were divided between programs presented by inter-American guests, war problems and general clinical medicine.

Gold Medal Awards for Scientific Exhibits were made to Eben J. Carey and Leo C. Massopust of Marquette University Medical School for their exhibit on Experimental Ameboid Motion of Motor End Plates and John C. Bugher and Manuel Roca-Garcia, National Department of Health, Bogota, Columbia, for their exhibit on Epidemiology of Jungle Fever.

President Elect
James E. Paullin, M.D

The honor of being elected to the office of President-Elect of the American Medical Association was conferred upon James E. Paullin, M.D., of Atlanta, Georgia, by unanimous vote of the House of Delegates.

Dr. Paullin is a graduate of Mercer University and Johns Hopkins University School of Medicine. He served in World War I in the Medical Corps of the United States Army.

At the out-break of World War II Dr. Paullin served on the Committee on Medical Preparedness of the American Medical Association and the directing board of Procurement and Assignment Service.

Distinguished Service Medal

The award of the Distinguished Service Medal was made to Ludvig Hektoen, M.D., of Chicago, Illinois. That Dr. Hektoen's contribution to medical science has merited this honor is well exemplified by his accomplishments as reported by the June, A. M. A. Journal.

Dr. Hektoen has been pathologist to the Presbyterian Hospital and head of the department in the University of Chicago and of pathology of St. Luke's Hospital. He established in 1902 the John McCormick Institute for Infectious Diseases and became its director. In 1932 he was made a member of the National Advisory Health Council of the U. S. Public Health Service and later became chairman of the Advisory Committee of the National Cancer Institute. In April 1915, he became

chairman of the Committee on Scientific Research of the American Medical Association, in which position he has been instrumental in determining grants of funds for research carried on throughout the country. In 1916 Dr. Hektoen gave the Cutter Lecture of the Harvard University Medical School and received the honorary degree of Doctor of Science from the University of Wisconsin. He was president of the American Society for Experimental Pathology. He received in 1920 the honorary degree of Doctor of Laws from the University of Cincinnati.

In 1924 he was chairman of the Division of Medical Sciences of the National Research Council and in the same year he was appointed consultant pathologist in the U. S. Public Health Service. In 1926 he served again as chairman of the Division of Medical Sciences of the National Research Council. The Norwegian government gave him its most distinguished recognition, The Order of St. Olaf, in 1929.

He has been editor of the Journal of Infectious Diseases since it was first established in 1904 and also editor of the Archives of Pathology since its first number in 1925. He has also been at various times editor of the Proceedings of the Institute of Medicine of Chicago, chairman of its board of governors and editor of the Transactions of the Chicago Pathological Society.

1945 Meeting

The House of Delegates at its final session voted to hold the 1945 session in New York City. There were only two invitations extended, the other being from the host city of Atlantic City.

Oklahomans Elected to Important Offices

That Oklahoma was well represented at the Atlantic City Session can be further substantiated by the fact that Mrs. W. K. West of Oklahoma City, was elected to the Board of Directors of Women's Auxiliary for a term of one year, Dr. Henry H. Turner becomes the new chairman of the Associated State Postgraduate Committees and Dr. A. S. Risser was appointed a Sergeant-at-Arms by the Speaker of the House of Delegates.

REHABILITATION PROGRAM AID TO DEPENDENT CHILDREN

Since the establishment of an Advisory Committee to the Public Welfare Department the Committee has endeavored to bring about Rehabilitations of as many applicants for aid as possible.

It is indeed interesting to report the results of this program as of April 12, 1942.

The following report of the program was made by Miss Oliva Hemphill of the Department of Public Welfare:

REPORT ON CASES RECOMMENDED BY MEDICAL ADVISORY COMMITTEE FOR REHABILITATION

Miss Hemphill reported the progress on rehabilitation on thirty-five (35) cases, covering the entire period from the time the committee first met to the present time. Of the thirty-five cases there are 13 in which the recommendation of the Medical Advisory Committee is now being followed. Treatment, as recommended, is actually being given. There are 12 cases in which arrangements and plans with the family have been made and they are waiting their turn, most of them in University Hospitals, but the patients themselves are willing to have the work done. In 2 cases out of the 35 the county worker has been unable to arrange any transportation. The worker has sent in her report indicating that there is no local resource through which this transportation can be provided. The Commissioners have not been able, and in some instances are unwilling, to arrange for transportation to the point of examination and treatment. This, of course, is something we want to give some thought to. The Department at present has no way of taking care of this situation. There is one case out of the 35 studied in which an operation was recommended; the work has been done and the family no longer needs assistance. One case was a service case, i.e., the recommendation of the county to deny was sustained by the committee; however, the committee recommended that certain work be done to help the man, and the county was planning to get this done when the man came in and said he had employment so that the Department need not make any further plans for him. Out of the 35 cases we found four were unwilling to follow the recommendations; (1) the patient had been unwilling because his doctor had advised that he could not live through an operation; (2) It had been recommended that the patient be sent to an institution and he is unwilling to go (his wife, however, has signed commitments papers to have him sent); (3) the patient was afraid of an operation; (He didn't refuse outright, but said he would give it some thought and would come back in to the county officer when he had decided definitely); (4) has tuberculosis and it had been recommended by the committee that he be given hospitalization. The man said that he had had a brother die in such a hospital and was afraid to go. The county department, however, had succeeded in getting the county commissioners to build a room so that he is isolated from his family and the public health nurse is supervising the family.

In one case out of the 35 the county has canceled the case because they have felt that a mistake was made in recommending assistance at all. The man is now working.

One case was referred to University Hospitals for operation but was advised by hospital not to have operation because of his age.

This report graphically pictures what can be accomplished when there is complete understanding and cooperation between public agencies and the medical profession.

Every member of the Association should take pride in assisting in this program and in knowing that it is only through his chosen profession, that such aid can be given. It is a service few are priviledged to give.

BEWARE!

The office of the Association has been advised by the Better Business Bureau of Oklahoma City that the Sheriff of Jackson County, Iowa, holds a warrant for the arrest of Frank W. Dugan of Des Moines, Iowa.

Dugan recently started a small business known as Specialty Forms Company, which was a proposition for the handling of professional accounts.

Any physician having contact with this man or any person representing Specialty Forms Company should immediately contact either the Sheriff of Jackson County, Iowa, or the Oklahoma City Better Business Bureau.

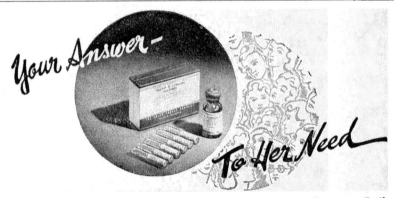

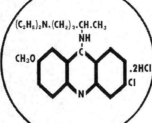
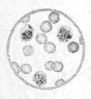

KANSAS AND OKLAHOMA WAR SESSIONS AMERICAN COLLEGE OF SURGEONS

Over four-hundred Oklahoma and Kansas physicians attended the War Session of the American College of Surgeons held in Oklahoma City, May 28.

Panel discussions were given concerning the Treatment and Management of War Injuries and the Organization and Functions of the Medical Departments of the Army and Navy.

Out of state physicians participating in these programs included John R. Paine, M.D., Minneapolis, Minn.; Clifford C. Nesselrode, M.D., Kansas City, Kansas; Lieutenant Colonel B. Noland Carter, Office of the Surgeon General, Washington, D. C.; Captain Frederick R. Hook, United States Naval Hospital, Washington, D. C.; Thomas G. Orr, M.D., Kansas City, Mo.; L. Haynes Fowler, M.D., Minneapolis, Minn.; Louis T. Byars, Jr., M.D., St. Louis, Mo.; and George S. Baker, M.D., Rochester, Minn.

In addition to the scientific program, Harold S. Diehl, M.D., Dean of the University of Minnesota School of Medicine, Minneapolis, Minn., and a member of the Directing Board of the Procurement and Assignment Service, discussed the activity of Procurement and Assignment and Lieutenant Colonel W. B. Russ, Medical Office, Eighth Civilian Defense Region, San Antonio, Texas, presented the subject "The Doctor and the Hospital in Civilian Defense."

The American College of Surgeons is to be complimented upon its foresightedness in conducting refresher courses of the type presented at the War Session.

PRESIDENT BRANDT ACKNOWLEDGES RESOLUTION IN SUPPORT OF UNIVERSITY SCHOOL OF MEDICINE

Acknowledging the resolution in support of the University of Oklahoma School of Medicine adopted at the last House of Delegates meeting of the Oklahoma State Medical Association, the following letter has been received by the President, James D. Osborn:

UNIVERSITY OF OKLAHOMA
Norman, Oklahoma
June 5, 1942

James D. Osborn, M.D., President,
Oklahoma State Medical Association,
Frederick, Oklahoma.

Dear Dr. Osborn:

Dean Patterson has sent me a copy of the resolution passed by the Oklahoma State Medical Association at its annual meeting held at Tulsa in April. We appreciate very must this expression of co-operation, and we hope that the State Medical Association will take an active interest in seeing that the School of Medicine is given the financial support needed to operate as a first class medical school should.

The training of doctors is of such vital importance that it cannot be regarded lightly. The funds that have been provided for the Medical School in Oklahoma have been far less than the funds of medical schools in other states, and it is a short-sighted policy to penalize ourselves when the young men that graduate year after year are to become guardians of our health in the future.

I know it is not necessary for me to tell you this, but I know of no more effective way to impress the citizens of the state of this fact than through the medical profession.

Sincerely yours,

Joseph A. Brandt, President.

B/b

REGISTRATION OF DIATHERMY APPARATUS ORDERED BY FEDERAL COMMUNICATIONS COMMISSION

Notice of the following action of the Federal Communications Commission was not received in time for publication in the May issue of the Journal.

Anyone owning apparatus coming in the confines of the Commission's Order and who has not complied with the orders, should do so at once.

*"'All possessors of apparatus designed, constructed or used for generating radio frequency energy for therapeutic purposes, described generally as diathermy apparatus, must register each such device with the Federal Communications Commission in Washington, D.C., by June 8, under Order No. 96, promulgated by the commission on May 18. Any person who wilfully violates any provision of the order or who falsifies any information required to be furnished to the commission becomes subject to a fine of not more than $10,000 or imprisonment for not more than ten years, or both, and any unregistered apparatus may be confiscated.

Application for registration must be on forms obtainable from the commission in Washington or from any of its field offices. Individual applications must be made for each set of diathermy apparatus to be registered, and physicians should keep this in mind when requesting application forms. The executed forms must be forwarded to the secretary of the Federal Communications Commission in Washington. On receipt of an application if the commission finds that sufficient and reliable information has been furnished, a nontransferable certificate of registration will be issued to the applicant, which must be conspicuously affixed to the apparatus for which it is issued.

Any person or organization hereafter in any manner coming into possession of apparatus required to be registered must apply for a certificate of registration within fifteen days after obtaining such apparatus. If registered apparatus is transferred, sold, assigned, leased, lent, stolen, destroyed or otherwise removed from the possession of the registrant the commission must, within five days, be notified of that fact and the name of recipient of the diathermy apparatus be furnished to the commission if such person is known to the registrant.

According to a news release issued by the commission, this order does not apply to persons owning sun lamps, infra-red lamps or ultraviolet ray devices. It applies only to apparatus generating electromagnetic energy at any frequency between the limits of 10 kilocycles and 10,000 megacycles. Apparatus in the possession of the United States government, its offices or agents, or apparatus which is under contract of delivery to the United States government is not subject to the registration order.

This order is a wartime security measure and its promulgation follows a determination previously reached by the Office for Emergency Management, Defense Commission Board, in Order No. 4, that the national security and defense and the successful conduct of the war demand that the government have knowledge of all persons who possess apparatus equipped for the transmission of radio frequency energy. Diathermy apparatus may not only interfere with radio transmitters and thus may be used to furnish valuable information to the enemy.

Oklahoma physicians should apply for application forms to the office of the Inspector in Charge, Federal Communications Commission, P. O. Box 5373, Dallas, Texas, or 809 U. S. Court House, Kansas City, Missouri.'"

*Taken from the A. M. A. Journal, page 354, May 23, 1942.

MEDICAL PREPAREDNESS

War Manpower Commission

Announcement has been received that Procurement and Assignment Service is now operating under the direct supervision of the War Manpower Commission with the Honorable Paul V. McNutt as Chairman.

Since there is a continued need for more physicians to enter the military service and especially those physicians under the age of thirty seven, the Procurement and Assignment Service of the W.M.C. will shortly send to every physician who indicated on his enrollment form that his first or second choice was service in United States Army Medical Department, the following letter:

Procurement and Assignment Service
Washington

Procurement and Assignment Service for
Physicians, Dentists and Veterinarians.

Dear Doctor:

You have indicated your willingness to serve the Nation in this great emergency. The Procurement and Assignment Service of the War Manpower Commission now calls on you to enter the Service. Please apply at once for a commission. You have been selected from among the available physicians in your community by a process that is believed to be fair and impartial.

Complete and mail the enclosed post cards immediately. The Office of the Sur-

geon General or his representative will provide the necessary application forms and authorize the time and the place for your physical examination.

Do not take any definite action regarding your practice until you receive specific instructions from the War Department. Each physician who is commissioned is routinely allowed fourteen days to wind up his affairs after receipt of orders from the War Department.

The rapidity of recruitment now in effect makes this communication necessary and requires your full cooperation. Please do not delay.

Sincerely yours,
Frank H. Lahey, M.D.,
Chairman, Directing Board
Procurement and Assignment Service.

Accompanying the letter will be two postal cards that may be used to secure application forms and notification of the action taken by the proper Governmental agency.

This announcement does not preclude or in any way change the present method of receiving a commission, but rather is a step to eliminate bottle-necks. All eligible and available physicians are still urged to contact the Recruiting Board located at 211 Plaza Court, 10th and Walker, Oklahoma City.

ARMY RECRUITING BOARD FOR OKLAHOMA

The recruiting board for physicians, dentists and doctors, of veterinary medicine is now located at 211 Plaza Court, 10th and Walker, Oklahoma City, telephone 7-0070, and is under the direction of Colonel Lee R. Wilhite, representing the Surgeon General, and Captain Oliver H. Cornelius of the Office of the Adjutant General.

The recruiting board has full authority to order physical examinations, waive physical defects, grant commissions, and administer the oath of office.

All physicians below the age of fifty-five, desiring to obtain commissions should immediately contact the board. An appointment is not necessary.

The board is particularly anxious to interview physicians under the age of forty-five.

The Procurement of Physicians*

A Statement for the Journal of the American Medical Association
Paul V. McNutt
Washington, D. C.

On June 8, I described to the American Medical Association at its Atlantic City meeting the acute need for physicians for the military services. I pointed out how far the recruitment of physicians lagged behind expected quotas. In conclusion I stated bluntly the fact, which could not have been evaded by any analysis, that unless voluntary recruitment progressed more rapidly some more rigorous form of selective service must be resorted to.

Those facts were necessary in order to permit the medical profession to diagnose its own case. And the case is urgent; physicians are members of what is probably the most indispensable of all professions. Despite the harshness of the facts and the bluntness with which I had to state them, I felt that the profession should be informed.

In fairness to the recruitment record of many of our states, it seems in order at this time to give the profession some further idea of how its problem is dis-

tributed. The failure of a sufficient number of physicians to volunteer for military service is not spread thinly over the whole country. There is an acute lag in certain populous states. Other states have supplied nearly all that they should supply.

We need more than twenty thousand additional physicians by the end of this year. But eight states—New York, Illinois, California, Massachusetts, New Jersey, Michigan and Ohio—should account for nearly sixteen thousand of that shortage.

By contrast, sixteen states have fewer than a hundred physicians to go to reach the total number they should supply. In order not to deplete unduly available medical service in those areas, we are asking that the Medical Officers Recruiting Boards be withdrawn and that further enlistments from those areas be then discouraged except in the case of the men under 37 in the urban areas. Those states are Alabama, Arizona, Delaware, Idaho, Louisiana, Mississippi, Montana, Nevada, New Mexico, North Dakota, South Carolina, Utah, Vermont, Wyoming and Virginia.

The acute problem for the next few months for those states is an equitable distribution of medical service

---

*Taken from the A.M.A. Journal, Vol. 119, No. 9, June 27, 1942, Page 715.

within their borders. This will avoid the necessity for any consideration of plans to allocate doctors from other states to meet civilian needs.

More than one hundred and thirty thousand physicians have returned their registration forms to the Roster for Scientific and Technical Personnel. Those forms are now being processed. When that work is complete we shall be able to give the profession a more comprehensive report on the relation of available medical service to wartime needs.

The seriousness of the deficit in the number of physicians available for armed forces should not be underestimated. The need must be met. It will be met by one method or another. Neither must we under-estimate the serious drain this puts on available medical service in civilian communities. It will mean long hours and hard work—sacrifices which will multiply the deep debt that every community owes to its physicians.

It cannot be met simply by multiplying the hours of the physicians who are left. There will be a real need to exercise every possible means for minimizing unnecessary medical services in order that the real needs may be met.

It is my belief that the lag in recruitment has been due chiefly to the fact that the individual physician has not realized the genuine urgency of the need. Measures must be taken which will bring those home to every individual. This means that there will have to be some education of the general public. Preventable illness must be reduced to a minimum. Unreasonable demands on the physician's time must be reduced to a minimum. Thus only may available medical service adequately cover the needs.

Effective, Convenient and Economical

THE effectiveness of Mercurochrome has been demonstrated by twenty years' extensive clinical use.

For the convenience of physicians Mercurochrome is supplied in four forms—Aqueous Solution for the treatment of wounds, Surgical Solution for preoperative skin disinfection, Tablets and Powder from which solutions of any desired concentration may readily be prepared.

Mercurochrome, H.W.&D.

(H. W. & D. Brand of dibrom-oxymercuri-fluorescein-sodium)

is economical because solutions may be dispensed at low cost. Stock solutions keep indefinitely.

 Mercurochrome is accepted by the Council on Pharmacy and Chemistry of the American Medical Association.

Literature furnished on request

HYNSON, WESTCOTT & DUNNING, INC.

BALTIMORE, MARYLAND

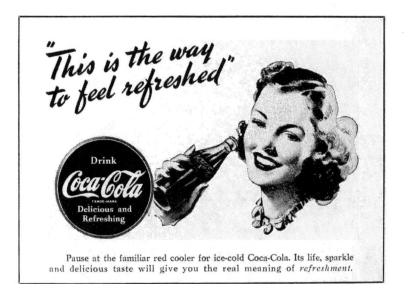

$\mathscr{A}$uxiliary News

Officers

1942-1943

President....................................Mrs Frank L. Flack, Tulsa
President-Elect............Mrs. Maxey Cooper, Oklahoma City
Vice-President...................Mrs. Jim L. Haddock, Norman
Secretary..............................Mrs. James Stevenson, Tulsa
Treasurer............................Mrs H. Lee Farris, Tulsa
Historian.............................Mrs. Clinton Gallaher, Shawnee
Parliamentarian..Mrs. Edward D. Greenberger, McAlester

Committee Chairmen

Public Relations................Mrs. Shade D. Neely, Muskogee
Program-Health Education........Mrs. Rush Wright, Poteau
Hygeia...........................Mrs. Maxey Cooper, Oklahoma City
Student Loan................................Mrs. C. F. Needham, Ada
Press & Publicity........................Mrs. Carl Hotz, Tulsa
Exhibits......................Mrs. Joseph Kelso, Oklahoma City
Convention............Mrs. Henry H. Turner, Oklahoma City
Tray....................Mrs. F. Redding Hood, Oklahoma City
Organization................Mrs. Jim L. Haddock, Norman
Legislative...............Mrs. George Garrison, Oklahoma City
Printing..........................Mrs. Thomas B. Coulter, Tulsa

During the summer months, the plans for the program for the year will be formulated. We expect to hear from the Woman's Auxiliary to the American Medical Association with suggestions for the year's work. Mrs. Frank Haggard, of San Antonio, Texas, as our new president, will direct the work of the States, and will undoubtedly be of great assistance in helping us complete our program.

Since this will be an unusual year with our country engaged in war, the activities of our organization will necessarily be enlarged to include war work, and we will need a special committee to head this work. This committee may be called "War Aid" or "War Work," and will include all Red Cross and O. C. D. work in which our members participate. Some of our members who are doctors or graduate nurses will be invaluable in formulating and carrying this forward. The tentative program for this war work has been recommended by our National President, Mrs. Haggard, in an article appearing in the "Convention" Bulletin, 1942, under the title of "The Woman's Auxiliary in War Time."

A complimentary copy of the "Bulletin," the official publication of the Woman's Auxiliary to the American Medical Association, which is published four times a year, will be sent to each State officer, Committee chairman, and to all County Presidents.

We have received word of the establishment of a central office for the Woman's Auxiliary to the American Medical Association, at 43 East Ohio Street, Chicago, Illinois, with Miss Margaret N. Wolfe as secretary, and any national news will be sent from this office.

At our annual meeting this year, we voted to award the Silver Tray for a permanent possession to the county who wins it three times (not necessarily in succession). Since the tray has not been won three times by any county, all have the opportunity to compete for this prize. The committee will judge according to the following points: Percentage of attendance at regular meetings and quality of annual report covering those objectives—Public Relations, Health Education, Hygeia, Membership, Organization, Program and Loan Fund. When the tray was purchased in 1936, the basis of award was voted to be on these things.

At the annual meeting of the Woman's Auxiliary to the American Medical Association in Atlantic City, Mrs Joseph Kelso, Oklahoma City, was the State delegate, and we anticipate carrying a report from her on the meeting in the near future.

Tulsa County News

The Auxiliary to the Tulsa County Medical Society held its last meeting until fall on June 2, 1942, with a 10 o'clock breakfast at the home of Mrs. James Stevenson, with 50 members present. A very interesting talk was given by Mrs. D. W. LeMaster on "Fun with Flowers." The hostesses for the breakfast were Mrs. M. O. Nelson, Mrs. J. C. Peden, Mrs. D. M. MacDonald, Mrs. Joseph Fulcher and Mrs. Ralph A. McGill. Mrs. Estelle Garebedian, a former Tulsan and member, now of Houston, Texas, was a special guest.

The following officers for the Woman's Auxiliary of the Tulsa County Medical Society for 1942-1943 were installed at the meeting: Mrs. J. W. Childs, President; Mrs. John Perry, President-Elect; Mrs. C. A. Pavy, Vice-President; Mrs John G. Matt, Secretary; Mrs. Fred Woodson, Treasurer; Mrs. C. C. Hoke, Corresponding Secretary; Mrs. L. C. Northrup, Historian; Mrs. A. W. Roth, Parliamentarian; and Dr. H. B. Stewart, Dr. A. Ray Wiley, and Dr. Ralph A. McGill, Advisory Council.

Following the installation of officers, the President announced her committee appointmnts for the coming year. Standing Committees—Mrs. Carl Hotz, Publicity; Mrs. S. J. Bradfield, Public Relations; Mrs. Ian MacKenzie, Philanthropie; Mrs. D. W. LeMaster, Program; Mrs. H. B. Stewart, Social; Mrs. H. W. Ford, Telephone; Mrs. H. C. Childs, Hygeia; Mrs. H. Lee Farris, Courtesy; and Mrs. M. O. Hart, Legislative. Special Committees—Mrs. John Perry, Year Book; Mrs. L. C. Northrup, Exhibits; and Mrs. C. C. Hoke, War Aid.

Muskogee-Sequoyah-Wagoner Counties

We are very pleased to report that the three counties of Muskogee, Sequoyah, and Wagoner have been organized into one County Medical Society, and that an Auxiliary has been formed from these three counties. Mrs. H. T. Ballentine, of Muskogee, was elected President for the year 1942-1943. We anticipate great work from these three counties, and shall be pleased to report their progress during the year.

As we go to press, we have not received the names of the publicity chairmen from the organized County Auxiliaries. Please forward these names to the State Publicity Chairman, as the rest of the State is interested in what you are doing, and we would like to contact these publicity chairmen before the next issue.

NEWS FROM THE COUNTY SOCIETIES

The Seminole County Medical Society met May 20, in Wewoka with 17 members present. The Scientific program was presented on the "Treatment of Burns." Dr. William R. Lytle gave a paper on the "Treatment of the Patient," and Dr. Max Van Sandt on "Treatment of the Burn."

The next meeting of the Society will be held June 17, at the home of Dr. Claude S. Chambers, the program to be announced later.

The April meeting of the Rogers County Medical Society was a farewell dinner held at the Will Rogers Hotel in Claremore, honoring Dr. P. S. Anderson and Dr. Earl E. Bigler, who are leaving for Military duty.

Dr. Anderson will be stationed at Miami, Florida, and Dr. Bigler at Ft. Sill. There were ten members present.

Dr. Coyne H. Campbell, Oklahoma City, was the guest speaker at the June 11, meeting of the Woodwarrd County Medical Society held at Supply.

Dr. Campbell read a paper on "The Relationship between Neurosis and Psychosis."

Following Dr. Campbell's paper, Dr. O. C. Templin, Alva, Councilor for District No. 1, gave a short address.

There were 20 members present with their wives and all enjoyed a chicken dinner as guests of Dr. John L. Day.

The Beckham County Medical Society met at Erick, Oklahoma, June 9, with nine members present.

Dr. P. J. Devanney of Sayre, read a paper on "Shock." It was followed by a round-table discussion. The July meeting of the Society will be held at Elk City, with Dr. H. K. Speed in charge of the program. It is contemplated that the Society will meet in conjunction with Dentists, Nurses and Doctors of Greer County.

Dr. L. R. Kirby, Okeene, Lt. M. P. Merryman, Enid, and Dr. Evans E. Tally, Enid, were speakers at the Woods-Alfalfa County Society meeting, May 26, at Alva. Fifteen members of the Society were present.

Dr. Kirby spoke on "The Surgical Gall Bladder," Lt. Merryman on "Catarrhal Jaundice," and Dr. Tally gave a discussion on these two papers.

The next meeting will be held September 29, at Cherokee, Oklahoma.

Members of the Pittsburg County Medical Society, met May 28, at Antlers to hear a program by a guest speaker, Dr. J. Speed of Memphis.

The topic for discussion was a Symposium on Fractures. The next meeting will be held June 25, at Dr. Edwin D. Greenberger's farm to honor Dr. Claude E. Lively who is leaving for Military service on July 1.

Twenty members of the Muskogee-Sequoyah-Wagoner Medical Societies, met at Dr. Charles Ed White's, "El Rancho," east of Muskogee for dinner.

The next meeting will be held September 7, at the Baptist Hospital in Muskogee, the program to be announced later.

Discussions on "Civilian Defense," were given by Mr. Wilson Wallace and Dr. F. W. Boadway of Ardmore, for members of the Carter County Medical Society, at a meeting May 19, at the Hardy Sanitarium in Ardmore, with 11 members present.

Dr. F. R. Hassler and Dr. John Battenfield of The State Health Department, Oklahoma City, will be the principle speakers at a meeting June 26, at the Hotel Ardmore. They will discuss "Rocky Mountain (Tick) Fever."

The Carter County Medical Society will have as its guests, all members from District No. 5.

The Craig County Medical Society met June 2, with six members present.

A bulletin was read on "Short Wave Therapy," and a report was given on Correspondence with Senator's Lee and Thomas about pending War Bill.

At a meeting of the Cherokee County Medical Society, held May 12, Dr. Eugene Gillis from the Oklahoma State Health Department, Oklahoma City, showed the U. S. P. H. film on "Syphilis."

A discussion on "Medicine During the Time of War," will be the topic for discussion at a meeting to be held June 29, in Muskogee.

The Creek County Medical Society met June 9, in Bristow, Oklahoma, with about ten members present.

A brief report on "Physician's Activity in the Technical End of the Air Corps," was given by Lt. White. Dr. Eugene Gillis of the Oklahoma State Health Department, presented a film on "Syphilis."

Dr. O. C. Coppedge of Bristow, was elected as Secretary, to fulfill the unexpired term of Dr. O. H. Cowart, who resigned to enter the army. The next meeting will be held October 13, in Sapulpa.

The Garvin County Medical Society, met in Pauls Valley, with ten members present.

The principal speaker for the evening was Dr. Hugh Monroe, Pauls Valley, who presented a paper on "Rocky Mountain Spotted Fever." Discussions of the paper were given by Dr. O. O. Dawson of Wayne, and Dr. M. E. Robberson, Jr., of Wynnewood.

The next meeting of the Society will be held September 16, at Pauls Valley, Oklahoma.

Captain James Hughes Reporting

The Journal reprints a letter received by the Executive Secretary from Captain James Hughes, M. C., who is now on active duty at the Station Hospital, Camp Gordon, Georgia.

Captain Hughes will be remembered as the State Association's instructor in Pediatrics.

Dear Dick:　　　　　　　　　　　　　May 17, 1942

It was nice to hear from you recently, and it brought back a lot of pleasant memories. There have been many occasions for me to wish I were back in Oklahoma again, not only for the work which I did enjoy so much but for the fine associations that went along, like dessert, with the work.

Little Jane is growing up already and is now six weeks of age. I haven't seen her since age 5 days but all reports are that she's a honey. Jane and both the children are going to come down to live with me June first, only two weeks away. We were fortunate enough to find a nice house, a difficult thing to do in this area where so many officers are.

I have no idea when I'll be sent off to foreign duty but it can't come too soon for me. In spite of having a family I feel very strongly that no doctor under 35 who is able to get around should be in station hospital work. Older men should have our places and we should be out with the field troops. I'm Chief of the Medical Service here, a good break in a way, with nine wards with over 200 patients to be responsible for. But still I'd like to get going and feel more as if I were helping win this thing.　　Sincerely yours,

　　　　　　　　　　　　　　Jim Hughes.

Group Hospital Service News

May, 1942, was a banner month for the Blue Cross Plan in Oklahoma, with 2,400 new members placing hospital care in the family budget. They can now say, "Worries Away," so far as their hospital bills are concerned.

The Midwest Air Depot of Oklahoma City formally approved the Blue Cross Plan for their employees. Present personnel will be enrolled during the month of June; others will be enrolled as they are added to the staff each month.

The Brown-Dunkin Department Store of Tulsa has added its name to the steadily growing family of Blue Cross members. The employees are enjoying splendid co-operation from the management by having dues paid through the payroll and arranging group management so that the service might be presented for their voluntary enrollment. Service for this group will be effective on June 15.

The Northeastern Oklahoma Hospital Council (numbering 32 hospitals) celebrated National Hospital Day in an impressive manner, with very satisfactory results. Mr. Elmer Pollock, Vice-President of the First National Bank of Tulsa, acted as general chairman, directing all activities. Work done by the hospitals in caring for patients from the recent Pryor tornado was emphasized through the local newspapers. Hospitals secured window space in downtown stores for display typifying some specific division of hospital work. Announcements of the National Hospital Day activities were made at local service clubs, and the Blue Cross movies, "The Common Defense," and, "The White Battalion," were shown to public schools, in the week preceding National Hospital Day. Milk bottle collars were attached to bottles on deliveries made on the preceding Sunday.

As a climax to the celebration, Dr. C. Rufus Rorem, Director of the Hospital Service Plan Commission, Chicago, addressed the Chamber of Commerce open forum on Friday, May 8, followed by a showing of the movie, "The Common Defense." On Friday afternoon Dr. Rorem gave a fifteen minute address over a local radio station. An informal dinner was given for Dr. Rorem that evening so that he might have the opportunity to become better acquainted with resident board members and civic leaders, who attended the dinner as guests of the Blue Cross Plan.

• OBITUARIES •

Dr. William C. Sain
1884-1942

Dr. William C. Sain, prominent Ardmore physician for many years, died March 7, 1942, at his home in Ardmore. Dr. Sain was born in Bolivar, Tenn., November 3, 1884. He was graduated from the Medical University of Tennessee, Memphis, in 1916, and he served one year at Memphis General hospital as an intern. Then, he served two years in the United States Army Medical corps, attaining the rank of Captain during World War I.

In 1919, Doctor Sain married Eloise Triplett of Macon, Miss., and the couple came to Ardmore in August of that year, where he established himself as a outstanding figure in his profession. He continued his practice until his death.

Doctor Sain was a member of the Rotary Club, and rendered signal service to the club and the community by his work on the Crippled Children's committee. He was also a member of the American Legion, the First Missionary Baptist church, and was active in Boy Scout work.

A member of the staff at Hardy sanitarium in Ardmore, Doctor Sain was a life member of the American Medical Association, and was active in the State Medical Association and Carter County Medical society.

Resolution

WHEREAS, It has pleased the Almighty to remove from our midst, by death, our esteemed friend and colaborer, Dr. W. C. Sain, who has for many years occupied a prominent rank in our midst, maintaining under all circumstances a character untarnished, and a reputation above reproach.

WHEREFORE, WE THE CARTER COUNTY MEDICAL SOCIETY, RESOLVED, That in the death of Dr. W. C. Sain, we have sustained the loss of a friend whose fellowship it was an honor and a pleasure to enjoy; that we bear willing testimony to his many virtues, to his unquestioned probity and stainless life; that we offer to his bereaved family and mourning friends, over whom sorrow has hung her sable mantle, our heartfelt condolence, and pray that Infinite Goodness may bring speedy relief to their burdened hearts and inspire them with the consolation that Hope in futurity and Faith in God give even in the shadow of the Tomb.

RESOLVED, That a copy of these resolutions, properly engrossed, be presented to the family of our deceased friends.

T. J. Jackson, M.D.
F. W. Broadway, M.D.
Lyman C. Veazey, M.D.

Dr. Henry J. Daily
1875-1942

Dr. Henry J. Daily, a practicing physician in Oklahoma county since 1929, died April 26, in Oklahoma City, following an illness of several months.

Born in Millersburg, Ky., Doctor Daily was graduated from Vanderbilt university in 1899, and studied medicine at Tufts college. He began the practice of medicine at Owingsville, Ky., in 1903, moving to Oklahoma City in 1929.

An active member of the County Medical Association and the State Medical Association, Doctor Daily was also a member of the Knights of Pythias, Odd Fellows, and was a Mason. He was active in the Linwood Methodist church.

Survivors include his wife, four sons, Paul and James, both of the home address; Frank, Cincinnati, Ohio, and Henry J. Daily, Jr., Lexington, Ky.; one daughter, Mrs. Lewis Dawson, Aruba, Netherland East Indies; three sisters, Mrs. Mable H. Green and Mrs. Bina McDowell of Oklahoma City, and Mrs. P. A. Tankersley, Putnam City; and two brothers, James Daily, Handsboro, Miss., and Wilson Daily, Elk City.

Dr. Allen C. Jenner
1874-1942

Dr. Allen C. Jenner was born June 4, 1874, at Noble, Ill. Doctor Jenner had been a practicing physician in Bryan county for 35 years, three years of which were at Bokchito before he moved in 1910 to Durant.

He was graduated from the Eclectic Medical school in Cincinnati and practiced medicine in Cincinnati until he moved to Bokchito in 1907.

He died at the Wilson N. Jones hospital in Sherman, Tex. Surviving him are his wife, one son, Lloyd Jenner, Durant; one daughter, Mrs. Dorothy Auld, Talera, Peru, South America, four brothers and two sisters.

Dr. Edward M. Harris
1872-1942

Dr. Edward M. Harris, well-known pioneer physician of Cushing, has passed away. He was a typical horse and buggy doctor, with an outstanding abundance of good horse sense, which was definitely an asset in the early days of this new state.

Doctor Harris was born May 16, 1872, on a farm near Tuscaloosa, Ala., of simple, rugged parentage, whose parents have produced three outstanding Oklahoma physicians since the turn of the century.

His early education was at a medical school at Fort Worth, Tex. He entered the practice of medicine during the Medical Practice Act in the Indian Territory. One year later he entered Grant University at Chattanooga, Tenn., where he graduated in 1901.

He came to Cushing in the fall of 1909, and has continued to administer to the wants of the sick and needy ever since.

Doctor Harris was married at Hamlin, Tex., in the year of 1908 to Miss Ida Belle Morrow, and to this union one son and two daughters were born. The son's passing away in early childhood was a staggering blow to the Doctor that was never entirely overcome. The two daughters, Mrs. Richard Hildebrand of Bartlesville, and Mrs. Robert Pearman of Santa Anna, California, with the wife, still survive him.

Doctor Harris' loyalty to his patients and to the medical profession was never questioned, and his innate judgment was counseled by all that knew him. He had the happy faculty of "hitting the nail on the head" interspersed with inborn, clean native wit that made all that knew, or contacted him "warm friends."

The Cushing community has lost a real practitioner, and the doctors a loyal friend in his passing, and his children a devoted father, with ever their interest in mind. Doctor Harris, in his later years, could not seem to slow down, and only with the constant efforts of his devoted wife was he able to carry on as he did.

He passed away on January 26, 1942, at the St. Anthony Hospital in Oklahoma City. Two days later, funeral services were conducted at the Presbyterian Church at Cushing, with an over-flowing crowd as his admirers.

Classified Advertisements

FOR SALE: To settle estate. Dr. Bently Squires Cystoscopic table with Wappler X-ray, one Victor fluroscope, steel X-Ray file, developing tank, lead chest, Cassettes, film hangers, Brown Buerger cystoscope, two Monel water sterilizers with stand, one Englen diathermy, one Hawley fracture and orthopedic table.
For further information contact the Executive office, 210 Plaza Court, Oklahoma City, Oklahoma.

FOR SALE—One Siebrandt Pivot Leg Splint Complete. For further information, contact the Bone and Joint Hospital, 605 N. W. Tenth, Oklahoma City, Oklahoma.

FOR SALE: Victor X-ray—30 millamperes, 2 tubes —table—movable bucky and Cassettes. For other information, write Dr. W. W. Kerley, Anadarko.

FOR SALE: Seven-piece white, enameled office furniture outfit, including operating table, glass shelf medicine or instrument cabinet, chair, stool, etc. This was originally over $100, but will be sold at half-price.

Instruments, including a gold (one foot long) obstetric tool, and other instruments too numerous to mention. A large stock of drugs also. For other information, write Mrs. A. C. Jenner, Durant.

FOR SALE: One Zimmer Leg and Arm Reduction Apparatus Complete. Bone and Joint Hospital, 605 N.W. 10th, Oklahoma City.

FOR SALE: One good G. E. Model F2 with table. Reasonable. Anyone interested in the above item, should contact Dr. C. E. Bradley, Medical Arts Building, Tulsa, Okla.

FOR SALE: Surplus used Hospital Equipment. For further information, see Dr. Fowler Border, 330 N.W. 10th Street, Oklahoma City.

Beckham County Adopts Resolution

The following resolution was passed by the Beckham County Medical Society at its May meeting. Its content is particularly apropos at thsi time.

The Beckham County Medical Society in open session the 12th day of May, 1942, voted unanimously the following resolution:

BE IT RESOLVED that after due consideration and deliberation this Society does wholeheartedly support the action of the State Board of Medical Examiners regarding their action in severing reciprocal relations with the State of New York for the following reasons:

1. To give proper protection to the doctors of our State.

2. Due to the fact that the qualifications of the reciprocal applicants could not be and were not obtainable.

3. That many of the applicants were refugees and their exact status of preparedness was not obtainable as many of the refugees' colleges only require two to three years; that the American Medical Association did not and could not give the Board definite information regarding qualifications and past professional standings of the applicants.

4. The loyalty to our Government of many of the refugees could not be substantiated.

5. The policy of the American Medical School has been to reduce the number and raise the standard of the Medical student, thereby eliminating many applicants.

THEREFORE, we, the members of the Beckham County Medical Society wish to commend the farsightedness and the resolute stand taken by the State Board of Medical Examiners and also commend the Governor of our State for his decision in the matter, which we feel was in no way discriminating or selfish from any point of view.

Signed:

H. K. Speed, M.D., President,
Beckham County Medical Society.

E. S. Kilpatrick, M.D., Secretary,
Beckham County Medical Society.

BOOK REVIEWS

"The chief glory of every people arises from its authors."—Dr. Samuel Johnson.

"NEPHRITIS." Leopold Lichwitz, Chief Medical Division, Montefiore Hospital; Clinical Professor of Medicine, Columbia University, New York. Published by Grune and Stratton, N. Y. (344 pages) (120 illustrations and tables.) Bibliography, index, cloth, $5.50. (1942).

This same author and publishing house brought out "Functional Pathology" late in 1941. The author published, some time ago, a "Practice of Diseases of the Kidneys," in three German editions, four Spanish, and one Portuguese edition. The edition completely rewritten, is the fruition of a more mature knowledge gleaned from the subject in a study of laboratory and bedside correlation, including the more recent and important conceptions. His approach to the subject is that of a physiologist, biochemist and endocrinologist, with "The basic condition that Clinical Medicine is a science in its own right, and not an appendix either to pathological anatomy or experimental physiology." He takes up the age old argument about the function of the kidneys, but brings it up to date by theories of the neuro-vascular-endocrine working basis. He clarifies the pathology by bringing out the important phase which the circulatory system has. According to A. R. Cushney, the kidneys get per minute an amount of blood corresponding to twice their weight, i.e., 1000 litres in 24 hours. Hence one gm. of kidney receives about eight to 12 times as much blood as one gram of resting striated muscle. The temperature of the urine entering the kidney pelvis was considerably higher than the blood in the renal artery. Experimentally, even a short time closure of the renal artery or renal vein is followed by albuminuria. An oxygen supply too small to meet the oxygen needs, results in albuminuria. His clarification of the Goldblatt ideas in which urinary system which consists of the renal parenchyma proper, and the vascular supply and nerve connections from the hypothalmus down to the last nerve ending, makes it a systemic rather than an isolated organ. Allergy he claims, plays a big part in these distorted functions.

He uses the time honored term "Bright's disease" liberally. He cautiously does not pin up a big nomenclature where pathologist and clinicians differ, but explains acute and chronic glomerulonephritis and nephrosis as a circulatory disfunction. One innovation in nomenclature is nephritis dolorosa, a painful nephritis. Uraemia is approached from a physiolgical and biochemical standpoint. His ideas of uraemia as a more generalized tissue changes with the dehydrating effects of acidosis and the water retention in alkalosis, and makes some very interesting creative deductions. The protean symptoms of uraemia are discussed from a clinical and chemical background. He classifies it as acute and chronic. The nervous symptomology is evidenced by some 18 different manifestations. The gastroenteric by some eight different symptoms, and the respiratory showing either kussmal's or Cheynes-Stokes' breathing. Symptoms of acute and chronic glomerulonephritis are almost identical. Renal acidosis does not develop in acute Bright's disease.—L.A.R.

"SCLEROSING THERAPY." Edited by Frank C. Yeomans, M.D., F.A.C.S., M.R.S.M. (London Hon.) with 185 Illustrations on 117 Figures. Published by Williams and Wilkins.

This book is a compilation of monographs by four different authors.

Part I, 135 pages. Injection Treatment of Hernia by Arthur F. Brathrud, M.D., F.A.C.S. First, there is a brief historical review followed by the anatomy, etiology, pathology, and differential diagnosis. The importance of proper fitting trusses when injection is done is stressed, and how to properly fit the truss clearly elucidated. This treatment is discussed for several different types of hernia and technic is well explained. He discusses the selection of cases for this type of treatment, and the legal aspects of the injection treatment of hernia.

Part II, 17 pages. Injection Treatment of Hydrocele by George F. Hoch, M.D., D. U. He first considers the embryology and anatomy of hydrocele. He then goes into the etiology and pathology. Injection treatment of hydrocele is highly recommended by the author, and the technic that he uses is clearly explained with the assistance of several illustrations.

Part III, 117 pages. Injection Treatment of Varicose Veins by Harold J. Shelley, M.D., F.A.C.S. The anatomy of the venous system of the legs is discussed at length. He quotes from many authors as to the etiology and pathology of this condition. One chapter is devoted to a symptomatology of the patient with varicose veins. Practically all of the accepted tests that are used in the examination of the patient are fully explained. He goes into great detail in the combined injection and surgical treatment. He discusses complications and means of avoiding complications. In our opinion, he is slightly optomistic as to the results that may be obtained to the injection treatment alone.

Part IV, 28 pages. Injection Treatment of Hemorrhoids by Frank C. Yeomans, M.D., F.A.C.S., M.R.S.M. (London Hon.) First, embryology and anatomy are considered. He mentions both the operative and injection treatment, and states that he prefers the injection treatment in selected cases, and this group consists of about 50 percent of all cases. He discusses various solutions that may be used for this treatment, and carefully explains the technic of injection.

This book is written by men who are competently doing the thing they are writing about. All four chapters are well reading by anyone who is interested in these subjects. We would recommend it as a book well worthy of purchase.—John Powers Wolff.

"TIME AND THE PHYSICIAN." The Autobiography of Lewellys F. Barker. 350 pages. New York: G. P. Putnam's Sons. Price $3.50.

"The writing of a biography is after all a very egocentric activity. It encourages one to put one's best foot forward and tempts one to reveal one's self to the point of self exhibition. Vanity is a personal quality from which few of us are entirely free."

Dr. Barker having been born of Quaker parents and faith, waited until he was 74 years of age before the spirit moved him to write about himself. This biography may have also been motivated by the physiological geriatries which revel in reminiscences. He very interestingly, and in his own inimitable language, has delineated his rise on the ladder of fame. The first rounds of this ladder was firmly planted in the basement in "the back shop of a drug store."

Like William Osler, he was Canadian born and of ministerial parents. He secured his first medical degree in the University of Toronto, and while interning there had the urge to go to Johns Hopkins (with Cullen), after having seen Howard Kelly operate. He was also lured there by the "four horsemen" whose energies and outstanding ability were making this College the mecca of ambitious young medical men.

After spending his last dollar while walking the wards with Osler, he was appointed Associate in anatomy, and then resident in pathology, laying a good foundation for the superstructure of Internal Medicine. His anatomy research was in neuro-anatomy. While spending five years in Rush Medical in Chicago as professor of anatomy, he published "Spalteholtz Hand Atlas of Human Anatomy in English," and also collaborated in publishing a "Laboratory Manuel of Human Anatomy." His studies in Europe under Mueller, His, et al and his association with Flexner at Hopkins gave him an opportunity for his odysseys on Federal Commissions to California to study the plague, and to the Philippines "to be of service to the American forces for the inhabitants of those islands and humanity at large." He also went to India to study the plague, accepted a visiting lecturship in the University of California, and the Peter Bient Brigham hospital.

When Osler tendered his resignation as Professor of Medicine in Hopkins, Lewellys Franklin Barker was called to take the chair (or settee). His growth with the institution, his voluminous writing of medical books, of articles for medical Journals, and his appointment on numerous medical programs, have made him one of the spokes in the Hopkins wheel of medical erudition. Fortunately this book is the repository of much knowledge of the history of Hopkins, including the human side of his confreres, as well as medical education and the development of medicine in this golden age. No other time in history has medicine made such strides. "The boundaries of your reputation are now world-wide." (Thayer)—Lea A. Riely, M.D.

Summer Diarrhea in Babies

Casec (calcium caseinate), which is almost wholly a combination of protein and calcium, offers a quickly effective method of treating all types of diarrhea, both in bottle-fed and breast-fed infants. For the former, the carbohydrate is temporarily omitted from the 24-hour formula and replaced with 8 level tablespoonfuls of Casec. Within a day or two the diarrhea will usually be arrested, and carbohydrate in the form of Dextri-Maltose may safely be added to the formula and the Casec gradually eliminated. Three to six teaspoonfuls of a thin paste of Casec and water, given before each nursing, is well indicated for loose stools in breast-fed babies.

Please send for samples to Mead Johnson & Company, Evansville, Indiana.

Watch War Tension As Trend To Alcoholism

War times can make drunkards unless people sip cautiously.

This is the warning of Dr. A. J. McGee of the Alcoholic Research Bureau of The Keeley Institute at Dwight, Ill., who says that overworked and nervous war workers should beware of the relaxation offered in an alcoholic drink, since alcoholism tends to get a firm grip on nervous persons in times of stress and tension.

"Executives in particular," said Dr. McGee, "tend to burn themselves out under the strain of wartime problems. Nervous fatigue, indigestion, insomnia—these are the wound stripes of civilization. Alcoholic indulgence aggravates rather than alleviates these conditions."

Two persons out of every hundred cannot take even one drink without danger of becoming alcoholics, said Dr. McGee. The statement is based on case histories of half a million patients treated at the Institute over a period of 65 years. The other 98, he said, may not become acute alcoholics and yet may drink enough to make them susceptible to gall bladder and kidney troubles, insomnia, acute nervousness and indigestion.

"The Red Cross warns every First Aider never to give an alcoholic drink to persons suffering from shock or injury," said Dr. McGee. "This warning is equally true for persons suffering from overwork. For an overworked mind or body there is no substitute for rest," he concluded.

"Soup Kitchen" for Bacteria

BACTERIA AND THEIR FELLOW TRAVELERS, the viruses, are epicures of the first order. Deny them the right ration and they refuse to go on living in the laboratory. Some subsist on daily dishes of milk and potatoes, while others thrive on beef tea and special mixtures of agar, gelatin and animal juices. The pneumococcus, a finicky fellow, must be fed the heart of the beef for the greatest proliferation. And we could go on citing many more cases of how science has satisfied their appetites.

A quarter of a million pounds of meat were consumed by bacteria at Lederle last year. Add to this a yearly consumption of two and a half million liters of agar solution, not to mention volumes and volumes of other culture media, and you have, we believe, the world's largest "soup kitchen" for bacteria. Here they are cultured under scientific control, allowed to thrive and then put to use for man's benefit.

Propagation of micro-organisms and viruses is a major feature of the art of biological production. At Lederle this important phase is under the direction of a staff of skilled bacteriologists, long experienced in making superior serums, antitoxins, vaccines and toxoids for the prevention and treatment of diseases of man and animals.

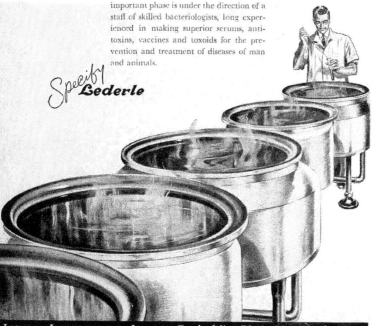

Specify **Lederle**

OFFICERS OF COUNTY SOCIETIES, 1942

COUNTY	PRESIDENT	SECRETARY	MEETING TIME
Alfalfa	Jack F. Parsons, Cherokee	L. T. Lancaster, Cherokee	Last Tues. Each 2nd Mo.
Atoka-Coal	J. B. Clark, Coalgate	J. S. Fulton, Atoka	
Beckham	H. K. Speed, Sayre	E. S. Kilpatrick, Elk City	Second Tues. eve.
Blaine	Virginia Olson Curtin, Watonga	W. F. Griffin, Watonga	
Bryan	A. J. Wells, Calera	W. K. Haynie, Durant	Second Tues. eve.
Caddo	Fred L. Patterson, Carnegie	C. B. Sullivan, Carnegie	
Canadian	P. F. Herod, El Reno	A. L. Johnson, El Reno	Subject to call
Carter	Walter Hardy, Ardmore	H. A. Higgins, Ardmore	
Cherokee	Park H. Medearis, Tahlequah	Isadore Dyer, Tahlequah	
Choctaw	C. H. Hale, Boswell	Fred D. Switzer, Hugo	
Cleveland	F. C. Buffington, Norman	Phil Haddock, Norman	Thursday nights
Comanche	George S. Barber, Lawton	W. F. Lewis, Lawton	
Cotton	George W. Baker, Walters	Mollie F. Scism, Walters	Third Friday
Craig	W. R. Marks, Vinita	J. M. McMillan, Vinita	
Creek	Frank Sisler, Bristow	O. H. Cowart, Bristow	
Custer	Richard M. Burke, Clinton	W. C. Tisdal, Clinton	Third Thursday
Garfield	D. S. Harris, Drummond	John R. Walker, Enid	Fourth Thursday
Garvin	T. F. Gross, Lindsay	John R. Callaway, Pauls Valley	Wed before 3rd Thurs.
Grady	D. S. Downey, Chickasha	Frank T. Joyce, Chickasha	3rd Thursday
Grant	I. V. Hardy, Medford	E. E. Lawson, Medford	
Greer	G. F. Border, Mangum	J. B. Hollis, Mangum	
Harmon	S. W. Hopkins, Hollis	W. M. Yeargan, Hollis	First Wednesday
Haskell	William Carson, Keota	N. K. Williams, McCurtain	
Hughes	Wm. L. Taylor, Holdenville	Imogene Mayfield, Holdenville	First Friday
Jackson	J. M. Allgood, Altus	Willard D. Holt, Altus	Last Monday
Jefferson	W. M. Browning, Waurika	J. I. Hollingsworth, Waurika	Second Monday
Kay	J. C. Wagner, Ponca City	J. Holland Howe, Ponca City	Third Thurs.
Kingfisher	C. M. Hodgson, Kingfisher	John R. Taylor, Kingfisher	
Kiowa	J. M. Bonham, Hobart	B. H. Watkins, Hobart	
LeFlore	G. R. Booth, LeFlore	Rush L. Wright, Poteau	
Lincoln	E. F. Hurlbut, Meeker	C. W. Robertson, Chandler	First Wednesday
Logan	William C. Miller, Guthrie	J. L. LeHew, Jr., Guthrie	Last Tuesday evening
Marshall	J. L. Holland, Madill	O. A. Cook, Madill	
Mayes	L. C. White, Adair	V. D. Herrington, Pryor	
McClain	B. W. Slover, Blanchard	R. L. Royster, Purcell	
McCurtain	R. D. Williams, Idabel	R. H. Sherrill, Broken Bow	Fourth Tues. eve.
McIntosh	F. R. First, Checotah	William A. Tolleson, Eufaula	Second Tuesday
Murray	P. V. Annadown, Sulphur	F. E. Sadler, Sulphur	
Muskogee	Shade D. Neely, Muskogee	J. T. McInnis, Muskogee	First & Third Mon.
Noble	J. W. Francis, Perry	C. H. Cooke, Perry	
Okfuskee	J. M. Pemberton, Okemah	L. J. Spickard, Okemah	Second Monday
Oklahoma	R. Q. Goodwin, Okla. City	Wm. E. Eastland, Okla. City	Fourth Tuesday
Okmulgee	J. G. Edwards, Okmulgee	John R. Cotteral, Henryetta	Second Monday
Osage	C. R. Weirich, Pawhuska	George K. Hemphill, Pawhuska	Second Monday
Ottawa	J. B. Hampton, Commerce	Walter Sanger, Picher	Third Thursday
Pawnee	E. T. Robinson, Cleveland	Robert L. Browning, Pawnee	
Payne	John W. Martin, Cushing	James D. Martin, Cushing	Third Thursday
Pittsburg	Austin R. Stough, McAlester	Edw. D. Greenberger, McAlester	Third Friday
Pontotoc	R. E. Cowling, Ada	E. R. Muntz, Ada	First Wednesday
Pottawatomie	John Carson, Shawnee	Clinton Gallaher, Shawnee	First & Third Sat.
Pushmataha	P. B. Rice, Antlers	John S. Lawson, Clayton	
Rogers	W. A. Howard, Chelsea	George D. Waller, Claremore	First Monday
Seminole	H. M. Reeder, Konawa	Mack I. Shanholtz, Wewoka	
Stephens	A. J. Weedn, Duncan	W. K. Walker, Marlow	
Texas	L. G. Blackmer, Hooker	Johnny A. Blue, Guymon	
Tillman	C. C. Allen, Frederick	O. G. Bacon, Frederick	
Tulsa	H. B. Stewart, Tulsa	E. O. Johnson, Tulsa	Second & Fourth Mon. eve.
Wagoner	J. H. Plunkett, Wagoner	H. K. Riddle, Coweta	
Washington-Nowata	R. W. Rucker, Bartlesville	J. V. Athey, Bartlesville	Second Wednesday
Washita	A. S. Neal, Cordell	James F. McMurry, Sentinel	
Woods	W. F. LaFon, Waynoka	O. E. Templin, Alva	Last Wednesday
Woodward	M. H. Newman, Shattuck	C. W. Tedrowe, Woodward	

THE JOURNAL
OF THE
OKLAHOMA STATE MEDICAL ASSOCIATION

| VOLUME XXXV | OKLAHOMA CITY, OKLAHOMA, AUGUST, 1942 | NUMBER 8 |

Influenzal Meningitis*
A Case Report

FRANCIS J. DAUGHERTY, M.D.
CARROLL M. POUNDERS, M.D.

OKLAHOMA CITY, OKLAHOMA

The prognosis in Influenzal Meningitis is not good, especially in very young children. It is interesting to compare the mortality rate before and after the advent of chemotherapy. In 1936, Wilkes-Weiss surveyed the literature and found 500 cases. In those patients under two years of age (373), the mortality rate was 97.6 percent. In those paients over two years of age (127), the rate was 79.5 percent. In 1940 Aleman collected 478 cases under two years of age who had been treated since 1936 and found the mortality rate to be 96.8 percent. Hence the death rate in patients of this age group has not been reduced significantly. Lindsay et al in 1940 reported a death rate of 54 percent in 33 patients of various ages. Other workers have reported a mortality rate as low as 33 percent in a small series of patients.

During the past 12 years fifteen cases of Influenzal Meningitis have been diagnosed and treated by the Pediatric Department of the Crippled Children's Hospital, Oklahoma City, Oklahoma. The ages of these patients ranged from four weeks to nine years and eleven were two years of age or younger. The duration of the disease was from two days to 43 days in the fatal cases. Five patients received chemotherapy but only recently has a patient with this disease recovered. The type of therapy used in this case differed from that previously employed and consisted of a modified form of the treatment recommended by Lindsay et al of Washington, D. C.

CASE REPORT

B. Mc., a three year old colored female,

*From the Pediatric Department of the Crippled Children's Hospital, Oklahoma City, Oklahoma.

was brought to this hospital on February 11, 1942 by her mother who stated that the patient had been well until ten days previously when she developed a common cold. No unusual symptoms were noted till the day before admission when the patient became irritable, disoriented, and would roll from side to side on the bed.

On physical examination, the child appeared well developed and well nourished but acutely ill. Her rectal temperature was 102°F., the pulse rate 148 and the respiratory rate 54. The nasal and pharyngeal mucosae were hyperemic. Her lungs were clear. She showed a mild degree of opisthotonos, a definite meningismus and positive Kernig and Brudzinski reflexes. The achilles tendon reflexes were either absent or hypoactive.

A lumbar puncture was done, and the cerebrospinal fluid was turbid and under pressure. On the basis that this was most likely a meningococcus meningitis 10 cc. of concentrated antimeningococcus serum was given intrathecally.

On the day following admission the laboratory findings were reported as follows: hemoglobin, 13.5 gms.; erythrocytes, 4,860,-000; leukocytes, 23,100 with 73 percent polymorphonuclear neutrophiles. The cerebrospinal fluid showed 4,500 leukocytes with 89 percent polymorphonuclear neutrophiles, 150 mg. protein, 10 mg. sugar and a negative Wassermann reaction. A smear from the cerebrospinal fluid showed long gram-negative bacilli and the culture was positive for Hemophilus Influenzae.

The plan of treatment consisted of daily lumbar punctures and drainage of cerebrospinal fluid to relieve the increased pressure. Following drainainge 15 cc. of a mixture of equal parts of anti-influenzal bacillus serum and two percent sodium sulfapyridine solution were injected intrathecally. The remaining 22 cc. of specific serum from one ampule was given intravenously or intramuscularly daily. Sodium sulfapyridine, 4 gms. in 500 cc. of .9 percent sodium chlodire solution, was injected subcutaneously daily. This amount kept the blood concentration around 10 mg. percent. 200 mg. of cevitamic acid was given daily by mouth. Supportive treatment consisted of a diet of 1,300 calories, adequate fluids, and four transfusions of 250 cc. of whole citrated blood each.

On the nineteenth day of her hospital course, the patient's spinal fluid was negative on culture and continued to be negative for three successive days. On the twenty-sixth day the cerebrospinal fluid was again examined and found to be negative for Hemophilus Influenzae.

The patient is now receiving a general diet with supportive treatment and apparently has no residual findings.

CONCLUSIONS

1. The prognosis of influenzal meningitis is not hopeless. ·
2. Early examination of spinal fluid by a competent bacteriologist, in doubtful cases, is essential.
3. Specific serum may be of. benefit and should be used.
4. Sulfapyridine is the drug of choice.
5. Early treatment of influenzal meningitis is essential.
6. Daily drainage of cerebrospinal fluid is indicated.
7. Even when recovery takes place, the course is rather long and not dramatic.

BIBLIOGRAPHY

1. Aleman, Ruth: Influenzal Meningitis, New Orleans Medical and Surgical Journal, 93:25-33, 1940.
2. Lindsoy, Janvier W.; Rice, E. Clarence, and Selinger, Maurice A.. Journal of Pediatrics, 17:220-227, 1940.

Problems of Behavior in Child Guidance*·

HAROLD J. BINDER, M.D.

OKLAHOMA CITY, OKLAHOMA

The problems of behavior adjustment in children are many and varied. To attempt to list all would be unnecessary. They run the gamut from feeding disturbances of infancy through complaints of enuresis, soiling, temper tantrums, speech disturbances, tics, spasms, to school and social maladjustment, running away from home, and stealing. Despite the apparent dissimilarity, they are all alike in that they are expressions of dissatisfaction or unmet needs of the child. The same factors which operate in the creation of early and mild problems continue to operate, though frequently in more exaggerated form, in the creation of later and more serious difficulties. With this in mind, the preventive aspects loom increasingly important

Leaving out for the moment the difficulties directly related to organic brain damage and to inherent intellectual deficiencies, it is generally accepted that the majority of problems result from conflicts in the parent-child relationship. The problem is merely a symp-

tom expressive of inner tension and anxiety. Thumbsucking, masturbation, or enuresis is not a problem to the young child. To the parent it is a source of irritation and a major complaint. To the child, it is a source of gratification. Treated symptomatically, by restraint, threats, and physical punishment, that particular symptom may be removed, but nothing has been done to understand and correct the deeper emotional problem which gave rise to the symptom. Instead, the child's tension and anxiety have been increased and may be expected to reveal themselves in other symptomatic behavior. Forcible removal of such neurotic manifestations, without substitution of adequate satisfactions, has frequently been of more harm than help to the child. In older children who are aware of the social implications of a particular habit and who are desirous of release from it, symptomatic treatment with his permission and understanding is frequently desirable since it may result in a better adjustment in other areas.

The role of the pediatrician has undergone considerable change in recent years. He is

*Presented at the Pediatric Session of the Oklahoma State Medical Association Meeting, April 23, 1942.

no longer concerned only with the physical care of the child. The "whole" child has become of increasing importance with the awareness of the inseparability of mind and body, of mental and physical growth. Routines for the physical management of infants and children have been glibly set forth and in too many instances mothers have interpreted such in a manner which best suited their own feelings. There is a dearth of sound information which parents have regarding the bringing up of children with reference to their emotional needs. The formulation and dissemination of psychologically sound suggestions for the management of children during the first five years is a current necessity. Parents require information on the different kinds of behavior which may normally be expected of the child at various stages during this period. A parent who is forewarned is less likely to become anxious and concerned or to make an issue over what they might otherwise regard as abnormal behavior. This presents an opportunity for the pediatrician which no one else is in so favorable a position to meet. On the part of the pediatrician it requires a thorough knowledge of habit formation, of emotional development and of personality growth. In addition, the time requirement is an element which cannot be overlooked in dealing with troubled parents and children. Behavior can neither be understood nor modified in one brief interview.

Psychiatry and mental hygiene have, unfortunately, no short cuts nor set of rules to offer in the treatment of problem behavior. What is offered is a point of view based upon certain general principles. The pediatrician is familiar with the use of the otoscope and ophthalmoscope and utilizes them in his daily practice, yet without claiming to be an otologist or an ophthalmologist. In similar fashion may he profit from becoming familiar with psychiatric methods of dealing with disturbed children, and concepts underlying these methods, without feeling the need to become a psychiatrist. These procedures may not be feasible for direct application in pediatric practice, but for orientation and guidance in developing to the fullest extent his relationship with parents and children, they should prove of value.

For the purpose of simplicity, we may consider the basic factors which influence personality development and behavior of children as falling into four categories or spheres; namely, the physical, intellectual, social, and emotional. However, the multiplicity of causative factors should be kept in mind since it is seldom that only one factor is involved. Yet, alleviation of one factor often serves to lighten the stress so that general improvement is observed.

Physical factors have been found to be both directly and indirectly responsible for the development of behavior disorders. Needless to say, a thorough physical examination is of prime importance in any study of the child. Symptoms of hyperactivity, restlessness, irritability, distractibility, inattention, school failure, belligerency, and even delinquency may be closely associated with diseased tonsils, dental caries, genito-urinary infection, defective vision or hearing, or endocrine dysfunction. The child with chronic infection or with defective vision fatigues more readily in the classroom and his restlessness and inattention may call forth the ire of the teacher. This may result in increased irritability and in active retaliation on the part of the child, or in sensitive withdrawal. A vicious circle is thus established, becoming more intolerable as time goes on. Such a chain of events is known, for example, to have been initiated by a scabetic infection which made the child restless and inattentive. Although physical factors initiate the disturbance, emotional reactions often set in which may well become so strong that treatment of the physical condition alone will not always suffice. Efforts directed toward an understanding of the individual case is frequently necessary both in the home and school to bring about acceptance of the child, and readjustment.

Physical complaints not infrequently mask underlying emotional problems. On the one hand, some parents feel less guilty if behavior can be explained on a physical basis, and they will take their children to the physician with specific diagnoses of their own or in search of some organic cause for the child's maladjustment. On the other hand, physical symptoms may be the child's only acceptable release for inner tensions. Recent studies, for example, on children with complaints of abdominal pain in whom no organic basis for such could be detected, have revealed interesting facts. From on intensive study of twenty-five such children, Dr. John Lambert concluded that the abdominal pain was the visceral accompaniment of emotional disturbance. The attitudes associated with the complaint were generally in the nature of fear, anxiety, and resentment and in most instances were directly related to the home setting. These emotional factors were not brought out by the parents, but in interviews with the children. These children did not seem able to express their feelings at home openly and directly to the same extent as most children. In the face of frustrating experiences, the child's hostility and rebellion appeared in the form of visceral sensations. One girl remarked, "When my mother wouldn't let me go, it made me excited inside and my tummy started hurting."

Serious problems may develop on an emotional basis following an illness or operation. The attitudes of parents and nurses during the actual illness, and especially during the convalescent period, may be too satisfying to the child for him readily to relinquish the extra attention. Added attention and love are necessary during the acute illness to maintain the security of the child, but this should be distinguished from giving in to unreasonable whims and demands on his part.

A child's first illness may result in a chronically overconcerned mother with an overprotective attitude which is a handicap to the child's continued emotional growth and maturation. Some parents have, through overprotective measures, succeeded in making veritable invalids out of their children, and the effects of this upon the adult personality are only too obvious. One cannot blame the young child for liking this expression of concern, for it may be his strongest emotional tie to the mother, and he may be unable, if not actually unwilling, to free himself of it as he grows.

Illness or an accident which results in physical handicap, such as heart disease, tuberculosis, paralysis, bone deformities and the like warrant a considerable amount of time and effort on the part of the physician in proper interpretation to child and parent. One should emphasize not the limitations and restrictions to be followed, but rather the things that can be done. Particular interests of the child should be utilized and built up so that he may achieve a sense of adequacy through accomplishment to make up for his inability to join in the usual pastimes of his friends. Too frequently, boys have been seen in correctional institutions who, as a result of "being different" from their fellows in not being able to do the things they did, sought and found ready acceptance in a delinquent group.

One should not overlook the possible traumatic elements inherent in hospitalization and operation. Children are often whisked away from home and to the hospital without any explanation by the parent of what is in store for them. Children should not be misinformed as to procedures for it results in loss of confidence and trust. Physicians and nurses, even though cognizant of this factor, are often prone to overlook it in the pressure of activities and because the child's apparent adjustment on the ward may be satisfactory.

Learning difficulties in school are not limited to retarded children. Children of average or superior intelligence may have specific disabilities in reading or arithmetic from the very start which will retard their progress and create emotional disturbances because they feel inferior to their classmates.

These disabilities must be accurately diagnosed by proper psychological tests before adequate remedial measures can be undertaken. There is also the child who is started in school without the desirable preparation, who regards the school as a hostile environment and as being responsible for his separation from mother. He may fear that a younger brother or sister, left at home, will completely usurp his place in the parental affections. These are some of the emotional barriers which can block the acquisition of knowledge. .

A comparatively large group of children will be found who are not feebleminded, but who fall in the range between borderline level of intelligence and average. Retardation of one to two years in their mental development will be sufficient to make it impossible for them to grasp the fundamentals in the early grades as do others of the same age group. Their schooling must be at a slower rate so that they may better absorb the instruction. Psychological tests help us to understand these cases by making us aware of their ability and capacity for learning.

Children in either of the above two groups will compensate for the sense of inadequacy they experience in accordance with their constitutional and personality make-up. Some will display aggressiveness of varying degrees; some will assume a veneer of indifference; others may withdraw within their own shell—a social recluse.

The mental defective or feebleminded child and the child with brain damage resulting from trauma or from residuals of encephalitis are brought to the physician for help. Unfortunately their parents have usually received little in the way of constructive suggestion. In most of these cases, even though a formal school program in the community is out of the question, there are various opportunities offered in handicrafts. These children can learn to do simple things with their hands and keeping them occupied and accomplishing something, even at a low level, helps both parent and child. Psychological tests help us appreciate at what mental level these children are ready to do things. Restlessness and distractibility are features which make it difficult to get them to concentrate on any one project, but the use of mild sedation may slow them down sufficiently to get their interest focused. Once the latter is accomplished, sedation can be withdrawn. Some of the behavior symptoms presented by these children are inherent in the brain damage suffered. Other symptoms, however, are superimposed upon this first group and are only indirectly connected with the organic illness. These latter symptoms are the result of faulty training, of parental rejection, of overprotection, and of veryprevalent faulty misconceptions as to what could be expected of these children in the way of independent initiative and achievement.

In considering the social and emotional phases of a child's development we are dealing with less obvious, less tangible material but none the less real. The child's first social contacts are within the home and remain predominantly so until entrance in school. It is in the home that he observes and takes on certain patterns of behavior, general attitudes and prejudices which may help or hinder him in his wider social relationships outside the home. In his social contacts outside he will first begin to feel keenly the differences from his fellows—differences in economic and cultural aspects of the family, differences in standards of living and standards of life. Some children find themselves unable to adjust these differences without help and encouragement and thereby unable to get along with their fellows. These experiences lead to emotional reactions which can mean the difference between success and failure. A good number of social misfits, on the other hand, have emotional problems which have developed in the home and which militate against successful adjustment outside. Some of these children, with more or less serious emotional conflicts in their family relationship, are able to compensate for their previous lack of satisfaction in the home through satisfying relationships in school and in the neighborhood. Too frequently, they are unable to do so without some help through a relationship with an adult in which they find acceptance.

Emotional problems of children developing directly and primarily as such, in contrast to those resulting from physical, intellectual or social factors, are usually based on failure to supply a fundamental need. Two basic needs are: (1) security (love and affection and awareness of being a wanted and integral part of the home) ; (2) development of independence and self-responsibility. (This entails recognition of the child's individuality and need for self-direction).

Lack of security results in feelings of rejection by the child and this is the most traumatic emotional experience possible. The rejection may be actual, as in the case of a parent who does not want the child, who is emotionally incapable of accepting the dependence of the child, or who projects his feelings toward someone else on the child. The rejection may be fancied as in the situation where the child feels another sibling is favored or where he is confused by the conflicting and inconsistent methods of discipline employed.

Many immature or neurotic parents make it difficult for a child to develop self-dependence. Such parents feel a strong unconscious need for keeping their children tied to them. The child may glory in this dependence or may be conflicted between a desire to remain in this blissful state and the desire to emancipate himself. The problem becomes increasingly serious as adolescence and adulthood are approached. Overt difficulties may first reveal themselves when such an individual goes off to college, gets a job or marries.

No two families react to their children alike. In fact, no set of parents reacts to each of their own children in exactly the same manner, at least in the eyes of the individual child. This difference in emotional feelings and reaction produces a different environment for the personality development of each individual child in spite of the fact that the parents, home and physical comforts are apparently identical. The mere presence of another child in the home produces a rivalry situation with resultant tensions between the children which call forth acts to which the parents may well be expected to react differently. To minimize rivalry and jealousy between siblings, there should be adequate preparation of an older child for the reception of a new arrival. In addition to being made to feel that he is going to be helpful in the care of the new child, it is important not to show excessive attention to the new infant in the presence of the other child.

Parental misunderstanding, immaturity and personal maladjustment are vital factors concerned with the behavior of the child. Misunderstanding can be corrected, and anxiety of the parent because of lack of knowledge can be alleviated. The neurotic parent, however, presents considerable difficulty in a treatment program. Parents have themselves come through a childhood of their own, charged with emotional gratifications' and frustrations. Their problems are of much longer duration than those of their children. Intellectually they may be able to accept the desirability of change in their attitudes and methods, but emotionally they may not. Many seriously neurotic adults are in need of psychiatric help.

Even though it is true that problems of children usually are indicative of "problem parents," I regret to see this latter term obtaining such wide circulation among the laity. The ultimate effect is to be feared. It makes it more difficult for a parent to seek help for the child since the term infers blame and creates a defensive attitude on the part of many parents. A parent feels a sense of failure and guilt before seeking help for his child. There is no place for blame or fault-finding in any treatment relationship with parent and child. Just as we have grown more understanding of the child with a problem and have progressed to the point of seeking an explanation for misbehavior, so should we begin to understand the difficulties besetting the parent. Scolding the parent is as destructive as scolding the child. ·Treatment for both is necessary through a tactful approach, with encouragement to the parent that he or she has done the best within his or her power under the circumstances.

BIBLIOGRAPHY

Pediatrics and Child Psychiatry: A Symposium. Amer. Journ. Orthopsychiatry. 11:428-451, July 1941.

Lambert, John P.: Psychiatric Observations on Children with Abdominal Pain. Amer. Journ. Psychiatry. 98:451-454, Nov. 1941.

Aldrich & Aldrich. Babies Are Human Beings. New York. The Macmillan Co., 1941.

Kanner, Leo: Child Psychiatry. Springfield Ill Charles C. Thomas, 1935.

Staff of the Institute for Juvenile Research Child Guidance Procedures. New York, D. Appleton, Century Co 1937.

Stevenson, George S.· Why Parents Consult the Pediatrician. New York The National Committee for Mental Hygiene.

Safety Factors in Cesarean Section

L. C. NORTHRUP, M.D.

TULSA, OKLAHOMA

In March 1941, I published a brief article on "Safety Factors in Obstetrics". In this paper mention was made of the universal improvement in mortality brought about by the adoption of the low cervical cesarean section. Since this paper appeared I have received many requests for detailed information about the technique of this operation as it is done today. This paper is in answer to those requests.

My interest in the low cervical cesarean section is founded on fourteen years of personal experience with the operation. During this time I have performed over 300 consecutive low cervical cesareans, without a single maternal death and with no injured babies. Some of the babies did not survive but their death was in no way associated with the operation. The average operating time for this entire series was 38 minutes. Average number of days in hospital was eight. There was not a single case of peritonitis or severe hemorrhage. The morbidity was confined to a few cases of pyelitis and a few cases of phlebitis. These were not in excess of the number encountered in any other type of delivery.

Since the adoption of the low segment operation, the indications for cesarean section have been greatly extended. For example, I am now doing low segment cesareans on almost all my breach positions, especially the full term primipara. This is because of the high mortality for this type when attempt is made to deliver them vaginally. The infant mortality rate for breach presentations at Hillcrest Memorial Hospital for the past fourteen years is over 16 percent. The indications have been summed up by Dr. McGilvery of New York as follows: "Whenever the obstetrician feels that a low cervical section will give his mother and her baby a better chance than a vaginal delivery, he has sufficient indication." For the past two years I have been doing low segment cesareans on all difficult cases. During these two years, I have not had a single infant death from any cause whatever.

The name "low cervical section" is not a good name, as the incision is not in the cervix at all. I much prefer the term "low segment operation". · The incision is in the lower uterine segment and not in the cervix. Any operation in which the incision extends into the contractile portion of the body of the uterus should not be classified as a low segment or low cervical operation. The safety of the low segment operation lies in the fact that the incision is confined to the lower uterine segment which is not contractile and is therefore not subjected to the churning action associated with the after pains during the process of involution. This low segment incision heals while at rest. The second safety factor is your ability to create two peritoneal flaps to suture, overlapping, over the incision. This prevents any leaking.

It is not the spill of amniotic fluid at the time of operation that causes peritonitis. Peritonitis is caused by the leaking of infected lochia thru the classical incision in the contractile portion of the uterus, which often gaps open as the uterus contracts after delivery. This also causes hemorrhage which never occurs in the low segment incision.

The primary factor in safe obstetrics is to have a safe patient to start with. If your patient has had adequate pre-natal care, she will be a good risk. She will not be anemic or toxic. She will be well nourished, having had plenty of calcium and vitamines. You will know about her heart, lungs and kidneys. You will know about the size and position of the baby. A good healthy patient will give you a lower mortality.

I wish now to take up some safety factors associated with the technique that have developed during the past fourteen years. No pre-operative medication is used except one hypodermic of 1/75 gr. atropine given one hour before surgery. The vulva is shaved and about one ounce of full strength plain Zephiran is instilled into vagina. The abdomen is painted with the Tincture of Zephiran.

Spinal anesthesia holds first place in safety for the baby but is about fourth place in safety for the mother. Cyclopropane is first choice for the mother and only second choice for the baby, so we use it exclusively. It is administered by an experienced specialist in anesthesia. At time of the incision, we give 1 cc. Pitutrin or Pitocin. This is timed so that it will take effect as soon as the head is ready to be delivered. The patient is placed in extreme Trendelenberg position. Don't attempt the operation with the patient flat. A fundamental principle of good surgery is to avoid trauma and mutilation, so keep the incision below five inches in length. Four inches is enough for most babies. Never go above umbilicus. I usually make a very short incision about two inches long, directly in the mid-line about half way between umbilicus and symphisis. This incision is carried directly into abdomen. Then, before enlarging the incision, inspect bladder and enlarge incision away from bladder so as not to cut into it. The completed incision should extend from the bladder up four or five inches.

No packs are used. I think they produce trauma and can serve no useful purpose. You will seldom see any intestine. Locate the place where the bladder is attached to the anterior surface of the uterus. There is us-

ually a white "V" shaped fold at this place which can be easily seen. Look also for the circular sinus, which is a large sinus that crosses the surface of the uterus from side to side, just under peritoneum. The incision thru the viseral peritoneum should be made just below this sinus and just above the bladder attachment. Make this incision in a semilunar direction, curving up at outer ends to avoid the vessels at each outer edge of uterus. Dissect peritoneal flaps up and down from this incision, about ½ inch only. These flaps will be large enough after the uterus contracts. The incision into the lower uterine segment follows parallel to and just beneath the incision in the viseral peritoneum. If your landmarks were right, you will be just above the junction of the lower uterine segment with the cervix. The uterus at this place is seldom more than ⅛ inch thick at full term. You will encounter very little bleeding. Make the incision just big enough to deliver the head and no bigger. I use bandage scissors for this incision into uterus so as not to cut the baby's face. Slip your right hand into uterus and lift the head up into incision. The assistant will now press on fundus and the head can be worked thru the incision. I use a special flat curved instrument to lift the head out. This instrument is called "Torpin Vectis", sold by Mueller Co. It is a curved blade 1½ inches wide and 9¾ inches long, with a handle. As soon as baby is delivered the placenta is delivered and then the uterus is delivered thru the incision in abdomen. A hot wet pack is wrapped around the uterus and it is grasped in right hand of assistant. The uterus, can, in this way, be pulled up out of pelvis so the incision can be accurately sutured. This is most important. Two rows of chromic gut are placed by continuous suture into the incision in lower uterine segment. The second row invaginates the first row. Then the peritoneal flaps are sutured over this incision. The upper flap first, then the lower flap, overlapping. The uterus is replaced into abdomen and the abdomen closed in usual manner. I am opposed to doing any other surgery at time of a cesarean section.

As soon as the baby is delivered the mother is given a hypodermic of morphine and ergotrate. The nurses on floor are instructed to repeat the ergotrate whenever necessary to check excessive flowing. This is seldom necessary in the elective cases. It is some times necessary in the cases that have had a long trial labor.

I am constantly amazed at the quick

smooth convalescence. In most cases food is given at end of 24 hours. Patient is allowed to get out in a chair on the sixth day and encouraged to walk about on the seventh. Early exercise helps to prevent phlebitis.

I believe that a low segment section is safer than a difficult vaginal delivery. You must have good help, a good anesthetic and above all a patient that has had adequate pre-natal care. If you are going to do a section, it is better to do it as an elective operation and avoid a trial labor if possible.

Complications of Duodenal Ulcer: Their Surgical Management*

R. L. Sanders, M.D.

MEMPHIS, TENNESSEE

Medical minds have been studying the problems of duodenal ulcer for twenty centuries, yet the further its mysteries are penetrated, the more mysterious it becomes. Especially is this true of its etiology. The many theories which have been advanced, all of which seem in a measure valid, lead one to believe that we are far from discovering the real truth, and certainly the whole truth. In the light of our present knowledge, diet, infection over-exertion, circulatory disturbances, and derangements of the nervous system, from intrinsic disorders or extrinsic influences, or both, are all active in more or less degree in the production of ulcer.

Questions of therapy are inseparably involved with those of etiology, and until we know the answers to the latter, we shall probably continue to have ulcers, many of which will require surgery. Until that time, therefore, we may well strive for a better understanding of the usage of the surgical procedures now available. It is not the way of progress to be content with any achievement, however seemingly perfect; nevertheless, certain of the operations thus far developed for duodenal ulcer, when properly applied, may ·be relied upon to insure patients, with rare exceptions, freedom from further difficulty from this source.

This discussion will deal with the operative treatment of duodenal ulcer in the presence of (1) acute perforation, (2) hemorrhage, (3) obstruction and (4) intractability, and of (5) gastrojejunal ulcer and gastrojejunocolic fistula, these being the only conditions in which surgery is recognized as indicated.

ACUTE PERFORATION

Acute perforations arise, as a rule, from ulcers on the anterior wall of the duodenum.

They are encountered most often in comparatively young individuals. The perforation occasionally occurs without previous warning, or with no more warning than a prodromal period of a few days, wherein the patient experiences some abdominal discomfort and digestive disturbance. Usually, however, a history of symptoms for weeks or months, or perhaps for years, is obtained. In the majority of cases, the perforation is brought about by some influence which causes intra-abdominal or intragastric pressure, such as eating, drinking carbonated waters, exertion or excitement.

The diagnosis should be readily made by anyone who has observed even one or two patients in this condition, the outstanding features being excruciating pain of sudden onset, and abdominal tenderness and rigidity. Usually, the pain is localized in the epigastrium, particularly on the right, though it may be generalized over the abdomen or referred to the left upper quadrant or to the shoulder region. In degree, it is out of all proportion to that of any other disorder. The patient's suffering is obvious: the expression is drawn and agonizing, beads of perspiration stand out on the brow, the skin is pale, cold and clammy, and the patient lies perfectly still, resenting the examining hand or any effort at movement. His appearance is that of one in great shock, yet the blood pressure is not elevated, the temperature is normal or subnormal, and the pulse is slow. Nausea and vomiting may or· may not be associated. Within a short while the abdominal muscles assume a rigidity which is so unyielding to pressure as to be characteristic of perforating ulcer.

After a few hours, these acute manifestations subside to some extent and the patient seems slightly more comfortable, though the abdominal tenderness and rigidity persist.

*Read before the Fiftieth Anniversary of the Oklahoma State Medical Association, Tulsa, April 24, 1942.

If surgery is not undertaken, however, this phase is soon followed by signs of bacterial peritonitis: the temperature and leukocyte count rise, the pulse rate is accelerated, the pulse volume is reduced, and the abdomen becomes increasingly distended. A plain film will often reveal gas beneath the diaphragm. This clinical picture is a definite indication for immediate operation.

Not all acute perforating ulcers present such an emergency. Many are of only pin point size, leakage is slight, and the opening is immediately protected by omentum or fat, or by the gallbladder, liver or other adjacent structures, and in a few days the patient recovers. Occasionally, the contents escape above the liver, producing a subdiaphragmatic abscess. In this event, the patient usually comes to surgery on account of the abscess and the ulcer is found only incidentally. Unless operated on promptly, a large quantity of fluid may accumulate beneath the diaphragm, increasing the risk and prolonging the convalescence. Just last month, a patient was referred to us four days following perforation of a duodenal ulcer. Although at operation the perforation was found to be partially protected, almost two quarts of fluid was removed from above the dome of the liver and beneath the diaphragm. The patient is still in the hospital, but is well on the way to recovery following a second drainage of the extensive subphrenic abscess.

Treatment.—It is our custom to approach the abdomen through an upper transverse incision. By this method, the danger of wound infection and disruption from escape of the chemically irritating and infectious fluid from the peritoneal cavity is minimized, in that the incision follows the course of the tissue fibers, thus permitting the edges of the wound to come together without strain upon the sutures. In addition, the nerve and blood supply are conserved and healing takes place rapidly and firmly. We have had no wound disruptions since beginning the use of this approach, ten years ago.

Formerly, we excised the ulcer and closed the perforation by purse-stringing the opening with Lembert sutures, or orthewise enfolding the perforating zone. During the past several years, however, we have made no effort to close the perforation itself; instead, by means of a series of sutures placed in the stomach and duodenum, the pyloric end of the stomach is folded over the ulcer, covering it completely, and omental fat is tied over the area. This method is based upon the presumption that a rapid and massive formation of fibrin effectually closes the opening. Dr. Willis Gatch, of Indianapolis, described practically the same procedure at a

meeting of the Southern Surgical Association in 1936.

There is still some discussion as to the necessity for gastroenterostomy in these cases. We once made a practice of performing a gastroenterostomy in addition to closure of the ulcer. There was a reason for it. Our effort to close the perforation completely by sutures usually obstructed the pylorus for several days. Since we have been using the suction syphon apparatus, as suggested by Wangensteen, thus putting the stomach at rest postoperatively, a simple closure by the method described has been found sufficient. Few of these patients require further surgery.

If the perforation is protected, the problem may be different. Often, one finds a large, edematous mass about the pylorus and the first portion of the duodenum, where the tissues are fixed because of this protection and the inflammatory reaction, producing a marked obstruction. In many such cases, a gastroenterostomy may be necessary as a life-saving measure.

After closure of the ulcer, it is our custom to pour from seven to 15 grams of one of the sulfonamide drugs into the peritoneal cavity and into the wound. We have observed no untoward effects from these drugs and are convinced that the peritoneal reaction is less, convalescence smoother, and the mortality lower.

If the operation is performed early, drainage is unnecessary. We practically never institute drainage unless more than twelve hours has elapsed since the perforation and bacterial peritonitis is present or imminent.

During the past nine and one-half years we have operated on 26 patients for protected and unprotected perforating duodenal ulcer. The unprotected perforations were simply closed, while a gastroenterostomy was performed for the protected perforations, with one exception; this patient had a gastrectomy for recurrent duodenal ulcer with perforation, following a pyloroplasty several years earlier. One of the group, for whom a gastroenterostomy was done, now has clinical and roentgenographic evidence of a recurrence.

HEMORRHAGE

Whereas ulcers on the anterior wall of the duodenum perforate into the peritoneal cavity, those on the posterior wall penetrate into the head of the pancreas, eroding the blood vessels and producing hemorrhage. In extent, the hemorrhage varies according to the size of the blood vessel which has become eroded. Usually, it appears as melena, though it may be presented as hematemesis, or again as both.

More than one-fourth of all duodenal ulcers are of the bleeding type. The majority give rise to a mild but recurrent hemorrhage with persistent symptoms of ulcer, especially pain referred to the back, from penetration into the head of the pancreas. There is another group, however, in which hemorrhage recurs often or is practically constant, obviously coming from a fairly large perforation of an artery, and keeping the blood pressure and hemoglobin at dangerously low levels despite repeated transfusions. Here, also resection should be undertaken as early as possible. The longer the delay, the graver the danger from damage to the liver, kidneys, heart, brain and other organs, and the greater the likelihood of a sudden massive hemorrhage.

Treatment.—In our opinion, the proper treatment for hemorrhagic ulcers is gastrectomy. Until a few years ago, it was our practice, if the patient was in poor condition, to open the duodenum, cauterize the ulcer, and do a pyloroplasty. This procedure is now seldom, if ever, employed, as it has been found that the radical operation, with few exceptions, may be safely carried out following adequate preparation.

Frequently, one may experience great difficulty in separating the duodenum from the pancreas without damaging the common duct and large vessels. With care, however, it may be freed three-fourth to one inch, which is sufficient to permit complete closure. Or, if the perforation is large, the duodenum may be divided at the level of the ulcer, Allis forceps placed on the distal stump (Fig. 1), and the pancreas and ulcer bed dissected free for the necessary distance. The stump

LEGENDS

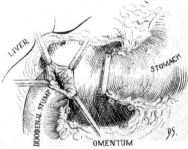

Fig. 1. Showing a safe method of handling the duodenal stump when the ulcer on the posterior wall has penetrated into the head of the pancreas, making separation of the duodenum and pancreas difficult. The duodenum is divided at the level of the ulcer and Allis forceps are placed on the stump. With gentle traction, the duodenal stump is separated from the pancreas for a distance of ½ to ¾ inch with comparative ease, making closure of the stump safe and satisfactory. To avoid spilling and soiling from the stomach, a small Furniss clamp is placed distal to the pylorus and just above the ulcer, and left with the clamp locked. The stomach can then be easily retracted to the left, permitting excellent exposure.

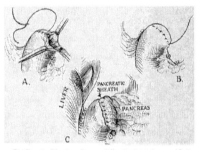

Fig. 2. *A*—Showing closure of the duodenal stump with the first row of sutures of fine chromic catgut.
B—Showing the second row of sutures completed, with satisfactory inversion and closure of the stump.
C—The sheath of the pancreas is sutured over the stump of the duodenum and fastened with several interrupted stitches of non-absorbable sutures. This prevents leakage and fixes the stump in a natural position without tension. In no case has leakage occurred following this procedure.

is then inverted and closed with two or three rows of catgut (Fig. 2A and B). As a further precaution against leakage, the sheath of the pancreas is sutured over the stump with a few interrupted silk sutures (Fig. 2C).

Formerly, we were hesitant about removing the lesion and disturbing the pylorus in poor risk cases, but with added experience we have found that this may be accomplished without materially increasing the hazard. Undoubtedly, if at all feasible, one should remove both the pylorus and the ulcer in order to eliminate pylorospasm and relieve the inflammatory reaction of the pancreas in the area of the penetration, as these are primary factors in the persistence of symptoms.

After liberation and closure of the duodenum and resection of an ample amount of the stomach, the continuity of the intestinal tract may be restored by one of several methods. We prefer the Polya anastomosis, uniting the entire end of the stomach to the side of the jejunum through the transverse mesocolon. The anterior anastomosis, after the method of Balfour, has been employed following high resections. The Hofmeister technic is preferred by a number of surgeons on the theory that it prevents too rapid emptying of the stomach. In our experience, however, function has been most satisfactory following the Polya and Balfour methods.

We do not supplement our resections by an entero-enterostomy. Such a procedure prevents reflux into the stomach of the alkaline duodenal secretions which aid in maintaining a low gastric acidity, and we have found no real indication for it.

One of the much discussed problems of gastrectomy for duodenal ulcer today has to do with the extent of the resection. Shall the stomach be removed to a point at which absolute achlorhydria to histamin stimulation is obtained? Total anacidity is likely to give rise to distressing symptoms, and, in our present opinion, is undesirable. We feel that, in the ma/ority of cases, resection of two-thirds of the stomach is ample; with the Polya anastomosis, which provides rapid emptying, more extensive resection is unnecessary unless the stomach acids are unusually high or the patient appears to be of the type who is likely to have further difficulty.

From October 1, 1932, to the present time we have employed the Polya gastrectomy in 20 cases of primary and recurrent bleeding duodenal ulcers, with one fatality, this being the first patient of the group, operated upon early in 1933. The immedate cause of death was pneumonia. Six of the resections were carried out for recurrent duodenal ulcer, one of them a third recurrence. In two of the six, a gastrojejunal ulcer was associated. An additional eight patients with bleeding ulcers have had either a gastroenterostomy or pyloroplasty during the same period; three of these have since experienced a return of ulcer symptoms. Functional results from gastrectomy have been uniformly excellent.

Massive Hemorrhage.—The indications for surgery in the presence of sudden massive hemorrhage from erosion of a large artery are less easily defined than those from repeated small hemorrhages. Surgeons are of different minds on this question. On the one hand are those who state that immediate operation is indicated only if the patient is, fifty years of age or beyond. In younger individuals whose vessels are elastic and in whom the clotting elements are practically normal, a clot usually forms and stops the hemorrhage, whereas in older persons, whose vessels have become sclerotic, this clot may form during the stage of shock, only to be dislodged by the force of the blood pressure after recovery from the shock; or, the clot may be dissolved by the stomach acids. Allen,[1] at the Massachusetts General Hospital, found only four deaths in a group of 90 patients under fifty years of age; in 42 over fifty, 14 or one-third bled to death. He concludes that all patients above the age of forty-five years with acute massive hemorrhage from duodenal ulcer should be carefully evaluated. Roscoe Graham[4] quotes a mortality of seven percent in 136 patients with massive hematemesis from duodenal ulcer, 70 percent of the fatalities having occurred in patients over fifty years of age. He reports that in the Toronto General Hospital the mortality from emergency operations for duodenal ulcer in patients beyond fifty has been forbidding, and therefore advocates waiting until the patient has recovered from the effects of the hemorrhage,

and then performing a resection. He further states, "No operation is advised for a young patient who has had but one massive hemorrhage from a duodenal ulcer, but should a second such hemorrhage occur, then operation is not only advisable, but is urgently indicated." Blackford,[2] from a survey of vital statistics of the city of Seattle, found that massive hemorrhage from older people was fatal in one-third of the cases; further, that three-fourths of all fatalities followed the first massive hemorrhage. From these investigations, he feels that the first massive hemorrhage in elderly people is by far the most dangerous. On the other hand, in his experience, emergency operations on young patients are unjustified, even for prostrating hemorrhage, as fatal bleeding is almost unknown in persons under forty-five years of age. In contrast to these opinions, Wangensteen[5] feels that a distinction based upon the age of the patient is not a safe criterion, and that young persons with flexible arteries may bleed briskly and die of hemorrhage as well as those beyond fifty.

The necessity for immediate surgery is probably more urgent in older patients, though operation, if done at all, should be carried out within forty-eight hours, as advocated by Finsterer.[3] If it becomes obvious that transfusion and other supportive measures will not control the hemorrhage and restore a satisfactory blood pressure, one should not wait until the loss of blood proves an insurmountable obstacle to recovery. Finsterer's mortality after early surgical intervention averages 5.1 percent, whereas the reported mortality following operations delayed after forty-eight hours has been, on the whole, exceedingly high.

OBSTRUCTION

Obstruction incident to healing and cicatrization of the doudenal ulcer, usually on the anterior wall, lends itself more readily to surgical cure than any of the other complications of this disease. The acid values being low and the ulcer having already healed, the pylorus need not be disturbed. A gastroenterostomy, if properly made, with a fairly large stoma, gives immediate and permanent relief practically without exception. The patient, previously in a state of malnutrition and dehydration from persistent vomiting over a long period of time, promptly regains normal weight and strength. There is, in fact, nothing more brilliant in all the domain of surgery than the relief obtained by a short-circuiting gastroenterostmy for cicatrization of a duodenal ulcer. Further, the probability of recurrence is remote, and of no significance as compared to the risk of the more radical operation.

Pyloric obstruction from edema and swelling associated with an active ulcer is a different matter. If the acid values are high, gastrectomy is indicated, as gastroenterostomy carries a not inconsiderable possibility of recurrence or of stomal ulcer. Should the patient be elderly or in poor condition, however, a gastroenterostomy may be the wiser course; if necessary, a resection may be performed later.

One should bear in mind that, in these cases, a low acid value at the first examination is likely to be misleading; the edema of the gastric wall may have interfered with secretion. In the event of such a finding, therefore, stomach lavage should be carried out continuously over a period of several days, until the edema and obstruction have subsided; with restored function, the acid values may be found excessive, indicating the need for gastrectomy.

INTRACTABILITY

It is axiomatic in our clinic that all ulcer patients, with the exception of those with acute perforation, obstruction or massive hemorrhage, shall be given the advantage of medical treatment. Many patients, however, are unable to adhere to a medical regimen because of their occupations, and thus are forced to seek relief through surgery. Others, particularly those who are highly nervous, do not respond to medical management, even under the most ideal conditions. The ulcer symptoms continue unabated and the patient remains disabled despite every effort, until both he and the doctor are exhausted. It is this status which we call intractability, and which we regard as a surgical problem.

We have observed that most of these patients have multiple ulcers and, strikingly, it is the posterior ulcer which produces the symptoms. The acid values are often high, and for this reason a gastroenterostomy is inadequate. A subtotal gastrectomy, including removal of the pylorus and the posterior ulcer, offers the surest promise of permanent relief. Even so, if the patient is of an unstable temperament, one may find it necessary to insist upon a regulation of diet for an indefinite period after operation.

GASTROJEJUNAL, MARGINAL, OR JEJUNAL ULCER; GASTROJEJUNOCOLIC FISTULA

Gastrojejunal, marginal or jejunal ulcers are observed, usually, in middle aged or fairly young individuals with high acid values who have previously had a gastroenterostomy for a duodenal ulcer. The reported incidence varies from two to 34 percent, the latter figure being reported by Lewisohn. The average is probably about six to ten percent.

The ulcer may appear within a few days after operation, or it may not become apparent for many years; the majority, however, develop within eighteen months. They are found, as a rule, on the margin of the stoma,

especially on the jejunal side. A few of them bleed, and many produce the original ulcer symptoms, though the picture is generally a little atypical, the pain being slightly lower and to the left, more constant and severe, and rarely completely controlled by food and alkali. Operation in such cases should be carried out without undue delay.

If the pylorus is not obstructed by cicatrization and one can do a good pyloroplasty to widen the outlet, lessen pylorospasm and permit a reflux of the jejunal contents into the stomach, this may be done, the gastroenterostomy detached, and the opening in both the stomach and jejunum closed, restoring the continuity of the gastrointestinal tract to its original condition. This procedure, however, is justified only when the patient is in no condition for the more radical operation.

In all our cases, we have found it possible to take down the gastroenterostomy and excise the gastrojejunal ulcer, or resect the jejunum and make an end-to-end anastomosis, and then perform a subtotal gastrectomy, including the pylorus and the ulcer-bearing zone. This is a formidable procedure under the circumstances, but relief is usually complete.

One of the reasons for early operation in the presence of gastrojejunal ulcer is the danger of perforation into the colon. This disaster occurs in approximately 11 percent of gastrojejunal ulcers and is the most serious of all the complications of duodenal ulcer. The mortality is exceedingly high. One should therefore bear in mind the possibility of a perforation when a gastrojejunal ulcer develops. If the condition is recognized in time, the gastroenterostomy should be disconnected, the colon freed at the site of the fistula, and closed, and the stomach resected.

We have operated upon a total of 47 patients with intractable and obstructive duodenal ulcers within the past nine and one-half years. Of this number, 15 had a gastroenterostomy, 12 a pyloroplasty, and 20 gastrectomy. Of the 15 who had gastroenterostomy, two have since developed clinical signs of recurrence, while four who had pyloroplasty have a reactivated ulcer. One patient for whom a gastrectomy was performed had persistent symptoms for several months, though he is now entirely free of any disturbance. This resection included only two-fifths of the stomach and was the only one in which less than half the organ was removed.

It may be mentioned that nine of the 20 patients with chronic ulcer who were treated by gastrectomy had had a previous operation: five a pyloroplasty, two a gastroenterostomy, and two a closure of a perforation. The last two patients had a gastrojejunal ulcer with an associated colon fistula. One of the two died, this being the only fatality in the entire group of 47 chronic ulcers. Another of the recurrences for which gastrectomy was done was that of a man who had previously had two gastroenterostomies, and at operation was found to have both a duodenal and a gastrojejunal ulcer.

COMMENT

As the years have gone by and the principles of the surgical treatment of duodenal ulcer have been more clearly determined, it has become obvious that removal of an ample amount of the acid bearing portion of the stomach, together with the pylorus and the lesion itself, is by far the procedure of choice for intractable and bleeding ulcers. As this fact is more widely appreciated in the future, fewer gastroenterostomies will be done in the presence of high acids and an open pylorus, and we shall have fewer recurrences.

REFERENCES

1 Allen, Arthur W.: Hemorrhage Associated with Ulcerating Lesions of the Stomach and Duodenum, Lahey Birthday Volume, Charles C. Thomas, Baltimore, p 13.

2. Blackford, J. M., and Williams, R H.: Fatal Hemorrhage from Peptic Ulcer, J. A M. A., 115:1774, Nov. 23, 1940.

3 Finsterer, H.: Surgical Treatment of Acute Profuse Gastric Hemorrhage, Surg, Gynec. & Obst, 69:291, Sept., 1939.

4. Graham, Roscoe R : Indications for Subtotal Gastrectomy for Duodenal Ulcer, Lahey Birthday Volume, Charles C. Thomas, Baltimore, p. 268.

5. Wangensteen, Owen H : The Problem of Surgical Arrest of Massive Hemorrhage in Duodenal Ulcer, Surgery, 8: 275, 1940.

Scarlet Fever Immunization: II The Dick's Injection Method

HUGH C. GRAHAM, M.D.

TULSA, OKLAHOMA

Scarlet fever immunization has been in use sufficiently long[1] to afford ample opportunity for critical evaluation and the only antigen to emerge from two or three decades of clinical experience is that of Dick and Dick which we have used exclusively for sixteen years. We[2] recently considered other methods than the subcutaneous injection method of the Dicks and concluded that all other methods were either inferior or had not been clinically proved. Only the Dicks' subcutaneous method has stood the critical clinical test of half a generation.

The use of the Dicks' toxin was early found to possess a number of defects which, while not at all peculiar to scarlet fever immunization, were negative aspects nevertheless, especially for a new and untried procedure. These criticisms we group under the following divisions: 1. Efficacy and duration of immunity, at first unknown, now fairly certain; 2. Adverse reactions; 3. Too many injections; and 4. Dependability of the Dick test. We attempt herein to answer, at least partially, some of these questions with reference to the Dicks' subcutaneous injection method.

EFFICACY AND DURATION OF IMMUNITY

Nearly all authors attest the satisfactory efficacy and specificity of scarlet fever immunization. Table 10 presents the findings of some of these authors' with reference to effectiveness. The results in each experiment are compared with a control group. The "control index" indicates the frequency, or incidence, of the disease in the non-immunized as compared with the Dick negatives, the non-immunized having the disease from four to 211 times as frequently as the immunized.

Table 1

Index of Scarlet Fever Incidence in Immunized
As Compared With Non-Immunized Controls.[3]

Authors	3	No. Cases Immunized	Percent Immunized	Having Scarlatina		Period Observed	Control Index
				Number	Percent		
Toomey	3(a)	1273 (nurses)	92.7	10	1.0	2.7 yrs.	(?)
Rappaport	3(b)	222 (nurses)	100	0	0	10 yrs.	(4)
Anderson Reinhardt	3(c)	1038 (nurses)	100	7	0.6	9 yrs.	4
Place	3(d)	1446 (nurses)	(?)	3	1.3		6
Platou	3(e)	164 (nurses)	100	0	0	4 yrs.	8 (?)
Anderson	3(f)	298 (nurses)	100	0	0		30 (?)
Toyoda et al	3(g)	7,000 (general)	60 to 85	1	0.1	6 yrs.	43 (gen. pop.)
Dick & Dick	3(h)	836 (school child.)	100	0.3	0.037	4½ yrs.	173 (2635)
Dick & Dick	3(h)	3,725 (school child.)	100	0.3	0.099	10 yrs.	211 (1595)

Some authors[4] recommend scarlet fever immunization for the control of epidemics, the same as small pox vaccination is used, and Dick and Dick[4] state that by the proper approach an epidemic of scarlet fever may be put under control in 48 hours. We have immunized completely or incompletely over 500 private cases, some few in the face of intimate exposures, and the results have been uniformly good. In no case of a negative Dick test, after immunization by the Dicks' method, have we ever found clinical scarlet fever. It should be remembered that in our area scarlet fever has declined in severity until recently, but even where the disease was rampant or fulminating the results are wonderfully good as reported by Toyoda and associates[5] in Manchuria. They report only 1/43 as many having scarlet fever in the immunized as among the non-immunized! The

highest total dosage used by these investigators was only 40,000 STD*!

In the early investigations it became apparent that the quantity of toxin employed was the most important factor in the immunity process, i e., the more the antigen the more the resulting immunity. Hence, The Scarlet Fever Committee has increased the antigen content of the toxin from time to time according to the following table, and in evaluating immunization efforts the lower dosage of the earlier years should be borne in mind:

We have used the above dosage with only occasional individual modifications from time to time since 1926 and have exclusively used toxin approved by the Committee and prepared by E. R. Squibb and Sons.[6] The following table shows our results to be 86 percent immunity for five to ten years and 84 percent from 13 to 15 years:

Table 2

Dosage of Scarlet Fever Toxin for Immunization[6]

Years	1st dose	Second	Third	Fourth	Fifth	Total STD* (Average)
1925-27	500	1,500	5,000	15,000	30,000 35,000	50,000
1927-36	500	2,000	8,000	25,000	80,000	116,000
1936-39	500	2,000	8,000	25,000	80,000 100,000	125,000
1939-42	650	2,500	10,000	30,000	100,000 120,000	150,000

*STD—Skin test dose.

Various authors (Table 4) report negative Dick Tests from 72 percent to 92 percent for four to 15 years. These figures indicate a very effective immunity over the years.

Table 3

Redicks from 5 to 15 Years After Immunization
(Subcutaneous Method)

5 to 10 Years			13 to 15 Years		
No. Dick Negative	No. Dick Doubtful or Positive	Percent Dirk Negative	No. Dick Negative	No. Dick Doubtful or Positive	Percent Dick Negative
43	7	86	25	5	84

and we have seen no report of diphtheria immunization any higher for a similar period of time, as shown in Table 5 for some recent authors:

Table 4

Degree of Scarlet Fever Immunization

Authors 7		Years	Type of Antigen	Percent Immunity
Veldee and associates	7(a)	4	Modified toxin	80%
Toomey	7(b)	5	Regular	72%
Dicks'	7(c)	12	Regular	92%
Author		15	Regular	84%

ADVERSE REACTIONS

Adverse reactions constitute the bane of any immunization procedure and we know of none without some such undesirable features. In our experience we should place them as follows: (1) small pox vaccination as the

Table 5

Degree of Diphtheria Immunization[s]

Authors	s	Years After Immunization	Number Cases	Number Positive	Type Antigen	Percent Negative
Schwartz & Janney (1938)	s(a)	8-9	145	32	Toxoid	78
Benjamin, Fleming and	s(b)	5-11	635	50	Toxoid 3 inj.	85.1
Ross (1940) Schwarz (1941)	s(c)	3-10	308	64	All types	79.2

worst and most consistent offender; (2) typhoid; (3) whooping cough and scarlet fever; (4) diphtheria-tetanus toxoid combined (alum pptd) ; (5) diphtheria toxoid; and (6) diphtheria toxoid-whooping cough vaccine (combined).

In vaccination against small pox and typhoid we have come to expect reactions of some moment while in diphtheria we are surprised when they do appear. In Table 6 we present a summary of reactions in 200 consecutive cases in ten years, 1926-1936.

Table 6

Reactions in Scarlet Fever Immunization

Total Number Cases	Local		General		Severe		Local & General (Incl. severe)	
	Number	Percent	Number	Percent	Number	Percent	Total Number	Total Percent
200	19	9%	32	16%	10	5%	61	30%

All the above immunizations were done with the old toxin. The new improved toxin was not available until about January 1, 1939, since then the incidence of reactions has been much reduced and we have had no severe reactions and only two or three of moderate severity have occurred, so that our percentage of reactions has been reduced to about ten percent including one percent moderate and the severe to nil. Some authors report reactions in only ten percent of patients and we have no satisfactory explanation for our higher rate of reaction, but are pleased with our reduction to the average generally reported.

We have noted certain characteristics of these moderate or severe reactions that are peculiar to scarlet fever immunization. The vomiting may become retching to disappear shortly. The depression may be lethargic in type, the same as in the disease, but for only a few hours after which it clears promptly.

The fever may rise to 104 to decline shortly to normal. This occasional intensity of reaction is peculiar, being due of course to great sensitivity to the toxin and is at times alarming to the parents and disturbing to the attending physician. In our experience no ill effects have resulted. We have previously pointed out the possibility of poor immunization results in those who have had bad reactions and we then "concluded that the more severe the reaction probably the poorer and more ephemeral will be the immunity."[2]

Whenever reactions occur the next dose of toxin should be reduced according to the severity of symptoms encountered and it may occasionally be necessary to give more than the usual five injections. Some authors feel that a large, strongly positive Dick test indicates directly, in addition to little or no immunity, one's cellular sensitivity to the toxin; hence they give smaller doses, at least at first, until such predisposition has been shown to be absent. In our experience, except for this intensity of reaction that occurs in about one percent or less of cases, the reactions in scarlet fever, immunization are much over-rated and do not occur as frequently or as severely as in small pox, and, of course, the intensity aspect is not to be compared to small pox vaccination encephalitis.

TOO MANY INJECTIONS

The five injections recommended for the regular immunization are one or two more than for any other such procedure. The single dose immunization is highly desirable, but small pox remains the only successful single-visit antigen. If too few injections of any antigen are given, even tho properl' spaced, a low or insufficient antitoxic titer results which is of short duration. The poor results of one shot alum precipitated toxoid have become apparent in recent years, and likewise the old diphtheria toxin-antitoxin was found to be quite inadequate. The effectiveness, present or future, of any immunization procedure should not be sacrificed upon the alter of an insufficient number of injections. The works of Veldee and associates[7] offers some promise. They are using a modified antigen and employing three injections. Methods of immunization other than hypodermic injection for scarlet fever are in our opinion, quite inferior as shown by our report.[2]

THE DICK TEST

The Dick test in our hands, when the proper precautions are observed, is just as reliable as the Schick test. In our opinion, much of the criticism against the test may be due to unfamiliarity with it by those who use it only occasionally. It must be kept in mind that the interpretation of the Dick test is quite different from that of the very familiar Schick test, for, as the Dicks[8] so ably state, *"The commonest error of all is interpreting positive reactions as negative.* The tendancy to regard slightly or even moderately positive reactions as negative is due to familiarity with the Schick test, which is usually interpreted as negative unless there is induration. *Skin reactions with Scarlet fever. toxin are never indurated.* They should be observed in bright light between 20 to 24 hours after the injection. Observations earlier than 18 hours or more than 24 hours are not reliable. The slightest flush or reddening, no matter how faint the color, constitutes a positive reaction if it measures as much as 10 mm. in any diameter. The color may be blanched by stretching the skin."

Whenever a Dick test is positive in an older child or adult, a control should always be used. Our procedure is to do the test and, if positive, repeat the test along with the control. This procedure affords a double check. Contrary to the Dick's findings that a positive Dick test is "never indurated," we found induration in about 15 percent of all positives and severer reactions (vesicle formation, painful edema, etc.) in one or two percent.

REMARKS

We have used the regular Dicks' subcutaneous method of immunization for over 15 years. From 1937 thru 1939 we largely used (on 59 cases) the intranasal spray method, but concluded it was rather inadequate and adopted the injection method. Also beginning in 1939, the improved toxin, made by a different method and containing less than one-sixth as much protein as the old, became available generally and with this material we have had a definite reduction in both the number of reactions (to ten percent) and in the severity (to less than one percent). We are pleased with the lack of known scarlet fever among those immunized by us. We place much reliance in the Dick test and use it frequently. While we recognize defects and imperfections in the immunization and the Dick test, we are trying to improve these by individual study and use. We are impelled to believe, from our experience and that of other authors, that scarlet fever immunization is as successful in its first 15 years as diphtheria immunization in nearly twice that period of time.

CONCLUSIONS

1. Scarlet fever immunization by the Dicks' subcutaneous injection method is quite effective and relatively safe.

2. The Dick test is quite dependable but its technical requirements are very exacting. It should not be used by the novice.

BIBLIOGRAPHY

1. July 1925, first license issued. Personal Communication from National Institute of Health to Author dated Sept 22, 1941 Approved by Council on Pharmacy and Chemistry, A. M. A., J A. M A, 86 199 (Jan. 16) 1926
2. Graham, Hugh C: Scarlet Fever Immunization, 1. An Evaluation of Some Methods of Immunization Over a Fifteen Year Period, Southern M J., 35:132 (Feb) 1942.
3. (a) Toomey, John A.: Scarlet Fever Immunization, In Press, Annals of Internal Med.; (b) Rappaport, Benjamin: Active Immunization to Scarlet Fever with Less Reactions, J. A. M. A., 106-107 (1936); (c) Anderson, Gaylord W and Reinhardt, Warren I.: Scarlet Fever Immunization of Nurses, J Infech, Dis 57-136 (1935); (d) Place, Edwin H.: Result of Active Immunization of Nurses Against Scarlet Fever, Am. J. Public Health, 28:137 (1938); (e) Platou, E. S.: Scarlet Fever Prevention by Immunization, J. Pediat, 5:551 (1934); (f) Anderson, Gaylord: Scarlet Fever Immunization with Toyoda, Taro, Moriwaki, Joji, Futagi, Yasuo, and Okumoto, Mosahito: Practical Value of Immunization Against Scarlet Fever with Streptococcus Toxin, J. Infect. Dis., 46:219 (1930); (h) Dick, George F. and Dick, Gladys H : Scarlet Fever, Yearbook Pub., Chicago, 1938.
4 Koehler, John P.: Recent Experiences in Scarlet Fever Control, Am. J. Pub. Health, 25:1859 (1935); Krumbiegel, Edward R.: Scarlet Fever Control, Am J. Pub. Health, 28: 1096 (1938); Dick and Dick (see 3 (h) above); Lempriere, L. R.: Attempted Immunization in Public Schools, Brit, M J 2:450 (1935).
5. Toyoda et al: see 3 (g) above.
6. As supplied routinely to the Drug trade: Personal communiation to author from E R. Squibb and Sons, dated June 24, 1941.
7. (a) Veldee, M V, Peck, E C., Franklin, J. P, and Dupuy, H. R : The Dick Reaction and Scarlet Fever Morbidity Following Injections of a Purified and Tannic Acid Precipitated Erythrogenic Toxin, Pub Health Reports 56:957 (May 9) 1941; (b) Toomey, John A. and Dick and Dick, see 3 (a) and (h) above.

8. (a) Schwartz, A B., and Jenney, F. R.: Need for Redetermining Schick Negativeness in School Children, J. A. M. A., 110:1754 (May 21) 1938; (b) Benjamin, Ben, Fleming, Grant, and Ross, M. A.: Results of Schick Test in Children One to Ten Years After Injections of Toxoid, Am. J. Dis Child., 60.1304 (Dec.) 1941; (c) Schwarz, Edwin G.: Immunity to Diphtheria, Following Immunizations, Texas J. Med., 37:292 (Aug.) 1941.
9. Dick and Dick (see 3 (h) above) page 80.

DISCUSSION

J. T. BELL, M.D.

OKLAHOMA CITY, OKLAHOMA

There has been, and still is, a difference of opinion regarding the use of scarlet fever toxin for active immunization of children against scarlet fever. This procedure has not been as favorably received as diphtheria immunization has been, primarily because of the number of doses necessary for protection and because of the number of severe reactions which appear after one or more of the toxin injections. .

However, as Dr. Graham's work demonstrated—that with refinement in the toxin has been a decrease in the proportion and severity of reactions. So now the question of which is worse—the risk of a reaction following inoculation with the Dick toxin, or the risk of contracting scarlet fever, can definitely be answered. It can be stated with certainty, that the incidence of scarlet fever is markedly less among inoculated persons than the non-inoculated. So I believe we can safely draw the conclusion that the reactions following the use of the new Dick toxin, should not influence our judgment against scarlet fever immunization.

At the present time we have another angle to consider, and that is the virulence of the present day type of scarlet fever organism, namely the mild type of scarlet fever that we have to deal with. I believe that all will agree that there has been a marked decrease in the virulence of the scarlet fever organism, and for the past ten years we see fewer and fewer cases of the severe type of scarlet fever.

The Oklahoma reports on morbidity and mortality bear this fact out.

In 1931, there were reported 1490 cases, with 37 deaths. Since that time there has been a progressive decline, except 1936 when there were 1160 cases reported with 41 deaths, to 1941 when 859 cases were reported with five death. We cannot conclude, however, that this present trend will continue in Oklahoma, and in view of the shifting population that we now have—as compared to a previously relatively stable population—it seems doubtful that this trend will continue.

To the general practitioner and the pediatrician, the question of induced immunity is a difficult one. I believe there can be no doubt as to the value and desirability of scarlet fever immunizations; but, at the present time, the necessity for it cannot be regarded as of the same order as protection against diphtheria and smallpox.

I think the medical profession owes Dr. Graham a vote of thanks and gratitude for his splendid work on this subject.

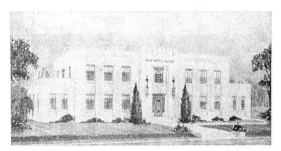

• THE PRESIDENT'S PAGE •

The demands being placed upon the medical profession during the present emergency must be given keen attention by organized medicine. Both State and County Medical Associations must take stock of their present medical personnel and the reserves that might be called up in the way of retired physicians and nurses.

The present emergency is and will continue to present a shifting population problem whose health must be given first consideration.

Small communities must continue to have medical attention for their inhabitants and yet the congregation in defense and war production areas of populations far in excess of the usual population will call for additional physicians for that area or well organized medical care by and through the members of the county society, acting individually and collectively.

Consider the problem analytically. There are ten cities of fifteen hundred population with one or two physicians. A hundred and fifty people move from these cities. This number leaving is not sufficient to warrant the removal of any of the medical personnel of that particular community. Now, assume that the hundred and fifty people from the ten cities all move into the defense areas of Oklahoma, Tulsa and Muskogee counties and you have a concentration of fifteen hundred people which must be rendered medical care.

These problems are the responsibilities of the medical profession, the same as the production of steel, rubber and all raw materials are the problems of their respective industries. Government aid is also being given the profession the same as industry through the Procurement and Assignment Service.

The problems of medical care must be solved and it will only be through the efforts of the county societies that it will be accomplished.

I urge the county societies to meet each month and take up this urgent condition as the first and only order of business.

Ask yourself, "What is my county society doing?"

Sincerely yours,

President.

• EDITORIALS •

COMA AND LUNG ABSCESS

The Comatose patient presents serious therapeutic problems, but modern knowledge of physiology, pharmacology and anesthesia has contributed much toward the solution of these problems. In spite of increased knowledge and skill in the management of Coma, too little attention is given to the respiratory hazards. The skill of the Bronchoscopist and the trained Anesthetist with their mechanical aids to respiratory therapy is often urgently needed.

Greene[1] has significantly said, "The character and usually fatal complications of the comatose state (whether the coma is due to alcohol, morphine, ether, cerebral hemorrhage, or pneumonia,) if the coma is deep and lasts more than a few hours, are pulmonary edema and pulmonary infection. The factors which favor their appearance are so many that in any individual case it is difficult to single out a specific cause. Usually the pulmonary edema and infection are the result of the interaction of several pathological processes. Chief among these causes are: Aspiration, Partial respiratory obstruction, Generalized tissue edema, Shock, Anoxia and Primary pulmonary infection."

In profound Coma regardless of the cause, the chief danger arises through the absence of the cough reflex and the unopposed aspiration of infectious material. The frequent occurrence of aspiration pneumonia and lung abscess following tonsillectomy, extraction of teeth and other operations about the mouth and nasopharynx is a matter of common knowledge. This is chiefly due to the fact that the cough reflex, which stands guard between the trachea and the pharynx, is depressed or oblitered by anesthesia. It should be remembered that the same hazards immediately arise in every case of coma. The General Practitioner who first makes contact with casualty cases, unconscious from trauma of the central nervous system or asphyxiation from various anesthetic gases, should bear in mind the fact that the laryngeal "watchdog" is off guard and that the gravity run of pharyngeal infection is not only unopposed but expedited by the suction of negative intrapulmonary pressure. Often the latter is increased by obstructive factors resulting from marked muscular relaxation leading to retrocession of the tongue, close approximation of the vocal cords and pharyngeal walls and soon the further narrowing of the respiratory channels by the edema which accompanies anoxia, and the increased suction due to obstruction.

When the physician first reaches a case of profound coma he should give prompt attention to the danger of aspiration of infectious material and try to obviate the same by favorable posture and detailed attention to the task of clearing the mouth and nasopharynx of accumulated material and keeping the airways open. Considering this task plus attention to the other possibilities listed by Greene[1] it is obvious that the attending physician carries a heavy responsibility. If he is wise he will employ all available preventive means and in cases not promptly responding to treatment he will seek the aid of the bronchoscopist or possibly the anethetist. If coma is due to trauma of the central nervous system the Neuro-surgeon may be of great assistance. The bronchoscopic dislodgment of mucous plugs or other materials obstructing the airways may prevent pneumonia and abscess through the removal of infectious material and the preservation of general and local resistance by clearing the way for adequate oxygenation. In some cases the retention of an endotracheal tube may be essential. This reduces the inhalation of accumulated secretions, keeps the airway open and makes it easy to remove bronchial secretions by suction through a bronchial catheter. Only the experienced bronchoscopist or the anesthetist with modern training should be entrusted with the intratracheal tube, as the introduction and retention of the same, without skill and sound judgment, may lead to serious consequences. In addition to the aspiration infection, each of the pathological conditions mentioned by Greene,[1] and quoted above presents its own therapeutic, pharmacological, anatomical and physiological problems, requiring careful discrimination for intelligent solution and occasionally highly technical therapeutic measures. All of the above mentioned factors are important because of their inter-relationship in the causation of the major pathology.

The physician who lacks initiative and enthusiasm in connection with the above recommendations should carefully consider the high mortality obtaining in the broncho pulmonary infections due to aspiration, and make sure he is doing all he can to achieve better results. In this connection the use of morphine in the treatment of shock should be carefully guarded. The danger of pulmonary infections may be greatly increased by the too free administration of morphine.

1. Greene, Barnett A.: Recent Advances in the Care of the Comatose Patient. Annals of Internal Medicine, 1942, XVI, 727.

MANY TIMES THEIR WEIGHT IN GOLD

Under "current comment," the Journal of The American Medical Association, July 11, sounds a warning against the theft of narcotics and urges all physicians, hospitals and clinics to safeguard the stock now on hand.

Attention is called to the fact that the United States is cut off from the sources of supply because of the war and that smuggling is virtually at an end, and the demand for illicit traffic must be met by theft. The necessity for accelerated vigilence is pointed out and it is suggested that all active supplies be closely guarded and all reserve supplies be secreted, under lock and key.

The Bureau of Narcotics considers these drugs "critical and strategical war materials" and because of urgent need for the relief of pain in the armed forces, replacement of stolen supplies for civilian needs ultimately may be impossible.

This important warning closes with the following statement, "Thefts should be promptly reported to the narcotic district supervisor having jurisdiction."

PROGRESS IN PEDIATRICS

In this issue of the Journal there are two scientific articles which justify the above title. One deals with induced immunity by Vaccination and the other with Chemotherapy in a case of influenzal Meningitis.

In no other field has preventive medicine approached the rapid strides made in pediatrics. Lest we forget, attention is called to a significant discourse by Dr. Henry A. Christian[1] containing this startling statement. "Perhaps after all, a very complete success of preventive medicine may not be a complete blessing." Dr. Christian points out the fact that the recurrence of an infectious disease in a race, or a community, confers an acquired immunity which will be lost when the disease fails to recur — Even though adequate immunity is conferred by vaccination, the implication is, that we may develop a sense of false security and relax our vigilence only to witness the return of infectious maladies in malignant form. Obviously this might happen to an unsuspecting, unprotected generation.

Therapeutic advances in this field are almost if not quite as remarkable—The advent of the sulfonamides in the treatment of the acute respiratory infections as well as many other infectious conditions has greatly augmented the therapeutic score.

The most potent factor in the advancement in child welfare is the educational program which has resulted in the close cooperation between the pediatrician and the mother in the childs behalf. The pediatrician has had the basic wisdom to see that the psychological inoculation of the mother is fully as important as induced immunization in the child. Again we must give credit to the art as well as the science of medicine. Before leaving this subject it is interesting to note that Voltaire was influential in introducing Jenner's method of Vaccination in France and it may be said that Benjamin Franklin and Thomas Jefferson should have credit for exerting a similar influence in America.

The following significant statement came from Franklin's pen approximately one hundred years ago.

"In 1736 I lost one of my sons, a fine boy four years old, by the smallpox, taken in the common way. I long regretted bitterly, and still regret that I had not given it to him by inoculation. This I mention for the sake of parents who omit that operation on the supposition that they should never forgive themselves if a child died under it, my example showing that regret may be the same either way, and that, therefore, the safer should be chosen."

1. Dr Henry A. Christian, Annals of Internal Medicine, Vol. 12, Page 1506, March, 1939.

THE NATIONAL PHYSICIANS COMMITTEE

It is the purpose of this Committee to see that Medicine in America continues to be American Medicine.

Those who appreciate present social and policital trends know that this Committee has a difficult task and that the successful performance of this task will depend upon the cooperation of the individual members of the Medical profession.

For the benefit of those who may not understand the relationship of this Committee to the American Medical Association, and for that reason may hesitate to lend their full support, attention is called to the fact that the Committee received the approval, commendation and support of the A. M. A. House of Delegates at the recent Atlantic City Meeting.

In addition to financial and moral support every doctor should forward the purposes of this Committee by his daily conduct and by taking advantage of every opportunity to instruct the average citizen in the principles of American Medicine, in the relationship of patient to doctor, in the freedom of choice and independence of action.

Thus the community doctor can wield a powerful influence. He should marshall his forces and employ his influence for the election of the candidates who have committed themselves to the task of preserving the fundamental principles of American Medicine, in order that the public may continue to have the full benefit of what medicine has to offer.

ASSOCIATION ACTIVITIES

PUBLIC WELFARE COMMISSION TO PAY FOR PHYSICAL EXAMINATION OF AID TO DEPENDENT CHILDREN APPLICANTS

The State Medical Association has been advised by Mr. Jess Harper, Director of the Public Welfare Commission, that beginning August 15, physicians will be paid a fee for the examination of applicants seeking assistance from the Aid to Dependent Children's Fund when such applicants are applying for reason of physical or mental incapacity.

The program worked out in cooperation with the Medical Advisory Committee to the department calls for the payment of a $3.00 fee for original examinations and $2.00 for subsequent re-examinations. Laboratoi y work will also be paid for when requested by the Medical Advisory Committee. The schedule of laboratory fees will be announced later.

Mr. Harper, in making the announcement, stated that applicants would at all times use their family physicians or the physician of their own choosing if they did not have a family physician. Mr. Harper also stressed the fact that arrangements for the examinations would be made through the County representative of the Welfare Department in such a manner as to cause the least possible disturbance in the individual physicians office time.

Full details of the program will be sent to all physicians as soon as possible.

The announcement as made by Mr. Harper also pointed out that the recommendations came from the Medical Advisory Committee and was adopted by the Commission in order to secure more complete examinations of the applicants by physicians where by in return, a more definite decision could be obtained as to whether the applicant was entitled to assistance.

It is believed that the new examination forms and payment of an examination fee will save many thousands of dollars for Oklahoma tax payers.

Members of the Medical Advisory Committee are: C. R. Rountree, M.D.; Walker Morledge, M.D.; A. R. Sugg, M.D.; Clinton Gallagher, M.D.; R. M. Shepard, M.D., and Moorman Prosser, M.D.

POSTGRADUATE COMMITTEE OPENS THIRD CIRCUIT IN INTERNAL MEDICINE

The postgraduate course in internal medicine has been a distinct success. Dr. L. W. Hunt, instructor, has proved to be a capable lecturer and demonstrator as well as a most practical and helpful consultant.

Detailed plans have been completed for lectures to the laity by Dr. Hunt. Officers of county medical societies and County Health Directors are urged to utilize these lay lectures among study and civic clubs and other groups wherever possible.

Postgraduate instruction has now been completed in ten teaching centers, as follows:

Circuit I		Circuit II	
Bartlesville	28	Ada	22
Miami	22	Durant	20
Pryor	15	Hugo	10
Vinita	12	Idabel	10
Claremore	8	Sulphur	8
Total	85	Total	70

Total number of physicians enrolled for two circuits 155.

The third circuit of five teaching centers will open in Muskogee, Okmulgee, Tahlequah, McAlester and Poteau the week of August 3. Total enrollments for these centers thus far are 73. Indications are that others will enroll during the first and second weeks of the course. This circuit will also include a teaching center at Camp Gruber where from 50 to 100 Medical Officers will attend.

The entrance into military service of so many physicians has increased the burden on those remaining. They are all too busy to leave their practice for postgraduate study away from home, but find our program very convenient and of great aid.

The Associated State Postgraduate Committees, in their deliberations this year at Atlantic City, met with the Council on Industrial Health of the American Medical Association. The latter suggested that the various states and agencies sponsoring postgraduate instruction under the extension plan consider including industrial medicine and surgery in their programs during the war period. This is necessitated by the rapid expansion of defense industry in smaller communities, which will require larger numbers of physicians adequately trained in industrial health. Incidentally, it should be known by the physicians of our state that Dr. Henry H. Turner, Chairman of our Oklahoma Postgraduate Committee, was elected Chairman of the National Associated State Postgraduate Committees this year.

SOUTHERN MEDICAL MEETING TO BE HELD

The Executive Committee of the Southern Medical Association, following its May 15 meeting in Richmond, Virginia, has announced that the 1942 meeting will be held November 10, 11 and 12.

Changes made in this year's program cut the number of days from four to three. The twenty one sections will conclude their programs in two days instead of three and the time alloted for the presentation of papers will be cut from twenty minutes to fifteen, with discussion reduced to three minutes instead of five.

The first day, Tuesday, will be Richmond Day and will be a series of clinical presentations by Richmond physicians. The sections of the Association will then convene the following two days.

The Executive Committee and officers of Southern Medical Association should have the wholehearted support of Oklahoma physicians in their determination to keep this outstanding scientific assembly available for continued postgraduate study particularly when the need is as great as it is in the present emergency.

Every Oklahoma physician who believes that he may be in a position to attend should make his reservation at once.

The Hotel John Marshall has been designated as headquarters.

MARRIAGE OF DR. WILLIAM L. TAYLOR. HOLDENVILLE, ANNOUNCED

The announcement of the marriage of Dr. W. L. "Bill" Taylor of Holdenville, was made to the office by the appearance of the bride and groom returning from their honeymoon in Texas.

Since we had not been fore-warned of the approaching event, we were a little excited and neglected to find out Mrs. Taylor's maiden name.

We sincerely hope that the new duties of the home will not prevent Dr. Taylor from continuing to be the first to register for both, The Annual Meeting and 1. Oklahoma City Clinical Society.

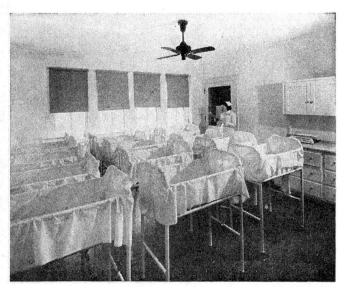

FIFTH ANNUAL EXHIBITION AMERICAN PHYSICIANS' ART ASSOCIATION

New Officers

President ....Samuel Gellert, M.D.
Vice-President ....Max Thorek, M.D.
Secretary-Treasurer ....F. H. Redewill, M.D.

The fifth annual exhibition of the American Physicians' Art Association was held June 8-12, 1942, at Atlantic City, N. J., in Convention Hall, under the same roof with the American Medical Association.

This exhibition was enthusiastically acclaimed the most attractive one of the entire convention, as evidenced by the fact that the 40′ x 60′ room was filled with visitors at all times. There were 350 original art works, a large number considering war time. Seventy-three prizes were awarded, so that every contestant felt that he had a chance to win an award, especially since the prizes were divided into four classes, according to the length of time the artist had been working: Class A, over eight years; Class B, three to eight years; Class C, eight months to three years; Class D, under eight months.

Under the new rules, no artist may receive more than one award in one year. No private or commercial prizes are permitted, all prizes being the Association's.

One of the interesting developments of the exhibition was that physicians returned again and again, bringing along friends and families. In many instances, doctors' wives brought the doctors. The estimated attendance was 15,000, and it is doubtful that a single visitor to the Convention missed viewing the art exhibit.

The annual banquet was attended by 130 members and friends of the Association, this number being many times larger than at previous meetings. A feature of the banquet was an illustrated talk by Mr. Fred Weber on "Newer Technic of Painting."

Many former members of the American Physicians' Art Association rejoined, and over 200 new members were enrolled. It is not obligatory for a physician to be an artist; he may join either in hope, or simply because he appreciates art and wishes to encourage the physicians' art movement.

Mead Johnson & Company's ambition to make the American Physicians' Art Association self-sustaining will probably be attained when the membership reaches 1,000. The outstanding success of the 1942 exhibition has assured a firm foundation and augurs well for the future.

OKLAHOMA SURGEONS ENTERTAIN VISITING GUESTS

An interesting program was recently conducted in Oklahoma City for visiting surgeons from Minneapolis, Omaha, Kansas City, Wichita, Dallas, Little Rock, Fort Worth and Los Angeles.

Radical resections of the terminal bowel were done in two cases of complicated malignancies and a new technique was demonstrated for operating on atresia ani vaginalis infants.

Those participating in the program were Dr. Hugh Jeter, Dr. Harry Wilkins, Dr. Neil Woodward and Dr. R. L. Murdoch.

The visiting surgeons were entertained by a buffet supper given by the Doctors Dinner Club.

MORE OKLAHOMA PHYSICIANS IN ARMED SERVICES

The Journal will attempt to keep its Roster of Oklahoma physicians serving in the Military Forces accurately to date. Since the last list published, the following have been granted commissions in the Armed Forces.

ALFALFA
PARSONS, JACK F. ....Cherokee

CARTER
CANTRELL, D. E., JR. ....Healdton
VEAZEY, LYMAN C. ....Ardmore

CHEROKEE
McINTOSH, R. K., JR. ....Tahlequah

CUSTER
TISDAL, WILLIAM C. ....Clinton
WOOD, J. GUILD ....Weatherford

GARFIELD
MERCER, J. WENDELL ....Enid
NEWELL, W. B., JR. ....Enid

HUGHES
MUNAL, JOHN ....Holdenville

KAY
HARMS, EDWIN M. ....Blackwell
KREGER, G. S. ....Tonkawa
NEAL, L. G. ....Ponca City

McINTOSH
STONER, RAYMOND W. ....Checotah

MUSKOGEE
DORWART, F. G. ....Muskogee
NEELY, SHADE ....Muskogee
SANDERS, H. U. ....Muskogee

NOBLE
EVANS, A. M. ....Perry

OKLAHOMA
ALLEN, GEORGE T. ....1200 N. Walker
BARB, T. J. ....318 S. W. 25th St.
BATTENFIELD, JOHN Y. ....State Health Dept.
BEDNAR, GERALD ....Medical Arts Bldg.
CHAFFIN, ZALE ....Municipal Bldg.
FRYER, SAM R. ....119 N. W. 5th St.
MESSINGER, R. P. ....807 N. W. 23rd St.
SNOW, J. B. ....1200 N. Walker

OKMULGEE
COTTERAL, J. R. ....Henryetta

PAYNE
MARTIN, JAS. D. ....Cushing

PITTSBURG
BARTHELD, FLOYD T. ....McAlester
MILLS, C. K. ....McAlester

STEPHENS
WATERS, CLAUDE B. ....Duncan

TULSA
BEST, RALPH L. ....Medical Arts Bldg.
BRANLEY, B. L. ....Medical Arts Bldg.
EDWARDS, JOHN ....Medical Arts Bldg.
KORNBLEE, A. T. ....1307 S. Main
MATT, JOHN G. ....Medical Arts Bldg.
MUNDING, L. A. ....Medical Arts Bldg.
PORTER, H. H. ....Medical Arts Bldg.
SWANSON, K. F. ....Springer Clinic

WASHINGTON
GENTRY, RAYMOND C. ....Bartlesville
RUCKER, RALPH W. ....Bartlesville

WOODWARD
RUTHERFORD, V. M. ....Woodward

The following physicians, not members of the Association, have also been called to the Military Forces.

CADDO
WILLIAMS, CLAUDE ....Anadarko

ELLIS
SMITH, JOSEPH JAMES ....Shattuck

LeFLORE
KLEIN, JACOB E. ....Talihina

OKLAHOMA
ARCHER, GEORGE P. ....Oklahoma City
BEATTIE, JAMES W. ....Oklahoma City
BROWN, SPENCER H. ....Oklahoma City
HARTFORD, WALTER K. ....Oklahoma City
MACKEY, ABNER ....Oklahoma City
MORGAN, VANCE ....Oklahoma City
READ, WILLIAM TOLBERT ....Oklahoma City
WINKELMAN, GEORGE WM. ....Oklahoma City

PAYNE
HAWLEY, HUGH H. ....Stillwater

TULSA
HOOVER, WILKIE D. ....Tulsa

Employ your time improving yourself by other men's documents: So shall you come easily by what others have labored hard for.—Socrates.

MEDICAL PREPAREDNESS

Medicine and the War*
CONSERVATION OF MEDICAL SUPPLIES

The medical profession and hospitals of the country must practice the most severe economy possible in the use of supplies containing materials essential to the conduct of the war. Rubber, metals, fixed equipment, chemicals and drugs must be conserved to the utmost to make the supply last for the duration of the war. Rubber gloves, when torn, should be patched; rubber drainage material should be resterialized and used again. Adhesive plaster contains rubber. Two pieces should not be used when one will suffice. Better, yet, none at all should be used if a cotton bandage will be an adequate substitute. Unnecessarily large dressings should be avoided. Catgut must be conserved. Alcohol and other chemicals should be used as sparingly as possible.

It is expected that hospital supplies will be available in sufficient amount to meet the need of civilian patients, but only if those needs are reduced to a minimum. Enormus quantities must be supplied to the military hospitals and to our allies, despite the fact that the materials from which most of the articles are made are in demand for other purposes. Waste, however slight, must be scrupulously avoided.

This program has the endorsement of the Health Supplies Branch of the War Production Board.

Committee on Drugs and Medical Supplies

W. W. Palmer, Chairman; Perrin H. Long, Vice Chairman; Morris Fishbein, Evarts A. Graham (ex officio), Ernest E. Irons, E. F. Kelly, George W. Merck, O. H. Perry Pepper (ex officio), John G. Searle.

Subcommittee on Hospital and Surgical Supplies.

Evarts A. Graham, Chairman; C. W. Munger, Mont R. Reid, Edward J. Sovatkin, G. W. Wallerich.

PROCUREMENT AND ASSIGNMENT SERVICE FOR PHYSICIANS, DENTISTS AND VETERINARIANS*

QUESTIONS FREQUENTLY ASKED WITH ANSWERS OFFICIALLY RELEASED BY THE BOARD
FRANK H. LAHEY, CHAIRMAN

GRADUATES OF FOREIGN MEDICAL SCHOOLS

1. Q. What can a graduate of a foreign medical school (aged 33, citizen) do to obtain a commission in some branch of the defense effort? What can he do to avoid being drafted as a private?

A. If such a man is willing to be dislocated for war effort, his best opportunity would be in industrial medicine and surgery or in some of the areas in which the department of public health is seeking to locate physicians. He might be able to obtain a commission with the Army if he complies with the recently formulated conditions for class B. medical school graduates.

MEN OVER 45—OVER 60

2. Q. What is the program for men of 60 years of age? For those between 45 and 60?

A. Men over 60 will be best utilized to take up the additional local load caused by the departure of younger men. Those between 45 and 60 would serve in this same fashion except in instances of specialists whose training makes them particularly desirable for the Army and who can obtain commissions granted for these special purposes.

OFFICE LEASES AND OTHER OBLIGATIONS

3. Q. What happens to office leases? Payments on instalment purchases. H. O. L. C. obligations?

A. The Soldiers' and Sailors' Civil Relief Act has been enacted by Congress to free persons in military service from harassment and injury to their civil rights during their terms of service and thus to enable them to devote their entire energy to the defense needs of the nation. The present law, however, does not apply to office leases; it applies to leases of property used for household purposes. Pending legislation does provide a method by which office leases may be canceled. Protection is afforded in the case of instalment contracts, mortgages, insurance premiums, taxes and the like. The law does not relieve you from liability but prevents the enforcement, to your detriment, of the terms of your agreement while you are in service. A detailed outline of the

*Taken from The Journal of A .M. A., Volume 119, Number 14, August 1, 1942, Page 1113.

present law was published in The Journal of The Oklahoma State Medical Association, February, 1942, page 75. The pending legislation, which has already passed the House of Representatives, will further safeguard the civil rights of persons in military service.

SELECTED APPOINTMENTS

4. Q. Can one select service under a certain doctor?

A. No, but one may ask for service in a certain outfit and will have to run his chances of getting it.

CALLED BY SELECTIVE SERVICE

5. Q. What happens if a man has given his name to "Procurement and Assignment" and his name is drawn by the draft but he has not been called by Procurement and Assignment?

A. This man should appeal to his state Procurement and Assignment chairman to intervene on his behalf.

ENROLMENT AND ENLISTMENT

6. Q. Is the word "enrolment" interpreted as an "enlistment" in the terms of the act?
A. No.

PLACES FOR SPECIALISTS

7. Q. For this emergency you speak of, there are many of us between 37 and 45 who are willing to go at once if needed but are not certified with any board as specialists but are nevertheless capable. Should we then wait for the Procurement and Assignment service to place us?

A. Procurement and Assignment cannot place men. Such men should request commissions, giving their professional qualifications, and they may ask that the state chairman of Procurement and Assignment write a confirmatory letter for them.

INTERNSHIPS OF TWO YEARS

8. Q. What is the attitude toward the intern in hospitals where two years' internship is regular appointment?

A. Deferment for one year's internship is all that is allowed at the present time.

RESIDENTS

9. Q. What will be the disposition of residents in teaching hospitals connected with medical schools?

A. Procurement and Assignment is making efforts to preserve enough residents in teaching hospitals to carry on the hospital service and to assure a continuing supply of specialists.

ESSENTIAL TEACHERS

10. Q. I want to get into active military service, but my medical school where I am teaching says that I am necessary for that school. What shall I do? Will I be looked on as a shirker if I stay at home when my associates go and risk their lives?

A. This man should stay home unless he can provide his medical school with some one capable of taking his place and thus be released as available.

ASSISTANT TO A SURGEON

11. Q. In what way does the Procurement Board evaluate one who has been assistant to a surgeon for eight years in his total practice?

A. The Procurement Board would consider such a man suitable for service with a station hospital as assistant surgeon or ward surgeon.

ESSENTIAL ON HOSPITAL STAFF

12. Q. On what basis do you call a man essential at a hospital. What yardstick do you use to call men essential to the hospital staff? What should the man who is 48 years of age and is on the essential list of a hospital do as to volunteering to the government service?

A. Each hospital is supposed to make its own list of essential men, which is submitted to the state chairman of Procurement and Assignment, If he agrees, they are considered essential; if he does not, the hospital will be required to modify its list. Men on the essential list over 45 years of age should not volunteer except for highly special service.

PHYSICAL QUALIFICATIONS OF MEDICAL STUDENTS

13. Q. Should students who are not physically up to the army and navy standards be admitted to medical schools?

A. Yes. Failure to meet physical standards should not exclude promising young persons from medical education. Furthermore, this type of student may be highly important in the next few years to carry on hospital and teaching work.

OBSTETRICIANS

14. Q. What should men doing obstetrics do?

A. Men doing obstetrics should conform to the general requirements of their age group laid down for the rest of the profession.

FAILURE OF PHYSICIANS TO APPLY FOR COMMISSION

15. Q. If a doctor has been notified through Procurement and Assignment service that he had been selected and to apply for a commission, is it compulsory that he apply immediately? What if I don't answer questionnaire and enrolment blanks?

A. It is not compulsory. Certainly it is expected that physicians will cooperate; if they fail to do so, they are not doing what they should to aid our nation in meeting our great emergency.

LIMITED SERVICE

16. Q. Do you wish applicants who have physical defects but could work under limited strain?

A. Yes, if they can meet the requirements for limited service.

SPECIALTY SERVICES

17. Q. I had intended going into a specialty this summer and have been taking postgraduate work in that direction with the intention of taking a residency in that specialty this summer. Is there any way in which I can possibly get into that specialty through the armed forces—such as taking courses or a residency in one of the government hospitals?

A. If a man is commissioned in the Medical Corps of the Army he may request assignment to positions where he could pursue a specialty, but there is no obligation, of course, on the Medical Corps to meet his request.

WAIVERS OF PHYSICAL DEFECTS

18. Q. If I have a physical defect and sign a statement to that effect in applying for a commission in the Army, do I thereby waive any benefits to which I might be justly entitled?

A. No. The Statement or affidavit does not constitute a waiver of any benefits. It is merely an acknowledgement of the existence of a physical disability which would, unless waived by the Army, preclude the granting of a commission to you. The statement you sign forms a basis of action by the Adjutant General's Office looking toward the waiver of your disability so that you may be accepted for military service.

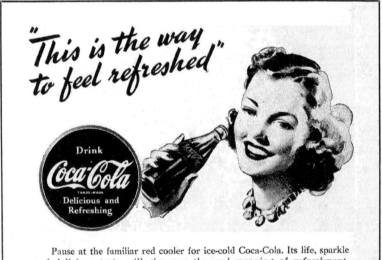

WOMEN'S AUXILIARY NEWS

Subscriptions to the "Bulletin," the official publication of the Woman's Auxiliary to the American Medical Association, have been ordered. The first issue of the fiscal year will be the Post-Convention number, which should be ready for distribution at this time. This periodical is published four times a year and not only contains information and suggestions from our National Officers but also has many interesting articles about our organization work in the forty other states which have auxiliaries. It is very beneficial in planning programs and furnishes many new ideas of ways to be of service to your community and to the medical profession. All county presidents, state officers and state committee chairmen receive their copies complimentary from the State Auxiliary. Please notify Mrs. James Stevenson, state secretary, if you have not received your Bulletin by September 1st.

OKLAHOMA COUNTY
OFFICERS AND COMMITTEE CHAIRMEN
1942-1943

President	Mrs. W. Floyd Keller	1213 Larchmont Lane, Oklahoma City
President-Elect	Mrs. G. E. Stanbro	220 Edgemere Court, Oklahoma City
Vice-President	Mrs. Walker Morledge	200 N. W. 18th St., Oklahoma City
Recording Secretary	Mrs. Allen G. Gibbs	2321 N. W. 25th St., Oklahoma City
Corresponding Secretary	Mrs. John S. Pine	423 N. E. 16th St., Oklahoma City
Treasurer	Mrs. Charles A. Smith	406 N. W. 22nd St., Oklahoma City
Assistant Treasurer	Mrs. B. E. Mulvey	2632 N. W. 27th St., Oklahoma City
Parliamentarian	Mrs. Neil Woodward	4301 Lincoln Blvd., Oklahoma City
Press & Publicity	Mrs. J. Powers Wolff	2816 N. W. 21st St., Oklahoma City
Program	Mrs. John F. Burton	1309 N. W. 19th St., Oklahoma City
Entertainment	Mrs. Gerald Rogers	220 N. W. 32nd St., Oklahoma City
Social Service	Mrs. R. Q. Goodwin	541 N. Hill St., Oklahoma City
Scrap Book	Mrs. Harvey Randle	413 W. Hill St., Oklahoma City
Membership & Visiting	Mrs. J. H. Robinson	836 N. W. 39th St., Oklahoma City
Transportation	Mrs. Wm. L. Bonham	536 N. W. 40th St., Oklahoma City
Flowers	Mrs. W .W. Rucks, Jr.	217 N. W. 19th St., Oklahoma City
Hygeia	Mrs. Jess D. Herrmann	1147 N. W. 38th St., Oklahoma City
Public Health & Relations	Mrs. Chas. R. Rountree	1215 Larchmont Lane, Oklahoma City
Historian	Mrs. M .M. Appleton	501 N. W. 35th St., Oklahoma City
Telephone	Mrs. John H. Lamb	4323 N. Georgia St., Oklahoma City
Emergency	Mrs. F. Maxey Cooper	248 N. W. 34th St., Oklahoma City

Oklahoma County

Under the leadership of Mrs. W. Floyd Keller, Oklahoma County is planning a very busy year. While a part of the membership, whose husbands are in the Service, will be away from home, there will be enough left to carry on the work of the auxiliary. The regular meetings do not start until October but the exectuive board and many of the committee chairmen will be busy during the summer months making plans for the winter. Mrs. Charles R. Rountree, chairman of Public Health and Relations, will also be the head of the war Work Committee. She and her committee will continue with the survey made last spring. This record will contain the information on all Red Cross and O. C. D. classes completed and the volunteer services given in the various phases of work of both organizations.

Tulsa County

Mrs. J. W. Childs, Tulsa County president, called an executive board meeting together in her home, 1616 S. Madison, on June 15. Mrs. Frank L. Flack, state president, was asked to meet with the board. Mrs Childs announced that her organization was complete, with all committees appointed. Although there is no regular auxiliary meeting until October, many of the committees are busy during the summer months planning their programs for the year. Mrs. C. C. Hoke, chairman of the War Aid Committee, has started a survey of the qualifications of all members. Each one is to report all Red Cross classes completed. Every member will be asked to keep a record of the number of hours of volunteer service they have contributed. This committee expects to complete the survey during the summer months but will keep it up to date by adding all classwork as it is finished. The Membership Committee, with Mrs. C. A. Pavy as chairman, are inviting all eligible doctor's wives to become members. They expect to have all dues collected before the Year Books go to press in September. Under the direction of Mrs. D. W. Le-Master, the Program Committee has met and discussed the work of their group. A Red Cross Nutrition Class has been meeting during the summer under the general supervision of one of the auxiliary members, Mrs. I. H. Nelson. Classes will be started in any other phase of Red Cross work, if enough show interest to warrant it. Mrs. N. Stewart White and Mrs. Frank L. Flack have successfully passed the Instructor's Course in First Aid but do not expect to be teaching before early fall.

Classified Advertisements

FOR SALE: Phorometer and Ophthalmometer Attached to Oculist's Chair, 40 Pair Trial Lens Set, New Project-O-Chart Complete, $650 Cash. Anyone interested should contact M. L. Whitney, M.D., Okemah, Oklahoma.

University of Oklahoma School of Medicine

At the annual meeting of the Faculty of the University of Oklahoma School of Medicine a Resolution was unanimously passed to the effect that the Faculty was in favor of accelerating the course in the School of Medicine and to take on additional duties. The recommendation of the Faculty was approved by the President of the University and the Board of Regents on June 1, 1942. As soon as the Legislature meets in 1943 and the additional funds which are required are made available, the school will begin to operate upon an accelerated basis, three semesters per annum, begining June 1, 1943.

The W. K. Kellogg Foundation has granted the sum of $10,000.00 for a loan and scholarship fund for students in the School of Medicine, and $4,000.00 for a loan and scholarship fund for students in the School of Nursing.

General Robert U. Patterson, Dean, addressed the students at the University of Texas School of Medicine at Galveston on June 5, on the subject "Military Medicine". General Patterson attended the meeting of the American Medical Association in Atlantic City June 8, to June 12.

Dr. Paul C. Colonna, Professor of Orthopaedic Surgery and Chief of the Orthopaedic Service in the University and Crippled Children's Hospitals has resigned his positions effective August 1, 1942, to accept the position of Professor of Orthopaedic Surgery in the University of Pennsylvania School of Medicine. Dr. Willis Kelly West, Associate Professor of Orthopaedic Surgery on the Faculty of the School of Medicine, has been appointed Acting Chairman of the Department of Orthopaedic Surgery and Acting Chief of the Orthopaedic Service in the Hospitals, replacing Dr. Colonna.

Dr. Bela Halpert has been appointed Director of the Laboratories of the University and Crippled Children's Hospitals, and Professor of Clinical Pathology in the School of Medicine. Dr. Halpert has held teaching positions in the Johns Hopkins University, the University of Chicago, Yale University, and more recently in the Department of Pathology and Bacteriology of the Louisiana State University School of Medicine.

Members of Evacuation Hospital No. 21, United States Army, received individual orders to report to Camp San Luis Obispo, California, on July 5, 1942. Personnel of this hospital unit is composed of members of the staff of the University and Crippled Children's Hospitals, many of whom are on the Faculty of the School of Medicine. The Unit will serve with Evacuation Hospital No. 53, United States Army, during maneuvers in that area during the summer months. The following is a complete list of the Professional Staff of Evacuation Hospital No. 21, United States Army:

Lt. Col. Herbert Dale Collins; Major Bert Ernest Mulvey; Major George Henry Kimball; Major John Powers Wolff; Major Ward Loren Shaffer, Dental Corps; Major Paul Brann Lingenfelter, Clinton, Oklahoma; Major Robert Leonard Noe; Major Jess Duval Herrman; Major Austin Holloway Bell; Captain Robert Bruce Howard, now on active duty at LaGrade General Hospital, New Orleans, La.; Captain Floyd Smith Newman, Shattuck, Okla.; Captain Cecil Willard Lemon; Captain Rudolph Joseph Reichert, Moore, Okla.; Captain John Frederick Kuhn, Jr; Captain Ray Harvey Lindsey, Pauls Valley, Oklahoma; Captain Evans Edward Talley, Enid, Oklahoma; Captain Samuel Ewing Franklin, Broken Arrow, Oklahoma; Captain Jim Mabury Taylor; Captain Everett Baker Neff; Captain Chester Randall Seba;

Captain William Ward Rucks, Jr.; Captain Allen Gilbert Gibbs; Captain John Millard Robertson; Lt. Felix M. Adams, Jr.; Lt. John Andrew Graham; Lt. Daniel Bester Pearson; Lt. John Dewitt Ashley; Lt. D. R. Bedford; Lt. Owen Royce, Jr.; Lt. Marion Allen Flesher; Lt. Harvey M. Richey.

Unfortunately, Lt. Col. Collins, Organizing Director of the unit, was ill and could not report for active duty with other members. Major Bert S. Mulvey, the next in rank, was appointed Acting Organizing Director and will act in that capacity until Lt. Col. Collins has recovered and is able to report for duty.

Dr. Irwin C. Winter, Associate Professor of Pharmacology, resigned effective June 30, 1942, to accept a position as Medical Consultant with the Council on Pharmacy and Chemistry of the American Medical Association.

Dr. A. A. Hellbaum, Associate Professor of Physiology, has been granted a leave of absence for further study at the University of Chicago.

Dr. Carl A. Bunde, Assistant Professor of Physiology, has resigned to accept the appointment of Assistant of Physiology at Baylor University School of Medicine, Dallas, Texas.

Dr. Irvin S. Danielson, Associate Professor of Biochemistry, has resigned to accept a position with the Lederle Laboratories, New York City.

• OBITUARIES •

Dr. Francis C. Myers
1880-1942

"If you wish the pick of men and women, take a good bachelor and a good wife."—R. L. Stevenson.

Dr. Francis Charles Myers, since 1920 a general practitioner of medicine and surgery in Tulsa, was found dead in his apartments on Sunday, June 7, by the maid who cared for his quarters in the Daniel Building.

Dr. Myers was 62 years of age and unmarried. He saw active service overseas in World War I, having the rank of Captain in the Medical Corps, and was attached to Field Hospital No. 5. When the period of hostilities was ended, he moved into Germany with the Army of Occupation, and served six months in Rhenish Prussia.

Returning to this State in 1919 he resumed his interrupted practice in Broken Arrow, from which city he enlisted, for one year prior to his move to Tulsa. Although his professional services were those of a general practitioner, his preference was Surgery, at which specialty he was very adept.

Of a quiet and retiring nature, a rather gruff manner concealed a kind heart and marked diagnostic skill. He was ever ready to answer the call of the sick and afflicted of our city, and was a staunch and loyal friend to many of us of the medical fraternity, who grieve at his passing.

Dr. Myers is survived by two brothers, Homer Myers of Boston, Mass., and M. T. Myers of Oklahoma City and one sister, Mrs. Homer Keegan, also of Oklahoma City.

Resolution

WHEREAS, Francis Charles Myers was for a period of 22 years an ethical and respected member of the Tulsa County Medical Society, and,

WHEREAS, the late Francis C. Myers was throughout this period a busy and skillful practitioner of the healing art in our city and county.

NOW, THEREFORE, BE IT RESOLVED by the Tulsa County Medical Society that in the death of Francis C. Myers the profession of Oklahoma and his associates of Tulsa have sustained a real and deep loss.

BE IT FURTHER RESOLVED that the Tulsa County Medical Society desires to publicly acknowledge the blameless career and professional ability of this valued member of our organization.

BE IT FURTHER RESOLVED that the foregoing Resolution be made an intimate part of Tulsa County Medical Society records and a copy of same be mailed to the near relatives of the deceased.

Roy W. Dunlap, M.D., Chairman
R. G. Ray, M.D.
S. C. Venable, M.D.—Committee.

Dr. Henry C. Childs
1878-1942

"My pity hath been balm to heal their wounds;
My mildness hath allayed their swelling griefs."
—Shakespeare.

Late on Thursday evening, at his attractive home, 2124 South Peoria, the final summons came to one of our veteran ear, nose and throat specialists, Dr. Henry C. Childs.

Ill for several years with a crippling heart lesion, he had been forced to drastically curtail his busy labors and proceed at a more leisurely pace. But just the week preceding his death he had attended the State Medical Convention at the Coliseum and had performed a number of tonsillectomies at the County Charity Clinic.

A lover of flowers, his home on South Peoria, with its rolling lawns and varigated blossoms was one of the showplaces of the Garden Club.

He carried his love of the beautiful also into his religion, that of Unitarian—whose belief include love of God; brotherly affection for our fellowmen; the diffusion of knowledge; meditation on the gems of literature; tolerance of the religious opinions of others; and the hope of eventual salvation of all humanity.

Thrice married, the worthy doctor leaves to mourn his passing, his widow, and a step-daughter, Betty, of the home; two sons—Dr. Darwin Childs of 2126 E. 15th Street and Dr. Jack Childs of 1205 S. Evanston; and six grandchildren.

Resolution

WHEREAS, Henry C. Childs was for over twenty-five years an active and capable member of the Tulsa County Medical Society, and

WHEREAS, during this long period, in addition to his busy practice he gave freely of his time and talents to the School Board, the Charity Medical Clinic and many other worthy causes.

NOW, THEREFORE, BE IT RESOLVED by the Tulsa County Medical Society that the passing of H. C. Childs is a distinct loss both to our local organization and to the city in which he practiced his profession.

BE IT FURTHER RESOLVED that the Tulsa County Medical Society takes this method of expressing to the medical profession of the State and to the bereaved family its sincere regret over the death of one of our untiring practitioners and faithful public servants.

BE IT FURTHER RESOLVED that a copy of this Resolution be spread upon the minutes of Tulsa County Medical Society and that a duplicate thereof be presented to the immediate relatives of Henry C. Childs.

Roy W. Dunlap, M.D., Chairman
R. G. Ray, M.D.
S. C. Venable, M.D.—Committee.

Robert M. Anderson
1870-1942

Robert M. Anderson, a pioneer physician of Shawnee, Oklahoma, died suddenly on July 16, 1942, while visiting his daughter in Marlow. Dr. Anderson had been apparently, in good health preceeding his death which came as he had always wished, in his sleep.

Dr. Anderson was born on December 29, 1870, in Bedford County, Tennessee, where he was raised and attended primary schools. He was graduated from the Medical Department of Vanderbilt University in 1894 and after his graduation he started the practice of medicine in Florida but shortly returned to Tennessee where he practiced in Pulaski until he moved to Shawnee in 1903.

When the Pottawatomie County Medical Society was oragnized in 1905, Dr. Anderson was one of the charter members and founders and has held the office of President of the Society on several occasions during the past thirty-seven years.

Dr. Anderson is a past-president of the Oklahoma State Medical Association, and at one time was Chairman of the Section on Obstetrics of the Southern Medical Association. At the time of his death he was Councilor for the state of Oklahoma for the Southern Medical Association.

He was a leader of the civic life of the community being a member of St. Paul's Methodist Church, Shawnee lodge No. 107 A. F. & A. M., the Shawnee Rotary Club, and the Board of Directors of the First Federal Building and Loan Association.

Dr. Anderson was associated in practice with two other pioneer Shawnee physicians, Drs. J. E. Hughes and F. L. Carson, since 1918.

The survivors include his wife, two daughters, four grandchildren, three brothers, one Dr. W. B. Anderson, a practicing physician in Nashville, Tenn., and two sisters.

Funeral services were conducted from the St. Paul's Methodist church in Shawnee on Saturday, June 18, which were conducted by Dr. Forney Hutchinson and Rev. R. E. L. Morgan, and were attended by many prominent physicians from over the entire state.

Dr. J. C. Bushyhead
1870-1942

Dr. Jesse C. Bushyhead of Claremore, the "Grand Old Man" of medicine in Northeast Oklahoma passed away at his home in Claremore, July 11, 1942, at the age of 72.

Dr. Bushyhead was known as Rogers County's most beloved citizen and was the original charter member of the Rogers County Medical Society.

Always preferring to be known as a country doctor he exemplified the highest traditions of the Medical profession.

He administered to the needs of the rich and the poor alike. Never was the storm too bad or the hour too late for Dr. Bushyhead to come to the bedside of the sick or injured.

In his passing, Oklahoma medicine loses a pioneer and a stalwart supporter. This loss can never be replaced though it may be superseded.

Dr. Bushyhead was born in Fort Gibson and moved to Claremore in 1891. He was a cousin of the late Will Rogers and a member of the Will Rogers Commission.

During his lifetime he had been honored by being elected to honorary membership in the Oklahoma State Medical Association and the Oklahoma Historical Society. He was the last treasurer of the Old Cherokee Indian nation.

He is survived by his widow, Mrs. Faye Bushyhead; one daughter, Mrs. H. C. Riggs; and three sons, Dennis Bushyhead, Jesse C. Bushyhead, Jr., and George Davis Bushyhead.

About eight members of the Beckham County Society met July 1, in Elk City. They had as their guests, Dentists, Druggists, their wives, Nurses and Doctor's office help.

A round-table discussion was held following a banquet at the Casa Grande Hotel.

The next meeting will be held August 11, at Sayre. Dr. R. M. Slaubaugh will discuss "Enemia".

Members of the Pittsburg County Society met June 26, at the country home of Dr. Edwin D. Greenberger, in McAlester with 25 members present.

The program consisted of a barbeque supper and an evening of fellowship to honor Dr. Floyd Bartheld and Dr. C. E. Lively, who are leaving McAlester to enter the Medical Corps of the U. S. Army.

The society will meet in August, to hear a lecture on Post Graduate Medicine.

Group Hospital Service News

Approved Blue Cross Plans are divided into four brackets, according to the number of applicants enrolled. Recently Oklahoma's plan passed a milestone and moved out of the lower bracket to the third division. This low cost family protection has now been extended to 27,000 in Oklahoma, from whom more than 2000 days of hospital care have been provided. The employees of five hundred and fifteen firms have voluntarily enrolled in this plan. Group Hospital Service has been given approval for a third time by and is an institutional member of The American Hospital Association.

Non Profit hospital service plans are now serving an area comprising more than 80 percent of the population of America. The member hospitals of this national health movement contain over two-thirds of the total bed capacity of non-governmental hospitals in this country. There are 72 approved plans with a total membership of almost 11,000,000. The American Hospital Association estimates that these plans will pay hospital bills to the extent of $50,000,000.00 during the year of 1942. This amount is considerably greater than the combined revenue of all endowment capital, individual philanthropy, and from county, city and community funds combined, for these hospitals.

Prepaid hospital care without profit is a part of a great voluntary health movement. One of the most significant of our time. It's performance, even thus far, not only justifies its continued existance but proclaims it a social necessity. While the enrollment in these non profit hospital service plans is now measured by each new million members enrolled, still it probably is in it's infancy. The solution to the problem will not have been approached until the 11,000,000 members approximate 80,000,000 who would probably be carried on a compulsory federal program.

Today America's free hospitals are overshadowed by clouds of fear that deceptive hopes of superior federal service and easy government money might lead to bureaucratic regimentation. That shadow must be dispelled if the American system of free hospitals is to be preserved.

Because a federal health program has not been presented to congress in legislative form, we must not adopt a "wait and see" attitude. Informed observers believe that the formal presentation is retarded only to determine to what extent a voluntary plan will be adopted.

Even now the Blue Cross in Oklahoma should be a source of satisfaction to every member of the Oklahoma State Medical Society. Daily the plea is made to leaders of industry and groups of employees, to perpetuate our voluntary health system. The medical profession, hospital representatives and civic leaders who direct our plan are giving their time without pay. The continued cooperation of the medical profession can accelerate our growth and retard social regimentation.

The Southwestern Oklahoma Medical Society met June 17, at Elk City, to hear a program given by Dr. Edwin A. Abernathy, Altus, and Dr. Richard M. Burke, Clinton. Dr. Abernathy spoke on "The Use of Sulfamides in the Treatment of Suppurative Conditions of the Ear," and Dr. Burke on "Trends in the Collapse Therapy of Pulmonary Tuberculosis."

The next meeting of the Society will be held September 19, in Clinton.

Dr. J. E. McDonald, Tulsa, who has recently returned from Minneapolis where he has been studying the Kenny Treatment of Infantile Paralysis, gave a discussion on this subject at the Osage County Society meeting, held June 15, in Pawhuska, with 13 members present.

Lt. Tommy R. Young, of the Medical Corps of the U. S. Army, presented the Need of Doctors in Technical Training Command in the Air Corps and the opportunities offered.

The next meeting of the society will be held July 13, at Pawhuska.

Office of Civilian Defense

Organization in the Control System of the State Civilian Defense Committee on Health and Housing, which includes Emergency Medical Service, has been completed in the seventy-seven counties of the state. These various county organizations are not perfect. As time goes by, they will become more highly organized, and, therefore, more proficient.

The three disasters that have occurred within the state; namely, Pryor, Guymon, and Oklahoma City, have afforded a wonderful opportunity for work-out in these areas, which has made apparent any defects that might exist so that they could be corrected, as well as the good qualities of the work. Many inquiries from doctors over the state relative to the functions, duties, and responsibilities of the Emergency Medical Relief Service of Civilian Defense prompt the giving of the following information which will aid materially in clarifying all of these different phases of the work.

This information is taken from a joint statement coming from Norman H. Davis, Chairman of the American Red Cross, and James M. Landis, Director of the Office of Civilian Defense, under date of May 19, 1942, which was received in Doctor Mathews' office on July 13, 1942.

"To secure unity of effort and avoid duplication of facilities in meeting civilian needs arising from enemy action, this statement is issued by the Office of Civilian Defense and the American National Red Cross for the guidance of Defense Councils and Red Cross Chapters."

"It is the responsibility of local Defense Councils to see that adequate provision is made for all services required in the event of bombing or other enemy attack. During an emergency period, the Commander of the Citizens' Defense Corps will exercise control over all such services."

Emergency Medical Services

"During bombing or other enemy attack, all services are directed from the Control Center in charge of the Commander of the Citizens' Defense Corps."

The local Chairman of the Health and Housing Committee, in case of enemy attack, will be stationed in the Control Room as an assistant to the Commander of the Citizens' Defense Corps.

"*Responsibility for the care of those injured as a result of enemy action rests with the Emergency Medical Service of the Citizens' Defense Corps under the direction of the Chief of Emergency Medical Service.*"

"Red Cross Chapters assist the Emergency Medical Service by (a) recruiting and training Volunteer Nurses' Aides who will be utilized by the Emergency Medical Service at Base and Casualty Hospitals, Casualty Stations, and First Aid Posts; (b) furnishing lists of persons trained in first aid to be enlisted by the Emergency Medical Service as members of its stretcher teams; (c) *providing dressings, bandages and supplementary equipment as the Chapter may decide in consultation with the Chief of Emergency Medical Service;* (d) equipping and operating emergency ambulances to be assigned to the Emergency Medical Service and to serve under its direction; (e) providing supplementary transportation for walking injured and for Emergency Medical Service personnel. During the emergency period, ambulances and motor units assigned to such transportation service will be under the direction of the Chief of Emergency Medical Service or the Transport Officer. The Emergency Medical Service of the Office of Civilian Defense will not be duplicated by the Red Cross, but will be utilized by the Red Cross in natural disasters."

BOOK REVIEWS

"The chief glory of every people arises from its authors."—Dr. Samuel Johnson.

"ANOXIA—ITS EFFECT ON THE BODY." 1942. Directing Editor, Edward L. Van Liere, M.D. Cloth. Price $3.00. Pp. 269. The University of Chicago Press—Chicago. 1942.

In this breath-taking, calamitous age when every thinking person comtemplates being up in the air, down under the sea, or possibly in the bomb shelter, oxygen becomes an important consideration and the question of Anoxia becomes a matter of grave significance. Modern methods of Warfare, modern transportation and modern industry call for a more general and comprehensive knowledge of oxygen and its relationship to the vital functions of the human organism.

This knowledge has been assembled and made available by the author of this attractive book, published by the University of Chicago Press under the title "Anoxia". A glance at the table of contents suggests the comprehensive scope of the text and its application to present needs. Following an interesting preface the chapters are listed as follows: Historical, Definition of Terms, Classification of Anoxia, Expression of the Degree of Anoxia, Experimental Methods of Producing Anoxia, General Considerations, Effect of Anoxia on the Blood, Chemical Changes in the Blood During Anoxia, Effect of Anoxia on the Heart and Circulation, Effect of Anoxia on the Blood Pressure, Effect of Anoxia on the Lymph, Effect of Anoxia on Respiration, Mountain Sickness and Altitude Sickness, Acclimatization, Effect of Anoxia on the Alimentary Tract, Anoxia and the Secretions of Urine, Effect of Anoxia on the Endocrine Glands, Metabolism and Anoxia, Anoxia and Heat Regulation, Anoxia and Nutrition, Effect of Anoxia on Water Distribution in the Body, Effect of Anoxia on the Nervous System, and Index.

One has only to note the effects of Anoxia on the various organs, symptoms, fluids and tissues of the body to be impressed with importance of oxygen in the body economy.

After clarifying the approach to the subject by giving definitions and discussing types and degrees of Anoxia, the author considers the response of the physiologic processes to low oxygen tension and the variables at high altitudes.

The succeeding chapters, particularly those dealing with the circulatory system, the respiratory and the nervous systems, are of the greatest interest and importance to all doctors. The knowledge contained in these chapters, plus that found in the section devoted to mountain sickness and altitude sickness, is indispensible for the doctors in the Army and Navy, Medical Corps.

The Author's attempt to assemble all the known facts having to do with oxygen want and to make them readily available to all who read is most commendable. His citation of unsolved problems and his discussion of controversial situations should stimulate further research in this field.—Lewis J. Moorman, M.D.

"CLINICAL IMMUNOLOGY, BIOTHERAPY AND CHEMOTHERAPY." John A. Koler, Professor of Medicine, Temple University School of Medicine, Philadelphia; Director, Research Institute of Cutaneous Medicine, and Louis Tuft, Assistant Professor of Medicine and Chief of Clinic and Allergy and Applied Immunology, Temple University School of Medicine. Published in July, 1941 by W. B. Saunders Company, Philadelphia, 941 pages and illustrations. Price $10.00.

Vis Medicatrix Naturae used by our fathers of old, by modern interpretation, may be called Immunology. The understanding of this phenomenon is put on a lucid basis by the bacteriologist, biotherapeutist, serologist, and the chemist.

The author does not go into the minute details of this procedure but leaves it to specialized details in their respective fields, i.e., it is not a laboratory book. The book is divided into two parts. Part I is used by the senior author in lecturing to the sophomore students, while Part II is used by the authors in junior and senior years. This is a book which I think should be in the library of every physician and surgeon, and especially one engaged in public health work.

The fundamental ground-work in Part I necessarily must be understood before applying it to the efficient use of chemotherapy and the biologies, both of which have had such dramatic development in the last few years. These measures are so powerful in their effect that a basic understanding is paramount in the intelligent use of the same.

The latency and chronicity of bacterial infections, why the tissue susceptibility and localization, the natural immunity of some people and animals and the means of acquiring an immunity are all very basic in understanding disease, especially bacterial infections, whether it be local, general, acute, chronic, bacteraemia, septicaemia, pyemia or toxemia, such as we get from certain diffusible toxines which circulate in the blood stream and are chemotoxic for certain tissues. Lengthy description of todays proved prophylactic and innumerological methods. Methods of diagnosis and treatment of allergy are discussed at length and it is shown that it is dominant in many phases due to split proteids, both exogenous and endogeneous, typical and atypical. That is not ordinarily considered. The junior author is especially interested in allergy and is Chief of the Allergy Clinic of Temple University.

The chapters on blood transfusion therapy and non-specific protein therapy which play such a role in the present treatment today, could have been given more space at the expense of subjects not so generally used. Fifty pages are devoted to the chemotherapy and is the last chapter of Part I.

Part II is devoted to "The Practical Applications of Immunity Biotherapy and Chemotherapy in Prophylaxis and Treatment of Disease." This having followed three basic principles and understanding when written by authors who practice bedside medicine, thus forming a liaison between research and clinical observation.

The chapters on the general considerations of septicaemia are worthy of thorough perusal. The ubiquitous streptococcus with its protein troubles, the testing of immunity as well as the many clinical symptoms, the chemotherapy and biologic therapy should be read by those in every special field of work. The same may be said about the staphlococci, meningococci, bacillary, virus, psitltacosis and richettsial diseases.

A good feature is the summary of each disease at the end of the chapter. This is an outline such as is often shown on a projector for classroom demonstration.

These authors have the best of standing in medical circles, are voluminous and practical writers. This book is entirely new, and the only one of any magnitude on this subject.—Lea A. Riley, M.D.

"MODERN MEDICINE: ITS PROGRESS AND OPPORTUNITIES." Netta W. Wilson, Minnesota Department of Health, and S. A. Weisman, M.D., F.A.C.P., Clinical Associate Professor of Medicine, University of Minnesota. Cloth, Price, $2.00 Pp. 218. New York: George W. Stewart, Inc., 1942.

In this handy volume, the authors have undertaken a difficult task. The difficulties have been augmented by an attempt to give the historical background and to indicate progress with suggestions as to opportunities for careers in various fields of scientific research. Naturally, much has been sacrificed in favor of brevity.

The historical approach is most commendable and in many sections of the text it has been employed with dramatic effect. But to one who reads with a knowledge of the history of medicine and even a meager understanding of the influence of disease upon the destiny of mankind, it appears that many opportunities to establish the continuity of medical progress have been overlooked. In addition, the well informed reader may wonder if the authors have not failed to adequately show the laborious methods and the untiring efforts which have motivated medical progress. The average layman would have a much better appreciation of the advantages which have accrued through modern medicine if he knew how it is steeped in the life blood of a long line of medical scientists, bent upon the acquisition of truth. In addition to certain omissions, there are a few historical errors. Among these are references to William Withering and William Osler. One page 94 we find the following:

But since Dr. William Withering in 1785 coaxed or bribed an old country woman of England to sell or give him a secret that she knew, we have possessed a way to prevent dropsy through the use of a powerful drug called "digitalis," made from the leaves of a flowering plant, the foxglove.

The following is quoted from Withering's own statement:

"In the year 1775, my opinion was asked concerning a family recipe for the cure of dropsy—."

It is true that Withering published his account of the foxglove in 1785, but the remarkable adequacy of his report is due to the fact that he devoted ten years to a careful experimental and clinical study of the action of digitalis before he assumed the responsibility of publication.

On page 11 we find the following:

After the Armistice we hasten back to America to see, if only for a moment, that great and beloved physician whose name is almost as meaningful in modern times as that of Hippocrates when the world was young. We find Sir William Osler—who will not long survive the loss of his only son in the war just ended—still chiefly concerned for the welfare of his patients.

At this time Sir William Osler was Reginus Professor of Medicine at Oxford University, where he had gone in 1905 after resigning his professorship at Johns Hopkins.

In justification of the task performed, it may be said that the text presents an interesting running story, containing a great store of valuable information about modern medicine made readily available for the lay reader, the prospective medical student and research worker, also for busy doctors who need a "refresher course" in the general progress of modern medicine.—Lewis J. Moorman, M.D.

"DISEASES OF THE RESPIRATORY TRACT." Jacob Segal, M.D., F.A.C.P., F.A.C.C.P., Attending Physician, Riverside Hospital; Associate Physician in Charge of Thoracic Diseases, Bronx Hospital; Formerly Physician in Charge of Fordham Hospital Tuberculosis Clinic. Cloth. Price $2.00. Pp. 172. New York: Oxford University Press, 1941.

The author has provided a valuable compendium on the diseases of the respiratory diseases. In this field, rapid development in diagnostic and therapeutic procedures keeps the medical student and the alert doctor constantly on the look-out for additional knowledge.

With the perennial prevalence of respiratory diseases and the seasonal accentuation of their importance constantly in mind, such a reference book should become the pocket companion of the medical student, the intern and the busy doctor. Those in need of immediate information and those who have read and forgotten, or who are too busy to read in great detail, will find in this handy volume the essential facts brought up-to-date.

On the other hand, this outline should not be considered as merely a short cut to knowledge. The author admits that isolated facts often suffer for want of amplification and proper association with related facts.

The following quotation from the Preface should serve as a guide for every one who makes use of this valuable outline. "One may read and absorb the descriptive text of a certain disease, yet fail to visualize the essential points clearly. The detailed exposition when read and reread attentively will leave a good general impression on the subject, but is apt to blur the salient and sequential delineation. An outline is calculated to help the reader systematize his thoughts on the subject matter he has read about extensively, and repeatedly in the textbook. It should be helpful to focus attention on essentials, and recall to memory the details in their proper proportion. I hope that the outline here presented will fulfill the aforementioned requirements."

The subject matter is presented in seven sections or chapters, with the following titles: *Diseases of the Nasal Cavities. Diseases of the Pharynx. Diseases of the Lymphatic Structures of the Pharynx. Diseases of the Larynx. Diseases of Trachea and Bronchi. Diseases of the Lungs. Diseases of the Pleura. Bibliography. Index.*

A careful perusal of the briefer but comprehensive text shows that the author, through a lucid style, has succeeded in giving us an accurate statement of facts in very few words. While the reader may occasionally regret the brevity necessary in such a book and note the omission of certain conditions, he must marvel at the store of knowledge made available in so few pages.—Lewis J. Moorman, M.D.

Columbia University announces Program

"Columbia University announces that begining September, 1942, a program of professional studies for the training of Physical Therapy technicians will be offered. This training and instruction will extend over a two-year period and has been organized in compliance with the requirements set down for such programs by the Council on Medical Education and Hospitals of the American Medical Association. The course is being set up in University Extension in close relationship with the College of Physicians and Surgeons of Columbia University, the Nursing Education and Health and Physical Education Departments of Teachers College. The Clinical and laboratory instruction will be given at the Vanderbilt Clinic, Neurological Institute, Presbyterian Hospital and New York Orthopedic Dispensary and Hospital."

"Two years or 60 semester hours of college, including courses in Physics and Biology, shall be required, or graduation for an accredited School of Nursing or an accredited School of Physical Education."

"A Certificate of Proficiency in Physical Therapy will be granted by Columbia University to those completing the course. Further information may be obtained by writing the Office of the Committee on Physical Therapy, Room 303B, School of Business, Columbia University, New York City."

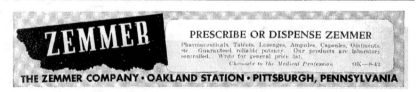

REVIEWS and CORRESPONDENCE

SURGERY AND GYNECOLOGY

Abstracts, Reviews and Comments From
LeRoy Long Clinic
714 Medical Arts Building, Oklahoma City

"INFECTIOUS LESIONS ABOUT THE EXTERNAL GENI-TALS." By Mortimer D. Speiser, M.D., American Journal of Obstetrics and Gynecology, April 1942. Page 681.

The incidence of the various infectious diseases about the external genitals in the Bellevue Hospital series is given. Since some of these patients are taken upon the dermatological service the incidence is given for both the gynecological and the female dermatological services. They include: (1) Primary Syphilis with 1.4 per 1,000 admissions on the gynecological service and 11 per 1,000 admissions upon the female dermatology service. (2) Secondary Syphilis 0.9 per 1,000 admissions on gynecology and 269 per 1,000 admissions mostly with genitalia lesions on dermatology. (3) Combined primary and secondary 39 per 1,000 admissions. (4) Lymphogranuloma venereum 5.2 per 1,000 admissions on gynecology and 34.4 per 1,000 admissions on dermatology. (5) Granuloma inguinale 0.4 per 1,000 admissions on gynecology and 6.9 per 1,000 admissions on female dermatology. (6) Chancroid 0.8 per 1,000 admissions on gynecology and 9.1 per 1,000 admissions on female dermatology. (7) Condylomata acuminata 2.0 per 1,000 admissions on gynecology.

Each one of these conditions as well as gonorrhea is carefully described as to diagnosis with the following important routine:

"A positive diagnosis should never be made solely on the appearance of infected lesions about the external genitals. Grossly similar lesions may result from different etiologic factors. A single agent may be capable of producing variable lesions. Combined infections may be present. Therefore, pathognomonic characteristics are lacking so that an unequivocal diagnosis can be established only by the employment of certain routine procedures. These must include dark-field examinations and serologic tests, smears for Donovan bodies, Ducrey bacilli and fusospirochetes, intradermal tests with the Ducrey bacillary antigen and the Frei antigen, and last microscopic examination of tissue obtained for biopsy."

COMMENT: This article has been abstracted because of the confusion that has existed about infectious lesions of the external genitalia, both as to diagnosis and treatment. The concluding paragraph of the authors is particularly important in that they emphasize that an unequivocal diagnosis can be established only by the employment of certain routine procedures which they then enumerate.—W. L., M.D.

"NYLON SUTURE." D. W. Melick, M.D. Annals of Surgery, March 1942, Page 475.

In the year 1938, it was learned that the DuPont Company had developed a synthetic substitute for silk, called Nylon. It was then that the suggestion that it might be used as a surgical suture was brought forward. Since many surgeons are advocates of silk, it was thought that Nylon might find equal favor, should it have the qualities attributed to silk.

The physical characteristics of Nylon as compared to silk appear in the following table:

	Nylon	Silk
Relative tensile strength	1.3%	1.0%
Elongation	25.7%	12.9%
Loss in strength when wet	14.7%	25.4%
Approximate moisture content under standard conditions	3.0%	15.0%
Elastic recovery under controlled conditions	77.0%	65.0%

Nylon sutures may be obtained either as a single strand suture called monofilament, or a multiple strand suture, called multifilament. The multifilament looks and feels very much like silk. The monofilament is comparable to the commonly known "dermal" or "tension" suture or heavy silk worm gut suture.

The author, under the direction of Dr. E. R. Schmidt, professor of surgery, University of Wisconsin, carried out experiments on dogs in order to study the effect of various sutures, (catgut and silk as well as Nylon) in relation to tissue reaction and to the process of wound healing as ascertained by gross and microscopic study. Nylon monofilament, Nylon multifilament, silk, plain and chromic catgut were imbedded in the anterior abdominal wall of dogs, and, at intervals between two days and 103 days, biopsies were taken and paraffin sections made. Intestinal anastomoses were also performed for comparison between fine cromic catgut (No. 00000) and Nylon multifilament (No. 000).

The author summarizes his animal experimentations as follows:

(1) Nylon multifilament causes less reaction in the tissues (of dogs) than does catgut. In the earlier stages of healing Nylon multifilament causes more reaction than does silk. The end-result of the healing process is practically the same for both Nylon multifilament and silk.

(2) Nylon multifilament is not completely noncapillary. Monocytes were heavily infiltrated between the interstices of the suture, when examined at the end of 34 days.

(3) Nylon multifilament is superior to silk in that it has a better tensile strength for comparable sizes.

(4) Nylon monofilament causes less tissue reaction than any of the sutures studied. It is not so flexible as Nylon multifilament, is more difficult to handle, and has a tendency to slip when tied with the usual surgical knot.

On the surgical service of Dr. Schmidt at the University of Wisconsin Hospital in Madison, 19 herniorrhaphies were performed by various surgeons, using Nylon multifilament suture. The opinions voiced, were favorable. It was agreed that the suture was comparable to silk in the way it handled. The greater tensile strength of the suture as compared with silk of a similar size was particularly noted by each operator. Wound healing was satisfactory in all of the patients upon whom Nylon multifilament was used as a suture. The incisions presented a minimal amount of reaction. The deep fascia and subcutaneous tissue was free of the diffuse induration noticed with catgut suture.

The author concluded that Nylon multifilament may be recommended as a satisfactory surgical suture. In this connection, he meant that it was satisfactory as a "buried suture."

COMMENT: We have been using Nylon monofilament for "stay or tension sutures" for the past two years. It has proved very satisfactory. Used as a stay suture, its tendency to slip when tied, can be overcome by multiple knots.

We have had no experience with Nylon multifilament as a buried suture, but, if inclined to use silk, we would not hesitate to employ this suture as a substitute.—L. D. L., M.D.

"AN EVALUATION OF INTESTINAL SUCTION IN IN-
TESTINAL OBSTRUCTION. J. B. Blodgett, M.D. Surgery, May 1942. Page 739.

The term "intestinal suction" does not mean "duodenal suction." As used here, intestinal suction applies
only to those cases in which the Miller-Abbott tube, or
other long tube, has definitely passed into the jejunum.

The author states that intestinal suction was introduced for the treatment of intestinal obstruction about four
years ago. He refers to the work of Abbott and Johnson who published an article entitled "Intubation Studies
of the Human Small Intestine" in Surgery, Gynecology,
and Obstetrics in the year 1938.

The cases reported in this article by Dr. Blodgett are
derived from a study of all cases of intestinal obstruction treated at the Peter Bent Brigham Hospital in
Boston from 1933 to July 1941. To these he has added
all available cases from the American Literature that
satisfied the requirements of the classification.

In order to compare similar types of intestinal obstruction, two distinct groups were chosen for analysis:
(1) Simple mechanical obstruction of the small or large
bowel; (2) Intestinal obstruction associated with peritonitis. The mortality of these two groups is so different
that it was necessary to consider them separately in
evaluating any therapy applied to them.

"Paralytic ileus" not associated with peritonitis is
too poorly defined a clinical entity to constitute a definite
group for an analysis of this sort, although individual
cases occasionally yield satisfactory results to intestinal
suction.

Three hundred and six cases of mechanical intestinal
obstruction were treated by the usual measures (including operation) but *Intestinal suction was not used*. This
was considered a controlled series of cases and resulted
in a mortality of 17.3 percent. One hundred and fifty-
one cases of mechanical intestinal obstruction were treated by the usual measures (including operation) and
intestinal suction was used. The mortality was 7.9 percent.

It appears, therefore, that when intestinal suction is
added to the usual measures of treatment of mechanical
intestinal obstruction, the mortality was reduced from
17.3 to 7.9 percent. This reduction in the mortality due
to the use of intestinal suction is of undeniable significance and is not a difference due to the results of
chance.

When peritonitis is associated with intestinal obstruction, the mortality is greatly increased. To evaluate the
effect of intestinal suction on this condition, the Peter
Bent Brigham Hospital cases were added to all acceptable cases appearing in the Literature. No distinction
was made on the basis of the extent of peritoneal involvement. The total number of cases treated without
intestinal suction and treated with intestinal suction is
not large, because authors seldom list their cases of
obstruction and peritonitis separately and satisfactory
intubation is difficult in the presence of peritonitis.
However, the difference in mortality percentages between these groups is highly significant. The mortality
in the controlled series of cases with obstruction is highly
significant. The mortality in the controlled series of
cases with obstruction and peritonitis that were not
treated with intestinal suction was found to be 73.1 percent. But the mortality in the same type of case when
treated with intestinal suction was found to be 25 percent.

This evidence that the use of intestinal suction is an
essential factor in reducing the mortality of intestinal
obstruction has been corroborated by other workers.

Intestinal suction is an ideal physiologic treatment because it produces an outlet for the intestinal contents at
a point just proximal to the obstruction. As the intestine
is decompressed, the circulation is improved, the smooth
muscle regains its normal tone, and the important function of nutrition may be resumed. When the pressure
within the intestine is released, the volume of circulating
plasma, which has been shown to be reduced in obstruc-

tion, is restored to normal. Reduction of the intra-
abdominal pressure by the decompression of the intestine
allows normal circulation in the great venous channels
and normal diaphragmatic excursion. Preoperative decompression of the alimentary tract by intestinal suction
may avoid the necessity of colostomy or enterostomy
and presents the operator with undistended bowel of
normal thickness and tone. Intestinal suction continued
into the postoperative period protects the anastomosis
by preventing intra-luminal pressure which might "blow-
out" the suture line or impair its circulation.

The author wisely points out the absolutely necessary
and all important point that the contraindications to
the use of intestinal suction for obstruction should be
emphasized.

There is danger in the routine use of intestinal suction.
When a reasonable possibility of vascular stangulation
exists, intestinal suction should not be resorted to except
as preparation for immediate operation. The danger is
that although decompression offers no relief for the
vascular obstruction, it may mask the symptoms to such
an extent as to minimize the urgency of operation which
is the essential therapy for intestinal strangulation. The
decision for immediate operation depends upon nice
clinical judgment of all facts at hand. If strangulation
cannot be ruled out, surgery should be advised. It is
pointed out that intestinal intubation should not be attempted in cases of obstruction of the large bowel which
show great distention of the colon and little or no
evidence of distention of the small bowel. In such
cases, the dangerous pressure on the colon cannot be
reduced until the tip of the long tube has passed
through the ileocecal valve. The passage of the tube
through the whole small bowel may not be complete for
days, and even then it may be impossible to get the
tip to pass through the competent ileocecal valve. Accordingly, intestinal intubation is not the treatment of
choice because the relief of pressure in the large bowel
may be unwisely delayed.

COMMENT: It is probable that intestinal suction
(as contrasted to duodenal suction) has not been used
as wisely as it should be used, because of the extreme
difficulty in successful intubation of the bowel beyond
the duodenum. As stated by Whipple, "the reason that
so many hospitals have failed to appreciate the value of
the Miller-Abbott tube in dealing with cases of ileus is
that no one person has learned the application and
technique of the method and acquired the experience
necessary to its success." I might add that the almost
constant attendence upon such a patient that is necessary is probably another reason why the method is not
in more universal use.

However, we must agree with the author that whatever
effort is involved in acquiring and applying the technique
is certainly justified by the fact that intestinal suction
is a life-saving procedure as an adjunct to the treatment
of obstruction.—L. D. L., M.D.

EYE, EAR, NOSE AND THROAT

Edited by Marvin D. Henley, M.D.
911 Medical Arts Building, Tulsa

"CANCER OF THE ESOPHAGUS." By W. A. Mill.
Laryngologist, Royal Cancer Hospital, London. Postgraduate Medical Journal, vol. 18, page 31-35, February, 1942.

Malignant disease of the esophagus is almost always
carcinoma. Sarcoma is exceedingly rare, and of no practical importance . Until recently, this disease laid claim to
a mortality of very nearly 100 percent.

More than half the patients complaining of esophageal
symptoms are found to be suffering from esophageal carcinoma, and most of them in the older age groups. Car-

cinoma of the esophagus comprises about 5 percent of all cases of cancer.

Men are much more commonly affected than women (80%). Chronic irritations of the esophageal mucosa by alcohol, tobacco, hot foods and drinks and by dental sepsis are considered of importance in the development of esophageal carcinoma. The growth tends to appear at levels in the esophagus where there is some anatomical narrowing;—at the upper end, at the levels of the aortic and left bronchial crossings and the diaphragmatic constriction. It has been observed that esophageal carcinoma may follow peptic ulcers, cardiospasm, diverticulum, cicatrical stenosis, or it may also occur in the congenitally short esophagus.

In women post-cricoid carcinoma is fairly common. The Plumber-Vinson syndrome also predisposes to disease in this situation. Yet, such cancers truly belong to the hypopharynx and not to the esophagus.

The common types of esophageal carcinoma are: (1) epitheliomatous ulcer, (2) a fungating mass, and (3) a hard scirrhous annular exulcerating growth. The esophageal carcinoma may be also secondary. Thus, cancer of the thyroid, the larynx, trachea or bronchus, even the cancer of the stomach may extend to the esophagus. Primary cancer may arise from glands in the esophageal wall or from isolated dystopic patches of gastric mucosa which occur there.

Most of the tumors are to be found in the middle part of the esophagus, fewer in the lower part, and still fewer in its upper part. The growth spreads round the esophageal wall and also longitudinally, and the various layers of the wall are successively involved until the surrounding structures become invaded.

In untreated cases metastases in the lymphatic glands are less common than might be expected (50%). The supraclavicular glands on both sides may be affected, also the glands round the left gastric artery and in the lesser omentum.

The main complaint of the patient is difficulty in swallowing. This symptom, however, appears too late after the disease has been present for some time Occasionally the onset of dysphagia is sudden owing to the blocking of the stricture by a pill or some hard food. More often the dysphagia develops gradually, and there is first some difficulty with solid food. A slight vague sense of something not being just right in the swallowing function may be present for a long time prior to actual difficulty in getting food down. The stricture may be very considerable when the first symptoms appear because any well-chewed solid food can be swallowed through a lumen 5 mm in diameter.

There may be also a feeling of weight or fullness behind the sternum. Or, the earliest complaint is of dyspepsia or flatulence. If the recurrent laryngeal nerve becomes involved, hoarseness may develop. This may be the first symptom of esophageal cancer. Other symptoms are salivation, blood-stained expectoration, coughing, regurgitation (usually a late symptom), actual pain, loss of weight and cachexia. Death may result from inanition and exaustion, or by some complication such as mediastinitis, broncho-pneumonia or hemorrhage from a large vessel. Fistula into the bronchial tree or trachea is mostly responsible for the development of pulmonary complications.

The diagnosis is made from the many symptoms and signs. There may be a collection of frothy saliva in the piriform sinuses at laryngeal examination. This indicates esophageal obstruction. Paralysis of some degree of the vocal cords may be noted. There may be enlarged glands in the neck, or a diffuse swelling pressing forward the trachea. This may be the first symptom of esophageal cancer. X-ray examination of the chest and esophagus should be carried out. A picture taken with the patient in the Trendelenburg position, just after swallowing the opaque meal, will show the lower limit of the stricture and will define its length. A very thick and heavy opaque meal will often show the length of the stricture, even in the upright position. The radiological appearances of a carcinomatous stricture are characteristic and diagnostic. During deglutition the opaque matter is seen to stop suddenly at the level of the upper end of the stricture and accumulate in the slightly dilated esophagus above while a little trickles through the narrow and irregular stricture.

Esophagoscopic examination will disclose one of the three types of lesion found. The degree of stenosis can be determined by the passage of bougies. A small piece of tissue should be removed for microscopical examination. The distance of the upper end of the stricture from the upper incisor teeth should be carefully noted.

Far too many cases are diagnosed too late for treatment to be anything but alleviative. The difficulty of early diagnosis has to be overcome. The prospect of cure is not so dark now as it was in the past. During any treatment it is important that attention be paid to diet and enough suitable and carefully sieved food must be given.

Gastrostomy is not practiced frequently nowadays. It enables sufficient nourishment for a long time, and it should not be postponed until the patient has become definitely cachectic. Yet, intubation is better than gastrostomy. Souttar's tubes of varying size may be introduced into the stricture through an esophagoscope. Such tubes are retained in position, and the patient may swallow practically normally for many months.

Nowadays the majority of cases received some form of radiation therapy. The results as regards alleviation are on the whole satisfactory and occasionally apparent cures result. Deep x-ray often gives relief and in certain cases cure seems to result. X-ray irradiation should be limited strictly to the esophagus, which needs special skill in roentgen therapeutical technic. Radon seeds introduced into the tumor itself are still in use. Alleviation results in most cases. Radium treatment is rather new for esophageal cancer. Guisez reported 270 cases, and life for most of them was greatly prolonged; there were also a few cases of apparent cure. The prognosis depends entirely on the early recognition of cancer.

Radical operation by some of the accepted methods is still a sensational operation, and the operative statistics still are varying according to the skill and experience of the operator. The main operations are the one-stage thoracico-cervical and the two-stage thoracico-abdominal. In spite of all treatment the prognosis is still extremely bad for esophageal cancer. The prognosis depends entirely on the early recognition of cancer.

"THE UTILIZATION OF PUS IN THE TREATMENT OF PYOGENIC DISORDERS." By Isaac J. Arnason, Buffalo, N. Y. New York State Journal of Medicine, vol. 42, p. 770-772, April 1942.

Pus represents the first and important line of defense which the body throws up against the invader. The idea of utilizing it for the offensive is not new in the history of medicine. The practical handicap was the form in which the pus could be used. In 1925, Orsos, of Hungary, reported on a method of preparation of an auto-pus vaccine which could be prepared by any practitioner in the routine office work and without an elaborate bacteriologic instrumentarium. He used this vaccine primarily in gonorrhea and furunculosis but recommended it for any staphylococcic or streptococcic infection. In 1926, Berde, also of Hungary, improved the autogenous pus vaccine by mixing it with a germicide called yatren. He added yatren to the vaccine in a ½ percent solution and advised the use of the vaccine not earlier than 24 hours after its preparation.

The present author followed the method of Orsos and Berde, and used the autogenous pus vaccine in 150 patients in private practice. The conditions in which it was used were: furunculosis, carbuncle, subaxillar abscess, panaritum, hordeolum, dacryocystitis suppurativa, also staphylococcic sepsis. For the group of furuncles the vaccine treatment gave a failure of only 3.25 percent.

Three cases of hordeolum were treated, all of a chronic type of over three months' duration. Treatment was successful in two cases. The third did not clear up after eight injections. One case of chronic dacryocystitis was sent by an ophthalmologist. Every conceivable previous therapeutic procedure, including repeated surgical draining, had failed. Six injections of autopus vaccine cleared up the condition. The vaccine was unsuccessful in staphylococcic septicemia, and it seems that septicemias are not the field for the Orsos vaccine.

A characteristic feature after the injection of the vaccine is the development of leukocytosis (15 to 25 thousand). Clinically, a profuse drainage sets in after the first and second injection. The healing process is a rapid one. As a rule, no untoward effects are observed. The temperature may rise one or two degrees after the first injection. A slight headache is complained of in about one fourth of all cases. No alarming symptoms of any kind were ever observed. Contraindications are the same as for any other intravenous injection.

Orsos prepares his vaccine by putting 0.06 gramme of the yatren powder into a sterile mortar, adding two to three platinum loops of pus to it grinding it for four to five minutes with a pestel, adding one to two drops of sterile water, grinding it again until a consistency of porridge is obtained, and adding, under constant stirring, the balance of water (8 cc.) The vaccine is ready for use in eight to ten minutes, and the injections are given intravenously every other day, beginning with 1 cc. for the first, followed by 2 cc. for the second and the third, and the balance for the last injection.

The vaccine may be prepared also so that after the first two drops of water are added it is ground thoroughly for five minutes; then one cc. of water is added, and the mixture stirred, and left to stand for 15 minutes. This method permits a saturated (5 percent) solution of yatren to work for 20 minutes on the microorganisms and carries the sterilization method further than in the original method.

"THE EFFECT OF FLIGHT UPON HEARING." By Major Paul A. Campbell, School of Aviation Medicine, Randolph Field, Texas. The Journal of Aviation Medicine, vol. 13, page 56-61, March 1942.

Already in 1773, when Pilatre de Rozier made a balloon journey reaching an altitude of 10,500 feet, it was noticed that descent from the air caused pain in the ear. Since that event there has been much study concerning the effect of flight upon the ears and hearing. The invention of audiometer made possible a more scientific approach to this problem.

It is definitely known today that the hearing of any flyer reflects in varying degree the influence of six forces any or all of which may be present in varying amount in individuals who have never been close to airplanes. The forces are: 1. the hearing apparatus which the flyer inherited, 2. his age, 3. the effect of noise to which he has been subjected during his life, 4. the ability of his tubo-tympanic apparatus to equalize barometric pressure changes to which he has been subjected, 5. disease past and present, 6. the effect of anoxia.

Superior acoustic mechanisms will withstand much of the insult coincident with life. Hence, more emphasis should be laid upon the family history of the flyer. The effect of age can be also demonstrated on every audiogram. Each decade of life brings a certain loss of hearing for the higher tones. It becomes measurable usually after the second decade and progresses with age both in degree and frequency range. At the age of 20 years there may be only a slight loss in the region of the 10,000 double vibration per second frequency but by the age of sixty this loss may have progressed to a point where it has involved all frequencies down to 1,000.

The perception portion of the hearing apparatus, the organ of Corti, with its connections to the brain, is susceptible to the phenomenon of fatigue. Noise or other vibratory energy, regardless of its origin, fatigues this neuro-sensory mechanism in direct relationship to its strength and the length of time it is applied. In flying, the energies which produce this effect are: engine explosions, propeller hum, noise produced by slip-stream effect on structures of the aircraft, sounds from moving parts, preaudible position and negative pressure changes from motion of the propeller, suprasonic vibratory frequencies produced by objects moving at high speed and their overtones. The effect is a notching of the 4,096

d.v. frequency area. This notch deepens and spreads fanwise as the insult is increased until it may involve the conversational range. Great and prolonged insults produce permanent damage to the ear of the aviator.

Faulty mechanism in the closing and opening of the Eustachian tube will result in a condition called aero-otitis media. It may become a rather serious factor because, in contrast to fatigue, it affects the conversational tone range as well as other portions of the curve of hearing.

Little is known concerning the effect of anoxia upon the ear. Yet, as fatigue and oxygenation are closely related, it seems reasonable to suppose that anoxia may account for some of the loss in the high tone levels which cannot be accounted for otherwise.

"MAXILLARY SINUSITIS OF DENTAL FRACTURE ORIGIN." Sobisca S. Hall, and Harry V. Thomas, Clarksburg, W. Va. The West Virginia Medical Journal, vol. 38, page 146-155, April 1942.

The authors analyze 48 patients co-operatively treated by a dentist and a rhinologist. The ages of the patients range from 16 to 65 years. The report suggests that a dental perforation into the maxillary sinus, unless adequate sinus treatment is instituted at once, will produce a serious maxillary sinusitis necessitating surgery for relief. It is also suggested that a spontaneous or surgical closure of the alveolar rent without adequate sinus attention is followed by a serious antral disease with all possible complications in a large percentage of the cases.

Residual patent alveolar fistulas were presented by 19 patients in this series, and 100 percent of them developed sinus disease. Twelve patients presented surgically closed alveolar fistulas without concurrent adequate sinus care. All of these patients developed sinus disease.

The authors believed that resection of part of the alveolar process and approximation of the lingual and buccal mucoperiosteum of the alveolar process with on-end mattress sutures is an ideal method of closure. They had 18 patients upon whom they performed this type of procedure, and 13 of them healed by primary intention. It is also possible to obtain a full thickness sliding graft from the palate and suture it over the area of perforation. Also, a sliding graft may be obtained from the buccal mucous membrane and sutured in place.

The aim of treatment should be prevention whenever possible. It is far better, when possible, to avoid fracture into an antrum than to face a prolonged course of sinus therapy. If the sinus alveolaris has been penetrated without rupturing the mucosa of a normal sinus, the condition should be treated with the greatest care, special care being taken not to rupture the mucosa. This means that no probing of this region should be done. Packs should be left out of the dental socket. If the mucosa has been ruptured, the fistula should be closed at once, and irrigation of the antrum either through the inferior meatus or through the normal ostium should be instituted and carried out for at least ten days. If at that time the x-ray does not show changes in the sinus, and there has been no collection of secretions, the sinus may be considered to have escaped infection.

In the case of fracture of the sinus alveolaris into an already infected antrum without rupture of the mucosa, the cavity should be treated without invading the antrum through the alveolus. Many disease of the antral mucosa are quiescent and do not require very extensive therapy for control. If, however, the rupture occurred into an infected sinus through the mucous membrane, treatment must be instituted immediately by closure of the process and antrotomy in the inferior meatus. Almost always, in such cases, the authors performed the Caldwell-Luc type of antrum operation. Later, they found that similar good results could be obtained by primary closure of the alveolar fistula, antral irrigations transnasally at once, and, only when necessary, should the antrotomy carried out for the maintenance of good nasal ventilation.

If adequate ventilation and drainage of the sinus

has been established, the prognosis is almost 100 percent for cure.

"TREATMENT OF OTOMYCOSIS." Merrill J. Reeh, M.D., Randolph Field, Texas. Annals of Otology, Rhinology, and Laryngology, March, 1942.

This disease is quite a problem in the Canal Zone. The relative high humidity and slight variation in temperature is a factor. Ninety cases were studied over a period of three months. Another one hundred twenty-five cases were studied over a period of four months. This study was preceded by sufficient laboratory and microscopic study to make the findings definite. As this is a valuable contribution to this unsatisfactory subject I am giving the author's summary in its entirety.

Before proper results can be obtained with any substance, the debris must be removed from the canal gently and thoroughly. Attention must be paid to the anterior acute angle. If removal cannot be effected mechanically, a gentle lavage with warm water usually will suffice. Medication is best applied on a wick for the first two or three days, leaving the wick for periods of twelve to twenty-four hours. When the wick is employed the medication is kept in constant contact with the infected surfaces, and undue swelling and obstruction of the canal are prevented.

Careful consideration was given to the work of McBurney and Searcy, Gill, Gill, Stokes, Minchew and co-workers, Whalen, and Lederman, before selecting agents for study. Many of the time-honored agents used in the tropics were found valueless during the preliminary four-month period. A few of the better ones were brought into study.

Thymol, 2 percent, in cresatin proved to be highly efficient as a fungicide. It did produce considerable burning and discomfort when used in raw canals. Thymol, 1 percent, in cresatin was found to be equally efficient as a fungicide. It did not produce burning, but proved to be a good local anesthetic and drying agent similar to cresatin alone. After the wick had remained twelve to twenty-four hours the canal walls were white, dry, and exfoliative. Much of the dry skin and debris could be removed with an applicator, thus expelling many spores. If the solution proved too strong, it was diluted with equal parts of olive oil. Occasionally the drops, used after wicks had been discontinued, were diluted. Cresatin alone proved to be excellent, but not as effective as 1 percent thymol in cresatin.

The result from Castelloni's solution was fair when it was used carefully. If used too frequently, it either unduly irritated the canal or caused drying of the skin with resulting pain.

Insufflation of 1 percent iodine and 1 percent thymol in boric acid powder produced fair results. It possessed some value as a medication to be used in resistant cases or in cases of chronic otitis media where an associated fungus infection is known or suspected to exist.

The time honored alcohol-boric solution was no better than the control. In general alcohol preparations proved to be painful and at times increased the inflammation.

The time honored icthyol-glycerine possessed value in early treatment of highly inflamed canals. It was found to be poor as a fungicide.

Glycerine preparations usually macerated the canal walls. Occasionally they aggravated a secondary bacterial infection which proved worse than the original condition.—M. D. H., M.D.

PLASTIC SURGERY

Edited by George H. Kimball, M.D., F.A.C.S.
912 Medical Arts Building, Oklahoma City

"THE NASAL ENTRANCE." W. Raymond McKenzie, M.D., F.A.C.S. Baltimore, Maryland. Southern Medical Journal Vol. 35, May 5, 1942.

The author estimated that 50, probably 75 percent of the men now being inducted into the armed forces have some deviation from the normal nasal entrance. He listed the deformities of the nasal entrance as follows:

1. Curling or curving of the anterior edge of the septal cartilage.
2. Deflection of the anterior edge of the septal cartilage.
3. Deflected columella.
4. Thickened columella.
5. Elongated columella.
6. Eversion of the medial crura of the alar cartilages.
7. Collapse of the lateral crura of the alar cartilages and the triangular cartilages.
8. Congenital atresia of the nares.
9. Any combination of two or more of the above named.

The author describes in detail the proper manner of examining the nose in order to discover these deformities.

Curling or Deflection of the Anterior Edge of the Septal Cartilage

These deformities are easily corrected either by shaving or removal of the anterior edge of the septal cartilage. The incision should be made at the anterior margin of the septal cartilage. Removal of one or two millimeters is usually all that is necessary. This amount can be removed safely, without altering the shape or interfere to do a submucous resection, that can be completed through the same incision, after which the wound is closed by two silk sutures.

Curving or Deflected Anterior Portion of the Septal Cartilage

These cases are really an exaggeration of the above mentioned in which the septum is either curved sharply or angulated acutely in such a shape or extent that it impinges against the outer wall or ala of the nose, either largely or completely occluding one nostril. Incision is made at the anterior edge of the cartilage and as much of the septum as is necessary to correct the deformity, even the entire anterior portion of the septal cartilage is removed, if nothing less will do. Then a straight piece of septal cartilage of proper size and shape is salvaged and transplanted in the columella to provide proper support for the nasal tip. The wound is closed by 2 silk sutures to protect the graft. If packs or splints are used after submucous resection they should be very lightly placed and not tightly packed. Too tight packing causes venous congestion, interfering with proper circulation, and may be responsible for loss of the cartilage transplant, for secondary infection and further deformity.

Thickened Columella

Most often this is due to some deformity of the anterior nasal spine or to an increase in the amount of fat or connective tissue in the columella or to both. The spine should be removed or shaving by chisel. No other method seems to be satisfactory or successful. Sufficient tissue is removed from the columella to reduce its size and a mattress suture is placed through and through the columella to eliminate the space produced by tissue removal.

Elongated Columella

This frequently interferes with nasal breathing because of the overhanging tip. A through-and-through or transfixion incision is made in the columella at the anterior margin of the septal cartilage; a triangular section with its base above, which includes the cartilage and its soft tissue covering, is removed from the fixed septum. In these cases it will also be necessary to remove a small section of the lower border of the upper lateral or triangular cartilages. The movable columella is sutured to the fixed septum on both sides to hold it in position. If the elongation of the columella is due to an enlargement or drooping of the medial crura of the alar cartilage, a marginal incision is made over the medial crus and sufficient skin and cartilage to correct the deformity are removed and the wound closed by sutures. Small adhesive strips are then placed around the tip of the nose to give added support, and to relieve tension on sutures.

Eversion of the Medial Crura

A marginal incision is made over the crus of the alar cartilage, the cartilage dissected free, the everted or deformed portion removed and the wound closed by fine silk sutures.

Collapse of the Triangular and Lateral Crura of the Alar Cartilages

Incision is made over the edge of the upper lateral or triangular cartilage, a small triangular portion removed and the wound allowed to fall together, making sure that none of the cartilage remains exposed. Sutures are not necessary in this location.

For lateral crus of the alar cartilage an eliptical incision is made on each side of the collapsed portion of the cartilage which includes mucous membrane and cartilage down to the overlying skin. This section is removed and the incision closed by one or two silk sutures. This does away with the redundant cartilage and enlarges the nasal entrance in proportion to the amount of tissue removed.

Deflected Columella

This deformity is most frequently due to a deflection of the septum together with some deformity of the anterior nasal spine, usually the result of fracture, at which time the spine was dislocated or deviated to one or the other side, or to an exostosis occurring on one side. Incision is made at the anterior margin of the septal cartilage and the deformity of the septum is corrected by shaving or removal. The nasal spine should be removed entirely or the exostosis removed from one side by a chisel so that the septal cartilage can be replaced in midline. If the nasal spine is not reshaped or removed the result will be disappointing and unsatisfactory.

Prominent or Bulbous Tip

This deformity is usually due to an enlargement of the alar cartilages. A marginal incision is made and by undermining, the cartilage is dissected free from the over-lying skin. A complete section two or three millimeters wide, including nasal mucosa, is removed from the upper inner portion near the nasal septum. Sutures are not necessary here, as the wound edges will fall together. Small adhesive strips are placed around the nasa ltip to maintain proper position of the severed ends of the alar cartilages.

Any or all of these operations can be done equally well under local or general anesthesia or a combination of both. I always inject a solution of 0.5 percent procaine hydrochloride to which is added one minim of epinephrine per dram of solution. This controls bleeding, makes inspection of the operative field easier and contributes greatly to accuracy.

Comment:

The author has pointed out some of the common conditions about the nasal tip which are correctible by Plastic Surgery. Cooperation with rhinologist is very essential in this type of work. Most of these cases can be done under local anesthetic without much time loss on the part of the patient.

Careful attention to detail in these cases is paramount. Most of the patients in this group are extremely grateful for improvement following operation.—G. H. K., M.D.

CARDIOLOGY

Edited by F. Redding Hood, M.D.
1200 North Walker, Oklahoma City

"TREATMENT OF CORONARY THROMBOSIS." Fred M. Smith, M.D., Iowa City, Iowa. Condensed from the Journal of the Indiana State Medical Association.

Despite a favorable condition during the early course of coronary thrombosis, the outlook is always in doubt. There is the possibility of extension of the infarct, or perhaps the development of a new one. Moreover, if the infarct involves the endocardium to a significant extent, mural thrombi usually develop. These often involve both the left and right ventricles and thus may be dislodged and pass to the lungs or into the greater circulation. It has been estimated that mural thrombi develop in about 50 percent of the cases, and that embolic manifestations occur in approximately 15 percent. Occasionally, the area of softening extends through the entire thickness of the wall of the left ventricle and may permit rupture and hemorrhage into the pericardial sac, resulting in death from cardiac compression. In those with extensive myocardial damage and as the result of wide-spread replacement of the muscle by fibrous tissue, the wall of the left ventricle may bulge, producing cardiac aneurysm.

It is apparent from the foregoing that left ventricular failure may be a conspicuous feature in certain instances during the early course of coronary thrombosis. This is usually manifested by periods of intense dyspnea and, if not combated promptly by energetic measures, may result in death.

Premature contractions are common during the first week to ten days. If these occur, there is the possibility of the onset of ventricular tachycardia. Occasionally auricular fibrillation occurs in paroxysms. Flutter, on the other hand, is more likely to be refractory to treatment.

The early stage, particularly the first ten days to two weeks, is the critical period of coronary thrombosis. Morphine should be given in sufficient amounts to control the pain and induce sleep. More recently the addition of atropine has been advocated in order to combat the possibility of associated spasm of the coronary vessels resulting from over activity of the vagus nerve. With the more severe and lasting pain, other measures, such as oxygen and aminophylline, should be employed. These agents contribute to the control of the pain by increasing the oxygen content and the amount of blood reaching the damaged myocardium. Moreover, one should endeavor to reduce the area of infarction to the minimum. My associates and I have demonstrated that it is possible to accomplish this in the dog with aminophylline. Consequently it has been our practice to institute the use of the drug early in the course of the disease. In some instances it is given intravenously in doses of 0.48 gm. twice daily during the first week. If plenty of time is allowed for the injection, there is seldom unfavorable reaction. After the first week, except in certain instances of left ventricular failure, this method of administration is discontinued and the drug is given by mouth in doses of grs. III, three to four times a day. In those with minimal cardiac damage the oral administration is employed from the onset. If the drug is too irritating to the gastro-intestinal tract, the enteric coated tablets are used.

After the pain has disappeared, unless there is dyspnea, a simple sedative such as phenobarbital, grs. ½, three to four times a day, is usually effective in promoting the desired relaxation and sleep. There are many individuals who would become very tired of the bed unless a sedative of this general nature is employed.

The diet should be simple in character and one calculated not to promote abdominal distention. Coffee is permissible, if desired. The fluid intake is not restricted except in the presence of cardiac failure, and then rarely below 2,000 cc. during the 24 hours.

During the first week or ten days in particular it is obvious that the patient should be spared all unnecessary physical effort. It is generally possible to regulate the bowels by simple measures, such as mineral oil and perhaps glycerin suppositories. Occasionally it may be advisable to employ a small warm water enema.

In many instances this, with the continuation of bed rest and the later management of the patient after he is allowed out of bed, constitutes the treatment. Certain complications, however, may arise. In presence of frequent premature beats, ventricular tachycardia may occur. The administration of quinidine sulfate grs. III, four to six times a day, affords the best means of eliminating the premature contractions. Ventricular tachycardia is a serious complication and, unless abolished, will ultimately terminate in death. Here again quinidine sulfate is the most effective remedy. However, large amounts are usually required and occasionally intravenous administration is necessary. When given intravenously the quinidine, usually in doses of grs. X to XX, is added to 100 cc. physiological salt solution, distilled water or glucose solution and is injected very slowly.

There seems to be considerable doubt regarding the use of digitalis. It is indicated where there is cardiac failure. If rapid action is desired, a preparation for intravenous use may be added to the solution containing aminophylline.

The duration of bed rest is determined by the circumstances. A period of four to six weeks is ordinarily advised; however, with extensive heart damage it should be longer. One should feel as certain as possible that the infarct has healed and that the maximum benefit has been derived from bed rest before the patient is allowed to be up and, particularly if he has been in bed for a long period, the legs and feet should be condition as much as possible by gentle massage.—F. R. H., M.D.

ORTHOPAEDIC SURGERY
Edited by Earl D. McBride, M.D., F.A.C.S.
605 N. W. 10th, Oklahoma City

"THREE PATIENTS SHOWING THE RESULT OF TREATMENT OF CARPAL DISLOCATION." F. A. Simmonds. Proceedings of the Royal Society of Medicine. XXXIV, 507.

The author presents three cases of anterior dislocation of the carpus, following hyperextension injury to the wrist, all three of which failed to respond to manual reduction. Symptomatology was characterized by swollen wrist, immobile fingers, and evidence of "median nerve irritation." The first case responded to skeletal traction by means of Kirschner wires through the metacarpal bases and the olecranon, and the use of the Zimmer apparatus. The dislocation was reduced by manipulation while the traction was active.

The other two cases failed to respond to this skeletal distraction method, and open reduction was necessary.

The author is also of the opinion that excision of the lunate alone gives a good result, but that removal of the scaphoid results invariably in a very poor wrist. He, therefore, feels that when excision of the scaphoid becomes necessary, the entire proximal carpal row should be removed. The latter procedure offers a prospect of a fair end result.

Compression Fractures of the Dorsolumbar vertebrae. John W. Gullikson and Edward R. Anderson. Western Journal of Surgery, Obstetrics & Gynecology, XLIX, 576, 1941.

The authors stress the importance of the "Soto-Hall" sign. This test is performed by acute flexion of the neck, and causes pain at the fracture site due to stretching of the ligamentous attachments of the vertebrae. By this test many fractures likely to be missed can be discovered.

In the treatment advocated, the patient is placed in bed and a sling is placed about him at the fracture site with a sulley arrangement and about forty to fifty pounds of overhead traction. This produces gradual hyperextension which the authors believe superior to rapid forceful methods, especially in patients with other injuries. The patient is allowed to rest in this apparatus for from four to ten days, and is then placed in a Rogers hammock frame in hyperextension. A body cast is then applied in this position, care being taken that a tight fit is secured about the pelvis. A window is cut in the abdomen to facilitate breathing. The patient is allowed up and about with the cast after two or three days. This is worn for at least two or three months, and is followed by a Taylor spinal brace for another two months, after which physiotherapy and graded exercises are started. The usual patient is able to discard his brace in from six to eight months, and is able to return to his usual work at that time.

Thirty-four cases of compression fracture were treated by this method. The average length of disability was eight and two-tenths months. There was one operation for compression symptoms of the cord to which the patient responded successfully. No development of Kummell's disease was seen in this series. Thirty-two patients were able to return to their regular work; twelve had occasional backaches, though not severe enough to cause loss of time; and sixteen were symptom-free.

Fractures of the Forearm and Elbow in Children. An Analysis of Three Hundred and Sixty-Four Consecutive Cases. Augustus Thorndike, Jr., and Charles L. Dimmler, Jr. New England Journal of Medicine, CCXXV, 475, 1941.

The author presents a valuable review of the methods of treating fractures of the forearm and elbow, and indicate that the incidence of such fractures in children under twelve years of age is high. They advise closed manipulative reduction; but if open reduction is necessary for alignment, it should be carried out within forty-eight hours. In their series, the incidence of open reduction was 1 percent in fractures of the distal forearm; none in the proximal two thirds; and 6 percent in fractures of the elbow. They discuss the well- accepted methods and position of fixation after reduction.

In fractures of the elbow, with the exception of those of the olecranon, the acute flexion position was used, with the position being maintained in the so-called "pistal holster" sling which permits ready inspection of fingers, hand, and radial pulse.

The authors condemn the indiscriminate use of open reduction, and the utilization of bone plates, screws, or other forms of advertised hardware, in treating fractures of the distal third of the forearm.—E. D. Mc., M.D.

INTERNAL MEDICINE
Edited by Hugh Jeter, M.D., F.A.C.P., A.S.C.P.
1260 North Walker, Oklahoma City

"SPECIFIC MORPHOLOGY OF CRYSTALS APPEARING IN THE URINE DURING ADMINISTRATION OF SULFANILAMIDE DERIVATIVES." By David Lehr and William Antopol. From the Laboratories of the Newark Beth Israel Hospital, Newark, N. J. American Journal of Clinical Pathology, Volume 12, Number 4, April 1942.

The authors have investigated and photographed crystals which occur in the human urine during the administration of sulfanilamide derivatives and have reviewed their findings as well as those of others representing the characteristic crystals for each derivative as follows:

Sulfapyridine crystals are described as "large jagged arrowhead-shaped," "crystals which resemble the cross section of a fairly thick convex lens with a peripheral portion of one are shorn off, as the most common form occurring singly or in spiky conglomeratoins," "whetstones" and "arrowhead's" may be present.

Sulfathiazole crystals are described as "dumbbell" or "shock of wheat" type, the dumbbell form being the most common. Occasionally they also form rosettes.

Sulfadiazine crystals are described as frequently of the "sheaves of wheat" type and in contradistinction to the acetylsulfathiazole "eccentric bindings" and "shell" forms.

Feather-like tufts or needle crystals, amber green in color were observed in a patient receiving sulfamethyl-thiazole.

Simple rectangular oblong plates with slight bulging in the long axis which tend to conglomeration and form a cross or star-like structures were found in cases taking acetylsulfaguanidine.

It has been noted that the frequency and quantity of the appearance of crystals in the urine is apparently closely related to the solubility of the sulfanilamide compounds and their acetylated derivatives.

In vitro formation of urinary crystals occurs most easily with acetylsulfadiazine and somewhat more difficulty with acetylsulfathiazole and most difficultly with acetylsulfapyridine.

A few types have been found in jaundiced patients and in others with concentrated urine which closely simulate crystals in sulfanilamide derivatives.

Interesting photomicrographs are shown.

"DIABETES YESTERDAY, TODAY AND TOMORROW."
Elliott P. Joslin. Proc. Am. Diabetes A., 1:119-37. 1941.

An accelerated tempo in treatment of the diabetic rules today as in the manufacture of munitions. We have the tools—diet and Insulin—and a beginning of treatment can usually be made at the first visit. It is good for the patient to leave the office knowing his improvement has begun, and this he recognizes at once if he takes his first dose of Insulin rather than talks about the first dose. The use of Protamine Zinc Insulin and the simple diet can be taught in half an hour and the patient realizes that he is getting results. Within a week a patient came to the office and related that at the first visit to his physician his disease was diagnosed, a diet given, and his injections begun. And besides that, he was also taught how to do a Benedict test.

What an opportunity for young doctors! Diabetes was twenty-seventh and is now eight hand almost inevitably soon to be sixth. Even if it is not the sixth cause of death, and that is quite possible because of statistical factors in reporting, at least it will rank sixth as the coincident disease. Diabetes is a disease for the doctor to follow throughout his whole medical career.

In the pituitary gland there is a hormone, not yet isolated, which injected into a dog will cause diabetes, but with each injection until the last massive dose there is a struggle for reversal of the process. There must be something like an antidiabetic hormone. Who will discover it?—H. J., M.D.

TRACHOMA CAN BE TREATED EFFECTIVELY

Acute trachoma, a contagious granular inflammation of the membrane that lines the yelids and covers the eyeball, can be treated so successfully that less than one percent of the eyes infected will become industrially blind, Harry S. Gradle, M.D., Chicago, declares in The Journal of the American Medical Association for July 4 in a report of the visual results obtained in the trachoma clinics of southern Illinois. His report lists the results from treating two groups of patients in stages one and two of the disease, 328 eyes in one group being treated with sulfanilamide and 493 eyes in the other group being treated by other means.

"From the final visual standpoint," he says, "systemic treatment with sulfanilamide is preferable to purely local treatment because: (a) twice as many eyes show definite improvement in vision and (b) less than half as many eyes show positive losses in vision."

Timely Hints on Immunization . . .

Diphtheria Toxoids Lederle
Smallpox Vaccine Lederle

COOPERATING WITH THE NATIONAL PLAN of having all children over six months of age immunized against diphtheria and smallpox, public health authorities of several states are undertaking intensive drives of their own to secure the protection of a maximum number of children from these infectious scourges of childhood.

Statistics† show that there was an increase of over 1,200 cases of diphtheria in the country in 1941 over the number reported for 1940. The median for the five preceding years was almost twice the number for 1940. Let us not lose valuable ground gained—the upward trend in the incidence of diphtheria must not continue in 1942!

The method of diphtheria immunization most generally favored at present is 2 doses of alum precipitated toxoid or 3 doses of plain toxoid. In addition, the Department of Health of New York City has adopted the plan of urging that a single supplemental dose of 1 cc. of plain toxoid be given shortly before entering school to all children who have previously been immunized during infancy.

Smallpox incidence in 1941 reached a new low,† and public health authorities and practitioners should be proud of this attainment! However, 1,363 cases of smallpox were reported in 1941. Since this is a preventable disease, it is obvious that the goal has not yet been reached.

†Pub. Health Rep. 57:23,24 (Jan. 2) 1942.

PACKAGES

"DIPHTHERIA TOXOID *Lederle*" (Plain)
1 and 10 immunizations

"DIPHTHERIA TOXOID *Lederle*" (Refined Alum Precipitated)
1, 5 and 10 immunizations

"SMALLPOX VACCINE *Lederle*" (U. S. P.)
1, 5 and 10 immunizations

"SMALLPOX VACCINE *Lederle*" (Preserved with Brilliant Green)
1, 5 and 10 immunizations

Pocket-size card, showing Lederle's Immunization Schedule and Chart of Vitamin requirements, on request.

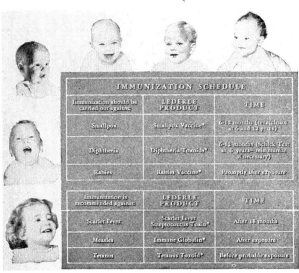

IMMUNIZATION SCHEDULE		
Immunization should be carried out against:	LEDERLE PRODUCT	TIME
Smallpox	Smallpox Vaccine*	6-12 months (revaccinate at 6 and 12 yrs.)
Diphtheria	Diphtheria Toxoids*	6-12 months (Schick Test at 6 years—reimmunize if necessary)
Rabies	Rabies Vaccine*	Promptly after exposure
Immunization is recommended against	LEDERLE PRODUCT	TIME
Scarlet Fever	Scarlet Fever Streptococcic Toxin*	After 18 months
Measles	Immune Globulin*	After exposure
Tetanus	Tetanus Toxoid*	Before probable exposure

Accepted by Council on Pharmacy and Chemistry of the American Medical Association.

Specify *Lederle*

OFFICERS OF COUNTY SOCIETIES, 1942

COUNTY	PRESIDENT	SECRETARY	MEETING TIME
Alfalfa	Jack F. Parsons, Cherokee	L. T. Lancaster, Cherokee	Last Tues. Each 2nd Mo.
Atoka-Coal	J. B. Clark, Coalgate	J. S. Fulton, Atoka	
Beckham	H. K. Speed, Sayre	E. S. Kilpatrick, Elk City	Second Tues. eve.
Blaine	Virginia Olson Curtin, Watonga	W. F. Griffin, Watonga	
Bryan	A. J. Wells, Calera	W. K. Haynie, Durant	Second Tues. eve.
Caddo	Fred L. Patterson, Carnegie	C. B. Sullivan, Carnegie	
Canadian	P. F. Herod, El Reno	A. L. Johnson, El Reno	Subject to call
Carter	Walter Hardy, Ardmore	H. A. Higgins, Ardmore	
Cherokee	Park H. Medearis, Tahlequah	Isadore Dyer, Tahlequah	
Choctaw	C. H. Hale, Boswell	Fred D. Switzer, Hugo	
Cleveland	F. C. Buffington, Norman	Phil Haddock, Norman	Thursday nights
Comanche	George S. Barber, Lawton	W. F. Lewis, Lawton	
Cotton	George W. Baker, Walters	Mollie F. Seism, Walters	Third Friday
Craig	W. R. Marks, Vinita	J. M. McMillan, Vinita	
Creek	Frank Sisler, Bristow	O. H. Cowart, Bristow	
Custer	Richard M. Burke, Clinton	W. C. Tisdal, Clinton	Third Thursday
Garfield	D. S. Harris, Drummond	John R. Walker, Enid	Fourth Thursday
Garvin	T. F. Gross, Lindsay	John R. Callaway, Pauls Valley	Wed before 3rd Thurs.
Grady	D. S. Downey, Chickasha	Frank T. Joyce, Chickasha	3rd Thursday
Grant	I. V. Hardy, Medford	E. E. Lawson, Medford	
Greer	G. F. Border, Mangum	J. B. Hollis, Mangum	
Harmon	S. W. Hopkins, Hollis	W. M. Yeargan, Hollis	First Wednesday
Haskell	William Carson, Keota	N. K. Williams, McCurtain	
Hughes	Wm. L. Taylor, Holdenville	Imogene Mayfield, Holdenville	First Friday
Jackson	J. M. Allgood, Altus	Willard D. Holt, Altus	Last Monday
Jefferson	W. M. Browning, Waurika	J. I. Hollingsworth, Waurika	Second Monday
Kay	J. C. Wagner, Ponca City	J. Holland Howe, Ponca City	Third Thurs.
Kingfisher	C. M. Hodgson, Kingfisher	John R. Taylor, Kingfisher	
Kiowa	J. M. Bonham, Hobart	B. H. Watkins, Hobart	
LeFlore	G. R. Booth, LeFlore	Rush L. Wright, Poteau	
Lincoln	E. F. Hurlbut, Meeker	C. W. Robertson, Chandler	First Wednesday
Logan	William C. Miller, Guthrie	J. L. LeHew, Jr., Guthrie	Last Tuesday evening
Marshall	J. L. Holland, Madill	O. A. Cook, Madill	
Mayes	L. C. White, Adair	V. D. Herrington, Pryor	
McClain	B. W. Slover, Blanchard	R. L. Royster, Purcell	
McCurtain	R. D. Williams, Idabel	R. H. Sherrill, Broken Bow	Fourth Tues. eve.
McIntosh	F. R. First, Checotah	William A. Tolleson, Eufaula	Second Tuesday
Murray	P. V. Annadown, Sulphur	F. E. Sadler, Sulphur	
Muskogee	Shade D. Neely, Muskogee	J. T. McInnis, Muskogee	First & Third Mon.
Noble	J. W. Francis, Perry	C. H. Cooke, Perry	
Okfuskee	J. M. Pemberton, Okemah	L. J. Spickard, Okemah	Second Monday
Oklahoma	R. Q. Goodwin, Okla. City	Wm. E. Eastland, Okla. City	Fourth Tuesday
Okmulgee	J. G. Edwards, Okmulgee	John R. Cotteral, Henryetta	Second Monday
Osage	C. R. Weirich, Pawhuska	George K. Hemphill, Pawhuska	Second Monday
Ottawa	J. B. Hampton, Commerce	Walter Sanger, Picher	Third Thursday
Pawnee	E. T. Robinson, Cleveland	Robert L. Browning, Pawnee	
Payne	John W. Martin, Cushing	James D. Martin, Cushing	Third Thursday
Pittsburg	Austin R. Stough, McAlester	Edw. D. Greenberger, McAlester	Third Friday
Pontotoc	R. E. Cowling, Ada	E. R. Muntz, Ada	First Wednesday
Pottawatomie	John Carson, Shawnee	Clinton Gallaher, Shawnee	First & Third Sat.
Pushmataha	P. B. Rice, Antlers	John S. Lawson, Clayton	
Rogers	W. A. Howard, Chelsea	George D. Waller, Claremore	First Monday
Seminole	H. M. Reeder, Konawa	Mack I. Shanheltz, Wewoka	
Stephens	A. J. Weedn, Duncan	W. K. Walker, Marlow	
Texas	L. G. Blackmer, Hooker	Johnny A. Blue, Guymon	
Tillman	C. C. Allen, Frederick	O. G. Bacon, Frederick	
Tulsa	H. B. Stewart, Tulsa	E. O. Johnson, Tulsa	Second & Fourth Mon. eve.
Wagoner	J. H. Plunkett, Wagoner	H. K. Riddle, Coweta	
Washington-Nowata	R. W. Rucker, Bartlesville	J. V. Athey, Bartlesville	Second Wednesday
Washita	A. S. Neal, Cordell	James F. McMurry, Sentinel	
Woods	W. F. LaFon, Wavnoka	O. E. Templin, Alva	Last Wednesday
Woodward	M. H. Newman, Shattuck	C. W. Tedrowe, Woodward	

THE JOURNAL
OF THE
OKLAHOMA STATE MEDICAL ASSOCIATION

| VOLUME XXXV | OKLAHOMA CITY, OKLAHOMA, SEPTEMBER, 1942 | NUMBER 9 |

Complications Following the Use of Sodium Diphenylhydantoinate (Dilantin) Therapy[*]

TITUS H. HARRIS, M.D. AND
JACK R. EWALT, M.D.

GALVESTON, TEXAS

A. Introduction.

Sodium Diphenylhydantoinate or Dilantin Sodium is the most effective anticonvulsant yet discovered by science. This preparation was developed by Houston Merritt and Tracy Putnam after a long series of animal (cats) experiments[1-2] in which they tested approximately 80 drugs for the property of raising the convulsive threshold to electrical stimulation. The drugs tested were phenyl derivatives, the experiments with this series apparently being prompted by the fact that phenobarbital is the most effective anticonvulsant of the barbituric acid derivatives now in use. Merritt & Putnam found ten of these compounds which effectively raised the threshold to convulsions in cats. Five compounds not previously considered ananticonvulsants were discovered to have a more profound anticonvulsant action than bromides or phenobarbital and further testing revealed that these preparations produced no sedative action, thus avoiding the drowsiness and lethargy which accompany the use of either phenobrabital or the bromide preparations.

Further experimentation revealed that of the five new preparations, sodium diphenylhydantoinate is most effective in raising the convulsive threshold to electric stimuli. The toxic reactions in animals were found to be minimal and transitory and the compound was then administered to the first of a series of 200 patients who suffered from one of the convulsive disorders. The first reports on the use of the drug in treating human patients was made one year after the series was started. In this paper they described complications referable to the nervous system, the gastro-intestinal system, and the skin. They caution against indescriminate

*Read before the Section on Neurology, Psychiatry and Endocrinology, Annual Session, Oklahoma State Medical Association, April 24, 1942.

use of the drug and state that it should be used only in cases who are not effectively treated with phenobarbital and they further note that it may be used only in patients who are under close medical supervision. These two statements have been to frequently disregarded by enthusiastic clinicians anxious to "use the new drug".

With more prolonged experience Merritt & Putnam report[4] that 60 percent of patients with grand mal attacks, 62 percent with psychic equivalent states and 39 percent with petit mal attacks are completely relieved of their malady as long as they stay on the medication. In addition to this number a respectable percentage of patients may be called improved. These results have been verified by numerous investigators.

This drug has one major disadvantage—it is toxic for some individuals and because of this requires rather careful supervision by the physician. The successful use of this drug requires some knowledge of the complications to be expected and the method of controlling them.

B. Toxic reactions.

The presence of toxic features were mentioned by Merritt & Putnam[3] in their original report on the use of the preparations in treating convulsive disorders in humans. In later[4-5] papers they discuss them more fully.

The complications are of many types and an occasional patient may show symptoms in more than one physiologic segment. For clarity in discussion the complications and their management will be discussed under the various bodily systems following in general the outline of Merritt & Putnam.[5]

I. Gastro-intestinal symptoms.

Dilantin sodium is a strongly alkaline preparation and the gastric distress is thought to be due to the ingestion of this preparation on an empty stomach. The symptoms consist of a feeling of nausea, some epigastric distress and in severe instances of vomiting after the medication is taken. The attacks are transitory but tend to recur with repeated dosage. The complication is avoided if the preparation is taken with food, either just before, during or just after eating. It is reported[5] that the simultaneous administration of dilute hydrochloric acid also prevents this complication. We will later discuss one instance in which severe gastrointestinal pathology resulted from the medication, the pathology consisting of a hemorrhagic enteritis and gastritis complicating a severe reaction in the skin.

II. Symptoms referable to the central nervous system.

Toxic reactions to dilantin with central nervous system manifestations were among the earliest[3] complications noted. They were at first thought to be due to overdosage but they do occur in adult patients who are taking the usual minimal dose, and are perhaps a manifestation of limited tolerance in that particular person. The occurrence of these toxic manifestations is not associated with any particular type or severity of epilepsy and is not any more prevalent in those individuals suffering from pathology of the central nervous system other than the epilepsy.

The symptoms are usually mild and transitory in type. They most often consist of tremors, ataxia, diplopia, vertigo and severe headaches. The symptoms are unpleasant but do not particularly incapacitate the patient and disappear promptly on withdrawal of the drug. In most persons they will recur if the previous dose is again prescribed and maintained for any prolonged period of time. This type of reaction is illustrated by the following case: E. D., age 19. There was a history of very mild petit mal attacks for the previous 18 months. Neurological study showed no cause for the convulsive attacks. Electroencephalogram showed typical changes, seen in petit mal conditions. She was placed on Dilantin, grs. 1½ four times daily in January, 1941. The spells were relieved completely. In May, 1941, she began to lose her appetite, in June seemed forgetful, became irritable, started vomiting, and then began experiencing double vision and ataxia. Examination in July, 1941, showed the patient to be extremely emaciated with a mild degree of hypertrophy of the gums, generalized muscular incoordination, horizontal nystagmus which was very pronounced. Mentally she was cheerful and cooperative, and manifested no behavior disturbance or change in sensorium. Dilantin was omitted, the vomiting ceased immediately, and the

symptoms entirely disappeared within ten days.

In more severe reactions the patient may show a marked confusion, a motor agitation and symptoms typical of an acute psychotic episode. These cases also improve upon withdrawal of the drug and may be regarded and treated as any other toxic reaction to medication. A reaction of this sort was shown by H. F., age 10. The patient had been having petit mal attacks about a year and a half. Usual neurological and laboratory investigations revealed no causative factor. Encephalogram showed nothing unusual. She left the hospital taking Dilantin grs. 1½ three times daily. She was free of seizures for the next ten months and then had an occasional seizure for the next several months. Dilantin was increased to grs. 1½ five times daily. Three weeks later she began to show unsteadiness in walking which progressed to a marked ataxia. Pronounced dysarthria and silly behavior were present, as well as dulling of the intellectual function. Examination showed considerable hypertrophy of the gums, very broad based ataxic gait, generalized muscular incoordination, dysarthric speech, nystagmus in all directions, with considerable clouding of the sensorium. The Dilantin was discontinued and she was placed on Phenobarbital, grs. 1½ twice daily. Her symptoms cleared up in two weeks, and there have been no more of the convulsive attacks.

Another syndrome is ataxia, aphasia, focal neurological signs, and confusion. In some instances the clinical picture resembles a brain tumor, but shows improvement upon withdrawal of the offending drug. An interesting case of this sort was seen in consultation by one of us. The patient was a 31 year old white male when he came to the Out Clinic first in March, 1941. At that time he complained of both petit mal and grand mal seizures. The usual routine laboratory tests, including blood count, uranalysis, blood serology and glucose tolerance tests, were negative. His physical and neurologic examinations at this time were also negative. On May 6, 1941, he was placed on phenobarbital, grains 1½, b.i.d., with dilantin, grains 1½, once daily. On June 3, 1941, his medication was changed to phenobarbital, grains 1½, b.i.d., and dilantin, grains 1½, b.i.d.

On September 16, 1941, he complained of some difficulty in his work which required considerable mentation and it was very apparent that he was suffering from an acute toxic, or organic, psychosis. He described visual and auditory hallucinations, as well as a great many "dream-like, nightmare-like sensations". His sensorium was grossly disturbed, and the question of brain tumor was raised. He was referred to one of us for an E.E.G. which gave evidence of idopathic epilepsy, poorly controlled by medication.

Repeated neurological examinations at this time revealed uniformly exaggerated deep reflexes throughout and a positive Babinski sign on the left. An air encephalogram was done with the following report: "Questionable slight displacement of inter-ventricular septum to the left. Right lateral ventricle shows less air filling than left. Appearance of cortical pathways practically is the same bilaterally." The E.E.G. was repeated but still gave no evidence of a tumor but was still typical of epilepsy. In spite of this on October 17, 1941, a craniotomy exploring the right frontal lobe was done and no gross or microscopic evidence of tumor was found.

He returned to the hospital on two or three occasions during November and December and seemed decidedly improved, returning to his work in the later part of December, but he still complained of some mental sluggishness with regard to his work.

The unusual feature in the above case is the small dose upon which the toxic symptoms developed, and the presence of what appeared to be a brain tumor with some signs pointing to localization of the pathology. Blair reports an analogous case in which a patient developed a hemiplegia from Dilantin 1½ grains t.i.d. The hemiplegia cleared completely and promptly upon withdrawal of the drug.

Levitt and Blonstein[6] report the case of a 27 year old male who developed a toxic amblyopia after taking dilantin sodium in a dose of 1½ grains t.i.d for four months. This patient's vision failed rapidly until he had 20/200 vision in the left eye and light preception only in the right. The vision returned to normal upon withdrawal of the drug.

On the other hand recovery has occurred after the suicidal ingestion of 67½ grains (45 capsules).[7] The symptoms in this case were drowsiness, dizziness, trembling, and unconsciousness. The patient was treated with stimulants, recovered within a few hours and was able to resume his normal activity in four days. Aring and Rosenbaum[8] report the case of a young man who took the drug for the "lift" he got from it, using it as a substitute for whiskey. On various occasions he took doses of 60 to 105 grains. Following a period of confusion he would develop nausea, vomiting, vertigo and nystagmus.

Gruber[9] and his co-workers in a series of animal experiments found the lethal dose to be three to four times the toxic dose under the conditions of their experiment. The animals receiving lethal doses had seizures and "died of central nervous system depression". It is interesting to note that Williamson[14] also noted that the idiots and imbeciles tolerate the drug less well than the feeble minded of comparatively greater intellectual development: He reports three deaths due to status epilepticus in this group of defective children. Blair[15] also reported an increased frequency of seizures in certain patients receiving sodium diphenylhydantoinate but his patients were adults of presumably normal intelligence. In these cases an increase in the dosage of the drug produced an increased frequency of seizures while a decrease in dosage brought about a reduction in the number of convulsions.

Finkelman and Arieff[16] have reported four cases showing a rather severe encephalopathy and confused paranoid irritable states in six individuals. They also report two children who developed temper tantrums while on the drug and two patients who developed a satus epilepticus while being treated with dilantin.

III. Complications involving the skin.

Cutaneous manifestations are among the most common toxic signs. About 5 percent of patients on this medication will at some time develop dermatologic pathology. The lesions usually develop within seven to 15 days but may occur at any stage of the administration of the drug. These cutaneous conditions are usually of mild generalized erythematous type similar to any drug intoxication and they subside spontaneously either with or without withdrawal of the drug. An occasional case will develop small hemorrhagic lesions of the skin and cases of severe exfoliation dermatitis with a generalized systemic reaction are reported. In these severe complications the drug should be withdrawn immediately. Withdrawal of the drug and general supportive measures are sufficient to bring about improvement and recovery from the complication. The lesions tend to reappear if the drug is again exhibited and in patients who develop the severe skin reactions the drug should be permanently discontinued. There are a few female patients who complain of an increased hair growth about the face and over the extremities. Such reactions are infrequent and in our experience very mild.

A severe cutaneous reaction of hemorrhagic erythema multiformi which resulted in death occurred on our service.

The patient was a 35 year old divorced white female waitress who had been under the care of the John Sealy Clinic for 10 years, for complaints of abortion, fracture, syphilis, salpingitis and seizures. During this time she received some treatment for syphilis but her attendance at clinic was irregular. The first convulsion occurred on November 8, 1937, at which time she was 31 years of age. At this time laboratory and neurologic studies including an air encephalogram revealed no cause for the seizure although it was felt the tertiary syphilis might have been contributory. No anticonvulsant was administered as the seizures were mild and infrequent at that time. On January 26, 1938, patient was started on phenobarbital grain 1½ daily which was increased to grains 1½ t.i.d. on April 4, 1938.

Dilantin sodium grains 1½ t.i.d., was prescribed on September 15, 1941 because she was having seizures with increasing frequency. She was next seen on September 29th at which time she entered complaining of vomiting, a sore mouth and a skin rash. She stated that after taking the drug for one week she had developed a pain in her leg and had increased the dose to 3 grains t.i.d. on her own initiative thinking it would relieve the pain. On the second day of this dose she began to have nausea, the skin rash appeared and her mouth became sore. She continued to take the drug however until the time of her admission.

Upon admission she was confused and lethargic, but cooperative. There were generalized hemorrhagic lesions of the skin subsequently diagnosed as hemorrhagic erythema multiformi. She had a temperature of 103.4°F. Her lips were red, swollen, sore and fissured. The gums were swollen and oosing blood. Her pharynx was acutely inflamed. She had a rather severe conjunctivitis. Vomiting occurred periodically, and the emesis was streaked with blood. (slide)

Laboratory studies revealed a positive Wassermann & Eagle, CO_2 combining power of blood 37.2 and 40, Platelets 175,000-200,-000. There was a moderate concentration of the blood. The drug was withdrawn and she was treated with fluids, glucose and sodium thiosulfate. The skin lesions improved and the temperature fell to 101° but subsequently returned to 102°. The conjuctivitis and sore mouth persisted. The confusion became more marked and she was semicomotose just preceeding her death. Post mortem report as follows:

Skin: Hemorrhagic dermatitis.

Respiratory: Hypostatic congestion.
 Pleural adhesions.

Gastro-Intestinal: Gingivitis.
 Stomatitis.
 Hemorrhagic gastritis.
 Hemorrhagic enteritis.
 Old appendectomy.

C.N.S.: Softening of right temporal lobe.

G. U.: Old panhysterectomy.

IV. Complications manifest in the mouth.

The most common toxic reaction to dilantin therapy is a reaction of the gums. This reaction may vary from a slight reddening of the dental margin to a marked hyperplasia of the membranes. Some type of gum reaction is seen in 20-30 percent of persons taking dilantin but five percent or less show reactions severe enough to warrant termination of treatment. The cause of this symptom, found only in cases receiving dilantin, is not known. Kimball reported a deficiency of Vitamin C in these patients but a more careful survey by Merritt & Foster[10] revealed this to be an erroneous observation.

Robinson[11] has classified the changes in the gums into five groups according to the severity of the reaction.

1. The gums are reddened at the dental margin but are not raised and do not bleed. This is the type of gum reaction seen in the majority of patients and treatment may be continued but observation should be frequent and the case closely followed.

2. Elevation of the tissue between adjacent teeth. This condition is painless and is not accompanied by bleeding. If patients have this complication and can be maintained on phenobarbital the dilantin should be discontinued. In cases uncontrolled by other measures the drug may be cautiously continued in the face of this pathology.

3. In this type of complication the area along the dental margin is raised. There is no bleeding and no pain. It is our belief that the medication should be withdrawn if this condition develops as a continuation of the drug usually produces one of the more severe stages.

4. Fungating, generalized overgrowth of the gums. The hypertrophied tissues may bleed but the condition is not painful and may go unnoticed by children.

5. An extensive overgrowth of the gums covering the anterior and posterior surface of the teeth. In this stage the teeth may be buried and chewing becomes a painful process. The tissues may bleed upon touch or where bitten by the underlying teeth.

The severe oral complications listed under 3, 4 and 5 are indications for prompt withdrawal of the drug. In most instances the gums return to normal with no treatment other than ceasation of the drug although one case is reported[11] in which the tissue remained after the drug was discontinued. The overgrowth tends to recur if the patient is again placed on dilantin therapy, and in individuals exhibiting severe reactions of the gums, the drug should be permanently discontinued. Progynon-B, Ascorbic acid, plastic operations and other measures suggested for this condition have proven ineffectual.

V. Complications of the Hemopietic System.

These complications are infrequent. In some persons a slight leucocytosis occurs and eosinophillia is often encountered. Aring[8] reports the development of an agranulocytic angina in a child who was in status epilepticus and who had ingested a total of 149¼ grains of dilantin sodium in a period of 67 days. Recovery was prompt upon withdrawal of the drug. In general it may be said that this type of complication is infrequent and inconsequental in the management of the epilepsies. Treatment is complete withdrawal of the drugs.

VI. Complications of the genito-urinary system.

Complications in this system are almost unknown. A few patients complain of an increase in libido. This may be an action of the drug or it may represent a reaction to the release from sedatives such a phenobarbital or the bromides which most of these patients had taken prior to institution of dilantin therapy. Williamson[14] mentions that two of his patients developed hematoporphyrinuria while on this medication and several authors noted albuminuria and a supression of urine in patients who were taking this drug. The findings are of course manifestations of general toxicity and not specific for dilantin.

VII. Cardiovascular complications.

These have been absent in our experience. Arieff in discussing a paper[12] on the use of this drug mentioned precordial distress and E.C.G. evidence of myocardial change in some of his cases.

Finkelman & Arieff[16] have reported a careful study of 27 patients with serial electrocardiograms before, during and after dilantin medication. Twenty-five of their patients showed some definite E.C.G. change. Fifty percent showed a prolonged P.R. interval and 78 percent showed a decreased amplitude in T-wave. In every instance discontinuation of the drug caused the E.C.G. pattern to return to the pre-treatment pattern for the particular patient. Williamson[14] also noted a slowing of the pulse rate in some of his patients while they were receiving this medication. This work should be investigated more extensively but in our experience cardiac complications have not been a significant factor in the management of patients with epilepsy.

VIII. Complications of the Respiratory System.

Complications of the respiratory organs appear to be rare. Frost[17] mentioned epistaxis as a complication to dilantin therapy but it has been generally observed.

Dickerson[12] reports a death in a child three years of age who had received dilantin 1½ t.i.d. for one month before the onset of toxic symptoms. The post mortem examination revealed a severe ulcerative, desquamative bronchitis, and bronchopneumonia. Other authors have reported deaths due to bronchopneumonia in patients receiving diphenylhydantoinate sodium but the role of the medication in the production of the pneumonic infection is uncertain.

C. Avoidance and Detection of Toxic Symptoms.

The milder toxic manifestations are so common that they can not be entirely avoided if the drug is to be used at all. Many persons develop these toxic symptoms on the usual therapeutic dose and the complications arise as a result of a poor tolerance for the drug or perhaps a hypersensitivity to some factor in the preparation. The reason for these severe reactions in some persons while others tolerate huge doses is not known and the selection of a particular body segment for development of the pathology is likewise unclear. It is not beyond the realm of expectation to assume that further experimentation with related synthetic products may reveal equally effective compounds with fewer toxic properties.

At present the drug may be used under the conditions originally outlined by Merritt & Putnam. That is the patient must be carefully supervised while receiving treatment with dilantin sodium. Almost all complications will quickly subside if treatment is discontinued immediately upon development of toxic signs. Patients placed on this anticonvulsant should be instructed to report to the physician immediately upon the development of any unusual or untoward reactions.

Some writers have mentioned prodromal signs of toxicity but these signs have not been found in enough patients to be of more than suggestive value in the management of these cases. McCarter and Carson[18] report that some of their patients developed twitching of the facial muscles for several days prior to the onset of the more severe signs of central nervous system complications. Finkelman and Arieff[16] believe "A loss of weight . . . was an indication of the development of toxic symptoms leading to an encephalopathy." In our experience a mild hyperplasia of the gums and a mild erythematous dermatitis are the most frequent early signs of toxicity.

D. Use of Diphenylhydantoinate Sodium.

Diphenylhydantoinate sodium should be reserved for use as an anticonvulsant medication in those patients who continue to have attacks in spite of heavy dosage with phenobarbital. These patients must be under strict medical supervision throughout the period of medication with this preparation. Patients who are adequately controlled with pheno-barbital should not be placed on the newer preparation as phenobarbital therapy is safer, produces few complications and requires less frequent check-ups of the patient. When dilantin is to be used the initial dose in adults is 1½ grains t.i.d. and ½ grain t.i.d. in small children. In all cases the minimal effective dose is the one of choice. The dosage is regulated by increasing by one dose daily until an effective level is reached, but patients who continue to have seizures on a daily dose of nine grains will probably not be benefited by this preparation and larger doses are prone to produce the early signs of central nervous system complications. All medication should be given with meals to prevent the development of nausea.

Caution is needed in changing patients from the bromides or phenobarbital to dilantin therapy or the reverse. In the absence of complications necessitating the prompt withdrawal of the medication, the replacing drug should be substituted one dose per day until the patient is taking only the newer drug. If the patient notes an increase in the frequency of seizures upon taking dilantin the drug should be promptly withdrawn, and phenobarbital again substituted because some of the above reports would at least suggest that this drug may percipitate a status epilepticus in certain individuals.

Certain persons suffering from sever epilepsy fail to respond satisfactorily to either phenobarbital, the bromides or sodium diphenylhydantoinate. The typical case of this type will show a decrease in the incidence of attacks on any of the preparations, but in spite of the improvement will be unable to continue in school or at work because of recurring seizures. Many of these patients may be almost or entirely protected from further attacks by using a combination of phenobarbital and diphenylhdantoinate sodium. Robinson and Osgood[19], Cohen and Showstack[20] and others report favorable results from a combination of the two drugs. Robinson and Osgood[19] noted that patients who responded to dilantin-phenobarbital therapy did so on relatively small doses and the increase in the size of the dose had little added effect on the patients who were refactory to the smaller amounts of drug. The reported experience of these workers coincides closely with our use of the combination of the two anticonvulsants. Cohen and Showstack[20] recommend the use of benzedrine in those patients who show signs of undue lethargy from the phenobarbital and also in those patients showing mild complications to the dilantin. In patients who are to receive the combined therapy the usual initial dose is phenobarbital grains 1 twice daily and sodium diphenylhydantoinate

grains 1½ twice daily. If this proves insufficient each drug should be increased by one dose daily until the seizures are controlled or to a maximum of dilantin grains nine daily and phenobarbital grains nine daily. In our experience almost all patients can be greatly benefited if not entirely controlled by this routine. If this dose proves ineffective larger doses will probably be of no further benefit. Patients on this combined routine of dosage are subject to all the complications of dilantin therapy outlined above and close supervision must be observed if serious reactions are to be avoided.

E. Summary.

Sodium diphenylhydantoinate is the most potent anticonvulsant medication now in use. It may produce toxic manifestations in certain susceptable persons and therefore requires careful medical supervision. Because of this toxic property its use should be reserved for those patients who cannot be controlled by phenobarbital medication. In patients who have convulsions in spite of either phenobarbital or dilantin therapy, a combination of the two drugs in smaller dosage is often effective. The complications first appear in a mild form and their detection and their management has been presented.

BIBLIOGRAPHY

1. Putnam, T. J. and Merritt, H. H.: Experimental Determination of the Anticonvulsant Properties of Some Phenyl Derivatives. Science, 85-525, 1937.
2. Merritt, H. H. and Putnam, T. J.: A New Series of Anticonvulsant Drugs Tested by Experiments on Animals. Arch. Neurol. & Psych. 39:1003, 1938.
3. Merritt, H. H. and Putnam, T. J: Sodium Diphenyl Hydantoinate in the Treatment of Convulsive Disorders. J.A. M.A. 111:1068, 1938.
4. Merritt, H H and Putnam, T. J.: Further Experience with Use of Sodium Diphenyl Hydantoinate in Treatment of Convulsive Disorders Am. Jour. Psychiat. 96.1023, 1940.
5. Merritt, H. H. and Putnam, T. J.: Sodium Diphenyl Hydantoinate in Treatment of Convulsive Seizures; Toxic Symptoms and Their Prevention. Arch. Neurol. and Psychiat. 42: 1053, 1939.
6. Levitt, J. M. and Blonstein, M.: Toxic Amblyopia Resulting from Sodium Diphenyl Hydantoinate. New York State Med. Journ. 40: 1538, 1940.
7. Robinson, L. J. Poisoning from Dilantin, with Recovery. J A M.A. 115:289, 1940.
8. Aring, C. D. and Rosenbaum, M.: Ingestion of Large Doses of Dilantin Sodium. Arch. Neurol & Psych. 43.265, 1941.
9. Gruber, C. M.; Haury, V. G and Drake, M. D.: The Toxic Action of Dilantin Sodium when Injected into Experimental Animals. J. Pharm. and Exper. Therap. 68.433, 1940.
10. Merritt, H. H. and Foster, A.: Vitamin C in Epilepsy, Dilantin Sodium Not a Cause of Vitamin C Deficiency. Am. J. Med Sc. 200:541, 1940
11 Robinson, Leon J Gingival Changes Produced by Dilantin Sodium. Diseases of the Nervous System. 3:88, March 1942
12 Dickerson, W. W.: Present Status of Dilantin Therapy. Am. Jour. Psychiat. 98:515, Jan. 1942
13 Blair, D.: Hemiplegia Complicating Sodium Diphenyl Hydantoinate Therapy in Epilepsy, Lancet, 1:269, 1940.
14. Williamson, J.: Severe Toxic Effects of Sodium Diphenyl Hydantoinate in Mentally Defective Epileptics. Journ. Ment. Science. 86:981, 1940.
15. Blair, D.: The Modern Treatment of Epilepsy. J. Ment. Science. 86:888, 1940
16. Finkelman, Isidore and Arieff, A. J.: Untoward Effects of Phenytoin Sodium in Epilepsy. J.A.M.A. 118:1209, April 4, 1942.
17. Frost: I, Sodium Diphenyl Hydantoinate in the Treatment of Severe Cases of Epilepsy. Journ. Ment. Science. 85: 956, 1939.
18. McCarter, W. and Carson, J.: The Uses of Diphenyl-hydantoinate. J. Ment Science. 85:965, 1939.
19. Robinson, L. J. and Osgood, R.: Comparative Effects of Phenobarbital and Dilantin Sodium in Treatment of Epilepsy. J.A M.A. 114:1334, 1940.
20. Cohen, B. and Showstack, and Myerson, A.: Synergism of Phenobarbital, Dilantin Sodium, and Other Drugs in Treatment of Institutional Epilepsy. J.A M.A. 114:484, 1940.

Typhoid Fever[*]

JOHN Y. BATTENFIELD, M.D.,
EPIDEMIOLOGIST
Oklahoma State Health Department
OKLAHOMA CITY, OKLAHOMA

In his classic of logical deduction William Budd, in 1873, stated that: "In connection with typhoid fever there are few things which concern the people of this country more deeply than to know the exact truth touching the mode in which this fatal fever is disseminated amongst them. Even in the highest class of society the introduction of this fever into the household is an event that generally long stands prominently out in the record of family afflictions. If this be true of the mansions of the rich, who have every means of alleviation which wealth can command, how much more true must it be of the cottages of the poor, which have scant provision even for the necessaries of life, and none for its great emergencies. Here, when fever once enters, then sorrow follows, and contagion is not slow to add its peculiar bitterness to the trial.

"How often have I seen in past days, in the single narrow chamber of the day laborer's cottage, the father in the coffin, the mother in the sick bed in muttering delirium, and nothing to relieve the desolation of the children but the devotion of some poor neighbor, who in too many cases paid the penalty of her kindness in becoming, herself, a victim of the same disorder."

"In its ordinary course, human life has few such consummations of misery as this."

Typhoid fever was confused for centuries with other continued fevers, such as recurrent fever, septic infections and typhus fever. Louis, the distinguished French clinician, in 1829, gave the name typhoid fever to the malady to distinguish it from typhus fever. Eberth, in 1880, saw the bacillus typhosus in the tissues, and four years later Gaffky grew it in pure culture. In 1894, Wright, Pfeiffer and Kolle began typhoid inoculations, but it took something over ten years to establish the prophylactic value of typhoid vaccines.

It is indeed fortunate that typhoid fever has practically disappeared from our larger cities.

Table I shows the degree of typhoid decline from the period 1910 to 1939, inclusive, for 78 cities of the United States:

TABLE I.

TOTAL TYPHOID RATE FOR 78 CITIES
1910-1939[†]

Year	Population	Typhoid Deaths	Typhoid Death Rate per 100,000
1910	22,573,435	4,637	20.54
1911	23,211,341	3,950	17.02
1912	23,835,399	3,132	13.14
1913	24,457,989	3,285	13.43
1914	25,091,112	2,781	11.08
1915	25,713,346	2,434	9.47
1916	26,257,550	2,191	8.34
1917	26,865,408	2,016	7.50
1918	27,086,696*	1,824*	6.73
1919	27,735,083*	1,151*	4.15
1920	28,244,878	1,088	3.85
1921	28,859,062	1,141	3.95
1922	29,473,246	963	3.26
1923	30,087,430	950	3.16
1924	30,701,614	943	3.07
1925	31,315,598	1,079	3.44
1926	31,929,782	907	2.84
1927	32,543,966	648	1.99
1928	33,158,150	628	1.89
1929	33,772,334	537	1.59
1930	34,386,717	554	1.61
1931	35,137,915	563	1.60
1932	35,691,815	442	1.24
1933	35,691,815	423	1.18
1934	35,401,715	413	1.17
1935	35,401,715	348	1.03
1936	36,216,404	336	0.96
1937	36,771,787	280	0.82
1938	36,972,985	248	0.74
1939	37,112,665	239	0.67

*Data for Fort Worth lacking

†The following 15 cities are omitted from this table because data for the full period are not available: Canton, Chattanooga, Dallas, Fort Wayne, Jacksonville, Knoxville, Long Beach, Miami, Oklahoma City, South Bend, Tampa, Tulsa, Utica, Wichita and Wilmington

Table II shows the total typhoid death rate per 100,000 of population for 93 cities according to geographic divisions:

[*]Read before the Section on General Medicine, Annual Session, Oklahoma State Medical Association, May 20, 1941.

TABLE II.

TOTAL TYPHOID DEATH RATE PER 100,000 OF POPULATION FOR 93 CITIES ACCORDING TO GEOGRAPHIC DIVISIONS

| | | Typhoid Deaths | | Typhoid Death Rates | | | | |
| | | | | | | | 1931-1935 | 1926-1930 |
	Population	1939	1938	1939	1938	1937	1935	1930
New England	2,657,824	6	12	0.23	0.45	0.45	0.70	1.31
Middle Atlantic	13,602,500	51	59	0.37	0.44	0.51	0.80	1.40
South Atlantic	2,622,237	27	46	1.03	1.74	1.96	2.70	4.50
East north-central	9,883,376	44	35	0.44	0.35	0.62	0.75	1.29*
East south-central	1,364,025	33	32	2.42	2.36	2.10	4.81	8.31
West north-central	2,809,679	14	11	0.50	0.40	0.76	1.24	1.83
West south-central	2,138,496	68	74	3.19	3.52	2.34	5.36	7.32†
Mountain & Pacific	4,276,412	22	22	0.51	0.52	0.68	0.88	1.80

*Data for South Bend for 1925-1929 are not available.
†Lacks data for Oklahoma City in 1926.

The west south-central group, which includes Oklahoma, shows a reduction in the death rate from 7.32 to 3.19. The causes of this improvement are the general cleanliness of water supplies, better milk supplies, more general use of pasteurization, typhoid preventive inoculations, the diffusion of information among the public concerning personal prophylaxis, the elimination of the great typhoid epidemic foci, and better public health administration, and the raising of the standard of general hygenic and sanitary measures.

Typhoid is not a vanishing disease. In 1939 there were 2,001 deaths in the United States from typhoid fever. Since the case fatality rate averages ten percent, there were approximately 20,010 needless cases of typhoid fever in the United States.

Typhoid fever is an acute, specific generalized infection due to the bacillus typhosus and characterized by a continued fever lasting about four weeks, a rose-colored eruption and diarrhea. The disease varies greatly in severity ranging from "walking typhoid," so mild that it may escape diagnosis to fatal infections. The symptoms are also quite inconstant. The lesions affect especially the lymphatic system, spleen and bone marrow. The lymph nodes in the intestines ulcerate and may lead to an intestinal hemorrhage, which is one of the complications. The bacilli are found in the blood early in the disease. A leukopenia soon develops. Leukocytosis in typhoid fever indicates some inflammatory complication such as intestinal perforation. One attack gives a fairly permanent immunity. The period of incubation is variable, usually ranging from seven to 23 days, commonly ten to 14 days. The extremes are three and 40 days. It differs in different epidemics, for the period of incubation depends upon the number of organisms ingested, their virulence and the resistance of the host.

Miner found the average periods of incubation in three epidemics due to infected water to be 13 and 19 days; whereas, the averages of milk-borne epidemics, in which the dose was probably more massive, were seven and nine days. Convalescence is deliberate; sequelae are few. An attack of typhoid fever, however, seems to leave the patient in a weakened state. For three years afterward the death rate of persons who have had typhoid fever is twice the normal rate for those of the same age who have not had typhoid.

From the standpoint of preventive medicine, it is proper to regard an outbreak of typhoid fever as a reproach to the sanitation and civilization of the community in which it occurs. It is clearly a disease of defective civilization, for communities that pay least attention to sanitation, as a rule, suffer most. The physician has a dual duty in the care of a case of typhoid fever. One is to assist the patient, the other is to protect the community. Every case of typhoid fever means a short circuit between the alvine discharges of one person and the mouth of another. The health authorities are charged with finding the origin of the infection and its mode of transmission in order to prevent further spread from that source.

It is the primary purpose of this paper to correlate the activities of the private physician and the health department so that needless infections may be avoided. With this in view a few practical suggestions are presented.

The importance of prompt reporting either by telephone or on the cards provided for that purpose cannot be over-estimated. To eliminate typhoid fever from any community every case should have a thorough epidemiological investigation. The purpose of this investigation is to ascertain, if possible, the source and route of infection responsible for the case. After convalescence, the possibility of a carrier state developing must be investigated and, if this has occurred, the carrier should be kept under health department control.

The typhoid bacillus enters by the mouth. Typhoid fever is generally thought of as a gastro-intestinal infection, although the disease itself does not occur without infection of the blood stream, the glands and other structures of the body. The disease is now regarded as primarily a blood infection or bacteriemia. The bacilli leave the body mainly in the feces and urine, occasionally in the sputum, and other discharges. They appear in the feces early in the disease, sometimes before the fever. Late in the disease they diminish in number and usually disappear during convalescence, although they may continue indefinitely.

Since typhoid bacilli appear in the blood early in the disease, perhaps occasionally during the prodromal symptoms the blood culture is the earliest laboratory aid to diagnosis. Rosenau obtained positive blood cultures from approximately 90 percent in the first week, 65-percent in the second, and 42 percent in the third. About 33 percent of cases continue to discharge typhoid bacilli in the feces or urine for three weeks after the onset of the disease and about 11 percent for eight to ten weeks. If the carrier state lasts a year it may be considered chronic. From two to four percent, and sometimes more, of all cases continue to discharge typhoid bacilli indefinitely; these are active chronic carriers.

Women seem to outnumber men as carriers and are more subject to involvement of the gallbladder and to gallstones. It is now well understood that typhoid bacilli localize and maintain themselves in the gallbladder and the bile ducts, which are the chief sources of typhoid bacilli found in fecal carriers. Children are less subject to gallbladded disease, and seldom become carriers. Typhoid carriers are either fecal or urinary, or both. The fecal type is more frequent than the urinary, and apparently more dangerous, since most outbreaks of typhoid fever are traced to this type of carrier.

The story of typhoid Mary is an epidemiological classic and was the first of its kind to be reported in America. Indifferent, indeed, must be the medical man or surgeon who is not fascinated by this interesting story recently told by Dr. George A. Soper. Fifty-three cases with three deaths were definitely traced to Mary Mallon. There were, doubtless, many others produced which were never recorded.

As has been stated, one of the principal sources of the spread of typhoid is milk produced under insanitary condition. The typhoid outbreak at Bartlesville in the summer of 1940, had certain characteristics pointing rather definitely toward a milk-born origin.

1. The incidence of the disease followed exactly the distribution of the suspected milk supply.

2. The better classes of homes were involved. There were none reported from families too poor to purchase milk.

3. Individuals who drank the most milk, such as children, were affected principally.

4. The incubation period was relatively short, probably on account of the large number of bacilli ingested.

5. More than one case occurred simultaneously in a home.

6. Clinically, some of the cases ran a very mild course owing to the fact, no doubt, that the organism became attentuated in the process of multiplication in the milk.

7. The outbreak was relatively small since the total number of persons drinking the suspected milk was small.

8. The sale of the milk in a nearby city where it had previously not been sold before, was followed in about two weeks by the appearance of several cases of the disease.

We may concern ourselves, principally, with the typhoid carrier and in this connection there have recently been some additions to our methods of carrier detection. In every suspected case of typhoid fever the physician should avail himself of all the laboratory procedures at his disposal. These may be obtained either through a private laboratory or a State Health Department laboratory. The clinical manifestations should always be confirmed by bacteriological examination of the blood, feces and urine, and by the Widal test. A positive culture is, of course, of much more significance than a positive Widal. However, cultures may sometimes be negative and a Widal reveal the nature of the disease. This is particularly true when there are two specimens taken, the second of which shows a higher titre than the first.

Every effort should be made to secure stool and urine cultures from all cases and their contacts. If there is reason to suspect a carrier, no limit should be placed upon the number of cultures obtained; that is, several negatives may be followed by a positive when least expected. In addition to the securing of cultures, it may now be definitely recommended that Widals be taken on all suspected cases, carriers and contacts. This recommendation may be made due to very recent refinements in the agglutination test.

S. S. Bhatnagar (1938) states that in the

laboratories of the army in India Wedal reactions have been carried out as a routine every fourth day throughout the course of a continued fever against standard O and H suspensions. From personal experience and from a study of the carefully kept records of the cases of typhoid fever for the past five years, he has observed that in a typhoid infection in the inoculated the trouble taken in estimating the O and H agglutinins could not be justified when the value of the results obtained was assessed. Reliance had, therefore, to be placed on the isolation of the infecting organism from the blood, the urine, or the feces. Where this failed, he was commonly confronted with a positive, clinical picture and doubtful serological findings. The results proved to be so disappointing that the practice of carrying out tests for the detection of H agglutinins has recently been entirely discontinued in the army of India.

It is now generally recognized that, apart from O and H antigens, the great majority of strains of bacterium typhosum contain a third antigen,—the Vi antigen described and designated as such by Felix and his coworkers.

1. The O or somatic antigen is present in the bacterial body and resists heating to 100°C.

2. The H antigen is present in the flagellum. It is thermolabile.

3. The Vi antigen is also present in the bacterial body, perhaps as a capsule about the O antigen. It is thermolabile and to it virulence has been attributed.

A new serological apporach was opened when Felix and Pitt (1934) described the Vi antigen of the typhoid bacillus. This antigen is present in all virulent typhoid cultures; hence designated as the Vi or virulence antigen, and is absent or much reduced in quantity in cultures of low virulence. The H antigen gives rise to H antibody which has no bearing on the infectiousness of the organism or the course of the disease. The somatic or so-called O antigen of the smooth culture is a surface carbohydrate which has been shown to be toxic when extracted and partially purified (Henderson and Morgan, 1938). The corresponding O antibody neutralizes toxicity and prevents disease under certain conditions. The Vi antigen is also a surface somatic carbohydrate (Eliot).

Up to the present, Bhatnagar has not failed to correlate a positive Vi agglutination reaction with either the isolation of the infecting organism or with a positive clinical picture of typhoid fever. The great advantage of this type of agglutination lies in the fact that a positive result clinches the diagnosis of typhoid fever.

Bensted expressed the opinion that typhoid paratyphoid inoculation does give rise to Vi antibody, but only in very small amounts, not large enough to be taken account of in Vi agglutination.

Bhatnagar further observed that during convalescence from typhoid fever, as a rule only traces of the Vi antibody could be found in the serum. In a certain number of cases, however, the Vi titre continued to be high in spite of the termination of the acute infection. He interprets this as a tendency toward the carrier condition. Bacterialogical examination of the stool and urine have confirmed this interpretation.

The suggestion that possibly Vi agglutination may be a useful method of detecting chronic typhoid carriers was made by Felix, Krikorian and Reitler (1935). In 1938 Felix published the results of the examination of a considerable number of chronic carriers, using this method with excellent results. It may be stated reliably that the detection of the Vi antibody in a serum is taken to be an indication for a thorough search for typhoid bacilli in the stools and urine.

Eliot, continuing this work, states that the carrier condition is manifested by demonstrable Vi agglutinin in the blood in 95 percent of proven chronic carriers. For practical purposes the isolation of the typhoid bacillus from feces is a laborious, expensive and uncertain procedure. This inadequacy of laboratory methods, coupled with the possible intermittency of excretion of typhoid bacilli by the cronic fecal carrier, makes a negative result on one or two specimens of doubtful diagnostic significance. Ultimate recognition of the carrier must, of course, depend on demonstration of the typhoid bacillus in feces, urine or duodenal fluid. But some surer, quicker method than isolation of the organism is urgently needed for the purpose of tracing the typhoid case to its source, or in detecting the potentially dangerous food handler. We feel that the Vi agglutination test may be a partial solution to this problem, and the Oklahoma State Health Department is planning to make this test available for special studies of typhoid carriers.

Craigie and Yen have reported 706 strains of bacillus typhosus of which 98.6 percent were typical Vi forms. The present paper will not concern itself with the typing of the various Vi forms with specific bacteriophage, since the health department is not ready to assume this additional burden at the present time. However, it is felt that the Vi agglutination test, as performed by the tube method, will be of considerable value in the diagnosis of typhoid fever and in the search for carriers when its technical difficulties have been overcome. Additional studies on the practicability of the Vi agglutination test in an endemic typhoid area, such as Oklahoma, are needed before this test can be released for general use by practitioners and health officers.

All State Health Departments should have a uniform method of procedure in the management and control of the carrier problem, which ideally would be incorporated in a central Federal bureau to preserve the records of the carriers, their movement, occupations, environments, and when available their classifications by phage typing.

SUMMARY

1. All typhoid fever cases, contacts and carrier suspects should have repeated stool and urine cultures.

2. The Widal agglutination tests as performed with O and H antigens is unsatisfactory in differentiating between a clinical case of the disease and a previously inoculated individual.

3. The Vi agglutination test is said to be a valuable means of differentiating between clinical typhoid and a previous vaccination, since the Vi agglutination titre is very low or negative following typhoid inoculation.

4. A positive Vi agglutination test is an indication for thorough culture examination of the stools and urine for typhoid bacilli.

5. The Vi agglutination tests is a valuable addition to blood, stool and urine cultures in the search for carriers and the diagnosis of the disease, but needs additional investigation in epidemic areas.

6. The Vi agglutination test is being added to the laboratory procedures of the State Health Department for special typhoid carrier studies.

7. Bacteriophage typing of bacillus typhosus is suggested as a desirable procedure in outbreaks of typhoid fever, and is being contemplated as a possible later addition to the Health Department laboratory.

BIBLIOGRAPHY

1. Milton J. Rosenau: Preventive Medicine and Hygiene, Sixth Edition, 1935.
2. Typhoid in the Large Cities of the U. S. in 1939. J.A. M A. 1940, 21:2103.
3. Bureau of Census, Vital Statistics, 1939 United States, 1941, 51:1516.
4. Miner: J. Infect. Dis. 1922, 31:296.
5. George A. Soper: Bull. New York Acad. Med. Oct. 1939, 15:698.
6. S. S. Bhatnagar: 1938. Vi Agglutination in the Diagnosis of Typhoid Fever and the Typhoid Carrier Condition, Brit. Med Jour. 2:1195-99.
7. Bensted, H. J.: 1937. J.R.A. M C. 68, 1.
8. Boyd, Mark F.: Preventive Medicine, Sixth Edition, 1940.
9. Eliot, Calista F.: Am. Jr. Hyg. 1940, 31:8.
10. Henderson, D. W. and Morgan, M. F.: J. 1938, The Isolation of Antigenic Substances for Strains of Z. Typhosus, B. J. Exp. Path. 19.82-94.
11. Craigie J. and Yen, C. H.: The Demonstration of Types of B. Typhosus by Means of Preparations of Type II Vi Phage, Canad. Pub. Health J. 30:37.

Eczema[*]

Modern Concepts of Treatment

HARRY GREEN, M.D.

TULSA, OKLAHOMA

Eczema is a sensitization dermatitis resulting from repeated exposure or contact with normally innocuous substances. It is not a scientific term but the word is so commonly used for the designation of any itching dermatosis of unknown etiology that the general practitioner unhesitatingly labels it eczema and the dermatologist arrives at the same conclusion rather doubtfully and reluctantly.

Eczema, however, is not the dermatologic waste basket that it once was. Investigative research has rescued, so to speak, many clinical and well defined entities such as seborrheic dermatitis, and certain characteristic eruptions involving the hands, feet and genito crural regions which are now known to be caused by fungi or monilia and are classified accordingly.

Food as the primary etiologic factor no longer holds sway and it is now known that its importance has been unduly emphasized. This holds true not only in adults but to a somewhat lesser extent in infantile eczema[1] as well, and it is to the allergic study of this condition that we are indebted for the more modern concept of eczema. Since this paper is primarily a resume of treatment, a discussion of allergy with its related concepts of sensitivity, hypersensitivity, hoposensitivity, immunology and idiosyncrasy will not be entered into. Nor will mention

*Read before the Section on Dermatology, Annual Session, Oklahoma State Medical Association, April 22, 1942.

be made of the various skin tests except to say that it is a much abused practice and of help only in a very small percentage of cases in establishing a causative agent. A carefully taken history will often disclose a family tendency toward hypersensitivity and will, in the industrial worker, or housewife, reveal such sensitizing agents as various chemicals, soaps, wool, silk, plants and so forth. The role of soap as an irritant and/or causative agent is discussed more at length later on. But, regardless of cause, the treatment is rather well defined.

Given a case of eczema in the acute stage when the skin is erythematous, vesicular and oozing, the treatment of choice is wet dressings. Nor is it material whether one uses a three percent aqueous solution of boric acid, a one to 15 solution of liquor aluminum acetate or a physiologic salt solution. What is important, however, is the method of application. Linen is preferable to gauze because it is not as irritating to a sensitive skin. The bandage must be wet at all times and the solution must under no circumstances be allowed to evaporate as the concentrate will act as an irritant. The bandage must be thick to permit of drainage and to do away with too frequent changes. An open bandage, one not covered with cellophane or oil silk, is preferable as it enhances slow evaporation, produces a cooling, soothing, antipruritic effect and has a lesser tendency to maceration. One can not emphasize too strongly the importance of a properly applied wet dressing as it oftentimes means the difference between success and failure. Time and again I have seen patients, even in hospitals, with one layer of gauze, half dried, loosely applied to an adherent skin. The patient or whoever is in charge is instructed to use clean, well washed linen, cut in strips three inches wide. The strips are saturated with any one of the aforementioned solutions and wrapped about the extremities five or six times. If on a flat surface the thickness of the linen should consist of five or six layers. The bandage need not be dripping wet. As already stated covered bandages are undesirable but where indicated as in the ambulatory case especially for the extremities, there is on the market at present a cellophane covering, known as dermotector which fits loosely over the dressing and is held in place by elastic bands protecting the patient's bed linen and clothes. Should a wet dressing, for various reasons, be undesirable, recourse may be had to lotions or pastes. Lotions are much cleaner and are more acceptable to patients than pastes, I hardly ever use the latter. The lotion most frequently used is the well known calamine formula. This formula may be greatly improved by adding six percent Ben-

tonite to the mixture, (Bentonite is a mineral clay associated with Fuller's earth and Kaolin. It is an aluminum-ferrous-magnesium-silicon hydrate. A two percent aqueous solution has a ph of 9.5-9.8) which forms a suspensoid and gives a more uniform dispersion to the solution. It may be added to any formula as it is not incompatible with anything. A prescription such as the following may then be used. Calamine eight percent, zinc oxide, eight percent, glycerine two percent, calcium hydroxide with six percent bentonite qs ad.

Lotions should be applied every two or three hours and should not be removed oftener than once a day and then only in the gentlest possible way, with olive oil or a boric acid solution. If the lotion adheres do not irritate the underlying sensitive skin by forcing its removal. There are details but most important ones and, as stated before, may well mean the difference between success or failure.

When the acute, exudative phase has subsided and the skin becomes dry and scaly, the wet bandages are discontinued and either lotions or salves are substituted. Here, too, my preference is for lotions because they are cleaner and easier of application and they save the patient the trouble and expense of bandaging. The following active ingredients can easily be incorporated, either alone or combined into the lotion previously described: chloralhydrate two to four percent, Ichthyol five to 15 percent, liquor carbonis détergens three to 10 percent. When more than one active ingredient is used it is advisable to reduce the strength of each. In addition, phenol ½ to one percent or menthol ¼ to ½ percent may be added, as these are well known antipruritic agents. A logical prescription then, for an itching dermatosis where there is but little or no exudation or inflammation would be: Phenol one percent, menthol ¼ of one percent, chloral hydrate two percent, liquor carbonis detergens 10 percent, liquor aluminum acetate qs.

A valuable aid in the extensive acute or subacute dermatosis is the use of the "colloid" bath. This is prepared by adding two cups of bulk oats to one quart of water and boiling it for 45 minutes in a double boiler. After cooling for 15 minutes one half cup of baking powder is added to the mass, all of it placed in a muslin sack and the top of the sack tied. This is placed in the bath where it is squeezed until the water becomes "soapy" from the contents. The water should be kept at a temperature of 98 to 100° F. and the patient may be kept in this for as long as it is comforting. On coming out from the bath the skin is patted dry and a soothing lotion applied.

The most invaluable agent in the treatment of some forms of eczema in the subacute stage which remains resistant to other forms of therapy is x-ray. The results are at times spectacular, especially in the cronic, lichenified type where the skin is leathery and pruritis. I am relying more and more on irradiation in the treatment of the subacute and cronic types of eczema. MacKee in his book "X-rays and Radium in the Treatment of Diseases of the Skin" says, "considered as one of the many remedies used in the treatment of eczema . . . and visualizing the disease in a very general way it is the author's opinion that x-rays are the best remedy that we have for eczema. In a general way it is our best antipruritic and our best resolvent agent for this purpose." That the use of x-ray as a therapeutic agent is not without its dangers is, of course, known to all and should not be attempted by the inexperienced. It is this type of eczema, with its tendency to chronicity that never fails to tax the skill of the physician and the patience of the victim. Of the topical remedies tar is the one commonly resorted to. Crude coal tar or any of its commoner preparations (Taraxide, taralba, liquor carbonis detergens, naftalan) are incorporated in an ointment containing an acid for keratolytic effect. In using tar one should begin with moderate strength and increase gradually to tolerance or until the desired effects are produced.

In eczema of the hands relapse is common in the winter months when the skin is naturally dried due to lessened sebaceous gland activity. The same may be said of other parts of the body. The use of soap in these individuals will cause an aggrevation of the eczematous process, due to the alkali action of the soap and the removal from the skin by its detergent properties what little of natural oil there may be present. Patients will, of course, react differently, to different soaps at different times but the reaction is invariably worse during the winter months. The number of skin eruptions directly traceable to the use of soap has increased in recent years due, I believe, to a gullible soap conscious public misled by a round the clock radio bombardment of tear jerking, nerve racking "washboard weepers" or soap operas. Good business for the soap manufacturers and broadcasting companies but bad for the skin. When one considers that there is also a neurogenic factor involved in most of these cases[3] the evil produced by these radio programs becomes even more apparent. That the presence of alkalis and saturated fatty acids in some soaps is responsible for skin irritation in certain individuals has been shown by Blank[4] and others.[5] Downing[6] in a report on two thousand cases of various skin diseases in industrial workers found that 249 of these were produced by soap. The use of sulfonated oils as a detergent in place of soap seems to be the answer to this vexing problem. There are a number of these on the market and their use is suggested in all cases of suspected soap eczemas because they have good cleansing actions and are free of eczematogenous factors. One[7] of these sulfonated oils in particular has been studied by Lane & Blank in the dermatologic clinic of the Massachusetts General Hospital and by dermatologists in the skin clinic of nine other cities and in a series of 350 cases of various skin dieasese 233 of which were eczemas, less than one percent showed hypersensitivity to the oil.

When eczema involves the lower extremities it is essential that the patient be kept in a recumbent posture with the foot of the bed in an elevated position as swelling will ensue and the course of the disease be unnecessarily prolonged if patient is permitted up and about. The treatment that I use in these cases is simple of application and is successful in a large majority. The leg or arm is painted with a five percent aqueous solution of gentian violet and permitted to dry. A two inch elastoplast or Ace adhensive bandage is then passed around the ankle, carried down over the foot, then upward in a spiral, overlapping turn to below the knee joint. The bandage is removed at the end of seven to 10 days. It is advisable to shave all hair over affected area prior to applying bandage. I have used the same method in the localized, vesicular patches of eczema — the so, called nummular type — when only small, isolated areas are seen on the dorsal surfaces of the hands or feet. Results are not due to the medical virtues of the bandage or the gentian violet as to the fact that the skin is immobilized, so to speak, patient cannot scratch and the skin does not come in contact with extraneous irritants.

Infantile eczema is deserving of more space and consideration than can be devoted to it in this paper. In contradistinction to adult eczema food may be an etiologic factor in some cases but its importance as a causative agent has been overemphasized while too little emphasis is given to contactants. The offending agents are usually wool, silk, mattress stuffing and other environmental agents. Of 124 children with eczema studied by Osborne, Jordon, and Hallett[1] about 50 percent were improved or entirely cured when hospitalization in a ward free of wool and feathers and fed a normal diet. In eczema of infants secondary infection is the rule rather than the exception and in these cases wet dressing of 1:4000 of potassium permanganate, or saturated solutions of boric acid are useful and may be applied six to eight hours during the day. With the onset of the dry state, or when the acuteness has subsided a mild tar[2] preparation may be used to advantage. This may be kept on at all times provided there is no tar sensitivity. I have also used x-ray therapy with excellent results in certain selected cases of atopic dermatitis in children.

What role do the vitamins play in the treatment of eczema? Finnerud and co-workers[8] report on a small series (18) of well controlled, hospitalized cases of eczema definitely improved when given lard by mouth, lard being rich in unsaturated fatty acids. Ginsberg and Bernstein[9] failed to see any specific benefits from feeding this type of cases with food rich in unsaturated fatty acids. Taub and Zakon[10] discouraged its use after trying it on eight cases. Cornbleet[11] reports gratifying results in a series of 87 patients from the internal administration of maize oil. M. Comel, quoted in the Year Book of Dermatology for 1935, cites good results in eczema when treated with vitamin D. Lever and Talbott[12] found "no direct correlation between the level of vitamin C in the blood and the development of the several diseases of the skin," including eczema. Ingestion of vitamin C by patients in this series had no influence.

S. N. Vendel of Copenhagen, Denmark, in the January, 1940, issue of the Lancet (quoted by The Year Book of Dermatology for 1940) states that "it is possible to cure most cases of eczema by administration of vitamin B complex." He reports on a series of more than 100 cases. The editors of The Year Book in commenting on the article observe that this "seems highly improbable" but add that "certain types of eczema, or eczematous eruptions, bordering on seborrheic dermatitis or subacute neurodermatitis seem to have been benefited by riboflavin or nicotinic acid and perhaps also by other constituents of the complex occurring in yeast or liver."

Paul Gross[3] reports that of 24 cases with nummular eczema treated with vitamin A satisfactory results were obtained in 18, two were greatly improved, one was improved to some extent, and three did not respond

consistently. He found in most of these cases an existing asteatosis (dry skin), and early sign of A avitaminosis. If his results can be duplicated by others in this chronically recurring, protracted dermatosis so frequently seen by dermatologists and general practitioners alike a valuable contribution will have been made.

From the above it will be seen that one has to resort to empiricism when prescribing any of the vitamins in the treatment of eczema. In my own experience a proper evaluation is difficult because the big majority of patients are in no experimental mood when they present themselves for treatment. They want to get well in the shortest possible time and while I have tried the various vitamins collaterally with other agents it is my belief that when a cure or a remission occurs it is the local medication and not the vitamins which are responsible. In the undernourished case where a true state of avitaminosis exists such as an associated cheilosis of riboflavin deficiency, the phrynoderma (toad skin) of vitamin A deficiency or the dermatitis of pellagra, immediate and almost spectacular results will follow when the deficient vitamin is restored.

BIBLIOGRAPHY

1. Osborne, E. D., Jordon, J W. and Hallett, J J.: The Practical Management of Eczema in Infants and Children. New York State J. Med. 42:47-50 (Jan.) 1942

3. Gross. P : Nummular Eczema. Its Clinical Picture and Successful Therapy. Arch. Dermat. & Syph. 44:1060 (Dec.) 1941

4 Blank, I. H : Action of Soap on Skin. Arch Dermat & Syph. 39.811-824 (May) 1939.

5. Jordon, J. W., Dolce, F A. and Osborne, E D.: Dermatitis of the Hands in Housewives: Role of Soap in Its Etiology and Methods for Its Prevention. J.A.M.A. 115:1001-1006 (Sept..21) 1940.

6. Downing, J. G.: Cutaneous Eruptions Among Industrial Workers: A Review of Two Thousand Claims for Compensation. Arch. Dermat. & Syph. 39:12 (Jan) 1939.

7. Lane, C. G. and Blank, I. H.: Sulfonated Oil As a Detergent for Disease of the Skin. Arch. Dermat. & Syph. 43: 435-443 (Mar.) 1941.

8. Finnerud, C. W., Kesler, R. L. and Wiese, H. F.: Ingestion of Lard in the Treatment of Eczema and Allied Dermatoses. A Clinical and Biochemical Study. Arch. Dermat. & Syph. 44:849 (Nov.) 1941.

9. Ginsberg, J. E and Bernstein, C., Jr.: Effects of Oils Containing Unsaturated Fatty Acids on Patients with Dermatitis. Arch. Dermat. & Syph. 36:1038 (Nov.) 1937.

10. Taub, S. J. and Zakon, S J.: The Use of Unsaturated Fatty Acids in the Treatment of Eczema.

11. Cornbleet, T.: Use of Maize Oil(unsaturated fatty acids) in the Treatment of Eczema. Arch. Dermat & Syph. 31: 1935

12. Lever, W. F. and Talbott, J. H.: Role of Vitamin C in Various Cutaneous Diseases. Arch. Dermat & Syph. 41:657 (April) 1940.

Dysentery Carriers

Since it is only slightly absorbed into the blood stream, succinylsulfathiazole, a sulfonamide compound, is much less likely to produce severe toxic or poisonous reactions from sulfaguanidine in the treatment of dysentery carriers, William M. M. Kirby, M.D., and Lowell A. Rantz, M.D., San Francisco, report in The Journal of the American Medical Association for June 20. They found succinylsulfathiazole to be as effective in treating dysentery carriers as sulfaguanidine and as ineffective in treating typhoid carriers.

Urolithiasis[*]

J. W. ROGERS, M.D.

TULSA, OKLAHOMA

The patients whom we see with urinary calculi are for the time being interested only in relief of the pain or the desire to get rid of the stone or both, but as soon as this is accomplished he will likely ask us why he had the stone and whether he may have another? In order to give an intelligent answer we will have to know a good deal about the patient, the type of stone, and make quite an extensive study of the individual, for there is so far as our present knowledge goes, no one cause for all urinary calculi. The etiology of urinary calculi has always been a controversal subject and it continues to be, in spite of a great amount of investigative work done in recent years. The Massachusetts General Hospital has had a stone clinic since 1935 and has done notable work in finding the cause in the individual patients in the clinic.

On some etiological factors all are agreed. All agree that parathyroid disease causes urinary calculi but the percentage of stones caused by parathyroid disease varies greatly in different clinics. In some it has been found to be the cause of as high as five percent of the calculi encountered, while in others with an equal number of patients with calculi, the percentage is as low as 1/10 of one percent. I am unable to find any reason for this discrepency. I presume as our diagnostic ability and methods become more settled there will be less difference. In any case, we can all accept the fact that parathyroid disease causes a small proportion of urinary calculi. Another etiological factor on which every one agrees is that long illnesses requiring the patient to remain in bed for long periods, such as fractures and Infantile paralysis, causes decalcification of the bones, increased calcium in the blood and urine and so formation of stones. In such cases stasis may become a contributory cause.

Another cause of stone formation of which there is no controversy is of recent origin. It has been found that the sulfa drugs, constitute a fairly common cause of stone formation, sulfapyidine being the chief offender. From these accepted causes we pass to the realm of controversial causes. Stasis is considered an important factor by most of us but many think that stasis is only indirectly a factor, in that it causes infection and infection is the cause of the calculis. There is a general agreement that infection is an etiological factor but just why it will cause stones in one patient and not in another is a question. The urea splitting organisms are the chief offenders, such as B. Proteus, influenza bacillus and certain strains of staphlococci and streptococci, other organisms may at times become urea splitting, such as B. Coli and B. Pyocyanous, Metabolic disturbances such as gout, cystinuria and endogenous oxaluria cannot be overlooked as possible causes. We now come to the subject of diet and the ever present vitamins. Certain localities are said to be relatively free of stones. It is said the negroes of South Africa rarely have calculi and even in this country, Livermore has made the observation that negroes in and around Memphis are less subject to calculi than the rest of the population in that locality and the conclusion is drawn that this difference should be attributed to the high acid ash Vitamin A, diet and not to racial differences. Higgins, in Cleveland, has done a tremendous amount of work both with animals and with patients on the effect of Vitamin A deficiency and acid and alkaline diets. He was able to produce and dissolve stones in animals at will but in the human being the results were less startling, but he has proven, at least to his own satisfaction, that Vitamin A is an important etiological factor. Some workers believe that infection is almost the sole cause of calculi. Kroll guotes Eisenstaedt as saying that in 55 consecutive cases of urinary calculi he found an infective nucleus in each calculus, staphlococci predominating. I don't believe other workers have found this to be true but at the Massachusetts General Hospital, 41 percent of the patients had urea splitting organisms present in the urine.

Heredity may play a minor role in that malformations may possibly be transmitted. Ureteral stones are most often stones that have been passed from the Kidney. We may occasionally have a primary ureteral calculus as a result of a foreign body or a malformed and saculated ureter. In the bladder, stasis certainly plays a major role in stone forma-

*Read before the Section on Urology and Syphilology, Annual Session, Oklahoma State Medical Association, April 24, 1942.

tion, it is a fairly common complication of prostatism, of course, infection is always present too. Stones from the kidneys may pass into the bladder and remain and grow if there is an obstruction, such as an enlarged prostate. Foreign bodies remaining in the bladder become incrusted. Prostatic calculi are not uncommon and here again stasis and infection are important etiological factors. Urethral stones may be primary or secondary. Stones may become lodged in the urethra on their passage from the bladder or primary stones may form in pockets caused by strictures. So it behooves us to study our patient as a whole before we try to answer his question as to why he has a stone or whether he may have another. Two or three decades ago 50 percent of the patients had recurrent stones, at the present time, due to increased knowledge as to causes and better surgical procedures only about ten percent have recurrence.

Diagnosis: We usually think that it is easy to diagnose urinary calculi where ever located but it isn't always so simple. A stone in the urethra is nearly always easy to diagnose whether retention is complete or partial. Instrumentation reveals the presence of the stone. I don't recall ever having failed to make the diagnosis of stone in this locality. Prostatic stones are easily overlooked. The patient may be treated for a long time for prostatitis and cystitis without the recognition of the presence of stones in the prostate. If we would always make a plain x-ray picture of the K. U. B. region, nearly all of these cases would be diagnosed at once. In all urological cases where the diagnosis is in question the x-ray should be employed. Even then one may get the cart before the horse. I recall a patient with pyuria and hematuria, pyogenic organisms were found in the urine and sulfathiazole administered, the bacterae dis appeared but not the pyuria. Repeated examinations for tubercle bacilli were negative and an x-ray picture showed a prostate full of stones. A resection of the prostate with the removal of the stones was done without relief. On further cystoscopic examination after the operation many tubercles were seen in the bladder, removal of an old tuberculous kidney cured the cystitis. Moral: Don't jump at conclusions. Too often we see a single pathological condition and assume that that is the sole cause of symptoms, while it may be only a secondary condition. Some years ago a patient came to me complaining that he had been treated for gonorrhea for over a year without results. In those days that wasn't such an unusual occurrence, but on examination the only find-

ing was pyuria and colon bacilli, he had had no urethral discharge for months but treatment for gonorrhea had been continued because of a cloudy urine. An x-ray picture showed a large stone in the right kidney and its removal promptly cured the pyuria. We should try to be alert and take nothing for granted. Ureteral calculi are not so easily diagnosed and here failure is sometimes excusable. A patient may have severe pain in the right lower abdomen, perhaps a slight elevation of temperature, urine clear or showing a few R. B. C. and a leucocytosis. A patient with such a syndrome may have a normal appendix removed and perhaps pass a stone the next day. I have seen a good many patients subject to right urinary calculi and in nearly all of them the appendix had been removed and I have always been suspicious that they had lost an appendix due to ureteral or renal colic. These cases often bear the marks of an emergency and it is perhaps more prudent to remove an inoffensive appendix than to spend too much time with diagnostic measures and allow a fulminating appendix to burst. Certainly a urinalysis should be made and if blood is found an x-ray picture should be made, as little time would be lost by such a procedure. Usually renal or ureteral colic is self-evident with pain radiating down the groin and into the bladder and genitalia, with urinary frequency. But all these symptoms might be caused by a retro-cecal appendicitis, including the hematuria. Renal calculi may be silent and only discovered by an x-ray examination for some other condition. These patients have a cloudy urine but this means nothing to many people, but if blood is passed they usually seek medical attention. More often they have recurrent attacks of renal and ureteral colic and frequently have pain in the lumbar region. Plain x-ray pictures will show about 95 percent of the calculi, Uretero-pyelograms will show a few additional percent of ureteral and renal calculi. In an article in the Journal of Urology of March 1942, Councill describes the use of the Teleprobe. By the use of this instrument he feels that these calculi can be found in 100 percent. How practical this method and instrument is for the neophyte, I am unable to say, but calculi would be found more often if we looked for them and could persuade our patients to have the necessary examinations made.

Having diagnosed a urinary calculus, what are we going to do about it? In many cases urinary calculi constitutes an emergency demanding prompt action. I had a patient brought in from a neighboring town with acute retention with a stone in the pendulus urethra. He was suffering intensely and the stone was palpable through the walls of the penis, but dislodging it was a problem. One doesn't like to open that portion of the urethra. After considerable probing with numerous instruments including a metal stone dislodger, I managed to loosen it and I have never seen a more grateful patient in spite of the discomfort attending its dislodgement. A doctor came into my office one afternoon suffering with renal colic. I gave him morphine and it eased him somewhat and later in the evening he passed the stone into his bladder. Years later he told me that the next morning it lodged in his urethra and he was unable to void. He said he drank two or three bottles of beer and gave a big push and out it came. This practice is not to be recommended, as one might get considerable back pressure before relief could be obtained.

Stones in the prostate may be silent and cause no trouble, if they break through into tne urethra, pockets form and cystitis and cystitis and urethritis arise. Perhaps the best form of treatment is prostatic resection. Stones in the bladder may be crushed or if too large, removed, suprapubically.

If accompanied by bladder incrustations it may be possible to dissolve both the stone and the incrustations by the use of a solution of sodium citrate and citric acid as described by Wilhelm and Levine.

Perhaps stone in the ureten constitutes the most common emergency. Most of these patients need relief and certainly want it quickly. Occasionally one is in doubt as to whether it is ureteral colic or appendicitis, but if the case is under close observation, it is fairly safe to give medicine for relief. I have usually resorted to morphine and atropine but Grayson Carrol has made a study of a pancreatic substance, on the market as Depropanex, that is said to stop ureteral contractions within three or four minutes, and usually the pain is relieved and does not recur quickly. A dose of two or three C.C. is injected intramuscularly. There are no ill effects noted. If one uses morphine, it usually takes from 15 to 30 minutes and often has to be repeated. After the pain is relieved the position and size of the stone should be ascertained and then the question is, what to do about it. About 66 percent pass without aid, the 33 or 34 percent have to have aid. Should we try by manipulation or resort to open operation? In some clinics over half the ureteral calculi are removed by open surgery. While in others, over 90 percent are removed by various engenious methods and instruments. Personally I've managed to dislodge those I've seen without resorting to open surgery but have regretted the occasional rather severe reactions, with

chills and fever, but with the modern drugs, one should have less trouble in this respect. There is some danger of puncturing the ureteral wall and I believe it hazardous to pass metal instruments very high up the ureter, R. P. Finney reports a large number of ureteral calculi removed by lassoing the stone and using traction of less than five pounds and gradually pulling them out. I believe he failed only one in fifty odd cases.

I am inclined to feel that we should try to remove the stones by manipulation before resorting to an open operation.

Renal calculi of any magnitude will have to be removed by surgery and here again the least trauma and least harm done to the kidney the better off the patient will be. Many surgeons believe that if a stone is in a calix the calix should be removed by the method advocated by Lowsley. One should leave no blood clots or gravel, otherwise, there is sure to be recurrence. Once the stones are removed, or even before, the patient as a whole should be studied, the type of stone ascertained, and the amount of calcium in the urine determined. Focci of infection, should be sought especially about the teeth. If the stones are of the alkaline group put the patient on an acid ash, high Vitamin A diet, if of the acid group use an alkaline ash diet with Vitamin A, always with large amounts of water, if parathyroid disease is present attend to that. If there are strictures dilate them, remove prostatic obstruction when indicated and do not dismiss the patient as soon as the stone or stones are removed, have him return for a check up once or twice a year for two or three years.

BIBLIOGRAPHY

George R. Livermore: Journal of Urology, March, 1939
J. Dillinger Barney and Hirsh W. Sulkowitch: Journal of Urology, Dec. 1936.
Charles Higgins. J.A.M.A., April 6, 1935.
Grayson Caroll: So. Med. Journal, March 1938.
S. F. Wilhelm and B. Levine: Journal of Urology, March 1942.
Francis Twinem: Journal of Urology, November 1940.
R. P. Finney: J.A.M.A., December 12, 1941.
H. P Winsbury: Year Book of Urology, 1938.

Restrictions on Quinine

The War Production Board has issued a conservation order affecting quinine and cinchona preparations. Physicians and pharmacists are advised that quinine or quinine salts and cinchona preparations are to be used only for the treatment of malaria fever and are to be dispensed for this purpose only upon a physician's prescription. Quinine may be used also for making urea or quinine hydrochloride.

Wholesale druggists and retail pharmacists will not be allowed to purchase the above mentioned products in quantities greater than 50 ounces. If your pharmacist is refusing to fill prescriptions for these drugs unless they are being used for the treatment of malarial fever, or, in the case of the exception, for making of urea and quinine hydrochloride, he is following the orders of the War Production Board.—Roland T. Lakey, Dean, College of Pharmacy, Wayne University, Detroit, Michigan.

• *THE PRESIDENT'S PAGE* •

The President's Page this month is dedicated to R. H. Graham, Executive Secretary of the Oklahoma State Medical Association, and is written in grateful recognition and acknowledgement of services well and faithfully rendered.

The Oklahoma State Medical Association has made a great contribution to our Government in the loan of our efficient Secretary, R. H. Graham, to the War Manpower Division, and it is a real sacrifice to the Association and its affairs.

At the present time, Dick is Administrative Assistant to Lieutenant Commander Max Lapham of the Procurement and Assignment Division of the War Manpower Commission. We do not doubt for one minute but that Dick will be of untold service to this important branch of the U. S. Government; for he will fit into this work like the glove fits the hand.

Dick has one of the brightest and most versatile minds it has ever been the writer's pleasure to know. He is a real fellow, a real red-blooded American, and in accepting this position, he does so at a real financial sacrifice to himself. But to this he gave no thought. He is anxious to serve where his services will benefit his Country the most.

We of the Oklahoma State Medical Association say to you Dick, "remember, we will not only miss you and your services greatly, but we all anxiously look forward to that day when you will be safely returned to us, and to the State of Oklahoma. You have done a great piece of work, both for the public and the profession. God speed the day of your return."

Sincerely yours,

James D Osborn

President.

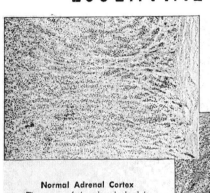
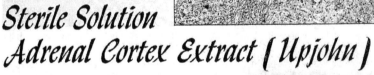
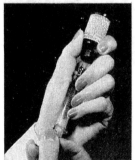

• EDITORIALS •

R. M. ANDERSON — J. C. BUSHYHEAD PIONEERS

The Medical profession of Oklahoma has recently lost two "old-timers" who stood as outstanding exponents of all that is good in Medicine.

Because of their exemplary lives, their professional attainments, their sound ethical principles and their long record of commendable service, their names are again placed before the readers of the Journal.

Those who knew them intimately will appreciate this added recognition and those who were not so fortunate will be glad to know that truly they were among the doctors of the old school, loved and revered by all who knew them and that they weathered the transition from the "horse and buggy" era into modern practice, appropriating all the good in the new, while holding fast to all endearing qualities of the old.

Through a long professional career they were continuously honored by being wanted at the bedside, and rewarded by their unfailing response to the call of those who needed them, and finally, they were chastened by the cumulative sense of duty well done.

What a fine example for modern young men engaged in the pursuit of a merciful profession.

Chronologically they lived to a good old age but if we deduct the time they gave to the sick, they died young. If we consider the years they added to the lives of others through their ministrations they are more alive today than we are.

While we regret their passing, we are grateful for what they contributed to Oklahoma medicine and we shall always cherish their memory.

LIVER SHOCK

Long standing biliary tract disease always causes liver damage and these cases are always serious surgical risks and it is not always possible to accurately determine the extent of this liver damage.

Many tests have been devised to obtain a general estimate of the amount of hepatic functional damage, but it is so often the case that grave hepatic insufficiency will be precipitated by operation in cases where the tests for hepatic function are normal.

In those cases where there has been long standing jaundice of any degree in conjunction with a history of hepatic duct colic with common duct obstruction there is always serious hepatic damage and these cases should be considered poor operative risks and it is advisable to prepare them for serious liver shock following the operation.

The best method of preparing the liver to withstand the operative shock and decompression of the bile ducts is to protect it against any possible exigencies by assuring a high glycogen storage and a low fat content by giving the patient a diet for at least one week preoperatively consisting mostly of carbohydrates with the usual amount of proteins while the fats are cut to a very minimum. It has also been found that Vitamin K will usually affect the prothrombin concentration and reduce the incidence of troublesome bleeding although the hepatic damage will in some cases be so severe that it will have no effect. Bile salts are given before operation to supply the deficiency that has been present over a period of time and are of particular value during the period of preoperative preparation when the proper assimilation of the diet is so essential.

Opening and exploration of the common duct must always be done in a patient who is icteric or who gives a history of jaundice and this disturbance of the dynamics of the biliary tract is in itself enough to precipitate serious liver shock.

So often there is a history of a patient with a common duct obstruction due to the presence of stones whose liver functions tests are nearly normal and who has been adequately prepared, to withstand the initial shock of the operative proceedure, then within twenty-four hours to develop a hyperpyrexia and to die within forty-eight hours due entirely to hepatic insufficiency. Postmortem examination on these cases reveals little changes except in the hepatic cells themselves which reveal extensive damage due entirely to biliary retention.

In all surgery of the biliary tract it is best to prepare the patient as though there was extensive hepatic damage even if the functional tests are normal and this is best done by means of a high carbohydrate and low fat diet, with vitamin K and bile salts added.—E. E. R., M.D.

PROMETHEUS AND PARE

If we accept the old oddage "Necessity is the Mother of Invention," we must admit that war has ever been the cruel father of necessity. Though at great cost, war does bring rare opportunities in the field of medicine and surgery.

We turn back the pages of history approximately four hundred years for a striking example. In the very beginning of his military career Pare was at Suse, a little place near Mont Cenis. It was in the year 1537. He was only 27 years old when he made a great discovery. Fortunately we have his own account of this experience: "The enemy within the castle, seeing our men come on them with great fury, did all that they could to defend themselves, and killed and wounded many of our soldiers with pikes, arquebuses, and stones: whereby the surgeons had all their work cut out for them. Now I was at this time a fresh-water soldier; I had not yet seen gunshot wounds at the first dressing. I had read in John de Vigo, book one, Of Wounds in General, chapter eight, that wounds made by fire-arms partake of venosity, by reason of the gunpowder; and for their cure he bids you cauterize them with oil of elders, scalding hot, mixed with a little treacle. And to make no mistake, before I would use the said oil, knowing that it was to bring great pain to the patient, I asked first, before I applied it, what the other surgeons used for a first-dressing; which was, to put the said oil, boiling well, into the wounds, with tents and setons: wherefore I took courage to do as they did. At last, my oil ran short; and I was compelled, instead of it, to apply a digestive made of yolks of eggs, oil of roses, and turpentine. In the night, I could not sleep in quiet, fearing some default in the not cauterizing, lest I should find those, to whom I had not applied the said oil, dead from the poison of their wounds; which made me rise very early to visit them: where, beyond my expectation, I found that they to whom I had applied my digestive had suffered but little pain, and their wounds without inflammation or swelling, having rested fairly well that night. The others, to whom the boiling oil was applied, I found feverish, with great pain, and swelling round the edges of their wounds. Then I resolved nevermore to burn thus cruelly poor men with gunshot wounds.

"When I was at Turin, I found a surgeon famed above all the rest for his treatment of gunshot wounds; into whose favor I found a way to insinuate myself, that I might have the recipe of his balm, as he called it, wherewith he dressed these wounds. And he made me pay my court to him for two years, before I could possibly get the recipe out of him. In the end, thanks to my gifts and presents, he gave it to me, which was this, to boil down, in oil of lilies, young whelps just born, and earthworms prepared

with Venice turpentine. Then was I joyful, and my heart made glad, that I had learned his remedy, which was like that which I had obtained by chance."

"See how I learned to treat gunshot wounds: not out of books."

Now that thousands of young American doctors are face to face with the necessity of meeting the emergencies of war in all parts of the world, they should take courage and be inspired by the opportunity to learn new lessons, in the hard school of necessity.

Prometheus brought fire to suffering mortals, Pare had the good fortune to discover its misguided application and saved much suffering by taking it away. Quoting from Garrison's *History of Medicine*. "Pare's greatest contribution to surgery hinges on the baneful effect which the pseudo-hippocratic aphonism that diseases not cureable by iron are cureable by fire exerted on the treatment of gunshot wounds, the new feature of Renaissance surgery."

Pare was born of hard working people in 1510. He was a country boy, uneducated except through apprenticeship. For three or four years he was resident at Hotel Dieu. He was an Army surgeon for approximately twenty years. Ultimately he had a lucrative practice, and many court appointments. He was highly regarded and wielded a profound influence. Garrison said, "In personality, Pare stands between his surgical peers, the rude, outspoken Hunter and the refined, self possessed Lister, as a man equally at home in the rigors of camp life and the slippery footing of courts."

Pare's life not only supplies a good example of the opportunities which war brings to the army doctor but might well be accepted as a model for those who are casting about for guidance and anchorage. "Here is one who can praise without offense his own performances, and chronicle with proper pride his own words, and score off a fool, and relish his meat and drink: a shrewd, happy, confident, business-like gentleman, not wholly free, in a vain and cruel age, from vanity, nor incapable of cruelty, but steadily compassionate, humble, wise and honorable: and a true lover of his country, his home, and his profession."

In his life of eighty years Pare exhibited what the word Prometheus stands for. "Forethought".

"THIS DISEASE IS BEYOND MY PRACTICE"

No wonder Macbeth said, "Throw physic to the dogs; I'll none of it." Lady Macbeth's physician lacked initiative and imagination. He also manifested mental cowardice. He admitted that his patient's disease was beyond his practice, and was content to say "infected minds to their deaf pillows will discharge their secrets. More needs she the divine, than the physician." Shirking his own responsibility he called upon God to "Look after her; remove from her the means of all annoyance, and still keep eyes upon her." Then he admitted, "My mind she has mated, and amazed by sight: I think, but dare not speak." Finally in answer to Macbeth's question he said she is "Not so sick my lord, as she is troubled with thick coming fancies, that keep her from rest."

This last provoked Macbeth's stinging indictment, "Canst thou not minister to a mind diseased; Pluck from the memory a rooted sorrow; Raze out the written troubles of the brain; And, with some sweet, oblivious antidote, cleanse the stuffed bosom of that perilous stuff, which weighs upon the heart?"

It was only after the doctor had bluntly replied "Therein the patient must minister to himself," that Macbeth threw the doctor and his physic to the dogs.

Even though we admit Lady Macbeth was demented, there is a lesson here for modern doctors who are called upon to meet the psychological problems arising out of these perilous times. Without fail we should call upon God for help but we should have powder and we should keep it dry. In other words we should be ready to meet mental aberations with patience, knowledge, skill and understanding. By so doing we may lift the burden "which weighs upon the heart".

The majority of neurotics must go untreated if they depend upon the specialists. Though it may sound like heresy to the experts, the family physician should be capable of analizing many of his psychological patients and interested in resolving their conflicts. At the same time he should be quick to recognize the need of institutional care and prompt in the recommendation of incarceration for the innocently hopeless and for those "possessed of the devil." It's amazing how a little common sense mixed with patience and experience may penetrate that mysterious realm which is never fully explored or actually charted even by the specialists.

"Are you a doctor?" asked the young lady, stepping into a drug store.

"Naw," replied the youth behind the white counter. "I'm just the fizzician."

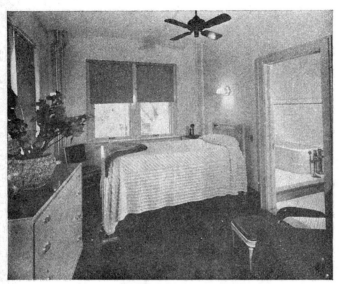

ASSOCIATION ACTIVITIES

OKLAHOMA CLINICAL CONFERENCE TO MEET OCTOBER 26-29

The Oklahoma City Clinical Society has completed its preparations for the twelfth annual conference to be held October 26, 27, 28, 29. In preparing the program this year, special effort has been necessary, and much additional work entailed because of the national emergency. The Society has been able, however, to secure speakers and teachers of unusual ability, and the caliber of the meeting is expected to exceed the excellent conferences of the past. Emphasis has been placed upon traumatic and industrial phases of medicine and surgery, which are particularly appropriate at this time. The guest speakers are:

Dr. James E. Paullin, President-Elect of the American Medical Association, of Atlanta, Georgia;

Dr. Isaac A. Bigger, Professor of Surgery and Surgeon-in-chief, Medical College of Virginia, Richmond, Virginia;

Dr. George M. Curtis, Professor of Surgery, Chairman of Department of Research Surgery, Ohio State University, Columbus, Ohio;

Dr. Frank H. Ewerhardt, Assistant Professor of Physical Therapy, Washington University School of Medicine, St. Louis, Missouri;

Dr. Frederick H. Falls, Professor and Head of Department of Obstetrics and Gynecology, University of Illinois College of Medicine, Chicago, Illinois;

Dr. Charles C. Higgins, Urology, Cleveland Clinic, Cleveland, Ohio;

Dr. Sara M. Jordan, Department of Gastro-Enterology, Lahey Clinic, Boston, Massachusetts;

Dr. John Albert Key, Clinical Professor of Orthopedic Surgery, Washington University School of Medicine, St. Louis, Missouri;

Dr. Byrl R. Kirklin, Professor of Radiology and Director of Division of Radiology, Mayo Foundation, University of Minnesota, Rochester, Minnesota;

Dr. Andrew W. McAlester, III, Ophthalmology, Kansas City, Missouri;

Dr. Donovan J. McCune, Associate Professor of Pediatrics, College of Physicians and Surgeons, Columbia University, New York, New York;

Dr. Frank J. Novak, Jr., Senior Attending Otolaryngologist, Henrotin Hospital, Chicago, Illinois;

Dr. Albert O. Singleton, Professor of Surgery, Medical Department, University of Texas, Galveston, Texas;

Dr. Tom D. Spies, Associate Professor of Medicine, University of Cincinnati College of Medicine, Cincinnati, Ohio;

Dr. Howard C. Taylor, Jr., Associate Professor of Obstetrics and Gynecology, New York University of Medicine;

Dr. Willard O. Thompson, Associate Professor of Medicine, University of Illinois Medical School, Chicago, Illinois;

Dr. Eugene F. Traub, Associate Clinical Professor of Dermatology and Syphilology, Skin and Cancer Unit, Post Graduate Medical School and Hospital, Columbia University, New York, New York.

Symposia presented by local physicians and discussed by guest speakers will continue to be most practical and stimulating.

Entertainment of the visiting physicians is not to be neglected, and the unique program for the annual smoker, "Hell's Broke Loose" promises to be a most hilarious evening.

Medical meetings of this type will necessarily be curtailed during the war period, and the Clinical Society therefore urges all physicians of the Southwest to avail themselves of these opportunities as they are presented.

The registration fee of $10.00 includes ALL the general assemblies, round table luncheons, dinner meetings, post graduate courses, and smoker, for registrants from outside Oklahoma City. Additional information may be obtained from the Secretary, 512 Medical Arts Building, Oklahoma City.

NORTHEASTERN OKLAHOMA CLINICAL SOCIETY HOLDS ANNUAL MEETING IN MUSKOGEE

The Northeastern Oklahoma Clinical Society held its annual meeting at the Severs Hotel in Muskogee on the evening of July 29, 1942, with approximately 70 members and guests in attendance. The Northeastern Society is comprised of the counties in the Eighth Councilor District: namely, Adair, Cherokee, Craig, Delaware, Mayes, Muskogee, Okmulgee, Ottawa, Sequoyah and Wagoner.

The program, which was conducted by the President of the Society, Dr. Isadore Dyer of Tahlequah, was centered around the problems confronting the practice of medicine in the present war emergency. The following speakers were presented: Lieutenant Colonel Robert A. Hale, Surgeon in Charge, Camp Hospital, Camp Gruber, Okla.; Dr. W. A. Moran, Medical Director, Oklahoma Ordnance Works, Chouteau, Okla., and Dr. Henry H. Turner, State Chairman, Procurement and Assignment Committee, Oklahoma City.

Colonel Hale discussed the function of a medical officer and the various tasks assigned to him in relation to the Army. The practice of medicine in industry with particular emphasis on problems concerning employees in a chemical plant was presented by Dr. Moran. Dr. Turner stressed the function of the Office of Procurement and Assignment and also pointed out the acute need of physicians for the Army.

Guests at the meeting included ten medical officers from Camp Gruber, among whom were Colonel E. A. Devers, Camp Surgeon, and Colonel Segard, Medical Commander of the 88th Infantry Division; physicians from the Oklahoma Ordnance Works at Chouteau; Dr. W. A. Howard of Chelsea, and Dr. Finis W. Ewing of Muskogee, both Past Presidents of the Oklahoma State Medical Association; Dr. Tom Lowry of Oklahoma City, Councilor of District No. 4, and Dr. L. C. Kuyrkendall of McAlester, Councilor of District No. 9, and Dr. James Stevenson of Tulsa, President-Elect of the State Medical Association.

Arrangements for the meeting were under the supervision of Dr. W. Jackson Sayles of Miami, Secretary of the Society, and Dr. Shade Neely of Muskogee made necessary arrangements for the banquet.

Officers elected to serve for the coming year are as follows: President, Dr. M. M. DeArman, Miami; Vice-President, Dr. J. S. Allison, Tahlequah, and Secretary, Dr. H. C. Ballantine, Muskogee.

TULSA COUNTY ANNUAL GOLF TOURNAMENT

Fifty guests were present at the Annual golf tournament and banquet of the Tulsa County Medical Society on Tuesday, July 28 at the Southern Hills Country Club, Tulsa.

The W. Albert Cook trophy was won by Dr. W. J. Bryan, Tulsa, and the Scotty Taylor trophy for runner-up was awarded to Dr. Paul Grosshart, also of Tulsa.

The committee responsible for all arrangements, in behalf of this entertaining event, was composed of Dr. Carl Simpson, chairman, Dr. W. A. Showman and Dr. W. Albert Cook.

MILITARY PHYSICIANS NOT EXEMPT FROM MALPRACTICE CLAIMS

The Judge Advocate General of the Army has held that members of the Army are entitled to the same civil rights of action between one another with reference to suits for malpractice and negligence as they would have been in civil life. Therefore, Doctors in the Service cannot safely discontinue such forms of malpractice insurance protection as they previously carried in civil practice.

The Medical Officer in the Army or Navy stands in no different position with respect to answerability to his patients than that of a Physician in civil practice.

A person in the Military Service may claim that an officer of the Medical Corps has in some manner been guilty of malpractice or negligence in treating or examining him in the line of duty. A similar claim may be pressed against an examining Physician for local Selective Service Board by a selectee called before that Board. The fact that a person is in the Military Service, or is in the course of being inducted therein, does not prevent him from asserting his civil rights as long as the interests of the National Defense are not concerned.

The Judge Advocate General of the Army has indicated that it is not customary for the War Department itself to defend a civil suit for malpractice brought against a member of the Medical Corps, but that the defendant medical officer has the right to have the case removed to a Federal Court and request the Department of Justice to furnish a United States Attorney to defend him.

If, however, a judgment was to be rendered against such a medical officer defendant, there is no provision by law by which the judgment could be paid by the government, or by which the defendant physician could be reimbursed by the government. The trial of such actions in Federal Courts is provided for in the 117th Article of War.

Therefore, since patriotic cooperation may be expected from all persons and malpractice suits in the Military Service are not as frequent as in civil life, the London & Lancashire Indemnity Company has agreed to reduce all malpractice premium rates 50 percent for Physicians while in the armed forces of the United States.

If a Doctor is planning to enter the Service and at the present time already has a London & Lancashire Indemnity Company Malpractice Policy or Certificate, please notify the local insurance agent who wrote the business, or address Eberle & Company, State Managers, Midwest Building, Oklahoma City, and a rider will be attached to the Policy or Certificate allowing the reduction, and refund will be made on a pro rata basis.

DR. GEORGE OSBORN NAMED COUNCILOR SOUTHERN MEDICAL

Dr. George R. Osborn, prominent Tulsa physician, has been named to fill the vacancy as Councilor of the Southern Medical Association occasioned by the death of Dr. Robert M. Anderson of Shawnee.

Dr. Osborn will serve the two unexpired years of the original five-year term of Dr. Anderson. He will represent the state of Oklahoma at the annual meetings, the next of which will be November 10-12 at Richmond, Virginia.

The appointment was made by Dr. M. Pinson Neal of Columbia, Missouri, President of the Association. Dr. Osborn is a graduate from the University of Illinois College of Medicine in 1906, and limits his pracitce to obstetrics and gynecology. He is a past president of the Oklahoma State Medical Association and the Tulsa County Medical Society.

Dr. Paul C. Gallaher of Shawnee reported for duty on September 3 as Lieutenant, junior grade, in the United States Naval Hospital at Oakland, California. Dr. Gallaher has been classified as an assistant surgeon in the Navy.

DICK GRAHAM IN WASHINGTON AT PRESENT TIME

In January of 1939, Mr. R. H. Graham came to Oklahoma from our neighboring state of Kansas as Executive Secretary of the Oklahoma State Medical Association.

Prior to the establishment of the executive office at 210 Plaza Court, Oklahoma City, in 1939, all records of the Association were maintained in the office of the Constitutional Secretary-Treasurer. Since that time the amount of service rendered through the full-time executive office to the doctors throughout the state as well as other states has continued to increase in volume.

During the first part of August, Dick was offered an appointment as assistant to Lieutenant Commander Max Lapham, Assistant Executive Director of Procurement and Assignment Service in the War Manpower Commission, Washington, D. C., and is serving in that capacity as a loan from the Oklahoma State Medical Association at the present time.

During his absence, Miss Anne Betche, who has been Mr. Graham's secretary for the past year and a half, will be in the office of the Association and will be willing, at all times, to assist and cooperate in every way possible in serving the doctors of the State. Correspondence requesting attention from the state office may be directed to either Mr. R. H. Graham or Miss Anne Betche.

CLEVELAND COUNTY MEDICAL SOCIETY ELECTS OFFICERS

At a special meeting of the Cleveland County Medical Society on August 2, 1942, in Norman, called by Dr. M. P. Prosser, an election of officers was held to fill the unexpired terms of those elected at the beginning of the year, but all of whom are now serving in the armed forces.

The following are the newly elected officers: President, Dr. Joseph A. Rieger; Vice-President, Dr. Felix Gastineau; Secretary-Treasurer, Dr. Curtis Berry; and Delegates, Dr. Joseph A. Rieger and Dr. Curtis Berry. According to the action of the Society, another election will be held in January at which time officers for 1943 will be elected.

Prior to the August meeting, Dr. F. C. Buffington was President, Dr. M. P. Prosser was Vice-President, Dr. Phil Haddock was Secretary-Treasurer and Dr. Buffington and Dr. Haddock were the Delegates. The above mentioned have been ordered to active duty at Jefferson Barracks, St. Louis, Mo., Camp Gruber, Okla.; and Camp Claiborne, Alexandria, La., respectively.

At a recent meeting of the Pottawatomie County Medical Society held at Shawnee on August 15, 1942, the following motion was unanimously adopted by the members of the Society: ''All members of Pottawatomie County Medical Society in good standing will be retained on the rolls without payment of dues when and if they assume duties with the armed forces of the United tSates.'' Motion carried. Ten members of the Society were present at the meeting.

CHANGES OF ADDRESS

Help your State Office to maintain an accurate mailing list. Send changes of address promptly to The Journal, 210 Plaza Court, Oklahoma City, Oklahoma.

COLORADO CANCELS ANNUAL MEETING

The Seventy-Second Annual Session of the Colorado State Medical Society, scheduled to be held in the Broadmoor Hotel, Colorado Springs, on September 23-26, 1942, has been cancelled by an order of the Board of Trustees.

The Society will be called to order at 4:00 P.M., September 23, in the Shirley-Savoy Hotel, Denver, for such part of the meeting as is legally necessary. The House of Delegates will meet the same evening at 8:00 P.M., and again the following morning to transact annual business. A noon luncheon on September 24 will conclude the meeting. The Women's Auxiliary was also asked to cancel all plans except necessary meetings of business bodies.

The decisions were made primarily because of government requests that all conventions not vitally necessary to the war effort be cancelled in order to reduce unnecessary travel. Further, it was the determination of the Trustees meeting jointly with the Committee on Scientific Work, after careful study, that 25 percent of the Society's membership would be in the military service by mid-September and that most of those remaining to care for the civilian population would be too busy to attend. It was also further determined that an exceptionally small registration would be an imposition to both the speakers as well as the exhibitors.

Central Association of Obstetricians and Gynecologists Will Meet in Des Moines

The fourteenth annual meeting of the Central Association of Obstetricians and Gynecologists, on invitation of the Iowa Obstetric and Gynecologic Society, will be held at the Hotel Fort Des Moines in Des Moines, October 22-24, 1942. The program will be conducted by national leaders in these two specialties.

AMERICAN BOARD OF OBSTETRICS AND GYNECOLOGY WILL HOLD EXAMINATIONS

The next written examination and review of case histories (Part I) for all candidates will be held in various cities of the United States and Canada on Saturday, February 13, 1943, at 2:00 P.M. Candidates who successfully complete the Part I examination proceed automatically to the Part II examination held later in the year. All applications must be in the office of the Secretary by November 16, 1942.

Effective this year there will be only one general classification of candidates, all now being required to have been out of medical school not less than eight years, having in that time completed an approved one year general rotating internship and at least three years of approved special formal training, or its equivalent, in the seven years following the interne year. This Board's requirements for internships and special training are similar to those of the American Medical Association since the Board and the A. M. A. are at present cooperating in a survey of acceptable institutions. All candidates must be full citizens of the United States or Canada before being eligible for admission to examinations.

All candidates will be required to take the Part I examination, which consists of a written examination and the submission of twenty-five (25) case history abstracts, and the Part II examination (oral-clinical and pathology examination). The Part I examination will be arranged so that the candidate may take it at or near his place of residence, while the Part II examination will be held late in May 1943, in that city nearest to the largest group of applicants. Time and place of this latter will be announced later.

For further information and application blanks, address Dr. Paul Titus, Secretary, 1015 Highland Building, Pittsburgh (6), Pennsylvania.

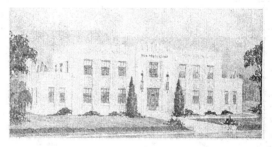

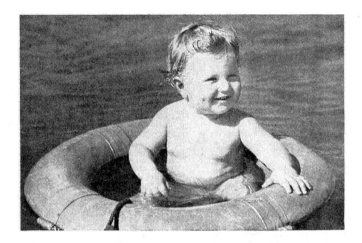

What's <u>completeness</u> got to do
with this baby's health?

THE COMPLETENESS of Biolac is a double health safeguard for infants.

Biolac provides for *all* nutritional needs of young infants, *except* vitamin C, and it requires simply dilution with boiled water. It thus minimizes the incidence of upsets arising from either formula contamination or unintentional omission by mothers of important formula ingredients.

This completeness of Biolac assures you that the baby will get *all* the nutritional elements you prescribe ... in amounts equal to or exceeding recognized requirements for optimal growth and health.

The advantages of Biolac's completeness extend also to the busy mother, whose time and energy are saved through the speed and simplicity of preparing Biolac formulas.

You'll fully appreciate the many advantages of Biolac when you prescribe it regularly in your own practice. For professional information, write Borden's Prescription Products Division, 350 Madison Avenue, New York City.

$\star$ $\star$ $\star$

Biolac is prepared from whole milk, skim milk, lactose, vitamin B_1, concentrate of vitamins A and D from cod liver oil, and ferric citrate. It is evaporated, homogenized, and sterilized.

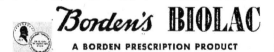

Borden's BIOLAC

A BORDEN PRESCRIPTION PRODUCT

WOMEN'S AUXILIARY NEWS

The Woman's Auxiliary is an affiliate of the American Medical Association, and is organized only to assist in its work and under its direction. The organizational structure of the Auxiliary is somewhat similar to that of the American Medical Association and its committees must of necessity outline their programs, but likewise of necessity must correlate their interlocking activities. Although there is more or less need for activities of various committees, yet each is essential to the organization. The officers and members of the board should attempt to correlate activities in order to meet the needs and the most important problems at any given time.

Auxiliary members must be familiar with the organization of the American Medical Association and with the accomplishments of the various councils, committees and bureaus, if they are to function in the true realm of an auxiliary organization and lend the greatest aid as such to the parent body. This familiarity will also permit them to be of greater assistance to their own County Medical Societies and State Medical Associations.

The national Woman's Auxiliary is now organized in 41 states and has been in existence since 1922. As early as 1917, there was an auxiliary organized in Shawnee, Oklahoma, and Oklahoma has had a state organization since 1928. At the present time, there are ten counties organized in the state, with a total membership of 360. One of the primary goals for the State Auxiliary this year is to form Auxiliaries in our unorganized counties.

TULSA COUNTY NEWS

Mrs. J. W. Childs, President of the Tulsa County Auxiliary, has been confined to her home the past month due to illness. We hope to be able to report soon that she has completely recovered.

Lieutenant-Commander and Mrs. Karl F. Swanson have moved to Corpus Christi, Texas, where Commander Swanson is serving with the United States Navy.

Dr. E. Rankin Denny, who has been commissioned a Major in the United States Army, is now stationed at Camp McCoy, Wisconsin, and Mrs. Denny and the children have joined him.

Dr. J. D. Shipp is now a Lieutenant Senior Grade, in the United States Navy, stationed at Oklahoma City, and Mrs. Shipp and the children are now making their home in Oklahoma City.

Mrs. D. L. Edwards and son expect to remain in Tulsa while Dr. Edwards is serving as a Captain in the United States Army at Will Rogers Field in Oklahoma City.

Dr. J. E. McDonald has been commissioned a Major in the United States Army Air Corps, to be located in Atlantic City, New Jersey, and Mrs. McDonald and the children will remain in Tulsa.

Dr. B. L. Branley has gone to Corpus Christi, Texas, where he is serving as Lieutenant-Commander in the United States Navy. Mrs. Branley and Judy will remain in Tulsa temporarily.

At this time, when many of our doctors and their wives are being transferred to various parts of the United States in the service of their country, it would be a fitting courtesy for our Auxiliaries to invite these "transplanted" wives to attend our Auxiliary meetings and to enjoy the fellowship of our members, as, they will be very much in need of all friendliness and courtesy we could possibly show them.

A nutrition class has been sponsored in Tulsa by the Tulsa County Auxiliary, during the summer months. Mrs. I. H. Nelson, one of the Auxiliary members, is general supervisor for the nutrition program for the Red Cross in Tulsa County. This nutrition course has been recommended by our National organization as an active part of this year's work.

LEFLORE COUNTY NEWS

The LeFlore County Auxiliary reports the following new officers: President, Mrs. E. L. Collins, Panama; President-Elect, Mrs. Neeson Rolle, Poteau; Vice-President, Mrs. S. D. Bevill, Poteau, and Secretary-Treasurer, Mrs. Earl M. Woodson, Poteau. This Auxiliary has been quite busy preparing a quota of Red Cross sweaters for shipment by August 15.

CLEVELAND COUNTY NEWS

The Cleveland County Auxiliary has sponsored a Red Cross course in home nursing, which has been taught by one of their members. This entire Auxiliary is very active in Red Cross work.

PONTOTOC COUNTY NEWS

The Pontotoc County Auxiliary reports the following new officers for the coming year: President, Mrs. M. L. Lewis, Ada; Vice-President, Mrs. W. F. Dean, Ada; Secretary, Mrs. Ollie McBride, Ada; Treasurer, Mrs. I. L. Cummings, Ada.

We have not yet received the names of the various publicity chairmen for the County Auxiliaries, and we should like very much to have these names, as well as any news they may have to send in. Please cooperate with us on this publicity, if you want your county represented on this page each month.

Two films, "The Warning" and "Defending the City's Health," are now available through the State Office of Civilian Defense for showing. These films may be utilized by County Medical Societies for their programs. For more detailed information see page 396.

Effective, Convenient and Economical

THE effectiveness of Mercurochrome has been demonstrated by twenty years' extensive clinical use.

For the convenience of physicians Mercurochrome is supplied in four forms—Aqueous Solution for the treatment of wounds, Surgical Solution for preoperative skin disinfection, Tablets and Powder from which solutions of any desired concentration may readily be prepared.

Mercurochrome, H. W. & D.

(H. W. & D. Brand of dibrom-oxymercuri-fluorescein-sodium)

is economical because solutions may be dispensed at low cost. Stock solutions keep indefinitely.

Mercurochrome is accepted by the Council on Pharmacy and Chemistry of the American Medical Association.

Literature furnished on request

HYNSON, WESTCOTT & DUNNING, INC.

BALTIMORE, MARYLAND

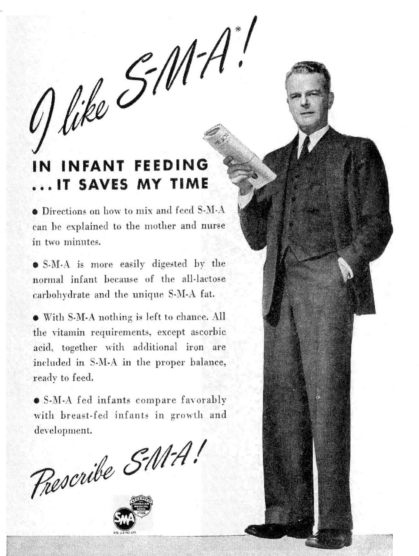

I like S-M-A*!

IN INFANT FEEDING ...IT SAVES MY TIME

● Directions on how to mix and feed S-M-A can be explained to the mother and nurse in two minutes.

● S-M-A is more easily digested by the normal infant because of the all-lactose carbohydrate and the unique S-M-A fat.

● With S-M-A nothing is left to chance. All the vitamin requirements, except ascorbic acid, together with additional iron are included in S-M-A in the proper balance, ready to feed.

● S-M-A fed infants compare favorably with breast-fed infants in growth and development.

Prescribe S-M-A!

*S-M-A, a trade mark of S.M.A. Corporation, for its brand of food especially prepared for infant feeding—derived from tuberculin-tested cow's milk, the fat of which is replaced by animal and vegetable fats, including biologically tested cod liver oil, with the addition of milk sugar and potassium chloride; altogether forming an antirachitic food. When diluted according to directions, it is essentially similar to human milk in percentages of protein, fat, carbohydrate and ash, in chemical constants of the fat and physical properties.

S. M. A. CORPORATION ▪ 8100 McCORMICK BOULEVARD ▪ CHICAGO, ILLINOIS

MEDICAL PREPAREDNESS

Questions and Answers on Procurement and Assignment Service*

Until special studies now under way are completed, it has been agreed by the Board of Procurement and Assignment Service for Physicians, Dentists and Veterinarians in answer to the question of how many people in a community can be served by one man, that for general medical service approximately one "effective" physician to fifteen hundred population is the minimum coverage that should be provided. Limited specialists are not included in the above basic figure. It is explained that a special committee of the Procurement and Assignment Service is making studies to serve as a basis for the determination of minimum quotas of medical service which should be retained for the civilian population.

The following are questions and answers contained in the special statement:

Q. Will the Procurement and Assignment Service protect a doctor from the draft?

A. The Procurement and Assignment Service was not established to protect anybody from anything. Its function is to enroll physicians, dentists and veterinarians and assign them to the positions in which their services will be of greatest value to the nation in the war emergency. This function obviously parallels the responsibilities of Selective Service, but the officials of the Selective Service have welcomed the co-operation of the Procurement and Assignment Service in dealing with these professional groups. To implement this cooperation, General Hershey issued a memorandum to Selective Service boards asking them to secure through the state director of Selective Service the recommendations of the Procurement and Assignment Service wherever they are considering the classification of a physician, dentist or veterinarian. Hence, if a doctor has enrolled with the Procurement and Assignment Service, his Selective Service board will be so advised and a recommendation for his deferment, until his services are needed in a professional capacity, will be made.

Q. Will men under 45 be called before men over that age will be considered?

A. The Army will consider applications for commission from men up to the age of 55 and the Navy up to the age of 50. The greatest need, however, is for younger men. Hence, the first call by the Procurement and Assignment Service will be for men under 36 and then men between 36 and 45 years of age.

Q. If a physician is physically disqualified for a commission, is he still subject to the draft?

A. The physical requirements for officers are higher than they are for enlisted men, but under the modified requirements for "limited service" in the Medical Corps most, if not all, physicians who meet the requirements for enlisted men will be eligible for commissions. If not, the physician concerned should consult the chairman of his State Procurement and Assignment Service Committee relative to service in a war industry or some other essential civilian service.

Q. How much consideration will be given to the choices of service listed on the enrolment form of the Procurement and Assignment Service?

A. So far as possible, the choices of service listed on the enrolment form will be given consideration. However, if the needs of the armed forces demand it, it may at times be necessary to ignore personal preferences.

Q. Do physicians in shipbuilding ad airplane factories receive any special consideration?

A. Essential medical service in vital war industries must be maintained. To do this, certain medical positions must be declared essential. Individual physicians who are of military age and physically fit for service should be declared essential in such positions only if it is impossible to replace them or have the necessary service provided by men not otherwise available for service with the armed forces.

Q. In determining the number of physicians needed to care for the civilian population, are rural communities considered on the same basis as larger cities?

A. A special committee is now working on the determination of minimum quotas of physicians for civilian medical care. In their studies consideration will be given to the density of the population, the ease of transportation, the availability of hospital service and other factors.

Q. Will doctors in draft age be called by the Procurement and Assignment Service on the basis of availability regardless of their Selective Service numbers?

A. In asking physicians to accept assignments, the Procurement and Assignment Service will select names by chance from alphabetical lists of the names of the physicians in the age group desired. Officials of national headquarters of Selective Service report that it is impossible to use Selective Service order numbers for this purpose. The first lists to be given assignments with the Army or Navy will be those who have indicated these services as their first choice.

Q. How many people in a community can be served by one man?

A. Studies are in progress by a special committee of the Procurement and Assignment Service to serve as a basis for the determination of minimum quotas of medical service which should be retained for the civilian population. Until these studies are completed it has been agreed that, for general medical service, approximately one "effective" doctor to fifteen hundred population is the minimum coverage that should be provided. Limited specialists are not included in this basic figure.

Q. Is it true that unless an intern for 1942-1943 has a commission in the Army or Navy he may be withdrawn at any time?

A. National headquarters of Selective Service has advised local boards that medical students and interns who wish deferment and are physically enabled should apply for the commissions which are available to them.

RECRUITING BOARD WITHDRAWN

The procurement of medical doctors for the Army in the State of Oklahoma has proceeded in a satisfactory manner. The Medical Recruiting Board, under the direction of Colonel Lee R. Willits, representing the Surgeon General, and Captain Oliver H. Cornelius of the Office of the Adjutant General, appointed by an order from the Adjutant General's office, Washington, D. C., as a full-time board, has been discontinued in this state and an immediate intensive recruiting drive is not anticipated.

All incomplete applications that were pending at the time of the discontinuance of the Board were forwarded to the Surgeon, Eighth Corps Service Command, Fort Sam Houston, San Antonio, Texas.

Should your application for a commission not have been completed, please address your inquiry to the Surgeon at San Antonio.

In view of this, interns who are physically fit and do not hold commissions may be subject to induction.

Q. What percentage of a man's time devoted to medical teaching is necessary to make him essential?

A. The determination as to whether an individual is an essential teacher cannot be put on a percentage basis. Some teachers on a full time basis cannot justifiably be considered essential, while others giving a much smaller proportion of time might be essential. In general, however, very special circumstances should exist to justify designating a physician of military age as an essential teacher unless he is devoting at least half time to teaching.

Q. Is the local draft board or the Procurement and Assignment Service to determine whether a doctor is necessary in his local community?

A. The legal responsibility for deciding whether any individual who is registered with Selective Service shall be given deferment rests with his local Selective Service board. However, General Hershey has directed local boards, when considering the classification of physicians, dentists or veterinarians, to secure the advice of the state committee of the Procurement and Assignment Service as to whether the individual under consideration is "essential" for the care of the civilian population in his community or whether he can be considered available for service elsewhere.

A. How many physicians are there in the United States under 35 years of age? Under 45?

A. Of the 152,923 physicians in private practice in the continental United States, 37,753, or 24.7 percent, are under 35 years of age, 35,240, or 23.0 percent, are 35-44 years of age, 24,573, or 17.4 percent are 45-54 years of age, 26,076, or 17.1 percent, are 55-64 years of age, 11,915, or 7.8 percent, are 65-69 years of age, 8,112, or 5.3 percent, are 70-74 years of age and 7,233, or 4.7 percent are 75 and over.

Q. Do you expect the needs of the armed forces to be filled by voluntary enlistment? If not, what is to be the procedure?

A. It is the firm conviction of the direction board of the Procurement and Assignment Service that the physicians of this country will willingly accept the assignments requested of them in meeting the medical needs of the nation during the war emergency. The executive order of the President establishing the Procurement and Assignment Service states that Mr. McNutt may "instruct the Agency to draft legislation, which may be necessary to submit to the Congress providing for the involuntary recruitment of medical, dental and veterinary personnel, in the event the exigencies of the national emergency appear to require it." The directing board, however, has given no thought to such legislation because it is convinced that it will not be necessary.

Q. In what grade may a doctor expect to receive a commission?

A. The policy which is being followed by the Office of the Surgeon General of the Army in making recommendations for commission is as follows:

1. All appointments must be limited to the quotas provided for medical personnel of various ranks in relation to the total over-all size of the Army.

2. All appointments in tactical units will be at minimum grades of first lieutenant, as no experience in civilian life qualifies a doctor for service in this capacity.

3. Appointments above the minimum grade will be made only on the basis of vacancies, special qualifications and there being no one qualified to fill the position by a promotion.

FIRST LIEUTENANT. All appointments under 37 will be in this rank except for individuals who possess special qualifications for a particular vacancy which exists. Certification by specialty board will be considered evidence of such special qualifications. Applicants who previously held appointments in the Medical Reserve Corps in the rank of captain may apply for reappointment at the same rank.

CAPTAIN. Initial appointees at the age of 37-45 may apply for this rank. Likewise, men under 37 with special qualifications.

MAJOR. Age 37-55. Eligible applicants must have the special qualifications required for appointment as captain and in addition experience and training which qualifies the individual as chief of a service or section, or executive of a large hospital.

LIEUTENANT COLONEL AND COLONEL. New applicants will be made in these ranks only for special assignments which cannot be filled by promotion.

Signed for the Board,

Procurement and Assignment Service,

Frank H. Lahey, M.D., Chairman.

*Taken from the Journal of the American Medical Association, Vol. 119, No. 11, July 11, 1942, Page 888.

SELECTIVE SERVICE AND ITS MEDICAL PROBLEMS

A recent announcement that a program for rehabilitation of those rejected by Selective Service as physically unfit is to be submitted to the War Manpower Commission rather than undertaken by Selective Service is commended by The Journal of the American Medical Association for August 8.

In papers presented at the annual session of the Association in Atlantic City in June and published in the August 8 issue of The Journal of the Association, Major Gen. Lewis B. Hershey, Director of Selective Service, and Col. Leonard G. Rowntree, M.D., Chief of the Medical Division of Selective Service, told of the rehabilitation program test which was conducted in Maryland, Virginia. They said that the results obtained there did not warrant the adoption of the program by Selective Service, but that rehabilitation is a method by which the nation's manpower may be made more efficient. Commenting on the announcement, The Journal says:

"Elsewhere in this issue appear two contributions of great importance to the medical profession. From the moment when Selective Service first began to function, the complete cooperation of physicians was tendered to it. The calm judgment of General Hershey and the work of his medical staff in the National Headquarters have been outstanding for their wisdom and efficiency. Although innumerable attempts have been made to stampede the Selective Service System into various welfare programs—venereal disease, prehabilitation, rehabilitation, physical fitness and what not—its leaders have held steadfastly to their main objective—the securing of a sufficient number of men sufficiently fit to meet the varying needs of the armed forces. As pointed out by both General Hershey and Colonel Rowntree, the Selective Service System has at the same time cooperated fully in maintaining both premedical and medical education, in retaining essential physicians for teaching and the civilian population, and in the conduct of pilot experiments to determine the worthiness of such programs as prehabilitation and rehabilitation is 'one of the methods by which our manpower may be made more efficient' but that 'the results obtained to date do not justify a program of physical rehabilitation by Selective Service.' The program is therefore being submitted by General Hershey to the War Manpower Commission. The medical profession will commend the type of scientific study and decision that have been exemplified by the leaders of Selective Service in this phase of their work. The procedure may well serve as a model for a functioning democracy."

E. R. Squibb and Sons of New York have recently forwarded a handbook to each of the Chiefs of Emergency Medical and Hospital Service through their field representatives. This reference book is entitled, "Physicians' Reference Book of Emergency Medical Service", and is a digest of first-hand medical experience in handling many news problems that have arisen in connection with aerial warfare.

Office of Civilian Defense

FILMS ON CIVILIAN DEFENSE AVAILABLE

The Chairman of the State Health and Housing Committee, Dr. Grady F. Mathews, has in a recent announcement to County Chiefs of Emergency Medical Service made known that two films are now available for showing without cost.

One film, entitled "*The Warning,*" portrays the reality of an air-raid on a typical British city and the destruction that accompanies it followed by the task of restoration as performed by the work of the military and organized civilian defense corps. The other film, "*Defending the City's Health,*" in which is stressed the role of the individual citizen in a health program, shows the work of a model city health department, including education, gathering statistics, nursing, supervising sanitation, laboratory analysis, child hygiene, and a comprehensive sequence on the control of communicable diseases.

The showing of these films should be under the auspices of the local Emergency Medical Service of each County Office of Civilian Defense, and need not be confined to individual groups. In addition to the personnel of the individual County Civilian Defense Committee, it is suggested that the general public be invited. In order to secure a large attendance, publicity may very nicely be conducted through the general county chairmen of civilian defense by the local publicity agent.

A representative from the State Office of Civilian Defense and necessary equipment will accompany the pictures to each county, and will do the showing unless arrangements for this service have been made through the local theaters. There is no limit to the number of showings of the films in a given county.

Showings in various counties will be scheduled according to the order in which they are received. All aplications should be sent to Committee on Health and Housing, 417 State Capitol, Oklahoma City.

RELATION OF EMERGENCY SERVICES TO INDUSTRIAL PLANTS*

The Office of Civilian Defense, Washington, D. C., in Medical Division memorandum No. 14, points out that the primary responsibility for the protection of industrial plants rests on the operators, owners and local and state governments. The War and Navy departments have included in their program the responsibility for recommending protection in certain civilian plants engaged in the production of war material. The War and Navy departments have requested all civilian manufacturing plants having important war contracts to cooperate with the local Emergency Medical Service of the U. S. Office of Civilian Defense.

All industrial plants are expected to provide medical services and first aid equipment within the plant for the care of the injured. The Office of Civilian Defense recommends that each industrial plant, in addition to providing its own medical staff and first aid equipment, should plan in collaboration with the chief of Emergency Medical Services of the locality for (1) services of ambulances and emergency medical field units when needed, (2) available beds at one or more hospitals to which the severe casualties may be transported, (3) the establishment of a casualty station of the Emergency Medical Service within a short distance of the plant and (4) obtaining the services of emergency medical field units if needed to supplement the plant medical service during an emergency.

If a plant is miles from a hospital and there is a possibility that the injured might be obliged to remain at the casualty station for hours before transfer to the hospital, the casualty station should be larger than the average for a given number of employees and be adequately equipped. It must have cots, blankets, water and heating facilities and be equipped at least with the emergency medical supplies outlined in Medical Division bulletin No. 2, equipment lists 1 and 2.

To implement these instructions, section V of Medical Division bulletin No. 4 is amended to include the following additional duties of the local chief of Emergency Medical Service:

During the period of preparation:

6. Protection of Industrial Plants. (a) Advising all employers concerning adequate emergency medical protection to be afforded within industrial, commercial and service installations, including location of casualty stations and medical supplies where needed. (b) Arranging for direct telephone lines between important installations and control center to facilitate evacuation of casualties and to provide emergency medical service with the minimum of delay.

*Taken from the Journal of the American Medical Association. Vol. 119, No. 16, Page 1378, August 15, 1942.

Conference on Venereal Disease Control Needs in Wartime

Venereal disease and America's war effort will be discussed by high-ranking medical officers of the War and the Navy Departments, prominent physicians, health officers and others at a Conference in Hot Springs National Park, Arkansas, October 21-24, 1942. Headquarters will be at the Arlington Hotel.

The Conference will be held under the auspices of the United States Public Health Service in conjunction with the Eighth Annual Meeting of the American Neisserian Medical Society, Surgeon General Thomas Parran will preside. State and local health officers, venereal disease control officers, practicing physicians, and all others engaged in venereal disease control activities are urged to attend.

Subjects for discussion will include venereal disease control measures influencing the war effort, epidemiology of syphilis and gonorrhea—1942, wartime venereal disease control education, research influencing the wartime venereal disease control program, and technics of venereal disease education.

Governmental, professional and health organizations to be represented at the Conference include: the War Department, the Navy Department, the Social Protection Section of the Office of Defense Health and Welfare Services, the American Medical Association, the American Neisserian Medical Society, the American Social Hygiene Association, State and local health departments, and the United States Public Health Service.

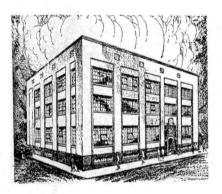

University of Oklahoma School of Medicine

There have been a number of changes in the Faculty of the School of Medicine, due to resignations and leaves of absence. Leaves of absence have been granted to all of the members of the Faculty who enter the Army or the Navy. The resignations from the Faculty have been among the full-time members. Dr. I. S. Danielson, Associate Professor of Biochemistry, has resigned to accept a position with Lederle Laboratories. Dr. Carl Bunde, Assistant Professor of Physiology, resigned to accept a similar position at Baylor University Medical School. Dr. Irwin C. Winter, Associate Professor of Pharmacology, resigned to accept a position with the Council on Pharmacy and Chemistry of the American Medical Association. Dr. Alton Clair Kurtz has been appointed as Assistant Professor of Biochemistry. Dr. Kurtz is coming here from the University of Pennsylvania, where he has been on the faculty of the school of medicine. Dr. O. Boyd Houchin has been appointed Instructor in Pharmacology. Dr. Houchin just recently completed his training at the State University of Iowa.

The first year class which will report for their physical examinations on September 10, 1942, and who will enroll on September 11 and 12, consists of seventy-five (75) residents of the State of Oklahoma. No non-residents have been admitted to the first year class on account of the large number of qualified residents of the State that have applied for admission. It is assumed that all of the accepted applicants will enroll.

A considerable number of repairs have been made to the School of Medicine Building during the summer months. One of the most important items was the correction of the acoustics in the auditorium of the Medical School Building.

General Robert U. Patterson, Dean of the School of Medicine, is vacationing in California during part of the month of August.

• OBITUARIES •

Resolution
Dr. J. C. Bushyhead
1870-1942

WHEREAS, Dr. J. C. Bushyhead had long been among us and had, at all times, taken a very active part in his chosen profession, and in all civic programs of our community, and

WHEREAS, Dr. J. C. Bushyhead has served his profession as President of our local organization at various and sundry times, and

WHEREAS, Dr. J. C. Bushyhead has given unstintingly of his time and ability to the people of our community regardless of financial conditions, and

WHEREAS, through his cheerful manner and gracious attention to his patients, everyone in and out of the profession had learned to love him,

THEREFORE; BE IT RESOLVED by the Rogers County Medical Association that in the death of Doctor Bushyhead the Medical Profession has lost a stalwart member, the community a great character, and his wife and family a devoted and loving husband and father.

BE IT FURTHER RESOLVED: That a copy of these resolutions be spread on the minutes of the Rogers County Medical Association, a copy furnished the family, and a copy given to the press.

George D. Waller, M.D.
Secretary.

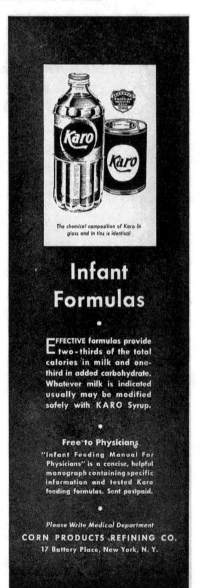

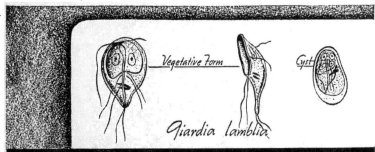

COUNTY HEALTH SUPERINTENDENTS

County	Superintendent	Address	Director Of County Unit Or District	Address	No. of Counties In Organized Unit Or District
Adair	Church, R. M.	Stilwell	Gray, James K.	Tahlequah	4
Alfalfa	Lancaster, L. T.	Cherokee	None		
Atoka	Huntley, H. C.	Atoka	Huntley, H. C.	Atoka	1
Beaver	Long, L. L.	Beaver	Nicholson, J. L.	Guymon	3
Beckham	Baker, L. V.	Elk City	None		
Blaine	Anderson, H. R.	Watonga	Anderson, H. R.	Watonga	1
Bryan	Sizemore, Paul	Durant	Sizemore, Paul	Durant	1
Caddo	Preston E. Wright	Anadarko	Preston E. Wright	Anadarko	1
Canadian	Johnson, A. L.	El Reno	None		
Carter	Canada, J. C.	Ardmore	Canada, J. C.	Ardmore	1
Cherokee		Tahlequah	Gray, James K.	Tahlequah	4
Choctaw	Gregg, O. R.	Hugo	Gregg, O. R.	Hugo	2
Cleveland	Gertrude Nielsen	Norman	Gertrude Nielsen	Norman	1
Cimarron	Hall, H. B.	Boise City	Nicholson, J. L.	Guymon	3
Coal	Hipes, J. J.	Coalgate	None		
Comanche	Gerchick, E. H.	Lawton	Gerchick, E. H.	Lawton	1
Cotton	Baker, G. W.	Walters	None		
Craig	McPike, Lloyd	Vinita	None		
Creek	Shryock, L. F.	Sapulpa	Shryock, L. F.	Sapulpa	1
Custer	Cushman, H. R.	Clinton	None		
Delware	Prowell, J. W.	Kansas	Gray, James K.	Tahlequah	4
Dewey	Seba, W. E.	Leedy	None		
Ellis	Beam, J. P.	Arnett	Murray, F. L.	Arnett	2
Garfield	Rempel, P. H.	Enid	None		
Garvin	Monroe, H. H.	Pauls Valley	None		
Grady	Renegar, J. F.	Tuttle	None		
Grant	Hardy, I. V.	Medford	None		
Greer	Lowe, J. T.	Mangum	None		
Harmon	Lynch, R. H.	Hollis	None		
Harper	Winchell, F. Z.	Buffalo		Woodward	2
Haskell	Rumley, J. C.	Stigler	None		
Hughes	Floyd, W. E.	Holdenville	None		
Jackson	Spears, C. G.	Altus	None		
Jefferson	Derr, J. I.	Waurika	Highfill, F. W.	Duncan	2
Johnston	Looney, J. T.	Tishomingo	Joseph, Phillip	Madill	3
Kay	Gardner, C. C.	Ponca City	None		
Kingfisher	Meredith, A. O.	Kingfisher	Meredith, A. O.	Kingfisher	1
Kiowa	Watkins, B. H.	Hobart	None		
Latimer	Harris, J. M.	Wilburton	None		
LeFlore	Wright, R. L.	Poteau	Wright, R. L.	Poteau	1
Lincoln	Norwood, F. H.	Prague	None		
Logan	Anderson, R. W.	Guthrie	Anderson, R. W.	Guthrie	1
Love	Gray, W. J.	Marietta	Joseph, Phillip	Madill	3
McClain	McCurdy, W. C.	Purcell		Purcell	1
McCurtain	Williams, R. D.	Idabel	Gregg, O. R.	Hugo	2
McIntosh	Little, D. E.	Eufaula	None		
Major	Johnson, B. F.	Fairview	None		
Marshall	Holland, J. L.	Madill	Joseph, Phillip	Madill	3
Mayes	Brown, J. W.	Pryor	Brown, J. W.	Pryor	1
Murray	Stover, G. W.	Sulphur	None		
Muskogee	William P. Parker	Muskogee		Muskogee	1
Noble	Frances, J. W.	Perry	None		
Nowata	Roberts, S. P.	Nowata	None		
Okfuskee	Spickard, L. J.	Okemah	None		
Oklahoma	Hunter, George	Okla. City	Hunter, George	Okla. City	1
Okmulgee	Peter, M. L.	Okmulgee	Peter, M. L.	Okmulgee	1
Osage	Aaron, Wm. H.	Pawhuska	None		
Ottawa	Hughes, A. R.	Miami	None		
Pawnee	Jones, R. E.	Pawnee	None		
Payne	Moore, C. W.	Stillwater	Moore, C. W.	Stillwater	1
Pittsburg	Dorrough, J.	McAlester	None		
Pontotoc	Mayes, R. H.	Ada	Mayes, R. H.	Ada	1
Pottawatomie	Haygood, C. W.	Shawnee	Haygood, C. W.	Shawnee	1
Pushmataha	Patterson, E. S.	Antlers	None		
Roger Mills	Cary, W. S.	Reydon	Murray, F. L.	Arnett	2
Rogers			None		
Seminole	Shanholtz, M. I.	Wewoka	Shanholtz, M. I.	Wewoka	1

County	Superintendent	Address	Director Of County Unit Or District	Address	No. of Counties In Organized Unit Or District
Sequoyah	Newlin, W. H.	Sallisaw	Gray, James K.	Tahlequah	4
Stephens	Highfill, F. W.	Duncan	Highfill, F. W.	Duncan	2
Texas	Lee, Daniel S.	Guymon	Nicholson, J. L.	Guymon	3
Tillman	Childers, J. E.	Frederick	None		
Tulsa	Presson, L. C.	Tulsa	None		
Wagoner	Riddle, R. K.	Coweta	None		
Washington	Shipman, W. H.	Bartlesville	None		
Washita	Weaver, E. S.	Cordell	None		
Woods	Templin, O. E.	Alva	None		
Woodward	Rutherford, V. M.	Woodward			2

Management of Cancer

The underlying principle of the modern management of cancer is coordinated team work. It is improbable that any one man can perform all the duties and carry out all the techniques required. Any organization that sets itself up to manage cancer must contain at least a surgeon, a roentgenologists and a pathologist. This is the minimum requirement in personnel. There should also be added to the group an internist to advise concerning the diagnosis of cancer in deeper organs, and specialists who devote attention to each particular part of the body for advice in connection with tumors in special locations. It would be well also to have on such a team a chemist and a physiologist. These could offer many helpful suggestions concerning special features of this disease. Each member of the team should have equal standing. Each should be considered as a consultant who is able to add something to the full understanding of cancer and to its management in any particular patient.—James P. Simonds, M.D., Chicago, Ill., Med. Jour., Vol. 81, No. 5.

Opportunities for Practice

An excellent opportunity for practice at Wetumka, Oklahoma, a town of 2500 population in Hughes county, has been reported to the office of the Association. Anyone interested in locating there and establishing a practice should communicate with Mr. Don C. Wright, Secretary, Chamber of Commerce, Wetumka.

A capable, well-trained physician in good health ineligible for military service is wanted to take charge of a well-established practice in a completely equipped office. No investment is required. For further information contact Nathan Horowitz, M.D., 2715 Jensen Drive, Houston, Texas.

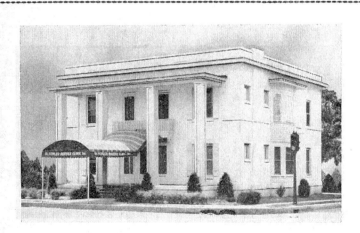

DR. FOWLER BORDER CLINIC

330 N. W. 10th Street — Phone 7-7777 — Oklahoma City, Oklahoma

BOOK REVIEWS

"The chief glory of every people arises from its authors."—Dr. Samuel Johnson.

"THE MODERN ATTACK ON TUBERCULOSIS." Henry D. Chadwick, M.D., and Alton S. Pope, M.D. Cloth. Pp. 95. The Commonwealth Fund, 41 East Fifty-Seventh Street, New York. Price $1.00.

This little volume of 95 pages constitutes a veritable compendium of the important facts having to do with the control of Tuberculosis. In the preface the Authors disclaim "any pretense of adding to the sum of our knowledge of Tuberculosis" but rather attempt to show that we have sufficient information to eradicate the disease in "a few generations if the established techniques are effectively applied."

In six streamlined chapters, stripped of all unnecessary details, the program proceeds with striking speed and simplicity and yet with the convincing promise of effectiveness.

In the reading, one is impressed with the authenticity and directness which comes only from personal experience supplimented by a profound knowledge of the accumulated experience of those who have gone before.

This valuable work should be read by every doctor and every individual interested in the control of Tuberculosis.—Lewis J. Moorman, M.D.

"STANDARD NOMENCLATURE OF DISEASE AND STANDARD NOMENCLATURE OF OPERATIONS." Edwin P. Jordon, M.D., American Medical Association, 535 North Dearborn Street, Chicago. 1942. Cloth. Pp. 1022.

The Third Edition of this important work presents accumulated knowledge and accepted standards to date.

Following the introduction, there is a short illustrated chapter designed for the instruction of Record Librarians.

One hundred pages are devoted to the Schema of Classification. Approximately 500 pages are devoted to the Nomenclature of Disease. This is followed by supplementary list and an index to the Nomenclature of Disease.

Following the index there is an alphabetical list of Eponymic Diseases. In the latter part of the book the Nomenclature of Operations is similarly treated. This section is also adequately indexed.

This volume should be in every doctors office, on the desk of every hospital record room and in the hands of every Medical Record Librarian.—Lewis J. Moorman, M.D.

"THE BIOLOGICAL ACTION OF THE VITAMINS." E. A. Evans, Jr. Cloth. Pp. 225. The University of Chicago Press, 5750 Ellis Avenue, Chicago, Illinois.

This volume edited by E. A. Evans, Jr., presents the Neutritional knowledge having to do with vitamins in Epitome. Fortunately it comes from the press at a time, when neutritional values are being recognized as of great importance not only by the Medical profession and other scientists but by the laity as well. It is

doubtful if anything of equal importance has come into the field of medicine since Pasteur's discovery of the bacterial cause of disease. One cannot read the scientific discussions assembled in this volume without being impressed with the vast amount of laboratory and clinical research, already devoted to this subject, and the tremendous store of accrued knowledge. Much of this knowledge is of practical value as clearly shown by the discussions on clinical application.

It is essential that the members of the medical profession keep abreast of the rapid progress in this field. Because of the present world crisis the average layman is rapidly accumulating knowledge of Neutrition through civilian defense neutrition classes. This growing store of information plus much misinformation about vitamins makes it essential for the average physician to acquire a working knowledge of vitamins and to develope a level vision with reference to their clinical application.

A careful perusal of the works presented in this little book will materially aid in the attainment of these two purposes.

The scope of these discussions may be partially appreciated by a glance at the table of contents. "The Biological Action of The Vitamins", by C. A. Elvehjem, Ph.D.; Cocarboxylase, by S. Ochoa, Ph.D.; Vitamin B: Clinical Aspects, by Norman Jolliffe, M.D.; Riboflavin, by Paul Gyorgy, M.D.; Human Riboflavin Deficiency (Ariboflavinosis), by W. H. Sebrell, M.D.; The Story of Pellagra and Its Treatment with Nicotinic Acid, by Davis T. Smith, M.D.; Pyridoxine, by S. Lepkovsky, Ph.D.; Pantothenic Acid and the Microbiological Approach to the Study, of Vitamins, by Roger J. Williams, Ph.D., D.Sc.; Pantothenic Acid in Human Nutrition, by Edgar S. Gordon, M.D.; Biotin, by Vincent du Vigneaud, Ph.D.; Chlorine, by Wendell H. Griffith, Ph.D.; The Economy of Phosphorus in the Animal Organism, by Franklin C. McLean, Ph.D., M.D.; Vitamin K, by D. W. MacCorquodale, Ph.D.; Vitamin K: Clinical Aspects, by H. P. Smith, M.D., and E. D. Warner, M.D.

Though much has been accomplished and much anticipated from investigations under way, the authors admit that the field lies fallow before them and that the future should bring valuable revelations.—Lewis J. Moorman, M.D.

"THE PREMATURE INFANT." Julius H. Hess, M.D.,Professor and Head of the Department of Pediatries, University of Illinois College of Medicine, and Evelyn C. Lundeen, R.N., Supervisor, Premature Infant Station, Sarah Morris Hospital, Chicago. Cloth. Price $3.50. Pp. 350, with 77 illustrations: Philadelphia: J. B. Lippincott, 1941.

This book should be in the library of every physician and nurse caring for prematures, in every training school and pediatric ward library, in fact it is a "must" book for every one doing any work with premature infants. The authors are doing outstanding work in

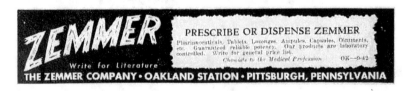

saving many of these small babies and in training others in their technic. In this book they discuss the physical development, growth of the infant and care both in the home and in the hospital entirely from the angle of the premature rather than the average infant. An important chapter is the one on transporting the baby from the home to the hospital. Every public health nurse should read this very carefully.

The methods of feeding the premature infants are carefully outlined, not only concerning the kind and amount of milk but also the complete procedure. This is something that is too often passed over with little thought, especially in hospitals giving no special care to the prematures.

This book is the most complete and satisfactory available on the premature. It should be available to everyone working with these small infants.—Clark H. Hall, M.D.

"WHITE EAGLE—CHIEF OF THE PONCAS." Charles LeRoy Zimmerman, M.D. Telegraph Press, Harrisburg, Pa. Pp. 273. Cloth. 1941.

Here is an interesting book with attractive format and many photographs and drawings. It is of genuine historic value and contains a wealth of information, not only about the Ponca Indians but about other tribes as well. It is of general interest to all Oklahomans because it is so intimately identified with the people and soil of this section. It is of particular interest to doctors because it is written by a doctor who once lived in Oklahoma and because it contains a chapter on The Medicine Man and a graphic description of his life, on the plains while serving as agency physician for the Poncas. Here again we see the combination of religion, magic and superstition as in primitive medicine.

In addition to treatment of the sick it was the duty of the medicine man to conduct the dances and paint the bodies of warriors before battle. He employed "roots, herbs, barks, twigs, seeds and flowers and some minerals. His treatment was partly mystic and partly medicinal and physical, while his supernatural incantations included in his medicine a bundle of certain sacred objects. He also used sweat or vapor baths made by dropping heated stones in water."

By placing his mouth over parts of the patient's body the evil spirits were sucked out and driven away by the rattling of gourds. The medicine man successfully treated injuries, fractures and wounds. Since the Indians accepted sickness as punishment for sins, their mental conditions usually responded to the medicine man's incantations. In the management of contagious disease they were lost as they knew nothing of isolation and prophylaxis.

Also of Medical interest is the chapter on "Peyote, Its History and Use." And, finally the "Personal Experiences of the Agency Doctor" gives a very good picture of country practice in the "horse and buggy" days.—Lewis J. Moorman, M.D.

Physicians Should Be Alert As Citizens

It is important for medical men and women to remember that the maintenance of high standards of medical practice and service—in unsettled times such as the present—requires that every physician shall not only be a competent Doctor of Medicine but that he and she shall also be high-class citizens, meaning, thereby, that every physician shall take a real interest in trends of a political nature—national, state, and local—and so be on guard against activities that might lead to a breaking down of public health and medical practice standards that have been proven of real value in the past.—California and Western Medicine.

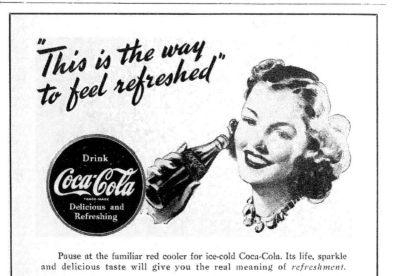

How One Should Select a Physician

"The Standards by which a physician can be measured are furnished by the medical profession. The way to judge a doctor is the way doctors judge each other. It is severe," Green Williams, Chicago, points out in the June issue of Hygeia, The Health Magazine, in an article enumerating some of the many factors that should be taken into consideration in selecting a physician. "The medical profession has set high standards for its members. . . .

"Let us first consider what we have a right to expect from a man who assumes the responsibility for health and disease. A noted specialist told me that he demands three things from his fellow physicians and surgeons in this order:

"1. Honesty. Faith in one's doctor is often more important to recovery than the treatment he prescribes, but it is false security if the physician is dishonest in his claims, intent, diagnosis, treatment, or fees. . . .

"2. Service. Careful examinations take time. You want a doctor who will give you enough attention to leave the smallest possible likelihood that he has missed some significant sign or symptom, as well as to relieve your psychologic anxieties.

"3. Knowledge. When you see a physician you want everything that is known in medical science about the detection, prevention and cure of your ailment to be brought to bear on your case. Some might place knowledge first, but the specialist put it third because you cannot get the benefit of existing knowledge unless the physician is honest (keeps within the limits of scientific knowledge) and gives you service (allows himself to apply his knowledge)."

To this list of characteristics Mr. Williams says that he would add a fourth quality—generosity. "While this is implicit in the humanitarian nature of medical care," he declares, "I know of no quality more desired by the patient in his doctor.

"The basic problem of the cost of medical care is economic, of course, but more patients would get what they can pay for if generosity, like honesty, did not suffer from selfishness. . . ."

In order to be most certain that a physician measuring up to these standards is selected, the author advises that "You should investigate the man you want to become your doctor, using the standards by which the medical profession judges its members.

"First there are the formal standards set by the American Medical Association. . . . The American Medical Association, more than any other agency, must be credited with raising the quality of medical practice in this country. It has set high standards of education, training, and experience for physicians. . . ."

In addition to the formal standards of the American Medical Association, such as graduation from a recognized medical school and membership on the staff of a hospital approved by the American Medical Association, Mr. Williams says that there are additional informal standards by which the physician can be judged. These include lack of advertising on the part of the physician of his name, specialty, methods, cures, or low fees in any commercial way; the dignity sobriety, and modesty with which he conducts himself before his patients; the neatness and cleanliness of his office and of his person; the efficiency with which he keeps his case records, and the amount of respect he receives from other doctors.

"A good doctor," Mr. Williams observes, "will not charge you too much. . . . Always ask the doctor his fees for any medical care he proposes to give you and always tell him your financial status. Doctors' fees are more or less standardized according to the patient's income, and the best is not likely to charge you more than the worst for a given treatment or operation. . . ."

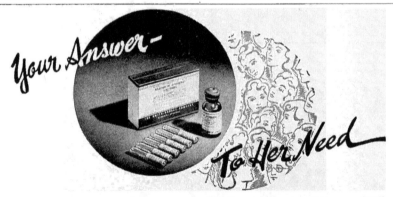

MEDICAL ABSTRACTS

"TRANSPLANTATION OF FIBULA FOR NONUNION OF TIBIA; REPORT OF CASE." M. S. Henderson and W. H. Bickel. Proceedings Staff Meetings Mayo Clinic. XVI, 510, 1941.

The authors report a case of a compound, comminuted fracture of the left tibia and fibula in the upper third, which was treated outside of the Clinic in 1937. In 1940 the roentgenogram of the left leg revealed a nonunion of an old comminuted fracture of the upper third of the tibia and fibula, with the loss of about one inch of bone, and that the head of the fibula was united by bony fusion to the superior lateral aspect of the tibia.

An osteotomy of the fibula was done, and it was swung against the tibia after the lateral surface had been freshened. It was held there by a Parham band. Five months later the leg felt solid. It was also stated that the Parham band was to be removed after there was solid union.

If there is non-union of the tibia, and the fibula is intact, there are two methods of choice: (1) an autogenous bone graft, (2) Huntington's operation.

Huntington's operation is the transplantation of the fibula to the tibia in two stages, fusing the upper end first.

"THE SEQUELAE TO INJURIES OF THE BONES AND JOINTS." St. J. D. Burton. The Medical Press and Circular. CCV, 376, 1941.

Early undesirable sequelae following injuries may be lessened by operative treatment as soon as shock is relieved, by better immobilization, and limitation of the wound dressings.

Wounds involving the shoulder joint may leave some stiffness, but even with complete bony ankylosis there remains little disability if it occurs in the ideal position (60 degrees abduction, 30 degrees external rotation, and elbow forward).

Elbow wounds frequently result in stiffness. If ankylosis is expected, the forearm and arm should form an angle of 120 degrees. The forearm should not be fixed in complete pronation. About half way between this and complete supination is preferable, and leaves the hand that can be used in most trades.

Hand wounds are always serious. Fingers, if ankylosed, should be in slight flexion.

Hip-joint injuries are always serious. Visceral complications, extensive suppuration, and, with healing, traumatic arthritis or anyklosis usually occur.—E. D. Mc., M.D.

"TREATMENT OF INTRACAPSULAR FRACTURES OF THE FEMORAL NECK." A. S. Blundell Bankard. The Lancet. I, 250, Feb. 28, 1942.

The author does not present a series of cases, but indicates some points which seem to call for further consideration if the Smith-Petersen nail or similar devices are to be placed on a surer basis. In discussing the selection of cases, the author points out several feasible contra-indications for nailing, and in some instances he feels that it is better to do a transtrochanteric osteotomy at once, rather than to wait for the failure of a nailing operation. He recalls that the impacted subcapital abduction fracture always heals with bony union if it is treated in a short walking plaster spica, and he suggests that weight-bearing on an impacted fracture is not in itself harmful, so long as the joint is

not moved, and he considers whether this has any bearing on the treatment of abduction fractures after internal fixation. He questions whether, in fact, the nailed abduction fracture should not be treated in the same way as the impacted abduction fracture,—in a short walking plaster spica. When cases unsuitable for nailing have been eliminated, the principal causes of failure are: imperfect reduction of the fracture, faulty application of the nail, and inappropriate after-care. In reducing the fracture, he feels that well-leg counter traction is the best method, as this can be adjusted at leisure, and when the reduction is perfect the patient can be lifted safely on the operating table with the traction still on the limb. In inserting the nail, he points out that the more vertically the nail is placed, the less will be the breaking strain across it, and the more will the proximal fragment be guided towards and pressed against the distal fragment by pressure from above, and he states that the best angle for the nail is one of 140 degrees with the long axis of the shaft of the femur. He points out that a nail can hold fragments apart as well as hold them together. He feels that the common practice of forbidding weight-bearing for some months after the operation while encouraging active movement of the hip should be reconsidered, and he gives reasons for believing that early weight-bearing should be encouraged while movement of the hip should be prevented until bony union has taken place. He outlines his technique for the nailing operation, and points out the importance of anchoring the proximal fragment to the pelvis while the nail is being driven in, in order to avoid displacement of the head by the oncoming nail. The article is most timely and contains many excellent suggestions.

"THE KENNY TREATMENT OF INFANTILE PARALYSIS DURING THE ACUTE STAGE." Philip Lewin. Illinois Medical Journal. LXXXI, 281, April, 1942.

In this article, Dr. Lewin gives a clear and accurate analysis of the Kenny method of treatment, to which he has given study and personal observation in different clinics in which it has been used. He states the principles and the method of application of the treatment, the technique of which he discusses in detail, and makes a fair and unprejudiced estimate of the results obtained. He discusses and interprets the theory of Miss Kenny's method, which is aimed at: the abolition of muscle spasm, the substitution of mental "awareness" for the pathological "alienation," and the restoration of co-ordination of muscle activity, and includes:

1. Proper bed placement—natural rest position.

2. A foot board to preserve the "standing reflex".

3. Hot fomentations to relieve pain and muscle spasm.

4. Special analysis, classification, and reeducation of muscles.

5. Passive movements.

6. Concentration of active movements on the insertions of muscles and tendons.

7. The abandonment of all splints, respirators, and artificial feeding.

Dr. Lewin's discussion of the theory of muscle spasm, rather than paralysis, is particularly helpful. He expresses a very favorable opinion of the Kenny treatment, as shown by her results, and in his summary he states that it is one of the outstanding advances in orthopaedic surgery.—E. D. Mc., M.D.

"HEMOLYTIC TRANSFUSION REACTIONS. II. PRE-VENTION, WITH SPECIAL REFERENCE TO A NEW BIOLOGICAL TEST." Alexander S. Wiener, I. Jerome Silverman and William Aronson. American Journal of Clinical Pathology, Volume 12, Number 5, May 1942.

In this the authors have added an additional step in connection with the problem of hemolysis following transfusion in instances where the ordinary cross matching and blood grouping tests have indicated compatibility. The authors insist that the old procedure sponsored particularly by Oehlecker, to inject a small amount of blood, about 10 cc. and then wait ten minutes before proceeding is not satisfactory in the case of hemolysis because clinical symptoms may be entirely absent or occur as long as one hour after the transfusion.

The following so-called biological test has been proposed. It has been used by the author for the past one year in cases in which the possibility of intragroup incompatibility was suspected.

One hundred cc. of the prospective donor's blood are drawn from the patient and divided between two tubes, one empty and the other containing 1 cc. of the citrate solution. Through the same needle 50 cc. of the donor's blood are injected by syringe. After one hour, 10 cc. of the blood are again drawn from the patient and treated in the same way as the pretransfusion sample. The citrated blood samples are centrifuged at once and the color of the plasma in the two tubes compared.

The serums from the clotted blood samples are later separated, after the blood has firmly clotted, this serving as a check on the results of the tests with the citrated blood samples. The purpose of the duplicate test is to avoid the occurrence of an artefact due to traumatization of the red blood cells, particularly when separating the clot from the wall of the tube. Naturally, care must be taken that the needles and syringes used for the test are perfectly dry.

If there is no change in the appearance of the patient's plasma, and the need for blood is urgent, one can then proceed with the transfusion of larger amounts of blood from the same donor. When time permits, however, it is preferable to inject another test dose of 50 cc. of the donor's blood and to draw a third sample of blood after an additional hour. In this way more reliable results can be obtained and the reaction in positive cases is more striking. A further refinement of the test, though this is not essential, is to select a donor who differs from the patient with respect to the M-N type. After 100 cc. of the donor's blood have been injected in the manner outlined above, it should be possible to determine the survival of the donor's cells by the method of differential agglutination where the biological test is negative, in patients having a red cell count of 2.5 million or less, as was previously pointed out.

In positive reactions, one hour after the test-injection of 50 cc. of blood, the patient may have a severe chill and rise in temperature, but the clinical symptoms may be quite mild and occasionally they may be entirely absent. Therefore more reliance is to be placed on the appearance of the patient's plasma, which will show a distinct rise in the icteric index as compared to the pretransfusion sample. Inasmuch as the rise in icteric index from the hemolysis of only 50 cc. of blood is relatively small, the final figure may still be within normal limits, even though it is twice as high as the pre-transfusion value.

The donor's blood used for the biological test should be fresh; if only bank blood is available, no sample more than three days old should be used. The reason for this is that blood stored for periods longer than seven to 10 days, even though apparently intact when transfused, often breaks down rapidly in the patient's circulaton. In this way a positive biological reaction might be obtained even with serologically compatible blood.

Two cases illustrating a positive and negative result each are reported and the question of multiple sensitization in patients having intragroup hemolytic reactions is discussed.

Comment: This is a very timely and important report. Much attention to the matter of intragroup hemolytic reactions is now being given by clinical pathologists and earnest endeavors are being made to devise tests which are practical and scientifically satisfy for the determination of the Rh and other isoagglutinin properties.—H. J., M.D.

"PRIMARY SPLENIC NEUTROPENIA." A Newly Recognized Syndrome, Closely Related to Congenital Hemolytic Icterus and Essential Thrombocytopenic Purpura. B. K. Wiseman and C. A. Doan. Annals of Internal Medicine, June, 1942, Vol. 16, Number 6, Page 1097.

This is a report of a condition which appears to have been previously unrecognized and in connection with the study of the so-called primary splenic neutropenia the authors have contributed considerable to the mystery and contraversies concerning the physiology of the spleen.

Anatomical facts are reviewed, the reticuloendothelium is discussed and that which appears to be a very ingenuous chart illustrating the function of the spleen is given. Five cases are reported in satisfactory detail.

These studies suggest that splenectomy is a definite indication and has proven to be curative. The condition is not to be confused with Banti's disease since in none of these has there been portal obstruction. The dominant findings are leucopenia, myeloid hyperplasia, hemolytic anemia and thrombocytopenia with splenomegaly. Purpur occasionally develops. Leukemia presents the most difficult differential diagnosis.

"THE CLINICAL VALUE OF STERNAL BONE MARROW PUNCTURE." Theodore H. Mendell, David R. Meranze and Theodore Meranze. Annals of Internal Medicine, June, 1942, Volume 16, Number 6, Page 1180.

The occasion for and the development of the more or less recent widespread application of sternal puncture and bone marrow studies is given. Different methods are mentioned and the results of a "three-fold" study analyzed. The studies are as follows: (1) To determine criteria of normal sternal marrow. (2) To study marrow of all cases showing disorders of the reticulo-endothelial system. (3) To correlate marrow studies with underlying disease. (4) The findings in 115 normal cases are tabulated and interesting reports are made in connection with the study of cases as pernicious anemia, anemia pregnancy, iron deficiency anemia, anemias due to hemorrhage, anemia of thrombocytopenic purpura, anemia in carcinoma, anemia due to sulfanilamide, anemias of infection, aplastic anemia, chronic benzol poisoning, Colley's anemia, polycythemia vera, splenic anemia, leukemia, infectious mononucleosis, amidopyrine granulopenia, multiple myelomata, Hodgkin's disease, trichinosis and malignancy. Negative marrow findings are also discussed.

Conclusions are as follows:

1. Bone marrow puncture is a simple, adequate and safe method of studying the living marrow. It is usable at all age periods and in all disease processes.

2. Bone marrow puncture is of inestimable value in the diagnosis and prognosis of diseases of the blood-forming organs.

3. It is of especial importance in excluding diseases of the blood-forming organs as a diagnostic possibility in many obscure conditions.

4. It provides material for an appraisal of the potentialities of the bone marrow.

5. It should, therefore, be considered as an essential adjunct in the study of any hematologic problem.

6. A series of 300 sternal punctures performed on nearly as many patients over a period of three years, chiefly in diagnostically uncertain cases, is presented to illustrate the above principles.—H. J., M.D.

"FAMILIAL DEGENERATION OF THE MACULA LUTEA. A REVIEW OF THE LITERATURE WITH A REPORT OF EIGHT ADDITIONAL CASES." Joseph William Crawford, San Francisco. American Journal of Ophthalmology, 1942, ser. 3, vol. 25, page 525-543, May.

Familial macular degeneration is the bilateral, symmetrical degeneration of the macular region of the eyes. It affects one or several children of a family, but the parents are usually free of the disease. Only exceptionally is another generation of the family affected. The disease is believed to be congenital, and is familial rather than hereditary in type.

The condition is chronic, manifesting a few signs or symptoms at the onset, and progressing to a serious impairment of central vision, after which it remains stationary. There is little impairment of peripheral vision, and complete blindness never occurs. It is strange that the vision is usually better in a dim light. The first case has been reported by Knapp in 1870. Later, other cases with definite familial character have been described by Batten, Stargardt, Lutz, Oatman, Stirling, and others.

The ophthalmoscopic picture is that of a localized retinal atrophy limited to the macular region. The early ophthalmoscopic signs indicate an alteration of the retinal pigment. In those in whom the condition had existed for some time there is in each macular area a region, usually horizontally oval, varying in size from 0.75 to 2 discs diameters, having well-demarcated borders, the entire area appearing to be slightly depressed. The background is of a salmon-pink color. In the well-advanced cases in which the depigmentation is complete, the choroidal vessels are exposed.

Scattered about the retina, and extending well beyond the area described, are small, pale, light spots, somewhat resembling drusen in appearance, lying beneath the retinal vessels situated in the deeper retinal layers. These probably represent colloid bodies. Optic atrophy may occur as a secondary manifestation of the retinal degeneration; it has been observed by others. There are no signs of inflammation, exudates, or hemorrhages, and the peripheral retina appears to be normal. The central vision of most patients is reduced to 6/60. Many of the patients are able to read newspaper print if it is held very close to the eyes.

No case has been reported that ended in blindness. In most patients, some central vision is retained, and in all cases normal peripheral vision remains. Vision with reduced illumination is amazingly good, and out of all proportion to the objective signs.

The etiology of the condition has not been determined. Consanguinity, race, the health of the parents, and the like could not be regarded as etiologic factors. The unaffected children in the family differ in no wise from their unfortunate brothers and sisters. The disease should be differentiated from four other conditions: cerebromacular degeneration, retinitis pigmentosa, retinitis punctata albescens, and central choroiditis. There is no successful treatment of this condition. In the author's series the disease appeared before the onset of puberty.
—M. D. H., M.D.

"CHEMOTHERAPY IN THE TREATMENT OF GONORRHEAL OPHTHALMIA; RELATIVE EFFECTIVENESS OF SULFANILAMIDE, SULFAPYRIDINE, AND SULFATHIAZOLE." Robert T. Wong, Honolulu. Archives of Ophthalmology, vol. 27, page 670-687, April, 1942.

For the past four years there have been numerous reports published describing the excellent effects of sulfanilamide therapy in gonorrheal ophthalmia. On the other hand, many reports mentioned unsatisfactory results.

The cases included in the author's study are only those in which the diagnosis of gonorrheal ophthalmia was confirmed by the demonstration of gram-negative intracellular diplococci of typical structure and distribution in stained smears of conjunctival secretions or epithelial scrapings.

Various compounds have been used for treating the cases. The dose of sulfanilamide and of sulfapyridine for infants and children was 0.2 gramm per kilogram of body weight per day. For infants the dose of sulfathiazole was 0.3 gramm per kilogram of body weight per day. There were only two adults in the entire series. They were treated with sulfapyridine and were given 4 grammes of the drug daily. The patients treated with sulfapyridine and sulfathiazole were given an initial dose of one-half the daily dose. It was considered best to give enough of the drug to maintain a level in the blood of 5 to 10 mg per 100 cc. Larger doses of sulfathiazole than of sulfanilamide and sulfapyridine were required to maintain an adequate concentration in the blood.

The drug was given at four hour intervals. In the case of infants it was dissolved and administered with the feedings. Alkalis were not given with the drug. The parenteral method of administration was not used. Sulfanilamide was given for three or four days and sulfapyridine and sulfathiazole for one or two days after all evidence of inflammation had subsided and three consecutive daily negative smears had been obtained, in order to forestall any possibility of recurrence.

The routine adjuvant treatment was as follows: (1) irrigations with warm boric acid solution were given often enough to keep the cul-de-sac free of secretion. These were usually done every three hours for the first two or three days and three or four times daily when the discharge began to subside.

(2) Metaphen in a dilution of 1:2,500 (aqueous) was instilled in the cul-de-sac after every irrigation. (3) Foreign protein in the form of sterile milk was administered in some cases but was omitted in others. (4) When corneal involvement was noted, atropine sulfate solution was given in sufficient dose and strength to keep the pupils dilated.

In the sulfathiazole group the only adjuvant treatment was boric acid irrigations given for four times a day for the first or second day and then only once or twice daily for the remaining two or three days of treatment.

The criteria of cure consisted of (1) arrest of discharge and subsidence of the inflammation, (2) obtaining three consecutive daily negative smears of the conjunctival secretion and (3) in the sulfathiazole group obtaining of one negative epithelial smear besides the negative smears of the secretion.

About a week after discharge from the hospital patients were seen again, and examined for evidence of recurrence.

The results of treatment with sulfanilamide are in agreement with those of previous reports. In 18 cases cure was effected within eight days. In two cases the condition was refractory. In one, 28 days of treatment was required, while in the second the cure was effected in 14 days. Such refractoriness is fairly common.

The results of treatment with sulfapyridine indicate that it was more effective than sulfanilamide. On the basis of this study, sulfathiazole seems to be superior to both sulfanilamide and sulfapyridine. In seven striking cases the gonococci disappeared from the secretion within twelve to twenty-four hours after treatment was instituted. In all cases the swelling and inflammation subsided and the discharge lessened within twelve hours. The average time required for cure was three and four-tenths days, and the maximum time was four days.

It can be concluded that sulfathiazole is the compound of choice not only because of its therapeutic efficiency but because of the low incidence of toxic reactions encountered in its use.—M. D. H., M.D.

"OTORHINOGENIC MENINGITIS; A REPORT OF FIFTY-EIGHT CASES." Herman J. Burman, Michael Rosenbluth, and Daniel Burman, Chicago. Archives of Otolaryngology, vol. 35, page 687-719, May, 1942.

Meningitis is still the most frequent fatal complication of suppurative disease of the ears and sinuses. In reviewing 160 consecutive cases of meningitis in patients seen at the Harlem Hospital, the authors found an otorhinogenic focus in 30.2 percent.

Rhinogenic intracranial complications result most frequently during the course of an acute lesion, in contradistinction to otogenic intracranial complications, which are said to occur most often during the course of chronic otitis media.

Infection of the meninges may result when microorganisms enter the arterial stream from the accessory sinuses or the temporal bone, are carried to all parts of the body and are arrested ·in the small pial arteries. When infection around the veins of the mucosa occurs, bacterial toxins transfuse through the vessel wall and, injuring the endothelial lining of the vessel, produce a thrombus, which becomes infected and advances by retrograde extension to cause meningitis.

Infection of the meninges may take place also through the ductus endolymphaticus, which connects the endolymphatic space of the labyrinth with the dura in the posterior cranial fossa, through the aqueduct of the cochlea. In only a small number of cases can a microscopic lesion in the paranasal sinuses be demonstrated as a probable focus of infection.

Microscopic bony defects, when they occur and produce an avenue for infection, are invariably traumatic in origin and most often result from intranasal operation.

Generally, the diagnosis of meningitis is not difficult because the clinical picture develops fairly rapidly and is rather impressive. In Type III Pneumococcus infection the clinical symptoms may be almost absent. The symptoms are influenced largely by whether actual systemic involvement, limited meningeal irritation or increased intracranial pressure predominates. The disease is frequently ushered in by a feeling of malaise. Headaches are common and are dull and persistent. Postauricular pain is moderate and persistent in cases of otitic origin, and there may be a dull, heavy sensation between the eyes in the case of rhinogenic infection. Transitory severe neuralgias are common, and various palsies of the cranial nerves and labyrinthine disturbances may appear.

When a discharge from the nose or ears has been present it frequently diminishes, although occasionally it may increase in quantity. Impaired hearing and tinnitus are often noted and may be severe. Vision may be impaired and examination of the eyegrounds show evidence of intracranial pressure. The patient may or may not complain of pain in the neck but does not have stiffness of neck until the cisterna magna becomes involved.

Of all the laboratory tests at one's disposal, examination of the spinal fluid is the most important. The type of meningitis present may be suspected from the appearance of the spinal fluid. But a cloudy fluid in itself does not mean generalized meningitis.

With the advent of chemotherapy the outlook in cases of bacterial meningitis has improved in spectacular fashion. The results in the authors' series show a 60 percent rate of cure in cases of otogenic and a 33 percent rate in cases of rhinogenic meningitis. In those cases of bacterial meningitis in which no other focus is apparent the infection should be suspected of emanating from the ear, nose or throat, and all pertinent clinical and laboratory investigations should be made.

Although cures have been reported from the use of chemotherapy alone, the best results have been obtained with the combination of surgical treatment, chemotherapy, and administration of serum in properly selected cases. The drainage of a demonstrable or suspected focus is an accepted surgical principle. The advice that the first symptom of meningitis is the last summons to operate is still an acceptable dictum. Operation should be carried out in every case of meningeal disease in which otologic or rhinologic involvement is suspected.

Intranasal operation on the sinuses in cases of meningitis is not as satisfactory as the external approach and the policy is now adopted of performing the so-called radical ethmo-spheno-frontal sinus operation whenever these sinuses are affected. The mastoid wound should not be left open but filled with sulfanilamide powder.

The efficacy of drug therapy depends largely on the extent of the pneumatization of the mastoid, and this accounts for its relative inefficiency in the treatment of the well ventilated accessory sinuses of the nose, the air cavities permitting the collection of large amount of infected inert exudate.

Because a complication frequently develops suddenly, the protection afforded by chemotherapy should be provided as an initial step in the treatment. The masking of symptoms which occurs with chemotherapy apparently can be interpreted as a desirable effect, indicating a definite limitation of the infectious process. The masking of symptoms by chemotherapy differs from the masking of pain by sedatives inasmuch as the disease itself is actually impeded.

With so many cases of recovery from meningitis, one must guard against presuming that the cure was effected by chemotherapy alone. One is likely to disregard the fact that a focus has been eradicated and surgical drainage established. Therefore, with the admitted benefit to be derived from chemotherapy, the patient is entitled to the additional advantage to be obtained from the elimination of a focus of infection.

It is to be emphasized that when there is bone necrosis, abscess formation or pooling of purulent material in air cavities, sulfanilamide and its derivatives will be ineffective unless the diseased areas are surgically evacuated.

In Pneumococcus meningitis serum may be also used. Such a treatment is always advisable. The specific type rabbit serum in average dose of from 250,000 to 725,000 U.S.P. units is administered intravenously. It may be found eventually that chemotherapy alone, that is without serum, may be equally effective. In influenzal meningitis, sulfanilamide seems to have given the best results. In staphylococcic meningitis, sulfathiazole is the most efficient.—M. D. H., M.D.

"NASOPHARYNGEAL FIBROMA." Hans Brunner, Chicago. Annals of Otology, Rhinology, and Laryngology, vol. 51, page 29-65, March, 1942.

In connection with reporting several cases, the author studies the pathogenesis of those tumors. The tumors originate in the nasopharynx as well as surrounding the choanae, and their matrix is probably the buccopharyngeal fascia. The microscopic picture of the tumors is approximately the same as that of the fascia basalis.

There is no existing treatment which could be called perfect. At present, the treatment consists chiefly of the application of radium and surgical diathermy. This combined treatment offers by far the most satisfactory therapeutic approach. The most important advantage of this type of treatment is the possibility to avoid severe hemorrhages.

The author favors surgery in the following types of cases: (1) in older individuals, (2) in very large tumors. More conservative measures seem to be indicated in the following cases: (1) patients who suffer from a severe hemorrhage in taking biopsy, pointing out the possible difficulties which might arise during an operation; (2) cases which offer a doubtful microscopic finding of biopsy suggesting a sarcomatous degeneration of the tumor; (3) a poor general condition of the patient, which would permit surgery only after a preliminary building-up of the patient; (4) recurrence of the tumor, which can be more readily managed by radium and surgical diathermy, provided it does not reach a considerable size; and (5) sign of intracranial involvement, making the outlook questionable for any form of treatment.—M. D. H., M.D.

KEY TO ABSTRACTORS

E. D. M. ....Earl D. McBride, M.D.
H. J. ....Hugh Jeter, M.D.
M. D. H. ....Marvin D. Healey, M.D.

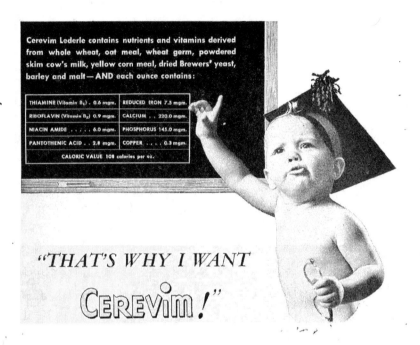

Cerevim Lederle contains nutrients and vitamins derived from whole wheat, oat meal, wheat germ, powdered skim cow's milk, yellow corn meal, dried Brewers' yeast, barley and malt—AND each ounce contains:

THIAMINE (Vitamin B_1) . . 0.6 mgm.	REDUCED IRON 7.5 mgm.
RIBOFLAVIN (Vitamin B_2) 0.9 mgm.	CALCIUM . . 220.0 mgm.
NIACIN AMIDE . . . . . 6.0 mgm.	PHOSPHORUS 145.0 mgm.
PANTOTHENIC ACID . . 2.8 mgm.	COPPER . . . . 0.3 mgm.
CALORIC VALUE 108 calories per oz.	

"THAT'S WHY I WANT CEREVIM!"

CEREVIM is enriched with thiamine, riboflavin, niacin, calcium pantothenate, calcium and iron; and contains in each one-ounce serving the complete daily recommended allowances* for thiamine, riboflavin, niacin and iron for infants and children 1 to 3 years of age, in addition to the other nutrients listed above.

The ingredients of Cerevim are blended uniformly in a precooking process. Cerevim is an excellent source of the vitamin B complex and iron. It is a good source of calcium. Cerevim contains 19.4% protein.

The chemical components and the vitamin content of CEREVIM are checked regularly at the Lederle Research Laboratories, where biological chemists collaborate in new investigations designed to keep pace with developments in the field of nutrition.

Specify *Lederle*

*As recommended by Committee on Foods & Nutrition, National Research Council, May, 1941.

OFFICERS OF COUNTY SOCIETIES, 1942

——Indicates serving in Armed Forces.

COUNTY	PRESIDENT	SECRETARY	MEETING TIME
Alfalfa	*Jack F. Parsons, Cherokee	L. T. Lancaster, Cherokee	Last Tues. Each 2nd Mo.
Atoka-Coal	J. B. Clark, Coalgate	J. S. Fulton, Atoka	
Beckham	H. K. Speed, Sayre	E. S. Kilpatrick, Elk City	Second Tues. eve.
Blaine	Virginia Olson Curtin, Watonga	W. F. Griffin, Watonga	
Bryan	A. J. Wells, Calera	W. K. Haynie, Durant	Second Tues. eve.
Caddo	Fred L. Patterson, Carnegie	C. B. Sullivan, Carnegie	
Canadian	P. F. Herod, El Reno	A. L. Johnson, El Reno	Subject to call
Carter	Walter Hardy, Ardmore	H. A. Higgins, Ardmore	
Cherokee	Park H. Medearis, Tahlequah	*Isadore Dyer, Tahlequah	
Choctaw	C. H. Hale, Boswell	Fred D. Switzer, Hugo	
Cleveland	Joseph A. Rieger, Norman	Curtis Berry, Norman	Thursday nights
Comanche	George S. Barber, Lawton	W. F. Lewis, Lawton	
Cotton	George W. Baker, Walters	Mollie F. Scism, Walters	Third Friday
Craig	W. R. Marks, Vinita	J. M. McMillan, Vinita	
Creek	Frank Sisler, Bristow	*O. H. Cowart, Bristow	
Custer	Richard M. Burke, Clinton	*W. C. Tisdal, Clinton	Third Thursday
Garfield	D. S. Harris, Drummond	John R. Walker, Enid	Fourth Thursday
Garvin	T. F. Gross, Lindsay	John R. Callaway, Pauls Valley	Wed before 3rd Thurs.
Grady	D. S. Downey, Chickasha	Frank T. Joyce, Chickasha	3rd Thursday
Grant	I. V. Hardy, Medford	E. E. Lawson, Medford	
Greer	G. F. Border, Mangum	J. B. Hollis, Mangum	
Harmon	S. W. Hopkins, Hollis	W. M. Yeargan, Hollis	First Wednesday
Haskell	William Carson, Keota	N. K. Williams, McCurtain	
Hughes	Wm. L. Taylor, Holdenville	Imogene Mayfield, Holdenville	First Friday
Jackson	J. M. Allgood, Altus	*Willard D. Holt, Altus	Last Monday
Jefferson	W. M. Browning, Waurika	J. I. Hollingsworth, Waurika	Second Monday
Kay	J. C. Wagner, Ponca City	J. Holland Howe, Ponca City	Third Thurs.
Kingfisher	C. M. Hodgson, Kingfisher	*John R. Taylor, Kingfisher	
Kiowa	J. M. Bonham, Hobart	B. H. Watkins, Hobart	
LeFlore	G. R. Booth, LeFlore	Rush L. Wright, Poteau	
Lincoln	E. F. Hurlbut, Meeker	C. W. Robertson, Chandler	First Wednesday
Logan	William C. Miller, Guthrie	J. L. LeHew, Jr., Guthrie	Last Tuesday evening
Marshall	J. L. Holland, Madill	O. A. Cook, Madill	
Mayes	L. C. White, Adair	V. D. Herrington, Pryor	
McClain	B. W. Slover, Blanchard	R. L. Royster, Purcell	
McCurtain	R. D. Williams, Idabel	R. H. Sherrill, Broken Bow	Fourth Tues. eve.
McIntosh	F. R. First, Checotah	William A. Tolleson, Eufaula	Second Tuesday
Murray	P. V. Annadown, Sulphur	F. E. Sadler, Sulphur	
Muskogee	L. S. McAlister, Muskogee	D. Evelyn Miller, Muskogee	First & Third Mon.
Noble	J. W. Francis, Perry	C. H. Cooke, Perry	
Okfuskee	J. M. Pemberton, Okemah	L. J. Spickard, Okemah	Second Monday
Oklahoma	R. Q. Goodwin. Okla. City	Wm. E. Eastland, Okla. City	Fourth Tuesday
Okmulgee	J. G. Edwards, Okmulgee	*John R. Cotteral, Henryetta	Second Monday
Osage	C. R. Weirich, Pawhuska	George K. Hemphill, Pawhuska	Second Monday
Ottawa	J. B. Hampton, Commerce	Walter Sanger, Picher	Third Thursday
Pawnee	E. T. Robinson, Cleveland	Robert L. Browning, Pawnee	
Payne	John W. Martin, Cushing	*James D. Martin, Cushing	Third Thursday
Pittsburg	Austin R. Stough, McAlester	Edw. D. Greenberger, McAlester	Third Friday
Pontotoc	R. E. Cowling, Ada	*E. R. Muntz, Ada	First Wednesday
Pottawatomie	John Carson, Shawnee	Clinton Gallaher, Shawnee	First & Third Sat.
Pushmataha	P. B. Rice, Antlers	John S. Lawson, Clayton	
Rogers	*W. A. Howard, Chelsea	George D. Waller, Claremore	First Monday
Seminole	H. M. Reeder, Konawa	Mack I. Shanholtz, Wewoka	
Stephens	A. J. Weedn, Duncan	W. K. Walker, Marlow	
Texas	L. G. Blackmer, Hooker	*Johnny A. Blue, Guymon	
Tillman	C. C. Allen, Frederick	O. G. Bacon, Frederick	
Tulsa	H. B. Stewart, Tulsa	E. O. Johnson, Tulsa	Second & Fourth Mon. eve.
Wagoner	J. H. Plunkett, Wagoner	H. K. Riddle, Coweta	
Washington-Nowata	*R. W. Rucker, Bartlesville	J. V. Athey, Bartlesville	Second Wednesday
Washita	A. S. Neal, Cordell	James F. McMurry. Sentinel	
Woods	W. F. LaFon, Waynoka	O. E. Templin, Alva	Last Wednesday
Woodward	M. H. Newman, Shattuck	C. W. Tedrowe, Woodward	

THE JOURNAL

OF THE

OKLAHOMA STATE MEDICAL ASSOCIATION

| VOLUME XXXV | OKLAHOMA CITY, OKLAHOMA, OCTOBER, 1942 | NUMBER 10 |

Isolation As An Aid in Treating a Mental Patient*

CHARLES E. LEONARD, M.D.

OKLAHOMA CITY, OKLAHOMA

It has been customary for many years to incarcerate people who are suffering from mental troubles in asylums especially built for that purpose.

At the beginning, the reason was primarily one of protecting the general public from a person possessed of the devil. As time passed it was found that this type of incarceration also protected the patients from themselves.

As psychiatry developed and scientific research advanced in the mental institution, it was discovered that the friendly neutral protective atmosphere of the institution was conducive to recovery of the mental patient.

It was not, however, well explained until the advent of Freud's dynamic psychology, how the early childhood environment of the patient was conducive of mental disorders and the isolation away from the family and the regular environmental situation was helpful in relieving the anxiety and tension of the patient, and thus favoring recovery.

Until the advent of shock therapy and psychotherapy, along with hydrotherapy, the isolation treatment was the only useful measure of the psychiatrist; and since the coming of the shock and psychotherapy, the value of isolation has increased. In psychiatry, even more than in general medicine, it is important to be able to treat the patient without the emotional interferences of the family.

Anna Freud, in her book on Child Analysis, makes the statement that unless the analyst has full cooperation of the parents, which is almost impossible to secure, the analysis is much more satisfactory if the child is removed from the home environment.

Doctor Weir Mitchell, in the early days of psychiatry discovered that rest and isolation

*Read before the Section on Neurology, Psychiatry and Endocrinology, Annual Session, Oklahoma State Medical Association, April 24, 1942.

of the patient were fundamental in the treatment of nervous disorders, and the so-called "rest cure" arose out of these findings.

It is also quite evident that the emotional reactions of different members of the family are quite often severe, and the patient's awareness of these reactions adds to the intensity of the symptoms, as seen in behavior problems in childhood. In fact, this influence is so obvious in work with children that the Institute for Juvenile Research at Chicago runs a social service child placement bureau to get the patient away from the home environment while under treatment.

In many instances, an abnormal dependent relationship to a mother or father is the dominant emotional factor in certain types of mental illnesses, especially in those in which the patient is suffering from an exaggerated childlike dependence upon the parent, and the anxiety pertaining to fear of being left alone arises out of this preverted dependence.

This was clearly shown in the case of an elderly lady who had been bed-ridden for seven years. She had been under the care of twenty doctors, and had been in ten different hospitals, one of these being a mental institution. She had developed various hypohondriacal complaints over the years, along with the inability to walk, except when the husband was behind to catch her if she fell. The husband and sister waited on her hand and foot and never left her alone. So even while suffering, she received an enormous amount of gratification, as her unconscious wishes for love and dependency were fulfilled. The recovery was facilitated when the husband's and sister's confidence was gained and they refrained from visiting the patient, until she could see that she was using her symptoms to gain a childlike gratification.

In other cases, there is an abnormal hostile

feeling toward a close acquaintance or relative, which in essence constitutes the illness per se. This is well demonstrated by the case of a young married woman who entered the hospital in an acute anxiety state, which was precipitated by her dog, who had developed rabies, being shot.

Her anxiety was associated with the fear that her two adopted children might have been bitten by the dog and maybe they would die. Under hospital routine and psychotherapy her anxiety was soon quieted until she saw her children one morning on her way to occupational therapy. The anxiety immediately returned and it was only with continued isolation that psychotherapy was able to continue until the patient gained insight into her hostility.

In other instances, obsessions, compulsions, phobias, and even hallucinatory experiences arise out of a perverted hostility directed toward a member of the family.

Another case that illustrates this is that of a fifty-year old male who developed anxiety over rather upsetting nightmares. He was taken for psychotherapy without hospitalization for a short time, but during this period the material he brought in was highly symbolic and disguised and could not be interpreted. Other than recognizing a strong competitive drive, the material was sterile for all useful purposes. Upon isolation in the hospial for a few weeks the unconscious material opened up and showed his strong jealousy of his son and his desire to compete with and dispose of his rival.

In some of Freud's earlier works, he cites a case of an extremely sick obsessive girl who came to him for psychoanalysis at the mother's request. The girl was very repressed and infantile and as soon as her life situation with reference to the mother was revealed by the analysis, she told the mother. The mother reacted with intense hostility, stopped the analytical treatment and shamed the girl for revealing the family secrets, until the girl finally became psychotic and was institutionalized and pointed to as another failure of analysis. If this case could have been isolated, the results probably would have been quite different.

In starting psychotherapeutic or analytic treatment on any case, it is always most important to evaluate the need of isolation in being away from relatives or family or in an institution. In fact, it may be stated that an important practical criterion with reference to prognosis in mental disorders consists of the attitude that relatives have toward the recommendation for isolation of the patient. For example, if a mother refuses to permit a daughter to enter a hospital for isolation but will permit the daughter to enter a hospital

for treatment, provided that she can have a bed in the same room with the patient; as a rule the illness in the daughter is one of insidious onset, usually of long standing, and the prognosis is unfavorable. The daughter is usually an inhibited character filled with hostility which she cannot express, except in her psychotic delusions.

On numerous occasions, it is the experience of any psychiatrist to be confronted with perhaps several members and even acquaintances who protest isolation of the patient. This likewise indicates the existence of a malignant and serious mental disturbance in the patient, with poor prognosis. On the other hand, proper cooperation and manifest emotional stability in the relatives toward psychiatric treatment of the patient contribute to a favorable prognosis. There are, of course, exceptions to the above, and the rule is applicable especially to the so-called "functional" types of nervous disorders.

It is, I think, the universal experience of all psychiatrists, that numerous mentally ill patients can be helped and would probably adjust to a fairly normal pattern of life if the environment that the patient must return to could be controlled.

I have in mind one girl who is now sitting in the back ward of one of our State Hospitals, because of the hostility and refusal of cooperation by the mother. The patient had made a nice remission to intensive insulin shock and psychotherapy. The home situation was studied. The mother was interviewed and found to have an enormous amount of jealousy and unconscious hostility toward the daughter. It was recommended that the patient be sent to an uncle in a different state where the environment would be more or less neutral and at least pleasant. The mother agreed, took the patient home and through various processes of rationalization, managed to keep the patient with her until the patient slipped back into her psychosis and had to be returned to the hospital.

It is a common experience of all psychiatrists to see a patient come out of a catatonic stupor only to return to it within an hour or so after a visit with the family or relatives.

In recommending isolation for a patient suffering from a mental illness one must be doubly cautious that he understand the unconscious dynamics of the case, or great harm can be done in certain types of cases when a so-called "rest cure" is recommended, and the patient is told to go on a fishing trip or vacation, with or without company. As a rule a patient who is sick enough for that advice, is sick enough for supervised isolation in a mental hospital. It is impossible for one to run away from one's own emotions, and unless the doctor is fully aware of what the unconscious emotional conflict is, it is best not to take a chance by permitting his patient to go on a vacation which may lead to his suicide.

One case that illustrates this very nicely is that of a brother of a nurse, who had developed an acute anxiety attack. Hospitalization was recommended, but the patient's family refused this, as he was not psychotic at that time, and they could not be convinced that a mental hospital was for all mental illnesses and not just the psychoses.

He was sent on a vacation with the sister on recommendation of the family and the second day out was found hanging by a bed sheet to a hook in the clothes closet.

I could cite numerous other cases, that, while not ending in suicide, returned with symptoms greatly intensified, which undoubtedly prolonged their stay in a mental hospital.

It has been our experience that the facilities of a general hospital are such that proper isolation in most instances cannot be executed. It has been suggested by some that the larger general hospitals should have psychiatric department and that facilities should be constructed in connection so that mental patients could be cared for there. Unfortunately, however, in accordance with the concept mentioned above, there continues to be such a fear of mental disease and such a persistent tendency on the part of relatives to deny the existence of mental disturbance; that the general hospital continues to indulge this attitude on the part of the general public and are of the opinion that the proximity to the surgical, obstetrical and the medical patients is exceedingly undesirable. Most general hospitals usually accept all patients, but as a rule call for help if psychiatric symptoms become manifest. Perhaps there is more than just the economic justification for this, because individuals suffering from major or even minor physical disturbances are concomitantly suffering from emotional reactions to the organic illness, hence, proximity of these potential psychiatric disorders to a ward of noisy patients would only serve to abet and exaggerate mental symptoms in the general hospital patient that might not otherwise occur.

Therefore, so long as the present attitude of general hospitals and physicians toward neuro-psychiatric disorders exists, mental hospitals would seem to be a necessity. By this it is meant those mental hospitals that actively engage in the treatment of psychiatric diseases exclusive of those patients who become custodial problems and must be relegated to mere custodial type of care. The large state institutions have shown great progress in recent years in the matter of properly isolating mental cases with a favorable prognosis from those who are incurable so that the patient who has been to a state institution can leave without carrying away unpleasant and traumatizing memories of his experience in the institution.

The mental hospital is a definite entity in the armamentarium of the psychiatrist in treatment of these disorders. It is striking to note how quickly many of the excruciating symptoms quickly disappear merely under the influence of sanatarium routine and isolation from the family. Recent studies are beginning to reveal that although shock treatment results in a shortening of the duration of the illness; that the ultimate recovery rate statisically remains about the same whether the patient is given shock treatment or whether the patient is subjected to routine sanitarium care without shock therapy.

It is quite often hazardous for the patient to be subjected to the home environment while attempting to carry out psychotherapeutic measures. This is especially true in the analytic types of psychotherapy in which the patient is burdened both with aggravation of the home environment in addition to material that is emerging under the technique of analytic treatment.

A careful appraisal of the intensity of symptoms arising out of a reaction of the patient to environment must be made.

Of course, there are selected types of character problems and neurotic disorders that can be cared for without resorting to institutional treatment. In fact some of these respond better to purely office treatment. In most instances, the general practitioner is successful in managing these cases. There are exceptions to this, but these are rather rare and it is for this reason that the extramural private practice of psychiatry necessitates such a high degree of specialization.

It is important that this type of psychiatric specialist be exceedingly cautious in selecting the patients for treatment without the aid of hospital facilities.

Many of the acute neuroses and psychoses and borderline states will be resolved quickly under hospital management whereas without the latter months or even years of treatment are carried out erroneously. The latter results in an unfortunate depreciation of the psychiatrist in the eyes of the general practitioner.

The elimination of these factors by hospital care in many instances result in a quick alleviation of symptoms and affords the opportunity of spontaneous recuperative powers so that the illness subsides in a matter of a few days or a few weeks, whereas without hospital care the illness might last for months or years or become incurable.

SUMMARY

This paper has been presented for the purpose of showing the importance of isolating certain types of mental cases from their environment while undergoing various types of treatment for emotional disorders.

Various cases have been presented to show the results of isolation during treatment, and the ill effects of procrastination.

While isolation in a mental institution is not necessary in every case, it is an important adjunct to the armamentarium of the psychotherapist.

Clinical Diagnosis of Ulcer of Meckel's Diverticulum*

JOHN G. MATT, M.D.

TULSA, OKLAHOMA

Uncomplicated Meckel's diverticulum has been described as occurring in 1.5 to 3 percent of all persons. Normally the vitelline duct undergoes complete obliteration during the seventh week of embryonic development, but the duct, or segments of it, may persist. When this remnant of the primitive duct ventral to the ileum persists, it forms what is called Meckel's diverticulum. The diverticulum is usually located on the anti-mesenteric surface of the ileum, from 12 to 50 inches proximal to the cecum. It most commonly runs from ½ to seven or more centimeters in length and its shape may vary from a mere out-pocketing of the ileum to that resembling the vermiform appendix. The diverticulum usually hangs free, but sometimes it may be found bound down to the surface of the ileum by adhesions or reduplication of the serosa. A few cases of intra-mesenteric diverticuli have been reported. Frequently a firm fibrous cord extends from the tip of the diverticulum to the umbilicus, or in the absence of the fibrous cord it may be directly attached to the navel which then often is the site of a tiny fistula or cyst. Heterotopic tissue is present in approximately 25 percent of all Meckel's diverticuli. When present, the heterotopic tissue usually lines the greater portion of the diverticulum, often involving the neck of the sac.

Numerous theories have been proposed in attempting to explain the presence of such aberrant tissues as gastric, duodenal and pancreatic tissue "rests". Albrecht[1] propounded the first and most commonly accepted theory which maintains that the entoderm lining the primitive intestinal tube possesses the ability to develop into any of the glandular tissues of the mature gastro-intestinal tract. Shaetz[2] theorized that during early

embryonic life there might be a transference of entodermal cells lining the primitive intestinal tube, due to the rotating movements of the embryo, causing reimplantation of these cells at narrowed points in the intestinal tract. Farr and Penke[3] suggest that the vitello-intestinal duct originally may have had a digestive function and hence constitutes a complete primitive digestive system. Greenblatt, Pund and Chaney[4] have proposed the theory of "dysembryoma" in which they agree with Albrecht that the entodermal lining does form cell groups which function as a distinct primitive digestive system such as Farr and Penke suggest. However, they go one step farther in stating that while normally this embryonic system retrogresses as soon as its function ceases, at approximately the seventh week of the life of the embryo, occasionally "a vestige of heterotopic tissue remains as a consequence of retarded embryological retrogression of the omphalo-mesenteric duct." Certainly the nutritive elements within the early yolk sac are assimilated by the embryo through the vitelline circulation, hence it would be reasonable to suppose that these elements must be acted upon by the cells of the vitelline duct in some manner analogous to passage of food through the upper digestive tract before it is absorbed by the cells of the jejunum and ileum of the fully matured intestinal tract.

Greenblatt and his associates emphasize the difficulty of making a correct diagnosis because the various symptom combinations of the different types of pathological diverticuli may closely imitate some of the more commonly encountered acute abdominal conditions. From an analysis of a series of cases observed at the University Hospital of the University of Georgia School of Medicine, they have classified Meckel's diverticuli into six groups, as shown in the following table:

*Read at Tulsa County Medical Society Meeting, May 11, 1942.

Group	Findings	Symptomatology
Peptic	Gastric Mucosa.................without ulcer / with ulcer / ulcer and hemorrhage / ulcer and perforation	May simulate duodenal ulcer. History of intestinal hemorrhage. Peritonitis due to perforation.
Obstructive	Intussusception / Volvulus / Bands and adhesions / Contents of inguinal or femoral hernia	Signs and symptoms of intestinal obstruction may vary from chronic to acute; partial to complete obstruction.
Diverticular	Simple acute inflammation / Acute with perforation and gangrene / Chronic inflammation	Symptomatology is essentially that of appendicitis.
Umbilical	Fecal fistula / Umbilical adenoma / Prolapse of intestine through umbilical fistula	Lesions of umbilicus often associated with underlying omphalomesenteric duct.
Tumor	Benign.................enterocystoma / carcinoid / adenoma / mesodermal tumors / Malignant.................carcinoma / sarcoma / Heterotopic.................pancreatic tissue / embryonal rests	
Incidental	Normal intestinal structure	None

Clinically, the diagnosis of groups two, three, five and naturally, six, is practically impossible because these conditions offer no clear cut differential sign that might enable one to rule out the more common abdominal conditions. The diagnosis of the umbilical group is often made possible because the presence of fistulas, cysts or tumors of the umbilicus so frequently accompany a patent omphalomesenteric duct within the abdominal cavity. The diagnosis of the lesions in the peptic group can frequently be made, as we will attempt to show. The cardinal symptoms and signs are: (1) a history of intermittent massive intestinal hemorrhage; (2) an average age of from one to 15 years; and (3) mild colicky abdominal pain developing *after* the appearance of the bloody stools.

Practically all authorities agree that the outstanding symptom of peptic ulcer of a Meckel's diverticulum is hemorrhage. It was present in 90 percent of the 34 cases reported by Greenwald and Steiner.[5] In five of these cases it was the only symptom noted, and extended over a period of from one day to nine months. In a second group of five cases the primary symptom was hemorrhage subsequently followed by abdominal pain. The hemorrhages were of longer duration in this group and were present for from two months to four years. Of a group of 77 histologically proven cases reviewed by the author[6], 16, or approximately 20 percent, contained no mention of intestinal hemorrhage having been present. An analysis of

these 16 cases revealed the interesting observation that in all but three of them the ulcers had perforated and either local or general peritonitis was present at the time the patients were first examined, so that very likely the emergency of an acute abdomen had so prejudiced the examiner's questioning that a cursory history had not elicited the presence of abdominal hemorrhage at some time prior to the existing grave condition.

The history given is usually that of previous intestinal hemorrhages followed by a relatively long period—months and even years—before recurrence. Usually the hemorrhage is massive and the stool is composed of bright red to black fluid or semi-clotted blood. It does not have the raspberry-jam appearance of bleeding from an intussusception, and it is not mixed with mucus as in acute bacillary or amoebic dysentery. The loss of blood may be so excessive that it is followed by shock and collapse. An important point in differentiating between diverticulum and intussusception is that hemorrhage from the latter condition most usually follows at some length of time after the onset of abdominal pain and the development of an abdominal mass, whereas hemorrhage from Meckel's diveritculum oftentimes is the first symptom noted and is either painless or followed by mild pain, and of course no mass may be palpated. In addition, the bloody stools are likely to be more frequent and greater in volume, whereas in intussusception there may be only two or three small movements of blood mixed with mucus or just some blood-stained mucus on the examiner's glove.

Conditions other than intussusception and the dysenteries from which diverticular ulcer must be differentiated are: Henoch's purpura; the absence of articular symptoms, the absence of purpuric spots, normal bleeding and clotting times, normal clot retraction and normal platelet count, and a blood picture of either acute or chronic secondary anaemia, all evidence favoring the diagnosis of diverticular ulcer. Bleeding peptic ulcer is somewhat more difficult to differentiate because some cases of diverticular ulcer do have a definite pain-food relation. However, the pain accompanying gastric or duodenal ulcer is usually epigastric in position rather than para-umbilical as in the case of diverticular ulcer; x-ray examination of the stomach and duodenum may be of value, and finally, the age of the patient offers a minor differential point. Ruptured rectal varicosities may cause sudden massive hemorrhage but here the proctoscope affords a means of differentiation. Rectal polyp may bleed profusely but there is usually a history of tenesmus, and here again the aid of the proctoscope enables us to make a proper differentiation. A number of other conditions must also be thought of despite their rarity. These are ascaridiasis, ileocecal tuberculosis, intestinal telangiectasis, and rectal fissure; the bleeding in these conditions is rarely, if ever, massive. It is our opinion that, irrespective of any other symptom, a history of massive semi-clotted hemorrhage from the rectum of a child followed by recovery and then recurrence of the hemorrhage after the lapse of weeks or months, may be considered pathognomonic of peptic ulcer of Meckel's diverticulum.

Peptic ulcer of a Meckel's diverticulum is an affection of childhood. The first two decades of life are most frequently involved, although the condition may be discovered in any age group. Kleinschmidt[7] reported a case in a patient 45 years old, and MacKeen[8] had a patient who was 53 in whom this condition was discovered. In a series of 77 cases analyzed approximately three-fourths were patients younger than 20 years with the greatest number occurring in the ages from one to 10 years.

Pain is present in most of the cases but it has no special features. It may vary from mild diffuse abdominal distress, on to the agonizing paroxyms of peritonitis. It may be permanently diffuse, or it may be colicky in nature. Very often it is referred to the para-umbilical or hypogastric region, very similar in nature to the pain complained of at the onset of acute appendicitis, and is probably due to distension of the small bowel

or cecum by the large quantity of blood and clots within their lumen. Of course the extreme degree of abdominal pain is found only after the anomalous viscus has perforated and, naturally, is of the peritonitic type. The pain, regardless of degree, usually bears no relationship to meals or season. Tenderness and rigidity are absent and palpation may either cause a moderate amount of discomfort or may be negative. Perforation of the ulcer is, after hemorrhage, the symptom complicating the clinical picture most frequently. The perforation may occur during the hemorrhagic phase or even some months after the last hemorrhage noted. Perforation of course yields a picture of peritonitis and an etiological diagnosis, except from the history, becomes impossible.

If a reasonable question exists as to whether the condition is an ulcer of the upper or the lower intestinal tract, an x-ray study can be done; however, only the first series of plates delineating the shape of the stomach and duodenum are of any value for the purpose of a differential diagnosis, because only in rare instances have the roentgenologists been able to outline the diverticulum.

The treatment of peptic ulcer of a Meckel's diverticulum is surgical. If operation is done after the ulcer has ruptured, the mortality rate is considerably over 50 percent, while the rate following operation which has been performed prior to rupture is only about four percent. If the condition has been undiagnosed the patient usually dies. The patient should receive an extremely restricted low residue diet over a period of several days if he is to be observed or prepared for operation. This period should be made as short as possible because of the danger of rupture of the ulcer during this time. If the patient is markedly anaemic, laparotomy should be deferred until one or more blood transfusions have been given to control the anaemia and lessen the risk of surgical shock. When heterotopic tissue is present it sometimes involves the neck of the sac and the ulcer quite commonly is found to have developed in the ileal mucosa. In this circumstance a small length of ileum extending to each side of the communicating sac should be removed and anastamosis performed. The type of resection performed must not be stereotyped but must depend upon the type of diverticulum present. In the great majority of cases, however, the anomaly may be seized close to its opening by two straight clamps placed diagonally to the long axis of the ileum and the diverticulum incised between the clamps; the incision then is closed by a running gastro-intestinal suture, reinforced by a row of Lembert or Halstead sutures; care being taken that the closure does not produce any marked angulation of the long axis of the intestine. Amputation of the diverticulum followed by ligation and purse string suture, in the manner of performing an appendectomy, cannot be too strongly condemned because of the marked angulation which is usually produced by this method of closure. The post-operative care is similar to that following any intestinal operation, except that one or more blood transfusions may be given if indicated.

CONCLUSIONS

Lesions of Meckel's diverticulum are present often enough that their possibility should be thought of in every case which presents unusual gastro-intestinal symptoms, particularly if bleeding is a part of the picture. Fortunately, examination of cases appearing each year in the literature shows that the medical profession is becoming more and more acquainted with this dangerous anomaly, so that it is being more frequently diagnosed and treated before perforation has

forced the puzzled surgeon to "open an acute abdomen."

The presence of the intermittent hemorrhage, age, pain, trilogy is almost as persumptive an indicator of diverticular peptic ulcer as the pain, vomiting, fever, leucocytosis syndrome, is of appendicitis. The history of hemorrhage only, if of the sudden, massive, recurrent type, even if the patient is an adult, is sufficient to require the positive exclusion of a diverticular ulcer.

BIBLIOGRAPHY

1. Albrecht, E. Munchen med Wehnschr, 48:2961, 1901.
2. Shaetz, E. Beitrage zur morphologie des Meckelschen Divertikels. Beitr. z. path. Anat. u.z allg Path, 74.115, 1925.
3. Farr, C. E., and Penke, M. Meckel's diverticulum. Ann. Surg., 101:1026, 1935.
4. Greenblatt, R. B., Pund, E. R., and Chaney, R. H., Meckel's diverticulum, Am. J. Surg., 31: 288, 1936.
5. Greenwald, H. M, and Steiner, M. Meckel's divertieulum in infancy and childhood. Am. J. Dis. Child., 42:1176, 1931.
6. Matt, J. G, and Timpone, P. J. Peptic Ulcer of Meckel's Diverticulum. Am. J. Surg, 47:612, 1940
7. Kleinschmidt, K. Das Uleus Peticum des Meckelschen Divertikels. Beitr. Z. Klin. Chir., 138:715, 1927.
8. McKeen, H.R., Bleeding ulcer of Meckel's diverticulum, Colorado Med., 29:258, 1932.

The Phrenic Nerve

F. P. BAKER, M.D.

TALIHINA, OKLAHOMA

We are told the phrenic nerve arises chiefly from the fourth cervical nerve with a few filaments from the third and a communicating branch from the fifth. It courses down the neck running obliquely across the Scalenus and Anticus muscles and beneath the Mastoid muscle, the posterior belly of the Omohyoid muscle and the Transversalis Colli and supra scapular vessels, passing over the subclavian artery, beneath it and the subclavian vein, and entering the chest close to the internal mammary artery near its origin. It then descends nearly vertically to the side of the roots of the lung and the pericardium between the pericardial and mediastinal portions of the pleura to the diaphragm where it divides into branches, a few of which are distributed to its thoracic surface, but most of which separately pierce that muscle and are distributed to the under surface.

There is some difference in the length and relations of the two phrenic nerves. The right is shorter and more vertical in direction. The left phrenic nerve is longer than

the right because of the inclination of the heart to the left side and the lower position of the diaphragm. The right phrenic nerve enters the thorax outside of the right innominate vein, while the left enters behind the innominate vein. Each phrenic nerve is accompanied in the thorax by a branch of the internal mammary artery. This nerve supplies filaments to the diaphragm, pericardium and the pleura. The phrenic nerve also receives some filaments from the subclavius muscle. Both nerves have filaments that join the small ganglia of the sympathetic nervous system.

From a surgical standpoint the phrenic nerve was not considered very seriously by anatomists until its interruption began to play a large part in the treatment of tuberculosis of the lungs. The tendency in the beginning was to do a phrenic avulsion on the side of the most affected lung but this produced a permanent paralysis of the diaphragm, and in recent years the nerve is rarely ever pulled from its bed. It has been found that phreniclasis, crushing anywhere from one-fourth to one-half cms. of the nerve with a hemostat produces a very satisfactory paralysis, with rise of the diaphragm, and may last from six months to a year or more.

The procedure for the phrenic nerve operation is as follows; the neck or the chosen field for operation is prepared in the usual manner from the ramus of the jaw to the clavicle and from the median line of the neck to the trapezius muscle. A point is selected about four cms. above the clavicle and immediately over the posterior triangle of the neck where an incision of four cms. in length is made parallel to the clavicle. This incision extends through the skin and down through the platysma muscle. A hemostat is then used to split the fascia and fat along the posterior border of the Sterno-mastoid muscle down to the Scalenus-Anticus muscle. An area of about five cms. is opened and a retractor is then pressed under the Sterno-mastoid muscle and is pulled toward the median line thereby exposing the Scalenus-Anticus where, if the nerve is in a normal position, it will be found to be running diagonally across the Scalenus-Anticus from above posteriorly, to the anterior border of this muscle below and is in the fascia and intigement covering the Scalenus-Anticus muscle. The nerve is then separated from this region and raised with a nerve hook.

After two or three centimeters of the nerve have been stripped, one to one and one-half centimeters are then crushed with a hemostat. The average length of the phrenic nerve is from 11 to 15 inches and its size varies considerably; however, the average normal nerve is about the size of the ordinary twine string. The size of the individual does not always determine the size of the nerve.

The operation described assumes that the phrenic nerve is normal and that it follows its normal course. Some of the anomolies of the phrenic nerve are; 1. It may divide into one, two or three filaments. 2. It may cross over the Scalenus-Anticus higher or lower, and should avulsion of the nerve be desired, it must be remembered that on rare occasions severe hemorrhage has resulted from this procedure when the nerve was looped around the internal mammary artery or some other blood vesssel along its course. This accident is very rare, but has been known to occur.

The indications for paralysis of the phrenic nerve are as follows; 1. When a lung cannot be collapsed by artificial pneumothorax and a certain amount of collapse is desired to close a tuberculous lesion. 2. When the lung is only partially collapsed with artificial pneumothorax and paralysis of the diaphragm would be of assistance in producing more collapse. 3. Phreniclasis may be used as a primary step toward a complete thoracoplasty. 4. Slight crushing of the phrenic nerve has been known to stop persistent hiccough, the patient having been fluoroscoped to determine which side of the diaphragm was producing the hiccough. 5. This operation has also been used successfully to allay persistent cough in tuberculosis which is sometimes due to irritation of the diaphragm.

The results obtained from phreniclasis are; 1. Paralysis of the diaphragm muscle on the side operated. This paralysis stops the excursion of the diaphragm, thereby producing a certain amount of rest to the lung. 2. If not prevented by pleural adhesions or other pathological conditions, the diaphragm will rise when the nerve is paralyzed, thereby reducing the cubic content of the thoracic cavity on the operated side.

It would appear that paralysis of the diaphragm would be much more applicable in a basal lesion than in any other parts of the lung, but acutally, the beneficial results of phrenic nerve interuption are exerted upon apical and upper lobe lesions with as good if not better affects than on basal lesions.

With the diaphragmatic rise, the lung tissue is naturally compressed and unless there are strong adhesions and thick cavity walls, the diseased portion is more apt to collapse than the healthy part of the lung, which will continue to function and the non-functioning part will retract and collapse.

There are a few contra-indications for phrenic nerve operations, the most important of which from the standpoint of the phthisiotherapists are bronchiectasis, lung abscess and malignancy. In these conditions, paralysis of the diaphragm may cause a kink in a bronchus or bronchiole and prevent proper drainage.

Among the possible untoward results following a phreniclasis is the possible injury to some other nerve if the phrenic nerve is not in its normal position. For instance, occasionally, we find tosis of the eye lid. Another is injury to the cervical plexus causing paralysis of the Deltoid muscle.

The anesthetic used is one-half of one percent novocain. The skin and underlying tissues are infiltrated with this solution, and when the nerve is reached this solution is used to infiltrate a portion of the nerve before crushing.

Before injecting the nerve, it is always well to determine its identity by pinching. This procedure should cause immediate twitching of the diaphragm. The patient will also complain of a severe pain in the shoulder, but rarely in the chest or about the diaphragm unless the nerve is extracted.

A Fluoroscopic Survey of Postnatal Syphilis In A Health Department Clinic*

DAVID V. HUDSON, M.D.

SIDNEY C. VENABLE, M.D.

TULSA, OKLAHOMA

The term prenatal syphilis was introduced by Kolmer[1] and recommended by Stokes[2] to indicate those infections contracted in utero through the maternal placenta previously known as congenital, heredofamilial, hereditary syphilis, etc. The logical term then for infections contracted after birth is postnatal syphilis and this term will be used to designate acquired syphilis.

The most important function of syphilis clinics is to find all early or infectious cases of syphilis and prevent the spread of the disease by prompt and adequate treatment. Since the Health Department has taken over the treatment of early syphilis it has been loaded down with the care of late or noninfectious syphilis. All cases of late syphilis do not require the same amount of treatment and unless some practical means is employed to sift out those requiring special or long continued treatment, relatively large numbers of individuals will either be over treated or receive inadequate treatment to prevent progression and ultimate disability. In all health department clinics in the State of

Oklahoma the records show a large number of individuals classified as having late latent syphilis (late asymptomatic syphilis). To give maximum treatment to this group would load the clinic beyond its capacity. Even moderate or minimal schedules of treatment require time which could be more profitably spent, from the standpoint of syphilis control, on the diagnosis and treatment of early infections.

History and physical examination will pick out the more obvious cases of cardiovascular, tertiary and neurosyphilis, but spinal fluid examination is necessary to detect asymptomatic neurosyphilis and the earlier this condition is found, the better are the chances for therapeutic success. The same is true of cardiovascular syphilis in that treatment of early aortitis is far more effective than the treatment of advanced aortitis complicated with regurgitation or aneurysm. Moore[3] shows the incidence and prognosis of the various grades of aortitis in the following table and emphasizes the necessity of early detection of this condition in order to secure the most favorable therapeutic results.

*Read before the Section on Public Health, Annual Session, Oklahoma State Medical Association, April 24, 1942.

TABLE 1

The Incidence and Prognosis of Various Types of Cardiovascular Syphilis (Moore)

Clinical Type of cardiovascular syphilis	Approximate percentage of patients with late syphilis affected	Prognosis in terms of probable average duration of life if	
		Untreated	Adequately treated
Uncomplicated aortitis clinically unrecognizable	70-90	Good—many years, no accurate data	Excellent—life probably not shortened
Uncomplicated aortitis, recognizable on the basis of symptoms and signs	5-10	5-10 years	10-20 years or better
Aortitis with saccular aneurysm	1-2	1-2 years	5-10 years
Aortitis with aortic regurgitation	2-3	2-3 years	4-10 years
Myocarditis; Coronary ostial stenosis	0.2-0.5	No accurate data	No accurate data

Since the majority of physicians in private practice do not consider a complete physical examination necessary in the diagnosis of syphilis and relatively few internists think in terms of uncomplicated aortitis, it is not surprising that this diagnosis is infrequently made. In checking over 3,000 admissions to the Tulsa Cooperative Clinic we found no patients referred with the diagnosis of uncomplicated aortitis. Two patients (without aortic regurgitation or aneurysm) were referred to the clinic with the notation "X-ray shows enlargement of the aorta". One came from an internist specializing in diseases of the chest and the other from a medical school hospital.

In the Tulsa Cooperative Clinic patients with late syphilis increased to such an extent that too much time was devoted to them and not enough time was available for interviews with patients with early syphilis. On the other hand disability from cardiovascular syphilis was very noticeable and the deaths from this condition were more numerous than those from neurosyphilis. Too frequently cardiovascular conditions would be found on subsequent examinations which were obviously present on admission but overlooked.

Dr. Joseph Earle Moore[4] suggested a minimal routine treatment for late latent syphilis for clinic use estimated to prevent development of aortitis in the majority of cases. This consists of preliminary bismuth and then twelve weekly doses of an arsenical, preferably mapharsen, followed by twelve weekly doses of bismuth. Thereafter the patient is examined once a year and treatment given if indicated. The requirements for the diagnosis of late latent (asymptomatic) syphilis are (1) serologic evidence of syphilis, (2) negative history of tertiary, cardiovascular or neurosyphilis, (3) negative physical-neurological examination, (4) negative fluoroscopic examination and (5) negative spinal fluid examination in an individual with an infection of over four years in duration. If the first four requirements are met and the patient refuses spinal fluid examination then the spinal fluid is arbitrarily considered negative and the patient assumes the responsibility for undetected asymptomatic neurosyphilis.

Moore and Metildi[5] list seven diagnostic criteria for uncomplicated aortitis and insist that to justify the diagnosis at least three must be present in an individual with proven syphilis but without mitral disease. The seven criteria are as follows:

1. Teleradiographic and fluoroscopic evidence of aortic dilatation.
2. Increased retromanubrial dullness.
3. A history of circulatory embarrassment.
4. A tympanitic bell-like, tambour accentuation of the aortic second sound.
5. Progressive cardiac failure.
6. Substernal pain.
7. Paroxysmal dyspnoea.

Fluoroscopic evidence of enlargement of the aorta is not per se pathognomonic of syphilitic aortitis. Kemp and Cochems[6] find that changes in the aortic shadow due to hypertension, arteriosclerosis and age are essentially the same in non-syphilitic individuals as in syphilitic individuals without syphilitic heart disease. They maintain that fluoroscopy and careful clinical evaluation of symptoms and physical signs are essential to establish the diagnosis of uncomplicated aortitis.

Fluoroscopic examinations were begun in the latter part of 1940 as an aid in the diagnosis of questionable cases of cardiovascular syphilis and later became a routine for all cases of late syphilis. Patients with early syphilis are fluoroscoped at the end of treatment and once a year throughout the period of observation which consists of at least five years. Prenatal syphilis is so infrequently complicated with aortitis that it is considered non-existant. In less than 50 cases in our clinic we have found no aortic enlargement from any cause. Later in life some of these patients will probably show evidence of enlargement due to hypertension or arteriosclerosis.

Patients are fluoroscoped in groups by sex, with white and colored on alternate days. It takes less time and "paper work" to fluoroscope twenty patients than to secure that many serological tests. The cardiac stripe is examined in the anterior-posterior, posterior-anterior and oblique positions. Degrees of enlargement of the aorta are arbitrarily recorded as 1, 2 and 3, with intermediate positions as 1+, or 2+ as follows in table 2:

TABLE 2

Normal aorta	A0 No enlargement
First degree enlargement of aorta	A1 Slight but definite enlargement
Second degree enlargement of aorta	A2 Marked enlargement
Third degree enlargement of aorta	A3 Extreme enlargement

Notations are made as to the size of the heart and comments as to pulsations, position and prominence of the arch, presence of sacculation, etc. Teleroentgenograms, proved too expensive for clinic or patients and in our opinion in the few instances used provided no more information than fluoroscopy afforded.

From October 1940 to April 16, 1942, 694 patients with late postnatal syphilis were examined fluoroscopically. Of this number 267 or approximately 38 percent showed some degree of aortic enlargement. The following table summarises the results of our examinations:

TABLE 3

Number of patients examined		694
No aortic enlargement	(A0)	427
1st. degree enlargement	(A1)	169
2d. degree enlargement	(A2)	84
3d. degree enlargement	(A3)	14

The individuals with normal aortas were classified as late latent syphilis (if the history and other examinations including the diagnostic criteria of Moore and Metildi were negative) and were given the minimal treatment suggested by Moore. Fluoroscopic and physical examinations were repeated at the end of the treatment(which takes approximately six months) and if found normal, the patient was placed on probation and instructed to report once a year for re-examination. We found a few individuals to show very definite changes at the end of this six months period and feel that the number developing signs of aortitis justifies re-examination before probation. One interesting case, a colored male, developed classical physical signs of aortic regurgitation at least twelve months before there was fluoroscopic evi-

dence of aortic enlargement. The fluoroscopic changes were, first, increased aortic pulsation, then marked pulsation, and finally, definite but moderate aortic enlargement.

Patients with fluoroscopic evidence of aortic enlargement but having less than three of the diagnostic criteria of Moore and Metildi for uncomplicated aortitis were placed on a modified cardiovascular routine. If progression took place the treatment was changed as indicated. If no progression was found, the treatment was continued for one year before placing the patient on probation.

Individuals with definite syphilitic aortitis (either uncomplicated or complicated with regurgitation or aneurysm) were placed on the appropriate routine and treatment continued for the customary two years before probation. Thereafter they receive periodic examinations and treatment as indicated. We are very much interested in finding an effective method of treating these patients so that adequate treatment may be given in a shorter period of time.

Persons with both aortitis and neurosyphilis presented problems and required more individualized treatment depending upon the relative severity of the two conditions. The greatest difficulty was giving adequate treatment for the neurosyphilis without damage to the cardiovascular system.

Table 4 which is a reproduction of a form on a colored front sheet for our charts provides a rapid and simple method of recording periodic examinations and serves to distinguish cardiovascular cases from other types of syphilis.

Symptomatic relief after treatment is usually present and practically amounts to corroboration of the diagnosis of uncomplicated aortitis. Some of our colored ladies insist that they can do "much bigger and better washings".

Approximately 38 percent of the 694 patients with late postnatal syphilis who were examined fluoroscopically showed some de-

TABLE 4

Duration of infection—4-+ years Date	Previous treatment— 7-1-41	1-7-41	None 7-7-42	1-6-42
1. X-ray	HOA1	HOA1	HOA1	HOA1
2. Retrosternal dullness	+	+	+	+
3. History of circulatory embarrassment or persistence of symptoms	+	+ +	—	—
4. Aortic second sound A2	+	+	+	+
5. Progressive cardiac failure	—	—	—	—
6. Substernal pain	—	—	—	—
7. Paroxysmal dyspnoea	—	—	—	—
Blood pressure	125-80	130-70	130-80	130-75
Symptomatic relief	+	—	+	+

gree of aortic enlargement (table 3). On clinical evaluation of signs and symptoms only about 20 percent of the total number of persons fluoroscoped were found to have definite syphilitic aortitis. This figure is too high since the first few hundred patients were fluoroscoped because of suspected cardiovascular disease and not as a routine.

As would be expected the majority of the grade two and three enlargements were found in the older age groups and appeared more frequently in colored than in white patients. In those which were studied for the relation of treatment previous to admission to the degree of enlargement it was found that no patient with a grade two or three aortic enlargement either syphilitic or presumably syphilitic had had adequate treatment early in the course of their infection and most of them had received no treatment at all.

Of 37 patients re-examined after the introduction of fluoroscopy and found to have three or more of the criteria of Moore and Matildi as well as a grade two or three enlargement, only two were diagnosed correctly on admission as aortitis and three as questionable aortitis. The remainder had "heart normal" recorded in the admission examination and were diagnosed as "late latency," "neurosyphilis" or "tertiary". This was obviously due in many cases to the habit of thinking of cardiovascular syphilis as aortic regurgitation. Frequently the only notation was "no murmurs". In other cases the examining physician in the absence of gross signs of cardiovascular disease records a provisional diagnosis of late latent syphilis and leaves the details for subsequent re-examination. Some are not interested. When cardiologists hesitate to commit themselves on retrosternal dullness by percussion and depend on the x-ray to determine aortic enlargement, it is reasonable to give the general practitioner or the examining physician in a syphilis clinic the benefit of fluoroscopic examinations in cases of late syphilis.

Since April 20, 1939, over 25 physicians have examined patients in the Tulsa Cooperative Clinic. Most of these are now with the armed forces. A new member on the staff at first misses the aortitis, then exaggerates the retrosternal dullness and quality of the aortic second sound, but soon settles down to a fairly accurate interpretation of the signs and symptoms present. The ones who observe the fluoroscopic examinations find their time well spent. The physician who never makes a mistake in diagnosis does not examine syphilis patients.

The authors are indebted to Miss Virginia Johnson for aid in tabulating material.

CONCLUSIONS

1. Routine fluoroscopic examinations in a health department syphilis clinic are essential in the consistent diagnosis of early uncomplicated aortitis, and screens out a large number of individuals with normal or presumably normal aortas who may be given minimal treatment decreasing the clinic load.

2. By examining patients in groups by sex, fluoroscopic examinations can be made, accurately, rapidly and economically.

3. All patients with uncomplicated aortitis having grade two or three enlargement of the aorta (fluoroscopically) either had had inadequate treatment or had received none at all during the early course of their infection.

BIBLIOGRAPHY

1. Kolmer, J. A., quoted by Stokes.
2. Stokes, John H., Modern Clinical Syphilology, 2d edition, 1934, W. B. Saunders.
3. Moore, J E., Modern Treatment of Syphilis, 2d edition, 1941, Charles C. Thomas, Springfield, Ill.
4. Moore, J. E., Personal communication.
5. Moore, J. E., and Matildi, P. F., Uncomplicated Syphilitic Aortitis-Diagnosis, Prognosis and Treatment, Archives of Internal Medicine, Vol. 52, p. 978.
6. Kemp, J. E., and Cochems, K. D., Teleroentgenography in the Diagnosis of Early Syphilitic Aortitis: A comparison of findings of 1,000 syphilitic and 600 nonsyphilitic individuals. The American Heart Journal, Vol. 13, p. 257, March, 1937.

DISCUSSION

EUGENE A. GILLIS, M.D., M.P.H.
Director Venereal Disease Division
Oklahoma State Health Department
OKLAHOMA CITY, OKLAHOMA

We venereal disease control officers look upon syphilis as two diseases:

The disease which we are earnestly trying to prevent, and treat promptly to obviate further spread, is early infectious syphilis. Health Department venereal disease programs and venereal disease clinics were established primarily to treat this disease in those unable to afford private medical care —that is, provide chemical quarantine for these individuals to prevent further spread.

This disease is most readily uncovered by educating the public to consult their private physician after exposure, or whenever suspicious lesions appear. If a sincere effort is made to find out where these individuals acquired their infectious syphilis and to whom they may have given it, many additional cases of early syphilis will be uncovered.

Late syphilis is not a major public health problem because of its lack of infectiousness, but it deserves attention because of the crippling and deaths, the public expense and loss of vitally needed man power which it causes. This type of syphilis is discovered by routine blood tests on all private patients, all hospital patients, all pregnant mothers, on pre-employment and periodic tests on all employees of industry, and by premarital blood tests. Doctors Hudson and Venable have shown us a practical and efficient way of screening and treating late syphilis without markedly sacrificing and interfering with our primary purpose of chemically quarantining those with infectious syphilis.

Doctor J. Earle Moore, in his 1941 edition of "The Modern Treatment of Syphilis" says: "The most promising field for immediate study lies in the earlier diagnosis of cardiovascular syphilis.

It cannot be too strongly emphasized that the diagnosis of latent syphilis depends on negative physical evidence, and that the more thorough and searching one's methods of clinical examinations become, the more frequently lesions of latent syphilis will be recognized, and fewer patients will be admitted to the classification of latency."

More and more spinal punctures are being done on syphilis patients in this country.

It has been very discouraging that some months in our State Health Laboratory as many as 25 percent of the spinal fluids examined are positive. As syphilis is treated earlier and more adequately, this percentage will undoubtedly decrease.

In the Tulsa Cooperative Venereal Disease Clinic, of which Doctor Hudson is director, only 15.2 percent of the 6,110 syphilis cases in State Health Department Sponsored Venereal Disease Clinics are being treated, but 59.2 percent of the reported cardiovascular syphilis is in this clinic.

This is certainly a challenge to all of us to do more thorough physical examinations of our syphilis patients, including fluoroscopic examinations of the cardiovascular stripe whenever possible.

If we examine our patients who have latent syphilis with sufficient care, to be certain they do not have cardiovascular or central nervous system syphilis, we need not be alarmed over sero-resistance, (so-called Wassermann Fastness), or an occasional serologic relapse.

These are in all probability merely an index of the sensitivity of the serologic tests employed. As serologic techniques become more sensitive, it may be difficult if not impossible, to ever obtain a negative serological test for syphilis from treatment in latent syphilis.

Winthrop Chemical Company Announces Appointment

Harold L. Hansen, Ph.D., has been appointed administrative assistant to the president of Winthrop Chemical Company, Inc., according to a recent announcement made by Dr. Theodore G. Klumpp, president. He takes up his new duties immediately.

Before joining Winthrop, Doctor Hansen was secretary of the Council on Dental Therapeutics of the American Dental Association, director of the A.D.A. Bureau of Chemistry, and consultant to the Federal Food and Drug Administration, the Federal Trade Commission and the Council on Pharmacy and Chemistry.

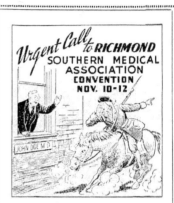

· THE PRESIDENT'S PAGE ·

In these perilous days, the President's Page is a liability. Under present conditions, declaring a policy or giving advice with reference to current issues is dangerous business. In every community, the ranks of the medical profession have been depleted through the voluntary response to Procurement and Assignment. The people are nervous and unsettled because of unusual mental and physical strain.

It seems a good time for every doctor to do as much as he can, as well as he can, for as many as he can, with the poise and dignity which so well becomes his profession. In this way, the time-honored traditions of his calling may be preserved and the age-old duties of the physician in relation to the patient may be duly discharged. While so many foundations are being shaken, the people must not lose faith in the medical profession.

Sincerely yours,

James D Osborn

President.

Antirabic Vaccine

SEMPLE METHOD

U. S. Government License No. 98

1. Patients bitten by suspected rabid animals, on any part of body other than Face and Wrist, usually require only 14 doses of Antirabic Vaccine.

    Ampoule Package......................$15.00

2. Patients bitten about Face or Wrist, or when treatment has been delayed, should receive at least 21 doses of Antirabic Vaccine. (Special instructions with each treatment.)

    Ampoule Package......................$22.50

Special Discounts to Doctors, Druggists, Hospitals and to County Health Officers for Indigent Cases.

Medical Arts Laboratory

1115 Medical Arts Building
Oklahoma City, Oklahoma

The JOURNAL Of The
OKLAHOMA STATE MEDICAL ASSOCIATION

EDITORIAL BOARD

L. J. MOORMAN, Oklahoma City, Editor-in-Chief

E. EUGENE RICE, Shawnee

NED R. SMITH, Tulsa

MR. R. H. GRAHAM, Oklahoma City, Business Manager

CONTRIBUTIONS: Articles accepted by this Journal for publication including those read at the annual meetings of the State Association are the sole property of this Journal.

The Editorial Department is not responsible for the opinions expressed in the original articles of contributors.

Manuscripts may be withdrawn by authors for publication elsewhere only upon the approval of the Editorial Board.

MANUSCRIPTS: Manuscripts should be typewritten, double-spaced, on white paper 8½ x 11 inches. The original copy, not the carbon copy, should be submitted.

Footnotes, bibliographies and legends for cuts should be typed on separate sheets in double space. Bibliography listing should follow this order: Name of author, title of article, name of periodical with volume, page and date of publication.

Manuscripts are accepted subject to the usual editorial revisions and with the understanding that they have not been published elsewhere.

NEWS: Local news of interest to the medical profession, changes of address, births, deaths and weddings will be gratefully received.

ADVERTISING: Advertising of articles, drugs or compounds unapproved by the Council on Pharmacy of the A.M.A. will not be accepted. Advertising rates will be supplied on application.

It is suggested that members of the State Association patronize our advertisers in preference to others.

SUBSCRIPTIONS: Failure to receive The Journal should call for immediate notification.

REPRINTS: Reprints of original articles will be supplied at actual cost provided request for them is attached to manuscripts or made in sufficient time before publication. Checks for reprints should be made payable to Industrial Printing Company, Oklahoma City.

Address all communications to THE JOURNAL OF THE OKLAHOMA STATE MEDICAL ASSOCIATION, 210 Plaza Court, Oklahoma City.

OFFICIAL PUBLICATION OF THE OKLAHOMA STATE MEDICAL ASSOCIATION

Copyrighted October, 1942

EDITORIALS

SAM F. SEELEY, M.D., LEAVES PROCUREMENT AND ASSIGNMENT SERVICE

The recent announcement that Lt. Colonel Sam F. Seeley has been recalled by the Office of the Surgeon General from the Procurement and Assignment Service as Executive Director to become the Commanding Officer of the new Army Hospital at White Sulphur Spring, West Virginia, will be accepted by the medical profession, but not without a tinge of regret and a sense of loss.

It is extremely doubtful if any physician in any capacity ever was given a greater task than the one assigned to Dr. Seeley.

His assignment, as every physician knows, was to mobilize the profession for war.

Had he only been confronted with a program of securing physicians for the military forces his task would not have been extremely difficult, but his was a two front offense, both military and civilian. An offense calling for a firm but level guiding hand, an understanding of supply and demand, diplomacy and tact, a sense of humor, and above all a will and desire to work twenty-four hours a day.

It is doubtful if any person ever spoke before the medical profession of Oklahoma and said so much in so few words and left a more firm and lasting impression of the responsibility of the medical profession in the present world conflict.

That Oklahoma physicians understood and had faith in the Procurement and Assignment Service under the leadership of Dr. Seeley is manifested in the record made by the physicians of this State in applying for commissions in such numbers that the Oklahoma quota was filled between May 15th and July 15th.

To you, Doctor Seeley, the medical profession of Oklahoma wishes health, happiness, and success.

Yours has been a job well done.

MEDICINE'S MARATHON

It is doubtful if our spirit in warfare has ever been surpassed, but for facility of expression we must go back to the Greeks.

The Battle of Marathon was initiated and sustained by the following battle cry: "On, sons of the Greeks! Strike for the freedom of your country—strike for the freedom of your children and your wives—for the shrine of your fathers' gods and for the sepulchres of your sires. All—all are now staked upon the strife."

The response of Oklahoma doctors to the call of Procurement and Assignment shows that those who daily experience the ultimate verities of life through intimate glances at bared souls, are in full possession of the spirit which encompassed the Plains of Marathon and engulfed the Medes and the Persians.

Like the Athenian youth, with the fatigue of battle upon him, may they bring the good news "Rejoice—we have conquered." After running thirty miles, this noble youth sprang to the center of the square and "throwing up his arms in an attitude of ecstasy he delivered the glorious message to the people of Athens"—then, amidst the shouts and cries of jubilation he reeled, sank to his knees, and fell dead.

If you ask—what has this to do with medicine, it should be remembered that fundamentally medicine is a matter of dealing soundly and tenderly with life and death. Today throughout America, it should be the hope and the prayer of every true American that our men in the Army and Navy Medical Corps may not only safeguard the lives of our soldiers but that they may save many a young man from an untimely death, even though his devotion to duty in action guarantees the posthumous halo of heroic deeds.

CORONARY CRITERIA

Modern Criteria concerning the coronary arteries, largely depend upon the work of American investigators. Though not generally known a fairly good clinical picture of the typical coronary syndrome may be dated back to Wm. Harvey (1578-1657) and it may be recognized in the recorded observations of many great clinicians who succeeded Harvey. Wm. Heberden (1710-1801) gave his original description of Angina Pectoris in 1768. In 1910 Wm. Osler,[1] in a lecture on Angina Pectoris, said, "Had Heberden listened to my first lecture he could have remarked very justly: 'Well they have not got much ahead since my day.'" The influence of mental strain and physical effect upon the clinical course of coronary disease was carefully noted. Everard Home's[2] account of John Hunters (1728-1793) case well illustrates this point. It is stated that his first attack was produced by mental irritation, "and although bodily exercise, or distention of the stomach, brought on slighter affections, it still required the mind to be affected to render them severe; and as his mind was irritated by trifles, these produced the most violent effects on the disease. His coachman being beyond his times, or a servant not attending to his directions, brought on the spasms, while a real misfortune produced no

effect. At the time of his death he was in the 65th year of his age, the same age at which his brother, the late Dr. Hunter, died."

Apparently his sudden death at St. George's Hospital was occasioned by an attempt to control his temper.

It is interesting to contrast the mental attitude of the two famous brothers. While John's spirit was so inflamable during the latter part of his life that he was consciously at the mercy of anybody who chose to cross him, his elder brother William, fostered a sustaining philosophy which in the last moments of his life enabled him to say to his attending physician, Dr. Combe, "If I had strength enough to hold a pen, I would write how easy and pleasant a thing it is to die."

The first clinical diagnosis of thrombotic coronary occlusion was made by Dr. A. Hammer[3] in St. Louis, Mo. (1876). The patient lived only a few hours after the diagnosis was made, and an autopsy revealed a thrombus "in the right sinus of Valsalva" finally reaching the coronary resulting in complete closure of its lumen.

In 1896 Dr. George Dock[4] reported a case of right coronary occlusion confirmed by autopsy. In his lecture on Angina published in 1910 Osler discusses the Coronary arteries and refers to 17 necropsies of which 13 showed different varieties of coronary disease.

James B. Herrick[5] gave his classical clinical discription of Sudden occlusion of the coronary arteries in 1912.

Since the publication of Herrick's clear cut clinical report with its convincing account of the autopsy findings, clinicians, in increasing numbers have learned to recognize the characteristic manifestations at the bed side. Confidence in the clinical syndrome has been established by successive Electrocardiographic and autopsy findings.

By the beginning of the 4th decade in this century we had virtually achieved universal acceptance of the above principles. But since then we have accumulated much additional knowledge, some of which may be classified as gratifying and some as disconcerting.

It is fortunate that our knowledge of diagnosis and therapy is constantly growing; that we know more about the compensatory physiologic processes and the life saving power of collateral circulation in the heart muscle which helps to restore lost function and to maintain a certain degree of myocardial integrity. Now that we develop mountain sickness on wings we are grateful for the recently discovered knowledge of the compensatory coronary response to high altitude. In the rarified air high above the earth the flow of blood in the coronary vessels is greatly increased otherwise the anoxic anoxemia would more quickly result in disturbed physiology and consequent pathologic changes. Wiggers[6] has written, "The pronounced anoxic vasodilatation is doubtless a providential mechanism by which the cardiac pump is sustained so well in progressive anoxia; indeed, it is probable that myocardial stimulation is converted into mycardial depression as soon as the angmentation of coronary blood flow cannot keep pace with the decreasing volume of oxygen carried by the blood."

Among the most gratifying results of our increasing knowledge of coronary disease is the growing tendency to offer a more hopeful prognosis.

Prominent among the disconcerting facts, stands the increasing incidence of Coronary disease and the mounting mortality statistics. But it must be remembered that in part this is due to enhanced diagnostic precision, also to increasing longevity which brings more susceptable individuals to the coronary morbidity age. There is a certain sense of defeatism in the thought that when we became skilled in the recognition of the Herrick syndrome we learned that silent or painless atypical coronary occlusion[7] is not uncommon.

In these days of financial stress and mounting taxes the observations of Swartz and Harvey[8] are disconcerting. In their analysis of 83 cases from a New York City financial area they make this interesting observation. As the activity of the stock market ticker varied in level, so did the occurence of coronary artery episodes. Individuals who rested over weekends or who enjoyed some quiet form of diversion were free from attacks during the early part of the week, whereas those who overstimulated themselves appeared to have their onset during the first two days of the business week. There was a steplike rise in incidence from 9:00 A. M. to noon. While discussing monetary considerations it is interesting to note that John Hunter's second severe attack of angina was occasioned by being obliged to pay a security debt.

BIBLIOGRAPHY

1. Osler, Wm.: The Lancet. 1910. Page 839.

2. "Life of John Hunter," by Evard Home, in John Hunter's er's Treatise on the Blood, Inflammation and gun-shot wounds. Philadelphia, 1796.

3. Wien. Med. Wchnschr. (1878), XXVIII, 102, Classical Description of Disease. Ralph H. Major.

4. Dock, George, Med. & Surg. Reporter (1896), LXXV, 1 Classical Description of Disease. Ralph H. Major.

5. J. A. M. A. 1912), LIX, 2015.

6. Wiggers, C. J., Ann. Int. Med., 14, 1237, 1941. Anoxia, Its Effect on the Body. Edward J. Van Liere, M D.

7. Stroud, Wm. D., & Wagner, Joseph A.: Silent or Atypical Coronary Occlusion. Ann. Int. Med. 15:25-32, July 1941.

8. Swartz, George and Harvey, Joseph: Coronary Artery Disease in a Financial Area. Med. Rec. 153:311-313, May 7, 1941.

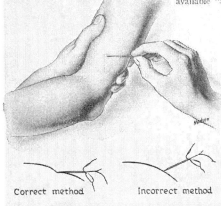

ASSOCIATION ACTIVITIES

NEW STATE PROCUREMENT AND ASSIGNMENT CHAIRMAN AND VICE-CHAIRMAN

Dr. W. W. Rucks, Sr., Oklahoma City, has been appointed by the Council of the Oklahoma State Medical Association to replace Dr. Henry H. Turner, Oklahoma City, who has recently resigned, as State Chairman of the Procurement and Assignment Committee.

In line with recent instructions received from the Chairman of the Directing Board of National Procurement and Assignment that the Vice-Chairman of each State Committee should reside in the same town as the Chairman, Dr. C. R. Rountree of Oklahoma City has been selected to replace Dr. L. S. Willour of McAlester.

The other members who comprise the State Committee are as follows: Council Chairmen in their respective Districts are No. 1, Dr. John L. Day, Supply; No. 2 Dr. J. M. Bonham, Hobart; No. 3, Dr. J. M. Watson, Enid; No. 4, Dr. Tom Lowry, Oklahoma City; No. 5, Dr. J. L. Patterson, Duncan; No. 6, Dr. W. Albert Cook, Tulsa; No. 7, Dr. W. M. Gallaher, Shawnee; No. 8, Dr. F. L. Wormington, Miami; No. 9, Dr. J. M. Harris, Wilburton, and No. 10, Dr. John A. Haynie, Durant. The following Advisory Members are all from Oklahoma City: Dr. Grady F. Mathews, Commissioner, Oklahoma State Health Department; Dean Robert U. Patterson, University of Oklahoma School of Medicine, and Major Louis H. Ritzhaupt, State Medical Officer of Selective Service.

The State Procurement and Assignment Committee, which was renamed in February, 1942, upon request from the Office of Procurement and Assignment, Washington, D. C., to replace the State Medical Preparedness Committee, functions through the County Medical Preparedness Representatives, who were appointed in 1940 in line with instructions issued by the American Medical Association at the time the first questionnaires were completed.

THIRD SECRETARIES CONFERENCE PLANNED FOR OCTOBER 25

The Third Annual Secretaries Conference of the Oklahoma State Medical Association will be held in Oklahoma City at the Biltmore hotel on October 25.

The Officers of the Conference are arranging for an interesting as well as instructive program which will deal with economic and political questions confronting the medical profession of today.

Dr. George K. Hemphill of Pawhuska is Chairman of the Conference; Dr. John R. Callaway of Pauls Valley is Vice-Chairman; and as Secretary-Treasurer, Dr. William E. Eastland of Oklahoma City replaces Dr. W. W. Rucks, Jr., Oklahoma City, who has been called to active military duty.

Dr. E. W. Hawkins Receives Honor

Meeting in conjunction with the 44th National Encampment of the United Spanish War Veterans in Cleveland, Ohio, during the latter part of August, Dr. E. W. Hawkins of Carnegie was elected Senior Vice-Commander of the Eighth Army Corps Veterans National Association.

Doctor Hawkins enlisted in the 29th United States Volunteers at the age of 18 years and served in the Philippines and was with the American troops in the Boxer Rebellion.

OKLAHOMA CITY CLINICAL SOCIETY

Information has come from the Surgeons General of the Army, Navy and Public Health Service in Washington, that strictly scientific professional meetings will contribute significantly to the war effort.

Older physicians who have been semi-retired are finding it necessary to increase their patient load. In order to do this, and in order to give their patients the proper kind of care, they are finding it necessary to brush up on the later developments and expanded fields of medicine. The Oklahoma City Clinical Society conference is the ideal place to do this. It is easily accessible to all physicians in the Southwest, and is in such concentrated form that a very thorough post graduate course may be obtained in the minimum of time.

While the meeting is primarily for the general practitioner, it also provides an opportunity for medical officers in service to meet and discuss their problems.

Emergency Medical Service for Civilian Defense, a subject of great importance to civilian physicians, will be discussed by Dr. Henry H. Ogilvie of San Antonio at the Clinic Dinner on Tuesday, October 27. Doctor Ogilvie is Regional Director of Emergency Medical Service for Civilian Defense, and is a brilliant speaker with a world of information at his finger tips.

The officers of the Oklahoma City Clinical Society have extended every effort to prepare a program that will be interesting and practical, and one which will be of essential value to preparations being made to adequately care for civilian and military needs during this emergency.

OPHTHALMOLOGY BOARD WILL GIVE ADDITIONAL EXAMINATIONS

Because of the War Emergency, the American Board of Ophthalmology announces the following additional examinations: New York City—December 13-16 and Los Angeles—January 15-16.

At the last meeting it was decided to cancel the 1943 written examination, to include in the oral examination all of the subjects previously covered by the written examination, and to temporarily dispense with the requirement of case reports. The oral examination is expected to require two or three days, and will cover the following subjects: External Diseases-Slit Lamp; Ophthalmoscopy; Histology-Pathology-Bacteriology; Ocular Motility; Refraction-Retinoscopy; Practical Surgery; Anatomy and Embryology; Perimetry; Therapeutics and Operations; Optics and Visual Physiology, and Relation of the Eye to General Diseases.

Formal application blanks must be filed with the Secretary not later than November and may be secured by writing to the American Board of Ophthalmology, 6830 Waterman Avenue, St. Louis, Mo.

NEW OFFICERS FOR MUSKOGEE, SEQUOYAH, WAGONER COUNTY MEDICAL SOCIETY

Dr. L. S. McAlister of Muskogee was elevated to the position of President of the Muskogee, Sequoyah, Wagoner County Medical Society to replace Dr. Shade D. Neely at a recently special called meeting. Dr. D. Evelyn Miller, also of Muskogee, was elected Secretary-Treasurer of the Society and will fill the unexpired term of Dr. J. T. McInnis. Dr. H. A. Scott is the newly elected Vice-President replacing Dr. McAlister.

Both Dr. Neely and Dr. McInnis have been ordered to active military duty. Dr. Neely is in the Navy and has reported for duty at Santa Ana, Calif., and Dr. McInnis is stationed at Camp Robinson, Ark.

DOCTOR EWING APPOINTED EIGHTH DISTRICT COUNCILOR

Dr. Finis W. Ewing of Muskogee, immediate past president of the Oklahoma State Medical Association, has been selected by the Council of the Association to replace Dr. Shade D. Neely, formerly of Muskogee, but now in the naval service of the United States.

As Councilor of District No. 8, Dr. Neely was re-elected to his post as Councilor at the time of the 1942 Annual Meeting in Tulsa, and Dr. Ewing will complete his three-year term. The duties of a Councilor are not altogether new to Dr. Ewing as he was the Eighth District Councilor for two years prior to his election as President-Elect of the Oklahoma State Medical Association in 1941.

The counties in Dr. Ewing's District are as follows: Adair, Cherokee, Craig, Delaware, Mayes, Muskogee, Okmulgee, Ottawa, Sequoyah and Wagoner.

RECENTLY LICENSED PHYSICIANS

J. D. Osborn, M.D., Secretary-Treasurer of the Oklahoma State Board of Medical Examiners, reports that licenses to practice medicine and surgery have been granted to 64 applicants during the period December 18, 1941, to August 12, 1942.

The following doctors of medicine were granted licenses:

Abshier, Alton Brooks, Oklahoma City; Asher, James Ottley, Oklahoma City; Bender, Herman Robert, Norman; Bradford, Vance Arthur, Syracuse, N. Y.; Brewer, Francis, Bookfield Center, Conn.; Brightwell, Richard Justice, Oklahoma City; Buford, Elvin Lee, Erie, Pa.; Bungardt, Alfred H., Jr., Camp Barkeley, Tex.; Campbell, John Moore, III, Oklahoma City; Chiasson, Emmerson Chaille, Stillwater; Cole, William Charles, Oklahoma City; Colvert, James Robert, Oklahoma City; Davis, Wesley Warren, Carlisle, Pa.; Denyer, Hillard Earl, Chandler; Dodson, Harrell Chandler, Oklahoma City; Drennan, Stanley Lewis, Oklahoma City; Farris, Edward Merhige, Baltimore, Md.; Fleetwood, Doyle H., Oklahoma City.

Flood, William Robert, Oakland, Calif.; Florence, Robert William, Seattle, Wash.; Hartford, Walter Kenneth, Oklahoma City; Haynes, William Madison, Henryetta; Heilman, Elwood Hess, Richmond, Va.; Hesser, James Matthew, Glencoe; Hubbard, William Ecton, Oklahoma City; Huber, Walter Arthur, Tulsa; Huntley, Henry Clay, Atoka; Jones, Delmas Bernard, Tulsa; Lester, Eugene Fay, Jr., Oklahoma City; Macrae, Donald Hanley, Tulsa; Mazzarella, Vincent, Tulsa; McCaleb, Philip Sheridan, Okemah; McClellan, Charles William, Claremore; McClure, Coye W., Oklahoma City; McCollum, Wiley Thomas, Kiowa, Kan.;

Mitchell, Wade Calhoon, Oklahoma City; Nelson, Willis Joret, Jr., Pryor; Norrick, John Howard, Oklahoma City; Overbey, Charles Brown, Jr., Mangum; Owens, Eugene Augustus, Lawton; Paul, Thomas Otis, Durant; Pearson, Daniel B., Oklahoma City; Phillips, James Gartrelle, Oklahoma City; Piatt, Louis Myer, Tulsa; Points, Thomas Craig, Oklahoma City; Powell, Paul Thurston, Norman; Reid, Roger James, Ardmore; Robinson, Ralph Dresden, Frederick; Rowland, Robert Hazel, Jr., Galveston, Tex.; Salkeld, Phil Lloyd, Vinita;

Sandlin, Dean Clifford, Oklahoma City; Sanford, Roy Keith, Perryton, Tex.; Schubert, Herbert Aloysius, Chickasha; Shofstall, William Howard, Tulsa; Smith, Paul Frederick, Tulsa; Swinburne, Mary Grace, Ardmore; Thomas, Charles Alfred, Coffeyville, Kan.; Threlkeld, Lal Dunean, Oklahoma City; Watson, Thomas Leonard, Tulsa; Wendel, William Eldon, Tulsa; Witt, Richard Earl, Oklahoma City; Wolff, John Powers, Oklahoma City; Word, Emery France, New Westminster, B. C., Can.; and Zeldes, Mary, Muskogee.

Dr. Philip C. Risser has recently returned to Blackwell after having served in the Navy. He is associated in practice with his father Dr. A. S. Risser.

ADDITIONAL MEMBERS IN MILITARY SERVICE

Below is a list of members of the Oklahoma State Medical Association who are now in active duty in some branch of the Armed Forces of the United States, in addition to those published in previous issues of the Journal.

In some instances, members enter the military service without notifying the State Association, therefore, it is very likely that the list is incomplete. The Journal will appreciate receiving notification concerning additional names that should be included in this list for publication each month.

Cherokee
DYER, ISADORE ....Tahlequah

Cleveland
LOY, WILLIAM A. ....Norman
PROSSER, MOORMAN P ....Norman

Creek
PICKHARDT, W. L. ....Sapulpa

Hughes
SHAW, JAMES F. ....Wetumka

Jackson
FOX, RAYMOND H. ....Altus

Kay
MORGAN, L. S. ....Ponca City
WHITE, M. S. ....Blackwell

Muskogee
McINNIS, J. T. ....Muskogee

Oklahoma
APPLETON, M. M. ....400 N. W. 10th St.
BIRGE, JACK P. ....Ramsey Tower
DILL, FRANCIS E. ....Medical Arts Bldg.
GINGLES, R. H. ....State Health Dept.
HUGGINS, J. R. ....2225 Exchange Ave.
HYROOP, GILBERT L. ....Medical Arts Bldg.
LITTLE, JOHN R. ....Ramsey Tower
MURDOCH, RAYMOND L. ....Medical Arts Bldg.
SHIRCLIFF, E. E., JR. ....128 N. W. 14th St.

Payne
BASSETT, CLIFFORD M. ....Cushing
ROBERTS, R. E. ....Stillwater

Pottawatomie
GALLAHER, PAUL C. ....Shawnee

Rogers
HOWARD, W. A. ....Chelsea

Seminole
RIPPY, O. M. ....Seminole

Tulsa
EADS, C. H. ....Medical Arts Bldg.
EDWARDS, D. L. ....Philcade Bldg.
HARDMAN, T. J. ....Medical Arts Bldg.
LUSK, E. M. ....915 S. Cincinnati
McDONALD, JOHN E. ....Nat'l Mutual Bldg.
MITCHELL, TOM HALL ......Nat'l Bank of Tulsa Bldg.
SPANN, LOGAN A. ....Braniff Bldg.
WHITE, ERIC M. ....Medical Arts Bldg.

Woodward
KING, FRANK M. ....Woodward

SPECIAL NOTICE!

The Oklahoma State Hospital Association is making an effort to place on its roster each Hospital operating in the state of Oklahoma.

In order to make this list of ethically operated hospitals accurate, the Secretary of the Hospital Association will contact each County Medical Society in the state, asking that they list all hospitals operating in their county in which members of their County Society practice.

This will not only give the Hospital Association a complete roster, but will increase the accuracy of ethically operated hospitals.

FEDERAL SOCIAL INSURANCE CONTRIBUTIONS ACT

(Editor's Note: The Public Policy Committee of the Oklahoma State Medical Association desires to present the following digest of certain portions of House Resolution 7534, by Dr. C. Rufus Rorem, Director, National Commission Office of the Blue Cross Plans, for your consideration as a member of the medical profession. The resolution was introduced before the present Congress by Mr. Eliot, Representative from Massachusetts, and it has been referred to the Committee on Ways and Means.)

This bill contemplates many important changes in the scope and administration of the Social Insurance provisions of the Social Security Act. It extends the coverage of Federal old-age and survivors insurance, provides insurance benefits for workers permanently and totally disabled, and establishes a Federal system of employment offices, unemployment compensation, temporary disability benefits, and hospitalization benefits.

Not all of the charges are of direct interest to persons concerned with hospitals and Blue Cross Plans. The following digest gives particular emphasis to the proposals to add hospitalization and temporary disability benefits to the coverage for insured workers and their dependents.

I. General Changes

The major changes in the Social Security Act which are of special interest to hospitals and Blue Cross Plans may be summarized as follows:

1. Extension of the social insurance provisions of the Social Security Act to essentially all employed persons, the new groups being agricultural labor, domestic service, employees of non-profit institutions, fishermen, insurance agents, etc.

2. Federalization of the unemployment compensation program, now administered by the various States.

3. Creation of provisions for insurance benefits during the workers' periods of temporary disability.

4. Creation of provisions for hospitalization benefits for insured workers and their dependents.

5. Liberalization of certain provisions for making old-age, survivors, and disability (total and permanent) insurance payments to the insured and his dependents or his estate; also authorization of expeditures for regular redetermination of disability and rehabilitation of disabled beneficiaries.

6. Waiver of payments for insured individuals who enter the military service (October 1, 1940 to termination of the emergency) and coverage of such persons for survivors or disability benefits, as well as unemployment compensation, when discharged.

II. Administrative Provisions of the New Law

A. *Trust Fund.* There is created on the books of the Treasury of the United States a trust fund to be known as the "Federal Social Insurance Trust Fund" (Title I A, Section 150,a,b), to be administered by a Board of Trustees composed of the Secretary of the Treasury, the Secretary of Labor, and the chairman of the Social Security Board. The Board will establish separate accounts as may seem necessary or desirable, and make reports to Congress of actual and estimated receipts and disbursements.

B. *Contributions for Social Insurance.* Contributions are based upon a percentage of "wages" paid and received, with each employer and employee (insured worker) making equal proportionate contributions to the Social Insurance Trust Fund. Benefits of the Federal Social Insurance System are shared alike by all workers in their capacities as employees, including the managers or owners of business or other establishments. There is no "earmarking" of stated percentages of the contributions for the different types of benefits, such as old-age and survivors insurance, unemployment, temporary disability, hospitalization, etc. But amounts are allocated for the various benefits upon recommendation of the Chairman of the Social Security Board.

TABLE I

PROPOSED FEDERAL SOCIAL INSURANCE CONTRIBUTIONS

(Percentages of Wages, not exceeding $3,000 annually)

Insured Classes	Year	By Employer	By Employee	Total
Groups Previously	1943-5	5%	5%	10%
Insured under So-	1946-8	5½%	5½%	11%
cial Security Act	After 1948	6%	6%	12%
Self-Employed	1943-5		4%	4%
Persons	1946-8		5%	5%
	After 1948		6%	6%
Agricultural Labor	1943-5	2%	2%	4%
Domestic Service	1946-8	2½%	2½%	5%
Non-Profit Insti-	After 1948	3%	3%	6%
tutions, etc.				

C. *Definitions.* The term "wages" is determined broadly to include all remuneration for employment (up to $3,000 annually) including commissions, salaries, market value of services of self-employed persons, etc.

The term "employment" means any service, of whatever nature, for wages or under any contract of hire, written or oral, expressed or employed, in the United States.

III. Hospitalization Benefits

A. *Eligible Persons* (Section 901).

1. Insured employee,
2. Dependent wife,
3. Dependent children (including adopted): (a) under 18 years of age; (b) unmarried; (c) not employed.

B. *Maximum Hospitalization Benefits* (Section 902).

Thirty days in any "benefit year" for the insured worker, and/or each dependent. If the hospitalization benefit account permits, the Board may increase benefits to 60 days.

"Benefit year" means the 52 weeks following the first day for which application for hospitalization benefits is made (and approved).

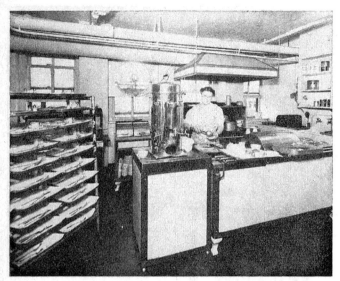

C. *Procedures.*

1. *Application.* Individual must apply for benefits within 90 days after entering a hospital (Section 903).

2. *Accredited hospitals.* Benefits are payable only for service in accredited hospitals (Section 904 and 908,b).

   a. The Board will establish a list of accredited hospitals by January 1, 1944.

   b. Hospitals may apply for accreditation, or may demand hearings if withdrawn from the list.

   c. Accredited hospitals must provide "at least" bed and board, general nursing, operating and delivery rooms, ordinary medications and dressings, laboratory and x-ray services, etc.; must afford "professional service, personnel, and equipment adequate to promote the health and safety of individuals customarily hospitalized therein"; and must have procedures for making reports and certifications to the Board.

   These requirements will not be enforced upon hospitals devoted chiefly to the care of persons afflicted with mental or nervous diseases, tuberculosis, or other chronic illnesses.

   Hospitals may be accredited for limited types of cases, and in every instance the Board may take into account the characteristics of the community which the hospital serves.

3. *National Advisory Hospital Benefits Council* (Section 905).

   This Council, appointed by the Board, will advise the Board on formulating standards for hospitals, making studies, etc.

   The members will be selected from the "professions and agencies concerned with the operations of hospitals, and other persons informed on the need for or provision of hospital services."

D. *Method of Payment.*

1. Payments will be made in cash, ordinarily to the insured worker.

2. Assignment will be permitted to an "accredited hospital, or to any other agency or institution utilized" (Section 907,a).

3. The Board will certify individuals who are entitled to payments, and the proper amounts will be paid by the Secretary of the Treasury (Section 907,c): (a) to any individual, agency or institution designated by the Board; (b) to the Board for its distribution.

E. *Use of Other Agencies* (Section 907,b).

   The Board may utilize the services and facilities of other agencies, "through agreements or cooperative working arrangements with appropriate agencies of the United States, or any State or political subdivision thereof, and with other appropriate public agencies and private persons, agencies or institutions".

F. *Amount of Per-Diem Hospitalization Benefits* (Section 908,d).

1. Benefits to the insured will be not less than $3.00, nor more than $6.00 per day of hospitalization.

2. "The Board may make arrangements with accredited hospitals for payments of the reasonable cost of hospital service".

G. *Types of Illnesses Covered.*

1. Application for benefits is not valid "with respect to any day of hospitalization for tuberculosis or for mental or nervous disease after such diagnosis has been made" (Section 903). There is no mention (directly or indirectly) of any other exclusions of any nature. By implication maternity hospitalization may be included with the maximum benefit-years allowance for an insured worker, or a dependent.

2. No payment shall be made for hospitalization "due to any injury or disability arising out of or in the course of any employment," that is for "any service, of whatever nature, performed by an employee for the person employing him" (Section 908, d).

IV. Temporary Disability Benefits

A. *Eligible individuals may receive weekly cash benefits* for 26 weeks in any benefit year if "unemployed", or absent from work because of temporary disability. (All part-time earning above $3,000 weekly are deducted.) (Section 801,a).

B. *The weekly benefits depends upon highest quarterly wage received* during the "base-period" preceding the application for unemployment or disability benefits. Additional payments are made for dependents, with weekly benefits ranging from a minimum of $5.00 for a single individual to a maximum of $23.00 for any employee with three or more dependents (Section 801,b).

C. There is an additional maternity benefit for employed women (equal to ordinary disability benefits) for 12 weeks maximum (six before and six after confinement), provided the insured women comply with rules concerning prenatal and postnatal care.

D. *Certification for disability benefits.*

   Individuals claiming or receiving temporary disability or maternity benefits must, if requested by the Board, "submit to an examination by such physician or expert as the Board may designate at such reasonable time and place as the Board may direct and any failure or refusal without good cause to submit to such examination or any obstruction thereof shall result in a forfeiture of such individual's right to such benefits until such examination has taken place".

E. *Eligibility for disability benefits.*

1. *Filing of claim* for benefits in proper manner.

2. *Certification* as to disability, and actual continuation of disability in accord with regulations.

3. *Waiting period of one week* prior to first week of benefits. This may be the same week as that required for unemployment benefits.

4. *Earnings of base period* must be thirty times the basic weekly benefit.

5. *Disqualifications.*

   Coverage under total disability provisions or workmen's compensation law.

"Guide to Therapy for Medical Officers," a technical manual based on material secured almost wholly from various committees of the Division of Medical Sciences of the National Research Council, has recently been issued by the Government Printing Office, Washington. Material covered includes general medicine, surgical emergencies, medical emergencies, diagnosis and treatment of venereal diseases, chemotherapy and serotherapy in certain infectious diseases, treatment and control of certain trophical diseases, and the rickettsial diseases.

News From The State Health Department

The following is a list of former full-time State and County Health Department personnel now on active duty in the armored forces of our Nation.

NAME	FORMER LOCATION
Edward Ashton	Oklahoma City
Dr. Paul N. Atkins	Muskogee County (Curative)
Dr. Harry E. Barnes	District 1, Tahlequah
Dr. J. Y. Battenfield	State Epidemiologist, Okla. City
Dr. T. T. Beeler	Atoka County
Dr. D. W. Branham	Oklahoma City
Dr. W. R. Cheatwood	Pontotoc County
Dr. C. D. Cunningham	Seminole County
Josephine Custer, R.N.	Carter County
Dr. R. H. Duewall	McCurtain County
Dr. Isadore Dyer	District 1, Tahlequah
Dr. R. F. Erdman	Oklahoma City
Martha Garson, R.N.	Payne County
Dr. James O. Hood	Cleveland County
Paul Hutchinson	Oklahoma City
Dr. Frank M. King	Harper-Woodward Counties
Gene King	Oklahoma City
Dr. Wm. A. Loy	Cleveland County
Dr. Glen W. McDonald	Pontotoc County
Dr. J. T. McInnis	Muskogee County
G. T. McNew	Oklahoma City
Essa Michel, R.N.	Payne County
Dr. V. F. Morgan	Comanche County
Dr. C. L. Oglesbee	Muskogee County (Curative)

Dr. W. L. Pickhardt	Creek County
Floyd Renshaw	Oklahoma City
Dr. O. M. Rippy	Seminole County
Eldon Rogers	Caddo County
Lester Settle	Creek County
Geneva Spencer, R.N.	Okmulgee County
Elbrege Sullivan	Comanche County
Dr. O. H. Tackett	McClain County
Fred Tharp	Oklahoma City
Gene White	Oklahoma City
Dr. Claude Williams	Caddo County
W. J. Wyatt	Oklahoma City
Dr. H. A. Zampetti	Comanche County

Steinmetz, of General Electric fame, defined a high-brow as "any person educated beyond his intelligence."
—N. Y. State Jour. of Med..

OMAHA MID-WEST CLINICAL SOCIETY MEETS OCTOBER 26-30

The tenth annual assembly of the Omaha Mid-West Clinical Society will convene October 26-30, 1942, in the Hotel Paxton. Though many obstacles and unpleasant factors have confronted the assembly, it is anticipated that this year's attendance will surpass all others as all physicians will readily recognize that this type of meeting, at which the care of the civilian population and military forces will be discussed, has much to offer at a minimum expense.

Interesting subjects for round table discussions have been selected, and an outstanding group of guest speakers have found it possible to accept the invitation of the assembly to attend.

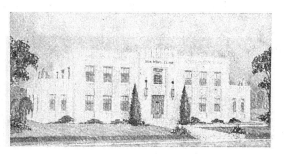

VON WEDEL CLINIC

PLASTIC and GENERAL SURGERY
Dr. Curt von Wedel

TRAUMATIC and INDUSTRIAL
SURGERY
Dr. Clarence A. Gallagher

INTERNAL MEDICINE and DIAGNOSIS
Dr. Harry A. Daniels

Special attention to cardiac and gastro intestinal diseases

Complete laboratory and X-ray facilities.
Electrocardiograph.

610 Northwest Ninth Street
Opposite St. Anthony's Hospital
Oklahoma City

TREND OF CAUSES OF DEATH DOWNWARD FOR
CERTAIN DISEASES IN OKLAHOMA

The Oklahoma State Health Department through its Vital Statistics Bureau and with the cooperation of the physicians in the State have just completed the following compilation of the causes of death from certain diseases in Oklahoma for the past five years.

	1941	1940	1939	1938	1937
Deaths, all causes (Rate per 1,000 population)	8.6	8.7	8.9	8.5	9.2
Births, exclusive of stillbirths (Rate per 1,000 population)	19.3	19.0	18.8	19.2	17.6
Infant Mortality (Rate per 1,000 live births)	49.0	50.0	52.0	43.0	59.0
Maternal Mortality (Rate per 1,000 live births)	3.0	3.5	4.2	4.0	6.9
Typhoid and Paratyphoid Fever (1,2) (Rate per 100,000 population)	1.5	2.5	3.4	4.1	5.8
Cerebrospinal Meningococcus Meningitis (Rate per 100,000 population)	.3	.9	.5	1.0	2.1
Scarlet Fever (8) (Rate per 100,000 population)	.2	.3	.7	.9	1.4
Whooping Cough (9) (Rate per 100,000 population)	5.0	2.4	1.0	7.9	3.6
Diphtheria (10) (Rate per 100,000 population)	2.9	3.2	3.3	5.2	4.1
Tuberculosis, all forms (13-22) (Rate per 100,000 population)	45.1	47.6	45.7	48.9	52.4
Malaria (28) (Rate per 100,000 population)	2.2	1.0	2.2	3.5	3.6
Influenza (Grippe) (33) (Rate per 100,000 population)	23.9	24.4	21.9	17.2	43.5
Measles (35) (Rate per 100,000 population)	.9	.2	3.2	2.4	1.0
Acute Poliomyelitis and Polioencephalitis (36) (Rate per 100,000 population)	.6	1.2	.4	1.0	2.5
Acute Infectious Encephalitis (Lethargic) (37) (Rate per 100,000 population)	.4	.6	.6	.3	.3
Cancer and Malignant Tumors (45-55) (Rate per 100,000 population)	82.9	82.6	78.6	75.3	77.9
Diabetes Mellitus (6) (Rate per 100,000 population)	14.7	14.0	14.7	13.8	13.8
Pellagra, except alcoholic (69) (Rate per 100,000 population)	2.1	2.2	4.2	4.5	4.3
Cerebral Hemorrhage, Embolism, and Thrombosis (83a,b) (Rate per 100,000 population)	78.3	80.6	85.9	68.0	67.5
Diseases of Heart (90-95) (Rate per 100,000 population)	182.9	162.4	152.1	140.1	140.5
Pneumonia, all forms (107-109) (Rate per 100,000 population)	49.5	57.4	61.3	62.1	78.6
Diseases of the Digestive System (115-129) (Rate per 100,000 population)	48.3	59.7	64.6	61.0	70.7
Diarrhea and Enteritis under two years (119) (Rate per 100,000 population)	4.7	10.4	9.4	10.3	14.1
Nephritis, all forms (130-132) (Rate per 100,000 population)	55.9	61.9	54.7	61.6	67.1

Lieutenant Glenn S. Kreger, formerly of Tonkawa, is now on active duty at Fort Bliss, Texas, where he is Battalion Surgeon.

A Clinic by Dr. Edward T. Shirley presenting a case of Addison's Disease, discussed by those in attendance, highlighted the meeting of the Garvin County Medical Society on Wednesday, September 16, at 8:00 P. M. Ten members of the Society were present at the meeting which was held in the Chamber of Commerce offices in Pauls Valley.

The date for the next meeting is scheduled for October 14.

Twenty-two members of the Woodward County Medical Society and their wives were guests of the Memorial Hospital Staff, at a regular meeting of the society on Thursday, September 10, at 7:30 P. M.

The program consisted of discussions by Dr. W. Floyd Keller and Dr. J. O. Asher, both of Oklahoma City, on "Shock and Its Treatment."

Dr. V. M. Rutherford of Woodward, who left for active military duty with the armed forces September 15, presided over the meeting in the absence of the President, Dr. M. H. Newman of Shattuck.

Eighteen members were present at the September 9 meeting of the Washington-Nowata County Medical Society in Bartlesville. Dr. Elizabeth M. Chamberlin presented a paper entitled "The Rh. Factor in Blood".

The October meeting will be held at Pawhuska at which time members from Osage, Kay and Washington-Nowata Counties will be in attendance. It is planned to have these Tri-County meetings throughout the year.

Word has been received by his friends in Oklahoma City that Dr. Edward D. McKay, a former city physician, has been commissioned an army captain and has reported to active duty at Fort Sam Houston, San Antonio, Texas.

Doctor McKay is a graduate of the University of Oklahoma Medical School in 1935, and practiced in the Oklahoma City Clinic during 1939-1940.

Classified Advertisements

University of Oklahoma School of Medicine

On September 10, 1942, 75 first-year medical students reported for physical examination. They subsequently enrolled and began their class work on Monday, September 14. There are 73 men and two women in this class. They come from all sections of the State of Oklahoma, as follows:

NAME	HOME TOWN
Edward Allphin Allgood	Altus
Cad Walder Arrendell	Ponca City
John Ahrens Blaschke	Norman
Broadway Broadrick	Chickasha
J. T. Brooks	Marlow
Arthur Merton Brown	Muskogee
Irwin Hubert Brown	Muskogee
Leonard Harold Brown	Muskogee
Nello DeLon Brown	Oklahoma City
Richard Herbert Burgtorf	Custer City
Martha Jene Burke	Hobart
Robert Elsworth Casey	Oklahoma City
Stanley Gray Childers	Tipton
Marvin Allen Childress	Webb City
James William Clopton	Oklahoma City
Charles Stewart Cunningham	Purcell
Walter Traynor Dardis, Jr.	Oklahoma City
Lawrence Albert Denney	Jenks
Robert Pinkerton Dennis	Oklahoma City
Walter Henry Dersch, Jr.	Oklahoma City
John Woodrow DeVore	Elk City
C. H. Dillingham, Jr.	Frederick
Loren Alonzo Dunton	Enid
Martin Dale Edwards	Cameron
Arthur Furman Elliott	Enid
Richard Allison Ellis	Duncan
James Burnette Askridge, III	Oklahoma City
Charles Louis Freede	Oklahoma City
Jack Birden Garlin	Bartlesville
Dorothy Elizabeth Gore	Blanchard
Jack L. Gregston	Marlow
Orville Lee Grigsby	Spiro
Arthur Edward Hale	Alva
James Dooley Hallenbeck	Guthrie
Richard Lowel Harris	Taloga
Marvin Bryant Hays	Vinita
Richard Guy Hobgood	Concho
Richard Davis Hoover	Oklahoma City
Joe Ben Hunsaker	Durant
Paul Kouri	Granite
William Pen Lerblance, Jr.	Checotah
Dave Bernard Lhevine	Tulsa
Dick Moss Lowry	Oklahoma City
Dalton Blue McInnis	Muskogee
Edward Daniel Mackenzie	Oklahoma City
Charles Robert Mathews	Britton
Vernon Conrad Merrifield	Norman
Raymond Delbert Niles Miller	Hollis
Walter Mason Moore	Muskogee
Nova Lemoine Morgan	Gate
Elmer Grant Murphy	Stillwater
Paul Joseph Ottis	Okarche
James William Parker	Elk City
Billy Raymond Paschal	Oklahoma City
Hugh William Payton	Shawnee
Sabin Crawford Perceefull	Miami
William Silvey Pugsley	Oklahoma City
Robert Fike Ranson	Hitchcock
Oren Creighton Reid	Lawton
Jean Earley Rorie	Oklahoma City
Clinton McKinley Shaw, Jr.	Durant
Charles Gibson Shellenberger	Yukon
Henry Clinton Smith	Lawton
John Byron Smith	Bristow
Newton Converse Smith	Cherokee
Walter Fred Speakman	Drumright
Gerald Matthew Steelman	Healdton
Byron Junior Tatlow	Oklahoma City
Lewis Albert Temple	Okmulgee
James Harold Tisdal	Clinton
Clyde Edward Tomlin	Tonkawa
Howard Grafflin Tozer	Muskogee
Milford Shael Ungerman	Tulsa
Ray Cecil Waterbury	Apache
James Riley Winterringer	Stillwater

Mr. Evan L. Copeland has been appointed Instructor in Physiology ad interim, and Dr. Samuel A. Corson has been appointed Assistant Professor of Physiology. Doctor Corson is transferring from the University of Texas.

Captain M. M. Appleton of Oklahoma City, a former reserve officer, has been assigned to duty at the William Beaumont Hospital, El Paso, Texas.

Blue Cross Reports

In war and in years of peace, an undeclared war—using the weapons illness and accident—is striking every minute of every day. And in this other kind of war, we find another use for our research, our science and our courage.

The hospital is the theater of the eternal war—the battlefield of the fight for health. In defense of our nation's health, this fight goes on endlessly. For no one is safe, no one knows when accident or illness will strike, nor the name of the next victim.

For years, American hospitals have housed the finest equipment and the best professional skills in the world. But even this wasn't enough. The people who needed care, and who couldn't afford to pay for it individually, constituted a serious problem.

The American Hospital Association studied a way to put necessary hospitalization within the reach of all. The Blue Cross Plans solved the problem. The story of their successful development is a "daily miracle"—all over America. Millions of people have grouped together in communities large and small to provide themselves with prompt, adequate hospital care.

The Blue Cross Plans are a distinctly American institution, a unique combination of individual initiative and social responsibility. They perform a public service without public compulsion, and exemplify private leadership without private gain. They prevent a drain upon the subscriber's savings, and stabilize the financial support of the community's hospitals which provide the services.

Through these plans, the services of the American hospitals are effectively distributed to meet the health needs of each individual and the entire nation.

Hospitalization is a problem that has received much attention, and many schemes have been suggested as solutions. Over ten million Americans, including 150,000 employers, believe that the Blue Cross Plans may be expanded to reach a major segment of the population without legislative compulsion or taxation.

The plans and member-hospitals are interested only in serving the public. But the expansion of that service will depend upon the increasing interest and cooperation of our doctors, civic and business leaders. Rapid growth of this voluntary method will assure the preservation of the voluntary system of hospitals.

MEDICAL PREPAREDNESS

Policies Governing Initial Appointment of Medical Officers*

The Surgeon General of the Army published detailed information concerning policies governing the inital appointment of physicians as medical officers on April 23, 1942. Necessary changes are given wide publicity, at his request, in order that the individual applicants, and all concerned in the procurement of medical officers, may know the status of such appointments.

The current military program provides for a definite number of position vacancies in the different grades. The number of such positions must necessarily determine the promotion of officers already on duty and, in addition, the appointment of new officers from civilian life. Such appointments are limited to qualified physicians required to fill the position vacancies for which no equally well qualified medical officers are available. Such positions calling for an increase in grade should be filled by promotion of those already in the service, insofar as possible, and not by new appointments.

If this policy is not followed, it would definitely penalize a large number of well qualified Lieutenants and Captains already on duty by blocking their promotions which have been earned by hard work. In view of these facts, it has been deemed necessary to raise the standards of training and experience for appointment in grades above that of First Lieutenant.

With this in view, The Surgeon General has announced the following policy which will govern action to be taken on all applications after September 15, 1942:

All appointments will be recommended in the grade of First Lieutenant with the following exceptions:

CAPTAIN. 1. Eligible applicants between the ages of 37 and 45 will be considered for appointment in the grade of Captain by reason of their age and general unclassified medical training and experience.

2. Below the age of 37 and above the age of 32, CONSIDERATION for appointment in the grade of Captain will be given to applicants who meet all of the following minimum requirements:
  a. Graduation from an approved medical school.
  b. Internship of not less than one year, preferably of the rotating type.
  c. Special training consisting of three years' residency in a recognized specialty.
  d. An additional period of not less than two years

of study and/or practice limited to the specialty.

3. Eligible applicants who previously held commissions in the grade of Captain in the Medical Corps (Regular Army, National Guard of the United States, or Officers Reserve Corps) MAY BE CONSIDERED for appointment in that grade provided they have not passed the age of 45 years.

MAJOR. 1. Eligible applicants between the ages of 37 and 55 MAY BE CONSIDERED for appointment under the following conditions:
  a. Graduation from an approved school.
  b. Internship of not less than one year, preferably of the rotating type.
  c. Special training consisting of three years' residency in a recognized specialty.
  d. An additional period of not less than seven years of study and/or practice limited to the specialty.
  e. The existence of appropriate position vacancies.
  f. Additional training of a special nature of value to the military service, in lieu of the above.

2. Applicants previously commissioned as Majors in the Medical Corps (Regular Army, National Guard of the United States, or Officers Reserve Corps) whose training and experience qualify them for appropriate assignments may be CONSIDERED for appointment in the grade of Major provided they have not passed the age of 55.

LIEUTENANT COLONEL AND COLONEL. In view of the small number of assignment vacancies for individuals of such grade, and the large number of Reserve Officers of these grades who are being called to duty, such appointments will be limited. Wherever possible, promotion of qualified officers on duty will be utilized

to fill the position vacancies.

Much misunderstanding has arisen concerning recognition by Specialty Boards and membership in specialty groups. It will be noted that mention is not made of these in the preceding paragraphs. This is due to the variation in requirements of the different Boards and organizations. Membership and recognition are definite factors in determining the professional background of the individual, but are NOT the deciding factor, as so many physicians have been led to believe.

Colonel Seeley Transferred to Military Duty

The Directing Board of the Procurement and Assignment Service for Physicians, Dentists, and Veterinarians, has formally expressed its appreciation of the services rendered by Colonel Sam F. Seeley, who has been transferred to military duty. Following is the text of the resolution adopted:

"The transfer of Lieutenant Colonel Sam F. Seeley from his connection with the Procurement and Assignment Service to active military duty causes a great loss. Colonel Seeley who has acted as Executive Officer since the beginning of this Service has been transferred to military duty, which is in keeping with the policy recently adopted by the War Department. His training and experience with the Medical Corps of the Army in his professional capacity amply justifies such a step.

"The Directing Board of the Procurement and Assignment Service wishes to take this opportunity of expressing to the Surgeon General of the United States Army its very deep appreciation for the valuable services which Colonel Seeley has rendered during its period of organization and functions.

"The Directing Board expresses to Colonel Seeley its deep appreciation for the great sacrifice which he has made in dislocating himself from actual military duty to serve with us in an executive capacity. He has been most unselfish, and has given unstintingly of his time, energy, and patience in helping to solve many of the problems connected with the functioning of the Procurement and Assignment Service. He has not only labored faithfully at our office in Washington, but he has traveled over the United States contacting many of his professional conferes and explaining to them the purpose for which the Procurement and Assignment Service was organized. His services have been most valuable and have helped to take us a long way in accomplishing the objectives for which it was created.

"The Directing Board expresses to Colonel Seeley its gratitude and thanks for his unselfish devotion to the organization of the Procurement and Assignment Service and wishes for him the greatest success in his new assignment."

Frank H. Lahey, M.D., Chairman,
Harvey B. Stone, M.D.,
Harold S. Diehl, M.D.,
James E. Paullin, M.D.,
C. Willard Camalier, D.D.S.

The action of the Grading Board, established by The Surgeon General in his office, is final in tendering inital appointments. Proper consideration must be given such factors as age, position vacancies, the functions of command, and original assignments. All questionable initial grades are decided by this Board. Due to the lack of time, no reconsideration can be given.

There are in the age group 24-45 more than a sufficient number of eligible, qualified physicians to meet the Medical Department requirements. It is upon this age group that the Congress has imposed a definite obligation of military service through the medium of the Selective Service Act. The physicians in this group are ones needed NOW for active duty. The requirements are immediate and imperative. Applications beyond 45 years may be considered for appointment only if they possess special qualifications for assignment to positions appropriate to the grade of MAJOR or above.

*Taken from The Journal of the A.M.A. Vol. 120, No. 2, Page 129, September 12, 1942.

DEDICATION OF NEW UNITED STATES NAVY MEDICAL CENTER

"On Monday, August 31," The Journal of the American Medical Association says in its September 5 issue, "the United States Navy celebrated the one hundredth anniversary of the establishment of its Bureau of Medicine and Surgery by dedicating the new Navy Medical Center at Bethesda, Maryland. The proceedings included an international broadcast by five networks, symbolic of the. worldwide scope of the work of this department of the Navy. The ceremony was featured by an address of President Franklin Delano Roosevelt and included messages to naval installations in Iceland, Ireland, Honolulu and Panama, with responses from Capt. Brython P. Davis, commanding officer of Destroyer Base Hospital No. 1, North Ireland; Capt. J. J. McMullin, commanding officer of the Pearl Harbor Naval Hospital; Capt. Lewis W. Johnson, senior naval medical officer in Iceland, and. Capt. Howard F. Lawrence of Panama. No celebration is contemplated at these remote points where the Navy is actively in service. 'The motto of the United States Naval Medical Department is:

"To keep as many men at as many guns as many days as possible." '

"The career of the United States Naval Medical Department over the century has been marked by many brilliant episodes, including several instances in which Naval medical officers took over command following the deaths of officers of the line. For example, a naval medical officer, Dr. Richard C. Edgar, was the recipient of those famous lines of Captain Lawrence, destined to become the motto of the Navy, 'Don't give up the ship.'

"The first chief of the new Bureau of Medicine and Surgery in 1842 was William Paul Crillon Barton of Philadelphia. Rear Admiral Ross T. McIntire is twenty-third in a long line of surgeon generals of the Bureau of Medicine and Surgery of the Navy.

"In the early days of the Navy a ship's surgeon received $25 a month and had the status of a hired hand. Today naval medical officers achieve high rank and are engaged in a multitude of scientific activities representative of the finest advancement of medicine. The func-

tions of the medical officers of the Navy include research on problems related to ships, airplanes and land warfare. Already notable contributions have been made on submarine warfare, aviation, treatment of burns, the effects of blast and the control of many types of epidemic disease. Naval medical officers have designed hospital ships, invented new appliances and contributed magnificiently to research in internal medicine and in surgery.

"A century ago the headquarters of the Bureau of Medicine and Surgery included a chief, an assistant chief and two clerks. Today the expanded Navy includes many hundred thousands of men and thousands of medical officers and medical personnel. Its responsibilities for medical care include the Marine Corps and Coast Guard as well as itself.

"The first century has been one of great achievement and high scientific endeavor. To the Surgeon General of the Navy, Rear Admiral Ross T. McIntire, and to the men whom he leads, our congratulations."

SURGEONS' CONGRESS SCHEDULED FOR CLEVELAND, NOVEMBER 17-20

The Thirty-second Annual Clinical Congress of the American College of Surgeons, originally scheduled for October in Chicago, will be held in Cleveland, with headquarters at the Cleveland Public Auditorium, from November 17-20, according to an announcement from College headquarters. The meeting was first scheduled for Los Angeles. The Twenty-fifth Annual Hospital Standardization Conference, sponsored by the College, will be held simultaneously.

The program of both meetings will begin with a Joint General Assembly on Tuesday morning, November 17, and will be based chiefly on wartime activities as they affect surgeons and hospital personnel in the rapidly expanding medical services of the Army and Navy. Special consideration will also be given to problems as related to the increasing activities of civilian defense. Dr. W. Edward Gallie of Toronto, Canada, is President of the College.

The Forum on Fundamental Surgical Problems, which was inaugurated at the 1941 Clinical Conference, will be repeated this year and will be conducted on three successive mornings.

For detailed information, address Secretary of the College, 40 East Erie Street, Chicago, Illinois.

Colonel Lee R. Wilhite, formerly of Perkins, is now commanding officer of the 134th Medical Regiment at Fort Bragg, North Carolina. As a representative of the Surgeon General's Office, he was in charge of the Medical Recruiting Board of Oklahoma until his transfer the first of August.

Two Ponca City physicians—Captain L. S. Morgan and Captain Laile G. Neal reported for active duty in the United States Army on September 29. Captain Morgan has been assigned to the Air Corps and reported for services at the Arrow Air Base, Santa Ana, California, and Captain Neal was assigned to Fort Sam Houston, San Antonio, Texas.

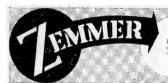

Great Opportunity Lies Ahead for American Women

"A great opportunity lies ahead for the women of America," R. R. Spencer, M.D., of the National Institute of Health, Bethesda, Md., declares in an article in the current issue of War Medicine, in which he urges "that college women of strong physique who have the will to serve humanity and who have special aptitudes in the biologic sciences be encouraged to major in such subjects with a view to earning a doctorate of philosophy or of medicine." War Medicine is published by the American Medical Association in cooperation with the Division of Medical Sciences of the National Research Council.

Pointing out that the nation at war requires the services of every available physician, Doctor Spencer says that while there are in the United States at this time over 160,000 physicians licensed to practice, only 7,000, or less than five percent of them, are women. The doctor says that the first wartime need for women physicians will be for those already trained who can step at once into positions now held by men physicians who will be thus freed for military service.

"I am sorry to say that as a rule women have not been encouraged to enter the medical profession," Doctor Spencer declares. "Now, when women physicians could be used to free men for military service, when they would be gratefully called on for civilian defense in the event of aerial bombardments and when they could be used in hospitals, medical schools, industrial plants, laboratories, public schools, clinics for venereal disease and many other places, the nation finds itself with only a handful of women physicians and surgeons. The policy has been short sighted and a bit ungenerous to those women who have had the urge to make their social contribution in the field of medicine. However, this is no time for postmortems. One must consider what can be done now and in the immediate future to meet the urgent needs for trained personnel. . . .

"At the National Institute of Health, which is engaged solely in medical and public health research, there is a fairly large number of women in the professional and scientific grades—four—in a total of 289 professional workers. . . .

"In medical research the quantity of workers needed may not be as great as in some other fields, but the quality of the workers must be high. However, medical research employs a composite group—embracing persons with only grade school education all the way up to those with the most highly specialized training offered by universities. . . .

"The personnel at the National Institute of Health both in the professional and in subprofessional groups is selected from Civil Service registers. Women and men have equal opportunities. The men called to military service from the subprofessional personnel are now rapidly being replaced by women wherever it can be done. . . .

"In the years ahead women physicians will be found in the service of their communities as general practitioners; as consultants in industrial hygiene—as directors of maternal and child health services in health and welfare agencies, where key positions are now held more often by men than by women; as directors of research, not merely as research assistants and laboratory technicians; as surgeons in hospitals for women and children and in general hospitals—in short, I believe that while many women physicians may not be used in this war for the simple reason that they are not available, they will be called on far more widely after the war than they have been in the past. And the time to begin training prospective women physicians is now. . . ."

A college professor has discovered that cockroaches have no vitamin A.—N. Y. State Jour. of Med.

Office of Civilian Defense

The Emergency Medical Service of the Office of Civilian Defense in Oklahoma made available a visual education program, consisting of two or more films to be shown in the various counties of the state under the auspices of the Emergency Medical Service.

The showing of these films has attracted a great deal of attention. The demand has been so great that the films have been scheduled out for some time in the future. In most cases, the Emergency Medical Service has extended an invitation to all of the local civilian defense organizations, as well as the general public, to attend these showings.

The response has been beyond the expectations of everyone. The first showing was made at Coalgate, where there was an attendance of better than 200. Most of the doctors of the county, and their wives, were in attendance. Usually presiding over the meeting where the showings are made, is the Chief of Emergency Medical Service or the physician who is the general chairman of the local Health and Housing Committee.

The second showing was made at Prague, with between three and four hundred in attendance. Showings have been made at Coalgate, Prague, Oklahoma City, Stigler, Hollis, Sapulpa, Shawnee, Hugo, Jay, and Miami.

The films shown consist of "The Warning," a 16 mm. sound film, 30 minutes in length, which pictures the overwhelming reality of an air-raid on a typical British city and the destruction that accompanies it. We see, too, the work of defense done by both the military and organized civilian defense corps, and the task of restoration as the tension slackens with the report, "Raiders passed". Another 16 mm. sound film, 15 minutes in length, entitled "Defending the City's Health," shows the work of a model city health department, including education, gathering statistics, nursing, supervising sanitation, laboratory analysis, child hygiene, and a comprehensive sequence on the control of communicable diseases. The role of the individual citizen in a health program is stressed. The third film that is shown is a 16 mm. sound film, 15 minutes in length, which shows the extent of America's efforts to arm against the threat of war, and then points out the problem of syphilis, gonorrhea, and prostitution as a threat to a strong nation. The need for adequate medical care, wholesome recreation, and guidance is clearly emphasized.

In order for the films to be shown in a county, it is necessary for the Chief of Emergency Medical Service to make a written application to Dr. G. F. Mathews, State Chief of Emergency Medical Service, State Health Department, Oklahoma City, Oklahoma. There is no cost attached to the showing of these films, and an operator will accompany the films with the necessary equipment for the showing. The publicity advertising the showings, and the place where the films are shown are arranged for locally by the Emergency Medical Service.

O. C. D. Urges Recruitment of More Nurses' Aides

The Civilian Mobilization Branch of the Office of Civilian Defense recently issued a memorandum to its regional representatives urging a concerted effort to stimulate the recruitment and enrollment of Nurses' Aides so as to relieve the serious shortage of nursing personnel in hospitals.

A report dated June 20, showed that 25,905 Nurses-Aides had been enrolled, of whom 12,890 had been certificated. This is only one-fourth of the 100,000 set as a goal at the beginning of the campaign in the summer of 1941. Reports from all parts of the country indicate that the training has been well carried out and the

Nurses' Aides are now giving valuable service in their assignments.

The memorandum reveals that some hospitals are reported to be accepting volunteer workers without training and permitting them to carry out many of the tasks usually performed by Nurses' Aides. Although several different types of volunteer assistants can be used in hospitals, untrained workers should not be assigned to duties similar to those of trained Nurses' Aides. Such a practice militates against the establishment of a reliable, disciplined corps of workers and deters enrollment of Nurses' Aides.

• OBITUARIES •

Dr. J. M. Denby
1877-1942

Dr. J. M. Denby, a prominent physician of Carter, Okla., passed away in San Bernardino, Calif., on August 22, 1942.

Dr. Denby is a graduate of the University of Nashville Medical Department in 1905. In 1910, following his marriage at Hillsboro, Texas, he moved to Carter, where he has since continued to practice.

Survivors include his wife, a son and daughter, all of the home address

He was an active member of the Beckham County Medical Society, State Medical Association, American Medical Association and the Southern Medical Association.

Resolution

WHEREAS, It has pleased the almighty to remove from our midst, by death, our esteemed friend and co-laborer, Dr. J. M. Denby, who has for many years occupied a prominent rank in our midst, maintaining under all circumstances a character untarnished, and a reputation above reproach.

WHEREFORE, WE THE BECKHAM COUNTY MEDICAL SOCIETY, RESOLVE, That in the death of Dr. J. M. Denby, we have sustained the loss of a friend whose fellowship it was an honor and a pleasure to enjoy; that we bear willing testimony to his many virtues, to his unquestioned probity and strainless life; that we offer to his bereaved family and mourning friends, over whom sorrow has hung her sable mantle our heartfelt condolence, and pray that Infinite Goodness may bring speedy relief to their burdened hearts and inspire them with the consolation, that Hope in futurity and Faith in God given even in the shadow of the Tomb.

RESOLVED, That a copy of this resolution, properly engrossed, be presented to the family of our deceased friend.

Dr. Thomas Tilden Norris
1876-1942

Dr. Thomas Tilden Norris, assistant superintendent of the Eastern Oklahoma hospital annex, and long a resident of Pittsburg county, passed away September 6, 1942, at his home in Krebs, Oklahoma.

Dr. S. R. Braden, Shawnee, former pastor of the McAlester church in which Dr. Norris held membership, officiated.

He had been ill for some time. For more than 40 years Dr. Norris administered to the community, having first practiced at Crowder before coming to Krebs.

He was born September 12, 1876, at Lagrange, Indiana, and was a graduate of the University of Nashville in 1901. From the Tennessee medical school, Dr. Norris went to Oklahoma City where only a year was spent before he settled at the then booming Fort Smith and Western railway town of Crowder.

Dr. Norris was a past president of the Pittsburg County Medical society. Since 1939, he officiated as physician for the state hospital, just west of the city. As a member of the Masonic fraternity and a political leader in the democratic party, Dr. Norris attained prominence. He also was a member of the Modern Woodmen of America.

Surviving besides his wife are their four children; Miss Helen Morris of the home; Mrs. Stanley B. Stuart, Brawley, Calif.; Thomas T. Norris, Jr., and John David Norris, of the home address. Two sisters and two brothers also are living. These are: Miss Ruth Norris, Lagrange, Ind.; Mrs. Flora Atwater, Topanga, Calif.; Hiram Norris and Rollin Norris, both of Lagrange, Ind.

Resolution

WHEREAS, on September 6, 1942, Thomas Tilden Norris of Krebs, Oklahoma, ceased his labors and

WHEREAS, Thomas Tilden Norris had been a practitioner in Pittsburg county for forty years and during that time was at all times on the side of orthodox medicine and the ethical practice of the same and

WHEREAS, in the death of Thomas Tilden Norris not only has Pittsburg county but Southeastern Oklahoma, as well as the Oklahoma State Medical Association, lost one of its most tireless and energetic physicians and one loved and respected by all who knew him. His place in our midst will indeed be hard to fill.

BE IT RESOLVED that Pittsburg County Medical Society desires to express its appreciation of the worth of our member to its organization.

THEREFORE BE IT FURTHER RESOLVED that the above resolution be spread upon the minutes of Pittsburg County Medical Society and a copy mailed to the family of our deceased member.

Dr. William Givens Ramsey
1872-1942

Dr. William Givens Ramsey, 69, Oklahoma State prison physician for nearly three years, died July 25, 1942, following an illness of several weeks.

He was a resident of Quinton from 1920 until 1939, when he accepted the prison office. At one time he was a member of the Pittsburg county election board.

Doctor Ramsey was born in Hackett, Ark., on November 14, 1872, but moved to Oklahoma in 1890. He married Miss Sophia Goode in Kansas City in 1902.

Doctor Ramsey graduated from the University Medical College of Kansas City in 1903 and the same year assumed the superintendency of All Saints hospital at McAlester and remained in that capacity until 1909. Doctor Ramsey was an officer in World War I. After the war he moved to Quinton.

Doctor Ramsey was a member of the Episcopal church and joined the Scottish Rite Masonic body in 1905. He was a member of Quinton lodge No. 213, A. F. and A. M.

Survivors include the widow, Mrs. Sophia Ramsey; one son, H. B. Ramsey of Okemah; one daughter, Mrs. Dorthea Peters of Muskogee, and one grandaughter, Sophia E. Ramsey of Okemah.

Funeral services for Doctor Ramsey were held at 2 o'clock Monday, July 27, at the Grand Avenue Methodist church with Rev. E. M. Lindgren of All Saints Episcopal church officiating.

Resolution

WHEREAS, William Givens Ramsey of McAlester passed into the Great Beyond on July 25, 1942, after having practiced the healing art for nearly 40 years in Pittsburg and Haskell counties, and

WHEREAS, his energetic devotion to his profession and high standards of ethics endeared him not only to his fellow practitioners but to his patients as well and

WHEREAS, in the death of William Givens Ramsey, Pittsburg County Medical Society has lost an ardent member and Oklahoma State Medical Association one of its bulwarks.

BE IT RESOLVED that Pittsburg County Medical Society desires to express its appreciation of the worth of our member to its organization and his labors in behalf of orthodox medicine.

BE IT FURTHER RESOLVED that the above resolution be spread upon the minutes of Pittsburg County Medical Society and a copy mailed to the family of our deceased member.

The Need of Uniform Standards of Medical Licensure Is Urgent

Immediate steps should be undertaken for the establishment of uniform standards, of licensure of physicians, The Journal of the American Medical Association declares in its May 9 issue, pointing out that war conditions emphasize the great need for such uniformity. The Journal says:

"The results of the state licensing examinations published in this issue of The Journal are striking evidence of the lack of uniformity of standards of licensure among the various states. Seven states reported not one failure in their 1941 licensing examinations; indeed, they had not had a failure in the past five years. Twelve additional states have reported failures of less than one percent during the same period. Other states, notably New York, have each year reported a high percentage of failures.

"In New York 21.8 percent of the graduates of the New York State medical colleges who tried the New York State licensing examinations failed, while 39.4 percent of the graduates of other approved medical colleges in the United States who tried these same examinations failed. Of the 145 graduates of New York State medical colleges who tried licensing examinations in other states, four or 2.8 percent, failed.

"The lack of uniformity of results in some states is made more obvious by the fact that a candidate is passed if he receives an average of 75 percent and is not below 50 percent in any subject. Furthermore, in case of failure in not more than two subjects the applicant may be entitled to another examination in the subjects failed and is considered conditioned and is not reported as a failure.

"Paradoxically, New York, which reported the highest percentage of failures among the graduates of approved medical colleges on its own examinations, issued a greater number of licenses on the basis of credentials without examination than did any other state.

"In spite of this lack of uniformity, the fact is striking that the graduates of the foreign medical schools and the unapproved schools in the United States showed the highest percentage of failures, 59.6 and 46.0 respectively. Six states licensed graduates of unapproved schools during 1941. Four states granted unlimited licenses to practice medicine to graduate of osteopathic schools.

"The best interests of the public and of the medical profession seem to demand serious thought right now on the establishment of uniform standards of licensure. These not only would facilitate the migration of qualified physicians from one state to another but would offer to the public greater assurance of the training and competence of practicing physicians. War conditions involving as they do the migration of great masses of the population including physicians, emphasize the great need for such uniformity.

"Is it unreasonable to hope that all states will sometime be willing to maintain standards high enough to make uniformity possible?"

Major Walter A. Howard of Chelsea is now stationed at Will Rogers Field, Oklahoma City. Major Howard was President of the Oklahoma State Medical Association in 1939 and 1940, and at the time he was called to active duty, he was President of the Rogers County Medical Society and Superintendent of Health of Rogers County. Major Howard also represents Oklahoma as Senior Delegate to the American Medical Association.

Dr. James A. Willie Opens Hospital

The office of the Association wishes to congratulate Dr. James A. Willie on the opening of his new hospital at 218 Northwest Seventh Street, Oklahoma City.

In the new hospital, Doctor Willie will carry on his regular practice of diagnosis, study and treatment of all types of neurological and psychiatric cases.

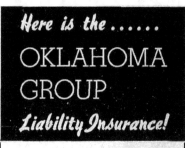

WOMEN'S AUXILIARY NEWS

The Woman's Auxiliary to the American Medical Association celebrated its Twentieth Anniversary at the convention held in Atlantic City from June 8 to June 12, 1942. It was organized in St. Louis, Missouri, on May 26, 1922, through the efforts of the late Mrs. Samuel Clarke Red, then President of the Auxiliary to the State Medical Association of Texas. Mrs. Frank N. Haggard, the new National President, stressed the fact that in the growth of the National Auxiliary during the past 20 years, full credit is due both the County and State organizations, as little could have been accomplished without their cooperation.

In Mrs. Haggard's address, "Our Challenge in This Crisis," she placed emphasis on the place of the Auxiliary in a world at war, and stated that every day our husbands are being called into Service, either into the armed forces or on civilian duty in the defense areas. They are being called upon to embrace the super-most concept of their most sacred oath, in sacrifice and endurance. Ours is the task of being worthy of the place we occupy as their wives. War has decided our program for us. As Auxiliary members we can take an active part in "Health for Defense". We can also cooperate with the Red Cross and Civilian Defense in their great effort. As an Auxiliary, we cannot affiliate with other organizations, but we are in a strategic position to acquaint the public with specific health issues. In stressing Public Relations, as has been done in the past few years, we are privileged to be of service to a country where one can still serve.

A very challenging address was given by Mrs. Augustus S. Kech, Director of the Division of Health Education for the Pennsylvania State Department of Health, in which she stated "We have a real task before us, a task that calls for our best reserves, and that is to educate the public in the best of modern public health. People are health hungry. They need authentic information, palatably served and digestible. You women can constitute a great civilian army that will carry the message of better health to the millions of our citizens engaged in this titanic struggle. YOU DARE NOT FAIL."

Dr. Morris Fishbein spoke on "A Program for the Auxiliary," and Dr. W. W. Bauer, Director of the Bureau of Health Education, also spoke on "The Woman's Auxiliary and the Bureau of Health Education."

The outstanding social event of the convention was the annual dinner on Thursday evening in the Rutland Room of Haddon Hall. The guest speakers were Dr. Ramindo DeCastro of Havana, Cuba, and Dr. Denio of the Philippines, and both addresses were very entertaining and interesting.

Mrs. William Hibbits, Chairman of the Program Committee, presented the Credo of the Doctor's Wife in Wartime, which is very worthy of adoption by every Auxiliary member.

We regret to report that our State President, Mrs. Frank L. Flack, of Tulsa, is confined to St. John's Hospital with a compression fracture of the second lumbar vertebra. It is our sincere hope that she will soon be able to return to her home, and we must all give her our full cooperation in carrying on the work of our State Organization.

Tulsa County News

Mrs. J. W. Childs, President of the Tulsa County Auxiliary, who has been ill most of the summer, is very much improved, and is anticipating her year of work with the Auxiliary.

The Tulsa County Auxiliary opened its fall program with a morning coffee on October 6, at the home of Mrs. H. B. Stewart.

We are again requesting the County Auxiliaries to send their news to the State Publicity Chairman, Mrs. Carl Hotz, 2234 East 22nd Place, Tulsa, as we are interested in just what your auxiliary is doing.

Thirty Pieces of Silver

There are certain physicians in this land of ours who have made no move on their own initiative to get into the service of the United States of America. Some of these men could qualify for duty with the armed services; others would be useful in civilian assignments. The point is that it behooves American medicine to volunteer to a man for service of some sort in this total peril our country now is facing.

Lest this writer be adjudged a common scold, and alone in his playing of this tune, read the following from the Journal of the Medical Society of New Jersey:

Some doctors have been reluctant to enroll with the Procurement and Assignment Service. The blank was published in the January issue of this Journal and a form will be mailed to each physician later this month. By signing, a doctor indicates that he is available for service to the Government in his own branch of medicine or surgery. It was expected that practically 100 percent of the physicians would respond to this call. Certainly it is hard to see how anyone can do otherwise.

At least one physician has said, however, that he felt under no obligation to sign the blank because he had received no individual request to do so. Its publication in a journal, he felt, was a hit-and-miss device which could not be meant to have any personal application to him.

Another doctor said: "Why should I stick my neck out?" Adding that if and when the Government wanted him it would get him without his inviting himself to be selected.

Perhaps the weirdest objection was this one: "No other profession in the country is expected to offer itself en masse in this way; no other group is being asked to dislocate itself completely; why should doctors be the victims of discrimination?"

Discriminated against? Is the offering of your services to your country a discrimination or a privilege? Is it to medicine's discredit or to medicine's pride that it was the first profession to offer itself? What other group now has the opportunity of securing officer's status in the Army immediately on entering from civilian life? The answer is none. This privilege—that of entering directly into the status of an officer—is given to the medical profession and only to them.

If American loses this war, few of us will be able to practice honest medicine at all; and many will not want to survive the holocaust of a Fascist America. Of all who have a stake in democratic victory, surely the intellectual, the scientist, the professional man has the largest. A physician who has to be coaxed into contributing his services to the winning of this war must indeed be troubled in conscience, narrow in vision, and mean in spirit.—Southwestern Medicine, June, 1942.

Lieutenant Isadore Dyer of Tahlequah, a former employee of the State Health Department in District 1, is now located at Hill Field, Ogden, Utah. Lieutenant Dyer reports that he has been assigned as "Group Surgeon" Headquarters and Headquarters Squadron for the 30th Air Depot Group. At the time he was called to active duty, Lieutenant Dyer was Secretary of the Cherokee County Medical Society.

BOOK REVIEWS

"The chief glory of every people arises from its authors."—Dr. Samuel Johnson.

"DIRECTORY OF MEDICAL SPECIALISTS." 1942. Columbia University Press, New York. Compiled By The Advisory Board for Medical Specialists. 2,500 Pp.

This directory devotes 2,500 pages to the task of listing 18,163 specialists occupying fifteen special fields, among the physicians of the United States and Canada. The otolaryngologists head the list with 2,971. Internists come next with 2,604, then the ophthalmologists with a total of 1,759 and the surgeons with 1,719. The radiologists constitute the fifth largest group with 1,638. Other groups are represented as follows: Pediatrics, 1,633; obstetrics and gynecology, 1,396; psychiatry and neurology, 1,202; pathology, 818; urology, 748; orthopaedic surgery, 734; dermatology and syphilology, 568; anesthesiology, 142; plastic surgeons, 124, and neurological surgeons, 107.

With the rapid shifting of population incident to the war, the value of this volume takes on added importance for the doctor who wishes to secure adequate care for his roving paients. On the other hand he must take into account the displacement of medical personnel in the special fields occasioned by Procurement and Assignment. —Lewis J. Moorman, M.D.

"CENTRAL AUTONOMIC REGULATIONS IN HEALTH AND DISEASE." Heymen R. Miller, M.D., Associate Attending Physician, Montefiore Hospital, New York City. Introduction by John F. Fulton, M.D. Fifteen Chapters, 440 pages, 64 illustrations, bibliography and index. Price $5.50.

Cartographers are certainly having a headache with the changing geographical names and boundaries, but so are neuroanatomists and neurophysiologists in the light of recent research. Our conception of the central autonomic and physiologic systems are quite kaleidioscopic in the light of modern observation. The hypothalmus and its regional control is considered the theostat of this anatomic nervous system, which was formerly considered a separate and distinct entity, apart from the cerebrol-spinal system. Recognition of the part played by the anatomic nervous system in the regulation of bodily functions may be ranked as one of the great milestones of modern medicine.

However his correlation of the relationship between the somatic and autonomic systems here helped to clarify the functional pathology back of nervous indigestion, cardiac and circulatory and many harmonal maladjustments. This book is timely because of the emotional and physical stress incident to this world-wide war. The cortical and subcortical liason as evidenced by the sham rage of Cannon's experimental animals is both of clinical and research interest, explaining many an explosive symptom.

This psychiatrist will note in the chapter on wake-sleep rhythm, that it is controlled primarily by autonomic function, possibly through an intermediate bio-chemical cause. Whether sleep is positive and awake is negative, the deponent sayeth not.

One of the most interesting chapters is on regulation of water and minerals, which rests on a neuroharmonal control. Investigators have found transient and permanent changes in this regulation by pathologic lesions, either surgical or tumor, showing most conclusively the hypothalmic-pituitary domination of that field. As a therapeutic demonstration, we note the specific relief in diabetes incipidus from the parenteral administration of posterior pituitary substance, or pitressin, in regulating the output of an abnormal urinary secretion. Pitressin Tannate in Oil acts by slow absorption, and is specific in most cases like Protamine Zinc Insulin in diabetes mellitus. It will bring the output down to a physiological amount but not below. The relationship between NACL intake and urinary output shows no parallel, hence polyuria is associated with deficiency of antiduretic harmone.

The chapter on central regulation of metabolism takes up what many think of the multiple harmonal action back of diabetes mellitus, aside from the Islands of Langerhans. Haussay's experiments show that an animal with the pituitary gland already extirpated subsequent to pancreatectomy, will not cause hyperglycaemia. Hence a hypersensitivity to insulin and a lowered sensitivity to adrenalin. Pituitary gland substance will produce diabetes if injected over a given time.

The chapter on the anatomy of the hypothalmos with its ill defined "cito-architecture" in the human and the changes in comparative anatomy excuses the neurophysiologists for the divergent views of its multiduous and errotic functions. Bibliography is voluminous and up to date because of the interest displayed in a system which is being understood more and more. Montefiore Hospital has given much time to this subject, as this is the third book on the subject within a year. Clinician and research investigation should be ever alert on this bizarre subject—Lea A. Riley, M.D.

"ENCEPHALITIS—A CLINICAL STUDY." Josephine B. Neal, Associate Director of Laboratories, Department of Health, New York; Clinical Professor of Neurology, College of Physicians and Surgeons, Columbia University. Grune and Stratton, New York. 1942. 562 Pages.

This encyclopedic volume on Encephalitis is the result of studies made possible by the William J. Matheson Commission of Encephalitis Research. These reports have been made in previous years: 1929, 1932 and 1939, but the present book summarizes all the knowledge of the encephalitides and brings this knowledge with its clinical applications down to date.

Not only Epidemic Encephalitis in its commonest forms discussed in details, but all other types of Encephalitis are also presented; each syndrome being presented under the classical heading of Ethiology, Symptomatology, and Prognosis, Laboratory aids, Differential diagnosis, and histories of both typical and atypical cases.

Among the disorders discussed are several which will be of especial interest to us in these days when Americans are scattered throughout the world. These are: "Louping Ill". A sheep borne encephalitis endemic in Northern England and Scotland; "Verno-estival tick borne encephalitis" found in Asiatic Russia; Australian X-Disease; and "Japanese B Encephalitis". All these syndromes present rather characteristic pictures, and undoubtedly many cases will appear in this country as our armed forces move about the globe.

In addition to the diseases mentioned, the St. Louis type encephalitis, Human encephalitis caused by the Viruses of Eastern and Western Equine Encephalomyelitis and lymphocytic Choriomeningitis receive detailed attention—also discussed are the encephalitides which are occasionally associated with common diseases such as measles, mumps, chickenpox, typhus, etc.

In considering the treatments of acute and subacute Epidemic Encephalitis, chemotherapy is reviewed and then a chapter is devoted to vaccine therapy. All known types of vaccine are compared and "Vaccine F" (obtainable from the Public Health Laboratory) is given favorable attention. There is considerable evidence that this vaccine serves to arrest the progress of the disease and affords much clinical relief.

Of particular interest to all physicians who have occasion to treat cases of chronic encephalitis is the chapter on the course and prognosis of this phase of the illness. Each symptom is weighed carefully, its pathology discussed, and therapy of symptoms as well as the disease is minutely outlined.

This book is written by a group who are exceedingly competent in the field, and the editor has devoted much of her life to research upon Encephalitis.—Moorman P. Prosser, M.D.

"PHYSICIANS' REFERENCE BOOK OF EMERGENCY MEDICAL SERVICE." 1942. E. R. Squibb & Sons, Publishers. New York. Pp. 270.

In this handy volume of 270 pages we find, in brief, the accumulated knowledge having to do with the civilian casualties arising through modern warfare.

Through this comprehensive compilation E. R. Squibb & Sons have rendered a genuine service. Every doctor in civilian practice should be well informed and ready for any emergency. Four fifths of the material found in this book has been gathered from foreign sources and represents the experience of those who have fought and suffered in this war.

The assembled material appears under the following heads: Section I. Precautionary Measures; The General Problem of Civilian Defense, Protection of Hospitals, Protection of Civilian Health. Section II. Hospital Services; Organization, Relation to First-Aid, Reception of Casualties. Section III. Management of Casualties; Shock, Burns, Wounds and Fractures, Wound Infection, Blast Injuries, Crush Injuries, War Gas Injuries.

The book is well indexed and suitable for ready reference.—Lewis J. Moorman, M.D.

Lieutenant Commander Don W. Branham reports that he has just been detached from the San Diego Naval Hospital to the recently constructed U. S. Naval Hospital at Seattle, Washington, and is in charge of the Urology Department. Prior to his entering the military service, Lieutenant Commander Branham practiced in Oklahoma City.

Word has been received in the office of the Association from Major Hervey A. Foerster, formerly of Oklahoma City, that he is now Venereal Disease Control Officer at the Station Hospital, Camp Maxey, Paris, Texas.

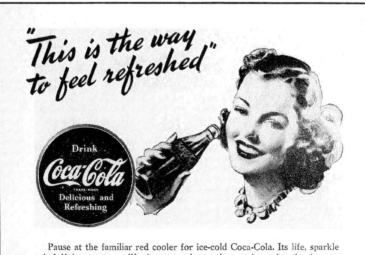

Medical Frauds Cost Victims Millions of Dollars Annually

Annually, victims of countless medical frauds hand over millions of dollars to the promoters of worthless gadgets, false cures and nostrums, R. M. Cunningham, Jr., Chicago, declares in Hygeia, The Health Magazine for September. "At best," he says, "these victims are defrauded of their money; their hopes of relief from suffering are cruelly crushed. But there are graver consequences. Their health is endangered by delaying the scientific diagnosis and treatment which hold their only real chance for recovery. Worse yet, in many instances they may have taken treatments or medications which were actually harmful. . . .

"Sufferers who know or suspect that they have an incurable disease will grasp at straws; thus patent mummery flourishes when promoted under the label of "cancer cure." . . . Tuberculosis cures for years were sure-fire money makers for the unscrupulous. Advertisements commonly seek the profit by the tuberculosis patient's reluctance to be confined in a sanatorium and his fear of surgery. An order by the Federal Trade Commission prohibiting false representations by the manufacturer of one of these nostrums reveals that it had been advertised as a compound that would cure tuberculosis, not only "without surgery or segregation"—the usual claims—but in this case "without diagnosis" as well. . . . Peddlers of nostrums were quick to recognize that the diabetic longs for some means of sustaining life without the necessity for daily injections of insulin. Today, many fakers are specializing in cures for diabetes, claiming that they can effect permanent cures regardless of the age or condition of the patient, and that the users may discontinue taking insulin. Actually, the science of medicine knows no substitute for insulin injections for the diabetic whose blood sugar cannot be regulated by dietary management. . . ."

Popular misconceptions about health, Mr. Cunningham declares, are an invitation for fraud. For example, he says, the widespread notion that backache indicates kidney disorder has created a market for herbs and drugs dispensed as cures for kidney trouble. While many of these are harmless, some of them may result in serious illness, even in those whose original backache was caused by simple muscular strain.

Venereal disease and disorders affecting the reproductive system create another market for swindlers, the author contends, because of the average patient's embarrassment at discussing his condition personally and his consequent susceptibility to any fraud offering home treatment. None of the numerous "cures" for these disease constitute competent treatment, and some are actually harmful. Also dangerous are many of the thousands of remedies whose appeal is based on the universality of the ailment they are supposed to prevent or relieve—the "reducing tonics" and the "cures" for baldness, the beautifiers and bust developers.

While the ignorant are most likely to be deceived by the more obvious medical frauds, Mr. Cunningham says that "the victims of medical frauds generally are by no means found only in uneducated groups; astonishing evidence of this can be seen in the medicine cabinets of many of the "best homes." No amount of education, apparently, will prevent ailing men and women from giving every proffered miracle a chance to perform. That hope persists in opposition to every reasonable possibility is well known to medical fakers, who work over the same lists time after time on the theory that a person who has been deceived by one swindle is a better, not a worse, prospect for the next one. The medicine cabinet, again, is proof: "There is seldom just one nostrum in the cabinet, either there are none or there is a whole shelf full."

MEDICAL ABSTRACTS

"VITAMINS AND DIABETES." Julian M. Freston, M.D., and Winifred C. Loughlin, M.D. Proceedings of the American Diabetes Association, Vol. 2, 1942.

This is a very timely and practical report on the much discussed case of vitamins in diabetes, summarized as follows.

The relationship of vitamin metabolism to diabetes is reviewed:

There is a disputed hypercarotenemia in diabetics. There is a tendency to hypovitaminosis A in dibeties. These are a function of the failure of the diabetic liver to convert carotene to Vitamin A.

The members of the B-complex are related to carbohydrate metabolism, normal and diabetic.

The reported incidence of polyneuritis, ariboflavinosis and pellagra in diabetes is discussed. All are low.

Ascorbic acid deficiency in diabetics is reportedly prevalent chemically and infrequent clinically.

Diagnostic criteria for the avitaminoses are set forth.

A report of a study of 93 diabetic children is given: the incidence of A and C deficiencies is low, that of B deficiency, especially B1, is high.

Prevention and treatment of "diabetic avitaminoses" is discussed.—H. J., M.D.

"THE ENDOCRINE CONTROL OF CARBOHYDRATE METABOLISM AND ITS RELATION TO DIABETES IN MAN." C. N. H. Long, M.D., D.Sc., New Haven, Conn. Proceedings of the American Diabetes Association, Vol. 2, 1942.

The authors admit the complexity of this subject and have discussed it by several different headings, such as Regulation of Carbohydrate Metabolism by Endocrine Glands, Insulin, The Adrenal Cortex, The Adrenal Medulla, The Thyroid, The Anterior Pituitary, Possible Causes of an Impairment of Carbohydrate Tolerance, and Factors Known to Be Associated with Appearance of Diabetes Mellitus in Man. Doctor Long concludes as follows:

"I would hazard the guess that it is unlikely that any at present unknown cause will be found to be of universal importance in the establishment of human diabetes. In consequence, our efforts in the control of the disease must be directed toward the education of the population in the dangers that lie not only in the physiological changes associated with certain periods of life, but also the consequences of excessive indulgence in food. The recent work from the Toronto Laboratories and those of the Cox Institute seem to be of particular significance in this regard and it is to be hoped that further studies on the circumstances and agents that influence insulin secretion will not be unduly delayed."

Interesting and very enlightening discussion of the paper by Drs. F. M. Allen of New York, Carlos P. Lamar, Miami, Fla., E. Perry McCullaugh of Cleveland, R. T. Woodyatt of Chicago, and the President of the association, Doctor Mosenthal, is given.—H. J., M.D.

"A CRITICAL SURVEY OF TEN YEARS' EXPERIENCE WITH FRACTURES OF THE NECK OF THE FEMUR." Mather Cleveland. Surg. Gyn. and Obst., LXXIV, 529, Feb. 15, 1942.

The author analyzes the results obtained in the treatment of 110 fractures of the neck of the femur at St. Luke's Hospital from 1930 to 1940. The first 50, already reported, are included for the sake of contrast.

Smith-Petersen's method of open reduction and internal fixation are used in 14 cases, with very little improvement in end-results over those obtained by non-operative means. Of the seven patients whose fractures united, results in only two were wholly satisfactory. There were three cases of extensive aseptic necrosis, and two of severe malunion with marked deformity.

Undisplaced fractures of the neck of the femur, treated by three to four weeks' rest in bed and weight-bearing after the application of a Thomas caliper brace, gave invariably optimum results. A number of undisplaced fractures have been nailed without reduction.

Accurate closed reduction by manipulation and the careful insertion of a three-phalanged nail has yielded surprisingly good results; union of the fracture occurred in 86 percent of the survivors.

When the circulatory disturbance occurred in the femoral head, it always appeared within the first year after the fracture. Seventy-five percent of the patients with nonunion of the fractures had extensive circulatory disturbance in the femoral head. Of those subjected to open reduction, whose fractures had united, 42.8 percent showed extensive aseptic necrosis of the femoral head. Of the 27 patients with united fractures, who had been treated by closed reduction and nailing, 18.5 percent showed some evidence of circulatory disturbance, for the most part very mild. The majority of all patients showing circulatory disturbance in the femoral head, whose fractures had united, had had an inadequate reduction of the fracture.

From experience with the last 60 patients the author found that the most important single factor in securing union and avoiding circulatory disturbance in the femoral head was adequate reduction of the fracture. The actual or so-called migration of the nail is usually due to failure to reduce properly the fracture, and occurs almost exclusively in ununited fractures.—E. D. M., M.D.

"THE USE OF VITALLIUM IN SURGERY WITH SPECIAL REFERENCE TO CUP ARTHROPLASTY." W. H. Cole. Proceedings of the Royal Society of Medicine, XXXIV, 779. Section of Orthopaedics, p. 29, 1941.

The author discusses the use of various metals prior to the development of vitallium, and feels that the latter is the most "silent" of all. He describes his findings in two cases in which he was able to examine the femoral heads six months and one month after cup arthroplasty has been done. In the first case, the cup split six months after surgery when the patient was up and about with an excellently functioning hip. In the other, where no weight-bearing and very little motion had taken place, the patient died one month postoperatively. No cartilage replacement was noted as contrasted to the findings reported by Smith-Petersen in two patients, 21 and 25 months postoperatively. In the author's first case, the cup had to be pried from the head. However, on removal of the cup, the head was excellently molded, smooth, and glistening, as was the acetabulum. Microscopically the head and acetabulum were lined with fibrous tissue. In the second case, the cup was loose and the stump of the neck (the head had been necrotic and therefore removed) was rounded and smooth, with irregular islands of what appeared to be cartilage but histologically revealed organizing fibrous tissue.

The author feels that removal of the cup two to three years postoperatively might result in a better hip. He also suggests that the cup fit loosely over the neck, so that motion may take place beneath it as well as between it and the acetabulum, in order to form a better new weight-bearing surface.

In postoperative treatment, the author places the extremity in balanced traction immediately following surgery, and a little swinging motion is attempted the very next day. This motion is increased gradually, and after two weeks is assisted by passive swinging, abduction, and adduction. A stationary bicycle is very worth while prior to weight-bearing, which can be started in five to eight weeks, if the bone in the femoral neck is not too cystic or atrophied. The author strongly advises against forcing too much motion at the start. He believes this should develop by continuous exercise and use. He also mentions the fact—and cites several cases—that these arthroplasties are remarkably free of pain on motion, despite previous arthritic involvement of the operated hip.—E. D. M., M.D.

"OTOLOGY AND AVIATION." Ralph A. Fenton. The Annals of Otology, Rhinology and Laryngology, vol. 51, pages 333-342, June, 1942.

At the time of the first World War, the U. S. Army Medical Corps began to investigate the physical and mental factors pertaining to military aviation. The investigation was carried on in a medical research laboratory at Mineola. In 1920, a school for flight surgeons was created at Mitchell Field. In 1926 the institution, known already as School of Aviation Medicine, moved to Brooks Field and in 1931 to Randolph Field, Texas. In addition, a research labatory was established in 1933 at Wright Field, Ohio, for intensive study of the effects of flight on the human organism.

In the early years of its existence, the School of Aviation Medicine did not pay much attention to the ear and the nasal sinuses. Lately, however, many practical observations have been made, and on the basis of these experiences many of the requirements in physical fitness of aviators have been standardized.

Applicants for flying training are rejected if any abnormality of either ear be present. Hearing is tested by whispering numerals, including 66, 18, and 23, from a distance of 20 feet, using residual air in the lungs at the end of an expiration. On original examination, 20/20 is required for each ear. Audiometric examination is made and recorded annually where such instruments are available; the average hearing loss permissible for pilots on original examination must not exceed 15 percent.

Patency of the eustachian tube is tested by the Politzer bag if the tympanic membranes are retracted and the light reflex of the tympanic membrane slants abnormally. Any obstructive lesion of the nose or pharynx (adenoids, aberrant lymphoid tissue, large tonsils, septal thickening or deviation, hypertrophied or allergic turbinates, nasal polypi or chronic sinusitis) may interfere with normal opening of the eustachian tube during swallowing, and thus with the aeration of the middle ear. Blocking of the eustachian tube disqualifies all classes of applicants.

For test of equilibrium, ordinarily, the self-balancing test is adequate; the applicant stands erect without shoes, heels and toes touching. He then flexes one knee backward to a right angle without bending the hip, thus avoiding support against the other leg, closes his eyes, and holds this position if possible for 15 seconds. The test is repeated on the other foot. The applicant fails when he cannot hold his position for 15 seconds, one out of three trials on each foot.

When there is unsteadiness on the self-balancing test, the vestibular test with a turning chair is made. Yet, the self-balancing tests have been found adequate for exclusion of almost all individuals with sensitive labyrinthine reactions. The caloric test, so much valued in civilian practice, is not ordinarily used in military examinations.

Good hearing is essential for the aviator, since he depends upon spoken or signaled orders by radio. Effects of flight upon hearing depend on noise and vibration,

and on changes in air pressure while ascending or descending. Noise and vibration from engine, propellers, and exhaust are somewhat masked by the pilot's helmet and rubber-cupped radio head set. Those others who do not have such helmets may use cotton or rubber ear plugs. Audiometer tests have shown gradual decrease in acuity for the higher frequencies in older pilots. Exposure to these noises produces acute fatigue, and a sudden drop around 4,096 double vibrations. This has been ascribed to the vulnerability of the basal turn of the cochlea, directly exposed to the force of vibration through the middle ear, ossicles and round window. Repeated exposure to such fatigue has produced permanent losses in many cases.

Changes in the air pressure interfere with hearing for the lower range of conversational tones. There may be severe pain, local congestion, especially of the drum membrane; transudation or hemorrhage into the middle ear; the low tone deafness of varying degrees, the condition known as acute aero-otitis media. Repeated exposure to this hazard will lead to chronic thickening of the tympanic membrane and eustachian linings, with eventual formation of connective tissue and considerable loss of hearing for low tones.

Rapid diving from a considerable height may cause minute hemorrhages in the end organs of hearing and equilibrium. These effects resemble those found in industrial workers doing job in compressed air locks. The same effects may be produced also by rapid climbing. Intratympanic pressure changes play a distinct role in the onset of fainting due to rapid ascent to critical altitudes.

Air sickness, with characteristic pallor and sweating followed by nausea, vertigo and vomiting, may be due to excessive labyrinthine stimulation in rapid turning, banking or sudden descent; visual impressions and visceral disturbances usually contribute to the clinical picture.

Persistence in flight through turbulent air or into a head wind way force the pilot into a wing-down position, due to faulty interpretation of his vestibular stimuli; he feels that he is sitting upright, but is actually leaning sidewise. Similarly, on recovery from a spin the sudden sense of reversal of motion may send the pilot into a second spin in an effort to recover his normal balance, unless he has learned to place entire confidence in his instruments and to disregard his own sensations. At high speed there is no time to allow faulty labyrinthine reactions to subside. Excessive vestibular sensations are always distinctly hazardous.

Acute upper respiratory disease, because of active hyperemia in the nose and throat, creates a flight hazard which might add infection to ordinary aero-otitis. Temporary psychic instability predisposes to circulatory upsets and thus to interference with tympanic and labyrinthine function.

Many more details might be included in the ear examination of pilots; but otologists have to remember that the psychic, cardiac and visual examinations are even more important. Flight surgeons contributed much to establish workable and simple standards for examination of the auditory and the vestibular apparatus, and they clarified many physiological problems of aviation.—M. D. H., M.D.

"USE IN OTOLARYNGOLOGY OF MICROCRYSTALS OF DRUGS OF THE SULFANILAMIDE GROUP." Louis E. Silcox and Harry P. Schenck. Archives of Otolaryngology, vol. 36, pages 171-186, August, 1942.

Most of the original experimental and clinical studies on sulfanilamide and its derivatives were concerned with the oral administration of the various drugs and the creation of an optimum level in the blood, thus bathing the infected tissues with these bacteriostatic agents. Local use of the drugs of the sulfanilamide group was started in 1936. It was found that sulfanilamide in the form of powders could be used effectively in the treatment of burns, infected wounds and sore throat.

The authors used microcrystals of various sulfanilamide drugs for local treatment of eye, ear, nose and throat conditions. Eighteen adult patients with unilateral acute maxillary sinusitis were treated by the installation through a Pierce cannula of a five percent suspension of microcrystals of sulfathiazole in physiologic solution of sodium chloride. The sinusitis subsided in from one to eight days after the therapy was started, with an average duration of three days.

In many patients who have acute sinusitis the discharge of infected secretions down through the nasopharynx sets up secondary pharyngitis. When the infection is of longer duration these secretions reach the larynx, trachea and bronchi and either start pulmonary complications or light up old pulmonary disease. In the present series of patients this complication of pharyngitis, laryngitis and pulmonary disease was reduced to a minimum.

Fifty-two patients with acute and chronic sinusitis were treated with a five percent suspension of microcrystals of sulfathiazole suspended in one percent aqueous solution of paredrine hydrobromide. This suspension was used in the form of drops, spray, Proetz displacement irrigations and intrasinal instillation, with uniformly good results. No untoward effects were noted, and many of the long standing conditions with foul-smelling discharges were completely cleared up with this therapy.

Fourteen patients with chronic maxillary sinusitis were operated on by the Caldwell-Luc technic and were treated postoperatively by the instillation of a five percent suspension of microcrystals of sulfathiazole daily. There was minimal postoperative swelling of the soft tissues over the sinus; healing was rapid, and unpleasant odor and crusting were almost completely eliminated. The patient was required to lie on the involved side for 15 minutes after the drug was introduced.

The preparation was also used in patients with chronic otitis media and acute suppurative otitis media. The results were satisfactory. The local application of the microcrystals is also recommended for treating mastoidectomy cavities or wounds after sinus operations. Microcrystals of drugs of the sulfanilamide group offer certain advantages when used in suspension, not the least of which is the elimination of caking which follows the introduction of the ordinary powdered drugs. Frequently the accumulation of the powdered drug acts as a foreign body. The penetration of microcrystals in suspension permits the medicament to reach the interstices of operatively traumatized tissues inaccessible to dry powders. When immediate action of the drug is desired, a mixture of microcrystals of sulfathiazole and sulfanilamide insures the more immediate action of the sulfanilamide.—M. D. H., M.D.

"TETANUS FOLLOWING EYE INJURY." John O. Wetzel. American Journal of Ophthalmology, vol. 25, pages 933-944, August, 1942.

Tetanus as a complication of eye injuries is of a very rare occurrence. The author reports such a case, and reviews 30 other cases found in the literature. His own patient was a farmer, with a perforating wound of the eyeball. Tetanus developed about a week after the eye injury, but the patient recovered.

In such cases the tetanus bacillus enters through the eye. In nine cases the agent was a horsewhip; in others it was a stable fork, or a broom, or a splinter from a horseshoe, a nail from a barn roof, or a top arrow which recently came in contact with the ground, etc. The actual amount of injury does not seem to have any relation to the liability to tetanus. It may be a deep injury or but a mere scratch.

Several authors are of the opinion that unless a panophthalmia takes place, the conditions essential for the propagation of the tetanus bacillus will be lacking. Records of several patients offer evidence in favor of radical removal of the injured eye as soon as signs of panophthalmia appear.

The lapse of time between the initial injury and the appearance of the first symptoms of tetanus varies considerably. In most instances the length of time is about 12 days. Trismus, the classic "lockjaw", is the first symptom to call attention to the condition in the majority of cases. Contraction of the jaw muscles causes "gritting" of the teeth, soon followed by stronger contractions which clamp the jaws so firmly together that it is quite impossible to separate them. When liquids could be forced through the teeth, a spasm of the glottis often prevents their being swallowed. Stiffness of the neck appears to be a less prominent and constant sign in tetanus of ophthalmic origin. Facial paralysis regularly supervenes promptly upon trismus, always taking place on the side of the injured eye.

Inasmuch as 80 percent of the cases proved fatal, whether or not antitoxin was administered *after* tetanic symptoms appeared, while the author's own patient, who received antitoxin *before* the tetanus developed, survived, the author recommends the routine use of prophylactic antitoxin administration for eye injuries, the same as is now the custom in wounds sustained by other parts of the body. In the majority of the recorded cases, death followed very rapidly the first symptoms of clinical tetanus.

The rapid spread of the infection is explained by the fact that the peripheral nerves convey it to the central nervous system, and when the wound of entrance is in the eye, the extremely rich nerve plexus of the cornea on the one hand, and the proximity of the ramifications of the optic nerve on the other hand, greatly facilitate the attack of the toxin upon the nerve centers.

In the few patients who survived, complete restoration to health did not take place for at least a month. Relapses seem to have been fairly frequent, but in the end all the tetanic manifestations disappeared completely without leaving permanent nerve alterations, as might have been expected in view of the severity of the complications.—M. D. H., M.D.

"INTRANASAL DRAINAGE FOR CURE OF CHRONIC TEAR SAC INFECTION; NEW TECHNIC AIDED BY ELECTROCOAGULATION SO SIMPLIFIED AS TO BE AN OFFICE PROCEDURE." David J. Morgenstern. Archives of Ophthalmology, vol. 27, pages 7-33-745, April, 1942.

Chronic tearing of the eye caused by obstruction in the tear conduction system may originate from either closed or misplaced puncta, from blocked canaliculi or from a blocked sac or nasolacrimal duct. Tearing is increased by exposure to cold, wind, dust, and fumes. Infection of the sac and its contents produces swelling and often a viscid, purulent fluid. This fluid, in passing through the puncta, causes chronic conjunctivitis, chiefly around the inner canthus; chronic swelling of the eyelids, which narrows the palpebral opening, and chronic swelling of the cheek. There were many efforts to relieve such infection. The author developed a simple and accurate surgical technic aided by the use of electrocoagulation.

Chronic rhinitis and sinusitis, particularly ethmoiditis, should be controlled and nasal polyps removed. Roentgen examination may reveal a mucocele of the ethmoid sinus causing pressure on the tear conduction apparatus. A nasal septum markedly deviated above to the affected side may require correction, although this is infrequently necessary. With the subsidence of postoperative swelling, the operation on the tear sac can be performed.

After local anesthetization, a dental root canal probe is passed into the punctum and through the canaliculus until the tip touches the medial wall of the sac, then the bottom of the sac is reached, and the probe is forced gently through the lacrimal bone and any intervening anterior ethmoid cells into the nasal cavity at an angle of 45 degrees. Various hooked instruments are then slid along the guiding probe from below, and the opening through the medial wall of the tear sac and through the lateral nasal wall is gradually enlarged. The tear sac is copiously irrigated with physiologic solution of sodium chloride through the newly formed opening into the nose. There is scarcely any bleeding. Then, by means of electrocoagulation, using the hooked instruments as electrodes, the opening made in the lacrimal sac is slightly coagulated. The coagulation can be repeated at subsequent visits of the patient. The sac has to be irrigated each week for the following few weeks. The newly formed pathway for tear conduction is a permanent, small fistula oval in shape, about 2.5 mm. by 3.5 mm.

The smallness of the final opening minimizes the danger that air or infected matter will be blown from the nose into the sac and through the canaliculi. By retrograde diathermic cauterization of the nasolacrimal duct (which may be all that is required in cases of stenosis without infection), complete eradication of infection from the tear conduction system is achieved.

Because of the slightness of the surgical intervention and the subsequent coagulating action of the electric current, bleeding and possible infection both operatively and postoperatively are reduced to a minimum. Hence, this method can be used as an office procedure.—M. D. H., M.D.

KEY TO ABSTRACTORS

H. J. ....Hugh Jeter, M.D.

E. D. M. ....Earl D. McBride, M.D.

M. D. H. ....Marvin D. Henley, M.D.

The Use and Abuse of the Barbiturates

The laity knows too much about the action of the barbiturates as sedatives, therefore a law should be enacted in every state prohibiting the sale of these drugs over the counter. Also to prevent abuse of his prescription, the practicing physicians should forbid the refilling of it.

It is an excellent drug for inhibiting convulsions as in strychnine poisoning, tetanus, and status epilepticus. Pediatricians use phenobarbital to allay spasms in children and to quiet a fretful crying baby. In such practice there is certainly a misuse of this drug.

The average dose used to produce sleep does not depress the respiration, but large doses especially such as may produce poisoning, cause death by respiratory failure. Overdoses of barbiturates affects the secretion of urine directly through the circulation, causing an oliguria and anuria. Since urine is the most important avenue for the excretion of these drugs, an anuria delays recovery.

Those destroyed by the liver are the short acting barbiturates. It is known that individuals with impaired hepatic function have remained deeply anesthetized for long periods of time from a hypnotic dose of evipal, which in a normal person would cause an anesthesia for only fifteen minutes. Consequently we are warned that barbiturates which depend upon the rapid destruction by the liver for their short action, should not be given to individuals with hepatic disease. Barbiturates should not be given in carbon tetrachloride poisoning, as this solvent itself damages the organ and it is adding insult to injury in this case because an impaired liver is unable to detoxify these drugs as efficiently as when normal.

The therapeutic dose does not cause death, but when fifteen times the ordinary hypnotic dose has been absorbed, the patient's life is in danger. In acute barbital poisoning, nothing characteristic is seen grossly at the postmortem.—William D. McNally, M.D., Chicago, August, 1942, issue of Michigan State Med. Jour.

NEW RECORD SCHEDULED BY MEDICAL COLLEGES

The Council on Medical Education and Hospitals of the American Medical Association has estimated in its forty-second Annual presentation of educational data, published in the August 15 issue of The Journal of the Association, that approved medical schools of the United States, operating under accelerated programs initiated to meet the unprecedented demand for physicians brought about by the war, will graduate a record total of 21,029 students during the next three years. This is "5,082 more than would have graduated without the adoption of the accelerated programs," the report states.

"Never before in the history of this country have as many as 21,000 physicians been graduated from its medical colleges within a three year period.

"In a previous issue of The Journal of the American Medical Association, it was estimated that the total number of deaths of physicians in the United States during 1941 was 3,460. It is difficult to determine what the over-all effect of the war will be on the annual deaths of physicians. However, the estimated number of graduates of the approved medical schools during the next three years, based on the annual deaths of physicians during recent years, provides more than two graduating physicians for every death.

"It is comforting to realize that, rather than permit this war to interfere with the education of physicians, the federal authorities in cooperation with medical schools have adopted programs which will increase the output of physicians and at the same time retain the normal curriculum without any material lowering of standards. . . .

"Medical schools of the United States have recognized that the national war emergency has created the need for a larger number of well qualified physicians. All but four medical schools have initiated an accelerated program to increase the supply of physicians for the Army, the Navy and the civilian population. The plan provides for the utilization of the long summer vacation as a teaching period, and, by continuing the schedule throughout the calendar year, the four year medical course is completed in three years. It should be possible for medical schools to maintain the quality and quantity of instruction which they have given in the past. The eligibility requirements for admission to medical schools have not been lowered from the present minimum standards set by the Association of American Medical Colleges and the Council on Medical Education and Hospitals of the American Medical Association.

"Fifty-three schools have adopted the accelerated curriculum involving both the acceptance of entering students and the graduation of a class every nine months. Ten schools will graduate a class every nine months during the next three years but will admit entering classes on an annual basis. . . . Eight schools of the basic medical sciences have adopted an accelerated program—Two schools—accelerated the senior year during 1941-1942 and graduated these students in March. The completion of the senior year was advanced from June to May, 1942, by 14 schools. . . .

"Licensure requirements in 41 states, the District of Columbia, Alaska and Puerto Rico permit the granting of licenses, or have been so modified as to permit admission to licensure, of graduates who have completed the accelerated courses of training in recognized medical schools. In seven states, Georgia, Illinois, Kansas, Michigan, Nebraska, New Jersey and South Carolina, existing statutory provisions require modification, probably by legislative action, before licenses can be granted to graduates who have completed the accelerated course of medical education. . . ."

Norman Anthony, brilliant writer and editor, who, through an acknowledged hypochondria, paradoxically enough shies from all doctors and things medical, is now editing a rare magazine. The Funny Bone is its title, and its mission is to keep impatient patients patient while waiting for the doctor to see them.

Health of the Army

The War Department announced June 29 that the Surgeon General reports that the health of the army is excellent. No general outbreak of acute respiratory disease occurred in the winter months, and compared to the previous winter, there was a reduction of 52 percent for all diseases and 70 percent for respiratory infections. Since the winter months, the admission rates to the army for all cases have showed a steady decline of nearly 25 percent, due chiefly to a falling off in respiratory infections. The venereal disease rates are now lower than at any time since the beginning of mobilization, and the syphilis rate for the first five months for 1942 is the lowest in the history of the army. There has been a steady decline of as much as 30 percent in cases of gonorrhea.

In recent weeks there have been numerous admissions to hospitals on account of jaundice, which has the characteristics, the War Department said, of catarrhal jaundice (epidemic hepatitis), but the total number of cases in the entire army has not been enough to appreciably increase the admission rate for all diseases. The War Department points out that this is definitely not yellow fever and it is not dangerous to the general public. The disease is being studied, however, by some of the outstanding medical scientists. Outside of the United States, health conditions in the army continue favorable. There have been no serious epidemics and only slight rises in admissions due to diseases peculiar to some of the new areas where the troops are established.

Mere bodily fitness is not the real thing we need most. If we could only develop a few military naval geniuses it would be much better for national security. A great many of the world's greatest officers have been rejected by the draft boards:

Name	Reason for Rejection
George Washington	False Teeth
Bismarck	Overweight
Napoleon	Ulcer of the Stomach
U. S. Grant	Alcoholism
Julius Caesar	Epilepsy
Horatio Nelson	One Eye, One Arm
Kaiser Wilhelm	Withered Arm
Genghis Khan	Paranoia
Duke of Wellington	Underweight

—Dr. Logan Clendening, "The State of the Nation's Health," Nation's Business.

Jaundice in Army Is Decreasing

The incidence of jaundice in the army, following vaccination against yellow fever, is decreasing, The Journal of the American Medical Association announces in its August 8 issue. The announcement says:

"As The Journal goes to press it may be announced that the incidence of cases of jaundice following vaccination against yellow fever is decreasing. Since such cases first appeared, investigators of the highest repute in the fields of epidemiology, pathology, infectious diseases and viruses have been intensively engaged in a study of the factors concerned. There is in the minds of those familiar with the situation the firm conviction that the condition concerned certainly is not yellow fever. There seems to be no reason to believe that it is yellow fever or any abortive or mild form of that disease. The vaccine concerned gives actual protection against yellow fever. Only a few batches of vaccine seem to have been involved, although obviously many thousands of men were inoculated with material from each batch. The investigators feel that the technic of preparation now in use will be followed shortly by a discontinuance of new cases. It must be remembered, however, that the incubation period may be months in duration. The jaundice concerned has not noticeably affected the civilian population. An official statement in the form of an army department circular will be issued in the near future."

American Soldier Is Best Fed Fighting Man in World Today

In an outline of the Army's nutritional problems, James A. Tobey, Dr. P.H., Lieutenant Colonel, Sanitary Corps Reserve, United States Army, New York, in a recent issue of War Medicine, published by the American Medical Association in cooperation with the Division of Medical Sciences of the National Research Council, declares that "For an army of 1,500,000 men, nearly 9,000,000 pounds of food must be procured, transported, stored, supplied, and prepared every day, the biggest catering job in the history of this country. With the expansion of the Army, this task will gradually become even greater." He explains that in camps and posts the American soldier eats about five pounds of food a day, or somewhat over 1,800 pounds a year whereas in the civilian population the average consumption of food is about 1,400 pounds a year.

Pointing out that good nutrition is a military necessity, Colonel Tobey says that "the American soldier can be, and generally is, the best fed fighting man in the world today. There is available to him an abundance of wholesome natural foods, and his menus are carefully selected and arranged by dietary experts who are thoroughly familiar with the newer knowledge of nutrition. . . .

"The fare of the American soldier is, in general, much superior to that of the Nazi and the Japanese soldier. Because of the shortage in natural foods, the Nazis depend in considerable measure on Ersatz, or substitute, foods, such as concentrates of soy bean flour mixed with dried vegetables and fruits. These concoctions are nourishing but not particularly appetizing. The Japanese subsist largely on polished rice, with soy beans, root vegetables, and a little fish. Staple foods common in America, such as bread, meat, milk and fruits, are almost totally lacking in the Japanese diet, although the military forces receive better rations than does the general populace."

Duty Performed Proves a Moral Tonic

Self-trust is the essence of heroism.—Emerson.

A hero is of distinguished courage, morale or physical —not born to heroism, but achieved through unswerving and unstinted devotion to duty in the interest of others. The essentials are here touched upon since the editor learned that a fellow member in practice seven years was recently commissioned in the Army Medical Corps in spite of an earlier refusal; in spite of being declared "essential" to his Alma Mater; in spite of being declared "not available" by Procurement and Assignment Service; and in spite of the loss of an eye several years ago.

Potential medical heroes of this global war will doubtless enter military service with singleness of purpose and continue to the triumphant end, having forgotten the oft-repeated excuses of those who hold back until their younger fellow practitioners have all preceded them into the nation's service.

The older physicians who remain at home will be tested too, through extraordinary calls upon their energies and professional skill and their application of the Golden Rule to the interests of their absent neighbor practitioners.

Men do less than they ought, unless they do all that they can.—Carlyle.

The "Keep Well Crusade," recently launched as an important contribution to the war effort by all life insurance companies, has won the unqualified support of men prominent in medical fields throughout the country.

The Crusade, though conducted by public-spirited insurance agents in their respective communities, was outlined by Holgar J. Johnson, President of the Institute of Life Insurance.

OFFICERS OF COUNTY SOCIETIES, 1942

—Indicates serving in Armed Forces.

COUNTY	PRESIDENT	SECRETARY	MEETING TIME
Alfalfa	*Jack F. Parsons, Cherokee	L. T. Lancaster, Cherokee	Last Tues. Each 2nd Mo.
Atoka-Coal	J. B. Clark, Coalgate	J. S. Fulton, Atoka	
Beckham	H. K. Speed, Sayre	E. S. Kilpatrick, Elk City	Second Tues. eve.
Blaine	Virginia Olson Curtin, Watonga	W. F. Griffin, Watonga	
Bryan	A. J. Wells, Calera	W. K. Haynie, Durant	Second Tues. eve.
Caddo	Fred L. Patterson, Carnegie	C. B. Sullivan, Carnegie	
Canadian	P. F. Herod, El Reno	A. L. Johnson, El Reno	Subject to call
Carter	Walter Hardy, Ardmore	H. A. Higgins, Ardmore	
Cherokee	Park H. Medearis, Tahlequah	*Isadore Dyer, Tahlequah	
Choctaw	C. H. Hale, Boswell	Fred D. Switzer, Hugo	
Cleveland	Joseph A. Rieger, Norman	Curtis Berry, Norman	Thursday nights
Comanche	George S. Barber, Lawton	W. F. Lewis, Lawton	
Cotton	George W. Baker, Walters	Mollie F. Scism, Walters	Third Friday
Craig	W. R. Marks, Vinita	J. M. McMillan, Vinita	
Creek	Frank Sisler, Bristow	*O. H. Cowart, Bristow	
Custer	Richard M. Burke, Clinton	*W. C. Tisdal, Clinton	Third Thursday
Garfield	D. S. Harris, Drummond	John R. Walker, Enid	Fourth Thursday
Garvin	T. F. Gross, Lindsay	John R. Callaway, Pauls Valley	Wed before 3rd Thurs.
Grady	D. S. Downey, Chickasha	Frank T. Joyce, Chickasha	3rd Thursday
Grant	I. V. Hardy, Medford	E. E. Lawson, Medford	
Greer	G. F. Border, Mangum	J. B. Hollis, Mangum	
Harmon	S. W. Hopkins, Hollis	W. M. Yeargan, Hollis	First Wednesday
Haskell	William Carson, Keota	N. K. Williams, McCurtain	
Hughes	Wm. L. Taylor, Holdenville	Imogene Mayfield, Holdenville	First Friday
Jackson	J. M. Allgood, Altus	*Willard D. Holt, Altus	Last Monday
Jefferson	W. M. Browning, Waurika	J. I. Hollingsworth, Waurika	Second Monday
Kay	J. C. Wagner, Ponca City	J. Holland Howe, Ponca City	Third Thurs.
Kingfisher	C. M. Hodgson, Kingfisher	*John R. Taylor, Kingfisher	
Kiowa	J. M. Bonham, Hobart	B. H. Watkins, Hobart	
LeFlore	G. R. Booth, LeFlore	Rush L. Wright, Poteau	
Lincoln	E. F. Hurlbut, Meeker	C. W. Robertson, Chandler	First Wednesday
Logan	William C. Miller, Guthrie	J. L. LeHew, Jr., Guthrie	Last Tuesday evening
Marshall	J. L. Holland, Madill	O. A. Cook, Madill	
Mayes	L. C. White, Adair	V. D. Herrington, Pryor	
McClain	B. W. Slover, Blanchard	R. L. Royster, Purcell	
McCurtain	R. D. Williams, Idabel	R. H. Sherrill, Broken Bow	Fourth Tues. eve.
McIntosh	F. R. First, Checotah	William A. Tolleson, Eufaula	Second Tuesday
Murray	P. V. Annadown, Sulphur	F. E. Sadler, Sulphur	
Muskogee	L. S. McAlister, Muskogee	D. Evelyn Miller, Muskogee	First & Third Mon.
Noble	J. W. Francis, Perry	C. H. Cooke, Perry	
Okfuskee	J. M. Pemberton, Okemah	L. J. Spickard, Okemah	Second Monday
Oklahoma	R. Q. Goodwin, Okla. City	Wm. E. Eastland, Okla. City	Fourth Tuesday
Okmulgee	J. G. Edwards, Okmulgee	*John R. Cotteral, Henryetta	Second Monday
Osage	C. R. Welrich, Pawhuska	George K. Hemphill, Pawhuska	Second Monday
Ottawa	J. B. Hampton, Commerce	Walter Sanger, Picher	Third Thursday
Pawnee	E. T. Robinson, Cleveland	Robert L. Browning, Pawnee	
Payne	John W. Martin, Cushing	Clifford W. Moore, Stillwater	Third Thursday
Pittsburg	Austin R. Stough, McAlester	Edw. D. Greenberger, McAlester	Third Friday
Pontotoc	R. E. Cowling, Ada	Alfred R. Sugg, Ada	First Wednesday
Pottawatomie	John Carson, Shawnee	Clinton Gallaher, Shawnee	First & Third Sat.
Pushmataha	P. B. Rice, Antlers	John S. Lawson, Clayton	
Rogers	*W. A. Howard, Chelsea	George D. Waller, Claremore	First Monday
Seminole	H. M. Reeder, Konawa	Mack I. Shanholtz, Wewoka	
Stephens	A. J. Weedn, Duncan	W. K. Walker, Marlow	
Texas	L. G. Blackmer, Hooker	*Johnny A. Blue, Guymon	
Tillman	C. C. Allen, Frederick	O. G. Bacon, Frederick	
Tulsa	H. B. Stewart, Tulsa	E. O. Johnson, Tulsa	Second & Fourth Mon. eve.
Wagoner	J. H. Plunkett, Wagoner	H. K. Riddle, Coweta	
Washington-Nowata	*R. W. Rucker, Bartlesville	J. V. Athey, Bartlesville	Second Wednesday
Washita	A. S. Neal, Cordell	James F. McMurry, Sentinel	
Woods	W. F. LaFon, Waynoka	O. E. Templin, Alva	Last Wednesday
Woodward	M. H. Newman, Shattuck	C. W. Tedrowe, Woodward	

THE JOURNAL

OF THE

OKLAHOMA STATE MEDICAL ASSOCIATION

| VOLUME XXXV | OKLAHOMA CITY, OKLAHOMA, NOVEMBER, 1942 | NUMBER 11 |

Delivery of the Sick Woman at or Near Term*

E. P. ALLEN, M.D.

OKLAHOMA CITY, OKLAHOMA

I have chosen this subject because of the increasing popularity of local anesthesia in obstetrical operations. I have in mind those suffering from acute upper respiratory infections, acute toxemia, bladder and kidney disturbances and acute exacerbations of chronic diseases. When the times comes for a patient to go in labor, regardless of her physical condition, she must be delivered.

The doctor's duty here is to conserve energy, relieve pain, support the patient, prevent the spread of infection, save time and above all save blood. Sick women are more apt to go into shock, they are more liable to bleed and, therefore, one must be prepared to meet emergencies.

It is my opinion that one should be more liberal with his analgesia during the first and second stages of labor. When the first stage is well under way, I give enough morphine with scopolamine to control pain and as far as possible, to relieve the nervous and physical strain. I hesitate to give the barbiturates in these cases as I do in normal cases, because I must have full cooperation. I think a patient who gets a barbiturate or scopolamine "jag" may suffer more injury than would result from the labor itself without any analgesia. I do not believe in over sedation for healthy women but I think in handling sick women, one must give sedation in quantity sufficient to control the pain and restlessness.

Supportive treatment such as food, fluid, glucose and blood transfusions, during labor and the delivery, should be employed as indicated.

When we come to the management of those suffering with the more chronic diseases, for example: the toxemias, Rheumatic Heart disease, blood dyscrasias, diabetes and active pulmonary tuberculosis, one has more time to treat the patient, more time to consult with the various specialists and more time to outline a definite line of treatment. At the present time, it seems to be the general opinion that it is best to treat the disease, allow these patients to go to term, go into labor naturally and be delivered by their own physical powers. This policy, I accept only in part. I believe that one can be more liberal with his indications for surgical delivery and if he decides to deliver by the abdominal route, he must use his judgment as to whether or not it would be good obstetrics to choose a time, say fourteen to ten days before term to make the delivery. It has been my idea for many years, with the help of the internist, to get these patients, chosen for surgical delivery, in as good condition as possible, and then, under local anesthesia, do a laparotrachelotomy (or Cesarean Section). Cesarean Section under local anesthesia may be done under the following conditions: 1. In primipara with floating head, in certain cases of occiput posterior, in breech and transverse presentations, and in cases with an oversize baby, and in elderly primiparas. 2. Even multiparas who give a history of having a long, hard, difficult previous delivery may be best delivered by the abdominal route. 3. The endocrine or distrophy dystocia syndrome types may demand surgical delivery.

If none of the above conditions are present and it seems wise to permit labor to pursue its normal course, then I think, the perineal forceps and episiotomy is indicated. This can be done quickly and easily and without pain under local infiltration of the perineum. I never ask sick patients to exert themselves. They are treated as above outlined until the

*Read before the Section on Obstetrics and Gynecology, Annual Session, Oklahoma State Medical Association, April 23, 1942

cervix is fully dilated and the head is on the perineum or well below the spines, then the perineum is infiltrated with one-half to one percent Novocaine, episiotomy is done, forceps applied, the baby lifted out and any resulting damage quickly repaired.

If and when we decide to deliver the patient from below, I believe she should be allowed to go in labor naturally. I am absolutely opposed, to some of the modern methods of inducing labor, namely, stripping the cervix, rupturing the bag of waters,

castor oil and quinine, pituitary extract and the Voorhees bag.

The main points I wish to stress in the delivery of any sick woman are the following: relieve pain, conserve energy, save blood, and support the patient. .

(Editor's Note: Following this discussion, Dr. Allen showed an interesting moving picture of his own work showing the successive steps in perineal infiltration episiotomy, forceps delivery and repair, also cesarean section under local anesthesia.)

Causes of Blindness in Oklahoma*

*An analysis of the blindness of recipients of
Aid to the Blind from the Oklahoma
Department of Public Welfare.*

TULLOS O. COSTON, M.D.

OKLAHOMA CITY, OKLAHOMA

In 1937 the Oklahoma Department of Public Welfare, in cooperation with the Federal Social Security Board, began granting financial assistance to properly qualified blind residents of the state. The present study represents an analysis of the 2,146 cases on the blind assistance roll as of March 31, 1941.

In addition to financial need, an approved applicant for blind assistance in Oklahoma must not have a corrected visual acuity greater than 20/200, unless there is a contraction of the visual field to a total diameter of 20° or less. Rare exceptions to these standards include cases of extreme photophobia during the acute stage of some ocular disease and cases of extreme ptosis.

It is to be noted in Table No. 1 that only 7.9 percent of the cases had a visual acuity as high as 20/200 and only 1.1 percent better than 20/200.

The classification of the causes of blindness used in this survey is that which was worked out by the National Committee on Statistics of the Blind and approved by the American Medical Association. This classification takes into account both the site (topography) and type of affection, as well as, the etiology.

*Read before the Section on Eye, Ear, Nose and Throat, Annual Session, Oklahoma State Medical Association, April 22, 1942.

Table I

Extent of Vision at Time of Last Examination of Recipients Of Aid to the Blind, March 31, 1941

Extent of Vision	Recipients	
	Number	Percent
Total	2,146	100.0
Absolute blindness	449	20.9
Light perception (and/or projection) only	488	22.7
Motion perception and form perception up to but not including 5/200	464	21.6
5/200 up to but not including 10/200	328	15.3
10/200 up to but not including 20/200	234	10.9
20/200	169	7.9
Better than 20/200, with peripheral limitation indicated	10	.5
Peripheral field 20° or less	9	.4
Peripheral field greater than 20°	1	.1
Better than 20/200 up to and including 20/70 with no peripheral limitation indicated	2	.1
Better than 20/70 with no peripheral limitation indicated	1	†
Not Reported	1	†

†—Less than one-tenth of one percent
Oklahoma Department of Public Welfare

Table No. 2 represents the topographical analysis and Table No. 3, the etiological factors. Table No. 4 is a composite, cross-classification, embracing both of these.

The comparison of the chief racial groups in Oklahoma is shown in Tables Nos. 5 and 6 and several interesting facts are observed. Glaucoma is the cause of blindness in 17.2 percent of the negroes; 10.1 percent of the Indians; and only 5.3 percent of the whites. This relatively high percentage for the negroes is in line with the well-known fact that

Table II

Site (Topography) and Type of Affection Among Recipients Of Aid to the Blind, March 31, 1941

Site (Topography) and Type of Affection	Recipients	
	Number	Percent
Total	2,146	100.0
Eyeball, in general	313	14.6
Hypertension (glaucoma)	148	6.9
Refractive errors	40	1.8
Myopia	39	1.8
Other refractive errors, specified	1	†
Panophthalmitis and acute endophthalmitis	10	.5
Structural anomalies	21	1.0
Albinism	10	.5
Anophthalmos (excluding surgical)	1	†
Microphthalmos	1	†
Coloboma, any part (excluding surgical)	4	.2
Other structural anomalies, specified	2	.1
Structural anomalies, not specified	3	.1
Degenerative changes	75	3.5
Disorganized eyeball (atrophic globe, phthisis bulbi)	75	3.5
Other affections of the eyeball, specified	4	.2
Affections of the eyeball, not specified	15	.7
Cornea	758	35.3
Keratitis, interstitial	12	.6
Keratitis, (keratoconjunctivitis), phlyctenular	1	†
Keratitis, ulcerative	196	9.1
Keratitis, not specified	85	4.0
Pannus	125	5.8
Ulceration and vascularization	317	14.8
Other affections of the cornea, specified	21	1.0
Affections of the cornea, not specified	1	†
Iris and ciliary body	110	5.1
Iritis	6	.3
Iridocyclitis and uveitis	74	3.4
Sympathetic ophthalmitis	30	1.4
Crystalline lens	390	18.2
Cataract	390	18.2
Choroid and retina	176	8.2
Choroiditis	36	
Retinitis	20	111	5.2
Chorioretinitis	55	
Detached retina	17	.8
Retinal hemorrhage	1	†
Retinal degeneration (including retinitis pigmentosa)	45	2.1
Arteriosclerotic disease of choroid and retina	2	.1
Optic nerve, visual pathway, and cortical visual centers	318	14.8
Optic nerve atrophy	300	14.0
Optic neuritis (papillitis)	7	.3
Papilledema (choked disc)	2	.1
Neuroretinitis	5	.2
Retrobulbar and intra-cranial lesions	3	.1
Other affections of the optic nerve, specified	1	†
Miscellaneous and ill-defined	81	3.8
Amblyopia, undefined	35	1.6
Lesions, not specified	46	2.2

†—Less than one-tenth of one percent
Oklahoma Department of Public Welfare

glaucoma in negroes is much less amenable to treatment than in whites. Corneal ulceration and pannus are much more common in the Indians as a result of the higher incidence of trachoma in that race (46.8 percent compared to 25.7 percent in whites and 2 percent in negroes). Optic nerve atrophy is reported as the type of affection in 23.2 percent of the negroes, compared to 13.0 percent in the whites and only 3.7 percent in the Indians. This is in keeping with the higher incidence of syphilis in negroes (7.2 percent as compared to 2.2 percent in whites and 1.8 percent in Indians). The incidence of syphilis in all groups is undoubtedly somewhat higher since only proven cases were classified as syphilitic in this study.

The principal causes of blindness (Chart No. 2) in the entire group of blind recipients, are trachoma (23.3 percent), cataract (18.1 percent), optic atrophy (14.8 percent), uveal disease (13.3 percent), keratitis (12.3 percent—excluding trachoma) and glaucoma (6.9 percent).

The geographical distribution of blind recipients, according to counties, is shown in Chart No. 3. This reveals the number of recipients per ten thousand population. The ten leading counties in order are as follows: Sequoyah, Atoka, Okfuskee, Adair, Cherokee, Haskell, Latimer, Leflore, Rogers, and Choctow. Only one county, Cimarron, has no resident receiving blind assistance.

The proportion of trachoma cases to the total number of blind cases is shown by counties in Chart No. 4. The following represent the first ten in order of highest incidence: Delaware, Greer, Cherokee, Pawnee, Cleveland, Marshall, Rogers, Leflore, Murray, Sequoyah and Washington.

The Oklahoma Department of Public Welfare has no funds available for the treatment

Table III

Etiology of Blindness Among Recipients of Aid to the Blind, March 31, 1941

Etiology	Recipients	
	Percent	Number
Total	2,146	100.0
Infectious diseases	663	30.9
Gonorrhea	7	.3
Measles	13	.6
Meningitis	19	.9
Ophthalmia neonatorum	40	1.9
Gonorrheal	5	.3
Type not specified	34	1.6
Scarlet fever	2	.1
Septicemia	1	†
Chronic	1	†
Smallpox	3	.1
Syphilis	63	2.9
Prenatal	11	.5
Acquired after birth	47	2.2
Origin not specified	5	.2
Trachoma	501	23.3
Typhoid fever	6	.3
Multiple infectious diseases	1	†
Other infectious diseases, specified	7	.3
Trauma (including chemical burns)	175	8.2
Nonoccupational activities	49	2.3
Medical and surgical procedures	3	.1
Play or sport	7	.3
Household activities	1	†
Traffic and transportation	3	.1
Other nonoccupational activities, specified	29	1.4
Nonoccupational activities, not specified	6	.3
Occupational activities	43	2.0
Activities, not specified	83	3.9
Poisonings	3	.1
Nonoccupational activities	3	.1
Neoplasms	19	.9
General diseases (not elsewhere classified)	44	2.0
Anemia and other blood diseases	1	†
Diabetes	5	.2
Nephritis and other kidney diseases	1	†
Vascular diseases	12	.6
Diseases of the central nervous system	23	1.1
Other general diseases, specified	1	†
General diseases, not specified	1	†
Prenatal origin (not elsewhere classified)	130	6.1
Hereditary origin, established	2	.1
Prenatal origin, cause not specified	128	6.0
Etiology undetermined or not specified	1,112	51.8
Unknown to science	524	24.4
Undetermined by physician	576	26.8
Not specified	12	.6

†—Less than one-tenth of one percent
Oklahoma Department of Public Welfare

Table IV

ETIOLOGY OF BLINDNESS BY SITE (TOPOGRAPHY) AND TYPE OF AFFECTION AMONG RECIPIENTS OF AID TO THE BLIND, MARCH 31, 1941

Table V

SITE (TOPOGRAPHY) AND TYPE OF AFFECTION AMONG RECIPIENTS OF AID TO THE BLIND CLASSIFIED BY RACE, MARCH 31, 1941

Site (Topography) and Type of Affection	Race of Recipients									
	Total		White		Negro		Indian		Other	
	No.	%	No.	%	No.	%	No.	%	No.	%
Total	2,146	100.0	1,728	100.0	308	100.0	109	100.0	1	100.0
Percent	100.0		80.5		14.4		5.1		†	
Eyeball, in general	313	14.6	225	13.0	77	25.0	11	10.1		
Hypertension (glaucoma)	148	6.9	91	5.3	53	17.2	4	3.7		
Myopia	39	1.8	33	1.9	6	2.0				
Panophthalmitis and acute endophthalmitis	10	.5	5	.3	4	1.3	1	.9		
Structural anomalies, all types	21	1.0	21	1.2						
Degenerative changes	75	3.5	56	3.2	13	4.2	6	5.5		
All other affections, and not specified	20	.9	19	1.1	1	.3				
Cornea	758	35.3	643	37.2	46	14.9	69	63.3		
Keratitis, interstitial	12	.6	7	.4	4	1.3	1	.9		
Keratitis, ulcerative	196	9.1	154	8.9	27	8.8	15	13.8		
Pannus	125	5.8	108	6.3	4	1.3	13	11.9		
Ulceration and vascularization	317	14.8	284	16.4	1	.3	32	29.4		
All other affections, and not specified	108	5.0	90	5.2	10	3.2	8	7.3		
Iris and ciliary body	110	5.1	89	5.2	16	5.2	5	4.6		
Iridocyclitis and uveitis	74	3.4	59	3.4	12	3.9	3	2.8		
Sympathetic ophthalmitis	30	1.4	25	1.5	3	1.0	2	1.8		
Iritis	6	.3	5	.3	1	.3				
Cataract	390	18.2	313	18.1	62	20.1	15	13.8		
Choroid and retina	176	8.2	151	8.7	21	6.8	4	3.6		
Choroiditis	36	1.7	30	1.7	5	1.6	1	.9		
Retinitis	20	.9	14	.8	5	1.6	1	.9		
Chorioretinitis	55	2.6	50	2.9	3	1.0	2	1.8		
Detached retina	17	.8	16	.9	1	.3				
Retinal degeneration (including pigmentosa)	45	2.1	38	2.2	7	2.3				
All other affections, and not specified	3	.1	3	.2						
Optic nerve, visual pathway, and cortical visual centers	318	14.8	238	13.8	75	24.4	4	3.7	1	100.0
Optic nerve atrophy	300	14.2	224	13.0	71	23.2	4	3.7	1	100.0
Optic neuritis (papillitis)	7	.3	5	.3	2	.6				
Neuroretinitis	5	.2	3	.2	2	.6				
All other affections, and not specified	6	.3	6	.3						
All other and not specified	81	3.8	69	4.0	11	3.6	1	.9		

†—Less than one-tenth of one percent
Oklahoma Department of Public Welfare

of blind recipients. Medical treatment or operation is advised in all cases who might expect improvement in vision by such measures. The Welfare Department does not have funds available even for transportation of recipients to the physician or hospital. As a result of this, and the recipients unwillingness to undergo treatment for fear of losing his grant, a relatively small percent of the 585 cases recommended for treatment have received same. The exact figures are not yet available. Many other states, Arkansas, Kansas, Colorado, and Iowa, to mention a few, supply ample funds for restorative methods in the hands of the properly qualified, private physicians. Recipients who

Table VI

ETIOLOGY OF BLINDNESS AMONG RECIPIENTS OF AID TO THE BLIND, CLASSIFIED BY RACE, MARCH 31, 1941

Etiology	Race of Recipients									
	Total		White		Negro		Indian		Other	
	No.	%	No.	%	No.	%	No.	%	No.	%
Total	2,146	100.0	1,728	100.0	308	100.0	109	100.0	1	100.0
Percent	100.0		80.5		14.4		5.1		†	
Infectious diseases	663	30.9	564	32.6	41	13.3	57	52.3	1	100.0
Ophthalmia neonatorum	40	1.9	28	1.6	9	2.9	3	2.8		
Gonorrhea	7	.3	7	.4						
Measles	13	.6	11	.6	2	.6				
Meningitis	19	.9	18	1.0	1	.3				
Syphilis	63	2.9	38	2.2	22	7.2	2	1.8	1	100.0
Trachoma	501	23.3	444	25.7	6	2.0	51	45.8		
Typhoid fever	6	.3	6	.4						
All others and not specified	14	.7	12	.7	1.	.3	1	.9		
Trauma	175	8.2	144	8.3	22	7.2	9	8.3		
Nonoccupational activities	49	2.3	37	2.1	8	2.7	4	3.7		
Occupational activities	43	2.0	39	2.3	2	.6	2	1.8		
Activities, not specified	83	3.9	68	3.9	12	3.9	3	2.8		
Poisonings	3	.1	1	.1	2	.6				
Neoplasms	19	.9	19	1.1						
General diseases	44	2.0	39	2.3	5	1.6				
Vascular diseases	12	.6	11	.6	1	.3				
Diseases of the central nervous system	23	1.0	20	1.2	3	1.0				
All others and not specified	9	.4	8	.5	1	.3				
Prenatal origin	130	6.1	118	6.8	11.	3.6	1	.9		
Hereditary origin, established	2	.1	2	.1						
Prenatal origin, cause not specified	128	6.0	116	6.7	11	3.6	1	.9		
Etiology undetermined or not specified	1,112	51.8	843	48.8	227	73.7	42	38.5		
Unknown to science	524	24.4	393	22.7	113	36.7	18	16.5		
Undetermined by physician	576	26.8	440	25.5	112	36.4	24	22.0		
Not specified	12	.6	10	.6	2	.6				

†—Less than one-tenth of one percent
Oklahoma Department of Public Welfare

Chart II

Principal Causes of Blindness Among Recipients of Aid to the Blind, March 31, 1941

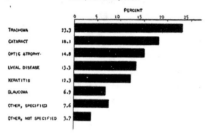

Oklahoma Department of Public Welfare.

refuse operation or treatment without good cause are dropped from the rolls.

Statistical studies of the causes of blindness are of value only in proportion to the needs, faults, possible preventative and rehabilitative measures which they point out.

The Oklahoma State Health Department has recently made a very encouraging start on the trachoma problem. Dr. J. A. Morrow, under whose guidance this work is progressing, will tell us some of the details.

I wish to compliment Miss McCollum and the Statistical Division of the Oklahoma Public Welfare Department on their excellent work in cataloguing and arranging the data presented here.

DISCUSSION

J. A. MORROW, M.D.
OKLAHOMA CITY, OKLAHOMA

As you have been advised by Dr. Coston, trachoma is the prevailing cause of blindness in Oklahoma. It being a communicable disease, it is of serious concern to the family, the state and the nation, for as a source of human suffering, as a cause of blindness and as a cause of economic loss it is second to none among diseases of the eye. Trachoma is responsible for 25 percent of the blind pensions in Oklahoma. Therefore from an economical, social and humanitarian standpoint, it is essential that something be done to control and eradicate it. Since it is a communicable disease, it becomes the responsibility of Public Health to take the initiative in the efforts at eradication. Like all other Public Health work the matter of education of the public is one of the major propositions.

While attending the Southern Medical Association in 1940 at Louisville, Kentucky, in company with Dr. Battenfield, our State Epidemiologist, we heard the programs as carried on in a few state that have Trachoma Control programs discussed, and became imbued with the idea of attempting such an effort in Oklahoma. After conferences with Dr. Mathews, State Commissioner of Health, and the Committee for Conservation of Vision, from the State Medical Association, a plan was outlined and submitted to the Children's Bureau at Washington, with a request for sufficient funds to carry on the work for a year. The result was granted and we were given a physician, a nurse, clerk and social medical worker.

We began our work in Sequoyah County, July 31, 1941, and since which time we have visited 13 counties, holding 62 clinics, examining 5,595 patients, (plus an uncounted number of school children in schools) finding 862 positive cases of trachoma which have been placed on treatment.

Our treatment has consisted of 1/5 gr. sulfanilamide per pound of body weight, each 24 hours for 10 days, reinforced by saturated solution of sulfanilamide dropped in the eyes several times daily or, sulfanilamide powder used in eye twice daily. If at the end of a 30 day period we have not had the improvement we think we should have had, another 10-day course of sulfanilamide is administered. Reactions from the drug have been practically nil, a few patients complaining of nausea, vertigo and two cases of slight cyanosis.

Sufficient time has not elapsed to warrant any definite conclusions as to permanent results, but upon the surface, results have been very gratifying to all concerned, and far superior to anything we have ever had at our command in the past. Of course heavy pannus, scarring of cornea, entropion, ectropion, trichiasis and such, are unaffected by treatment except these patients may be rendered more comfortable and non-infectious. Cases of entropion or trichiasis that keep the patients in constant pain and discomfort and contribute to ultimate blindness are being relieved by surgery.

We sincerely hope, gentlemen, that each of you may acquire an interest in this disease and lend full support to controlling it, which we have every reason to believe can be done. Of course, as you all know, it is a disease, confined mostly to those in the lower income brackets and with poor hygienic surroundings. You cannot expect much in the way of material remuneration for your services but, for the community as a whole, the control of this disease is a splendid investment.

Chart III

RECIPIENTS OF AID TO THE BLIND MARCH 31, 1941, AND
NUMBER PER 10,000 POPULATION

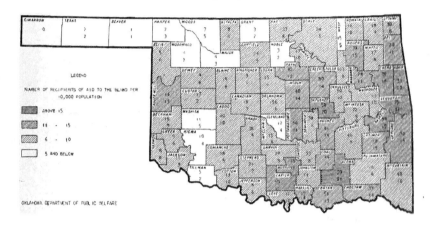

The 501 blind persons in Oklahoma, who are receiving Blind Assistance, due to trachoma, are costing the tax payers approximately $120,000 annually. Give us concerted action upon the part of the Medical profession of this state in the war against this disease, and in a few years it will be as rare as diphtheria or typhoid fever.

Chart IV

PROPORTION OF BLIND RECIPIENTS WITH ETIOLOGY OF BLINDNESS AS
TRACHOMA TO TOTAL AID TO THE BLIND RECIPIENTS, MARCH 31, 1941

(Percentage)

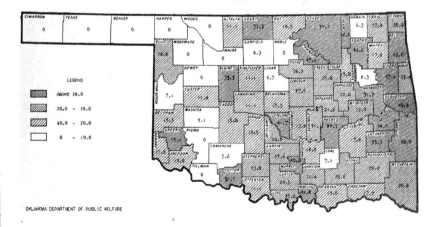

Medicine and Pharmacy in War[*]

Orville L. Prather, Ph.C.

TULSA, OKLAHOMA

Ever since Medicine and Pharmacy were discovered in the Middle Ages, there has been need for closer collaboration between the two. I would not intimate that they have quarreled, although there has been occasional bickering. On the whole, they have remained on friendly terms with each other, but they have failed to work together as they should. Each has been disposed to go his own way, to do his own work, and to leave the other alone.

This would perhaps be of small concern but for the fact that there is a third party to be considered—the general public. The public is entitled to the closest team-work between the physician and the pharmacist; for unless there is such team-work the people cannot have that adequate medical care to which they are entitled.

Modern science has so extended the field of what the physician must know about disease, its diagnosis, its treatment and its control, that no doctor can possibly know everything within the scope of his own work. Likewise, Science has discovered so much concerning medication, its sources, its extraction and purification, the means of determining its potency and of maintaining exact standards, that pharmaceutical practice now includes much more than the technique of filling prescriptions.

Diagnosis and treatment have become such complicated problems that no conscientious pharmacist would think of counter-prescribing, even though the law allowed it; and likewise new pharmaceutical discoveries have come so thick and fast that the busy doctor, more than ever, needs the assistance of his natural partner, the practicing pharmacist.

Just now, under the impact of a global war, the knowledge of the pharmacist is needed to supplement that of the physician, for new and special reasons. For the time is past when a physician can sit down and write a prescription without up-to-the-minute information.

Assuming that he has had time to keep abreast of pharmaceutical as well as strictly

medical developments—and that is a big order—and knows all about the new drugs and preparations which research pharmacists have found and developed, the physician can no longer prescribe anything he would like to prescribe, for the drug may no longer be available.

The sources of supply of many important drugs, drugs frequently prescribed, have been cut off by the War. The countries which produce them may be in the hands of the enemy, or the need for using all shipping for war supplies may have made it impossible to procure them. Also materials used in medicine, even though produced within our own country, may not be available because they are needed for the manufacture of munitions. The Government has impounded many drugs for use by the armed forces, leaving, of some of them, none, or almost none, for the civilian population.

Prescribing is the doctor's business, but finding and supplying the things prescribed is the druggist's business—and it is of no use to prescribe anything the druggist cannot obtain. Hence, there needs to be closer collaboration than ever between doctor and druggist.

So it becomes the proper function of the pharmacist to stress the use of drugs known to have therapeutic merit, which are plentiful or at least obtainable, and to advise against the use of others which are scarce; likewise to discourage the use of preparations of doubtful or unproved efficacy, which only serve to deplete the supply of the materials from which they are made; and to recommend the prescribing of medicines in the form of tablets or powders, instead of in liquid form, when the latter calls for such scarce materials as glycerin, alcohol and sugar.

It may be like carrying coals to Newcastle to enumerate the chemicals of which there is a shortage; furthermore, the list is lengthening from day to day and therefore can never be considered complete. I can mention Ethyl Alcohol, Methyl Alcohol, Isopropyl Alcohol, Chloroform, Ether, Acetone, Formaldehyde, Acetic Acid, Ammonia, Chlorine,

---

[*]Read before Staff Meeting, Hillcrest Memorial Hospital, September 7, 1942.

Phenol, Mercury, Toluene, Creosote, Carbon Tetrachloride, Glycerin, Sugar, Citric Acid, Tartaric Acid, Alum Salts, Borax, Boric Acid, Iodine, Phosphorus, Potassium Permanganate, Camphor, Menthol, Theophylline, Theobromine, Caffiene, Tannic Acid, Potassium Salts, Nitrates, and all mineral acids.

In the classification of botanical drugs, the list of shortages is even longer. It includes Cinchona from Java, which produces 90 percent of it, and from Peru; Opium for India, China, Persia and Turkey; Belladonna from Central and Southern Europe; Acacia, Buchu, Strophantus and Cudbear from Africa; Tragacanth from Persia and Asia Minor; Squill from India and the Mediterranean area; Senna from India and Egypt; Camphor, Menthol, Oil of Peppermint, and Agar from Japan; Strychnine from India; Hyoscyamus from Europe, Asia and Africa; Glycyrrhiza from Spain; Olive Oil from Spain and the Mediterranean area; Castor Oil from India, China and Brazil; Expressed Oil of Almond and Oil of Bitter Almond from Asia Minor and southern Europe; Oil of Eucalyptus from Spain, France and Australia; Oil of Lavender and Psyllium Seed from France and Spain; Oil of Citronella from Java and Ceylon; Rhubarb from China; Pilocarpus from Central and South America; Ipecac from Brazil; Lycopodium from Poland and Russia; Oil of Rose from the Balkans; Santal Oil from the Malayan Archipelago; Sesame Oil from India; Aloe from Africa and the West Indies; Asafedita from India and Persia; Benzoin from Thailand, Sumatra and Java; Ergot from Russia, Germany and Spain; Anise from Spain and China; Clove from the Philippines; Cassia from many tropical region; Copra from the Philippines; Karaya Gum from the Far East —and this list of scarce botanicals is by no means complete.

The scarcity of these essential drugs and chemicals places on our two professions the joint responsibility of finding substitutes—products which have the same, or nearly the same values, as those which are no longer available. That is our duty to the public we serve.

The items I have just listed are becoming scarce due to the all-out war that we are now in. There are many more and will be more so long as this condition exists.

If we were able to load our ships at the shores of supply with the goods that I have just mentioned, it would still be practically impossible to secure them due to the shortage of transportation. Still another reason would be the extreme hazard from the possible loss by Axis submarines.

I do not like to use the word substitutes; it has a bad thought. It is needless to say that I do not condone that form of substitution which takes place when a pharmacist takes liberties with a doctor's prescription. That kind of substitution is condemned by my profession as much as it is by yours. A prescription should be filled as written, unless a change is directed or authorized, in writing, by the physician who wrote it.

That kind of substitution which I am thinking of, and the only kind of which either you or I would approve, is the substitution or replacement mutually agreed upon by the doctor and the pharmacist, which may have been made necessary by conditions during the war emergency. The need for that kind of replacement already has been recognized in the United States Pharmacopoeia and the National Formulary, which have accepted certain products in lieu of those formerly indicated.

I have already referred to one kind of substitution or replacement, which can be made without hurting anything but the patient's sense of taste—the dispensing of medicines in the form of tablets and capsules instead of elixirs, tinctures and fluid extracts, and the use of saccharine instead of sugar for sweetening. If this were done generally, it would save no end of sugar, alcohol and glycerin for other uses. To be more specific, there seems to be no reason why tablets of Phenobarbital and capsules of Terpin Hydrate and Codeine would not serve just as well as the elixirs generally prescribed in the past.

Further, coal tar analgesics would serve in place of codeine for relief of muscular aches and pains, headaches and colds; and Bromides and steam inhalations containing Menthol for coughs. If we cut down on the use of Morphine derivatives, we leave just that much more Morphine for the relief of pain on the battlefield and thereby make a real contribution to the Nation's war effort.

Belladonna and its alkaloids are on the scarce list. Why should we not use such synthetics as Novathropine, Eumydrine, Syntropan, Trasentin or Pavatrine as antispasmodics? The synthetic Atabrine is almost as good as Quinine for purposes for which the latter has been used. For emulsifying purposes, Gelatin, Methyl Cellulose, Pecton and Irish Moss, as well as many synthetic products, will serve almost as well as Agar, Acacia, Tragacanth and Gum Karaya. For purposes of suspension Bentonite may be used quite successfully. Oils of Spearmint, Lemon and Orange, and the synthetic Methyl Salicylate will easily take the place of Menthol. Instead of natural Camphor we can employ synthetic Camphor made from Oil of Turpentine, of which there is an abundance. As counter-irritants Methyl Salicylate or the more abundant Volatile Oil of Mustard, Oil of Turpentine, and many of the Pine Oils, are available.

Benzoic Acid, Sodium Benzoate, Methyl p-Hydroxybenzoate, Propyl p-Hydroxybenzoate and Butyl p-Hydroxybenzoate will do instead of Glycerin, as preservatives. The Sulfa drugs are displacing Mercury and Mercury compounds in medication, and in many instances where the use of Mercury is still indicated, such as Blue Ointment and Ointment of Ammoniated Mercury, it has been found that the amount of Mercury may be reduced without impairing effectiveness. Combinations of Starch, Kaolin, Talc, Calcium Carbonate and Bentonite will serve as covering and protective agents, when Zinc Oxide is scarce. In the field of Herbal Laxatives, replacement for Cascara Sagrada are the various mineral or saline salts and the synthetic Phenolphthaelin; and one can always fall back on Mineral Oil.

It has not been my purpose to catalog all the alternatives to which the War is driving us, but only to indicate that new conditions make new methods imperative and that there needs to be the closest cooperation henceforth between the doctor who prescribes and the pharmacist who compounds and dispenses. Out of such cooperation each profession will gain, for each has much to learn. The public also will gain, for it will be assured of adequate medication even during a period of scarcities.

Out of such a relationship I can see coming a new conception by the retail druggist of his proper function. Economic conditions have forced him to become a merchant as well as a professional man. A fault which I willingly admit is that his mercantile interest in too many instances has been predominant, and that he has often gone far afield. Physicians have deplored this, and sometimes it has caused them to have less confidence in the pharmacist than they have wished to have.

I am not blaming physicians for this attitude, but I believe I shall be pardoned for suggesting that the Medical profession may not be entirely without blame for the situation which prompted the attitude. If the doctor himself would discontinue dispensing the ready-made products of pharmaceutical manufacturers, which may or may not be exactly what the individual patient should have; if he would write prescriptions calling for Official remedies and thereby actually save his patients money; if he would consult the pharmacist on problems specifically within the latter's province and in turn encourage the pharmacist to consult him; I say if these things were done, the prescription department would soon seem more important to the retail pharmacist, he would strive harder to keep abreast with the phenomenal advances of knowledge in his own profession, he would be awakened to a keener sense of his own place in the Medical-Pharmaceutical partnership and be less disposed to engage in counter-prescribing and other practices, far too prevalent, to which the physician has full right to object—aye, even to resent with righteous indignation.

Some of the deprivations of the war will, in my opinion, help the retail druggist more than they will hurt him. The scarcity of trinkets and notions—of pots and pans and gadgets—will force him to fall back on his prescription business and to cultivate it. Thereby he will make his store what it should be—a drug store. Perhaps then he will not only regain, but justify your confidence.

The trend toward commercialism, initiated and followed chiefly by multiple-store systems owned by non-pharmacists and promoted for gain, has not been universal. There are still in this country tens of thousands of drug stores which are drug stores. One valuable by-product of the war, it seems to me, will be that these whom I would denominate the ethical branch of the business, who still constitute the majority numerically and even in volume, will gain unquestioned honor. When the operators of questionable drug stores no longer are able to get the racket-store merchandise in which they deal, the ethical druggist will come into his own.

The rank and file of druggists must come to realize that they are truly professional men; and the rank and file of pharmacists must come to realize that even in their professional capacity they are not mere fillers of prescriptions. They need to be familiar with, and be able to give information upon, not only drugs and chemicals but all medical supplies. They should be the physician's first source of information.

The hospitals of the country have begun to recognize their need for the pharmacist. The American College of Surgeons is directing hospitals to have proper pharmaceutical service; it is even going further—it is recommending that pharmacists be called into the various conferences; that they be represented on the staff; and that, at least, they should have the same status as the pathologist and the head of the X-ray department. This means that the pharmacist's function in the treatment of the sick is definitely recognized by the very elite of the medical profession. My assurance to you is that the pharmacists of the United States are trying to justify that recognition.

Recent Advances in the Treatment of Acute and Chronic Sinus Infection*

MARVIN D. HENLEY, M.D.

TULSA, OKLAHOMA

How do you treat infections of the nasal accessory sinuses?

This is a frequent question asked because of the fact that there is a mass of confusion regarding this subject; first, there is little unanimity of opinion among the members of our profession; second, treatments advocated today are changed tomorrow; third, proponents of specific therapeutic measures do not always practice what they recommend; fourth, there is an appalling lack of sustained conviction on the subject of sinus disease in general. Many who have expounded their own opinions have often been looked upon contemptuously by students of different thought. The conclusion then to which one is inevitably driven is that there are an inordinate variety of methods of treatment in sinus disease and that no specific cure, either medicinal, surgical or biological, has yet been discovered.

This paper is a cross-section of a recapitulation of the views of about forty different rhinologists.

Discussion of sinus infection is a favorite topic of the rhinologist, especially when talking to general practitioners. This is probably so because the nasal accessory sinuses are still considered as somewhat mysterious parts of the human anatomy, the physiological function of which is still unrevealed. Even their development is still a matter of speculation among the embryologists. Some of them are present already at time of birth; others will develop during the early years of childhood.

At birth, the maxillary sinus is the furthest developed of all the nasal air cavities, although it is still a slitlike recess. Its growth, however, is very rapid, and it will become the largest of the sinuses. The frontal sinus develops after birth; in children of one or two years of age it is still rudimentary, and sometimes it may remain undeveloped during the whole life. The labyrinth of ethmoid cells attain their final form only by the twelfth or fourteenth year. The sphenoid sinuses are recognizable only at three years of age, and reach their final form at the twelfth or the sixteenth year of age. By these developmental differences we may expect a great variety of sinus disease both in children and in adults. And, since the sinuses are lined with the same mucosa as the nasal fossa, and since the sinuses are in continuity with the nasal fossa, any infection of the nose itself will readily travel from one cavity to the other through the natural passageways of the ostia.

There is practically little for the natural defense of the sinuses. The nasal secretion itself contains certain germicidal qualities in the form of the protective antibacterial enzyme called lysozyme. There are also the cilia in the sinuses which are the brooms for the backyards of the nose, and which sweep toward the sinus ostia. Lymphatic drainage and certain vasomotor reactions are further protections against bacterial invasion of the accessory nasal cavities. Yet, the natural defense often fails, especially by non-physiological measures used for the treatment of the common cold, and an acute sinus infection develops.

Sinus infection is the most frequent nasal disease. In a series of 526 rhinological cases, Bowers found 64 percent to be sinus infection. There have been many suggestions for its treatment, and many failures so that an unfortunate slogan originated: "once a sinus, always a sinus." Lack of success was partly due to the inexperience of the rhinologist and his unwillingness to perform a radical surgical operation when indicated, or to do the other extreme: treating every case of sinusitis by radical measures.

At the present time, most of the rhinologists have returned to more conservative and more physiological forms of treatment, and with a few exceptions, they attempt to rely upon the natural defense mechanism of the sinus system, and by all available therapeutic measures they tend to support or to restore the normal physiological functions of the nose and the sinuses.

Before any treatment is initiated, it is first decided whether the sinus inflammation is due to real invasion of pathogenic bacteria

*Read before the Section on Eye, Ear, Nose and Throat, Annual Session, Oklahoma State Medical Association, April 22, 1942.

into the nasal accessory cavities, or is it a non-infectious inflammation produced by allergy, dietetic errors, improper water balance, endocrine disorders, improper balance in the action of the autonomic nervous system, and similar other factors. A true infection of the sinuses is most commonly the result of a neglected common cold, especially a cold self-treated with various advertised nasal drops. Recent investigations indicate that such drops paralyze the motion of the cilia of the mucosal lining and tend to defeat the natural defenses. Other circumstances in which bacteria may be forced into the sinuses are swimming and diving, or a nasal operation such as irrigation of the maxillary sinus, etc. Any condition that makes natural drainage through the normal ostia difficult will predispose to sinus infection. Swelling of the mucosa of the nasal fossa whether inflammatory or of other nature serves as an example. Cook pointed out that repeated swelling of the erectile tissue of the nose and the resulting nasal obstructions will make erotic individuals especially prone to sinus infection. Deformity of the nasal septum, of course, is a predisposing condition, yet neither deformity of a sinus itself or difference in the size of sinuses of the two sides is particularly apt to make the sinus more vulnerable to infection.

The invading bacteria may come from the nose itself, or from some distant foci of infection through the bloodstream. Such types of sinus infection are, however, rare. Chronic bronchiectasis may act as a focus of re-infection, and circulus vitiosus may become established. Acute infections of childhood may be accompanied by a sinus infection caused by specific pathogenic organisms. Some of these infections are especially vicious; e.g., scarlet fever may cause necrotic sphenoiditis. The bacteria responsible for the sinus disease are chiefly streptococci and staphylococci. The more specific infections due to fungi (actinomycosis), spirochaetes (syphilis) or to acid-fast bacteria (tuberculosis, leprosy) are rather infrequent. Occasionally, one may observe a sinus infection resulting from a dental disease. It should be repeated, however, that the common cold is the most frequent cause of sinus infection. It should be remarked here that every common cold or every nasal inflammation is accompanied by a secondary inflammation in the nasal accessory sinuses just as much as every otitis media is accompanied by secondary reactive mastoiditis. Such a reactive sinusitis is not yet a sinus infection, though it predisposes to an infection. As general experience shows, the reactive sinusitis will disappear together with the cold in most of the cases; infection will develop only when other predisposing and debilitating influences are present.

Most cases of acute sinusitis are such types of reactive inflammation. In children, we usually have a pansinusitis according to Cone. The treatment should stimulate natural defenses, and nothing should be done to harm the activity of the cilia. The chief purpose is to maintain aeration and drainage. Nasal drops should not be used, except saline and ephedrine. No surgery is allowed, neither turbinectomy nor sinusectomy. Thus, treatment of an acute sinusitis consists chiefly of many don'ts.

Van Alyea recommends vasoconstrictors for shrinkage of the swollen linings of the nose and sinuses in order to promote adequate drainage. Other harmless measures, such as bed rest in a warm and moist room, sedatives against the symptomatic pain and headache, infrared or other type of heat, occasionally foreign protein injection to produce fever and phagocytosis, also increased intake of vitamin C in the diet are useful adjuncts of the conservative therapy. Chemotherapeutic measures, such as the sulfonamides are also advocated, but their value in acute sinusitis is still under discussion.

The conservative treatment of an acute sinusitis is so important that Nodine advises "hands-off" in such cases. Yet, the above mentioned measures may be safely used. For shrinkage of the mucous linings we have a number of vasoconstrictor substances. Recently, benzedrine insufflation has been introduced, and it is especially recommended for young infants.

Rarely one encounters a highly virulent and fulminating type of sinus infection. For such cases, blood transfusions in small doses and given repeatedly are useful. Greenwood considers chemotherapeutical remedies only as adjuncts to the regular treatment including adequate drainage, rest and sedatives.

In true acute infection of the sinuses, irrigation of the sinus cavity and Proetz's displacement therapy are generally advisable. Cone cautions, however, that irrigation and displacement therapy may be injurious in the acute stage of sinus infection. There is no objection to irrigate in the subacute stage of sinusitis. Gundrum used ephedrine, neosynephrine, bacterial antigens and foreign proteins for washing the sinuses. Parkinson has obtained good results from a one percent solution of ephedrine sulfate in a .68 percent solution of sodium chloride. Black tried a one percent solution of sulfanilamide for irrigation fluid. Szilagyi used a one percent solution of hydrogen peroxide for washing the sinus, and five percent trypaflavin solution for filling the sinus by displacement.

Irrigation of any sinus should be done with great care, and under as little pressure as possible. There have been cases of cerebral air embolism reported due to irrigation of the sinuses under high pressure. The fluid for irrigation can be introduced either through the natural ostium of the sinus, or through a hole artificially punctured at the most advantageous point in the sinus wall. Sometimes, e.g. in the maxillary sinus, a puncture is better than leaving drainage to the natural ostium.

I mention ionization only to point out that it is not a treatment for sinusitis. Indeed, success of ionization as properly recommended for the treatment of vasomotor rhinitis depends chiefly on the freedom of sinuses from any disease.

Two other recent methods should be recorded: one is radiothermy, the other is roentgen irradiation. Both are relatively new methods for treatment of sinus infection, and not enough evidence has so far accumulated either to condemn or to recommend them.

Radiothermy is a form of thermotherapy by penetrating shortwaves. It is supposed to produce hyperemia, local edema, and, thereby, to increase the natural protective inflammatory reaction of the organism against infection. It may be indicated in cases of acute sinus infection. Hollender says that radiothermy is indicated only in acute sinusitis; it has no value in chronic sinus infection, or in cases complicated by allergy and hyperplasia of the mucosa. Others, however, use radiothermy also in chronic cases after operations on the sinuses, but for such instances long waves (600 to 2,000 meters) may be more effective. Wahrer found that ten meter waves with parallelly spaced, air-spaced electrodes are effective in acute sinus infection. He gave daily treatments of ten minutes duration. He claims that the course of acute sinusitis is shortened. Yet, Teed asserts that radiothermy has very little value against sinusitis, even if used as an adjunct. Certainly, it should not be anything but an adjunct to the regular measures.

Roentgen irradiation, used as an adjunct, has been proved of much more value than short-wave therapy in acute sinusitis. It has been employed for sinus treatment since 1916. The usual factors are: 130 kilovolts, 6 mm. aluminum filter, and 40 cm. distance, with portals covering the affected sinuses. Success of roentgen irradiation depends on preliminary shrinkage of the mucosa, and establishment of proper drainage. No good can be expected if there is pus in the sinus. The stage in which roentgen irradiation should be tried is the acute stage of infection.

Roentgen irradiation stimulates phagocytosis and increases the signs of inflammation for about 24 hours. Thereafter, it hastens the convalescence. Already after the first irradiation, the pain and headache is relieved, and this symptomatic relief alone would justify roentgen irradiation in the treatment of sinus infection. Levin found that the younger the patient the more ready the response to roentgen irradiation. Williams treated 56 acute cases with from 50r to 100r (roentgen unit) doses, and gave one to three treatments on alternate days until full recovery from the sinus infection. Cherubino treated 39 acute and subacute cases of sinusitis, and claimed a cure for all of them; he gave 75r to 100r units one or two daily in the acute cases, and one or two weekly in the chronic cases.

An interesting observation has been made recently on the effect of reduced air pressure upon sinus infection and sinusitis. Andrews experimented with 16 patients who had sinusitis, put them in airplanes, and when he reached 8,000 feet altitude, he began to fly up and down between 6,000 feet and 8,000 feet altitude, making his changes of altitude at a rate of from 100 to 1,000 feet a minute. The sinusitis patients were in the air about an hour. Nine of the patients found temporary complete relief; five patients felt partial relief, but two had no relief. Next day after the experiment in the air all patients reported that they had a much more copious discharge from the nose.

The maxillary sinus is often the first of the sinuses that becomes infected. In fact, this sinus is the keystone of the entire accessory sinus system, and, alone or in combination, is affected in at least 95 percent of the sinusitis cases. Prevention of maxillary sinuse infection would reduce sinus ailments greatly. Surveys of children between one and six years of age show that 35.5 percent of them have a maxillary sinus infection; those between six and 12 years of age have pathological maxillary sinuses in about 16 percent of the cases. Maxillary sinusitis in its subacute stage requires irrigation and displacement therapy. Certain rhinologists advocate the puncture by way of the inferior meatus and not through the natural ostium, which is too high for a good drainage. Irrigation of the maxillary sinus often improves drainage from the ethmoid sinus. In frontal sinusitis, irrigation is not advisable according to Bombelli.

The time to correct all predisposing factors of sinus infection is after acute sinus infections have subsided. This may include some surgery for the elimination of predisposing nasal deformities (septum deviation, nasal polyps, turbinate hypertrophy, etc.). It should also include the proper care of an existing bronchiectasis, of tonsillitis, removal of adenoids, etc. Bronchiectasis, as stated before, may be a constant source of reinfection. Goodale reported that 24 percent in a series of 150 cases of bronchiectasis showed recurrent acute sinusitis.

While acute sinus infection is treated chiefly along conservative lines, and with medical measures, the treatment of chronic sinus infections should be definitely radical and chiefly surgical. When should we consider a sinusitis or a sinus infection chronic? Or when should we decide that surgery should no longer be delayed? Surgery is indicated if the symptoms do not subside in four or five weeks on conservative treatment; or, if there is no drainage from the sinus; or, if polpi are present, or if three or four conservative treatments do not help.

In case of maxillary sinusitis Hosen follows a combined plan of treatment: weekly irrigations for six weeks, and autogenus vaccine injections every three to five days for 15 doses. If after this treatment there is still pus in the maxillary sinus, he prepares a permanent window for drainage.

Before any sinus surgery is instituted, an active allergy should be first relieved, and the swelling of the mucosa should be corrected by shrinkage, which is a prerequisite for the successful treatment of chronic sinus infection. The surgical intervention should be accurate and well planned, radical rather than a sort of timid intervention.

That a chronic unyielding sinus infection has to be treated radically there is no doubt, if one remembers all the possible dangers, the great many intracranial complications, and other systemic illnesses which may result from an infectious focus in an accessory nasal sinus. Recently, the long list of complications (asthma, respiratory disorders, bronchiectasis, rheumatism, gastrointestinal disease, recurrent colds, fibrositis, nephritis, trigeminal neuralgia) has been increased by mental diseases as they have been brought into definite connection with chronic sinusitis by Bedford Russell.

On the other hand, we must consider the danger of nasal operation, or of operations on the sinuses, which include intracranial diseases, and osteomyelitis of the skull. Such an osteomyelitis may result even from a minor surgical intervention on a sinus. It is especially frequent after the Killian operation, but its development depends entirely on the resistance of the perisinusal bone, and not on the rhinologist's skill. Zoltan gave us a number of rules by which the surgical risk of sinus operations can be reduced to a minimum, or to a point where the advantages of a surgical intervention on a sinus for chronic infection will greatly overwhelm the possibility of postoperative complications.

These rules include the following: avoid always the danger zones of the nose; do not operate in acute rhinitis or in acute sinusitis (except in fulminating infection in order to avoid an osteomyelitis); make wide drainage towards the nose in all intranasal operations; operate externally if the face of the patient is edematous; do not remove the lining of the sinus with sharp instruments; examine all sinuses, and operate on all infected sinuses.

The operation to be performed depends upon the sinus or sinuses affected, the etiology of the disease, the age and general constitution of the patient, and upon social-economic factors as well.

For the maxillary sinus, the Caldwell-Luc operation is still a favorite of many. Out of 285 operations on the maxillary sinus, Kolba used the Caldwell-Luc method in 268 cases. The Denker operation is now abandoned because there is too much danger to the lacrimal apparatus. Similarly, the Stuhrmann operation is no longer practiced. The Claoue-Lothrop operation is very useful, especially if the patient is weak, or if the sinus infection was secondary.

For the drainage of the upper group of sinuses various technics and approaches are in use. Recently, Hogg and others advocated the transantral approach to the upper group of sinuses, which is probably the best. This is an external operation. There is still much discussion whether the operation should be chiefly intranasal or chiefly external. In the opinion of many, the intranasal approach is unsatisfactory and results in the greatest number of postoperative complications. Regardless of the advantages and disadvantages of the external or intranasal methods, it is true that an external operation is much more radical than the intranasal technic. Most rhinologists, however, object to making it a routine procedure in the treatment of chronic sinus infection.

BIBLIOGRAPHY

1. Andrews, A. H.: Quar. Bulletin Northwestern Univ. Med. School, 1941, 15: 46-52.
2. Bedford Russell, H. G.: Jour. Ment. Sci., 1941, 87: 479-528.
3. Black, W. B.: Jour. Missouri Med. Assn., 1941, 38: 41-45.
4. Bombelli, U.: Acta Otolar., 1940, 28: 376-379.
5. Bowers, W. C.: Virginia Med. Monthly, 1940, 67: 660-668.
6. Cherubino, M.: Bulletin Mal. Orecchio, 1940, 58: 201-213.
7. Cone, A. J.: Tr. Am. Acad. Ophth. Otolar., 1941, 46: 79-94.
8. Cooke, G. C.: North Carolina Med. Jour., 1940, 1: 657-661.
9. Del Piano, J. Rev.: As. Med. Argent., 1940, 40: 868-870.
10. Goodale, R. L.: New England Jour. Med., 1940, 223: 654-656.
11. Graham, H. B.: Pacific Coast Medicine, 1941, 8: No. 2.
12. Greenwood, G. J.: Illinois Med. Jour., 1940, 78: 410-418.
13. Gundrum, L. K.: Laryngoscope, 1940, 50: 989-1001.

14. Hochfilzer, J. J.: Laryngoscope, 1940, 50: 792-795.
15. Hogg, J. C.: Proceedings Royal Society Medicine, London, 1941, 34: 117-124.
16. Hollender, A. R.: Arch. Phys. Ther., 1941, 22: 12-16.
17. Hosen, H.: Texas Jour. Med., 1941, 36: 633-637.
18. Kolba, V.: Orvosi Hetilap, 1940, 84: 611-613.
19. Levin, A. G.: Arch. Phys. Ther., 1941, 22: 217-219.
20. Littell, J. J.: Jour. Indiana Med. Assn., 1940, 33: 412-414.
21. Livereiro, E.: Acta Otolar., 1940, 28: 387-392.
22. Lothrop, O. A.: Arch. Otolar., 1941, 33: 72-77.
23. McGovern, F. H.: Arch. Otolar., 1941, 34: 593-595.
24. Maresh, M. M.: Am. Jour. Dis. Children, 1940, 60: 55-78
25. Maresh, M. M.: Am. Jour. Dis. Children, 1940, 60: 841-861.
26. Miller, H. A.: Arch. Otolar., 1940, 32: 1107.
27. Mood, G. F.: Medical Record, Houston, 1941, 35: 913-915.
28. Nodine, R. R.: Texas Jour. Med., 1941, 37: 478-481.
29. Rich, B. S.: Bulletin Med. School Univ. Maryland, 1941, 25: 181-183.
30. Sato, T.: Tr. Soc. Path. Jap., 1940, 30: 367-378.
31. Skillern, S. R.: Medical World, 1940, 58: 455-457.
32. Solo, D. H.: Medical Record, New York, 1941, 154: 101.
33. Steffensen, W. H.: Jour. Michigan Med. Soc., 1941, 40: 30-32.
34. Stamm, C.: Laryngoscope, 1941, 51: 77-86.
35. Stroud, E. F.: Texas Jour. Med., 1941, 37: 478-481.
36. Szilagyi, L.: Orvosi Hetilap, 1940, 84: 370.
37. Teed, R. W.: Guthrie Clinical Bulletin, 1940, 10: 47-58
38. Tremble, G. E.: Arch. Otolar., 1940, 32: 952-957.
39. Turnbull, F. M.: Jour. Am. Med. Assn., 1941, 116: 1899.
40. Tyler, A. F.: Eye & C. Monthly, 1941, 20: 78-82.
41. Van Alyea, O. E.: Tr. Am. Acad. Ophth. Otolar., 1941, 46: 69-78.
42. Wahrer, F. L.: Arch. Phys. Ther., 1940, 21: 410-413.
43. White, F. W.: Pennsylvania Med. Jour., 1940, 44: 141-147.
44. Williams, H. L.: Ann. Otol. Rhinol., 1940, 49: 749-754.
45. Zoltan, I.: Acta Otolar., 1941, 29: 184-215.

Importance of General Practitioner

The general practitioner is again taking his rightful place in the practice of medicine—and with a background of study and training that justifies the highest confidence in his ability, John Joseph Nutt, M.D., New York, declares in Hygeia, The Health Magazine for November, asserting that "If specialists would accept no patients except those referred by family physicians it would benefit the patient, the family physician and the specialist.

"The patient would, of necessity, have a physician who would be friend and adviser in all things pertaining to health. The prevention of illness has become a large part of the practice of medicine, and surely this is work for the family physician, who knows his patient from top to toe. He also should be the judge of the good or evil of treatments, drugs foods, exercise and climates. . . . No matter where he lives, the most recent advances in science are available to the family doctor through medical journals, circulating medical libraries and medical societies. By consulting him in small matters his patients may often avoid serious consequences. . . . The specialist would not be called on to treat conditions which the family physician can treat exactly as well; he would be consulted only for those conditions which come within his special field. The final result would be the thinning out of the ranks of the specialists —only the really fit surviving—and the return of the family physician to his own. . . ."

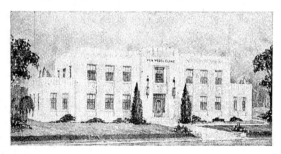

· THE PRESIDENT'S PAGE ·

The Third Annual Secretaries Conference of the Oklahoma State Medical Association and the Twelfth Annual Fall Conference of the Oklahoma City Clinical Society have recently been held with the usual amount of interest by physicians of this state.

In this period of world emergency and economic unrest, it is a tribute to any organization that will endeavor to continue to know and study its problems in order that a better service might be rendered the public. That medicine has a greater obligation to keep abreast of the times is apparent from the everyday releases read in the newspapers of both the American and controlled foreign press. Disease and famine are daily taking as great a toll in Europe as the defense of Stalingrad.

Every physician, no matter whether he is located in a remote locality or in a metropolitan center, should so arrange his time that he may constantly keep abreast of the latest achievements in the prevention and treatment of disease. Unless our profession assumes the obligation of giving the people of our country healthful bodies and minds, there will be a retarding of the war effort.

During the coming months, there will be many changes take place in the economic life of the entire country with the adoption of gasoline rationing, and where families could, in a very short time, be in a doctor's office, they will shortly, of necessity, have to depend upon a greater amount of the doctor's time in bringing medicine to their door.

County Medical Societies should immediately accept this responsibility and attempt to work out, with other interested organizations, a broad plan of medical care for the community that will take into consideration these factors.

Sincerely yours,

James D Osborn

President.

The JOURNAL Of The
OKLAHOMA STATE MEDICAL ASSOCIATION

EDITORIAL BOARD

L. J. MOORMAN, Oklahoma City, Editor-in-Chief

E. EUGENE RICE, Shawnee   NED R. SMITH, Tulsa

MR. R. H. GRAHAM, Oklahoma City, Business Manager

CONTRIBUTIONS: Articles accepted by this Journal for publication including those read at the annual meetings of the State Association are the sole property of this Journal.

The Editorial Department is not responsible for the opinions expressed in the original articles of contributors.

Manuscripts may be withdrawn by authors for publication elsewhere only upon the approval of the Editorial Board.

MANUSCRIPTS: Manuscripts should be typewritten, double-spaced, on white paper 8½ x 11 inches. The original copy, not the carbon copy, should be submitted.

Footnotes, bibliographies and legends for cuts should be typed on separate sheets in double space. Bibliography listing should follow this order: Name of author, title of article, name of periodical with volume, page and date of publication.

Manuscripts are accepted subject to the usual editorial revisions and with the understanding that they have not been published elsewhere.

NEWS: Local news of interest to the medical profession, changes of address, births, deaths and weddings will be gratefully received.

ADVERTISING: Advertising of articles, drugs or compounds unapproved by the Council on Pharmacy of the A.M.A. will not be accepted. Advertising rates will be supplied on application.

It is suggested that members of the State Association patronize our advertisers in preference to others.

SUBSCRIPTIONS: Failure to receive The Journal should call for immediate notification.

REPRINTS: Reprints of original articles will be supplied at actual cost provided request for them is attached to manuscripts or made in sufficient time before publication. Checks for reprints should be made payable to Industrial Printing Company, Oklahoma City.

Address all communications to THE JOURNAL OF THE OKLAHOMA STATE MEDICAL ASSOCIATION, 210 Plaza Court, Oklahoma City.

OFFICIAL PUBLICATION OF THE OKLAHOMA STATE MEDICAL ASSOCIATION
Copyrighted October, 1942

EDITORIALS

THE CHRISTMAS SEAL SALE

In this issue of the Journal, there are a number of quotations and abstracts from the recent literature dealing with tuberculosis. Your attention is being called to the present status of the tuberculosis problem because the season for the Christmas Seal sale is now upon us.

Interest in tuberculosis and its discovery and control are greatly augmented by organized agencies. Attention is called to the fact that money raised through the sale of Christmas Seals is not devoted to the care of tuberculosis patients, but is employed in the dissemination of knowledge, the discovery of active cases and the proper disposal of the same. Those who are not able to pay for private care are advised to go to one of the state sanatoria where the taxpayers provide proper care. Those who are able to pay are urged to see their family doctor who should see that they have the best available private care.

Every doctor should be interested in the Christmas Seal sale and should do everything possible to make it a success. The remarkable progress in the control of tuberculosis in this country during the past few decades may be attributed largely to the educational value of the Christmas Seal sale and the wise expenditure of the funds raised.

On account of the strain and stress of the present war, there is great danger of an increase in tuberculosis. Because of this danger, we must be on guard, but, since there can be no increased vigilance without adequate funds, we must be diligent in the sale of Christmas Seals.

If called upon to lend a helping hand, roll up your sleeves and make this a part of your war work.

ONLY MEDICINE CAN TURN THE TRICK

In another section of this issue of the Journal, the reader will find a review of *Ambassadors in White* by Charles Morrow Wilson. In this timely discussion, the author points out the fact that "Hemispheric solidarity cannot be built on a sick man's society. Latin America cannot live as a contributing factor in the Western Hemisphere on world civilization until it has conquered its health problems."

With our rapidly growing inter-communications, we should ever keep in mind the fact that not only is South-America subject to all the diseases which afflict our own people, including tuberculosis with a death rate five times that in the United States, but it has a long list of tropical diseases which, for us, may prove more deadly than the despicable Japanese.

In spite of all our knowledge and all our known preventive measures, we have no assurance that these diseases may not become epidemic in our own country. Even yellow fever may again spread its ominous pall over the land.

Let us hope the United States government will have the good sense to see that our political, economic and war defense interests in the South American countries are bound up with the health and the physical well being of their people. We are entering a new era in our inter-American relationships, and our success will depend largely upon medical and sanitary vision similar to that which characterized the building of the Panama Canal.

Bureaucratic control, political expediency and economic shortcuts are the most deadly enemies of scientific, social and cultural progress. The Panama Canal adventure barely escaped their annuling influence. Only the appeals of the American Medical Association and Theodore Roosevelt's confidence in General Gorgas saved the day.

PLACING THE RESPONSIBILITY

If individual doctors would carefully search their hearts with frank recognition of their personal shortcomings, politicians would have fewer excuses to plead legislative expediency with reference to things medical and the administration would not dare advocate bureaucratic control of medical service.

When socialized medicine, in some form, seems imminent and members of the medical profession are blaming Congress, the administration and the common people, they should think seriously on the quality of human nature which has to do with the molding of mass psychology and in the stillness of the night, with keen awareness of the existing danger, they should ask—What is the matter; why do people run after false Gods?

An adequate knowledge of the history and the traditions of the medical profession should cause every doctor to ask the long neglected question—Is it I? Have I failed to practice medicine as it should be practiced; have I failed to teach medicine as it should be taught; have I failed to preserve the ideal

patient and doctor relationship; have I failed to inspire public esteem?

The doctor who does not respond to the needs of the worthy poor, regardless of the question of remuneration, is helping the cause of socialized medicine; the doctor who exacts the price of a big game hunt; a pack-in fishing trip or an expensive stay at a fashionable resort, for the care of a patient who cannot afford to leave his work for a simple vacation, is adding fuel to the fire; the doctor who has neither time nor disposition to win his patients' confidence and to meet his psychological needs, is fanning the flame; the doctor whose selfish ego prompts him to seek a colorful career at the expense of his colleagues augments the danger of conflagration.

In the last analysis the doctor who serves well, who inspires confidence and finds an abiding place in the hearts of his people makes unfavorable legislation improbable if not impossible.

Though the science of medicine has made rapid strides and, in a manner, usurped much of the time and thought formerly devoted to the art of caring for the sick, we must remember that human nature has not changed. We must temper the wind to the shorn lamb. In other words, we must season science with sense and sentiment. We must remember that, after all is said and done, good medicine is an art—not a trade.

On a gray afternoon seventy-five years ago an intellectual invalid with unusual insight and keen analytical powers beautifutly, lovingly and hopefully placed this stinging indictment against the medical profession. In the merky atmosphere now enveloping our great profession let us follow this representative patient to the altar and humbly make our confessions and renew our vows.

"Why do doctors so often make mistakes? Because they are not sufficiently individual in their diagnoses or their treatment. They class a sick man under some given department of their nosology, whereas every invalid is really a special case, a unique example. How is it possible that so coarse a method of sifting should produce judicious therapeutics? Every illness is a factor simple or complex, which is multiplied by a second factor, invariably complex—the individual, that is to say, who is suffering from it, so that the result is a special problem, demanding a special solution, the more so the greater the remoteness of the patient from childhood or from country life.

"The principal grievance which I have against the doctors is that they neglect the real problem, which is to seize the unity of the individual who claims their care. Their methods of investigation are far too elementary; a doctor who does not read you to the bottom is ignorant of essentials. To me the ideal doctor would be a man endowed with profound knowledge of life and of the soul, intuitively divining any suffering or disorder of whatever kind, and restoring peace by his mere presence. Such a doctor is possible, but the greater number of them lack the higher and inner life, they know nothing of the transcendent laboratories of nature; they seem to me superficial, profane, strangers to divine things, destitute of intuition and sympathy."

CLINICS

The office of the State Medical Association welcomes the new publication, "CLINICS," Volume I, No. 1, J. B. Lippincott Company,

This bi-monthly publication replaces the International Clinics which came quarterly. The change is designed to speed up medical reporting to meet the present crisis.

The editor, George Morris Piersol with a long list of competent collaborators, should be able to choose wisely medical grist from all sections of the country and give it ready distribution in practical form through this new medium.

Included in this issue is an interesting symposium on burns and shock.

In addition, it contains original contributions, clinics and a review on recent progress.

Hospital Growth Tripled Over Thirty-One Year Average

American hospitals grew three times as fast last year as during the previous thirty-one years, according to the twenty-first annual hospital survey of the Council on Medical Education and Hospitals of the American Medical Association.

For thirty-one years, the report says, the average net increase in hospital facilities was around 25,000 to 30 000 beds each year. The increase between the censuses of 1940 and 1941 was 98,136 beds, which is "astonishing even for this unusual period."

This growth, the report continued, is equal to construction of one 269 bed hospital every day, Sundays and holidays included, for a year.

Total capacity of registered hospitals was 1,324,381 beds and 66,163 bassinets. There are 98,136 more beds and 4,224 more bassinets than a year ago; reports were received for 6,318 registered hospitals out of a total of 6,358.

Results of a survey in January of this year of blood and plasma banks in approved hospitals showed that 462 of 1,070 such hospitals either had one or the other of these facilities or were in the process of establishing them.

Two hundred and six hospitals maintain both blood and plasma banks, with seventeen others in the process of development. In addition, there are 171 hospitals operating plasma banks and thirty-three separate institutions with blood banks.—Science News Letter.

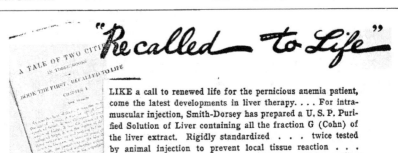
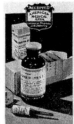

The up-to-the-minute man
fights on two fronts!

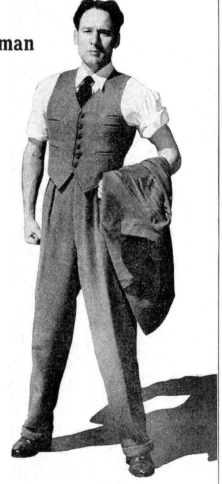

YOU WOULDN'T THINK Jim Norris was a fighter. He's not in uniform. But he's buying plenty of War Bonds . . . and Christmas Seals.

Since 1907, Jim Norris and many millions of other Americans have helped us cut the TB death rate 75%! But they're not stopping now. They know TB still kills more people between 15 and 45 than any other disease . . . and that it strikes out hard in wartime.

So get behind us in our victory effort, won't you? Send in your contribution today.

Buy
WAR BONDS
and
CHRISTMAS SEALS

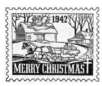

BUY
CHRISTMAS
The National, State and Local
Tuberculosis Associations in **SEALS**
the United States.

ASSOCIATION ACTIVITIES

THIRD ANNUAL SECRETARIES CONFERENCE HELD OCTOBER 25

The Third Annual Secretaries Conference of the Oklahoma State Medical Association was held at the Biltmore hotel in Oklahoma City on October 25. Approximately ninety doctors and guests were present at the afternoon meeting and the evening meeting which was preceded by a Buffet Dinner at 6:30.

The Conference, designed in 1940 to bring about a closer cooperation and a more thorough understanding of mutual problems of the county societies and the Executive Office of the Association, opened the afternoon session at 2:15 P. M. with Dr. George K. Hemphill of Pawhuska, President of the Conference, presiding. Other officers of the Third Annual Secretaries Conference were Vice-President, Dr. John R. Callaway of Pauls Valley, and Dr. W. E. Eastland of Oklahoma City replaced Dr. W. W. Rucks, Jr., Oklahoma City, who had been called to military duty, as Secretary-Treasurer.

Dr. C. R. Rountree of Oklahoma City, Chairman of the Medical Advisory Committee to the Public Welfare Department, opened the program by giving a report of the work accomplished by his committee during the last fifteen months. Dr. Lewis J. Moorman, Secretary of the Oklahoma State Medical Association, next appeared on the program. Other numbers on the program consisted of "Malpractice Insurance in Oklahoma," by Dr. V. K. Allen of Tulsa, Chairman of the State Committee; "The Present Postgraduate Program," by Dr. Henry H. Turner, Chairman of the Committee on Postgraduate Medical Teaching; Dr. L. W. Hunt of the University of Chicago, present instructor in Internal Medicine, added several supplementary remarks following Dr. Turner's appearance; Dr. J. D. Osborn, Frederick, President of the Oklahoma State Medical Association, next appeared on the program.

Major Joseph D. Stafford, a representative from the Office of the Director of State Selective Service, concluded the afternoon session and discussed "The Relationship of the Physician to Selective Service." Following his discussion, Major Stafford answered questions from those in attendance.

The following were elected to serve as Officers of the Conference for the coming year: President, Dr. Alfred R. Sugg, Ada; Vice-President, Dr. E. S. Kilpatrick, Elk City, and Secretary-Treasurer, Dr. D. Evelyn Miller, Muskogee.

Following the Buffet Dinner, Dick Graham, Executive Secretary of the Oklahoma State Medical Association, who has been in Washington, D. C., in the central office of Procurement and Assignment for the past several months, appeared before those in attendance and discussed "Recent Developments in the Procurement and Assignment of Physicians, Dentists and Veterinarians."

Mr. Robert S. Kerr, Democratic nominee for Governor of Oklahoma concluded the Secretaries Conference by discussing "Physicians and Their Relationship to the Present Emergency."

Guests of the Conference included Secretaries and Presidents of component county medical societies; Officers and Councilors of the Oklahoma State Medical Association; State Procurement and Assignment Committee; Advisory Committee to the State Procurement and Assignment Committee and Medical Preparedness Chairmen of the committees of the local county medical societies. In addition to physicians, those invited to the evening session included the Officers of the Oklahoma State Dental and the Oklahoma Veterinary Medical Associations.

DR. TOM LOWRY NAMED DEAN OKLAHOMA MEDICAL SCHOOL

Dr. Tom Lowry, prominent Oklahoma City physician for twenty-five years, has been named Dean of the University of Oklahoma Medical School and Superintendent of the University and Crippled Children's Hospitals by the University Board of Regents to become effective November 15.

Doctor Lowry is the first University alumnus to occupy the Deanship of the Medical School, and succeeds General Robert U. Patterson, who resigned several months ago to become Dean of the University of Maryland Medical School at Baltimore.

Although medical deans are usually appointed for seven years, Doctor Lowry's appointment will terminate in compliance with his request July 1. During the interim, a permanent dean will be secured. In addition to his new duties, Doctor Lowry, who is widely known over the state and who has gained a high reputation among his fellow associates, will continue in private practice.

Doctor Lowry is a graduate of the University of Oklahoma Medical School. Since 1920, he has been a member of the Medical School staff and presently holds the rank of Professor of Clinical Medicine in which capacity he presents tri-weekly lectures to the medical students.

At the time of writing, Dr. Tom Lowry is ill at his home and has been ordered to take a complete rest for several weeks. No further announcement has been made by the Board of Regents.

DR. T. C. BLACK NAMED HEAD OF CLINTON SANATORIUM

Dr. Thomas C. Black, assistant physician at the Florida Tuberculosis Sanatorium, Orlando, Fla., and a graduate of the University of Kansas, has recently accepted the position as physician in charge of the Western Oklahoma Tuberculosis Sanatorium at Clinton.

Doctor Black, who succeeds Dr. Richard M. Burke, arrived in the state October 15 to begin his new duties. Doctor Burke, who resigned at Clinton September 15, has established his practice in Oklahoma City in the Medical Arts Building.

The new medical director was approached through the National Tuberculosis Association with headquarters in New York City. He is a former Staff physician of the Kansas State Sanatorium for Tuberculosis at Norton and was on the staff of Glen Lake Sanitarium at Minneapolis, Minn., prior to his Florida position.

Dr. and Mrs. Milton J. Serwer at Home

Dr. and Mrs. Milton J. Serwer, Oklahoma City, following a brief wedding trip, have established a home at 3512 North Robinson.

Mrs. Serwer, the former Miss Ora Bucknum of Oklahoma City, daughter of Mr. and Mrs. Frank W. Bucknum of Chandler, is a graduate of the University of Oklahoma Nursing School and is presently employed by the Southwestern Bell Telephone Company. Dr. Serwer, son of Mr. and Mrs. William S. Serwer, Detroit, Mich., is a graduate of the University of Chicago and Rush Medical College, Chicago.

The marriage was an event of October 9 in the home of Rabbi Joseph Blatt, 901 Northwest Twenty-fourth Street, who officiated.

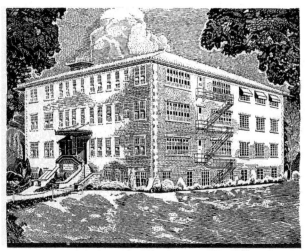

1943 ANNUAL A. M. A. SESSION CANCELED

"The American Medical Association will not hold its ninety-fourth annual session, scheduled to convene in San Francisco in 1943," The Journal of the Association announces in its September 26 issue. The editorial on the action by the Association's Board of Trustees explains that: "This is the third time in the history of the Association that an annual session has been canceled. In 1861 the session was postponed for a year because of the outbreak of the war between the states, and in 1862 it was again postponed for a year because of the demands of the war on the medical profession. The House of Delegates, the Board of Trustees, the scientific councils and the officials of the Association will be called into session to deal with the affairs of the Association, particularly the many wartime responsibilities being borne by the medical profession.

"The tremendous demands on the medical profession of the United States in association with the war, including the provision of physicians for the armed forces, for the care of veterans, for industry and for the care of the civilian population, has caused the Board of Trustees of the American Medical Association to give special consideration to problems associated with the holding of the session.

"The annual session of the Association with the attendance usually assembled on such occasions would take away from medical practice at the time from six to ten thousand doctors, together with many persons in associated professions concerned with the Scientific Exhibit, the Technical Exhibit and other features. The demands on the time of physicians are already innumerable. Moreover, the holding of the session in San Francisco would involve transportation in large part from other sections of the country, calling particularly on the railroads and also on all other means of transportation.

"The Board of Trustees has given special attention to statements issued by the Office of Defense Transportation, the War Department, the Navy Department and other governmental agencies concerning the holding of conventions.

"The primary consideration involved particularly relating to the annual session is the call that would be made on the time and work of physicians. Already the utmost that the medical profession can do to provide medical services for the Selective Service System, the Army, the Navy, the Public Health Service, industry and the civilian population is in some places being severely strained. These demands will no doubt be intensified by next June.

"While the Scientific Assembly and the Scientific and Technical exhibits will not be held in 1943, the many significant problems of the medical profession occasioned by war, particularly such as concern the provision and distribution of physicians and the provision of medical service, are of such moment that the House of Delegates, the Board of Trustees, the various scientific councils and officials will be called into session in June, 1943. This meeting will be held in Chicago in order to place the minimum stress on the time of the physicians concerned and on the transportation facilities of the nation.

"In making these decisions, the Board of Trustees has kept in mind the solemn obligation entered into by the House of Delegates and the Board of Trustees of the American Medical Association to give to the nation every possible contribution that the Association can make to aid the war effort."

Word has been received that, somewhere in New Guinea, Major D. J. Lyons of Seminole has been in consultation on the case of the Associated Press Correspondent Vern Haugland, who is recovering from exhaustion and fever after having spent 43 days fighting his way out of the mountainous jungle into which he parachuted from a storm-spent bomber on August 7.

TWENTY-SECOND ANNUAL MEETING OF SOUTH CENTRAL SECTION OF AMERICAN UROLOGICAL ASSOCIATION HELD IN OKLAHOMA CITY

Approximately sixty out-of-state, in addition to a number of state, physicians attended the Twenty-second Annual Meeting of the South Central Section of the American Urological Association which was held in Oklahoma City, September 24-26, 1942, at the Biltmore hotel.

Proving to be one of the most successful meetings of the Association, the first day was devoted to registration of the members and the annual golf tournament, which was played at the Twin Hills Golf and Country Club. A stag dinner followed the golf tournament at which time prizes were awarded.

The scientific program, beginning on September 25, was opened with a paper by Dr. J. R. Reagan of Wichita Falls, Texas. On Friday, other papers were presented by Drs. J. Robert Rinker, Fort Worth; Charles B. Taylor, Oklahoma City; Hjalmar S. Carlson, Kansas City, Mo.; Alfonso E. Guerra, Monterrey, Mexico; Linwood Keyser, Roanoke, Va.; Alfred R. Sugg, Ada; Harold E. Neptune, Salina, Kans., and Arbor D. Munger, Lincoln, Nebr. Friday's discussions were led by Drs. H. A. O'Brien, Dallas; Robert E. Cone, Galveston, and Otto J. Wilhelmi, St. Louis, Mo.

Papers were read Sunday by Drs. Basil A. Hayes and J. D. Ashley, Oklahoma City; John M. Pace, Dallas; Samuel B. Potter and Harold T. Low, Pueblo, Colo.; Robert H. Akin, Oklahoma City; Carl A. Wattenberg and D. K. Rose, St. Louis, Mo., and Lt. Col. Roy Lee Smith and Captain J. F. Harrold, Denver, Col. Discussions were opened by Drs. R. Lee Hoffman, Kansas City, Mo.; Rex E. Van Duzen, Dallas, and Clinton K. Smith, Kansas City, Mo.

The President's Reception was at 6:30 p.m. Friday, and was followed by the Annual Dinner at 7:30 in the Dining Room of the Biltmore. Dr. Everett E. Angle of Lincoln, Nebr., succeeds Dr. Henry S. Browne of Tulsa as President of the Association for the coming year.

Dr. Linwood Keyser of Roanoka, Va., an authority on Urinary Lithiasis, was Guest Speaker at the meeting. Dr. C. E. Burford of St. Louis, Mo., President of the American Urological Association, attended the convention, and Dr. Thomas B. Moore of Memphis, Tenn., Secretary of the National Association, was also present.

Dr. T. Leon Howard of Denver, Colo., past president of the American Urological Associatoin, attended the convention and closed the session with his annual T. Leon Howard Hour, which is a clinical case discussion conference.

Dr. McBride Attends Meeting in Washington

Dr. Earl D. McBride of the McBride Clinic in Oklahoma City has recently returned from a trip to Washington, D. C., where he went on Presidential request to serve as a Professional Consultant to the Federal Social Security Board.

The meeting was held on October 1 and 2, and was called for the purpose of establishing a disability rating schedule for civilians disabled through enemy action. This procedure will become effective through the Pepper Bill No. 2412.

The schedule is to be patterned after that adopted in the United States Veterans' Pension bill. Civilian defense workers and any civilian man, woman or child actually injured by enemy action will be covered under this action. Many cases of this type have already been reported in Hawaii and Alaska.

Dr. McBride will return to Washington for further consultation in November.

Dr. Messenbaugh Opens New Offices

Dr. Joseph F. Messenbaugh has recently announced the removal of his offices to 1102 Medical Arts Building from the Colcord Building.

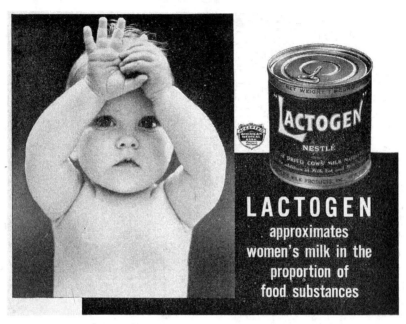

LACTOGEN
approximates women's milk in the proportion of food substances

The cow's milk used for Lactogen is scientifically modified for infant feeding. This modification is effected by the addition of milk fat and milk sugar in definite proportions. When Lactogen is properly diluted with water it results in a formula containing the food substances—fat, carbohydrate, protein, and ash—in approximately the same proportion as they exist in woman's milk.

No advertising or feeding directions, except to physicians. For free samples and literature, send your professional blank to "Lactogen Dept." Nestle's Milk Products, Inc., 155 East 44th St., New York, N. Y.

"My own belief is, as already stated, that the average well baby thrives best on artificial foods in which the relations of the fat, sugar, and protein in the mixture are similar to those in human milk."

John Lovett Morse, A. M., M. D. Clinical Pediatrics, p. 156.

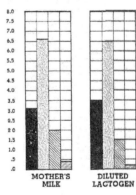

MOTHER'S MILK   DILUTED LACTOGEN

Fat   Carb.   Protein   Ash

NESTLÉ'S MILK PRODUCTS, INC.
155 EAST 44TH ST., NEW YORK, N. Y.

AMERICAN BOARD OF OBSTETRICS AND GYNE-COLOGY WILL CONDUCT EXAMINATIONS

The next written examination and review of case histories (Part I) for all candidates will be held in various cities of the United States and Canada on Saturday, February 13, 1943 at 2:00 P.M.

Arrangements will be made so far as possible for candidates in military service to take the Part I examination (written paper and submission of case records) at their places of duty, the written examination to be proctored by the Commanding Officer (medical) or some responsible person designated by him. Material for the written examination will be sent to the proctor several weeks in advance of the examination date. Case records may be submitted in advance of the above date, only by candidates in Service, by forwarding these to the office of the Board Secretary by the candidate upon entering military service, or in the event of assignment to foreign duty. All other candidates should present their case records to the examiner at the time and place of taking the written examination.

The Office of the Surgeon-General (U. S. Army) has issued instructions that men in Service, eligible for Board examinations, be encouraged to apply and that they may be ordered to Detached Duty for the purpose of taking these examinations whenever possible. The Office of the Surgeon-General of the U. S. Navy presumably takes a similar attitude on this matter.

All candidates will be required to take both the Part I examination, and the Part II examination (oral-clinical and pathology examination). Candidates who successfully complete the Part I examination proceed automatically to the Part II examination to be held later in the year.

The Part II examination for 1943 will be held late in May. Because of the cancellation of the American Medical Association's annual convention, the place of the Board's Part II examination has not yet been decided, but it will be held in that city nearest to the largest group of candidates. The exact time and place will be announced later.

If a candidate in Service finds it impossible to proceed with the examinations of the Board, deferment without time penalty will be granted under a waiver of our published regulations covering civilian examinations.

Applications for this year's examinations must be in the office of the Secretary not later than November 16, 1942.

For further information and application blanks, address Dr. Paul Titus, Secretary, 1015 Highland Building, Pittsburgh (6), Pennsylvania.

AMERICAN COLLEGE OF SURGEONS CANCELS CLINICAL CONGRESS

The annual Clinic Congress of the American College of Surgeons which was scheduled to be held in Cleveland November 17-20, 1942, was cancelled by the Board of Regents of the College at a meeting held in Chicago, Wednesday morning, October 14. Motivated primarily by patriotism, the Regents were influenced by the present conditions surrounding the general war program which have led to a greater burden on the members of the surgical profession in their local communities as a result of the large proportion of the profession which is serving with the armed forces. The Regents by this action took cognizance of the desire of the profession to do nothing which would interfere with the successful prosecution of the war program such as would be caused by temporary absence of its members from civilian duties during the period of the Congress, embarrassment of the transportation system, and interference with the work of the local profession in Cleveland in preparations and presentations incident to such a meeting.

Another transfer in location is that of Lieutenant Roy J. Baze of Chickasha. Dr. Baze is presently stationed at Camp Gruber, Oklahoma.

1943 TEXAS MEETING CHANGED

The Executive Council of the State Medical Association of Texas has made a recent announcement to the effect that the coming annual meeting will be held in Fort Worth, May 3-6, 1943, instead of San Antonio, May 10-13, 1943, as previously planned.

The Committee on Arrangements, upon investigation, found that it would be impossible to hold the meeting in San Antonio inasmuch as rooms in hotels, which would ordinarily be available for meeting places, were practically all in war service, and such a large proportion of the guest rooms of the hotel were under permanent occupancy by military and governmental authorities, that it was evident hotel accommodations were not available, hence the change.

The 1941 meeting was held in Fort Worth and practically the same arrangements will be worked out for the 1943 session.

PUBLIC HEALTH NURSES NEEDED

The U. S. Civil Service Commission recently issued a call to Public Health Nurses through the pages of this journal. The Commission has now asked that we print a correction regarding a statement made in their press release regarding the omission of high school education as a requirement for Public Health Nurse positions. This statement was made in error by the Commission. In effect the educational requirements for Public Health Nurse cannot be obtained without completion of high school education.

The Public Health Nurse positions pay $2,000 a year. The requirements are: Completion, subsequent to January 1, 1920, of a full course in a recognized school of nursing including two years in a general hospital having a daily average of 50 bed patients or more; registration as a graduate nurse; and completion of one year of study in public health nursing at a college giving a course of study approved by the National Organization for Public Health Nursing. One year of public health nursing experience is also necessary.

Other nursing opportunities open in the Federal service include the following: Junior Public Health Nurse, $1,800 a year; Graduate Nurse, $1,800 a year; Junior Graduate Nurse, $1,620; Graduate Nurse for the Panama Canal service, $168.75 a month; Nursing Education Consultant, $2,600 to $4,600 a year; and Public Health Nursing Consultant, $2,600 to $5,000 a year.

Except for Panama Canal service, there are no age limits for any of these positions. Applications will be accepted at the Commission's Washington office until the needs of the service have been met.

FOURTH BIENNIAL MEETING OF ROCKY MOUNTAIN MEDICAL CONFERENCE POSTPONED

The Executive Committte of the Rocky Mountain Medical Conference has, by unanimous vote, directed that the Fourth Biennial Meeting of the Conference, originally scheduled for May 19-21, 1943, at Albuquerque, N. Mex., be postponed indefinitely on account of war conditions.

The current organization of the Conference will be retained subject to further advice from the Continuing Committee, and current funds of the Conference will be invested in United States War Bonds in so far as is practicable.

The Executive Committee of this Conference is elected biennially by the Continuing Committee, which in turn consists of five representatives from each participating state medical society. It is the hope of the Executive Committee, subject to unforseen future contingencies, that the tentative plans for conduct of the Fourth Meeting may be so retained that, at the conclusion of the War or at any earlier time that governmental authority so advises, these plans may be reactivated at Albuquerque.

PLANS TO MEET NEED FOR MEDICAL CARE

The following proposed plan appeared in the American Medical Association Journal, October 10, 1942:

"Plans for meeting the need for medical care in communities where a shortage of physicians has developed, The Journal of the American Medical Association reports in its October 10 issue, are being made now by the U. S. Public Health Service and the Procurement and Assignment Service of the War Manpower Commission, according to an announcement by Paul V. McNutt, chairman of the Commission, who said the two services are cooperating closely in the planning of this emergency action. The announcement in The Journal says:

"Mr. McNutt explained that in many areas an acute need for medical service has arisen as a result of extraordinary increases in population brought about by expansion of war industries or other war activities. In other areas there is shortage of medical service resulting from the entry of physicians into the armed forces.

"Distributed throughout the industrial areas of the country are more than three hundred communities in which the lack of medical care is being felt. The chairman pointed out that among the most critical of these localities are Baltimore County (around Glenn L. Martin Company); Valpariso, Fla.; Huntsville, Ala.; Childersburg, Ala.; LaPorte, Ind.; Charleston, Ind.; Fort Knox, Ky.; Rantoul, Ill.; Texarkana area; Bremerton, Wash.; Pryor-Choteau, Okla.; Vallejo, Calif.; Velasco, Texas; Waynesville, Mo.; Wichita Falls, Texas, and Norfolk, Va.

"Mr. McNutt also announced his approval of a statement of policy adopted by the directing board of the Procurement and Assignment Service in which the Procurement and Assignment Service accepts the responsibility of ascertaining the needs of the civilian population for medical service and providing the medical personnel to meet them.

"The principles set forth in this policy statement, Mr. McNutt said, were developed in cooperation with the federal officials concerned and have the approval of the Surgeon General of the United States Public Health Service. The statment has been approved by the boards of trustees of the American Medical Association, the American Dental Association and the war service committees of the two associations, and the executive committee representing the State and Territorial Health Officers Association.

"Following are the principles recommended by the directing board of the Procurement and Assignment Service for meeting the emergency needs:

"1. That it is a responsibility of the Procurement and Assignment Service to ascertain the needs of the civilian population—nonmilitary—for medical service.

"2. That it is the responsibility of the Procurement and Assignment Service to aid in providing the medical personnel to meet these needs.

"3. That, as now constituted, the Procurement and Assignment Service is not in a position to deal with the financial and administrative problems involved in the provision of medical care.

"4. That as fas as possible these problems should be met at the state level in view of the many different types of problems and needs and the relation to these and their solution to local situations.

"5. That a survey of these needs should be made by the existing committees of the Procurement and Assignment Service with the aid of such technical assistance as may be necessary. It is especially desirable that in determining these needs the state procurment and assignment committee seek the cooperation of the state health department, of the state medical society and of the state dental society, of industry, of organized labor and of other agencies, such as the state defense council, which should be able to make significant contributions to the solution of this problem.

"6. That whenever possible the civilian needs as determined by these committees should be met through local arrangements, resources and agencies. In case assistance is needed for the organization, administration or financing of necessary medical or dental services in these areas, the responsibility should devolve on an agency which should include representatives of the state health department, the state medical society and the state dental society, with the cooperation and support—financial and technical—of the appropriate federal agencies, the administration of funds being delegated to the appropriate state agency.

"7. That, since these problems have been occasioned by the war and in many instances transcend state lines, the federal government has a definite responsibility to cooperate with the states in meeting these needs by the provision, when necessary, of financial and technical assistance.

"8. That the needs for medical care in certain areas are so acute and the pressure from various sources so great that it is imperative to have prompt action for implementation of this program. It appears to the directing board that the responsibility for the initiation of such action rests with the War Manpower Commission."

Attention is called to paragraphs 4 and 6 which definitely open the way for local arrangements, resources and agencies to provide the best possible medical care or to actively participate in any plans which may be evolved.

Organized medicine should not permit this opportunity to pass unheeded. If we are to escape regimented medicine, we must be on the alert and ready to work out comprehensive methods of giving adequate voluntary medical care whenever and wherever the need arises.

This is something for the State Medical Association and the County Society to seriously take into consideration.

State E.E.N.T. Group Attends Chicago Meeting

Numbered among the Oklahoma specialists who attended the Annual Meeting of the American Academy of Ophthalmology and Otolaryngology at Chicago, October 11 to 14, were Dr. O. Alton Watson, Dr. E. Gordon Ferguson, Dr. William L. Bonham, Dr. Harvey O. Randel, Dr. L. Chester McHenry, Dr. Joseph C. Macdonald, Dr. F. Maxey Cooper, all of Oklahoma City, Dr. C. H. Haralson, Dr. W. Albert Cook and Dr. Ruric N. Smith, of Tulsa, and Dr. E. H. Coachman of Muskogee.

NEWS FROM THE COUNTY SOCIETIES

"Earlier Cataract Extraction" was the topic of discussion by Dr. F. Maxey Cooper, Oklahoma City, guest speaker at the meeting of the Muskogee-Sequoyah-Wagoner Medical Society on October 5, at 8:00 o'clock. Twelve members and four guests were in attendance.

The next meeting of the tri-county society is scheduled for November 2 at which time Dr. John Rafter will discuss the subject "Emergency Surgery." Invited guests will be the medical officers from Camp Gruber.

Twenty members of Pottawatomie County attended a dinner meeting of the Society on September 19 at Shawnee. Dr. T. D. Rowland presented a paper entitled "Undulant Fever." Discussions by Dr. Earl D. McBride of Oklahoma City, Dr. Charles W. Haygood, Dr. J. M. Bynum and Dr. G. S. Baxter followed.

In business session, the Society moved to approve a plan that would provide obstetric, hospital and pediatric care for wives and infants of noncommissioned men in the armed forces. Volunteer Nurses' Aide Corps examinations at no charge were discussed.

The next meeting of the Society will be October 17, at which time Dr. Eugene Gillis, Venereal Disease Officer, State Health Department, will present the picture "Syphilis."

One hundred and fifty members of the Oklahoma County Medical Association were present at the regular meeting on October 20 at the Oklahoma Club.

Following a buffet dinner at 6:30, the scientific program consisted of a "Clinical-Pathological Conference"

with Dr. Walker Morledge, Dr. John E. Heatley and Dr. Bela Halpert, Professor of Clinical Pathology at the University Medical School, participating.

The November meeting is scheduled for the 24th at the Oklahoma Club.

The Osage County Medical Society met in Pawhuska, September 14, at 7:00 P. M., with twelve members in attendance.

Guest speakers for the evening were Dr. Fred E. Woodson of Tulsa, who spoke on "Newer Developments in Anesthesia," and Dr. H. D. Murdock, also of Tulsa, who discussed "Facia Transplant." The two talks were preceeded by a dinner and business meeting of the Society at which time was discussed the purchasing of a resuscitator with the Infantile Paralysis Fund in Osage County.

Inasmuch as a postgraduate course in Internal Medicine, under the instruction of Dr. L. W. Hunt of Chicago, is now being conducted in Pawhuska once each week, the Society will not meet in regular session again until December.

Eight members of the Stephens County Medical Society met in regular session at Duncan, Tuesday, September 29, at 8:00 P. M.

This was the first meeting since the summer recess, and following dinner at the Wade Hotel, a general business meeting was held.

The coming meeting is scheduled for 7:30 P. M., October 20, at Duncan.

Because of the various contributing factors—gasoline rationing, rubber shortage, distance, scarcity of physicians, etc., the Woodward County Medical Society has disbanded regular monthly medical meetings for the duration. However, the annual society meeting scheduled for December 3 will be held.

The scientific program of the Tulsa County Medical Society, meeting in regular session at 8:00 P. M., September 14, at the Mayo Hotel, consisted of a "Symposium on Toxic Goitre" by Dr. Eugene Wolfe, Dr. Frank Nelson, Dr. I. A. Nelson, Dr. H. A. Reprecht and Dr. C. C. Hoke. Approximately fifty members were in attendance.

The October meeting is scheduled for October 12 at which time Dr. James Stevenson, Dr. David V. Hudson, Dr. M. O. Nelson and Dr. M. D. Spottswood will present a "Symposium on Syphilis."

Dr. E. E. Beechwood of Bartlesville presented a paper entitled "Hypothyroidism" at the September 14 meeting of the Washington-Nowata County Medical Society. Ten members were present at the meeting which was held at the Hospital.

The November meeting will be held at the Hospital at 7:30 P. M., on November 11.

Dr. K. D. Davis of Nowata, vice-president of the Society, has taken over the president's duties since Dr. R. W. Rucker of Bartlesville has gone to the Army.

Seven members of the Garvin County Medical Society were in attendance at the October 14 meeting, which was held at the Chamber of Commerce in Pauls Valley. The membership discussed topics of general interest to the profession.

The November 18 meeting of the Society is scheduled for 7:30 P. M., at the Chamber of Commerce in Pauls Valley, and is open to the public.

The Tri-county Medical Society composed of Grady, Caddo and Stephens counties met October 15, in Chickasha, at which time twenty members were in attendance.

The evening program consisted of a paper ''Rocky Mountain Spotted Fever,'' presented by Dr. Frank T. Joyce of Chickasha; Dr. Roy E. Emanuel of Chickasha presented ''Pregnancy Mistaken for Tumor,'' and a moving picture on peptic ulcer sponsored by Dr. Emanuel. Medical men associated with the Borden General Hospital at Chickasha were invited guests.

News From The State Health Department

The big job now facing the Venereal Disease Control Division is getting under treatment those selectees who have been rejected for army service due to infection by syphilis. In round numbers, there are about 8,000 of these in Oklahoma, and according to figures compiled in the Oklahoma State Health Department Central Registry only about 60 percent, or 4,800, of them are now taking treatment.

Many of these men would now be available for military service if they had started taking treatment for their syphilis as soon as they were rejected. As it is, many state that they did not know why they were rejected, others say they did know they were supposed to take treatment, and then, of course, there are always the indigents who cannot afford treatment? and have not taken the trouble to find out how to get it. It is difficult to say just how many of these do not want treatment so as to stay out of the army, but there is no question that there are some who are avoiding induction by failing to take treatment.

The Oklahoma Headquarters for Selective Service has requested the State Health Department to keep close ''tab'' on all selectees with syphilis, not only for the purpose of betting them under treatment but also to make sure that they do not take injections for a few weeks and then become delinquent. Several preliminary steps have already been taken toward getting this task done.

Questionnaires have been sent to all selectees who had positive blood tests. These ask if the selectee had ever had reason to believe that he had syphilis prior to his army physical, if he had ever taken treatment for syphilis before the army examination, if he has taken treatment since and, if so, from whom. In the event he is not taking regular treatment, he is asked to outline the reason for not having done so.

Replies to these questionnaires are divided into two groups: one, consisting of those already under treatment by private physicians or clinics, and the other, containing the names of all those who are not under treatment. These latter are divided into a number of groups, depending on the nature of the reply and either form or individual letters are sent out on each one. All of these are advisory in content, but there is also a factful yet firm paragraph which reads:

''You are required by the State Laws of Oklahoma to receive treatment for your infection. In order for us to know that you are receiving treatment regularly, have your physician fill out the lower portion of this form, and return to us immediately in the enclosed, postage-free envelope.''

These letters are proving very effective, but when they do not get the desired result, there is no alternative except to turn the case over to the county health officer for disposition which should include the cooperation of police enforcement officers if necessary.

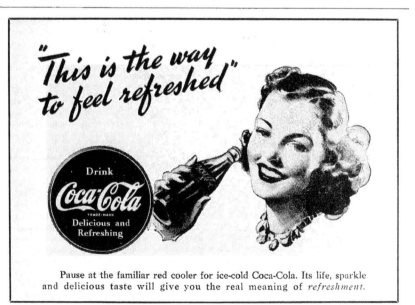

WOMEN'S AUXILIARY NEWS

We are very happy to report that our State President, Mrs. Frank L. Flack, who has been confined to the hospital in Tulsa, has returned to her home, and is very much improved. She will appreciate the continued cooperation of all the County Auxiliaries in carrying out the State program for the year.

Oklahoma County

The first meeting of the Oklahoma County Auxiliary was a Registration Coffee held on October 2 at the home of Mrs. Walker Morledge, with the Executive Board acting as hostesses.

Oklahoma County reports two changes in the Executive Board: Recording Secretary, Mrs. T. L. Wainwright, 2221 N. W. 28th Street, replacing Mrs. Allen G. Gibbs; and Flower Committee Chairman, Mrs. Brunel D. Faris, 2212 N. W. 29th Street, replacing Mrs. W. W. Rucks, Jr.

It is with regret that we report the death of Mrs. S. E. Frierson on August 2, 1942. She was a member of the Oklahoma County Auxiliary.

Pittsburg County

The first meeting for the year of the Pittsburg County Auxiliary was held in McAlester in October. The following officers and committee chairmen were elected and appointed last spring to serve for the present year:

President ....Mrs. L. S. Willour
Vice-President ....Mrs. C. K. Mills
Recording Secretary ....Mrs. Walter J. Dell
Corresponding Secretary ....Mrs. E. H. Shuller
Treasurer ....Mrs. Graham Street
Historian ....Mrs. J. F. Park

Committee Chairmen

Public Relations ....Mrs. C. E. Lively
Program ....Mrs. Floyd T. Bartheld
Hygeia ....Mrs. Edward Greenberger
Student Loan ....Mrs. J. F. Park
Press and Publicity ....Mrs. Walter J. Dell
Exhibits ....Mrs. T. T. Norris

Cleveland County

The Cleveland County Auxiliary reports the following new officers who will serve for the coming year:

President ....Mrs. M. P. Prosser
Vice-President ....Mrs. W. B. Carroll
Secretary ....Mrs. Curtis Berry
Treasurer ....Mrs. W. H. Atkins

Committee Chairmen

Program-Health Education ....Mrs. William A. Loy
Public Relations ....Mrs. M. M. Wickham
Hygeia ....Mrs. F. T. Gastineau

Pottawatomie County

The new president for the Pottawatomie County Auxiliary is Mrs. Frank M. Keen, 15 East Independence, Shawnee, Oklahoma, and the Committee Chairmen are as follows:

Program ....Mrs. Chas. W. Haygood
Public Relations ....Mrs. W. M. Gallaher
Legislative ....Mrs. T. C. Sanders
Hygeia ....Mrs. Paul Gallaher

Muskogee-Sequoyah-Wagoner Counties

Mrs. Shade Neely of Muskogee has joined her husband on the Pacific Coast, where Dr. Neely is in the Medical Corps of the Navy.

Tulsa County

The Tulsa County Auxiliary opened its fall program with a morning coffee held in the home of Mrs. H. B. Stewart on October 6, 1942. The Social Committee assisted Mrs. Stewart in receiving the members, and the year books were distributed at this coffee.

There have been two changes made in the Executive Board of the Tulsa County Auxiliary, as follows: Recording Secretary, Mrs. A. H. Ungerman, replacing Mrs. John G. Matt; Hygeia Committee Chairman, Mrs. A. W. Pigford, replacing Mrs. H. C. Childs.

Dr. F. D. Sinclair leaves on October 27 for San Antonio, Texas, where he will be stationed with the Army Air Force at the Brooks General Hospital, Fort Sam Houston. Mrs. Sinclair and their two sons, Franklin and Johnson, will remain in Tulsa at present.

University of Oklahoma School of Medicine

Major General Robert U. Patterson, Dean of the School of Medicine, has resigned as Dean, having reached the retirement age of 65. He has been appointed Dean of the University of Maryland, Baltimore, Maryland, and will assume his duties at the University of Maryland early in November. The faculty and staff of the School of Medicine and the staff of the University and Crippled Children's Hospitals will miss him a great deal. Dr. Tom Lowry has been appointed Dean of the School of Medicine until July 1, 1943, thus giving a faculty committee of the school ample time to find a successor for Dean Patterson.

The faculty and staff of the School of Medicine lost a valuable member on October 12, 1942, by the death of Dr. H. Dale Collins. Dr. Collins was associate in surgery and was Commanding Officer of Evacuation Hospital No. 21. He became ill on May 15, 1942, and was unable to go into active service with his unit when it was called for duty.

The Admissions Committee of the School of Medicine is making selections for the class to enter in June, 1943. It is expected that by the end of December all members for admission to the Freshman class will have been selected.

The Third Annual Meeting of the National Foundation for Infantile Paralysis will be held in New York City on December 3 and 4, 1942.

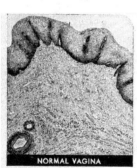
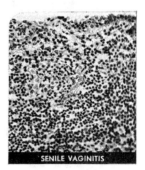

MEDICAL PREPAREDNESS

Soldiers' and Sailors' Civil Relief Act Amendments[*]

The Soldiers' and Sailors' Civil Relief Act was approved on October 17, 1940. Its purpose as indicated in an analysis of it that was published in The Journal, January 24, 1942, page 306, was to free persons in military service from harassment and injury to their civil rights during their term of military service and thus to enable them to devote their entire energy to the national defense. Experience under the act, however, has disclosed many defects and shortcomings, and numerous bills have been introduced in the Congress dealing with specific problems that have arisen. A subcommittee of the House Committee on Military Affairs was appointed to study the various proposals and as a result of that study legislation was drafted, H. R. 7164, to extend the relief and benefits provided under the original act. This bill has now passed the House and Senate and was approved by the President on October 6.

In General

The new law extends benefits to transactions that have occurred since October 17, 1940. It extends benefits to persons who serve with the forces of any nation with which the United States may be allied in the prosecution of the war and who immediately prior to such service were citizens of the United States. Persons who have been ordered to report for induction under the Selective Training and Service Act will be entitled to benefits during the period beginning on the date of receipt of such an order and ending on the date on which such person reports for induction. Any member of the Enlisted Reserve Corps who is ordered to report for military service will be entitled to benefits during the period beginning on the date of receipt of such order and ending on the date on which he reports for such service. The Secretary of War and the Secretary of the Navy are required to make provision in such manner as each may deem appropriate for his respective department, to insure the giving of notice of the benefits accorded by the act to persons in and to the persons entering military service.

Leases

Of particular interest to physicians is the new provision relating to leases. Under the original act no provision was made for the cancellation of leases, nor did the section relating to leases apply to leases on property used for office purposes. The new law applies to any lease covering premises occupied for dwelling, professional, business, agricultural or similar purposes in any case in which (a) such lease was executed by or on the behalf of a person who, after the execution of such lease, enters military service and (b) the premises so leased have been occupied for such purpose or for a combination of such purposes by such persons or by him and his dependents.

Any such lease may be terminated by notice in writing delivered to the lessor (or his grantee) or to the lessor's (or his grantee's) agent by the lessee at any time following the date of the beginning of his period of military service. Delivery of such notice may be accomplished by placing it in an envelope properly stamped and duly addressed to the lessor (or his grantee) or to the lessor's (or his grantee's) agent and depositing the notice in the mails. Termination of any such lease providing for monthly payment of rent will not be effective until thirty days after the first date on which the next rental payment is due and payable subsequent to the date when such notice is delivered or mailed. In the case of all other leases, termination will be effected on the last day of the month following the month in which the notice is delivered or mailed, and in such case any unpaid rental for a period preceding termination shall be proratably computed and any rental paid in advance for a period succeeding termination must be refunded by the lessor (or his assignee).

On application by the lessor to an appropriate court prior to the termination period provided for in the notice, any relief granted by the act will be subject to such modifications or restrictions as, in the opinion of the court, justice and equity may in the circumstances require.

Any person who knowingly seizes, holds or detains the personal effects, clothing, furniture or other property of any person who has lawfully terminated a lease covered by the act or in any manner interferes with the removal of such property from the premises covered by the lease, for the purpose of subjecting or attempting to subject any of the property to a claim for rent accruing subsequent to the date of termination of the lease, or attempts so to do, will be guilty of a misdemeanor and punishable by imprisonment not to exceed one year or by fine not to exceed $1,000 or both.

Storage Liens

A new section clarifies the original act in connection with the protection of persons coming into service from foreclosure of storage liens on household goods stored for the period of military service. No person may exercise any right to foreclose or enforce any lien for storage of household goods, furniture or personal effects of a person in military service during such person's period of service and for three months thereafter except on an order previously granted by a court. In such a proceeding the court may, unless in the opinion of the court the ability of the defendant to pay the storage charges due is not materially affected by reason of his military service, (a) stay the proceedings or (b) make such other disposition of the case as may be equitable to conserve the interests of all parties.

Benefits Accorded Dependents

The dependents of a person in military service will be

EIGHTH SERVICE COMMAND RECRUITING BOARD WITHDRAWN

Inasmuch as the quota for physicians in the Eighth Corps for 1942 has been obtained, the Eighth Service Command Medical Officer Recruiting Board, 515 Calcasieu Building, San Antonio, Texas, under the direction of Major Oliver C. Seastrunk of the Medical Corps, has been discontinued. The states included under the jurisdiction of this Board were Texas, Louisiana, Arkansas, New Mexico and Oklahoma.

All of the records of this Board have been transferred to the Chief, Medical Branch, Personnel Division, Eighth Service Command, San Antonio, and all inquiries and communications concerning applications should be forwarded to the above address, attention of Lieutenant James W. Dean.

entitled, on application to a court therefor, to the benefits accorded to persons in military service in connection with rents, instalment contracts, mortgages, liens, assignments and leases, unless in the opinion of the court the ability of such dependents to comply with the terms thereof has not been materially impaired by reason of the military service of the person on whom the applicants are dependent.

Insurance Premiums

The benefits of the act in connection with insurance premiums are extended to policies up to $10,000 face value. In order to obtain the benefits, the insured must make written application to the Administrator of Veterans' Affairs. If the insured is outside the continental United States, excluding Alaska and the Panama Canal Zone, the beneficiary may apply for the benefits. The term "policy" is defined to include any contract of life insurance or policy on a life, endowment or term plan, including any benefits in the nature of life insurance arising out of membership in any fraternal or beneficial association. The policy must not provide for the payment of any sum less than the face value thereof or for the payment of an additional amount as premiums if the insured engages in military service. It must not contain any limitation or restriction on coverage relating to engagement in or pursuit of certain types of activities which a person might be required to engage in by virtue of his being in military service. The policy must (1) have been in force on a premium-paying basis at the time of application for benefits and (2) must have been made and a premium paid thereon before October 6, 1942, and not less than thirty days before the date the insured entered into military service. The benefits are not applicable to policies or contracts issued under the War Risk Insurance Act, the World War Veterans Act or the National Service Life Insurance Act of 1940.

The Veterans' Administration is required to give notice to the military and naval authorities of the provisions of the act and must include in such notice an explanation of the provisions for the information of those desiring to make application for the benefits. An insured will have two years after the period of military service to repay premiums guaranteed by the government under the act. Interest on such premiums will be payable at the same interest rate as fixed in the policy for policy loans.

Miscellaneous Benefits

The section of the original act which authorized in certain circumstances the repossession of automobiles of persons in military service is repealed. A new section prohibits interest at a rate in excess of six percent on obligations of persons in military service incurred prior to his entry therein. A court may grant certain relief with respect to mortgages and taxes on property owned by persons not in military service when the rent for such property is not paid by dependents of persons in military service. The protection provided by the original act in respect of taxes on real property is extended to include taxes (other than income taxes) on personal property. The requirement that such taxes must have fallen due during the period of military service has been eliminated, as has also been the requirement that the person in military service must file an affidavit with the tax collector in order to prevent sale for delinquency without court action. A new section grants to persons in military service relief for a specified period after military service in order to enable them to liquidate their liabilities in an orderly fashion and not be subjected to the accrual and payment of the liabilities all at one time. The court may grant an order staying enforcement of obligations either for a period of time equal to the period of military service or, in the case of certain real estate mortgages and contracts, for a period of time equal to the remaining life of the contract plus the period of military service.

*Taken from A. M. A. Journal, Vol. 120, No. 7, Page 539, October 17, 1942.

95 PERCENT 1942 QUOTA OBTAINED

"The Directing Board of the Procurement and Assignment Service is pleased to announce that 95 percent of the 1942 procurement objective of medical officers for the armed forces has already been met. Toward this total a number of States have supplied more than their share of physicians and only a few States are lagging behind in their quotas. It is from these States that the additional physicians needed during the current year should come.

"The recruitment of such a large number of physicians in a few months is a remarkable achievement and another demonstration of the traditional patriotism and unselfishness of the medical profession. In this achievement, and particularly in those of its members who are 'in service,' the profession can justifiably take pride.

"The end, of course, is not yet. Increases in the armed forces will necessitate more medical officers and additional demands will be made upon the profession for medical services in critical war production areas. The Directing Board is convinced, however, that the physicians of this country will respond to future calls for service, whatever they may be, in the same splendid manner with which they have already volunteered for service with the armed forces."

> Frank H. Lahey, M.D., Chairman
> Harold S. Diehl, M.D.
> Harvey B. Stone, M.D.
> James E. Paullin, M.D.
> C. Willard Camalier, D.D.S.

Dr. A. M. Evans, formerly of Perry, is now addressed as Lieutenant Commander Evans, and his address is U. S. N. A. S. Dispensary, Corpus Christi, Texas.

Major Howard B. Shorbe, who was associated with the McBride Clinic in Oklahoma City prior to his entrance into the Army, has recently been transferred from the Station Hospital at Fort Sill to the Lawson General Hospital in Atlanta, Ga.

Dr. John R. Cotteral of Henryetta, recently commissioned as a Captain in the Army, is now located at Santa Ana, Calif.

Lieutenant J. D. Shipp of Tulsa is presently stationed at San Antonio, Texas, where he is on duty at the School of Aviation Medicine, Randolph Field.

Lieutenant Commander Russell C. Pigford of Tulsa reported for active duty at Corpus Christi, Texas, as of November 9.

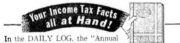

I like S·M·A!

IN INFANT FEEDING
...IT SAVES MY TIME

● Directions on how to mix and feed S-M-A can be explained to the mother and nurse in two minutes.

● S-M-A is more easily digested by the normal infant because of the all-lactose carbohydrate and the unique S-M-A fat.

● With S-M-A nothing is left to chance. All the vitamin requirements, except ascorbic acid, together with additional iron are included in S-M-A in the proper balance, ready to feed.

● S-M-A fed infants compare favorably with breast-fed infants in growth and development.

Prescribe S·M·A!

• OBITUARIES •

Dr. Herbert Dale Collins
(1901-1942)

With the death of Herbert Dale Collins, Oklahoma Medicine has lost one of its most promising members. Seldom indeed has the course of one's illness been followed with more keen interest and more growing concern by doctor and layman alike. His host of friends were grieved when he finally lost the fight he had carried on so valiantly over so many weeks and months.

Dr. Dale's achievements were legion. He was a leader in his profession, a sincere personality, a keen promoter of all that provided benefit for the community; he stood head and shoulders above the mass and pointed the way toward advancement.

The students at the medical school respected his knowledge, admired his ability and enjoyed the warmth of his nature. He served as a sincere and sympathetic preceptor guiding them by advice and example. He was truly "the young man's friend".

Long interested in affairs military, Lt. Col. Collins served in a key capacity in the organization of Evacuation Hospital Unit No. 21 and soon moved to its active command. He keenly anticipated going into active service with the rest of the unit and would have been an able leader, had not his illness interfered. One of the major stimulants in his fight for recovery was the hope of joining his confreres in active military service. He will be sorely missed by his friends in this Unit.

Dr. Herbert Dale Collins was born at Panama, Oklahoma, August 13, 1901, and died at Oklahoma City, October 12, 1942. He is survived by his immediate family; wife, Dorothy Brandle Collins; son, Michael Alan Collins; parents, Dr. and Mrs. E. L. Collins, and one brother, Robert L. Collins of the U. S. Army.

After completing his preliminary education at Panama, Oklahoma, and Pittsburg, Kansas, he attended Kansas University for two years and then matriculated in the University of Oklahoma School of Medicine, graduating in 1926. He served a one year rotating internship at University Hospitals, Oklahoma City. The following year he received an appointment as Surgical resident in the same institution. During his residency he was married to Miss Dorothy Brandle, to whom he had been engaged since their scholastic days at Kansas University.

He entered private practice in Oklahoma City, associated with Dr. .S R. Cunningham, and in 1930 completed postgraduate training in Surgery at Pennsylvania University. In 1934 he opened his own office for the practice of surgery which he continued until the onset of his fatal illness.

He was a member of many outstanding medical organizations including the American College of Surgeons and was a Diplomat of the American Board of Surgery. He was also a member of the American Medical Association and the Oklahoma State Medical Association. Local activities included, The Oklahoma City Clinical Society, of which he was President in 1939; The Oklahoma County Medical Association; The Academy of Medicine; The Doctor's Dinner Club; and The Doctor's Luncheon Club. He, also, belonged to the Men's Dinner Club and Rotary. His fraternal affiliations were Delta Upsilon and Phi Beta Pi.

No record of Dale Collins would be complete without some personal tribute to him. To those of us that knew him best it will be increasingly evident how great a place he filled in our every day lives, and how much a part of us he had actually become. It seems in retrospection that many of our most pleasant moments included Dale, and his passing has left a void that no one can fill. He was a man that enjoyed living; his 41 years were crowded with many activities. He was in the prime of life and had the innate ability to do even greater things. When measured by the common yardstick of human endeavor his accomplished deeds were equivalent to a full and successful life. We are too prone to think of what he could have done, rather than what he has accomplished. If we all can do, during our short span of life, what Dale has done in his, the world will become a better place in which to live.

Dr. George S. Barger
(1876-1942)

Dr. George S. Barger, pioneer McClain County, physician, collapsed in his office Tuesday morning, September 15, and died almost instantly as a result of a heart attack.

Doctor Barger was born in Eddyville, Ill., in 1876, and after receiving his degree from the Marion-Sims College of Medicine, St. Louis, Mo., came to Wayne, Okla., in 1904. After practicing medicine in that community for a number of years, he later returned to Illinois and then moved to Casper, Wyo. Upon his return to Oklahoma, Doctor Barger established his residence at Purcell, where he has continued in active practice. At the time of his death, Doctor Barger was 66 years of age.

Funeral services were conducted Thursday afternoon in the Rackley Chapel with the Rev. Harry Anderson officiating. Interment was made in the Hillside cemetery.

Survivors include his wife of the home address; three sons, Dr. Blanchard Barger, somewhere in the Pacific war area; Bill Barger, stationed at the naval base at Los Angeles, Calif., and Blaine Barger of Purcell. Also surviving are three brothers, Marion of Harrisburg, Ill.; Lee of Poplar Bluff, Mo.; Berry of Sheldon, Wash; and two sisters, Mrs. J. W. F. Davis of Harrisburg, Ill., and Mrs. Syd Jenkins of Mounds, Ill.

Dr. W. D. Baird, Jr.
(1901-1942)

Dr. Wilson Davis, Jr., prominent Oklahoma City physician, who had practiced medicine in Capitol Hill for the past ten years, died of septicemia and pneumonia Wednesday, August 19, following a month's illness. Doctor Baird was owner of the South Robinson Avenue clinic.

Doctor Baird was born August 22, 1901, at Altus, Oklahoma. He was graduated from the Stroud High School in 1919, and in 1926, he received his degree from the Oklahoma School of Medicine. Prior to establishing a permanent residency in Oklahoma City, Doctor Baird practiced in Seminole and Stroud.

Doctor Baird was a member of the American Medical, Oklahoma County and Oklahoma State Medical Associations. His fraternal affiliations were Phi Chi, medical and Pi Kappa Phi, social. He was also a member of the Oklahoma club.

Funeral services were conducted at 2:00 P. M., Friday, at the Hunter funeral home. Survivors include his parents, Dr. and Mrs. W. D. Baird, Sr., 321 Southwest Twenty-fourth Street, and a sister, Mrs. John S. Fogarty, 2800 Northwest Twentieth Street, all of Oklahoma City, and a brother, Dr. J. Byron Baird of Houston, Texas.

Use of Saccharin for Sweetening

"Sugar rationing and new emphasis on weight reduction have doubtless increased the use of saccharin for sweetening purposes," The Journal of the American Medical Association for July 25 says. "Renewed interest in the possible harmful effect of this substance is an apparent corollary. Earlier investigations of saccharin, however, have failed to reveal dangerous side-actions except from extremely large doses. Likewise the evidence does not reveal any reason why saccharin cannot be used continuously in average sweetening doses for an indefinite period. Many patients have taken saccharin for years without harmful effect."

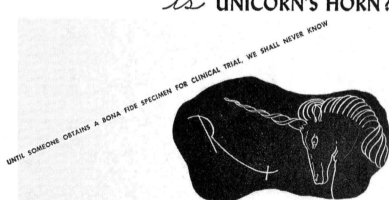

Blue Cross Reports

A few years ago there were less than 10,000 subscribers to non-profit hospital service plans throughout the United States. At the American Hospital Association convention in 1937, C. Rufus Rorem, M.D., Director of the Commission reported 1,000,000 members. At the same time he astonished many of his colleagues by predicting 10,000,000 subscribers within five years. Plan directors and hospital representatives listened to this prediction with skepticism. Today, five years later, this incredible enrollment has not only been achieved, but has been exceeded.

Directors of Blue Cross Plans from all over America met this month in St. Louis in connection with the American Hospital Association convention. Today Blue Cross Directors are looking to the future with optimism. While only five years ago an enrollment of 10,000,000 was almost inconceivable, today the ultimate enrollment is thought of in terms of 50,000,000 or 60,000,000.

More than at any previous convention, there was manifest a spirit of complete harmony among Blue Cross Plan directors. The national emergency has presented problems common to all plans—problems that necessitate correlation of all our efforts toward presenting a more unified program.

At the St. Louis convention five new non-profit hospital service plans were approved and given institutional membership in the American Hospital Association. This brings the number of approved plans to seventy-five. Of particular interest to Oklahoma was the approval of plans for the states of Texas and Kansas, both operating on a state-wide basis.

Throughout America our doctors, hospital administrators and the public at large are becoming more and more convinced that The Blue Cross Plans are very satisfactorily solving a serious economic problem. Civic and industrial leadership have made a splendid contribution to this national health service. This response has been eager and spontaneous because The Blue Cross Plans operate on a sound and practical basis, and without a selfish motive.

Classified Advertisements

FOR SALE: Well-equipped, 25-bed hospital in Western Oklahoma in county seat town of over 5,000 population. Good location for clinic.

For further information, contact the Executive Office, 210 Plaza Court, Oklahoma City.

FOR SALE: Office equipment consisting of one treating table, instrument cabinet, roll top desk and chair, optical equipment, a complete set of tonsil instruments, an electrical nose and throat spray and other instruments. For further information, contact Mrs. G. S. Barger, 430 West Adams Street, Purcell, Oklahoma.

Opportunities for Practice

There is an excellent opportunity for practice at Stilwell, Okla. The town of Stilwell has a population of 1,800 and is the county seat of Adair county.

Office of Civilian Defense

This is to advise that the State Health and Housing Committee and the State Emergency Medical Service have made available the services of a full-time, well-trained, graduate, registered nurse as nurse deputy in the State Emergency Medical Service; namely, Mrs. Virginia Fowler, R.N. The duties of the State Nurse Deputy are:

1. To assist the State Chief of Emergency Medical Service and the local Nurse Deputies in the state in mobilizing all members of the nursing profession for duty in the Emergency Medical Service during and after an enemy attack or other war-time disaster.

2. To aid the American Red Cross and the hospitals to carry through a full program of training of Nurses' Aides so that the depleted ranks of hospital and public health nursing services may be assisted in carrying the heavy burden of war-time service in civilian hospitals and health departments, as well as in the casualty stations and first aid posts of the Emergency Medical Service.

3. To assist the State Hospital Officer and State Chief of Emergency Medical Service in the emergency assignment of private duty nurses, and of nurses from local and state hospitals and health agencies to base hospitals, if the need arises for the evacuation of patients from casualty receiving hospitals of the costal cities.

Correspondence requesting the Nurse Deputy's services should be address to Dr. G. F. Mathews, State Chief, Emergency Medical Service, State Health Department, Oklahoma City, Oklahoma. Her appointment is effective October 1, 1942, and her services will be avialable beginning October 16, 1942.

Dallas New Civilian Defense Headquarters

Headquarters of the Office of Civilian Defense of the Eighth Defense Region have been moved from San Antonio to Dallas, as of November 15. This procedure was established following the removal of the Eighth Service Command to Dallas.

The Eighth Regional Defense area is composed of five states; namely, Texas, Louisiana, Arkansas, Oklahoma and New Mexico.

Civilians in Target Areas of Country Should Carry Identification Tags

"To facilitate identification, each civilian in target areas of the country should be encouraged to carry an identification bracelet or necklace or metal identification pocket piece." The Journal of the American Medical Association advises in its October 17 issue in a condensation of Bulletin No. 5 on Emergency Mortuary Services, to be issued by the Medical Division of the United States Office of Civilian Defense. It is pointed out that in some air raids 40 percent of the casualties may be fatal and that although the wounded require first attention, the dead should also be cared for promptly and inconspicuously.

The staff of the emergency mortuary service, according to the bulletin as condensed in The Journal, should include a physician to confirm deaths and a coroner or other medical examiner's representative who has authority to sign death certificates and order disposal of unidentified bodies. Volunteer members of an emergency mortuary organization are to enroll with the Volunteer Civilian Defense Office and are entitled to wear the armband and insignia of the Emergency Medical Service, of which the Mortuary Service is a part.

Among the other point brought out in the condensation by The Journal is that it is important that the identification tags on gas contaminated bodies be distinctly marked "gas case" in order that persons handl-

Anniversaries of Progress . . .

SULFADIAZINE
Lederle

ONE YEAR AGO *Lederle* made available to the medical profession a new sulfonamide which represented at that moment the highest development achieved by synthetic chemists in their search for perfection in the sulfonamide field. During that year "SULFADIAZINE *Lederle*" has been hailed throughout the civilized world—the world of free peoples and free scientists—as a medicament of unusually low toxicity, exceptionally high effectiveness and uncommonly broad applicability. Sulfadiazine is a "drug of choice" in many instances.

TWO YEARS AGO physicians in the United States, Canada and England were investigating "SULFADIAZINE *Lederle*" with the keenest interest. The most concentrated study yielded results that exceeded all previous expectations. The names of these physicians was a roster of the great in medicine.

THREE YEARS AGO the chemical and pharmacological investigations upon this new drug were being conducted with exceptional intensity by the Lederle-American Cyanamid research group. The brilliant collaboration of synthetic chemists and pharmacologists established the firm foundation upon which the structure of the final product was reared.

FUTURE YEARS will yield many such anniversaries of scientific progress for the benefit of mankind. We pledge ourselves to the future development of chemotherapy and we shall judge our success by the recognition given to the services we render for the masses of common men.

PACKAGES:

"SULFADIAZINE TABLETS *Lederle*"
  Bottles of 50, 100, 1,000 tablets—0.5 Gm. (7.7 grains) each
  Sterile Powder: Bottles of 5 Gm.

"SODIUM SULFADIAZINE STERILE *Lederle*" (Powder)
  Bottles of 5 Gm.

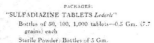

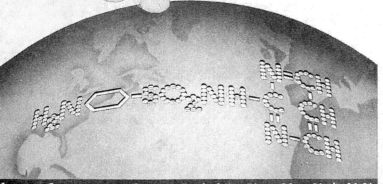

ing them will be warned to give them special treatment. Such bodies should be handled only by workers wearing protective clothing and masks and these workers must subsequently go through the cleansing prescribed for decontamination squad members.

HOW TO PROTECT YOURSELF AGAINST GAS

The following information on war gases is supplied for general publication from the office of James M. Landis, Director, Civilian Defense, because of the possibility that they may at some time be used by the enemy. If people will remember a few simple facts, they will have no unreasonable fear of this agent.

I. War gases stay close to the ground, for they are heavier than air. To get out of a gassed area, simply walk against the wind or go upstairs.

II. Gas is irritating and annoying to the eyes, nose, lungs, or to the skin, but it is usually harmless if you do not become panicky but promptly leave the gas area and cleanse yourself. A soldier must put on a mask where it is necessary to remain in the contaminated area, but a civilian can go up on the second or third floor and literally ignore it if the windows are kept closed.

III. If the gas should get on your skin, you can prevent it from doing much harm by sponging it off as quickly as possible with a piece of clothing, such as a handkerchief, and applying some neutralizing substance, followed by a thorough bath, preferably a shower, with common laundry soap and water.

IV. If you are indoors, stay there with doors and windows closed, and go up to the second or third story. Stay out of basements. Turn off the air conditioning, and stop up fireplaces and any other large openings.

V. Some gases are spread as oily droplets which blister and burn the skin and eyes. If you are outside when gas is used, do not look up. Tear off a piece of clothing or use a handkerchief to blot any drops or liquid from your skin and throw the contaminated cloth away. Blot; do not rub, as rubbing will spread the liquid. Then go home, if it is nearby, or to the nearest place where you can wash immediately with soap and water and cleanse yourself in the following manner:

1. Remove all outer clothing outside the house, since gas can be transmitted to others from contaminated clothing. Put it preferably in a covered garbage pail.

2. Apply one of the following effective household remedies to the part of your skin that has been contaminated: Chlorox or similar household bleach (for mustard); peroxide of hydrogen (for Lewisite); paste or solution of baking soda if you have no peroxide or bleach. If you do not know the gas, use both peroxide and bleach. Keep bleach and peroxide out of the eyes. Do not waste time looking for these remedies; bathe immediately if they are not at hand.

3. After entering the house, wash the bleach or peroxide from hands with laundry soap and water and then wash the face. Remove the underclothing, place it in a covered garbage pail, and enter the bathroom.

4. Irrigate the eyes with large amounts of lukewarm 2 percent solution of baking soda (one tablespoonful to a quart of water), or else with plain water. Use an ordinary irrigating douch bag or an eye irrigator. If you do not have these, let plain warm water pour into the eyes from the shower, washing them thoroughly. Do not press or rub the eyes.

5. Lastly, take a shower, using soap and hot water.

6. If the nose and throat feel irritated, wash them out also with baking soda solution.

7. If your chest feels heavy and oppressed, if you have any trouble breathing, or if cigarette smoke becomes distasteful, lie down and stay perfectly still until a doctor sees you.

8. If blisters develop, be careful not to break them and call a doctor.

REMEMBER: Soldiers require gas masks because they must remain in the contaminated area. Civilians can get out of the gassed area or get above the level of the gas, where they do not need gas masks or protective clothing.

Injured persons, who are gassed, require decontamination before they can be admitted to hospitals. All other civilians can best prevent any serious injury by promptly helping themselves in the manner outlined, using a kitchen or bathroom, laundry soap and water, and a few materials found in every household.

Word has been received in the office of the Association that Dr. Myron C. England, formerly of Woodward, is now in foreign service. His address is Captain Myron C. England, 12th Station Hospital, A. P. O. 922, San Francisco, Calif.

Dr. Raymond M. Slabaugh, Jr., of Sayre, recently commissioned in the Navy as Lieutenant, junior grade, has reported for duty as commandant of the Mare Island, Calif., Naval Yard.

Dr. Sam R. Fryer of Oklahoma City has recently been commissioned a lieutenant in the medical division of the army air corps, and is now stationed at Randolph Field, San Antonio, Texas.

Word has recently been received in the office of the Association from Lieutenant Colonel Roscoe C. Baker that he is now stationed at Station Hospital, Lordsburg Internment Camp, Lordsburg, New Mexico. Lt. Col. Baker is a former resident of Enid.

Lieutenant Johnny A. Blue, U. S. N., formerly of Guymon, has recently received an appointment for postgraduate work in allergy at the National Naval Medical Center hospital, Bethesda, Maryland. For the past several months, Lieutenant Blue has been chief medical examiner at the Oklahoma City naval recruiting center.

Lieutenant Powell E. Fry, formerly of Stillwater, is now stationed at the Chico Army Flying School, Chico, Calif.

Captain James M. Gordon has reported for active duty in the medical division of the army air corps and is stationed at Luke Field, Phoenix, Arizona. Captain Gordon formerly practiced at Ardmore.

Captain Wm. Jackson Sayles of Miami is now on duty with the medical corps of the Army Air Forces and is stationed at Salt Lake City, Uath.

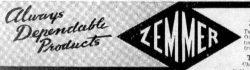

BOOK REVIEWS

"The chief glory of every people arises from its authors."—Dr. Samuel Johnson.

AMBASSADORS IN WHITE. Charles Morrow Wilson. Cloth. Pp. 372. 14 chapters. 42 illustrations. Henry Holt and Company, 257 Fourth Avenue, New York City. Price $3.50.

Here is a well written true story crammed with mystery and adventure, full of searching investigations and rich in discovery. While it is a story of great promise it presents grave potentialities. It not only points out our political, economic and defensive opportunities through friendly cooperation with our South American neighbors but it spotlights the ominous hazards arising through the danger of tropical diseases in epidemic form, a danger immeasurably augmented by modern transportation and the exigencies of war.

With a world conflict encircling the globe and pressing hard upon the equator this story of medicine in the American tropics is of phenominal importance and the knowledge it contains should be made available to every intelligent American citizen. "As never before, the American health front is a community problem. As never before, the threat of migratory diseases must be studied. Microbes are still tourists and tourist-like success among them encourages new waves of migration. As Pan-American union becomes more close and boundaries come to mean less, the exploits of disease as well as the inter-communication of men will be facilitated. Americans must realize that if their efforts toward the eventual solidarity of the hemisphere are to meet with durable success the warfare against disease must be increased and its battle lines better solidified." It stands as a shining monument to American medicine and pays due tribue to Carlos Finlay, Walter Reed, and William Gorgas, their collaborators and their successors.

In the light of present trends toward bureaucratic control of medical service it is significant that the author boldly points out the fact that the Isthmian canal commission authorized by congress did not contain a single doctor and that lay ignorance and stupidity plus political interference came near robbing the United States of the world's outstanding monument to preventive medicine. After refusing the American Medical Association's request for representation on the commission President Theodore Roosevelt had the good sense to send Gorgas along as "Sanitary Advisor" and to his everlasting credit he had the wisdom and fortitude to keep him on when the politicians on the commission "issued an urgent recommendation that Gorgas and his associates be dismissed and men of more practical views appointed."

Aside from certain omissions, the author over-emphasizes the work of some of the investigators. But these errors do not alter the general significance of the theme.

Every doctor should read "Ambassadors in White" and it should be in the library of every military post, every medical corps station, every army and navy camp and every battleship.—Lewis J. Moorman, M.D.

THE MANAGEMENT OF FRACTURES, DISLOCATIONS AND SPRAINS. John Albert Key, B.S., M.D., St. Louis, Mo., and H. Earle Conwell, M.D., F.A.C.S., Birmingham, Ala. Third Edition. The C. V. Mosby Company, St. Louis, 1942.

The third edition of this very worthwhile book is indeed a welcome addition to the library of anyone who has to do any traumatic surgery. The original edition filled a very important place in that it presented an extremely practical viewpoint in conjunction with excellent scientific background. The succeeding editions have maintained this point of view and the present one is no exception. This book is equally fitted for the specialist, or for one treating an occasional case, since there is often a very complete discussion of the various phases of a certain problem and at the same time a practical presentation of the exact technique and method which has been found by the authors to be more suited to its care.

There are so many worthy additions that in a short review, it is impossible to go over them all. They have presented two excellent chapters by collaborators which are worthy of mention. Dr. Edgar F. Fincher has completely revised the discussion on fractures of the skull and brain trauma, and presents the subject in an extremely interesting and useful way. Dr. James B. Brown, who has been a pioneer in the treatment of fractures about the face and jaws, has contributed a chapter on treatment of these conditions, including excellent illustrations which, in themselves, are almost self-explanatory.

Another improvement is the chapter on compound fractures and war wounds. This extremely current subject has been brought up to date by a very able discussion which should be of great value to anyone who is suddenly called on to treat war injuries, without a long background of training in this work. This all-inclusive section bears an able discussion of the various factors to be considered in shock; the routine of care for open wounds; the use of chemotherapy as opposed to, or in conjunction to other methods, such as, bacteriophage, etc. Here, again, several viewpoints are presented, along with the conclusions of the authors and their reason for the selection of one particular method in preference to others.

There are several chapters which have been completely rewritten, since the subjects under consideration have undergone such marked advancement in the past few years. Worthy of mention is the discussion on intervertebral disk which at the time of the last edition, was in a state of flux and not well understood. The authors present a conservative and valuable point of view which should enable one to rationalize the very interesting field of low back pain. The revision of the chapter on treatment of fractures of the neck of the femur, as compared to the original chapter on the same subject is extremely enlightening and calls to mind the very rapid advancement taken place in this particular field within a few years. It is worth the careful scrutiny of anyone treating this condition. The discussion of the use of chemotherapy has been brought up to date by the inclusion of the various sulfonamides which have so completely altered the prognosis in many grave situations.

We must congratulate Drs. Key and Conwell for continuing the very happy collaboration which combines the utilitarian with the scientific. It is an extremely valuable book for reference. It is organized ideally for use as a text and should be included in the library of every practicing physician.—D. H. O'Donoghue, M.D.

SYNOPSIS OF PATHOLOGY. W. A. D. Anderson, M.A., M.D., Assistant Professor of Pathology, St. Louis University School of Medicine; Pathologist, St. Mary's Group of Hospitals. Cloth. Pp. 661. The C. V. Mosby Company, St. Louis, Mo.

This is a small, convenient size book, elegantly and profusely illustrated with both color and black and white plates. The illustrations are very clear and apropos and seem to represent equally the gross and microscopic pathology. It is concise, remarkably well-condensed and simplified. Many of the old and unsubstantiated ideas and theories are pleasingly conspicuous by their absence. Sufficient reference is made. Modern concepts of allergy, biochemistry, vitamins and endocrines, this in itself making the book an exceptional and satisfactory reference or handbook, are included.

A glance at the references or bibliography impresses one with the idea that not all references on the subject covered are given, but that key references representing modern authors and up to date reports, many of which are abstracts, are listed.

Ample description of virus and rickettsial diseases, spirochetal and venereal disease, mycotic, protozoal and helminthic infections are given. These are remarkably well condensed and at the same time practical considerations are, in most instances, fully covered.

None of the book is set aside for the particular description of neoplasms. These are mentioned under the heading of the various anatomical systems. Oncology probably occupies a smaller percentage of space than in the average textbook of pathology. Adequate space is given to the more recently studied embryonal tumors of the ovary, which have direct bearing in connection with the endocrine studies.

The book seems to be an ideal one for medical school and nurses training schools. It contains modern fundamentals and much of the chaff handed down from period to period in the past, has been eliminated. This should make it ideal for students.

The following, from the authors preface, is in principal an accurate key to the type of book he has written:

"Knowledge of the seemingly endless, finer details and variations in the patterns of disease will continue to be acquired as long as an individual remains a student of a medical science. The process of learning is most efficiently and pleasurably accomplished by acquiring first the essentials and the broad outlines, with the addition of greater and greater detail as the subject is pursued further, rather than by adding minute fact to minute fact until the required mass is accumulated."

The clinician cannot hope to find a book or "synopsis" more convenient and practical. The author appears to have had clinical medicine more uppermost in his mind than the average professor of pathology ordinarily manifests in his writings, and therein lies unusual practiceability as a handbook of handy reference.—Hugh Jeter, M.D.

Its Now Sterling Drug, Inc., But Same Sales Policies Hold

The name of Sterling Products (Inc.) was changed to Sterling Drug Inc. at a special meeting of stockholders held October 15 in Wilmington, Delaware. Of the number of shares voted, only 1/6th of 1 percent were against the proposal. Sterling Drug Inc. includes among its subsidiaries the manufacturers of such products as Bayer's Aspirin, Phillips' Milk of Magnesia and Dr. Lyon's Tooth Powder.

Explaining the move, James Hill, Jr., president, said that the change of name would leave "entirely undisturbed the sales policies, management and personnel of the company's subsidiaries. Sterling's many well-known brand names will be retained, and advertising programs remain unaffected. Of course, the listing of the company's stock on the New York Stock Exchange will be under the new name."

At the same time, it was pointed out that "subject to the passage of pending tax legislation, the corporation may deem it advisable to simplify its subsidiary corporate structure and to operate some of the business now being conducted through subsidiaries." If this change is effected, the "Sterling" name will appear for the first time on packages containing many of the company's well advertised popular drug products.

The change of name was recommended by the Board of Directors to make possible transformation of the company from a "holding" to an operating company. Sterling Products (Incorporated) as a corporate name is similar to the corporate names of other corporations already organized or licensed to do business in a number of States, thereby making it impossible for the corporation to obtain a license to do business under that name in several States.

A survey of corporate names available throughout the United States led the management to select Sterling Drug, Inc., "as the most appropriate."

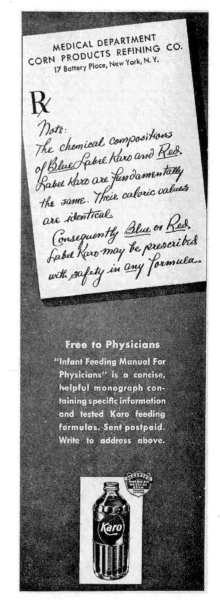

APROPOS CHRISTMAS SEAL SALE TUBERCULOSIS ABSTRACTS

Civilian physicians need feel no chagrin when they see their colleagues in uniform. They can serve their country with the same high patriotism and with more lasting benefit to its health if they will solemnly agree to press relentlessly and with reborn ardor the fight along the home front for the conquest of tuberculosis. —Kendall Emerson, M.D.

The source of the great bulk of infections with tuberculosis is a human carrier with a pulmonary cavity. While the home is probably the place of most childhood and some adults contacts, many primary infections and more reinfections must occur in the place of work. Nurses, physicians and attendents on the sick encounter a real occupational hazard from infection itself and this hazard should be accepted as incidental to the professional life while hospital management should assume the obligation of minimizing opportunities for mass infection. —Saranac Lake Symposium on Tuberculosis in Industry, Saranac Lake, June, 1941.

All evidence indicates that tubercle bacilli live a very short time in rooms well supplied with unfiltered daylight. In the dosages in which they are apt to be spread by trained patients of a well-run institution, they probably do not survive in infectious quantities more than a few hours. In absolute darkness they may live several months.—C. Richard Smith, Amer. Rev. of Tuber., March, 1942.

Illness may be a social disaster—the head of a family develops pulmonary tuberculosis. Suddenly, the whole course of his life is changed; to adjust him to his altered status requires more than the direction that he be resigned to an indefinite furlough from active work or that he leave his home for institutional care. Friendly, detailed inquiry may indicate that he is disturbed more by unselfish thoughts than by concern for his own well-being. If his fears for the health of his family are not allayed by careful examination of those who were exposed to his infection, if this anxiety as to how they will get on while he is ill or away is not relieved, if his disappointment and his depression, induced by a gloomy outlook on the future, are not lessened by a better estimate of his condition, he may refuse to accept good therapeutic advice, or if he does accept it, an uneasy mind and nervous tension during the period of enforced invalidism may slow or even prevent his recovery.—Chas. R. Austrian, M.D., Diplomate, Jan., 1941.

To find anything one should look for it. Every case of tuberculosis found and put under treatment stops short a possible source of the spread of this disease whose ramifications are more widespread than a chain-letter. Every case of tuberculosis found in the early stage gives that person a much greater chance for recovery than if it is a late stage of the disease.—J. L. Gompertz, M.D., Bull. Alameda Co. Tuber. and Health Assn., March, 1942.

The plague of tuberculosis is not one of the irresistible scourges of nature, to which we must bow as to the inevitable; the remedy and the means of prevention are known, the difficulty is to prevail upon the public to avail themselves of this knowledge, and thus protect their homes from avoidable loss of life.—From a letter received by the Canadian Tuberculosis Assn., in 1912 from the Duke of Connaught, late Governor-General of Canada.

It is well to remember that during one year tuberculosis among the veterans of the World War cost the United States government more than 40 million dollars, exclusive of the cost of hospitalization. One-third of the total amount paid out for compensation to the services was for tuberculosis and 61,330 veterans were in hospitals at government expense. In this day of pensions and augmented government health services, every known scientific procedure should be used to cut down this enormous burden on the taxpayer. Tuberculosis can be detected by the use of the x-ray. The experience of twenty odd years ago need not be repeated.

The National Tuberculosis Association has recently reported that the death rate for tuberculosis among unskilled workers is seven times higher than that among professional workers.

In the United States, tuberculosis is responsible for the death of more than 2,500 children under the age of 10 years annually.

Tuberculosis is the remaining arch-foe of childhood, harbored unwittingly by many adult associates and calling for special attack, although the principles applicable to its control are identical in the main with those pertaining to contact infections in general.—Wise, Assn. for the Disabled, June, 1942.

Boys and girls in secondary schools, technical schools, colleges and universities are at a period of life where physical and mental strain is great, and the risk of tuberculosis serious. The disease at these age periods shows a tendency to increase. Regular X-ray examinations are advisable. Doctors responsible for the health of such institutions are asked to encourage their wider use.—Tubercle, February, 1942.

Sixty thousand Americans, most of them young, die each year of tuberculosis. Compared with the loss of life from this cause a century ago, it is a triumph that there are only 60,000. Compared with the number who could be saved by the prompt application of modern knowledge, it shows gross neglect that there are so many.—Surgeon General Thomas Parran, Survey-Graphic, March, 1942.

The tuberculin test should be a part of the pre-school examination. Tuberculosis seldom develops in its clinically serious forms in children but they are easily infected with the germs of the disease, which may remain dormant until they reach the teen age or early adult life, and then cause trouble. Through the tuberculin test it is possible to determine whether or not a child has been infected. When the test is positive every effort should be made to find the source of infection and to protect the child from further exposure to the disease. It is important to point out here that precaution should be taken to make sure that maids and other household employees are free from tuberculosis by having them tuberculin tested and X-rayed if positive to the test.— Chester A. Stewart, M.D., Louisiana News in Brief, Sept.-Oct., 1941.

For years the after-care attention meted out to post-sanatorium cases has been the Cinderella of the Tuberculosis Service. This has been due to a variety of reasons. In the main, the results were less spectacular than those of the operating theater and hense never achieved the same popularity in the lay mind; and again with the floating peacetime unemployed population of about three million, healthy labor was at a premium.

Information about tuberculosis disease or previous treatment at a sanatorium or dispensary should be made compulsory for all persons entering industry. This is the practice at military boards and there appears no legitimate reason why this should not be incorporated into the civilian industrial life of the country. Such a measure would insure the control of infection in the interests of the health of the community. Naturally, such a course will occasion opposition. It will be argued that this represents an encroachment on the freedom of the individual; however, freedom would be an intolerable institution if it permitted an individual indiscriminately to infect with disease his fellow creatures.

An etremely strong case can be made out in view of the recent extension of the defense orders making the treatment of scabies compulsory in the interests of national health. The extension of such a defense regulation to incorporate tuberculosis should prove a relatively simple legal measure.—Some Reflections on the Tuberculosis in Industry, Bertram Mann, B.M., Tubercle, March, 1942.

The role of the general practitioner in the eradication of tuberculosis cannot be overemphasized. Mass programs of case finding in high school, colleges, industry and racial groups are public health functions. But there are other categories that such drag-nets do not reach. One of these is the older third of the population. They constitute no single group to be rounded up for mass examination. Yet, they contain a higher percentage of infectious cases than any other age. The family doctor alone has direct access to this reservoir of community infection. To train it effectively and speedily his aid is indispensable.—Editorial, Tuber. Abstracts, Nov., 1942.

Tuberculosis already appears on the increase in the warring nations in the second world conflict. No single cause is apparent. All the factors concerned in the other world war again operate. Malnutrition is known to be serious in certain countries—Esmond R. Long., M.D., Amer. Rev. of Tuber., June, 1942.

Deaths from tuberculosis in Scotland have been increasing in number since the war began. The increases are in every instance larger for females than for males and the proportionate increases are greatest for tuberculous meningitis, a form of the disease which reacts quickly, to increase in the amount of infection present in the community.—Editorial, Tubercle, June, 1942.

Even after 1,000 days of war the health of the nation is in many respects better than it was in peacetime. Tuberculosis, however, is an exception.—The Minister of Health for Great Britain. Bulletin, Canadian Tuber. Assn., Sept., 1942.

Despite the precaution of a supplementary diet for persons with active tuberculosis, the march of the disease has been ominously progressive in France, the figures for 1941 compared with corresponding ones for 1939 show a 10 percent increase in mortality from tuberculosis. In children from one to nine, the increase was 28 percent.—Marcel Moine, M.D., Academie de Medecin de Paris, Sept., 1941.

Tuberculosis remains the most deadly saboteur in our midst. Sixty thousand Americans will perish by the disease this year.—C. M. Wylie, Mich. Tuber. Assn.

Sources of Infection in Tuberculosis

The prevalence of tuberculosis in any community is determined by the general standard of living and by the number of open carriers. In particular occupations the factors of selective employment and unfavorable environment modify the picture.

The source of the great bulk of infections is a human carrier with a pulmonary cavity. While the home is probably the place of most childhood and some adult contacts, many primary infections and more reinfections must occur in the place of work. Nurses, physicians and attendants on the sick encounter a real occupational hazard from infection itself and this hazard should be accepted as incidental to the professional life while hospital management should assume the obligation of minimizing opportunities for mass infection.

Fumes and gases are inhalable and many of them are sufficiently irritating to provoke severe inflammatory reaction. Mature judgment on the effects of gas used by the armies during the last war reversed the early opinion that this agent was responsible for the excess of tuberculosis that developed. Routine annual examination of a large group of employees engaged in the manufacture of chlorine, phosgene, hydrofluoric acid and other irritating gases, supports the view that exposure to irritant gasses is not responsible for excess tuberculosis.

WAR SAVINGS STAMPS AND BONDS

The United States Treasury Department has recently prepared a condensed explanation of the various types of war savings stamps and bonds. This will be of interest to physicians since they, like all other citizens, should assist the war effort by lending their dollars to the government through the purchase of war stamps and bonds. Likewise, the physician has a wonderful opportunity of influencing those he might contact during his daily rounds, and in this way encourage others to participate in the War Savings Program.

The following points taken from the memorandum are of interest:

"The Treasury Department offers three series of War Savings Bonds: Series E, F and G. Series E Bonds are "The People's Bonds." They cannot be purchased by banks or corporations, a restriction adopted so that they will be People's Bonds. These are "appreciation bonds," meaning that you buy the bond for less than the amount printed on its face. For example, a $25.00 face value bond costs only $18.75. At the end of the ten year maturity period, the Government pays back to you the full $25.00. This is an increase in value of 33 1/3 percent, equivalent to an average interest rate over the life of the bond of almost 3 percent—2.9 to be exact. It is the highest interest rate the Government is paying anybody today on new securities.

"The smallest of the People's Bonds costs $18.75 but this is not the smallest amount that can be put into War Savings. Smaller sums of money purchase War Savings Stamps which range in price from 10c to $5.00. Money invested in stamps does not bring interest as do the bonds, but when as much as $18.75 has been invested in them, they can be turned in for one of the registered, interest-bearing bonds. People's Bonds may be purchased at any post office and almost any bank. War Stamps may be obtained at post offices, banks, many retail stores and other locations. Just look for the War Stamps sales window or booth.

"Series F Bonds, like the Series E, are appreciation bonds, but these may be bought by corporations and associations as well as individuals. These are twelve-year bonds, which provide a return equivalent to an annual interest rate of 2.53 percent. The smallest of this series costs $18.50 and pays $25.00 at the end of twelve years; the largest costs $7,400 and pays $10,000 at maturity.

"The bonds of Series G, unlike those of Series E and F, are sold at par; that is, the cost is the same as their face value. But also unlike Series E and F, Series G Bonds pay interest semiannually at the rate of 2½ percent throughout their twelve-year maturity period. Bonds of this series are issued in denominations ranging from $100 to $10,000. Only the Treasury and Federal Reserve Banks issue F and G Bonds, but most commercial banks accept applications for them."

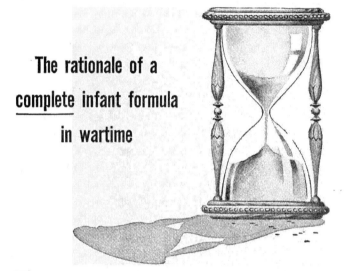

OFFICERS OF COUNTY SOCIETIES, 1942

——Indicates serving in Armed Forces.

COUNTY	PRESIDENT	SECRETARY	MEETING TIME
Alfalfa	*Jack F. Parsons, Cherokee	L. T. Lancaster, Cherokee	Last Tues. Each 2nd Mo.
Atoka-Coal	J. B. Clark, Coalgate	J. S. Fulton, Atoka	
Beckham	H. K. Speed, Sayre	E. S. Kilpatrick, Elk City	Second Tues. eve.
Blaine	Virginia Olson Curtin, Watonga	W. F. Griffin, Watonga	
Bryan	A. J. Wells, Calera	W. K. Haynie, Durant	Second Tues. eve.
Caddo	Fred L. Patterson, Carnegie	C. B. Sullivan, Carnegie	
Canadian	P. F. Herod, El Reno	A. L. Johnson, El Reno	Subject to call
Carter	Walter Hardy, Ardmore	H. A. Higgins, Ardmore	
Cherokee	Park H. Medearis, Tahlequah	*Isadore Dyer, Tahlequah	
Choctaw	C. H. Hale, Boswell	Fred D. Switzer, Hugo	
Cleveland	Joseph A. Rieger, Norman	Curtis Berry, Norman	Thursday nights
Comanche	George S. Barber, Lawton	W. F. Lewis, Lawton	
Cotton	George W. Baker, Walters	Mollie F. Seism, Walters	Third Friday
Craig	W. R. Marks, Vinita	J. M. McMillan, Vinita	
Creek	Frank Sisler, Bristow	O. C. Coppedge, Bristow	
Custer		*W. C. Tisdal, Clinton	Third Thursday
Garfield	D. S. Harris, Drummond	John R. Walker, Enid	Fourth Thursday
Garvin	T. F. Gross, Lindsay	John R. Callaway, Pauls Valley	Wed. before 3d Thurs.
Grady	D. S. Downey, Chickasha	*Frank T. Joyce, Chickasha	3rd Thursday
Grant	I. V. Hardy, Medford	E. E. Lawson, Medford	
Greer	G. F. Border, Mangum	J. B. Hollis, Mangum	
Harmon	S. W. Hopkins, Hollis	W. M. Yeargan, Hollis	First Wednesday
Haskell	William Carson, Keota	N. K. Williams, McCurtain	
Hughes	Wm. L. Taylor, Holdenville	Imogene Mayfield, Holdenville	First Friday
Jackson	J. M. Allgood, Altus	E. W. Mabry, Altus	Last Monday
Jefferson	W. M. Browning, Waurika	J. I. Hollingsworth, Waurika	Second Monday
Kay	J. C. Wagner, Ponca City	J. Holland Howe, Ponca City	Third Thurs.
Kingfisher	C. M. Hodgson, Kingfisher	*John R. Taylor, Kingfisher	
Kiowa	J. M. Bonham, Hobart	B. H. Watkins, Hobart	
LeFlore	G. R. Booth, LeFlore	Rush L. Wright, Poteau	
Lincoln	E. F. Hurlbut, Meeker	C. W. Robertson, Chandler	First Wednesday
Logan	William C. Miller, Guthrie	J. L. LeHew, Jr., Guthrie	Last Tuesday evening
Marshall	J. L. Holland, Madill	O. A. Cook, Madill	
Mayes	L. C. White, Adair	V. D. Herrington, Pryor	
McClain	B. W. Slover, Blanchard	R. L. Royster, Purcell	
McCurtain	R. D. Williams, Idabel	R. H. Sherrill, Broken Bow	Fourth Tues. eve.
McIntosh	F. R. First, Checotah	William A. Tolleson, Eufaula	Second Tuesday
Murray	P. V. Annadown, Sulphur	F. E. Sadler, Sulphur	
Muskogee	L. S. McAlister, Muskogee	D. Evelyn Miller, Muskogee	First & Third Mon.
Noble	J. W. Francis, Perry	C. H. Cooke, Perry	
Okfuskee	J. M. Pemberton, Okemah	L. J. Spickard, Okemah	Second Monday
Oklahoma	R. Q. Goodwin, Okla. City	Wm. E. Eastland, Okla. City	Fourth Tuesday
Okmulgee	J. G. Edwards, Okmulgee	*John R. Cotteral, Henryetta	Second Monday
Osage	C. R. Weirich, Pawhuska	George K. Hemphill, Pawhuska	Second Monday
Ottawa	J. B. Hampton, Commerce	Walter Sanger, Picher	Third Thursday
Pawnee	E. T. Robinson, Cleveland	Robert L. Browning, Pawnee	
Payne	John W. Martin, Cushing	Clifford W. Moore, Stillwater	Third Thursday
Pittsburg	Austin R. Stough, McAlester	Edw. D. Greenberger, McAlester	Third Friday
Pontotoc	R. E. Cowling, Ada	Alfred R. Sugg, Ada	First Wednesday
Pottawatomie	John Carson, Shawnee	Clinton Graham, Shawnee	First & Third Sat.
Pushmataha	P. B. Rice, Antlers	John S. Lawson, Clayton	
Rogers	*W. A. Howard, Chelsea	George D. Waller, Claremore	First Monday
Seminole	H. M. Reeder, Konawa	Mack I. Shanholtz, Wewoka	
Stephens	A. J. Weedn, Duncan	W. K. Walker, Marlow	
Texas	L. G. Blackmer, Hooker	*Johnny A. Blue, Guymon	
Tillman	C. C. Allen, Frederick	O. G. Bacon, Frederick	
Tulsa	H. B. Stewart, Tulsa	E. O. Johnson, Tulsa	Second & Fourth Mon. eve.
Wagoner	J. H. Plunkett, Wagoner	H. K. Riddle, Coweta	
Washington-Nowata	K. D. Davis, Nowata	J. V. Athey, Bartlesville	Second Wednesday
Washita	A. S. Neal, Cordell	James F. McMurry, Sentinel	
Woods	W. F. LaFon, Waynoka	O. E. Templin, Alva	Last Wednesday
Woodward	M. H. Newman, Shattuck	C. W. Tedrowe, Woodward	

THE JOURNAL

OF THE

OKLAHOMA STATE MEDICAL ASSOCIATION

| VOLUME XXXV | OKLAHOMA CITY, OKLAHOMA, DECEMBER, 1942 | NUMBER 12 |

Functional Cardiovascular Disorders Including The Soldier's Heart*

GEORGE HERRMANN, M.D.**

GALVESTON, TEXAS

The functional disorders of the cardiovascular system present different etiological factors and mechanisms for the various clinical types. The causes may be purely psychogenic or neurogenic or vegetative and may affect the heart or the peripheral vascular system and may give rise to severe or mild symptoms or be entirely asymptomatic. Malingering is a totally different sort of psychological problem and should not be accorded the recognition of being considered along with neuroses.

There are overlappings of the borderlines of the various closely related conditions that are to be taken under consideration in this paper and both psychogenic and neurogenic disturbances may be present. The predominating factor and condition should be singled out and the clinical picture as clearly delineated and classified as possible. The primary source and secondary related conditions should be established.

The diagnosis of purely functional cardiovascular disorders should be made only in the patient who presents no sign whatsoever of organic heart disease. A functional or psychogenic exaggeration of symptoms occurs fairly frequently in patients with organic heart disease, but such a clinical picture should not be included in the group designated generally as "Functional Disorders." Functional, as here used, is not exactly synonymous with physiological but must include psychological, as well. The latter factors disturb the normal function very often. The absence of organic changes in the cardiovascular system is indicated by the designation "functional" as used in this discussion.

In civilian life, women make up the large proportion of functional cardiovascular cases and far more come from the leisure class than from among those who must work to earn a living. Some of these may present hysteria and show major stigmata if these are sought out. Many are pure neurasthenia, partly constitutional, partly post infectious. A fair number of anxiety and fatigue neuroses are encountered and relatively few civilians present true neurocirculatory asthenia. In civilians such secondary factors as partial starvation, avitaminosis, overwork, worry, and exhaustion cause fatigue neuroses. The beginning insufficiency of otherwise asymptomatic heart disease may be a most significant factor in the precipitation of a cardiovascular neurosis. Convalescence from severe infectious diseases as tonsillitis or pneumonia, or absorption from definite foci of sub-clinical infection produce symptoms of neurasthenia. Perplexing private circumstances may arise, creating a situation of distress with which the patient is at a loss adequately to cope. Fear, anxiety, and worry, play perhaps a greater role in precipitating neuroses in hard pressed individual workers in every field of sharp competition than overworking or underfeeding. In the opinion of many, it is nervous exhaustion rather than physical fatigue that is the chief etiological condition.

Theories As to the Etiology

Eppinger and Hess identified all cardiovascular neuroses with functional autonomic nervous system disease and included cases of hysteria and neurasthenia as "vagotonic neurosis."

Oswald Schwarz taught that cardiac neuroses were all purely psychogenic forms of psychasthenia or neurasthenia, due to depressed aggressive tendencies and the spiritual conflict that they engender, an escape or

*Presented before the General Assembly, Annual Meeting, Oklahoma State Medical Association, Tulsa, April 23, 1942.
**Professor of Medicine, University of Texas Medical School.

rebellion from, an incomprehension of or apathy toward, decisive action. The heightened psychic irritability and a sensitized neurovegetative effector system then, he concluded, produced the neuroses.

Teofilo Ortiz Ramirez of Mexico agrees with Schwarz in that he feels emotional disequilibrium produces mental and vegetative nervous fatigue, and that the patients inferior organic vegetative constitution, amplifies or distorts the bodily expressions of mental activity. Ortiz accepts Effinger and Hess's classification term "neurotonia cardiaca" but includes in it: 1. dyspnea without reliable criteria of heart diseases. 2. Precordial pain likewise without unequivocal signs. 3. Capricious, disproportionate, theatrical "cardiac" syndromes without organic heart disease. 4. Pure psychogenic or fictitious symptoms referred by patient to his "heart" representing "cardiophobia." He excluded from the "neurotonia cardiaca" group, those with temporary 1. Emotional storms; 2. Carotid sinus syndrome; 3. Sinus bradycardia (60-70) or 4. Febrile tachycardia, or 5. Other cardiac manifestations of systemic disease. Ortiz thus included conditions that could all be considered psychogenic in our terminology and the excluded, except for the first condition, would be neurogenic.

Recently, P. G. Wood pointed out that the symptoms and signs of neurocirculatory asthenia, effort syndrome (Lewis), soldier's heart (Da. Costa) resemble those of emotion especially fear rather than of effort. He felt that the mechanism of the somatic manifestation depends upon central, emotional or fear stimulation, not upon hypersensitivity of the peripheral automonic system.

The reaction becomes linked to· effort, Wood argues, by a variety of devices which include misinterpretation of emotional symptoms, certain vicious circular patterns, the growth of a conviction that the heart is to blame. Upon this is based a fear of sudden dissolution on exertion, conditioning and hysteria. Incapacity tends to be exaggerated consciously or subconsciously to protect the individual from further painful emotional experiences.

The neurocirculatory asthenia symptom complex apparently may appear as the result of fatigue alone in certain individuals without any recognized neurosis. It may be accepted as such although there must have been a latent neurosis of the sympathetic nervous system that cannot be recognized alone. There is often, however, a strong suggestion of a general neurosis. A differentiation from neurasthenia, fatigue or anxiety neuroses requires great ability and infinite care. Anxiety can bring on considerable trouble particularly when accompanied by changed heart action. Many cases designated in the previous world war as D.A.H. (disordered action of the heart), were complicated in many instances by the addition of cardiac neuroses. These should be clearly defined and separated from neurocirculatory asthenia in which condition the heart action is usually rapid and therefore usually regular.

Pure induced cardiac psychoneuroses may develop in some nervous individuals as the result of suggestion without any basis, with or without, regular or irregular pulse, palpitation and tachycardia. It is the anxiety on the part of the patient, rather than the disturbed heart action, that precipitates the trouble but the mechanism disorder keeps the patient heart conscious and maintains the vicious circle. There need be no other psychogenic factors. Again, irregular heart actions as isolated short or long runs of premature contractions, may be first felt during an examination. If the disorder is enthusiastically announced by an overzealous examiner and calls forth much attention the incident may serve as the basis for the development of ·a mild psychosis. In some individuals who have some latent asymptomatic valvular deformity or other lesions with little or no functional disturbances, the loudly heralded discovery of the condition may precipitate a symptom complex of increasing gravity.

Functional mechanism disorders or irritability of the heart and functional non-valvulitis, non-significant murmurs are among the commonest sources of worry but at the same time these groups constitute the most innocuous troubles of the heart or in the circulatory system. Functional must not be considered as synonomous with physiological or with hysterical. In the cardiovascular field, in addition to psychogenic, there are definite neurogenic disorders. Neurogenic factors may in time contribute to the production of anatomic lesions. The designation functional disorders in cardiovascular practice implies that there are no primary or symptom responsible organic or anatomical changes. If some are accidentally presented they are ruled out as not necessarily direct etiological factors in the situation under discussion.

Functional cardiac mechanism disorders give the patient trouble when he gets anxious about them. This is particularly true if the examining physician betrays any uncertainty in the recognition of the disorder and of its innocuousness. Any suggestion of lack of confidence in the physician's ability to make the diagnosis and/or his own ability to tolerate the condition and carry on, will demoralize the nervous patient and create a vicious circle. An anxiety neurosis with the heart as the sensor organ is easily precipitated in nervous individuals. The neurosis, so easily engendered, is more difficult to uproot.

Murmurs as such cannot give rise to symptoms whether they are of the relative, accidental or organic types. Even valvular heart lesions are asymptomatic until heart failure intervenes. The knowledge of the presence of any type murmur may give rise to worry and the development of a cardiac neurosis.

Functional cardiac murmurs in the nervous patient unceremoniously apprised of the presence of some sort of "heart leakage" naturally causes the patient to begin to worry about the consequences. Murmurs in themselves do not give rise to any symptoms. It is the erroneous interpretation or the inadvertent careless announcement that precipitates trouble. A differentiation of totally insignificant murmurs from those of organic valvulitis might be gone into. It is important that the physician be able to reassure the patient without reservations whatsoever. This is of great help in "curing" the patient. Functional murmurs are characteristically systolic in time, variable in position, most frequently in the pulmonary area and usually soft but changeable in intensity with respiratory maneuvers and changes in position.

Individuals with significant murmurs who have gone along for years with unrecognized and generally asymptomatic valvular lesions may experience anxiety when the findings are heralded by an immature examiner and given undue attention. Any findings excitedly exaggerated and enthusiastically corroborated by other consultants aggravate matters. The medical examiners must always take time to explain and to reassure the examinee to avoid creating in him any anxiety. Thoughtlessness will precipitate a very definite cardiac neurosis, which perhaps is more troublesome than some of the latent organic conditions.

Cardiac Neuroses— The Pure Psychoneuroses

We could take into consideration under the title of cardiac neuroses, functional murmurs, heart pain, disordered heart action, mechanism disturbances, neurocirculatory asthenia, and peripheral vascular disorders. We can do little more than touch upon an outline of these broad divisions and omit entirely the discussion of some of them. We might elaborate upon one division or upon an individual topic and not be able to complete it to the satisfaction of all or of a critical reader.

The cardiac neuroses or psychoses are de-pendent upon psychic influences presenting capricious tendencies and various other factors. It is generally accepted that anxiety, apprehension and persistent introspective and pathological imagination contribute to the development of phobias. There may result symptoms that mimick closely those of organic disease in any system. These psychogenic symptoms tend to increase the patient's anxiety which in turn further aggravates the situation. The vicious circle created tends to establish in the patient the absolute belief that he is suffering from an organic disease.

Psychogenic Heart Pain— Pseudoangina Innocens

Pain that is often indistinguishable from cardiac coronary or aortic pain may occur in some individuals with a gastro-intestinal neurosis. It may originate in esophageal, gastric or intestinal constrictions or other affections. The neurotic's chief complaints are of heaviness or aching in the left chest, a sense of fullness or constriction, which really is in a gut with distention; in the transverse colon, or in the high placed stomach with a dilated fundus or in the lower esophagus. This may be aggravated by aerophagia. A hyperactive gastrocardiac reflex may give rise to subxiphoid distress and pain.

As a rule, in functional cardiac pain there are no progressive increases in the severity of attacks and no vascular deterioration. Instead there occur cyclic periods of steady improvement and sudden reversal. Major stigmata of hysteria may be present. A severe spasmodic attack may be associated with some disturbance in the coronary circulation yet no definite evidence of such a change can be electrocardiographically or otherwise established. An overly sensitive central nervous system, psychologic, physiologic, pathologic and endocrine factors may contribute. There may sometimes be an associated active focal infection that seems to produce an irritable nervous system of the heart. Just how focal pathology has an effect is still obscure.

Functional cardiac pain is twice as frequent in females as in males but may be present in individuals of all ages from ten years to sixty-five years. It occurs in those who have psychological disorders or disturbances but may be found among those who have had rheumatic fever, tonsillitis or other infections. The chief complaints are of a heaviness or aching in the left chest, a sense of fullness or constriction and a sharply localized pain. Common accompanying factors are slight shortness of breath, dyspnea, but only rarely is orthopnea purely functional in origin.

The Irritable Heart

The designation irritable heart might well be limited to the disorders of actions of the heart. Actual functional derangement for which the term irritable heart is applied may be entirely psychogenic. Under or after nervous strain, premature contractions may occur at occasional or frequent intervals or in runs as paroxysms of auricular or atrial tachycardia; more rarely auricular or atrial flutter or fibrillation may appear after a shock. There are no other physical findings in the heart except that faint distant apical systolic murmurs may develop under stress.

Psychoneurotics with symptoms such as those described and no pathognomonic signs of organic heart disease may suffer more acutely than more stolid individuals with organic heart disease. The mechanism disorder of premature contractions only rarely occurs with neurocirculatory asthenia which is accompanied by a sinus tachycardia as a rule. The irritable heart should therefore be differentiated from neurocirculatory asthenia.

In some cases, there may be a complaint of troublesome palpitation of the heart at rest. The sensations of a simple cardiac irregularity may be most disturbing. The patient feels as though his heart stopped, skipped a beat and turned over, or as though the heart were jumping into the throat, or drawn together in a knot, as though it were about to burst.

There may be with these angioneurotic complaints such as hot flushes, tenseness of the skin, throbbing hot or icy cold extremities, bursting headaches or extreme vertigo. All including heart action are described with much greater emphasis than is usually employed by patients with cardiovascular disease.

Treatment

The treatment of cardiac neuroses should be thorough. The use of all well known heart drugs should be, if possible, scrupulously avoided lest the alert patient begin to doubt the profuse reassurance. However, myocardial sedatives and alteratives as potassium iodide and quinidine may be very valuable adjuvants. The action should be explained and the patient duly reassured.

Psychotherapy or suggestion will often relieve the distress temporarily but such alleviation is only temporary. The patient must be brought to face the facts in his situation and an external open and frank adjustment must be made and acknowledged. In those in whom the neurosis is engrafted upon an organic lesion the management must be carefully maneuvered with guarded reassurance and partial restriction of activity insisted upon.

Observations must be made unostentatiously and without much ado at rather frequent intervals. Psychotherapy is, according to Ortiz, bagatellizitic, destructive, pedagogic and moral, persuasive and re-educative as well as psychoanalytic. Sedatives may aggravate the lowered vegetative inhibitory tone. Hence, psychotherapy in itself it not medicamentation sufficient.

Neurocirculatory Asthenia, Lewis' Effort Syndrome or Da Costa's Soldier's Heart

All cardiovascular neuroses are most significant in war times. This is particularly true of the syndrome, irritable heart and of the soldier's heart which warrants careful consideration. It cannot be said that this is a proven single clinical entity. It may, however, occur in apparently pure form particularly in draftees. Then again it seems to accompany or follow some infectious disease, as well as sometimes following physical exhaustion or a psychic shock or an emotional upset. A demoralizing mental conflict, the fear of disfigurement, and the terror of death and destruction are most important etiological factors. There are certain types of individuals who are seemingly predisposed to this stubborn disabling condition. These should be recognized and disqualified at the first draft examination. They are unfit for military service and if inducted they become liabilities rather than assets.

The constitutionally inadequate, undersized, undernourished, frail, flat chested, nervous, introspective, sedentary individuals, thus physically and mentally subnormal, with a basic nervous instability, are easy victims of this disorder. They have usually suffered from repeated partially disabling upper respiratory infections or general pyogenic, or focal lesions and have been suspected of having atypical tuberculous lesions and have shown definitely low tolerance for physical activities. Every effort should be made to prevent the precipitation of this symptom complex by disqualifying obviously susceptible individuals for the rigors of army life. In susceptible civilians we must also prevent the development of symptoms of the "Effort Syndrome."

The *symptoms* of neurocirculatory asthenia may be almost indistinguishable from those of organic origin and are quite as disabling and apparently as distressing as those of structural heart disease. The clinical pattern consists of a group of several symptoms which on close studying may be somewhat bizarre. There may be persisting heartache, precordial rather than substernal, distress of an atypical type may be brought on by the slightest exertion and is sometimes accompanied by headache usually also dizziness, faintness and even syncope. Insignificant effort or inadequate excitement is followed by a form of breathlessness that is more of a tachypnea or may be a sighing respiratory action, palpitation, or a sense of increased heart action is usually complained of, weakness, and exhaustion. At times the patient may become panicy, jittery, tremulous, and sweating. A more or less constant or persistent status may develop in severe cases. Hyperventilation may produce alkalosis and tetany.

The *signs* are usually few and nonpathognomonic. Some definite color changes such as blanching or flushing or dermatographism and cold perspiration especially in the hands as well as tachypnea, tachycardia and rapid blood pressure fluctuations with a slight tendency to elevation are usually present. The heart action is usually regular, an incidental irregularity may be present and aggravate matters. Course tremors and generally flabby musculature and low exercise tolerance are characteristic along with the hypotonic heart and vascular system. The reliable signs of organic heart disease are usually all absent. Electrocardiographic and roentgenographic studies reveal no abnormalities unless over ventilation has produced tetany and T waves changes. There are no significant pathognomonic findings in any physical or laboratory examination. The responses to exercise tests, none of which are very satisfactory, are of course, greatly exaggerated. The physical findings are not as abnormal as the psychic reactions of the victim.

The course and prognosis depend upon the makeup of the patient. In an exceptional case, it may be transient; usually, it is persistent, partially or completely disabling the individual, occasionally subsiding partially only to recur in varying degrees, throughout many years of life.

TREATMENT

In the treatment of neurocirculatory asthenia, the first step is to remove, if possible , the distressing environmental factors which have caused or have aggravated the breakdown. The patient must be convincingly and completely reassured. He must squarely face the facts concerning his neurovascular system. A life of even tenure with minimum physical and mental strain must be adhered to. Re-education will help to prevent relapses in intelligent individuals. The patients clear understanding of the "condition" will help him to adjust his life to his condition. The successful handling of such cases requires personal, skillful management of individuals.

Wood recently concluded that in the army, successful treatment is impossible since it is

difficult to establish the necessary intimate contact between patient and the assigned and unchosen medical officer. The medical officer's duty is to serve the state first and the patient secondly. The circumstances tend to thwart success at the outset. It is therefore highly desirable to prevent the development of this condition.

Careful differentiation of the various closely allied conditions must be carried out. All of these must be accorded primary attention and careful consideration. All removable aggravating factors as overwork and undue stimulation as intoxications or smoking to excess should all be taken care of. Heart disease thyrotoxicosis and tuberculosis are usually easily ruled out. Reassurance with re-education and carefully graduated exercises will yield some measure of cure in many cases.

Summary

The increase in functional cardiovascular disorders incident to the war effort is discussed.

The relationships of Da Costa's soldier's heart, Lewis' Effort syndrome, the irritable heart or disordered action of the heart to cardiac neuroses or psychoneurosis due to anxiety or depression, have been touched upon.

Functional heart pain or distress, mechanism disorders and murmurs are considered.

The soldier's heart is described in some detail, as a psychoneurotic complex.

The many peripheral vascular disorders of neurogenic origin have been omitted.

BIBLIOGRAPHY

1. Ortiz Ramirez, Teofilo, Tratamiento de la Neurotonia Cardiaca. Archivos Lat. Amer. De Cardiologia Y. Hematologia, IX: 287, 1939.
2. Eppinger, Hans, and Hess, Leo. Vagotonia. A Clinical Study in Vegetative Neurology. Nervous and Mental Disease Publishing Co., New York, 1915.
3. Schwarz, O., Vienna. Psycogenesis y Psicoterapia de los Sintomas Corporales. Trad. Dr. Ramon Sarro. Editorial Labor, S. A. Madrid, 1932.
4. Lewis, T. The Soldier's Heart and the Effort Syndrome. Paul B. Hoeber, N. Y. 1919. 2nd Edition, Shaw & Sons, 1940.
5. Da Costa, J. M. On the Irritable Heart: A Clinical Study of a Form of Functional Cardiac Disorder. Am. Jour. Med. Sc., 61:17, 1871.
6. Wood, P. H. El Sindrome de Da Costa. Archivos Lat. Amer. De Cardiologia Y Hematologia. ii:241-264, 1941.
7. Wood, Paul. Goulstonian Lecture to R.C.P. of London. British Medical Journal. 1:767, 1941.
8. White, P. D. The Soldier's Irritable Heart. Jour. A.M.A 118:270-271, 1942.

A bandage that can be contracted and stiffened to any desired degree for use in place of a cast, tourniquet, or elastic stocking, has just been patented. It is made of rubber strands which have been coated with a plastic. After the bandage has been wound about the part affected, the plastic can be hardened to the extent desired by treatment with chemicals. The patent specifically covers the process of coating the rubber strands, which previously had not been successful, the inventor states.
—Science News Letter, September 26, 1942.

Atypical Pneumonia*

SAMUEL GOODMAN, M.D., F.A.C.P.

TULSA, OKLAHOMA

Within the past decade there has occurred in this vicinity three successive and distinct forms of penumonia. These pneumonias have differed from each other in etiology, clinical picture, course and laboratory findings.

In the first phase, prior to 1935, broncho-pneumonia, due chiefly to various strepto-cocci, was the predominant type. In a survey which I made on 612 cases of pneumonia occurring here from January, 1930, to April, 1936, the incidence of pneumococcal lobar pneumonia was extremely low, comprising but 10.6 percent of the total number.

Beginning with January, 1935, an upward trend in the incidence of the pneumococcus pneumonias and a corresponding decrease in the incidence of broncho pneumonia and atypical lobar pneumonia due to bacteria other than pneumococci occurred. In the period from January, 1935, which might be termed the beginning of the second pneumonia phase, to May, 1936, 25.5 percent of all the pneumonias were due to the pneumococcus. In the following year, the incidence of the pneumococcal pneumonias had risen to 46.8 percent of a total number of 109 cases admitted to St. John's Hospital. From May, 1937, to May, 1938, there was a decline in both the number of all pneumonias and in the incidence of pneumococcus pneumonias. The latter comprised 45.3 percent of a total number of 81 cases admitted to the hospital. Excluding infants and children under the age of seven years, a total number of 258 pneumonias were admitted into the hospital from May, 1938, to March, 1942. Of this number, 161 or about 64 percent were caused by the various types of pneumococci. Without further detailed comment on these pneumonias, I think it might be of more than passing interest to compare the mortality rate prior to the institution of chemotherapy and the present time. From 1935 to 1938, the death rate due to the pneumococcus pneumonias was 27.6 percent. During the years of 1940 and 1941, the death rate had dropped to 8.1 percent.

In May, 1940, which may be termed the beginning of the third pneumonia phase, we observed for the first time a patient with a type of pneumonia which differed rather strikingly from the ordinary broncho-pneumonias and the typical pneumococcus lobar pneumonias.

The patient, a business man, entered St. John's Hospital with a history that for about three days prior to his entry he had felt weak, developed a headache and a harsh dry cough associated with retrosernal soreness. He had a moderate temperature elevation. On admission his temperature was 101, pulse rate was 84, and respirations were 20. He did not appear to be acutely ill. The physical examination was negative except for questionably decreased breath sounds over a small area in the right base near the spine. The white blood count was 8,100 with 73 percent neutrophils. Sputum examination showed a predominance of gram positive diplococci in pairs and short chains. The Neufeld was negative. A roentgen ray film (Fig. 1) showed an area of infiltration in the right base at the cardio phrenic angle. For the

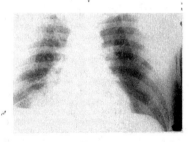

Fig. 1

next two days his temperature varied from 98.6 to 100.2. The symptoms became somewhat aggravated. On the third hospital day, for the first time, crepitant rales could be heard at the right base along the vertebral column. At this time the patient became afebrile although the chest findings remained unchanged for several more days. He was dismissed on the tenth hospital day. During

*Read before the Section on General Medicine, Annual Session, Oklahoma State Medical Association, April 22, 1942.

his stay in the hospital he perspired profusely.

This case represents a typical mild type. Of striking interest is the scarcity of physical signs and the roentgen ray findings which are indistinguishable from those of an early lobar pneumonic process.

The following case seen by another physician represents a severe type of the disease.

The patient, a nurse age 23 years, was admitted to St. John's Hospital November 15, 1941, with the history that for eight days she had been having several chills daily, headache and temperature elevation. For four days she had had severe paroxysms of coughing which was productive of a frothy white mucous. Her past history was irrelevant. For six days she had been taking sulfanilamide. On admission, the patient appeared to be acutely ill. Her temperature was 103, pulse rate was 120 and respirations were 20. She complained of pain in the right side of the chest, severe headache, and vomiting. Physical signs were essentially negative except for decreased expansion of the right side of the chest and fine rales over the right middle part of the chest anteriorly. A roentgen ray film (Fig. 2) of the chest on admission revealed an area of increased density about one by two inches situated in the lower part of the right upper lobe which, although not distinctive, was suggestive of a very early solidification of lobar pneumonia. A white blood count was 10,750 of which 68 percent were neutrophils. Sputum examination showed the presence of long chain streptococci but no pneumococci were found. For the next four days the patient had signs of increasing toxemia, there was frequent vomiting, increased cough, severe headache and chest pain. Her temperature ranged from 98.6 in the mornings to 103.6 in the afternoons, respirations were 20 and 28 and the pulse rate varied between 80 and 112.

A roentgen ray film (Fig. 3) of the chest twenty-four hours after admission showed the previously reported area of increased density to be considerably larger. The white blood count was now 8,600. On the sixth hospital day, the patient developed a severe chill and became extremely apprehensive. Her temperature rose to 105. At this time the chest physical signs indicated consolidation of the right upper lobe. A roentgen ray film (Fig. 4) showed infiltration of the entire right upper lobe and part of the middle lobe. The white blood count was 8,950 with 75 percent neutrophils.

There was but little change in her condition until the eighth day when she went into a mild collapse. The heart became irregular, the sounds weaker and there was a drop in blood pressure. She became quite cyanotic and perspired freely. She was given intravenously 250 cc. of convalescent blood. Following this, she began to improve. On the eleventh day, her temperature became subnormal and remained within a normal range until she was discharged a week later. With the fall in temperature the symptoms subsided although sweating, which was quite profuse at times, persisted during the entire period.

A roentgen ray film, on November 30, fif-

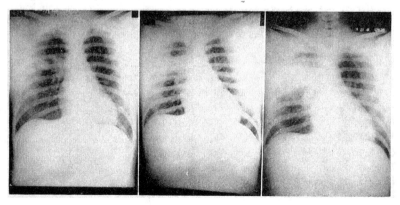

Fig. 2   Fig. 3   Fig. 4

teen days after admission showed that the area of consolidation had assumed its normal transparency.

These cases resemble in detail those described by various clinicians[1,2,3,4] and have been referred to as atypical pronbro-pneumonia, virus pneumonias, virus pneumonitis, and atypical broncho-pneumonia of unknown etiology. While no virus has been isolated in reported cases, the clinical picture, at least, suggests that the etiological agent is a pneumotropic virus.

The disease may be mild or severe in character although the mortality rate is extremely low. There is frequently a history suggesting the onset of a mild infection characterized by malaise, headache, chilly sensations, and mild temperature elevation. The complaint of sore throat is frequent. Within twenty-four to seventy-two hours the patient develops a paroxysmal type of harsh nonproductive cough which increases in severity. There is very little sputum even during or after resolution of the pneumonic process has taken place. Examination at the onset reveals but little. Occasionally injection of the pharynx is observed. The temperature elevation is of a swinging type and accompanied at the low point with sweating of various degrees. Within the period of a week or two the temperature elevation falls by lysis. In many cases the pulse is relatively slow and the respiration is not as rapid as is seen in other pneumonias. Abnormal physical signs related to the chest in the first few days are conspicuous by their absence. If a roentgen ray film is made at this period one is surprised to se that an infiltrative process is present.

Later on as the infiltrative process becomes more extensive subcrepitant and sibilant rales may be heard together with alteration in the breath sounds, vocal fremitus and resonance. These findings are almost always localized to a rather small and circumscribed area. If the pneumonic process remains localized in a small area, there may be no abnormal physical chest signs during the entire course of the disease. Physical examination otherwise is essentially negative although occasionally the spleen may be palpated.

A normal leukocyte count or leukopenia with a relative neutropenia is commonly present. The white blood count may vary from three to twelve thousand. In some instances a leukocytosis up to twenty thousand may occur during convalescence[5] without any evidence of complications.

During the course of the illness the patient, as a rule, does not appear to be acutely ill. Severe prostration such as is seen in

influenza does not occur. Recovery is generally rapid and without after effects.

Diagnosis: While the history and clinical picture of these atypical pneumonias seem to follow a definite and characteristic pattern, the diagnosis in the early stage is not easy. It is only when the clinical picture and radiological evidence of infiltration in the lung exists that the diagnosis is definite. Since radiological evidence of infiltration is usually present before attention is directed to the possibility of a pneumonic process it is advisable to have a roentgenogram done routinely in all patients as soon as they are admitted to the hospital.

Treatment: There is no specific treatment known at this time. Ordinary measures, such as bed rest, plenty of fluids, a general diet if tolerated, mild sedation and some form of the salicylates together with measures to combat symptoms which may arise during the course of the disease are generally sufficient. Chemotherapy in the form of sulfonamides is wholly without benefit and is not indicated.

From May 11, 1940, to March, 1942, twenty-two patients were admitted to St. John's Hospital with the diagnosis of virus pneumonia or virus pneumonitis. Of this group, nineteen cases which fulfilled the criteria of this new form of pneumonia were selected for analysis. Three of the twenty-two cases were not acceptable because of insufficient data. Of the nineteen cases, three occurred in the last half of 1940; fifteen occurred during the year of 1941, and only one has occurred in the first two months of this year. Ten of the nineteen cases occurred during the months of November and December. In this group there were ten females and nine males. All were white.

The onset as will be noted in Table No. 1

Table 1

Onset	Number of cases
Sudden	5
Gradual	14
Total	19

was sudden, i.e., within thirty-six hours in five and gradual in fourteen. Symptoms preceding admission to the hospital suggested some mild type of acute infection characterized by generalized aching, headache, chilliness, temperature elevation of moderate degree and slight non-productive cough.

Symptoms on admission to the hospital are shown in Table No. 2. All cases had a cough which in fifteen was non-productive. Headache was present in eleven, frank chills or chilliness was present in eleven, sore throat was complained of by four, coryza was

Table 2

Symptoms

	Yes	No	Total
Cough	19	0	19
Productive	4	15	19
Headache	11	8	19
Chill	11	8	19
Sore throat	4	15	19
Coryza	7	12	19
Chest pain	7	12	19
Nausea	2	17	19
Weakness	4	15	19
Sweating	6	13	19

present in seven; nausea was complained of by two patients. Weakness in various degrees was present in four. Sweating was present in only six cases. Physical findings at the onset revealed little or no signs except for temperature elevation, a disproportionately slow pulse and respiration. The relatively slow pulse and respiratory rate prevailed in a majority of the cases throughout the course of the illness. The temperature elevation during the course of the illness was unsustained and of a swinging type. In Table No. 3 are listed the physical signs related to the chest on admission. It is of

Table 3

Physical Findings

Rales	Crepitant	Subcrepitant	None	Total
	4	7	9	20*

*One patient had both crepitant and subcrepitant rales

Cyanosis		Yes	No	Total
		2*	17	19

*One patient had congestive heart failure.

	Decreased	Increased	Unchanged	Total
Breath sounds	9	2	8	19
Respiration				
24 and above		13	6	19
Pulse rate		2	17	19
Resonance			Number of Cases	
Impaired			9	
Unchanged			10	
Total			19	

interest to note that in nine cases there were no rales, in eight cases the breath sounds were unchanged and in ten cases there was no dullness or impaired resonance on percussion. After a progression of the disease for a few days and in some cases during resolution only was there evidence that consolidation of a part of a lobe was present. Tubular breathing was heard in but a few patients. The scarcity of physical signs in the chest was not difficult to explain in view of the roentgen ray findings. The early roentgenalogical findings (Fig. 5) are limited to a small area of increased density poorly defined and beginning at or near the hilus of the lung. This infiltration spreads gradually toward the periphery in a wedge shaped

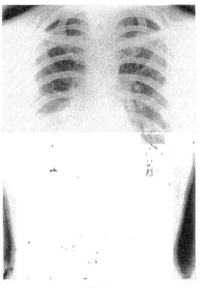

Fig. 5

manner, suggesting, when complete, the picture of an infarction. Early, the lesion cannot be distinguished from that of an early lobar pneumonia. The infiltration extends, after a few days, to the periphery of the lung and rarely involves a whole lobe. When fully developed the infiltration does not present the density which is found in lobar pneumonia. In a few instances the initial lesion does not spread and remains limited to a rather small area such as indicated in the first case presented. When this occurs the course of the disease is rather mild. In the severe case which was presented in detail the progession of the pneumonic process is clearly shown in the x-ray films (Fig. 2, 3 and 4). In this instance, it will be noted that the process was extensive and involved parts of the middle and upper lobe. In the nineteen cases, the pneumonic process was localized in the lower left lobe in seven; in the right lower lobe in five; in the right upper lobe in four; in the middle lobe in two; and unknown in one.

In a few cases the spleen was palpable but no other evidence of a generalized recticulo endothelial reaction was obvious.

The laboratory findings are shown in the Table No. 4. The majority of cases on ad-

Table 4

Leukocyte count

2,000 to 3,000	0
3,000 to 4,000	1
4,000 to 5,000	0
5,000 to 6,000	2
6,000 to 7,000	2
7,000 to 8,000	3
8,000 to 9 000	4
9,000 to 10,000	5
10,000 to 11,000	2
Above 11,000	0

Polymorphonuclear

50 to 60%	2
60 to 70%	7
70 to 80%	8
Above 80%	2

Sputum

Typed	17
Not typed	2

Sputum typed-Neufeld

Negative	16
Positive	1

mission had a normal or slightly elevated leukocyte count, the largest number having a count from five to ten thousand. There was one with a pronounced leukopenia and but two with a count between ten and eleven thousand. Fifteen of the nineteen cases had a polynuclear count between 60 and 80 percent.

In seventeen out of the nineteen cases, the sputum was examined. In sixteen no pneumococci were found. In one a specific pneumococcus of type thirteen was found. Inasmuch as this is one of the higher types, it is improbable that it was of any etiological significance.

On the whole, the course of the illness in this series was mild and there were no complications. Six patients had less than three febrile days in the hospital, six had three to seven days of temperature elevation and only five had seven to fourteen days of temperature elevation.

Sulfonamide therapy was tried on fifteen patients. No obvious effect on the course of the disease was noted. It is certain that the sulfonamides did not influence the course of the disease, in some instances the patients while receiving the drugs felt worse until the drugs were discontinued. The lack of results obtained with the sulfonamides in this group confirms the conclusion reached by others in reported cases that the sulfonamides in the virus pneumonias are ineffective.

CONCLUSIONS

Within the past ten years three different forms of pneumonia have been observed. In the first phase, before 1935, atypical pneumonias due chiefly to the various streptococci prevailed. In the second phase, typical pneumococcus pneumonias at first amounting to only 10.6 percent of the total number of pneumonias increased almost without interruption until within the past three years the incidence had reached a high of 64 percent. Beginning in May of 1940, a new form of atypical pneumonia made its appearance. The similarity of this group of cases to those described by other observers suggests that the etiological agent was a pneumotropic virus.

An analytical study of nineteen cases of atypical pneumonia showing sex, seasonal incidence, symptoms, physical signs, roentgen ray and laboratory findings and course is presented. The importance of early radiological examination in order to verify diagnosis is stressed. Attention is directed to the fact that there is nothing specific as far as treatment is concerned. The sulfonamide group of drugs are not only ineffective but in most instances tend to aggravate certain symptoms. They are not indicated unless complications due to susceptible organisms occur.

BIBLIOGRAPHY

1. Reimann, H. A.: Journal of American Medical Association, 111:2377, 1938.

2. Longcope, W. T: Bulletin of John Hopkins Hospital, 67:269, 1940.

3. Murray, M. E, Jr: New England Journal of Medical Sciences, 222:No. 14:565.

4. Daniels, M. D.: American Journal of Medical Sciences, 203:2:263, 1942

5. Murray, M. E., Jr.: New England Journal of Medicine, 222:No. 14:565, 1940.

The Weight Gain of Pregnancy*

JOE L. DUER, M.D.*

WOODWARD, OKLAHOMA

All textbooks, articles and lectures that mention the subject remark on the significance of the weight gain of pregnancy and glibly state that the pregnant woman should limit her weight gain to twenty or twenty-five pounds. Clinicians pass this information on to the patient, just as glibly, with no further explanation of the whys and wherefores of this gain. Unfortunately, there are some clinicians who still retain the old idea advanced by Prochownik that the size of the baby can be influenced by diet, often to the distinct detriment of the mother. Judging from the paucity of the information on this subject and the difficulty in finding adequate determinations of just what the gain amounts to or how it arises, it seems that a more careful consideration of the various factors involved is in order.

The developing fetus is an individual, even as you and I. Its size is determined by the admixture of chromosomes, endocrines and metabolic factors that all individuals have. Its nourishment comes from the maternal blood that is constantly present, and the demands of the individual determine the quantity utilized—not the amount that is present in the circulating maternal blood stream. All who have delivered babies have seen large, fat babies from starving, sick women and small, skinny babies from fat, over-fed mothers. Stoeckel reports that the size of babies even increased a little under the war rations in Germany during the last war. Controlling the size of the baby should not be given as a reason for controlling the weight of the mother.

*Doctor Duer is now a Lieutenant in the Navy and is stationed at the Naval Base Hospital, Norman, Oklahoma.

Mothers, as well as many clinicians, are in the dark as to where this increase of "20 to 25 pounds" comes from. The average full-term baby weighs about 7½ pounds. This varies slightly with sex, males averaging a little more. The average placenta weighs about one-sixth that of the baby, or about one pound. The pregnant uterus weighs about two pounds whereas the non-pregnant uterus weighs from one to two ounces. The amount of amniotic fluid varies a great deal but will average about two quarts with an average weight of four pounds. Just so does the weight gain of the breasts vary so that no adequate figure can be presented. Nevertheless, to estimate an average of one pound per breast seems not to be out of order. In addition there is some increase in the blood volume of the mother and a slight hypertrophy of the heart which adds a variable amount of weight. No adequate figures for this latter are available. The table below shows graphically what has just been presented.

It will be noted that the above figures are estimates and averages and that any of the factors might vary considerably in a given individual. For instance, the increase in the breast weight is noticeably variable in different individuals and the figure given is merely a guess.

Likewise, the increase in blood volume, although proven, cannot be stated with exactness. Hobbauer states: "The preponderance of evidence indicates a remarkable increase of the blood volume in pregnant women." Although the amount of increase seems to be questionable it is agreed that it is sufficient to increase the cardiac output as much

Wt. Factor	Normal	Wt. at Term	Gain
New Born	——	7½ lbs.	7½ lbs.
Placenta	——	1-1½ lbs.	1-1½ lbs.
Amniotic fluid	——	2 lbs.	2 lbs.
Uterus	1-2 oz.	2 lbs.	2 lbs.
Breasts	Variable	Variable	Est. ave. 2 lbs.
Blood Vol. Etc.	?	?	?
Known totals	1-2 oz.	13 lbs.	15 lbs.

as from 50 percent to 60 percent of the normal non-pregnant volume. Consequently, it seems not unreasonable to ascribe an appreciable weight gain to this factor.

The amount of amniotic fluid is also a very variable factor. It is usually averaged at about one quart. Orey (Curtis) states that more than 2,000 cc. may be considered as polyhydramnios, while less than 500 cc. is oligohydramnios.

Since it was previously stated that the control of the baby's size is not a reason for controlling the mother's weight, other reasons must necessarily follow. They can be summarized as follows:

First, and most important, controlling the mother's weight reduces the load on the circulatory and excretory systems and lessens toxemia.

Second, the over-weight woman with flabby muscles may expect gestation and labor to be somewhat more difficult and inconvenient.

Third, the over-weight woman is less likely to be able to nurse the baby.

Fourth, an appealing point to most women is the preservation of graceful feminine lines.

Experience has shown that the over-weight woman is more susceptable to toxemia. Much of the extra weight present in toxic individuals is usually due to edema, but it must be remembered that even before edema develops, either in occult or manifest proportions, every extra ounce of fat requires an increase in circulation for its maintenance. Likewise, these same extra ounces have metabolic products that must be excreted. In an individual whose circulatory and excretory systems are doing extra work because of the pregnancy, this extra work may easily become the deciding factor between a toxic and non-toxic condition. Especially is this true in individuals whose circulatory and excretory organs have been damaged by previous diseases.

Polyhydramnion and multiple pregnancy naturally augment the weight gain. These conditions are also more commonly associated with the toxic state than is the normal hydramnion or the single pregnancy, and they must be considered in the patient who has gained a great deal of weight.

A case that illustrates the association of many factors is that of Mrs. W. L., age 32. Third pregnancy. History of having "kidney poison" and considerable edema in each of the previous pregnancies but had gone through labor uneventfully. Her usual weight was about 240.

She was brought to the hospital at the beginning of the last month of pregnancy in an extremely toxic condition, having blindness, convulsions, generalized heavy pitting edema, blood pressure 160/110, and the urine heavily loaded with albumin, casts, red and white cells. She had had no prenatal care whatsoever. A diagnosis of advanced eclampsia, with albuminuric retinitis and convulsions, and multiple pregnancy was made.

After hospitalization and treatment had controlled the toxic symptoms and reduced the edema, her weight was still 337 pounds. Close observation and care for 12 days succeeded in getting her condition on a relatively safe basis and labor was induced (I say "induced" with reservations) by two ounces of castor oil given orally and she spontaneously and precipitously delivered full-term twins, weight 7¾ and 4¾ pounds. Being of opposite sex, each was in a separate amnion with about the usual amount of fluid in each (one quart). The post-partum course was uneventful thereafter.

This case represents: (1) Uncontrolled diet and exercise, in fact, the absence of all the usual accepted ante-partum care; (2) History suggestive of pre-existing renal damage; (3) Multiple pregnancy with an increased total amount of amniotic fluid, though not an actual polyhydramnion; (4) A marked increase in weight due to diet, multiple pregnancy, increase of amniotic fluid, and severe edema; (5) An evident glandular type of obesity; (6) The toxemia, convulsions, etc., which were probably inevitable in the face of the other existing conditions.

You may answer as you will, why she and her babies are still living and thriving after a year, having been just turned loose down in the black-jacks with one post-partum call since they were dismissed from the hospital. This patient returned to the office eleven months after delivery in the first trimester of her fourth pregnancy. Weight 237 pounds. Urine normal. Blood Pressure 130/80.

The previous case represents the unusual. As a rule, the patient continues on her way gaining fairly regularly. Suddenly it is noted that she has gained twice or three times as much as usual between visits. The urine and blood pressure may still be normal. On the next visit, if the weight persists, it will most likely be noted that albumin appears in the urine and that the blood pressure rises considerably. So often has this sequence been noted that I am beginning to believe that the scales are better indicators of impending toxic states than either the test tube or the sphygmomanometer.

A rather striking illustration is shown by the case of Mrs. W.P., age 17. A primiparous woman who had gained 23 pounds up to the beginning of the last month of pregnancy and had shown no signs or symptoms of trouble. She neglected to report during the last month of pregnancy until the day before delivery. It was found that she had gained 18 pounds during the last month. Blood pressure was 130/80. The urine showed a slight trace of albumin with no cellular elements. There was a slight amount of edema of the feet and ankles. She was having slight, irregular pains at the time. More regular labor pains started after about six hours, and within eight hours she had delivered a normal seven pound and fourteen ounce boy without hemorrhage or laceration. Her condition was quite good. Two hours after delivery she vomited profusely and immediately went into the first of three post-partum convulsions. These were controlled and further progress was uneventful, except for the rapid changes in her blood pressure which ranged from 118/80 to 160/110 with hourly fluctuations. This continued for four days and then became steady at about 120/80. I have no explanation of these phenomena. Her urine remained normal and she has since gone through her second pregnancy quite normally. Needless to say her regime was much more rigid than during her first pregnancy. No such fluctuation of blood pressure occurred following the second delivery, nor have I observed it in other convulsive patients.

Most women know very little about pregnancy and, as a rule, they are very willing to learn. If they are interested enough to present themselves for prenatal care sometime during the earlier months of pregnancy, it is the doctor's duty to help maintain that interest and encourage cooperation by proper instruction. Among other things, they should be told how much they may expect to gain and why they should keep their weight within bounds.

No one likes a rigid diet and since pregnancy is supposed to be a normal physiological process, the pregnant woman should not be rationed unless it becomes quite necessary. She should be taught the caloric value of food, the importance of a well balanced diet and the necessity for an adequate supply of minerals and vitamins. The basic diet should consist of milk, green vegetables, some lean meat, eggs, fruits and fruit juices. Other foods should be eaten sparingly and not in various combinations. This basic diet has the advantage of being well supplied with the minerals and vitamins—except D which should be given in the form of cod liver oil.

Exercise should be encouraged so long as there are no contraindications. This should be well within the usual limits of the particular patient's habits and stamina.

CONCLUSIONS

This paper was prepared with a view of presenting some of the salient factors in the weight gain of pregnancy. The factors involved in the normal gain in weight have been presented and some of the important reasons for controlling the weight during pregnancy have been outlined. Methods of control have been suggested.

BIBLIOGRAPHY

1. Gray's Anatomy.
2. Williams' Obstetrics.
3. Danforth, Wm. G.: The Management of Normal Pregnancy—Curtis, Ob. and Gyn., Vol 1, Chap XXI.
4. Hofbauer, J. I.: Maternal Changes Incident to Pregnancy—Curtis, Ob. and Gyn., Vol. I, Pp. 613-143, 1934.
5. Gammeltaft, R.: Surgery, Gynecology and Obstetrics. Chap. XIVI, P. 382, 1928.
6. Douglas, R. G.: Treatment of Pregnancy and Labor—Reiman, Treatment in General Medicine, Vol II, Chapter XXXIX, 1939.
7. Smith, E. N.: Abstract of Lectures in Obstetrics, Oklahoma State Medical Association. 1938-1939.
8. Dannreuther, W. T. and Hyams, M. N.: Bridges—Dietetics for the Clinician, Third Edition, Pp. 414-445, 1937.

Vital Banana Diet to Celiac Suffers Assured

The United Fruit Company has announced that it has made provisions so that all children suffering from celiac, a nutritional disturbance of late infancy and early childhood for which a diet of bananas is the indicated therapy, will receive priority for necessary supply of bananas, despite the present shortage of bananas brought about by the U-boat activity in the Caribbean.

The Company, in response to queries from physicians and anxious mothers, has arranged to give priority on bananas to all celiac cases. In face of the scarcity caused by war conditions and lack of ships, the Company states that so long as there are bananas at all in this country, they will make every effort to see that such patients are supplied.

Anyone who is unable to obtain bananas for celiac sufferers is advised to have their doctor write or telegraph the Fruit Dispatch Company, Pier 3, North River, New York City.

Give me health and a day and I will make the pomp of emperors ridiculous.—Ralph Waldo Emerson.

Do not forget that of all the countless remedies, rest, alone, has stood the test of time.—Gerald B. Webb, M.D.

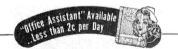

• *THE PRESIDENT'S PAGE* •

The October 31 issue of the American Medical Association Journal contains an article on Gasoline and Tire Rationing written by John R. Richards, Chief Gasoline Rationing Branch Office of Price Administration. The statements made in this article are highly complimentary and very flattering to the medical profession. The statements contained therein are not only complimentary, but absolutely true. When these regulations were framed the medical profession was one of the first to be provided for, due of course to its importance to the public.

Mr. Richards states, "Without question or hesitation, doctors have been and will be granted all the gasoline needed to carry out their professional work. We hope that they will regard their concrete symbol of their indispensability, the C book, as a moral obligation and not a personal privilege. From another point of view, the C book is a part of a doctor's equipment; it should not be used for anything but the work of humanity."

The article goes on to show the doctor how he can set a splendid example for others in the saving of gasoline, thus saving precious rubber. Conversely, if granted a C book, see how many unused coupons you can return to your local board. The moral affect of such an act on your fellow citizens will be incalculable. Doctors are the leaders and molders of public opinion in their community.

Now let's set the example by scrupulously observing the thirty-five mile speed limit, except in cases of emergencies. Refrain from any kind of driving whatever which might appear to be non-essential in the eyes of the public. Let the doctors, as a group, observe the letter and spirit of the Regulations. If you can find time, read the article in full.

May it be the lot of each one of you to spend a most Happy Christmas and a Prosperous 1943.

Sincerely yours,

James D Osborn

President.

We squeezed into this bottle...

a TON of

LIVER

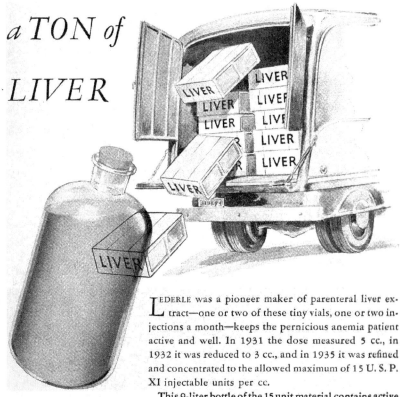

LEDERLE was a pioneer maker of parenteral liver extract—one or two of these tiny vials, one or two injections a month—keeps the pernicious anemia patient active and well. In 1931 the dose measured 5 cc., in 1932 it was reduced to 3 cc., and in 1935 it was refined and concentrated to the allowed maximum of 15 U. S. P. XI injectable units per cc.

This 9-liter bottle of the 15 unit material contains active material obtained from 2000 pounds of beef liver. Its concentration to so fine a point is the fruit of eleven years of progress and experience (1931-1942) which has kept Lederle out among the leaders in this field.

Specify ***Lederle***

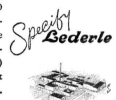

The JOURNAL Of The
OKLAHOMA STATE MEDICAL ASSOCIATION

EDITORIAL BOARD
L. J. MOORMAN, Oklahoma City, Editor-in-Chief

E. EUGENE RICE, Shawnee

NED R. SMITH, Tulsa

MR. R. H. GRAHAM, Oklahoma City, Business Manager

CONTRIBUTIONS: Articles accepted by this Journal for publication including those read at the annual meetings of the State Association are the sole property of this Journal.

The Editorial Department is not responsible for the opinions expressed in the original articles of contributors.

Manuscripts may be withdrawn by authors for publication elsewhere only upon the approval of the Editorial Board.

MANUSCRIPTS: Manuscripts should be typewritten, double-spaced, on white paper 8½ x 11 inches. The original copy, not the carbon copy, should be submitted.

Footnotes, bibliographies and legends for cuts should be typed on separate sheets in double space. Bibliography listing should follow this order: Name of author, title of article, name of periodical with volume, page and date of publication.

Manuscripts are accepted subject to the usual editorial revisions and with the understanding that they have not been published elsewhere.

NEWS: Local news of interest to the medical profession, changes of address, births, deaths and weddings will be gratefully received.

ADVERTISING: Advertising of articles, drugs or compounds unapproved by the Council on Pharmacy of the A.M.A. will not be accepted. Advertising rates will be supplied on application.

It is suggested that members of the State Association patronize our advertisers in preference to others.

SUBSCRIPTIONS: Failure to receive The Journal should call for immediate notification.

REPRINTS: Reprints of original articles will be supplied at actual cost provided request for them is attached to manuscripts or made in sufficient time before publication. Checks for reprints should be made payable to Industrial Printing Company, Oklahoma City.

Address all communications to THE JOURNAL OF THE OKLAHOMA STATE MEDICAL ASSOCIATION, 210 Plaza Court, Oklahoma City.

OFFICIAL PUBLICATION OF THE OKLAHOMA STATE MEDICAL ASSOCIATION
Copyrighted October, 1942

EDITORIALS

"THE MASTER-WORD IN MEDICINE"

In one of Osler's matchless essays, he indicates that the master-word is *work*.

Perhaps the outstanding verification of this statement is to be found in his textbook *The Principles and Practice of Medicine*, the first edition of which came from the press in 1892. After more than forty years of preparation, this monumental work was prepared for publication in less than eighteen months.

For a long time the writing of this great book had been on Osler's mind, but he had "continually procrastinated on the plea that up to the fortieth year a man was fit for better things than textbooks." As he passed this age, he made the following confession: "I began to feel that the energy and persistence necessary for the task were lacking." It is interesting to note that even Osler, with his knowledge and experience plus a God given facility for expression, needed a little prodding. But what is of greater importance is the fact that Osler's conscience was quite sensative, he felt the sharp thrust of duty, marshalled the energy and mastered the difficult task. Relatively few doctors realize the full significance of this accomplishment.

For approximately forty years, Watson's celebrated *Practice* had been the student's guide. Other texts had been published, but none fully met the need. It should be remembered that Osler's decision came when medical science was in a state of flux; in that notable decade of 1880 to 1890, which initiated a period of remarkable scientific development and which needed conservative consideration and sane recording. This was a critical period, and America was most fortunate in having a man so well fitted for the task. Harvey Cushing said, "He was, all things considered, extraordinarily well equipped to undertake the task. The one 'weakness' which has been mentioned proved in a curious way, as will be seen, an unexpected and most important service to medicine in general. For it led, in an indirect way, to the rescue of the hospital from its financial embarrassment after the Baltimore fire in 1903; to the establishment of the Rockefeller Institute a few years later; and, finally, to the incalculable benefit to humanity which the General Education Board has rendered with Mr. Rockefeller's money, owing to its interest in the prevention and cure of disease. Indeed, the present position of his colleague Welch, as Director of the Institute of Hygiene, is remotely due to the fact that Osler set himself thirty years before to write a textbook of Medicine, and, as Falconer Madan said years later, 'succeeded in making a scientific treatise literature.' "

Every student and every doctor, who consults this great textbook, should know what Fielding H. Garrison thought of its illustrious author. "When he came to die, Osler was, in a very real sense, the greatest physician of our time. He was one of Nature's chosen. Good looks, distinction, blithe, benignant manners, a sunbright personality, radiant with kind feeling and good will toward his fellow men, an Apollonian poise, swiftness and surety of thought and speech, every gift of the Gods was his; and to these were added careful training, unsurpassed clinical ability, the widest knowledge of his subject, the deepest interest in everything human, and a serene hold upon his fellows that was as a seal set upon them. His enthusiasm for his calling was boundless. As Hare says, 'Osler went into the post-mortem room with the joyous demeanor of the youthful Sophocles leading the chorus of victory after the battle of Salamis.' All young English and American physicians who have followed the science and art of medicine in this spirit have been 'pupils of Osler.' His writings have been aptly described as belonging to the true 'literature of power.' "

Eighteen years ago, Garrison said "Osler's *Principles and Practice of Medicine* is the best English textbook on the subject in our time."

The cloak of responsibility has successively descended upon the shoulders of sound editors. The Fourteenth Edition, which is reviewed in this issue of the Journal, indicates that McCrae and Christian have faithfully preserved the spirit of the author and that the text continues to merit Garrison's appraisal of eighteen years ago.

Aside from the fact that Osler's textbook merits this editorial mention, the Fourteenth Edition possesses an additional appeal for all loyal Oklahoma doctors. Twenty-two years ago, in the basement of St. Anthony's Hospital, an Oklahoma boy, then a student extern, was introduced to the present editor, Doctor Christian, with the recommendation that he be permitted to take the examinations for intern service at Peter Bent Brigham Hospital in Boston. This boy, Charles L. Brown, a graduate of the University of Oklahoma School of Medicine, now stands among the three outstanding internists to whom this edition of Osler is dedicated.

THE WARY TUBERCULE BACILLUS

The tubercle bacillus has ever been the research worker's enigma. The fractional analysis of this micro-organism has shown that the saccharides are among the important toxic elements. It has been shown that when these saccharides are introduced into the blood of the healthy animal, they promptly appear in the urine; but when introduced into the blood of an animal suffering from tuberculosis, they do not appear in demonstrable form and it must be assumed that they are present but bound in such a way as to evade present methods of detection.

If a simple method of detection is discovered and the significance of their presence properly appraised, it may be discovered that they have great clinical and diagnostic value. The research committee of the National Tuberculosis Association has had this under consideration, and it is to be hoped that something practical may come out of the interesting studies constantly in progress.

Truly, the tubercle bacillus continues to merit the term "a bug full of tricks." No doubt the average doctor wonders why tuberculosis does not respond to chemotherapy. Perhaps the tubercle bacillus anticipated chemotherapy ten thousand years ago and, through some strange, intuitive sense, developed a waxy capsule and planned its onslaught in the cells and its more permanent residence in caseous material away from the circulation. In this way, it escapes chemical agents which are conveyed by body fluids to the field of battle.

So the fight on the tubercle bacillus must go on with no assurance of a short cut to victory.

IMPORTANCE OF LOCAL AND REGIONAL MEETINGS

The Oklahoma City Clinical Society conducted its Twelfth Annual Clinical assembly the last week in October.

The program was of the usual high order and the attendance exceptionally good considering the fact that so many of the younger men are in the war and that the urgent demands upon those remaining at home make it difficult for them to attend meetings. This post-graduate assembly has rendered a great service and because of it, the doctors who were in attendance are better prepared to serve the people of Oklahoma.

It was gratifying to hear Dr. James E. Paullin, President-Elect of the American Medical Association, assert his approval of such regional medical meetings.

The necessity of keeping up with the development of "War Medicine" alone should justify the continuation of local and regional meetings.

TO LIVE IN HEARTS

(*Editor's Note*: The following Editorial was inspired by the death of a faithful family physician. It appeared in a Virginia Daily Newspaper and is so representative of what a physician's life should be, it is reproduced for the benefit of those who read the Journal. The author was well acquainted with this beloved exponent of the medical profession, and it is his opinion that the high place he held in the hearts of his people was largely due to strict adherence to the fundamental principles found in the Hippocratic oath. This type of individual integrity with such widespread recognition and acclaim could never come to a doctor working under any form of socialized medicine.

He was in active practice in one location 56 years. Not many ministers of the gospel remain with one church a full lifetime. This "incomparable citizen" visited the poor and the rich alike and cared for the small and the great without discrimination. For more than 50 years he served as physician to a famous woman's college, thus extending his service and his influence from coast to coast.)

"In every community there are citizens who stand out from the mass because of some special performances in the line of civic duty, of some special quality that makes them valuable members of the society. Some of these are great, some are good, some merely important, but all of them have made their contribution. They are prominent citizens.

"Sometimes to a community there comes one who stands out among those who are known and esteemed, who is universally respected, admired, loved. He is unique in that community. Asked by a stranger for some example of concrete achievement by this esteemed citizen, those who speak his praises do not respond promptly and unanimously to tell of some beautiful building of which he was the inspiration, or of some great business giving employment to thousands and known for its integrity in operation, or of some quality of superiority in his chosen profession, or of a long line of activities in community affairs. Some of these things, or others, he has done. It is not for

lack of specific contribution to community welfare or community happiness or community beauty that those who are asked to specify pause before replying, or do not wholly agree when they do reply. It is because what the man has done is obscured in what the man is.

"What is the quality that overshadows performance? Pat to mind comes the word character. That, yes, but something more than that, something in addition to that Humanity? That sometimes abused word does not suffice. Devotion to his work did not blind him, rather it opened his eyes, to the humanities of life, but the picture is not complete, does not end the search of the stranger for the explanation of this man's hold upon his fellow citizens. Sweetness of soul, kindliness of thought, charity and tolerance which altogether do not undermine strength. "He that walketh uprightly . . . and speaketh the truth in his heart. He that backbiteth not with his tongue. . . . He that sweareth to his own heart and changeth not . . . nor taketh reward against the innocent." The seeker after knowledge of what manner of man is this is impressed. He has acquired knowledge. But full understanding is not his. It can't be—yet.

"For this man has lived long, and the years have made the pattern. And years are required to know it. This man did not catapult himself upon the community with a flaming perforance or a flaming personality. His entry into the hearts of his people was by slow penetration, and it is by slow process only, and by familiarity, that the miracle can be understood. The stranger gets a glimpse when he first sees this man, for the secret shines in his face, but it is only in time that this first impression is confirmed and made lasting. It is only by association, by unconscious absorption, that full understanding comes, and the stranger finds himself at last among those who know and enjoy and are comforted but who are inarticulate when they are asked to tell why in words which can not be found. Then, he is a stranger no more.

"When such a man, after a long life that is a benediction, dies there is mourning, but not too much. For such a man does not die, and the people know it. They will have him with them as long as memory lasts."

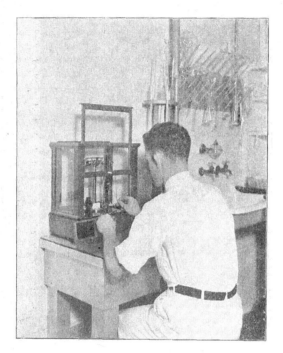

ASSOCIATION ACTIVITIES

THE NEED FOR DOCTORS' COOPERATION WITH "BLUE CROSS PLAN"

In May, 1940, the Oklahoma State Medical Association with the cooperation of the Oklahoma Hospital Association started the Blue Cross Plan. Two and one-half years have now passed, 30,000 members have been enrolled, 65 hospitals in the state have signed as member hospitals guaranteeing the service of the plan. Each month the plan pays out $10,000.00 to these hospitals in care for these members. By so doing, the plan fills a long felt need for the average family.

The management of the plan, however, now finds itself faced with the problem that only the doctors can solve if we are to maintain our standards.

The fundamental principle of all the 76 Blue Cross Plans in the United States is that *the attending physician shall determine when the patient shall enter the hospital and when he shall be dismissed.* The rates our members pay and the benefits they receive are based on the promise:

1. That only cases be admitted to the hospital which would normally be hospitalized if the plan did not exist.

2. That conditions be excluded which are known to require hospital care before the date of application for Blue Cross.

3. That the patient be dismissed by the attending physician, when in the physician's opinion, the patient is able to go home, and that the patient not be permitted to stay as long as he wishes, unless he pays for the extra days himself.

One of the main reasons for starting the Oklahoma plan was to discourage undesirable procedures from getting started, particularly a federal program of health care. Under a federal program there would be a great deal of regimentation of doctor, hospital, and patient. We believe it is a fair statement to say that the 76 nonprofit Blue Cross Hospital Plans in the United States with 11,000,000 people enrolled have so far played a very important role in keeping a federal program from getting under way. However, in order to enjoy this freedom, with no alteration in the doctor, hospital, and patient relationship, it is necessary that the proper responsibility be assumed by the physicians who attend the Blue Cross patients. The following comparison as to length of stay by Blue Cross patients and those who do not belong to the plan will demonstrate the point.

	Blue Cross Patients	Patients Who Pay Their Own Bills
Maternity	10.6 days	5 to 7 days
Appendectomy	11.0 days	6 to 7 days
Tonsillectomy	2.0 days	1 day
Hernia	15.0 days	8 to 10 days

The purpose of Blue Cross is to make it possible for the members of a family to go to the hospital when they need hospital care without delay, without red tape, and without financial embarrassment. It is capable of doing so in a fine way, but only if they are dismissed when care is no longer necessary.

The contract issued to Blue Cross members clearly states that the obligation of the plan ceases when, in the opinion of the attending physician, hospital care is no longer needed for the patient. If the attending physician gives this information to the hospital, it is a simple matter for the hospital to notify the patient that financial arrangements for a longer stay will have to be made.

We realize that there may be cases where the patient will tease the doctor to stay longer when the plan is paying the bill, but during these trying times it is easy to explain that it is a patriotic duty of every patient to make room for other people needing care. During the past year it has become common practice in many sections of the country to arbitrarily establish a limit on the length of stay for the normal cases, in order to provide beds for other patients and keep the hospital occupancy at a point where efficient service may be rendered by the hospital.

When the patient's hospital bill is paid by the Blue Cross Plan, he is then in a much better position to pay the doctor. If the patient were to pay the hospital first in cash, he seldom has enough funds left to pay the doctor.

"Let us not kill the goose that laid the golden egg."

OKLAHOMA CITY CLINICAL SOCIETY

On numerous occasions throughout the year the officers of the Oklahoma City Clinical Society met and discussed the advisability of holding the twelfth annual conference of the society, and each time, with some misgiving, decided to proceed with the preparations. Their decision was thoroughly justified with the successful culmination of the meeting.

It was particularly gratifying to note that the lecture rooms were consistently well attended. Evidently the doctors attending the conference came for the serious purpose of obtaining information from the guest speakers. The society was particularly fortunate in obtaining teachers who presented excellent, practical material, and the entire program was outstanding from an academic standpoint.

The registration was about 15 percent under that of last year. Considering the number of physicians in the Southwest who have entered military service, the registration was considered exceptional.

Dr. James E. Paullin, President-Elect of the American Medical Association, in a letter received since the meeting adjourned, stated: "I was very much impressed with the seriousness of your organization, with the quality of men whom you had on the program, and with their eagerness to teach those who attended their lectures a lesson, and the earnestness in carrying out this purpose. . . . I do hope you will not abandon your meetings. . . ." The Oklahoma City Clinical Society appreciates this tribute, and will extend every effort to continue presenting clinics of scientific worth.

Dr. Galbraith Appointed Member of Medical Advisory Committee

Dr. Hugh M. Galbraith of Oklahoma City has been appointed by Mr. J. B. Harper, Director of the Oklahoma Department of Public Welfare, to replace Dr. Moorman P. Prosser of Norman, who has been called to duty with the Armed Forces, as a member of the Medical Advisory Committee of the Oklahoma State Medical Association to the Public Welfare Department.

Other members of the Committee are: Dr. C. R. Rountree, Oklahoma City, Chairman; Dr. Walker Morledge, Oklahoma City; Dr. Alfred R. Sugg, Ada; Dr. Clinton Gallaher, Shawnee, and Dr. R. M. Shepard, Tulsa.

Dr. Prosser is the second of the original six-member Committee to be called into Service. Dr. F. Redding Hood of Oklahoma City left in June and was replaced by Dr. Morledge.

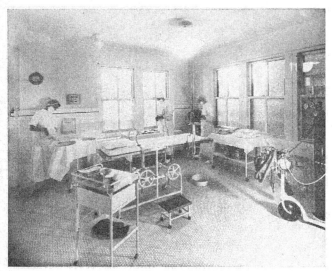

SUPPLEMENTARY ROSTER

(*Indicates serving in armed forces).

The following is the list of 1942 memberships that have been received in the Executive Office of the Association since the publication of the roster in the July issue of the Journal:

Bryan
BOLINGER, E. W. ....Achille
HYDE, W. A. ....Durant
RUTHERFORD, J. P. ....Bennington
WEBB, JAMES P. ....Durant

Choctaw
SWITZER, FRED D. ....Hugo

Hughes
*SHAW, JAMES F. ....Wetumka

Jefferson
YEATS, H. WESLEY ....Ringling
(member Bryan Co. Medical Society)

Johnston
LOONEY, J. T. ....Tishomingo

McClain
COCHRAN, J. E. ....Byars

Oklahoma
*BIRGE, JACK P. ....Ramsey Tower
CRICK, L. E. ....Britton
*DILL, FRANCIS E. ....Medical Arts Bldg.
ELEY, N. PRICE ....1200 N. Walker
EPLEY, C. O. ....1200 N. Walker
MOTH, M. V. ....American Nat'l Bldg.
SMITH, L. L. ....220 S. W. 29th
WILLIAMS, LEONARD C. ....1200 N. Walker

Payne
CLEVERDON, L. A. ....Stillwater

Pittsburg
PACKARD, LOUIS A. ....McAlester

Seminole
PRICE, J. T. ....Seminole
WRIGHT, HERBERT L. ....Sasakwa

Tillman
ROBINSON, R. D. ....Frederick

Tulsa
*STUARD, C. G. ....Jefferson Barracks, Mo.

APPRECIATION OF JOURNAL EXPRESSED

The following letter has been received in the office of the Editor-in-Chief of the Journal. Prior to Dr. Seeley's transfer to active duty, he was Executive Director of the Procurement and Assignment Service, Washington, D. C.

ASHFORD GENERAL HOSPITAL
White Sulphur Springs, West Virginia
November 3, 1942

Editor
Journal of the Oklahoma State Medical Association
Oklahoma City, Oklahoma

Dear Sir:

Please accept my thanks for the marked copy of the October Journal of the Oklahoma State Medical Association and for the generous statements included in your editorial with reference to my assignment back to the Office of the Surgeon General for duty.

Please convey to my many friends in Oklahoma my sincere thanks for the hospitality and care which I received at their hands during my tour of office with the Procurement and Assignment Service. No single individual can be deserving of the honors attendant to the assignment which I enjoyed so much. My congratulations to your State for fulfilling its quota so readily.

Sincerely yours,
Sam F. Seeley
Lt. Col., M. C.

Word has been received that Dr. H. A. Schubert of Chickasha is presently stationed with the 396th Medical Sanitary Company, Camp Maxey, Texas.

FIFTH CIRCUIT IN POSTGRADUATE INTERNAL MEDICINE OPENS

The next circuit, or fifth, in postgraduate medicine will open in Oklahoma City, Norman, Pauls Valley, Shawnee and Wewoka or Holdenville the week of January 11. Dr. L. W. Hunt, from the Medical Faculty, University of Chicago, is now giving his lectures in the fourth circuit with the following number enrolled:

Tulsa	75
Sapulpa	21
Ponca City	19
Stillwater	10
Pawhuska	18

A total of 400 physicians have enrolled and taken the course in the first four circuits. It is significant to observe that the total enrollments have exceeded both the programs in obstetrics and pediatrics up to the present, and this has occurred during the war time when many physicians state that their Medical Societies are finding it difficult to maintain a quorum for meetings. There is an occasional physician who says he is too busy to attend these courses, but the vast majority insists that they are more important now than in the past because they cannot go away for post study.

Doctor Hunt has already given more than 500 consultations. Apparently physicians have confidence in his practical ability over cases in practice.

It should be understood by all that the course in medicine, by Doctor Hunt, is being received with much enthusiasm by physicians in all sections.

Those interested in enrolling for the fifth circuit may turn in their enrollments to the Secretary of the County Medical Society (in Oklahoma City to the Chairman of the Committee on Organization) or mail them direct to the Postgraduate Committee, 210 Plaza Court, Oklahoma City.

PRELIMINARY REPORT OF THE PUBLIC POLICY COMMITTEE

As Chairman of your Committee on Public Policies, I wish to report that on the eve of the convening legislature we know of no medical legislation that, in this war time, is of importance to bring to the attention of our law making body, but there is a matter of paramount importance to us, as physicians, at this moment. It is proper that we supply our armed forces with sufficient medical personnel.

The Sub-Committee on Manpower of the Senate Committee on Education and Labor of the United States Senate has submitted a report to the Committee in respect to the supply of physicians available to meet the military, industrial and civilian needs. This report is a rather lengthy document and I will summarize some of the salient points.

First, there is a scarcity of physicians to fill all three needs; namely, that of the armed forces, industrial demands and civilian needs. Second, the distribution of physicians entering the armed forces has been uneven throughout the country. Third, the demands of industry are concentrated in some areas much more than in others, and lastly, the civilian needs in certain localities have become acute.

In regard to the first point, I am proud to state that our Oklahoma physicians have volunteered for medical service very patriotically and to quote from this report "the armed services, the Federal Government and the public should know now that certain states as South Carolina and Oklahoma have produced from three to four times as many doctors for the armed services in proportion to peace time supplies as such states as New York and Illinois."

The industrial demands in Oklahoma are undoubtedly much less than those of many of our states more favored by war industries, but these demands in our state are increasing as is now evident at the Chouteau plant and in the Douglas Bomber plant at Tulsa and soon will be evident in the Cargo Plane plant in Oklahoma City. Some of our communities are being stripped dangerously bare of medical personnel.

In view of these facts, I think it would behoove the Secretaries and Presidents of every County Medical Society in the state to make a careful survey and have the results available at all times, because in the very near future the country is to be surveyed at the request of this Committee of the Senate to ascertain the present status of medical service to the civilian and industrial population therein. If the officers of each County Medical Society could make such information available for compilation in the office of our State Medical Association, the action of the Senate Committee should be greatly facilitated.

J. T. Martin, M.D., Chairman,
Public Policy Committee.

COMMONWEALTH FUND ANNOUNCES FELLOWSHIPS AVAILABLE FOR POSTGRADUATE STUDY

Announcement has just been received from Dr. Harry E. Handley, Assistant Director of the Division of Public Health of the Commonwealth Fund, that the Fund is planning to make available a limited number of fellowships to qualified physicians during 1943 despite the fact that postgraduate instruction has been drastically reduced in most of the medical schools.

As in the past, perference will be given to physicians in the younger age group and those practicing in the smaller communities. Dr. Handley states, however, that it is his opinion that the general practitioners who have not reached the age of 55 will be given favorable consideration as well as those physicians who are practicing in larger communities, and that it is probable that work which is of a somewhat more special character will be considered than has been available in the past.

The duration of the fellowships will be determined by the work which is available in the teaching centers selected, and the needs of the individual. At the present time, the only postgraduate instruction being planned at Tulane in 1943 is concerned with short intensive courses. A course in pediatrics is planned for the period January 25-28 and tentative plans are under consideration for courses in internal medicine and obstetrics and gynecology. Harvard is planning a refresher course in medicine of a month's duration to be given in October, 1943.

Those awarded fellowships will receive a modest stipend plus a reimbursement for tuition and travel expense.

Interested physicians should make application directly to the Commonwealth Fund, 41 East 57th Street, New York City.

Public Health Doctors Attend Meeting

Representatives from the Oklahoma State Health Department, who attended the meeting of the American Public Health Association held in St. Louis, Mo., October 26 to 28, 1942, were Dr. Grady F. Mathews, Commissioner, Dr. James T. Bell, Dr. John W. Shackelford, and Dr. John F. Hackler, all of Oklahoma City.

County Health officials attending the National meeting included Dr. H. C. Huntley of Atoka, Dr. F. W. Highfill of Duncan, and Dr. Paul Sizemore of Durant.

Dr. Turner Attends Meeting in Chicago

"Persistence of Estrogen Induced Sexual Development" was the topic selected for presentation by Dr. Henry H. Turner of Oklahoma City before the Regional Meeting of the American College of Physicians at the Drake Hotel in Chicago, Saturday, November 21.

The meeting included the states of Illinois, Indiana, Iowa, Michigan and Wisconsin and followed "Postgraduate Nights" at Camp Grant, November 19, and at Great Lakes Naval Training Station, November 20.

RECORD OF BIRTH CERTIFICATE REQUESTS

The entry of our Nation in war on December 8, 1941, brought about an unanticipated and unknown demand on the Division of Vital Statistics of the Oklahoma State Health Department for birth certificates. Birth certificates are required for employment in the vast manufacturing war program, as well as for various phases of the armored forces. Dealing with this large number of applications for certificates has clearly and definitely demonstrated and shown that in the past years in our state we did not have complete of accurate birth records.

Dr. G. F. Mathews, Commissioner of the Oklahoma State Health Department, gives the following facts, as well as the following suggestions to improve birth reporting within the state.

Total Number of Certified Copies of Birth Certificates Issued since December 7—Pearl Harbor	334,299
Number of Delayed Certificates Filed, where either doctor, parents, or registrar failed to put record on file	164,000
Of the above number, Births Occurring in Oklahoma prior to 1908	27,000
Affidavits Correcting Birth Certificates on file Incomplete by doctor, parents, or registrar	6,782
Delayed Certificates Filed for July, 1942 Births prior to 1908	3,618
Since 1908, where either doctor, parents, or registrar failed to file original certificate	5,562
June Affidavits of Correction; original birth certificates Incomplete (This costs the parent an additional 50 cents)	1,181

Checking the applications for 334,299 birth certificates clearly shows that the failure in the past to have complete and accurate birth certificate reporting within our state rests (1) with the doctor, (2) with the parents, and (3) with State Health Department local registrars.

Suggestions for Improving Birth Reporting Within the State

1. All birth certificates should be completed in unfading black ink or typewritten.
2. Check as to whether child was born *alive* or *stillborn.*
3. Always give place of birth (Some doctors write in the county, and give the place of birth as *rural.*)
4. Give the mother's mailing address.
5. When twins are born, make a birth certificate for each child.
6. Insist on getting the name of child when completing the history of parents.
7. Birth certificates are transcribed and mailed to the Bureau of Census, Washington, D. C., and if they are not complete, they are returned to the State Health Department for further and complete information.

Delay in getting birth certificates has led up to loss of many man hours in the great industrial armament program.

It is mandatory under the laws of our State that all births be promptly reported. Birth certificates under law should be completed by the attending physician and filed with the local registrar by the first day of each month. It is further mandatory that the local registrars have all of the birth certificates in the hands of the State Health Department not later than the tenth day of each month.

Major Onis G. Hazel, formerly of Oklahoma City, is presently stationed with the U. S. Army Air Forces at Benjamin Field, Tampa, Fla.

Dr. Joe Leslie Duer of Woodward has been called to duty with the Navy, effective December 7, as a Lieutenant, senior grade, and is stationed at the new Naval Base Hospital, Norman, Okla.

NINE-YEAR REPORT OF OKLAHOMA STATE INSURANCE FUND RELEASED

The following report of the State Insurance Fund's expenditures covering a period of nine years, beginning with the creation of the Fund by an Act of the Oklahoma Legislature in July, 1933, until July, 1942, has been received in the office of the Association and should be of especial interest to the profession. It should also be noted that, at present, the commissioner of the Fund is Mr. Mott Keys, who has been responsible for its operation since April 15, 1940.

HISTORY: Created by an Act of the Oklahoma Legislature July 1, 1933.

PURPOSE: There was created and established a "Fund" known as "The State Insurance Fund" to be administered by the State Insurance Fund Commissioner without liability on the part of the State beyond the amount of said Fund, for the purpose of insuring employers against liability for compensation under the Oklahoma Workmen's Compensation Act, and for assuring for the persons entitled thereto Compensation as provided by the Workmen's Compensation Law, and for the further purpose of insuring persons, firms and corporations against loss, expense, or liability by reason of bodily injury, death by accident, etc., for which the insured may be liable or have assumed liability.

APPROPRIATION: For the purpose of paying awards from the State Insurance Fund in the first instance, and the necessary expense in putting the State Fund Act into operation, the sum of Twenty-Five Thousand ($25,000.00) Dollars was appropriated out of the General Revenue Fund of the State. This $25,000.00 was never used by the State Insurance Fund, and the entire amount so appropriated was returned, and put back into the General Revenue Fund of the State, thereby eliminating any cost by the State Insurance Fund to the taxpayers of Oklahoma.

FACTS WORTH KNOWING: The State Insurance Fund in its nine (9) years of service to Oklahoma employers, July 1, 1933 to July 1, 1942, has paid out by check or voucher the following sums of money:

Medical and hospital bills to Oklahoma Doctors, hospitals and drug stores ....$ 814,500.00

Compensation and Attorney fees to injured employees and Attorneys 2,171,700.00

Operating, Salaries, Supplies, to office employees and business firms 462,800.00

Total in nine years $3,499,000.00

The fund was the first institution in Oklahoma to purchase its limit in War Bonds when the War Bond drive was started in Oklahoma. War Bonds purchased out of "Fund's" Surplus Account are as follows: June, 1941, the Fund purchased $50,000.00 Series G Bonds; January, 1942, the Fund purchased $50,000.00 Series G Bonds; and July, 1942, the Fund purchased $50,000.00 Series G Bonds. Total purchased to date equals $150,000.00. These bonds are earning 2.5 percent interest for the State Insurance Fund.

In addition to these War Bonds, the State Insurance Fund has in cash on deposit with the Oklahoma State Treasurer as of this date $76,000.00.

As of January 1, 1943, these War Bonds will have earned for the State Insurance Fund $4,375.00 in interest. By the end of the same year (1943), this Bond investment alone will have earned $8,125.00 in interest. Under the present management of the State Insurance Fund effected April 15, 1940, by the Governor and the Board of Managers, The State Insurance Fund had a known liability on seventy (70) cases of approximately $298,000.00.

These 70 cases, plus 168 other cases with an unknown or nuisance value, were settled by the State Fund's Claim Department on Joint Petition for $148,310.00, to say nothing of the 168 cases, a portion of which is left to run unsettled, would no doubt have developed into orders from the Industrial Commission, and would have proved quite costly.

There were 238 cases settled by the Claims Department on Joint Petition from April 15, 1940, to April 1, 1942, as follows: 52 cases of 300 week orders at $10.00 per week totaling $156,000.00; 13 cases of 500 week orders at $9,000 per case totaling $117,000.00; and five death cases at $5,000 per case totaling $25,000.00. The combined total of 70 cases produced a known liability of $298,000.00, and there was a total of 168 cases with an unknown liability, making a total of 238 cases settled at approximately 50 cents on the dollar, thus eliminating forever any further liability on the State Insurance Fund.

As of April 15, 1940, under present management, the State Insurance Fund had outstanding and unpaid medical bills in the approximate amount of $70,000.00. These bills, as have all other outstanding obligations of the State Insurance Fund, been paid, and to date all bills and obligations of the Fund are being paid currently, and the State Insurance Fund has a nest egg in the Surplus Accounts of $150,000.00 in War Bonds alone, and will increase this amount to $200,000.00 by January, 1943.

Your State Insurance Fund has kept the faith with the employers, employees, doctors and hospitals of Oklahoma, and such accomplishments have been made in spite of a tremendous decline in premium value brought about by the National Emergency and the War Production Board's curtailment of smaller industries and insureds composed a majority of the Fund's premium income.

In April, 1940, the Fund had 1,629 open claims with reserves set up to cover liability on these claims of $277,730.00. As of June 30, 1942, the Fund has reduced these 1,629 open claims to 302 with reserves set up to cover liability of $154,895.00, thereby closing 1,327 claims and reducing The State Insurance Fund's liability from $277,730.00 to $154,895.00, or a total reduction in liability to the Fund of $122,835.00.

Fifth Annual Forum on Allergy

The international postgraduate society will meet in the Hotel Statler in Cleveland, Ohio, the week end of January 9-10, 1943. This Forum will offer in most intensive presentation both the new and the old in Allergy. The meeting will be characterized by its use of all the various types of instruction. Formal lectures, special talks, dry clinics, study groups, moving pictures, Kodachromes, panel discussions, ending with an "Information on Allergy, Please," will all be used to teach the physicians of the United States and Canada. Not only will specialists in this new field of Internal Medicine gather but also those whose interests are in allied fields of medicine will be welcome, for in war time every physician is called upon to advise and treat allergic patients. This is especially true of those in Internal Medicine, Diseases of Children, Diseases of the Skin, Diseases of the Eye, Diseases of the Nose and Throat, as well as those engaged in basic research in Immunology. A course in Immunology as it applies to Allergy will be given the week before Dr. Eckers to a limited number of physicians and associates. Any physician interested in either or both of the foregoing is invited to write Dr. Jonathan Forman, 956 Bryden Road, Columbus, Ohio, for copies of the printed program and registration blanks.

Among the 58 Allergists participating in the program are most of the leaders in this field. Arthur Coca, M.D., of New York, will receive the Forum's Gold Medal and will give the annual Forum Lecture on Sunday afternoon.

Dr. Marvin Elkins of Muskogee has recently been called to active duty with the Army, and is at the Station Hospital, Fort Sill.

Major Thomas H. Davis of Tulsa reports that his present address is Medical Detachment, 157th Infantry, A. P. O. No. 45, c/o Postmaster, New York, N. Y.

Loan Scholarships for Medical Students

The federal government has recently announced that funds amounting to $5,000,000 have been appropriated to provide loan scholarships for about 10,000 students now enrolled in a 12-month accelerated course, including medicine, chemistry, veterinary science, dentistry, pharmacy, and engineering.

Students eligible to borrow this money, in addition to fees and tuition, will receive $25 a month, but not more than $500 in any 12-month period. The students agree, in addition to participating in courses of study in authorized fields, and maintaining satisfactory standards, to accept, after graduation, such employment or service as might be assigned by officers or agencies designated by the chairman of the War Manpower Commission.

Students may obtain loans through the colleges or universities which they are attending, and arrangements for repayment may be made directly with the institutions. The students may make notes payable to the United States treasury at 2½ percent interest. This arrangement will be beneficial for students who continue their studies for 12 consecutive months as they will have no opportunity for summer employment to help defray college expenses.

WPB Freezes Quinine

A recent order of the War Production Board freezes quinine, cinchonine and their salts, and prohibits the dispensing or sale of quinine upon any prescription other than for malaria. Even if combined with other ingredients, the pharmacist is not permitted to dispense a prescription containing quinine. However, if the physician certifies on the prescription that the quinine he is prescribing is for malaria, or the quinidine is for a cardiac, it may be filled by the pharmacist.

ALLOCATION OF NARCOTIC DRUGS

Under a directive issued by the chairman of the War Production Board, October 6, the U. S. Bureau of Narcotics is authorized to allocate narcotic drugs in such manner and to such extent as it may deem necessary or appropriate in the public interest and to promote the national defense, according to the October 17th issue of the Journal of the American Medical Association.

The bureau may regulate or prohibit the production, manufacture, sale, transfer or other disposition of narcotic drugs by any person who has acted in violation of any regulation or order prescribed by it pursuant to the directive and may require such reports and the keeping of such records and may make such investigations as it deems necessary or appropriate.

The chairman of the War Production Board may from time to time delegate to the bureau such additional powers with respect to the exercise of control over narcotic drugs or may amend or revoke the delegation contained in the directive in such manner and to such extent as he may determine to be necessary or appropriate. No preference rating heretofore or hereafter assigned, applied or extended will have any binding effect with respect to any transaction in narcotic drugs unless the Bureau of Narcotics expressly so orders. For the purpose of the directive, the term ''narcotic drugs'' is defined to mean opium, coca leaves, cocaine or any salt, derivative or preparation of opium, coca leaves or cocaine.

Major W. A. Howard of Chelsea reports that his present address is Station Hospital, Fort Sill.

Captain Shade D. Neely of Muskogee has recently been transferred, and his present address is Station Hospital, Williams Field, Chandler, Ariz.

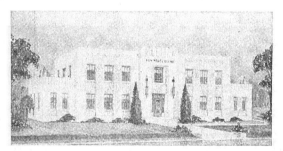

Affiliation Links Three Medical Institutions

A professional affiliation between the Department of Nursing of the College of Physicians and Surgeons of Columbia University (Presbyterian Hospital School of Nursing in the city of New York) and the Neuro-Psychiatric Institute of the Hartford Retreat is announced jointly by Miss Margaret E. Conrad, Professor and Executive Officer of the Department of Nursing of Columbia's College of Physicians and Surgeons, and Dr. C. Charles Burlingame, Psychiatrist-in-Chief of the Neuro-Psychiatric Institute. The affiliation has been approved by the Columbia University Council and the Board of Directors of the Institute.

Under this affiliation, students with university degrees who are receiving advanced time credit in the Department of Nursing, College of Physicians and Surgeons of Columbia, will undertake an intensive two months' course in neuro-psychiatric nursing at the Institute, under the direction of the Institute's medical and nursing staffs. The curriculum will include instruction in all branches of psychiatric nursing, as well as clinical experience on both the hall and cottage services.

The affiliation is limited to those students who have received university degrees and whose qualifications have permitted them to undertake to complete their basic training course in Columbia's Department of Nursing in twenty-eight months, instead of the usual three years. These students are being trained to fill administrative positions and positions of leadership in the field of nursing.

Fifteen students are expected to begin classes in December.

The affiliation marks the educational linking of three of the nation's oldest and most distinguished medical institutions—Columbia University, founded in 1754; the Neuro-Psychiatric Institute, founded in 1822 and the Presbyterian Hospital, opened in 1868. The Nursing School of the Presbyterian Hospital received university status in 1937, and the Hospital celebrated its fiftieth anniversary in June, 1941.

Members of the Board of Nursing Advisors of the Neuro-Psychiatric Institute are: Miss Helen Young, chairman, Directors of the Nursing Service, Presbyterian Hospital in the city of New York; Miss Margaret E. Conrad, Professor and Executive Officer, Department of Nursing, College of Physicians and Surgeons, Columbia University (Presbyterian Hospital in the city of New York); Miss Annie W. Goodrich, Dean Emerita, Yale University School of Nursing, New Haven; Miss Effie J. Taylor, Dean, Yale School of Nursing; Dr. Nolan D. C. Lewis, Professor of Psychiatry, Faculty of Medicine, Columbia University and Dr. Willard C. Rappleye, Dean, College of Physicians and Surgeons, Columbia University.

Inter-American Publication

The simultaneous publication of the June issue of *Annals of Surgery* in Philadelphia by the J. B. Lippincott Company and in Buenos Aires by the Guillermo Kraft Company was a new step toward the consolidation of medical interests here and in South America.

The *Annals of Surgery* is the oldest surgical journal in the English language. Its appearance in Spanish marks a high spot in the Lippincott Company's celebration of its sesquicentennial this year.

As the result of negotiations and with the assistance of the Coordinator of Inter-American Affairs, and Mr. Lewis Hanke, Director of the Hispanic Foundation, Guillermo Kraft Company, one of the oldest and most respected publishing firms in Buenos Aires, is translating the *Annals of Surgery* each month for South American physicians and surgeons.

The medical profession in this country has become increasingly aware of its obligations and responsibilities in South America. No better symbolic demonstration could be given of its sincere willingness to develop permanent intellectual fraternization between the surgeons of the two continents.

• OBITUARIES •

Dr. John Marion McFarling
1903-1942

John Marion McFarling, 39, one of the youngest and prominent physicians of Shawnee, died suddenly on Tuesday, October 27, 1942, at 6 P. M., of coronary occlusion.

Previous to the terminal attack, Dr. McFarling had apparently been in good health when on Tuesday morning he suffered an acute coronary episode and was apparently recovering from the initial attack when he was again stricken.

Dr. John was the son of Dr. A. C. McFarling, a practicing physician who is a specialist in epthoromogy and otolaryngology and a resident of this community since 1915, having moved here from Texas with his parents.

He was secretary of the Staff of the Shawnee City Hospital and a former Secretary of the Pottawatomie County Medical Society, as well as being a member of the Oklahoma State Medical Association and the American Medical Association.

He was a member of the Presbyterian Church, the Shawnee Lodge No. 107 A. F. and A. M. and of the Indian Consistory No. 2 of the Masonic Lodge at McAlester.

Dr. John attended public schools in this community and later attended the Terrell Texas Military School from which he graduated. His higher education was obtained at the Oklahoma Baptist University here and his medical education was obtained at the University of Oklahoma Medical School from which he graduated in 1935.

His internship was spent in the Hollywood Hospital in Hollywood, Calif., and for one year was the studio physician for Metro-Goldwyn-Mayre Co., there.

He has been engaged in the general practice of medicine in Shawnee since returning from California, being associated with his father, Dr. A. C. McFarling, and with Dr. Alpha McAdams Williams.

He is survived by his wife, Mrs. Justine McFarling, son, Robert McFarling, father and mother, Dr. and Mrs. A. C. McFarling, a sister, Mrs. Ted S. Bland, Keniston, Md., a brother, Pvt. Alonzo McFarling, in the air corps of the U. S. army stationed at Lowry Field, Denver, Colo.

Dr. John, as he was known to all, was respected by the medical fraternity as well as the entire community, and his sudden and unexpected death was a great shock to his friends and associates and the Society expresses its deepest regrets that a young and useful member should be taken from us in the prime of his life.

Industrial Hygiene Manual To Be Published

A manual on "Industrial Hygiene and Mental Service in War Industries" is being prepared by the Division of Industrial Hygiene of the National Institute of Health and will be released for distribution among industrial physicians and the medical profession generally in the near future. This brochure is being compiled and edited by the Division's full-time and consultant staff, following a recommendation by the Committee on Industrial Medicine of the National Research Council. According to the resolution initiating the project, the manual will embrace discussions of "toxicity and potential dangers of organic and inorganic substances in the war industries, occupational cutaneous diseases in war industries, engineering control, industrial medical services, nursing in industry, dental services, fatigue, women in industry, medical control of diseases of the respiratory tract, nutrition in war industries, available governmental industrial hygiene services, and integration of plan and community emergency medical services."

Office of Civilian Defense

O. C. D. Mobile Emergency Medical Hospital Units

The Emergency Medical Service of the Oklahoma State Defense Committee has equipped, or has in the process of equipping, four mobile emergency medical hospital units. This service was made possible by an agreement between the Highway Patrol and the Emergency Medical Service. The Highway Patrol furnished the trailers, and is to keep in storage and transport the trailers to the scene of disaster. These trailer units have been put in shape and equipped by the Emergency Medical Service. Money to buy the equipment was especially allocated by the State for this specific and definite purpose.

One unit has been completed. Each unit is complete in detail for this type of emergency medical service. Each unit has its own lighting facility, run by storage batteries. Each unit has one operating table. Each unit carries its own water supply in storage tanks. Each unit also has its own sterilizing equipment. Each unit is equipped with a reasonable supply of drugs, dressings, instruments, biologics, etc.

The following is the way each of the units is labeled and identified:

OKLAHOMA
O. C. D.
MOBILE EMERGENCY
MEDICAL HOSPITAL
UNIT

These units were designated primarily to take care of any emergency due to enemy activity, or for any emergency that might be caused by water or other natural disaster.

Where will the trailer units be located? These trailer units will be strategically located over the State of Oklahoma; so located that no part of the State will be a greater distance than two and one-half hours away. Who will man the units? These emergency medical units will be manned by the county emergency medical service in the county where the disaster occurs; which means that if a disaster occurs, the mobil emergency medical hospital units will be wheeled to the point of disaster and then manned by the nurses and doctors of the county emergency medical organization.

Dr. Wile Commissioned in U. S. Public Health Service

Dr. Udo J. Wile, Professor of Dermatology and Syphilology in the School of Medicine, University of Michigan, has been commissioned Medical Director (R) in the U. S. Public Health Service for active duty with the Division of Venereal Disease Control, Surgeon General Thomas Parran announced recently.

Dr. Wile will conduct a study of all new methods described in recent years by various clinicians for the intensive treatment of syphilis.

He will also supervise the quarantine hospitals which the Public Health Service and the States are developing in a number of critical war areas. These hospitals are for the treatment of prostitutes and recalcitrant persons who are infected with syphilis and who are capable of spreading the disease. Through quarantine and intensive treatment of infectious cases under controlled conditions, it is expected that the most effective and economical methods for the clinical management of syphilis will be demonstrated and their prompt adoption insured.

The hospitals will be staffed by physicians, nurses, and record analysts of the Public Health Service, who will be given special training in rapid therapy under the supervision of Dr. Wile. The first training course will begin in November, with headquarters at Ann Arbor. Some 20 physicians, 60 nurses, and 20 record analysts are expected to report for training in the first class.

University of Oklahoma School of Medicine

The Hospitality Club held its thirteenth annual circus for crippled children in the Lew Wentz Auditorium of the Crippled Children's Hospital, on Friday, October 30.

On Saturday, October 31, Colonel Frank S. Gillespie, of the British Army Medical Corps, spoke to members of the County Medical Society on medical aspects of the war in the Middle East.

Dr. Moorman P. Prosser, Associate in Psychiatry, University of Oklahoma School of Medicine, has been granted a leave of absence for the duration. Doctor Prosser is now stationed at Camp Gruber, Oklahoma.

Dr. Donald B. McMullen, Assistant Professor of Bacteriology and Associate Professor of Hygiene and Public Health, attended a meeting of the American Public Health Association at St. Louis, Missouri, from October 24-30.

Dr. Bela Halpert, Professor of Clinical Pathology and Director of Laboratories in the University and Crippled Children's Hospitals, attended a meeting of the Southern Medical Association in Richmond, Virginia, November 10-12. Dr. Halpert had an exhibit on "Incidence of Carcinoma of the Lung" at this meeting.

NEW JOURNAL TO BE PUBLISHED MONTHLY

The American Gastroenterological Association on January 1, 1943, will publish the first issue of a new Journal to be called, *Gastroenterology*. The new Journal will be owned by the Association, will be the official publication of the Association, and will be published by Williams and Wilkins Company. It will appear monthly, and the subscription price will be $6.00 per year.

Dr. W. C. Alvarez will be the Editor after June, 1943, and Dr. A. C. Ivy will be the Assistant Editor. The Editorial Board will consist of Doctors A. H. Aaron, Buffalo; J. A. Bargen, Rochester; H. L. Bockus, Philadelphia; W. C. Boeck, Los Angeles; B. B. Crohn, New York; R. Elman, St. Louis; F. Hollander, New York; Sara Jordan, Boston; J. L. Kantor, New York; B. R. Kirklin, Rochester; P. Klemperer, New York; F. H. Lahey, Boston; F. C. Mann, Rochester; H. J. Moersch, Rochester; V. C. Myers, Cleveland; W. L. Palmer, Chicago; J. M. Ruffin, Durham; R. Schindler, Chicago, and D. L. Wilbur, San Francisco.

Gastroenterology invites for publication clinical and investigative contributions which are of interest to the general practitioner as well as the specialist and which deal with the diseases of digestion and nutrition, including their physiological, biochemical, pathological, parasitological, radiological and surgical aspects.

Manuscripts should be sent to Dr. A. C. Ivy, 303 East Chicago Avenue, Chicago, Illinois. Letters regarding subscriptions and business matters should be addressed to Mr. R. S. Gill, Williams and Wilkins Company, Baltimore, Maryland.

A new address reported for Dr. C. E. Hollingsworth of Oklahoma City is A. P. O. 942, c/o Postmaster, Seattle, Wash.

Dr. Maurice D. Spottswood of Tulsa reported for duty as a Lieutenant, junior grade, in the Navy at Washington, D. C., on November 1.

Captain William K. Ishmael of Oklahoma City is now located at the Station Hospital, Harding Field, Baton Rouge, La. Prior to his transfer Dr. Ishmael was stationed at Will Rogers Field, Oklahoma City.

NEWS FROM THE COUNTY SOCIETIES

Members of the Carter County Medical Society met October 27, in the Hardy Sanitarium at Ardmore. The meeting was a business session for the reports of committees regarding their activities during the past year.

Dr. H. A. Higgins, Secretary of the Society, gave a report of the Third Annual Secretaries Conference which was held in Oklahoma City, October 25. Other members of the Society attending the Secretaries Conference were Dr. Walter Hardy, President, and Dr. F. W. Boadway, Chairman of the Medical Preparedness Committee.

Fifteen members of the Pottawatomie County Society attended the dinner and regular meeting of the Society on October 17, 1942, at 7:00 P. M., in Shawnee.

Following the dinner, the program consisted of a technicolor motion picture with sound entitled "Syphilis," presented by Dr. Eugene A. Gillis, Venereal Disease Control Officer of the Oklahoma State Health Department, Oklahoma City. Dr. Clinton Gallaher and Dr. Charles W. Haygood also presented a paper "Interstitial (Luetic) Keratitis."

Colonel Frank S. Gillespie of the British Army Medical Corps appeared before the Oklahoma County Medical Association as guest speaker at its regular meeting Saturday, October 31, 7:30 P. M., in the Medical School Auditorium.

For his discussion, Colonel Gillespie chose the subject "Medicine in the Near East."

"Diagnosis of Common Skin Diseases" was the subject of discussion by Dr. James Stevenson of Tulsa, guest speaker of the Washington-Nowata County Medical Society, at its meeting on November 11 in Bartlesville when 16 members of the Society were in attendance. As a second subject for discussion, Dr. K. D. Davis of Nowata, President of the Society, presented a paper entitled "Caesarean Section: Indications for Same."

At the meeting of the Society on December 9, Dr. J. V. Athey and Dr. H. G. Crawford will present papers.

Members of the Rogers County Medical Society met at the Claremore Indian Hospital in regular monthly session on Wednesday, October 28, at 8:00 P.M. The program consisted of presentation and discussion of six varied types of cases.

The November meeting is scheduled for 7:30 P. M., November 18.

The Beckham County Medical Society met November 10 at 7:30 P.M., in Sayre, in the offices of Dr. H. K. Speed, President of the Society. Following a discussion of general topics of interest, the host served refreshments to those in attendance.

On December 8, the Society will meet at Elk City.

"Aviation Medicine" was the subject selected by the guest speaker of the Tulsa County Medical Society, Lieutenant Edward J. Gallagher, Flight Surgeon, Spartan School of Aeronautics, Tulsa, at its regular meeting on November 9 at the Mayo Hotel. Approximately 55 members of the Society were in attendance.

The next meeting of the Society is scheduled for December 14, Mayo Hotel, at which time the annual election of officers will be the order of business. Yearly committee reports will likewise be presented.

At a regular bi-monthly meeting of the Pottawatomie County Medical Society at the Shawnee City Hospital on Saturday, November 7, 1942, nomination of Officers for 1943 was the order of business.

The nomination of Officers will not close until the time of the election, which will occur at the regular November meeting of the Society on the 21st at the Aldridge Hotel.

The proper place to install a Blood Plasma Bank in Ardmore was the subject of discussion at the meeting of the Carter County Medical Society at the Hardy Sanitarium on November 16.

At a meeting of the Society a week later, November 23, Dr. Eugene A. Gillis, Director of the Venereal Disease Division of the Oklahoma State Health Department, Oklahoma City, presented the film "Syphilis" to the members of the Society.

"Estrogens" was the subject of discussion by Dr. William Finch of Hobart, guest speaker of the Tri-County Society composed of Grady, Caddo and Stephens counties at its meeting in Chickasha, November 19. Staff members of the Borden General Hospital, a new Army hospital in Chickasha, were special guests.

Dr. Frank T. Joyce, Secretary of the Grady County Medical Society, has been called to duty with the Air Corps and is stationed at San Antonio. His duties for the remainder of the year will be assumed by Dr. Turner Bynum.

Mr. Harold Howell of the State Health and Housing Committee was presented as guest speaker of the Garvin County Medical Society at its meeting in Pauls Valley, at the High School Building, on November 18. Mr. Howell was introduced by Dr. Hugh Monroe, Chairman of the program committee. Ten members attended the meeting.

Election of officers and payment of dues is the scheduled order of business for the Society at its meeting on December 16.

Dr. M. D. Glismann of Oklahoma City has moved his offices from 911 Northwest 23rd Street to 1021 North Lee.

News From The State Health Department

War and Tuberculosis

Tuberculosis control has made tremendous strides since World War I. The death rate in the United States has dropped from 150 per one hundred thousand, in 1918, to 44, in 1941 (Oklahoma's rate was 45 in 1941). A question which confronts us now is whether World War II is going to nullify many of our hard-fought gains. War has always left in its wake an increase in tuberculosis. England is experiencing this rise now. In this country, it is presumed we are in position to hold the tuberculosis mortality in check. To do this though we must keep in full operation the public health machinery we now have. To maintain the public health, we all admit is most vital to the war effort. The armed services are seeing to it that no tuberculosis develops among our soldiers. They are profiting by the unhappy experience of World War I and x-raying every recruit. Industry, too, has seen the need for the routine chest film, which is now used by the majority of large industrial organizations. It is among the general civilian population that we must need especially concern ourselves and augment, if necessary, the existing facilities.

Let us examine the tuberculosis control machinery in Oklahoma. The State Tuberculosis Association which is financed by Christmas Seals has been very active in recent years. There are now 45 county-wide tuberculosis associations. Among their activities they stress education as to the nature of tuberculosis and initiate early diagnosis campaigns and programs. The bulk of the active case-finding is carried on by the State Health Department, under the Division of Tuberculosis Control. This case-finding program is an integrated part of the general health program of the full-time county health units, of which there are thirty-eight. Regular clinics are held, with the efforts of the doctors and nurses being concentrated on examination of contacts (those exposed to known active tuberculosis).

Some 5,000 chest films were taken last year by the two portable x-ray units maintained by the department. Four hundred new cases of tuberculosis were discovered. Incidentally, a good share of these films were paid for by Christmas Seal funds. Both Tulsa and Oklahoma Counties have exceptionally well operated tuberculosis clinics. An outstanding example of a rural county health unit is furnished by Seminole County, where twenty-seven new cases of tuberculosis were discovered last year. Both state sanatoria have outpatient departments, where diagnostic facilities are available and follow-up examinations of ex-patients are carried on.

How then can we keep the death rate from rising despite the war? We can help by buying Christmas Seals. We can support legislation for adequate appropriations for maintaining and advancing the state tuberculosis control program. One of the big needs is to expand our diagnostic facilities so that all the counties in the state may be reached. Only 66 percent of the population is now reached by regularly conducted clinics. As physicians, we should continue to be ever alert for tuberculosis. Furthermore, it is our responsibility after the diagnosis is made to see that all contacts are examined.

Dr. F. G. Dorwart of Muskogee has been called to active duty with the Army and is stationed at the General Hospital, Vancouver, Wash.

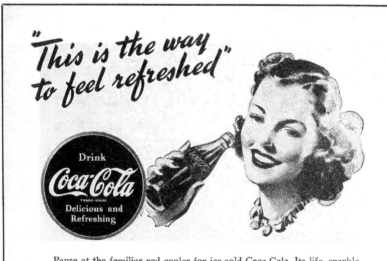

WOMEN'S AUXILIARY NEWS

Cleveland County

Mrs. M. P. Prosser, of Norman, President of the Cleveland County Auxiliary, has resigned to join her husband, where he is stationed at Camp Gruber, and the Secretary, Mrs. Curtis Berry, of Norman, will act as President for the balance of this year.

Tulsa County

The Tulsa County Auxiliary held its regular monthly luncheon on Tuesday, November 3, in the home of Mrs. J. F. Gorrell. A total of 56 members attended this luncheon, and a very interesting program was presented. The speakers were Mrs. Louis P. Cummings, from the Office of Civilian Defense, Dr. M. O. Hart, an Auxiliary member, Mrs. C. C. Hoke, and Mrs. Wade Sisler, both of whom are Auxiliary members. The entire program concerned the work of the Auxiliary in defense and war projects.

The following Credo was presented at the National Convention by Mrs. William Hibbitts, and we feel it is worthy of repetition here:

Credo of the Doctor's Wife in Wartime

I am the American doctor's wife. I am anxious to render my best service to America and believe this can be done by helping to maintain her present high standard of health. I feel that the most effectual way to do this is through my Auxiliary to the County Medical Society. My doctor husband is serving America through his profession and his medical association. My part shall be to serve through my Auxiliary. Health education is one of the main objectives of the Woman's Auxiliary to the American Medical Association. Furtherance of this program shall be our wartime program.

I shall urge every member of my Auxiliary to have a complete physical examination, for soon our doctors will be too busy to give us the special attention which we have enjoyed in the past. Such an examination is an individual responsibility which each of us must assume. I feel that now more than ever it is vitally important to me, to my family and to the servants in my household to be examined. I shall ask my Auxiliary to sponsor such a check-up for everyone and to present programs on "What is a physical health examination, anyway?" and "Rules of the Game."

My Auxiliary will give special study to local health problems and cooperate with local health authorities in correcting any conditions which could prove to be a hazard to public health; particularly those made acute by military and defense plants. My Auxiliary shall do everything within its power to preserve the health of women in defense work and to remind constantly that local neglect is the basis for national health problems.

I shall ask my Auxiliary to appoint a nutrition council this year with a trained instructor from our own group, if one is qualified. This council shall urge all members to take a standard course in nutrition and to study the advanced course for canteen workers. Food conservation too, and how to plan a well balanced diet despite the restrictions of certain foods occasioned by emergency rationing, shall be stressed.

I shall urge our members to work with the Red Cross, to take a course in first aid, home nursing or nurses aid, so that we shall be ready to replace the nurses who are being called to serve with our armed forces.

I shall attempt to build and try ever to maintain a high state of morale in my community, and stress simplicity in our social gatherings of our medical group through timely book reviews and through public relations meetings to instruct the laity on matters of health with particular emphasis on mental hygiene.

Each day brings new changes in our government. It shall be my duty to be better informed on legislative matters, particularly medical legislation. I believe we should study facts about inflation this year and do what we can to prevent this disaster.

If I am to be a good neighbor to South America and to Canada, I must know something about these countries and their practice of medicine. I believe we should profit greatly through studying the effects of war on the health of the English people.

I shall keep abreast of the changes taking place in American medicine, and be informed on what the American doctor is doing to help win the war.

I shall subscribe to and carefully read the Bulletin. It will keep me informed as to the plans and accomplishments of other Auxiliaries and serve as a measuring stick for my own group.

I shall seek to have more Auxiliary quiz programs this year, as these contests are always very enjoyable. In turn I shall be very glad to assist in preparing other quiz programs for my county and state auxiliary from the excellent material contained in Hygeia and the Hand Book. A review of "Be Informed," which gives information about the American Medical Association, the Woman's Auxiliary, Public Relations and Legislation, shall be a feature of this year's program.

Panel discussions, always a source of valuable information, shall be an aim during the year, and if possible I shall have county or state health officials as guest leaders.

I shall urge my Auxiliary to have a public speaking class twice a month, so I may become a well informed and interesting speaker on topics of health and medical economics.

I shall urge our Auxiliary to read and promote the sale of Hygeia and to use the valuable material presented in this authentic health magazine. I shall encourage our members to request articles from the Health Bureau of the American Medical Association and to study the survey of Women's health interests which has been compiled by the Bureau of Health Education of the American Medical Association.

I shall always insist that our Advisory Committee be consulted about all of our plans and policies.

My Auxiliary shall become a training school where I shall strive to learn to be a leader in health work and thus I shall serve my community and my country.

Lieutenant J. F. Curry of Sapulpa has reported for duty with the medical corps of the Army and is stationed at Paris, Texas.

On October 27, Dr. F. D. Sinclair of Tulsa reported for duty with the Army Air Force and is presently located at the Brooks General Hospital, Fort Sam Houston, San Antonio, Texas.

Dr. J. E. Levick, formerly of Elk City, is stationed at the Army Base Hospital, Sioux City, Iowa.

Word has been received in the office of the Association that Dr. Raymond L. Murdock of Oklahoma City is presently stationed at the 27th Field Hospital, Camp Campbell, Ky.

The U. S. Secret Service, Post Office Inspectors
and Your Police Warn You

BEFORE YOU ACCEPT COMMERCIAL AND
GOVERNMENT CHECKS

Demand and Receive
Absolute and Positive Identification

MAIL THIEVES . . . CHECK FORGERS
MAKE POOR PATIENTS

"KNOW YOUR ENDORSERS"

MEDICAL PREPAREDNESS

ADDITIONAL OKLAHOMA PHYSICIANS IN MILITARY SERVICE

The following supplementary list are those physicians who have reported for duty in one of the branches of service since the publication of previous lists in the Journal:

Beckham

DAVANNEY, P. J. ....*Sayre*
LEVICK, J. E. ....*Elk City*
SLABAUGH, RAYMOND M. ....*Sayre*

Craig

DARROUGH, JAMES B. ....*Vinita*

Grady

JOYCE, FRANK T. ....*Chickasha*
SCHUBERT, H. A. ....*Chickasha*

Jackson

ALLGOOD, J. M. ....*Altus*

Muskogee

ELKINS, MARVIN ....*Muskogee*
SCHNOEBELEN, R. E. ....*Muskogee*

Osage

SMITH, R. O. ....*Hominy*

Ottawa

CHESNUT, WYLIE G. ....*Miami*
SAYLES, W. JACKSON ....*Miami*

Payne

PUCKETT, H. L. ....*Stillwater*

Tulsa

McDONALD, J. E. ....619 *S. Main*
PIGFORD, RUSSELL C. ....*Medical Arts Bldg.*
SINCLAIR, F. D. ....*Springer Clinic*
SPOTTSWOOD, MAURICE B. ....*Medical Arts Bldg.*
STUART, FRANK A. ....619 *S. Main*

Woodward

DUER, JOE L. ....*Woodward*

Army Takes Over Red Cross-Harvard Hospital in England

The U. S. Army headquarters for the European theater of operations has announced that the American Red Cross-Harvard University Hospital in southern England has been taken over by the army and will be the central laboratory for U. S. armed forces in Britain. This hospital was established in 1940 and operated jointly by the American Red Cross, Harvard University and the British Ministry of Health for the study of wartime epidemics. Its twenty-two buildings were all fabricated in the United States, from which the sixty-six thousand pieces of fabricated building material were shipped to England to be erected by British workmen. The director of the hospital was Dr. John E. Gordon, professor of preventive medicine and epidemiology at Harvard University Medical School. The staff comprised ten doctors, sixty-two nurses, six technicians and eight administrative members. Secretary of War Stimson said that it was a truly splendid addition to the U. S. Army's medical facilities. The hospital will be turned over to the British Ministry of Health at the end of the war.—A. M. A. Journal, October 3, 1942.

Major Frank A. Stuart of Tulsa has reported to the office that he is now stationed at the Station Hospital, Amarillo Field, Amarillo, Texas. Dr. J. E. McDonald of the McDonald and Stuart partnership is also on duty with the Army Air Force, and is presently located in Atlantic City, New Jersey.

TRIBUTE TO MEDICAL SOLDIERS

The Medical Soldier, published at Carlisle Barracks, Pa., in its August 22 issue, carried an article by Raymond Clapper, the well known Washington correspondent and columnist, relative to the heroic deeds of medical soldiers. Permission was given by Mr. Clapper for reprinting the article, and it follows in full text:

"As this war goes along I hope some way will be found to give due credit before the American people to the medical soldier and the work of the Medical Corps.

"For centuries the medical man has shunned the public eye. He is content to do his noble work. He cares only to do his best and to retain the respect of his colleagues. For that reason, I suppose, the medical officer and the medical soldier do not receive in war time the recognition and appreciation which is due them. The work of the medical men is overlooked in the official communiques and in the news reports which the war correspondents send back. Yet the medical units are on the front line, functioning with every combat arm. In the last war per capita casualties were larger in the Medical Department than in the Infantry. The medical soldier and officer, armed only with his litter and first aid pouches, must work under fire, evacuating casualties and conserving fighting strength. He fights not with guns, grenades and bayonets, but with sulfanilimide, sterile dressings, leg splints, and a strong back to carry a litter.

"True, the medical soldier has assailed no stronghold, he has planted no flag in enemy territory, he has not killed one of the enemy. But, he has been aiding our own wounded, keeping up their morale, saving their lives, thereby doing his heroic part in strengthening our own side.

"Not only at the front and in the shell-torn aid stations and back at the base hospitals is the Medical Corps doing its work, but in laboratories the Medical Corps is pioneering in finding new ways to save lives. It is a shining historical circumstance that out of the death and destruction of war the Medical Corps has salvaged countless human lives and found ways which save civilian human life, and thus put all humanity in its debt. Yellow fever was conquered by Army medicine. Typhoid fever was conquered by Army medicine. Hookworm, one of peacetime's deadliest enemies, was conquered by Army medicine, Malaria, cholera, plague fevers of many kinds have been defeated by the valiant scientific work of the Medical Corps.

"These are victories which in the long life of civilization must count along with the decisive military battles of the world. Yet, for the lack of imagination, and because of the self-effacing character of all medical men, this story of the Medical Corps has been lightly passed over by war historians. It is being passed over now by those whose job it is to paint a portrait of the United States Army in action in this war. I know this is not intentional, but I hope, as I know anyone would who stops to think about it, that some way will be found whereby the public is constantly told about the great work which medical men in the Army are doing to help with this war for freedom and humanity."—Army and Navy Register, Sept. 12, 1942.

Major Dan R. Sewell has recently been transferred to Pecos, Texas, from the Army Air Base, Station Hospital, Albuquerque, New Mex. Prior to his entry into active service, Dr. Sewell practiced in Oklahoma City.

EMERGENCY BASE HOSPITALS

The Medical Division of the U. S. Office of Civilian Defense, through its Regional Medical Officers and State Chiefs of Emergency Medical Service, has now made emergency provision for the establishment of a chain of Emergency Base Hospitals in the interior of all the coastal States. They will be activated only in the event of an enemy attack upon our coast which necessitates the evacuation of coastal hospitals. Each base hospital will be related to the casualty receiving hospital which has been evacuated and it is expected that the staff will be recruited largely from the parent institution.

In order to meet a sudden and unexpected crisis without delay, arrangements have been completed with State authorities for the prompt taking over of appropriate institutions in the interior of the State for this purpose and with local military establishments for the transportation of casualties and other hospitalized persons along appropriate lines of evacuation.

More than 150 hospitals in the coastal cities are in the process of organizing small affiliated units of physicians and surgeons, which will be prepared to staff the Emergency Base Hospitals if they should be needed. These units are composed of the older members of the staff and those with physical disabilities which render them ineligible for military service, and of women physicians. In order that a balanced professional team may be immediately available the doctors comprising units are being commissioned in the inactive Reserve of the U. S. Public Health Service so that, if called to duty, they may receive the rank, pay and allowances equivalent to that of an officer in the armed forces.

Dr. George Baehr, Chief Medical Officer of the U. S. Office of Civilian Defense, states that the members of these affiliated hospital units will continue to remain on an inactive status for the duration of the war, unless a serious enemy attack occurs in their Region which necessitates the transfer of casualties to protected sites in the interior. Their commissions may be terminated upon their request six months after the end of the war, or sooner if approved by the Surgeon General. Such approval will be given in the event such officer desires active duty in the Army or Navy.

Dr. L. A. Munding of Tulsa has recently been commissioned a first Lieutenant in the medical corps of the Army Air Force and has reported for duty at the Cadet Training Center, Kelly Field, Texas.

Captain Lyman C. Veazey of Ardmore has recently been transferred from Santa Ana, Calif., to Marana, Ariz.

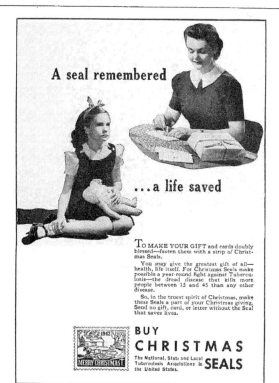

HOSPITALS TO BE REIMBURSED FOR CARE OF CIVILIAN CASUALTIES

Payment for temporary hospitalization of civilians injured as the result of enemy action has been made possible by a recent agreement between Administrator Paul V. McNutt of the Federal Security Agency and Director James M. Landis of the Office of Civilian Defense. The funds have been allocated to the U. S. Public Health Service by the Federal Security Administrator from funds made available to him from the President's emergency fund. A joint memorandum embodying the details of the program has been issued by Surgeon General Thomas Parran of the U. S. Public Health Service and Dr. George Baehr, Chief Medical Officer of the Office of Civilian Defense.

The plan provides that all hospitals caring for civilian casualties in the event of air raids or other enemy action will be reimbursed by the federal government at a rate of $3.75 a day. This is the rate of reimbursement established by the Federal Board of Hospitalization for federal beneficiaries in government hospitals and may be changed as conditions require, it was stated.

Any hospital in the nation, voluntary or governmental, may be used as a casualty receiving hospital in the Emergency Medical Service established by the Medical Division of the Office of Civilian Defense. In addition, certain hospitals and other institutions in "safe areas" may be used as emergency base hospitals for casualties or other patients whom it may be necessary to evacuate from urban hospitals in exposed areas. The new agreement provides that federally owned equipment may be loaned to the base hospitals and that their staffs will be supplemented by physicians of the region who will be commissioned in the reserve corps of the U. S. Public Health Service. It was emphasized that management and control of all hospitals, both local casualty receiving hospitals and emergency base hospitals, will remain the responsibility of the local or state authorities.

In the establishment of emergency base hospitals, emphasis will be placed on the relative safety of the area and the availability of existing hospitals and other institutions. Hospitals are now being surveyed for this purpose and will be classified on a basis of size, equipment and standards of operation.

It is proposed to begin immediately the organization of medical staffs for future base hospitals as hospital units affiliated with casualty hospitals similar to the affiliated general hospitals of the Army. The physicians, surgeons, specialists and dentists who are to be commissioned in the Public Health Service Reserve for service in these hospitals will receive rank, pay and allowance equivalent to those of the Medical Corps of the U. S. Army. They will be selected from older age groups, from physicians with disabilities that make them ineligible for military service, and from women physicians. As far as possible, they will be assigned to service in the regions in which they live. Because they are to function as balanced professional staffs, they will be recruited from the staffs of civilian hospitals and cleared through the Procurement and Assignment Service.

Regional Medical Officers of O.C.D. who are appointed in the Public Health Service will be the regional representatives of both agencies for this program. State Chiefs of Emergency Medical Service or their deputies may also be appointed consultants or commissioned in the Public Health Service in order that they may act as state representatives for the two agencies in the organization of emergency hospital facilities and the reimbursement of hospitals for the care of civilian casualties. In the more populous coastal states a full-time State Hospital Officer may be needed, who will also be eligible for appointment in the Public Health Service.

Appointment of a state hospital officer as an official of Emergency Medical Service has been recommended by the Medical Division for densely populated states in the target areas. These areas are the First, Second, Third, Fourth, Eighth and Ninth Defense Regions.

The principal function of the hospital officer will be the planning of emergency base hospitals for the reception of civilian casualties and other hospital evacuees. An official memorandum sets forth his duties as follows:

1. To survey the hospitals throughout the state (excluding those in the exposed cities) to determine how many beds can be put into immediate use in emergency with existing kitchen, laundry, sanitation and other engineering facilities:

   (a) By clearing patients to their homes
   (b) By restricting admissions
   (c) By use of rooms not normally used for patients
   (d) By rehousing medical and nursing staff and other hospital personnel outside the hospital
   (e) By use of neighboring building (schools, hotels, etc.), for patients (or staff)
   (f) By extra bed accomodation in temporary structures erected on available grounds adjacent to the hospital.

2. To assist in designing for each casualty hospital or group of hospitals in each exposed city:

   (a) The line of evacuation to the base
   (b) The transport arrangement
   (c) The emergency base hospitals provisionally alloted to each casualty unit.

3. To keep constantly informed of the bed state of every hospital in his area by weekly returns.

4. To advise the Office of Civilian Defense, through the Regional Medical Officer, on the need for providing additional accommodations, e.g., by temporary construction or by converting convalescent homes, hotels, school dormitories or other structures into hospitals.

5. To report to the Regional Medical Officer of the Office of Civilian Defense any exceptional conditions requiring action (e.g., beyond state boundaries, or required by the need of the military situation) and to forward to him copies of a monthly summary report on the state's emergency hospital program. Where a hospital outside a state boundary is readily accessible for the reception of casualties from an exposed city, this fact should also be noted.

6. To maintain constant touch with the other service departments of the State Defense Council (e.g., evacuation, etc.).

7. To supervise the distribution of medical and hospital supplies under the direction of the State Civilian Defense Property Officer and report any threatened deficiency to the Regional Medical Officer.

8. To supervise staff arrangement for emergency base hospitals and for reception areas.

9. To control movements of medical and nursing staff, as well as of casualties in any situation affecting emergency base hospitals.

The hospital officer must work in close collaboration with the state evacuation authority, the memorandum points out. In addition, he may find it necessary to collaborate with the state officer in charge of institutions for the care of mental patients, if such hospitals are to be used as emergency base hospitals for the reception of casualties and other patients evacuated from urban hospitals. Transport arrangements are to be handled in collaboration with the evacuation authorities of the state and the military authorities of the area.

Heat-Resistant Butter Developed by Army

A new "butter" developed by the Army Quartermaster Corps can be shipped without refrigeration and will resist temperatures up to 110 degrees Fahrenheit. Ten thousand pounds have already been shipped to U. S. troops overseas.

Named "Carter spread" after its inventor, Lt. Col. Robert F. Carter of the Quartermaster Corps, the new butter consists of dairy butter fortified with hydrogenated cotton seed oil flakes to raise its melting point. Quartermaster Corps officers say it still tastes like butter. —Science News Letter.

BOOK REVIEWS

"The chief glory of every people arises from its authors."—Dr. Samuel Johnson.

OSLER'S PRINCIPLES AND PRACTICE OF MEDI-CINE. Fourteenth Edition. Semicentennial (1892-1942). Henry A. Christian, A.M., M.D., LL.D., Hon. Sc.D., Hon. F.R.C.P. (Can.), F.A.C.P. D. Appleton-Century Co., New York. 1475 Pp.

The fourteenth and semicentennial edition of the above well known text is ready for students and practitioners of medicine. This great textbook on medicine represents the knowledge and experience of three of the modern world's outstanding internists. The present editor, a pupil of Osler and the friend and colleague of McCrae, points out the fact that Thomas McCrae, as "pupil and junior colleague of Osler, collaborating with him in editorial work, naturally continued the Oslerian tradition when he became editor." This teacher-pupil-colleague relationship has assured preservatoin of original merit and continuity of thought and method through successive editions in spite of rapidly increasing knowledge.

This edition has been largely rewritten in order to bring the text in line with modern medical thought and to incorporate much that is new. At this moment progress in medical science is almost as phenomenal as it was fifty years ago when the first edition greeted the profession and it is comforting to have Osler's conservativism supplemented by this apothegm from Dr. Christian. "The editor believes that this is a book in which the new should not appear, because it is new, but because its value has seemed to have been demonstrated by experienced clinicians—"

In this day of haste and high pressure, when the tempting voice of expediency is ever assailing the ears of the overworked student, it is good to have the wisdom and experience of Osler shining through his clinical and pathological observations. Of equal importance is the inclusion of modern advances assayed by the level vision and clinical judgment of McCrae and Christian.

This edition merits the following quotation from Plato which the master employed in the first edition and which now appears in the fourteenth:

"And I said of medicine, that this is an art which considers the constitution of the patient, and has principles of action and reasons in each case."—Lewis J. Moorman, M.D.

TEXTBOOK OF MEDICAL TREATMENT. Second Edition. D. M. Dunlap, M.D., L. S. P. Davidson, M.D., and J. W. McNee, M.D. The Williams and Wilkins Company, Baltimore, Md. Cloth. Price $8.00.

This useful volume of twelve hundred pages comprises 24 separate categories with many subdivisions. This book on treatment should prove a valuable supplement to the average textbook on medicine. An adequate discussion of therapeutic measures often requires more space than the text allows.

The size and weight of the volume, the arrangement of the text and the comprehensive index makes it a handy reference book.

The following from the preface to the second edition suggests the scope and purposes of the work and its favorable reception:

"The hope entertained by the editors that a book of this nature on rational therapeutics would prove to be of some service to medical practitioners and students has been realized by the fact that the first edition and large amended reprint have been exhausted in approximately two years. An opportunity was taken to insert in the reprint a section on the sex hormones because of the growing importance of this subject in medical practice, and, in addition, a section on the treatment of alcoholism and drug addiction, which had been omitted in the first edition."

The chapters on "Psychotherapy in General Practice" and "Technical Procedures and Oxygen Therapy" deserve special mention.—Lewis J. Moorman, M.D.

MACLEOD'S PHYSIOLOGY IN MODERN MEDI-CINE. Edited by Philip Bard. Ninth edition. 1256 pages. Price $10.00. C. V. Mosby Company, St. Louis, 1941.

The eighth edition of this textbook was largely written by a group of authors each a specialist in his field of physiology. The present edition (ninth) has continued this arrangement and ten individuals have contributed, including the editor Philip Bard. Such an approach to the subject offers many advantages and also some disadvantages. The advantages are evident if one desires a reference book which covers the subject authoritatively and more completely than any other textbook. However, from the viewpoint of the average medical student, who has had practically no elementary training in the subject, the book shares the disadvantage of other similar texts. The modern tendency seems to be to produce the largest book possible and to forget that the beginning student wants a unified, fundamental, and working conception of the subject. The arrangement of the material in this book lacks the sequence and continuity necessary to give the average student a comprehension of the interrelationship of the various physiological systems.

The practicing physician will find the book a splendid reference volume if he is interested in scientific physiology but "In the interest of candor it should be stated that the present volume makes no pretense of being a textbook of 'applied' physiology."

The publishers have used a quality of paper which makes it possible to present the splendid illustrations including several color plates. It is another good example of high class book building so characteristic of C. V. Mosby Company.—Edward C. Mason, M.D.

"I insist that it is the duty of the whole people never to intrust to any hands but their own the preservation of their own liberties and institutions."—Lincoln.

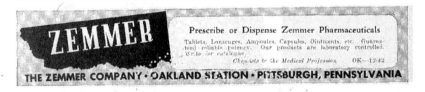

XXXV INDEX TO CONTENTS 1942

The use of the index will be greatly facilitated by remembering that articles are often listed under more than one head. Scientific articles may be found under both the name of the author and the subject discussed. Editorials, Book Reviews and Obituaries are listed under the special headings as well as alphabetically.

KEY TO ABBREVIATIONS

(S)—Scientific articles (E)—Editorial (M)—Miscellaneous (abs)—Abstract
(A)—Association Activities (br)—Book Review (MP)—Medical Preparedness (o)—Obituary

Quinine Substitute

There is no shortage of atabrine, the synthetic substitute for quinine.

But if more is needed, the atabrine patents will be available, royalty free, to a score of pharmaceutical manufacturers who can step up production to astronomical figures. Equipment priorities for this purpose have not been granted because production is already far in excess of needs.

These facts emerged last week in answer to questions of California's Representative Bertrand W. Gearhart in the House. Said he: "Is it true that our soldiers, sailors and marines are today threatened with disablement because of a scarcity of this indispensable medicine? The American people are entitled to know, to know right now."

Winthrop Chemical Company makes atabrine by a former German process under U. S. patents. Since 1933 Winthrop has gradually increased its atabrine production in stiff competition with natural quinine, generally reduced its price (to the Government) from $66 to $6 per thousand tablets. By 1941, it produced 90 million tablets a year, enough for six million malaria cases. Even before Pearl Harbor this had been increased to 227 million tablets.

With quinine imports from the Orient shut off, Winthrop contracted with Merck & Company, Inc., to manufacture atabrine. Present production of the two firms is 500 million tablets, enough for 33 million cases of malaria. But both could produce several hundred million more in case of need.

Atabrine, however, is not a complete substitute for quinine since it attacks only one of the two forms of the malaria germ. Quinine attacks both. To make atabrine as effective as quinine it must be administered together with plasmochin (another synthetic). But, the amount of plasmochin needed is small, and Winthrop has already increased its production 10,000 percent.—*Time*, Sept., 1942.

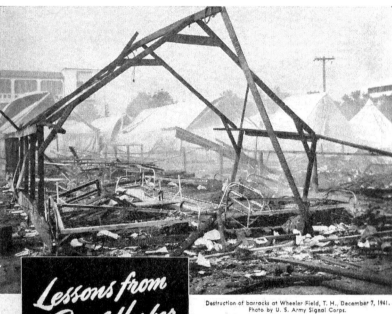

Lessons from Pearl Harbor

Destruction of barracks at Wheeler Field, T. H., December 7, 1941.
Photo by U. S. Army Signal Corps.

OUT of the chaos and confusion—the burns, lacerated wounds and compound fractures—that was Pearl Harbor on that first Sunday of December, 1941 — have come many lessons. Not the least among them is the value of the sulfonamides—used topically for the management of the potentially infected traumata.

Field conditions were ideal for the production of Clostridial infections—yet the incidence of gas gangrene was remarkably low and resulted in no deaths. Hospital facilities and surgical skill were hard-pressed and surgical operations were delayed from hours to days. Due in no small measure to the use of the sulfonamides, postoperative mortality was only 3.8 per cent, and most of these fatalities were from shock and hemorrhage.

Topical use of sulfonamides is assuming increasing importance not alone in military practice but in industry and civil life. These compounds should be regarded as an important adjunct to surgery, regardless of whether the surgeon is dealing with grossly contaminated wounds or maintaining asepsis in his operative field. Further studies must, of course, be made to determine the method of application best suited for each type of wound.

The Squibb Laboratories have available many of the sulfonamide compounds. There are several dosage forms under laboratory and clinical investigation and these will be provided as the need arises and results prove favorable.

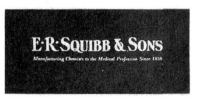

OFFICERS OF COUNTY SOCIETIES, 1942

—Indicates serving in Armed Forces.

COUNTY	PRESIDENT	SECRETARY	MEETING TIME
Alfalfa	*Jack F. Parsons, Cherokee	L. T. Lancaster, Cherokee	Last Tues. Each 2nd Mo.
Atoka-Coal	J. B. Clark, Coalgate	J. S. Fulton, Atoka	
Beckham	H. K. Speed, Sayre	E. S. Kilpatrick, Elk City	Second Tues. eve.
Blaine	Virginia Olson Curtin, Watonga	W. F. Griflin, Watonga	
Bryan	A. J. Wells, Calera	W. K. Haynie, Durant	Second Tues. eve.
Caddo	Fred L. Patterson, Carnegie	C. B. Sullivan, Carnegie	
Canadian	P. F. Herod, El Reno	A. L. Johnson, El Reno	Subject to call
Carter	Walter Hardy, Ardmore	H. A. Higgins, Ardmore	
Cherokee	Park H. Medearis, Tahlequah	*Isadore Dyer, Tahlequah	
Choctaw	C. H. Hale, Boswell	Fred D. Switzer, Hugo	
Cleveland	Joseph A. Rieger, Norman	Curtis Berry, Norman	Thursday nights
Comanche	George S. Barber, Lawton	W. F. Lewis, Lawton	
Cotton	George W. Baker, Walters	Mollie F. Seism, Walters	Third Friday
Craig	W. R. Marks, Vinita	J. M. McMillan, Vinita	
Creek	Frank Sisler, Bristow	O. C. Coppedge, Bristow	
Custer		*W. C. Tisdal, Clinton	Third Thursday
Garfield	D. S. Harris, Drummond	John R. Walker, Enid	Fourth Thursday
Garvin	T. F. Gross, Lindsay	John R. Callaway, Pauls Valley	Wed. before 3d Thurs.
Grady	D. S. Downey, Chickasha	*Frank T. Joyce, Chickasha	3rd Thursday
Grant	I. V. Hardy, Medford	E. E. Lawson, Medford	
Greer	G. F. Border, Mangum	J. B. Hollis, Mangum	
Harmon	S. W. Hopkins, Hollis	W. M. Yeargan, Hollis	First Wednesday
Haskell	William Carson, Keota	N. K. Williams, McCurtain	
Hughes	Wm. L. Taylor, Holdenville	Imogene Mayfield, Holdenville	First Friday
Jackson	J. M. Allgood, Altus	E. W. Mabry, Altus	Last Monday
Jefferson	W. M. Browning, Waurika	J. L. Hollingsworth, Waurika	Second Monday
Kay	I. C. Wagner, Ponca City	J. Holland Howe, Ponca City	Third Thurs.
Kingfisher	C. M. Hodgson, Kingfisher	*John R. Taylor, Kingfisher	
Kiowa	J. M. Bonham, Hobart	B. H. Watkins, Hobart	
LeFlore	G. R. Booth, LeFlore	Rush L. Wright, Poteau	
Lincoln	E. F. Hurlbut, Meeker	C. W. Robertson, Chandler	First Wednesday
Logan	William C. Miller, Guthrie	J. L. LeHew, Jr., Guthrie	Last Tuesday evening
Marshall	J. L. Holland, Madill	O. A. Cook, Madill	
Mayes	L. C. White, Adair	V. D. Herrington, Pryor	
McClain	B. W. Slover, Blanchard	R. L. Royster, Purcell	
McCurtain	R. D. Williams, Idabel	R. H. Sherrill, Broken Bow	Fourth Tues. eve.
McIntosh	F. R. First, Checotah	William A. Tolleson, Eufaula	Second Tuesday
Murray	P. V. Annadown, Sulphur	F. E. Sadler, Sulphur	
Muskogee	L. S. McAlister, Muskogee	D. Evelyn Miller, Muskogee	First & Third Mon.
Noble	J. W. Francis, Perry	C. H. Cooke, Perry	
Okfuskee	I. M. Pemberton, Okemah	L. J. Spickard, Okemah	Second Monday
Oklahoma	R. Q. Goodwin, Okla. City	Wm. E. Eastland, Okla. City	Fourth Tuesday
Okmulgee	J. G. Edwards, Okmulgee	*John R. Cotteral, Henryetta	Second Monday
Osage	C. R. Weirich, Pawhuska	George K. Hemphill, Pawhuska	Second Monday
Ottawa	J. B. Hampton, Commerce	Walter Sanger, Picher	Third Thursday
Pawnee	E. T. Robinson, Cleveland	Robert L. Browning, Pawnee	
Payne	John W. Martin, Cushing	Clifford W. Moore, Stillwater	Third Thursday
Pittsburg	Austin R. Stough, McAlester	Edw. D. Greenberger, McAlester	Third Friday
Pontotoc	R. E. Cowling, Ada	Alfred R. Sugg, Ada	First Wednesday
Pottawatomie	John Carson, Shawnee	Clinton Gallaher, Shawnee	First & Third Sat.
Pushmataha	P. B. Rice, Antlers	John S. Lawson, Clayton	
Rogers	*W. A. Howard, Chelsea	George D. Waller, Claremore	First Monday
Seminole	H. M. Reeder, Konawa	Mack I. Shanholtz ,Wewoka	
Stephens	A. J. Weedn, Duncan	W. K. Walker, Marlow	
Texas	L. G. Blackmer, Hooker	*Johnny A. Blue, Guymon	
Tillman	C. C. Allen, Frederick	O. G. Bacon, Frederick	
Tulsa	H. B. Stewart, Tulsa	E. O. Johnson, Tulsa	Second & Fourth Mon. eve.
Wagoner	J. H. Plunkett, Wagoner	H. K. Biddle, Coweta	
Washington-Nowata	K. D. Davis, Nowata	J. V. Athey, Bartlesville	Second Wednesday
Washita	A. S. Neal, Cordell	James F. McMurry, Sentinel	
Woods	W. F. LaFon, Waynoka	O. E. Templin, Alva	Last Wednesday
Woodward	M. H. Newman, Shattuck	C. W. Tedrowe, Woodward	

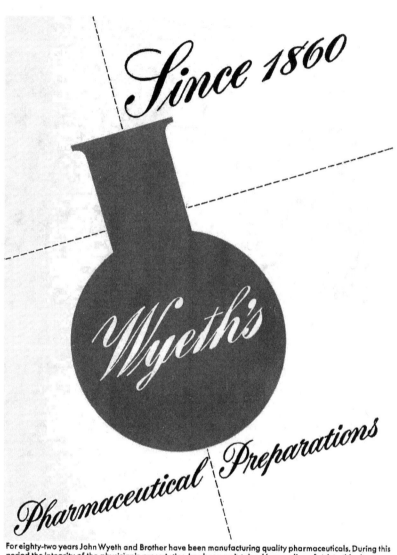

Since 1860

Wyeth's

Pharmaceutical Preparations

For eighty-two years John Wyeth and Brother have been manufacturing quality pharmaceuticals. During this period the integrity of the physician's prescription has been maintained by a policy of strict ethical promotion. Wyeth products are not known to the laity. Emphasis is placed on research and production control so that standardized potency and therapeutic effect are always obtained when the physician writes "Wyeth's."

The name Wyeth's is Reg. U. S. Pat. Off.

John Wyeth and Brother, Inc., Philadelphia

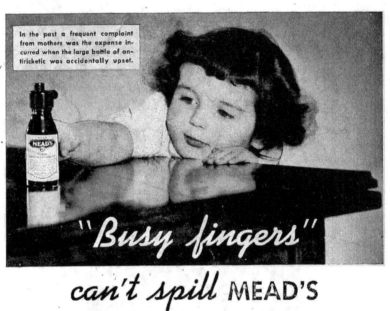

In the past a frequent complaint from mothers was the expense incurred when the large bottle of antiricketic was accidentally upset.

"Busy fingers"
can't spill MEAD'S
OLEUM PERCOMORPHUM

Even if the bottle of Mead's Oleum Percomorphum is accidentally tipped over, there is no loss of precious oil nor damage to clothing and furnishings. The unique Mead's Vacap-Dropper* is a tight seal which remains attached to the bottle, even while the antiricketic is being measured out. Mead's Vacap-Dropper offers these extra advantages also, at no increase in price:

Unbreakable
Mead's Vacap-Dropper will not break even when bottle is tipped over or dropped. No glass dropper to become rough or serrated.

No "messiness"
Mead's Vacap-Dropper protects against dust and rancidity. (Rancidity reduces vitamin potency.) Surface of oil need never be exposed to light and dust. This dropper cannot roll about and collect bacteria.

Accurate
This unique device, after the patient becomes accustomed to using it, delivers drops of uniform size.

No deterioration
Made of bakelite, Mead's Vacap-Dropper is impervious to oil. No chance of oil rising into rubber bulb, as with ordinary droppers, and deteriorating both oil and rubber. No glass or bulb to become separated while in use.

How to Use MEAD'S Vacap-Dropper
Remove both top and side caps. Wipe dropper tip. Place forefinger firmly over top opening and regulate rate of flow by varying the degree of pressure. Oleum Percomorphum is best measured into the child's tomato juice. This is just as convenient and much safer than dropping the oil directly into the baby's mouth, a practice which may provoke a coughing spasm.

*Supplied only on the 50 c.c. size. the 10 c.c. size is still supplied with the ordinary type of dropper.

MEAD'S OLEUM PERCOMORPHUM
More Economical Now Than Ever

MEAD JOHNSON & COMPANY, EVANSVILLE, INDIANA, U. S. A.

Please enclose professional card when requesting samples of Mead Johnson products to co-operate in preventing their reaching unauthorized persons

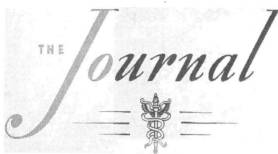

OF THE OKLAHOMA STATE MEDICAL ASSOCIATION

VOLUME XXXV • OKLAHOMA CITY, OKLAHOMA, DECEMBER, 1942 • NUMBER 12

★ *Published Monthly at Oklahoma City, Oklahoma, Under Direction of the Council*

Terrell's Laboratories

North Texas and Oklahoma Pasteur Institutes

PATHOLOGICAL BACTERIOLOGICAL SEROLOGICAL CHEMICAL

Ft. Worth   Abilene   Muskogee   Amarillo   Corpus Christi

X-RAY *and* RADIUM DEPT.
FORT WORTH

Lain-Eastland-Lamb Clinic

*Dermatology, Syphilology,
Radium and X-Ray
Therapy*

Everett S. Lain, M.D.   Wm. E. Eastland, M.D.

John H. Lamb, M.D.

Medical Arts Building

Oklahoma City, Oklahoma

Throw out your chest!

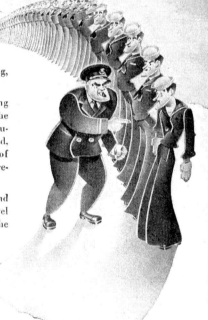

● Navy training helps to build strong, healthy bodies.

First in command of establishing health habits in civilian life is the family physician. When the daily routine for regular bowel habits is disturbed, the physician's recommendation of Petrogalar* frequently facilitates a return to normal.

Petrogalar helps soften the stool and renders it mobile for comfortable bowel movement. Consider Petrogalar for the treatment of constipation.

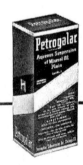

FOR THE TREATMENT OF CONSTIPATION

Petrogalar

Reg. U. S. Pat. Off. Petrogalar is an aqueous suspension of pure mineral oil each 100 cc. of which contains 65 cc. pure mineral oil suspended in an aqueous jelly containing agar and acacia.

Petrogalar Laboratories, Inc. • 8134 McCormick Boulevard • Chicago, Illinois

Antirabic Vaccine

SEMPLE METHOD

U. S. Government License No. 98

1. Patients bitten by suspected rabid animals, on any part of body other than Face and Wrist, usually require only 14 doses of Antirabic Vaccine.

   Ampoule Package......................$15.00

2. Patients bitten about Face or Wrist, or when treatment has been delayed, should receive at least 21 doses of Antirabic Vaccine. (Special instructions with each treatment.)

   Ampoule Package......................$22.50

Special Discounts to Doctors, Druggists, Hospitals and to County Health Officers for Indigent Cases.

Medical Arts Laboratory

1115 Medical Arts Building
Oklahoma City, Oklahoma

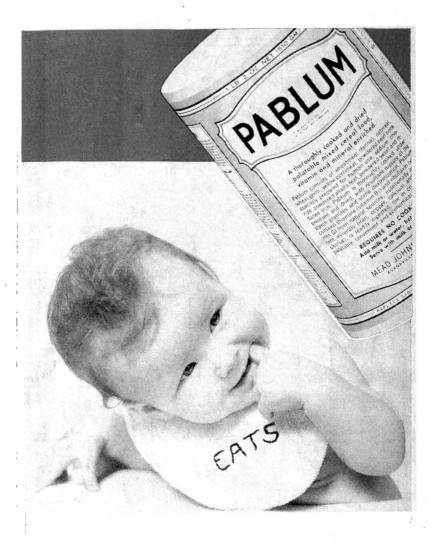